This book is due for return on or before the last date shown below.

PRINCIPLES OF
Clinical
Gastroenterology

EDITED BY

Tadataka Yamada, MD

President, Global Health Program
Bill & Melinda Gates Foundation
Seattle, Washington;
Adjunct Professor
Department of Internal Medicine
Division of Gastroenterology
University of Michigan Health System
Ann Arbor, Michigan, USA

ASSOCIATE EDITORS

David H. Alpers, MD

William B. Kountz Professor of Medicine
Department of Internal Medicine
Division of Gastroenterology
Washington University School of Medicine
St Louis, Missouri, USA

Anthony N. Kalloo, MD

Professor of Medicine
Johns Hopkins University School of Medicine;
Director, Division of Gastroenterology and Hepatology
Johns Hopkins Hospital
Baltimore, Maryland, USA

Neil Kaplowitz, MD

Brem Professor of Medicine and Chief
Division of Gastrointestinal and Liver Diseases
Director, Liver Disease Research Center
Keck School of Medicine
University of Southern California
Los Angeles, California, USA

Chung Owyang, MD

Professor of Internal Medicine
H. Marvin Pollard Collegiate Professor and Chief
Division of Gastroenterology
University of Michigan Health System
Ann Arbor, Michigan, USA

Don W. Powell, MD

The Bassel and Frances Blanton Distinguished Professor of Internal Medicine
Professor, Neuroscience and Cell Biology
Program Director, General Clinical Research Center
Director, Division of Gastroenterology and Hepatology
The University of Texas Medical Branch
Galveston, Texas, USA

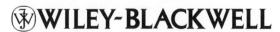

A John Wiley & Sons, Ltd., Publication

This edition first published 2008, © 2008 by Blackwell Publishing Ltd

Blackwell Publishing was acquired by John Wiley & Sons in February 2007. Blackwell's publishing program has been merged with Wiley's global Scientific, Technical and Medical business to form Wiley-Blackwell.

Registered office: John Wiley & Sons Ltd, The Atrium, Southern Gate, Chichester, West Sussex, PO19 8SQ, UK

Editorial offices: 9600 Garsington Road, Oxford, OX4 2DQ, UK
The Atrium, Southern Gate, Chichester, West Sussex, PO19 8SQ, UK
111 River Street, Hoboken, NJ 07030-5774, USA

For details of our global editorial offices, for customer services and for information about how to apply for permission to reuse the copyright material in this book please see our website at www.wiley.com/wiley-blackwell.

The right of the author to be identified as the author of this work has been asserted in accordance with the Copyright, Designs and Patents Act 1988.

Wiley also publishes its books in a variety of electronic formats. Some content that appears in print may not be available as electronic books.

Designations used by companies to distinguish their products are often claimed as trademarks. All brand names and product names used in this book are trade names, service marks, trademarks or registered trademarks of their respective owners. The publisher is not associated with any product or vendor mentioned in this book. This publication is designed to provide accurate and authoritative information in regard to the subject matter covered. It is sold on the understanding that the publisher is not engaged in rendering professional services. If professional advice or other expert assistance is required, the services of a competent professional should be sought.

The contents of this work are intended to further general scientific research, understanding, and discussion only and are not intended and should not be relied upon as recommending or promoting a specific method, diagnosis, or treatment by physicians for any particular patient. The publisher and the author make no representations or warranties with respect to the accuracy or completeness of the contents of this work and specifically disclaim all warranties, including without limitation any implied warranties of fitness for a particular purpose. In view of ongoing research, equipment modifications, changes in governmental regulations, and the constant flow of information relating to the use of medicines, equipment, and devices, the reader is urged to review and evaluate the information provided in the package insert or instructions for each medicine, equipment, or device for, among other things, any changes in the instructions or indication of usage and for added warnings and precautions. Readers should consult with a specialist where appropriate. The fact that an organization or website is referred to in this work as a citation and/or a potential source of further information does not mean that the author or the publisher endorses the information the organization or website may provide or recommendations it may make. Further, readers should be aware that Internet websites listed in this work may have changed or disappeared between when this work was written and when it is read. No warranty may be created or extended by any promotional statements for this work. Neither the publisher nor the author shall be liable for any damages arising herefrom.

Library of Congress Cataloguing-in-Publication Data
Principles of clinical gastroenterology / edited by Tadataka Yamada ; associate editors, David H. Alpers . . . [et al.].
    p. ; cm.
  Includes bibliographical references and index.
  ISBN 978-1-4051-6910-3
  1. Gastrointestinal system—Diseases.   2. Liver—Diseases.   3. Gastroenterology.
I. Yamada, Tadataka.   II. Alpers, David H.
[DNLM: 1. Gastrointestinal Diseases.   2. Liver Diseases.   WI 140 P957 2008]
RC801.P753 2008
616.3'3—dc22
                                                                            2008000954

ISBN: 978-1-4051-6910-3

A catalogue record for this book is available from the British Library

Set in 9/12pt Palatino/Frutiger by Graphicraft Limited, Hong Kong
Printed in Singapore by COS Printers Pte Ltd

1   2008

Contents

Contributors, vii

Preface, ix

1 Clinical decision making, 1
Philip S. Schoenfeld

2 Economic analysis in the diagnosis and treatment of gastrointestinal diseases, 14
John M. Inadomi

3 Psychosocial factors in the care of patients with functional gastrointestinal disorders, 20
Bruce D. Naliboff, Jeffrey M. Lackner, Emeran A. Mayer

4 Approach to the patient with dyspepsia and related functional gastrointestinal complaints, 38
Nicholas J. Talley, Gerald Holtmann

5 Approach to the patient with dysphagia, odynophagia, or noncardiac chest pain, 62
Chandra Prakash Gyawali, Ray E. Clouse

6 Approach to the patient with gastroesophageal reflux disease, 83
Joel E. Richter

7 Approach to the patient with dyspepsia and peptic ulcer disease, 99
Andrew H. Soll, David Y. Graham

8 Approach to the patient with gross gastrointestinal bleeding, 122
Grace H. Elta, Mimi Takami

9 Approach to the patient with occult gastrointestinal bleeding, 152
David A. Ahlquist, Graeme P. Young

10 Approach to screening for colorectal cancer, 170
Graeme P. Young, James E. Allison

11 Approach to the patient with unintentional weight loss, 183
Andrew W. DuPont

12 Approach to the patient with obesity, 191
Louis A. Chaptini, Steven R. Peikin

13 Approach to the patient with nausea and vomiting, 205
William L. Hasler

14 Approach to the patient with abdominal pain, 228
Pankaj Jay Pasricha

15 Approach to the patient with gas and bloating, 255
William L. Hasler

16 Approach to the patient with acute abdomen, 271
Rebecca M. Minter, Michael W. Mulholland

17 Approach to the patient with ileus and obstruction, 287
Klaus Bielefeldt, Anthony J. Bauer

18 Approach to the patient with diarrhea, 304
Don W. Powell

19 Approach to the patient with suspected acute infectious diarrhea, 360
John D. Long, Ralph A. Giannella

20 Approach to the patient with constipation, 373
Satish S.C. Rao

21 Approach to the patient with abnormal liver chemistries, 399
Richard H. Moseley

22 Approach to the patient with jaundice, 422
Raphael B. Merriman, Marion G. Peters

23 Approach to the patient with ascites and its complications, 442
Guadalupe Garcia-Tsao

24 Approach to the patient with central nervous system and pulmonary complications of end-stage liver disease, 467
Javier Vaquero, Andres T. Blei, Roger F. Butterworth

25 Approach to the patient with acute liver failure, 492
Ryan M. Taylor, Robert J. Fontana

26 Approach to the patient with chronic viral hepatitis B or C, 516
Sammy Saab, Hugo Rosen

27 Approach to the patient with a liver mass, 526
John A. Donovan, Edward G. Grant

28 Approach to gastrointestinal and liver diseases in pregnancy, 534
Willemijntje A. Hoogerwerf

29 General nutritional principles, 557
David H. Alpers, Beth Taylor, Samuel Klein

30 Approach to the patient requiring nutritional supplementation, 588
David H. Alpers, Beth Taylor, Samuel Klein

31 Genetic counseling for gastrointestinal patients, 624
Cindy Solomon, Deborah W. Neklason, Angela Schwab, Randall W. Burt

Index, 645

Contributors

David A. Ahlquist, MD
Professor of Medicine
Mayo Clinic College of Medicine;
Consultant, Division of Gastroenterology
and Hepatology
Mayo Clinic
Rochester, Minnesota, USA

James E. Allison, MD, FACP, AGAF
Clinical Professor of Medicine Emeritus
University of California, San Francisco;
Division of Gastroenterology
San Francisco General Hospital;
Adjunct Investigator, Kaiser Division of Research
San Francisco, California, USA

Anthony J. Bauer, PhD
Associate Professor of Medicine
Division of Gastroenterology
University of Pittsburgh
Pittsburgh, Pennsylvania, USA

Klaus Bielefeldt, MD, PhD
Associate Professor of Medicine
Division of Gastroenterology
University of Pittsburgh
Pittsburgh, Pennsylvania, USA

Andres T. Blei, MD
Professor of Medicine
Division of Hepatology
Feinberg School of Medicine
Northwestern University
Chicago, Illinois, USA

Randall W. Burt, MD
Professor of Medicine
Division of Gastroenterology
University of Utah School of Medicine;
Senior Director for Prevention and Outreach
Huntsman Cancer Institute
University of Utah
Salt Lake City, Utah, USA

Roger F. Butterworth, PhD, DSc
Director, Neuroscience Research Unit
Hôpital Saint-Luc
University of Montreal
Montreal, Quebec, Canada

Louis A. Chaptini, MD
Assistant Professor of Medicine
Division of Gastroenterology and Liver Diseases
Cooper University Hospital
Robert Wood Johnson Medical School
University of Medicine and Dentistry of New Jersey
Camden, New Jersey, USA

Ray E. Clouse, MD
Professor of Medicine and Psychiatry
Late of Division of Gastroenterology
Washington University School of Medicine;
Physician, late of Department of Medicine
Barnes-Jewish Hospital
St Louis, Missouri, USA

John A. Donovan, MD
Assistant Professor of Clinical Medicine
Division of Gastrointestinal and Liver Diseases
Keck School of Medicine
University of Southern California
Los Angeles, California, USA

Andrew W. DuPont, MD, MSPH
Assistant Professor, Internal Medicine
Division of Gastroenterology and Hepatology
The University of Texas Medical Branch
Galveston, Texas, USA

Grace H. Elta, MD
Professor
Department of Internal Medicine
Division of Gastroenterology
University of Michigan Health System
Ann Arbor, Michigan, USA

Robert J. Fontana, MD
Associate Professor
Department of Internal Medicine
Division of Gastroenterology
University of Michigan Health System
Ann Arbor, Michigan, USA

Guadalupe Garcia-Tsao, MD
Professor of Medicine
Section of Digestive Diseases
Yale School of Medicine
New Haven, Connecticut;
Veterans Affairs Connecticut Healthcare System
West Haven, Connecticut, USA

Ralph A. Giannella, MD
Mark Brown Professor of Medicine
Division of Digestive Diseases
University of Cincinnati College of Medicine
Cincinnati, Ohio, USA

David Y. Graham, MD
Professor of Medicine and Molecular Virology
and Microbiology
Michael E. DeBakey Veterans Affairs Medical
Center
Baylor College of Medicine
Houston, Texas, USA

Edward G. Grant, MD
Professor and Chair
Department of Radiology
Keck School of Medicine
University of Southern California
Los Angeles, California, USA

Chandra Prakash Gyawali, MD, MRCP
Associate Professor of Medicine
Associate Program Director
Division of Gastroenterology
Washington University School of Medicine
St Louis, Missouri, USA

William L. Hasler, MD
Professor
Department of Internal Medicine
Division of Gastroenterology
University of Michigan Health System
Ann Arbor, Michigan, USA

Gerald Holtmann, MD, PhD
Professor of Medicine
University of Adelaide;
Director, Department of Gastroenterology
and Hepatology
Royal Adelaide Hospital
Adelaide, South Australia, Australia

Willemijntje A. Hoogerwerf, MD
Assistant Professor
Department of Internal Medicine
Division of Gastroenterology
University of Michigan Health System
Ann Arbor, Michigan, USA

CONTRIBUTORS

John M. Inadomi, MD
Dean M. Craig Endowed Chair in
Gastrointestinal Medicine
Director, GI Health Outcomes, Policy and
Economics (HOPE) Research Program
University of California, San Francisco;
Chief, Clinical Gastroenterology
San Francisco General Hospital
San Francisco, California, USA

Samuel Klein, MD
William H. Danforth Professor of Medicine and
Nutritional Science
Center for Human Nutrition
Washington University School of Medicine
St Louis, Missouri, USA

Jeffrey M. Lackner, PsyD
Assistant Professor
University at Buffalo
The State University of New York
Buffalo, New York, USA

John D. Long, MD
Associate Professor of Medicine
Section on Gastroenterology
Wake Forest University School of Medicine
Winston-Salem, North Carolina, USA

Emeran A. Mayer, MD
UCLA Center for Neurovisceral Sciences and
Women's Health
David Geffen School of Medicine
University of California, Los Angeles
Los Angeles, California, USA

Raphael B. Merriman, MD, MRCPI
Assistant Professor of Medicine
Division of Gastroenterology
University of California, San Francisco
San Francisco, California, USA

Rebecca M. Minter, MD
Assistant Professor
Department of Surgery
University of Michigan Health System
Ann Arbor, Michigan, USA

Richard H. Moseley, MD
Professor
Department of Internal Medicine
Division of Gastroenterology
University of Michigan Health System;
Chief, Medical Service
Veterans Affairs Ann Arbor
Healthcare System
Ann Arbor, Michigan, USA

Michael W. Mulholland, MD, PhD
Professor and Chair
Department of Surgery
University of Michigan Health System
Ann Arbor, Michigan, USA

Bruce D. Naliboff, PhD
UCLA Center for Neurovisceral Sciences and
Women's Health
David Geffen School of Medicine
University of California, Los Angeles
Los Angeles, California, USA

Deborah W. Neklason, PhD
Research Assistant Professor
Department of Oncological Sciences
Huntsman Cancer Institute
University of Utah
Salt Lake City, Utah, USA

Pankaj Jay Pasricha, MD
Professor of Medicine
Chief, Division of Gastroenterology
and Hepatology
Stanford University School of Medicine
Stanford, California, USA

Steven R. Peikin, MD
Professor of Medicine
Division of Gastroenterology and Liver Diseases
Cooper University Hospital
Robert Wood Johnson Medical School
University of Medicine and Dentistry of New Jersey
Camden, New Jersey, USA

Marion G. Peters, MD
John V. Carbone, MD, Endowed Chair in Medicine
Division of Gastroenterology
University of California, San Francisco
San Francisco, California, USA

Satish S.C. Rao, MD, PhD, FRCP
Professor of Medicine
Director, Neurogastroenterology and
Gastrointestinal Motility
University of Iowa Carver College of Medicine
Iowa City, Iowa, USA

Joel E. Richter, MD
Richard L. Evans Chair and Professor
Department of Medicine
Temple University School of Medicine
Philadelphia, Pennsylvania, USA

Hugo Rosen, MD, FACP
Waterman Professor of Medicine and Immunology
Endowed Chair in Liver Research
Division Head, Gastroenterology and Hepatology
University of Colorado Health Sciences Center
Aurora, Colorado, USA

Sammy Saab, MD, MPH
Head, Outcomes Research in Hepatology
Associate Professor of Medicine and Surgery
David Geffen School of Medicine
University of California, Los Angeles
Los Angeles, California, USA

Philip S. Schoenfeld, MD, MSEd,
MSc(Epi)
Associate Professor
Department of Internal Medicine

Division of Gastroenterology;
Director, Training Program in Gastrointestinal
Epidemiology
University of Michigan Health System
Ann Arbor, Michigan, USA

Angela Schwab, MS, CGC
Cardiovascular Research Manager
Intermountain Healthcare
Salt Lake City, Utah, USA

Andrew H. Soll, MD
Professor, David Geffen School of Medicine
University of California, Los Angeles;
Attending Physician, Veterans Affairs Greater
Los Angeles Healthcare System
Los Angeles, California, USA

Cindy Solomon, MS, CGC
MELARIS Product Manager
Myriad Genetic Laboratories
Salt Lake City, Utah, USA

Mimi Takami, MD
Assistant Professor
Department of Internal Medicine
Division of Gastroenterology
University of Michigan Health System
Ann Arbor, Michigan, USA

Nicholas J. Talley, MD, PhD
Chair, Department of Internal Medicine
Mayo Clinic Jacksonville
Jacksonville, Florida;
Professor of Medicine and Epidemiology
Consultant, Division of Gastroenterology
and Hepatology
Mayo Clinic College of Medicine
Rochester, Minnesota, USA

Beth Taylor, MS, RD, CNSD
Nutrition Support Specialist
Barnes-Jewish Hospital
St Louis, Missouri, USA

Ryan M. Taylor, MD, MSc
Fellow
Department of Internal Medicine
Division of Gastroenterology
University of Michigan Health System
Ann Arbor, Michigan, USA

Javier Vaquero, MD
Postdoctoral Research Fellow
Neuroscience Research Unit
Hôpital Saint-Luc
University of Montreal
Montreal, Quebec, Canada

Graeme P. Young, MD, FRACP
Professor of Gastroenterology
Department of Medicine
Flinders University of South Australia;
Director, Department of Gastroenterology
Flinders Medical Centre
Adelaide, South Australia, Australia

Preface

The *Textbook of Gastroenterology* was launched over 20 years ago, and from the beginning it was designed to be an encyclopedic discussion of all of the disease states encountered in clinical practice by gastroenterologists, internists, surgeons, and other clinicians who see patients with gastrointestinal and liver disorders. A major component of the *Textbook* was a section that described the approaches a clinician might take to common symptoms and signs presented by patients with such disorders. This section has proved to be an invaluable resource for students, house officers, and practitioners who are not primarily gastroenterologists. To meet the needs of these readers more effectively we have expanded on the concept embodied in the chapters comprising that section of the *Textbook* and formatted them into a separate textbook in its own right, which we have titled *Principles of Clinical Gastroenterology*. It is designed to inform the reader on the features of the major clinical disorders in gastroenterology and hepatology, from the point of view of the clinician observing signs and symptoms of a patient under care and management. We hope that the *Principles* will be a practical guide to diagnosis and decision making in clinical practice and provide a rich source of information on diseases of the gastrointestinal tract and the liver. Of course, we refer the reader of the *Principles* to the *Textbook* for in-depth discussion of the basic science underlying these diseases, as well as the many diagnostic and therapeutic modalities available to the patients who suffer from them.

We are delighted to have a new publisher, Wiley-Blackwell, for this edition. Their keen insight into the publishing industry and the way in which textbooks are utilized today has been the basis for creating the *Principles*. We are also grateful for their knowledge of the international world of medicine, which will help us to distribute the contents of the *Principles* to a global audience. The editors would like especially to thank Elisabeth Dodds at Wiley-Blackwell, whose commitment to excellence has contributed materially to the quality of the book. In addition, without the assistance of Alison Brown the *Principles* would not have been published.

Our efforts were especially facilitated by the expert assistance of Lori Ennis and Barbara Boughen, who collaborated as a team complementing editorial talents with interpersonal skills, to maintain the high quality of the text and deliver the manuscripts in a timely fashion. The editors are indebted to their administrative and secretarial assistants, Patricia Lai, Terri Astin, Jennifer Mayes, Sue Sparrow, Patty Poole, Gracie Bernal-Muñoz, and Maria L. Vidrio.

Tadataka Yamada, MD

1 Clinical decision making

Philip S. Schoenfeld

What is evidence-based medicine? 1
Critical appraisal of an article about a diagnostic test, 2
Critical appraisal of an article about a therapy, 7
Conclusions, 12

What is evidence-based medicine?

David Sackett, the "father" of evidence-based medicine (EBM) stated that EBM is "the conscientious and judicious use of current best evidence from clinical care research in the management of individual patients" [1]. Terms used in this definition can be explained as follows.

• *Conscientious use* implies that physicians review articles about clinical research and apply this information to clinical decision making.

• *Current best evidence from clinical care research* implies that physicians systematically appraise the methods and results of clinical research articles using EBM tools. With these tools, physicians can separate the "wheat from the chaff" when reading medical journals and identify poorly designed studies that will produce biased results and should be discarded before being applied to patient care. This chapter will focus on techniques to identify and interpret the best evidence from properly designed research articles.

• *Judicious use* implies that a physician's experience and patient's preferences are crucial components of decision making and that these judgments must be balanced with the data from best evidence.

Judicious use of best evidence is a particularly important concept to understand [2]. Many critics state that the practice of EBM is "cookbook" medicine that devalues the judgment of a clinician and the values of an individual patient. This interpretation is inaccurate. Physicians must consider a patient's preferences about the potential benefits and side effects and costs of a medication when deciding a specific treatment. Also, a specific patient may not fit the criteria for enrollment of patients into a randomized controlled trial (RCT). For example, an RCT demonstrated that rifaximin, a nonabsorbable antibiotic, improved bloating in Lebanese patients [3]. Will bloating (and other gastrointestinal symptoms) improve if rifaximin is used in patients with irritable bowel syndrome (IBS) in the United States? If we assume that these results are applicable to patients with IBS in the United States, then is it worthwhile to use a treatment that may only produce a temporary relief of symptoms? What if the patient had a past history of *Clostridium difficile* colitis after a course of ciprofloxacin? Would the patient be willing to risk another case of *C. difficile* colitis? What if the patient does not have insurance and would have to pay $200 for this prescription? These questions are qualitative questions that require clinical judgments on the part of the patient and the physician [4]. Although the best evidence from an RCT [3] may identify an effective treatment for bloating, both physician judgment and patient preferences must also be used for effective clinical decision making. Thus, EBM and a reliance on best evidence is not intended to be "cookbook" medicine [2].

Nevertheless, EBM is a helpful tool for the quantitative aspect of clinical decision making, which arises from a systematic examination of study methodology and study results [2]. The medical literature is expanding at an exponential rate [5], and the time available for reading may be hurried and fragmented. Physicians need tools to build a framework for the rapid evaluation of the methodology and results of published studies, and EBM provides these tools (Tables 1.1 and 1.2). With these frameworks, physicians can rapidly identify well-designed studies that produce accurate and unbiased results and should be applied to patient care. Studies using improper methodology and biased results are quickly identified and ignored.

Principles of Clinical Gastroenterology. Edited by Tadataka Yamada, David H. Alpers, Anthony N. Kalloo, Neil Kaplowitz, Chung Owyang, and Don W. Powell. © 2008 Blackwell Publishing. ISBN 978-1-4051-69103

Table 1.1 Critical approach to an article about a diagnostic test

1. When are diagnostic tests necessary?
   a. Is the pretest probability of disease so high or so low that further diagnostic tests are not needed?
   b. How is pretest probability estimated?
2. Assessing study design
   a. Was there a blinded comparison of the diagnostic test to a gold standard test?
   b. Were negative study tests verified by performing the gold standard test?
   c. Was the diagnostic study tested in patients similar to the population in which the test will be used?
3. Getting from pretest probability to posttest probability
   a. Interpret and apply data about sensitivity and specificity.
   b. Use likelihood ratios to maximize the data from a diagnostic test.
4. Applying the results of clinical research to your patient
   a. Are the results applicable to your patient?
   b. Is the test available with reproducible accuracy?

From Schoenfeld et al. [6].

Table 1.2 Critical approach to an article about a therapy

1. Assessing study design
   a. Did the study use concealed random allocation?
   b. Were patients and physicians blinded about allocation to treatment or placebo groups?
   c. Did groups receive equal treatment (cointerventions) except for the experimental study treatment?
   d. Did the study use an intention-to-treat analysis?
   e. Was follow-up of study patients complete?
2. Clinically significant results and statistically significant results
   a. Estimating treatment-effect size: relative risk reduction, absolute risk reduction, and number needed to treat
   b. Evaluating the sample size in a non-statistically significant study: were enough patients entered into the study?
   c. What is the precision of the treatment effect: how large are the 95% confidence intervals?
3. Applying the results of clinical research to your patient
   a. Are the results applicable to your patient?
   b. Are the potential treatment benefits worth the potential side effects, cost, and inconvenience to your patient?

From Guyatt et al. [19].

This chapter outlines systematic frameworks for the evaluation of methodology and results of studies about diagnostic tests and therapies; it reviews different statistical presentations of study results and discusses the use of physicians' clinical judgments and patients' preferences when applying these results to patient care.

Critical appraisal of an article about a diagnostic test

Case scenario A – part I

A 65-year-old woman presents for colon cancer screening. The patient has never been screened for colon cancer. She is asymptomatic and she denies weight loss, hematochezia, abdominal pain, or family history of colon cancer. You proceed to describe the benefits and risks of colonoscopy. However, the patient has heard radio advertisements for a *virtual colonoscopy* that uses a computed tomography (CT) scanner to look for polyps (this procedure is more appropriately called "CT colonography"). This radio advertisement emphasized that colon perforations can occur during colonoscopy. To provide adequate guidance to this woman, you consider the following questions:
- What is the probability of colon polyps in this woman?
- How accurate is virtual or CT colonography for the diagnosis of colon polyps?

You decide to apply EBM frameworks [6] to appraise a recent study [7] that examines the accuracy of CT colonography and answers these questions.

When are diagnostic tests necessary?
Is the pretest probability of disease so high or so low that further diagnostic tests are not needed?

Pretest probability defines the likelihood that a patient has a specific disorder before any diagnostic test result is available. Diagnostic tests should be ordered when the pretest probability is intermediate. If the pretest probability of a specific disorder is 50%, then accurate diagnostic tests may rule out the disorder or definitively confirm the presence of the disorder. Conversely, if the pretest probability is very high or very low, then ordering additional diagnostic tests may be unnecessary.

Several examples illustrate the concept of pretest probability. What diagnostic tests would you order for a hospitalized patient who suddenly develops diarrhea? Stool tests for ova and parasites are routinely ordered to evaluate diarrhea, but the pretest probability of a parasitic infection in a hospitalized patient with new-onset diarrhea approaches zero [8]. In this situation, the pretest probability is so low that stool tests for ova and parasites should not be obtained. Conversely, patients with peptic ulcers are rarely tested for *Helicobacter pylori* in some countries (e.g., Armenia) because the prevalence of *H. pylori* approaches 100%. These patients are automatically treated for *H. pylori* after identification of peptic ulcers without testing for *H. pylori*. What level of pretest probability is intermediate and suggests the need for diagnostic tests? Would it be 25% likelihood of disease being present or 75% likelihood of disease being present? A physician must use clinical judgment here and consider the cost, accuracy, and side effects of the diagnostic test, the consequences of a "missed" diagnosis (i.e., if a missed diagnosis may have fatal consequences, then clinicians will have a lower threshold to order diagnostic tests), and a patient's preferences. Patient preference is an important concept with respect to diagnostic tests. For example, many patients may be particularly anxious that their symptoms represent the signs of a fatal disease. These patients may need to be reassured by the results of a negative diagnostic test, and physicians may have a lower threshold to order diagnostic tests in this situation.

How is pretest probability estimated?

When physicians evaluate a patient's complaint, they intuitively use their experience and clues from the history and physical examination to estimate pretest probabilities for different medical disorders. However, these estimates are often inaccurate [9]. The prevalence of a disorder (the proportion of patients with a specific disorder at a distinct point in time) provides a more accurate estimate of pretest probability.

Valid studies about the prevalence of a particular diagnosis should meet several methodological criteria [10]. First, the technique for confirming the diagnosis should be explicit and credible. For example, colonoscopy would be an explicit and credible test to estimate the prevalence of colon polyps. However, flexible sigmoidoscopy, which does not examine the right side of the colon, would not be a credible test. Second, the technique for confirming the diagnosis should be applied to consecutive patients who present with a specific complex of symptoms, physical examination signs, or laboratory results. For example, an appropriate study about prevalence of colon polyps could be applied to our case scenario if the study enrolled patients who were women 50 years of age or older, who were asymptomatic (e.g., no hematochezia or abdominal pain), and who were undergoing colorectal cancer screening. Finally, clinicians should determine whether the characteristics of their patients are similar to those of the patients examined in the study. For example, if a study estimated the prevalence of colon polyps in women with a family history of colon cancer, then the results from this study might not apply to the patient in our case scenario because the prevalence of colon polyps in patients with a family history of colon cancer is higher than the prevalence of colon polyps in patients with no family history of colon cancer.

Case scenario A – part II

A recent publication in the *New England Journal of Medicine* estimates the pretest probability for colon polyps in asymptomatic, average-risk women referred for colon cancer screening [11]. In this study, asymptomatic women referred for colon cancer screening underwent colonoscopy. Colonoscopy is a credible diagnostic test to define the prevalence of colon polyps. Consecutive women referred for colon cancer screening were offered colonoscopy. Patients were asymptomatic (e.g., denied history of hematochezia, change in bowel habits, or abdominal pain) and were screened with complete blood cell counts and fecal occult blood tests to rule out anemia or occult gastrointestinal (GI) bleeding. In this

trial, the prevalence of colon polyps among asymptomatic women was 21%, and the prevalence of advanced colon polyps (i.e., polyps larger than 10 mm, villous adenomas, adenomas with high-grade dysplasia, or colorectal carcinoma) was approximately 8% among women aged 60–69 years. Although the prevalence of advanced colon polyps is not very high, you recognize that a missed diagnosis of advanced colon polyps could lead to a fatal colon cancer. This study also demonstrates that evaluation of the left side of the colon with flexible sigmoidoscopy is a very poor predictor of polyps in the right side of the colon. Therefore, it is clear that it is crucial to evaluate the entire colon despite guideline recommendations which suggest that flexible sigmoidoscopy is still a reasonable alternative for colon cancer screening [12]. With this knowledge, you proceed to review the study about the diagnostic accuracy of CT colonography [7].

Assessing study design
Was there a blinded comparison of a diagnostic test to a gold standard test?

A *gold standard* or reference standard refers to a diagnostic test that definitively establishes the presence or absence of disease. For example, a study examining the diagnostic accuracy of magnetic resonance cholangiography (MRC) for the diagnosis of choledocholithiasis used endoscopic retrograde cholangiopancreatography (ERCP) as the reference test [13]. Reference standards are usually costlier, riskier, or more inconvenient than new diagnostic tests being studied. Otherwise, performing the reference standard would be more sensible. Biopsies, autopsies, surgical pathology, or even prolonged patient follow-up may also be reference standards that determine the presence or absence of disease.

The results from the reference standard and the diagnostic test should be examined by investigators who do not know the patient's history or the results of other tests. This *blinded* comparison is especially important when the interpretation of test results is subjective. For example, in the study assessing the diagnostic accuracy of MRC [13], the radiologist's interpretation of the MRC would be biased if he or she knew that the ERCP demonstrated choledocholithiasis.

Establishing a reference standard test may be an elusive goal. New technologies may be more accurate than the established reference standard test. If a potentially poor diagnostic test is being used as the reference standard, then the diagnostic accuracy of the new test may appear worse than it truly is. For example, one study evaluated the accuracy of ultrasonography to diagnose cholelithiasis but used oral cholecystograms as the gold standard test [14]. In this study, only patients with abnormal results on cholecystography were referred for surgery. Five patients in this study had ultrasounds that showed evidence of cholelithiasis, but normal-appearing cholecystograms. Based on this study's analysis, these positive ultrasound results were false-positive test results (i.e., patients did not truly have disease). Ultimately, several of these patients underwent cholecystectomy because of recurrent symptoms, confirming the presence of cholelithiasis and demonstrating that oral cholecystograms may not be an adequate gold standard test.

Were negative study results verified by performing the gold standard test?

Study results will be distorted if investigators use the results of the new diagnostic test to decide whether or not to perform the gold standard test. This *verification bias* may produce biased study results in more than 50% of diagnostic test studies [15]. For example, in the study about the accuracy of MRC for choledocholithiasis [13], a few patients with normal MRCs actually had choledocholithiasis on ERCP. If ERCPs were withheld from these patients (because investigators assumed choledocholithiasis was absent based on the normal MRCs), then MRC would appear more accurate than it truly is.

Was the diagnostic study tested in patients similar to the population in which the test will be used?

Patients with end-stage disease may have grossly abnormal diagnostic test results, making it easy to differentiate healthy people from ill patients. For example, virtual colonoscopy might easily differentiate patients with normal colons from patients with end-stage, near-obstructing colon cancer. The real value of a diagnostic test is its ability to identify patients with early manifestations of disease (e.g., colon polyps) that could be easily confused with a normal finding (e.g., stool). To assess the accuracy of a diagnostic test properly, the test should be studied in a broad range of patients, similar to the patients seen in clinical practice [16]. The best example of this *spectrum bias* may be carcinoembryonic antigen (CEA).

Measurement of CEA was evaluated as a diagnostic test for colorectal cancer. Initially, the test was studied in patients with advanced colorectal cancer and in healthy controls [17]. The results demonstrated that almost all (98%) of the patients with advanced colorectal cancer had elevated CEA, whereas almost all healthy controls had low levels of CEA. These initial results raised hope that CEA might be a useful screening tool for colorectal cancer. However, when this test was studied in a broad population of patients with early-stage colorectal cancer and patients with other GI disorders, the test was inaccurate and unable to differentiate patients with early cancer from patients with other disorders [18].

Case scenario A – part III

The study assessing the diagnostic accuracy of CT colonography used conventional colonoscopy as a gold standard, which is appropriate. Conventional colonoscopy was performed in all patients who underwent CT colonography, which eliminates verification bias. Patients were average-risk, asymptomatic men and women referred for colorectal cancer screening, so CT colonography was being evaluated in a population of patients that was similar to the population

in which it would be used. So, there was no spectrum bias. All study patients proceeded to conventional colonoscopy even if their CT colonography did not show any polyps. In other words, negative study results were verified by performing the gold standard test (i.e., conventional colonoscopy) and verification bias was avoided. Finally, the comparison of the CT colonography results with the conventional colonoscopy results was completely blinded using a segmental unblinding technique. After completion of the CT colonography, the radiological examination was immediately examined by a radiologist who reported the results for the cecum, ascending colon, transverse colon, descending colon–sigmoid colon, and rectum. The patient then immediately went for conventional colonoscopy. During the colonoscopy, the colonoscopist would complete the evaluation of a given segment of colon (e.g., ascending colon). Then, a study coordinator would reveal the results of the CT colonography for that segment of the colon. If a polyp was seen on CT colonography, but not seen on conventional colonoscopy, then the colonoscopist would carefully reexamine that portion of the colon. If no polyps were found, then the result was a false-positive finding on CT colonography. If a polyp was found on reexamination of the colon, then the result would be a false-negative for conventional colonoscopy. This is a particularly elegant technique to compare the new diagnostic test, CT colonography, to the gold standard, conventional colonoscopy, because the gold standard test is not perfect for identification of all polyps and the new diagnostic test, CT colonography, may occasionally identify polyps that are missed by conventional colonoscopy. Overall, you determine that the article has adequate methodology and you proceed to review the results.

Getting from pretest probability to posttest probability

Interpret and apply data about sensitivity and specificity

Sensitivity and specificity can be calculated from the classic 2×2 table (see Fig. 1.1). The 2×2 table is completed by filling in the true-positive test results (positive test result when disease is present), false-positive test results (positive test result when disease is absent), true-negative test results (negative test result when disease is absent), and false-negative test results (negative test result when disease is present). For example, a recent study assessed the accuracy of ferritin for the diagnosis of iron deficiency anemia, using bone marrow aspirates as a gold standard for the diagnosis of iron deficiency [19]. This trial found that 150 patients had high ferritin levels (more than 45 µg/L) and 85 patients had low ferritin levels (45 µg/L or less). Of the 85 patients with low ferritin levels, 70 had iron deficiency anemia (true-positive test results) and 15 did not (false-positive test results). Of the 150 patients with high ferritin levels, 135 patients did not have iron deficiency anemia (true-negative test results), and 15 did (false-negative test results).

	Iron deficiency anemia		
	Anemia present	Anemia absent	
Test positive (Ferritin ≤ 45 μg/L)	70 (TP)	15 (FP)	PPV: TP/(TP + FP) = 70/(70 + 15) = 82%
Test negative (Ferritin > 45 μg/L)	15 (FN)	135 (TN)	NPV: TN/(FN + TN) = 135/(135 + 15) = 90%
	Sensitivity: TP/(TP + FN) = 70/(70 + 15) = 82%	Specificity: TN/(FP + TN) = 135/(135 + 15) = 90%	

TP: True positive = test positive and disease present
FP: False positive = test positive and disease absent
FN: False negative = test negative and disease present
TN: True negative = test negative and disease absent
PPV: Positive predictive value
NPV: Negative predictive value

Figure 1.1 Sensitivity and specificity of ferritin for the diagnosis of iron deficiency anemia (36% prevalence of iron deficiency anemia) in an elderly population. Data from Guyatt et al. [19].

In the 2×2 table (see Fig. 1.1), the formulas for sensitivity (the percentage of patients with the disease in whom the test results are positive) and specificity (the percentage of patients without the disease in whom the test results are negative) are defined. Using these formulas, the sensitivity of ferritin (with a cutoff point of 45 μg/L of ferritin) for iron deficiency anemia is 82%, and the specificity is 90%.

Unfortunately, sensitivity and specificity "work backwards" from clinical practice, evaluating patients with known disease and providing data about the presence or absence of certain diagnostic test results. However, patients present with symptoms and diagnostic test results, and we "work forwards" with these results to determine the likelihood of disease. The positive predictive value (PPV) and negative predictive value (NPV) from the 2×2 table (see Fig. 1.1) provide these data. The formulas for PPV (the proportion of patients with positive test results who have the disease) and NPV (the proportion of patients with negative test results who do not have the disease) are also provided in the 2×2 table. Using these formulas, the PPV for low ferritin level (45 μg/L or less) in the diagnosis of iron deficiency anemia is 82%. Hence, 82% of patients with ferritin levels of 45 μg/L or less had iron deficiency anemia. The NPV for high ferritin level is 90%, or 90% of patients with ferritin levels of more than 45 μg/L did not have iron deficiency anemia. Before clinicians apply PPV and NPV to their individual patients, the limitations of these statistics must be recognized. Sensitivity and specificity usually remain relatively constant, although they may vary slightly depending on the severity of disease in a specific patient population. However, PPV and NPV vary widely depending on the prevalence of the disease. For example, consider if all internal medicine admissions to a hospital were screened with ferritin for iron deficiency anemia. In this diverse population, the prevalence of iron deficiency anemia might only be 5%, although the prevalence of iron deficiency anemia was 36% among the elderly anemic patients in the ferritin–iron deficiency anemia study [19]. Assuming that the sensitivity and specificity remain constant, a new 2×2 table (Fig. 1.2) can be constructed, producing a significantly lower PPV of 32% and a significantly higher NPV of 99%. Hence, when prevalence of a disease decreases, the PPV decreases and the NPV increases.

Use likelihood ratios to maximize the data from a diagnostic test

Likelihood ratios express the likelihood that a particular range of values for a diagnostic test will be found in a patient with a specific disease. They overcome two weaknesses of sensitivity/specificity and PPV/NPV. First, likelihood ratios predict the presence of disease based on a diagnostic test result (similar to PPV/NPV), but likelihood ratios do not change with different disease prevalence (unlike PPV/NPV). Second, studies reporting sensitivity and specificity usually provide data about the accuracy of a diagnostic test around

	Iron deficiency anemia		
	Anemia present	Anemia absent	
Test positive (Ferritin ≤ 45 μg/L)	8 (TP)	17 (FP)	PPV: TP/(TP + FP) = 8/(8 + 17) = 32%
Test negative (Ferritin > 45 μg/L)	2 (FN)	173 (TN)	NPV: TN/(FN + TN) = 173/(173 + 2) = 99%
	Sensitivity: TP/(TP + FN) = 8/(8 + 2) = 80%	Specificity: TN/(FP + TN) = 173/(173 + 17) = 91%	

Figure 1.2 Positive and negative predictive value of ferritin in the diagnosis of iron deficiency anemia in a hypothetical population of 200 hospitalized patients (5% prevalence of iron deficiency anemia).

Table 1.3 Likelihood ratios for ferritin in the diagnosis of iron deficiency anemia

Ferritin	Likelihood ratio
> 100 μg/L	0.13
> 45 to ≤ 100 μg/L	0.46
> 18 to ≤ 45 μg/L	3.12
≤ 18 μg/L	41.47

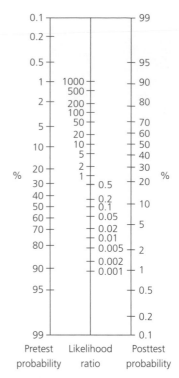

Figure 1.3 Nomogram for interpreting diagnostic test results. Adapted from Fagan [20], with permission from the Massachusetts Medical Society.

only one value. For example, the ferritin–iron deficiency anemia study [19] calculated sensitivity and specificity of ferritin around a cutoff point of 45 μg/L (i.e., ferritin level less than or equal to 45 μg/L is consistent with iron deficiency anemia and ferritin level greater than 45 μg/L is not consistent with iron deficiency anemia). Intuitively, a patient with a ferritin level of 5 μg/L is more likely to have iron deficiency anemia than a patient with a ferritin level of 40 μg/L, but the sensitivity and specificity cannot differentiate between these two patients. However, likelihood ratios are usually calculated for multiple ranges of diagnostic test results, thereby maximizing the information from a diagnostic test. Thus, likelihood ratios may facilitate the application of diagnostic test results to patient care.

Mathematically, the likelihood ratio for a positive test result is as follows: sensitivity / (1 – specificity), or true-positive rate/false-positive rate.

The likelihood ratio for a negative test result is as follows: (1 – sensitivity) / specificity, or false-negative rate/true-negative rate.

In the ferritin–iron deficiency anemia study [15], likelihood ratios were calculated for four ranges of ferritin: less than or equal to 18 μg/L, 19–45 μg/L, 46–100 μg/L, and more than 100 μg/L (Table 1.3).

By using a nomogram [20], likelihood ratios easily convert pretest probabilities to posttest probabilities (Fig. 1.3). Simply place the base of a ruler at the pretest probability and angle the ruler through the likelihood ratio to find the posttest probability. For example, clinicians might assume that a 70-year-old patient with a history of myocardial infarction, daily use of aspirin, a mean corpuscular volume of 78, and a hemoglobin level of 11 g/dL has a 50% pretest probability of iron deficiency anemia (moderately higher than the prevalence of iron deficiency anemia among a general population of elderly anemic patients). If this patient has a ferritin level of 5 μg/L, then the pretest probability of 50% and the likelihood ratio of 41 produces a 98% posttest probability that iron deficiency anemia is present. Conversely, if this patient has a ferritin level of 110 μg/L, then the posttest probability is 10%.

Case scenario A – part IV

For patients with large polyps (at least 10 mm), CT colonography produced sensitivity of 93.8% and specificity of 96% with a likelihood ratio for a positive test of 23 and a likelihood ratio for a negative test of 0.06. For patients with polyps larger than 5 mm in size, CT colonography produced sensitivity of 88.7% and specificity of 79.6% with likelihood ratios of 4 for a positive test and 0.1 for a negative test. Based on the data from the screening colonoscopy study in women [11], the prevalence of large (more than 10 mm) polyps in 65-year-old women is 5%, and the prevalence of colon polyps of larger than 5 mm is about 10%. Therefore, using likelihood ratios, positive results on CT colonography for large polyps predicts a 55% posttest probability of large polyps in our 65-year-old woman. Positive results on CT colonography for colon polyps larger than 5 mm predicts a 33% posttest probability of colon polyps in our patient.

The CT colonography is not very accurate for polyps that are 5 mm or less in size. However, this may not be a significant concern because fewer than 1% of these polyps have villous architecture or high-grade dysplasia contained within them [21]. Therefore, these diminutive polyps are very unlikely to develop into colorectal cancer.

Applying the results of clinical research to your patient

Are the results applicable to your patient?

A study may have valid methodology, and the results may indicate that the diagnostic test is accurate. However, if the study patient population is much different from your patient population (e.g., geriatric vs pediatric patients, symptomatic vs asymptomatic patients), then the diagnostic test may perform differently in your patients. If your own patient meets all the inclusion criteria of a study and the prevalence of disease is similar in your setting, the results are probably applicable to your patient.

Physicians need to use their own judgment when there are no definitive research data about the accuracy of the diagnostic test in specific patients. For example, the study being evaluated in the case scenario does not provide specific data about the diagnostic accuracy of CT colonography in 60- to 69-year-old women. However, there is no obvious pathological or physiological reason why CT colonography should be less accurate among women aged 60–69 years compared to other patients in this study. Thus, results from the CT colonoscopy study [7] should be applicable to the case scenario patient.

Is the test available with reproducible accuracy?

Even when a diagnostic test is adequately described to permit replication in your clinical setting, the test may not be available. Some diagnostic tests require special equipment or skilled examiners, which may not be widely available. For example, CT colonography is not widely available outside academic medical centers in 2007. Many diagnostic tests, including CT colonography, require subjective interpretation. A well-designed study of a diagnostic test will have the diagnostic test results reviewed by examiners with different levels of expertise. If experienced and inexperienced practitioners produce similar interpretations of diagnostic test results, then you may be assured that study results may be reproduced in your own clinical setting. For example, previous studies [22] have demonstrated that both experienced and inexperienced radiologists can accurately diagnose choledocholithiasis on MRC. Recent studies [23] demonstrate that properly trained radiologists and gastroenterologists produce reproducible and accurate interpretations of CT colonography when the three-dimensional "fly-through" technique is used. The three-dimensional fly-through technique produces an image that is similar to the endoscopic view of the colon produced during conventional colonoscopy.

Case scenario A – part V

Based on the radio advertisement that she heard, CT colonography is available to the patient and the study that examined the accuracy of CT colonoscopy indicates that it is very accurate for polyps larger than 5 mm in diameter. Although you do not know about the experience of radiologists at this specific CT colonography center, you recognize that properly trained radiologists appear to produce accurate and reproducible evaluations of CT colonography if they use the three-dimensional fly-through technique. Overall, you decide that CT colonography may be a reasonable

alternative based on the quantitative data from this particular study [7]. However, you also review several qualitative issues that the patient should consider before scheduling the CT colonography.

CT colonography requires a full preparation to evacuate stool from the colon. In fact, the study from the case scenario also had patients drink a barium-based solution to tag any remaining stool or water in the colon, and then used digital subtraction to remove these wastes from the three-dimensional fly-through image. If the local CT colonography center does not include this in their protocol, then they may not be able to reproduce the accurate polyp detection reported here [7]. Even if the local CT colonography center does add barium-based solutions to their protocol, then patients still need to go through two separate bowel preparations if they are found to have colon polyps (i.e., one bowel preparation for the CT colonography and then a second bowel preparation for the conventional colonoscopy that is subsequently performed to remove polyps identified on CT colonography). Many patients will not want to undergo two separate bowel preparations. Also, CT colonography is not reimbursed by most insurance policies, so the patient will probably have to pay $800–$1000 for the procedure. Finally, you reassure your patient that the reported rate of colon perforation during colonoscopy in asymptomatic individuals undergoing colorectal cancer screening appears to be less than 1 in 10 000 [23]. Given these issues, your patient decides that she would prefer to proceed directly to colonoscopy.

In the future, you recognize that CT colonography may become widespread when Medicare and insurance companies reimburse for this service. Proof-of-concept studies have demonstrated that CT colonography may be possible without evacuation of stool with bowel preparation [24]. (i.e., consumption of barium-based solution alone may be adequate to perform digital subtraction of stool during CT colonography.) If CT colonography is accurate, is reimbursed by insurance, and is performed without evacuation of stool by bowel preparation, then CT colonography could become the preferred tool for colorectal cancer screening. You are glad that recent research [22] demonstrates that gastroenterologists can also be taught to accurately interpret CT colonography images.

Critical appraisal of an article about a therapy

Case scenario B – part I

You are seeing a 75-year-old man with osteoarthritis of the hip and a past history of a nonsteroidal antiinflammatory drug (NSAID)-associated bleeding ulcer. His test results were negative for *H. pylori* infection during the evaluation of his bleeding ulcer. The primary care physician has referred this patient because treatment of osteoarthritis with acetaminophen and physical therapy has been ineffective. The primary care physician wants to restart the patient on an NSAID, but she is still concerned about the risk for recurrent NSAID-associated bleeding ulcers. Specifically, she asks the following questions.

• Among patients using NSAIDs, does the addition of proton pump inhibitors (PPIs) reduce the frequency of GI bleeding?

• If the addition of PPIs does reduce GI bleeding, how large is the reduction?

• Would it be more appropriate to place the patient on a cyclooxygenase-2 (COX-2) -selective NSAID or on a combination of PPI and conventional NSAID.

You recently saw an article [25] that may address the first two questions. This trial randomized patients with a history of *H. pylori* infection and NSAID-associated bleeding peptic ulcers to receive NSAID + PPI vs NSAID + *H. pylori* eradication. You apply EBM frameworks [26] to determine whether the study has appropriate methodology that is likely to produce accurate results (see Table 1.2).

Assessing study design

Did the study use concealed random allocation?

A patient's response to treatment may be influenced by many factors other than treatment. Age, severity of illness, and comorbid medical problems will affect a patient's prognosis and limit the effect of treatment. Therefore, these factors should be distributed equally between the treatment and placebo groups (or between a "new" treatment group and a control group) to identify a "true" or accurate estimate about the effectiveness of the treatment. In an RCT, every patient has an equal chance of receiving treatment or placebo when they enter the trial, so that these factors are usually distributed equally between the treatment and placebo groups.

In a nonrandomized trial, physicians determine which patients enter the treatment group and which patients enter the placebo group. For unclear reasons, patients with a good prognosis are disproportionately entered into the treatment group in a nonrandomized trial. Patients with a good prognosis are more likely to have a favorable outcome, regardless of the effectiveness of treatment [27]. Nonrandomized trials illustrate that these studies demonstrate larger treatment effects than randomized trials and are more likely to demonstrate a false-positive result [27].

Concealment of allocation maintains the integrity of randomization. In concealed random allocation, researchers who obtain informed consent and enroll patients into a trial do not know whether the next study patient will receive treatment or placebo. If concealment of allocation was used, then the methods section of a study should indicate this (e.g., sealed, opaque, sequentially numbered envelopes were opened after patients gave informed consent; a central coordinating center was called for treatment assignment after a patient gave informed consent). Researchers may subconsciously wish to show that the therapy being studied is superior to the control therapy. Therefore, without concealed allocation, researchers may subconsciously assess a patient's prognosis and guide patients with good prognosis into the treatment or new therapy group and guide patients with a bad prognosis into the placebo or control therapy group.

Were patients and physicians blinded about allocation to treatment or placebo groups?

Blinding simply means that the patients and physicians do not know if the patient received placebo or treatment. This is particularly important when the outcome is subjective. For example, another study [28] compared rates of peptic ulcer bleeding among patients with rheumatoid arthritis who took a COX-2-selective NSAID or naproxen. As part of this study, the VIGOR trial, the frequency of dyspepsia among study patients was assessed. However, the assessment of dyspepsia is quite subjective and variable. Both the patient and the study physicians may assume that COX-2 inhibitors are less likely to cause dyspepsia than conventional NSAIDs, like naproxen, possibly introducing bias into their subjective assessment of dyspepsia. Blinding both the patients and the health-care personnel (double blinding) is the best method to avoid this bias. Double blinding has been demonstrated to prevent inflated estimates of treatment benefit in randomized trials [29]. Randomization, concealed allocation, and double blinding are the only techniques that have been shown to reduce inflated estimates of treatment benefit in epidemiological studies [27,29].

The importance of blinding is self-evident, but it may be difficult to ensure. For example, a recent double-blind, randomized controlled trial compared lubiprostone with placebo among patients with constipation-predominant IBS [30]. In this trial, the study end point was global assessment of improvement in IBS symptoms, which is clearly a subjective outcome. However, lubiprostone, a calcium channel agonist, stimulates intestinal secretion of water and rapidly increases the frequency of bowel movements in constipated patients. Thus, patients using lubiprostone may have noted the rapid increase in frequency of bowel movements and assumed that they were using lubiprostone. This knowledge may have *unmasked* the blinding process and biased the subjective assessment of improvement in IBS symptoms. One possible resolution would be to ask patients to guess whether they had received lubiprostone or placebo at the end of the trial. If 50% of patients receiving lubiprostone guess correctly and 50% of patients using tegaserod guess incorrectly, then the blinding process still worked.

Even when the study outcome is objective, it is still helpful to maintain double blinding. For example, one study of primary prevention of bleeding esophageal varices with β-blockers examined overall mortality as a study outcome [31]. This is certainly an objective outcome, but double blinding was still maintained in this study because of the risk for co-interventions. Cointerventions are treatments other than the study treatment that may affect the outcome, especially when the cointerventions are unequally distributed between the treatment and placebo groups. For example, isosorbide-5-mononitrate has been shown to reduce variceal bleeding [32]. Without double blinding, the physician or the patient might be tempted to start isosorbide-5-mononitrate in one group more than the other group. Double blinding limits the unequal use of cointerventions.

Did the groups receive equal treatment (cointerventions) except for the experimental study treatment?

Additional treatments or cointerventions are most problematic when they are very effective, such as the additional use of isosorbide-5-mononitrate in a study about the effectiveness of β-blockers to prevent variceal bleeding. Although the methodology of a study may be strengthened if all cointerventions are withheld, it may be unethical to withhold effective treatment from patients enrolled in a study. Research does not occur in a vacuum, and patients receive additional treatments or cointerventions to optimize their health while participating in a study. To balance this conflict, the indications to use cointerventions should be clearly described in the Methods section, their use should be limited, and their use should be recorded for later analysis.

The VIGOR trial [28], which compared a COX-2-selective NSAID with naproxen in patients with isosorbide-5-mononitrate, clearly described the use of cointerventions in the Methods section. Patients were allowed to take other treatments for rheumatoid arthritis, including acetaminophen, methotrexate, and corticosteroids, even though concurrent use of corticosteroids with NSAIDs increases the risk for serious NSAID-associated GI complications [33]. The frequency of serious NSAID-associated GI complications among corticosteroid-using patients who used rofecoxib or naproxen was recorded for subgroup analysis. Concurrent use of other NSAIDs was forbidden because use of multiple NSAIDs increases the risk for NSAID-associated GI complications [33]. Patients on NSAIDs develop dyspepsia, and over-the-counter preparations to treat dyspepsia are readily available. So, recognizing that trials do not occur in a vacuum, researchers allowed patients to use antacids or *limited* doses of H_2-receptor antagonists. In limited doses, these medications are unlikely to affect the occurrence of serious NSAID-associated GI complications, but allowing use of these medications will treat dyspepsia.

Did the study trial use an intention-to-treat analysis?

In almost every study, some patients stop taking the study medication (treatment or placebo). They are noncompliant, or they believe that the study medication is causing side effects. An intention-to-treat analysis includes all randomized patients in the final data analysis, regardless of whether the patients completed the study or were compliant. An adherence-to-protocol analysis excludes patients who did not complete the study owing to noncompliance or side effects. An intention-to-treat analysis preserves the value of randomization because some patients with a poor prognosis may not be able to complete the study, but these patients should be included to understand fully the true effectiveness of a treatment.

An example best illustrates the concept of intention-to-treat analysis. A randomized trial compared desipramine, a tricyclic antidepressant, with placebo in patients with moderate to severe symptoms of functional bowel disease [34]. Some patients randomized to receive desipramine withdrew from the trial because they experienced severe side effects, including constipation, which is a well-known complication of anticholinergic drugs including tricyclic antidepressants. In the intention-to-treat analysis, these patients must be considered *treatment failures*, and the intention-to-treat analysis did not demonstrate that patients using desipramine were significantly more likely to experience global relief of symptoms compared to patients using placebo (60% vs 47%, $P = 0.13$).

An adherence-to-protocol analysis only includes patients who complete therapy, estimating the likelihood of a good outcome for patients who complete therapy. However, an adherence-to-protocol analysis may lose the value of randomization because patients unlikely to have a good outcome are eliminated from analysis. In the adherence-to-protocol analysis of patients with functional bowel disease, desipramine-treated patients were significantly more likely to experience global symptom relief (73% vs 49%, $P = 0.006$). Therefore, if a patient with functional bowel disease can tolerate desipramine without side effects, then they are more likely to experience global symptom relief compared to placebo-treated patients.

Robust studies will present both an intention-to-treat analysis and an adherence-to-protocol analysis, allowing readers to assess fully the results and to make up their own minds about the benefits of treatment. Because an intention-to-treat analysis includes compliant patients and patients who discontinue therapy as a result of side effects, it estimates the likelihood of achieving a desired outcome when a patient first starts a treatment, consistent with "real-world" medical practice. The adherence-to-protocol analysis estimates the likelihood of achieving a desired outcome when a patient can tolerate therapy without severe side effects. Notably, the study from our example [34] recognized that patients with constipation-predominant IBS were more likely to have side effects, while patients with diarrhea-predominant IBS would benefit from the constipation induced by desipramine. Therefore, the investigators performed a subgroup analysis of diarrhea-predominant IBS patients and demonstrated that desipramine was superior to placebo using an intention-to-treat analysis. Therefore, it appears that desipramine is most appropriate for patients with functional bowel disease who have diarrhea as their predominant bowel habit.

Was follow-up of study patients complete?

When patients drop out of studies, several explanations are possible. The patients may have disappeared because they experienced a side effect or even died from the study treatment, or they may stop follow-up because their symptoms have resolved. How can you determine whether the loss to follow-up biased the study's results? In a treatment study with a positive result, the study results could be recalculated, assuming that all treatment group patients lost to follow-up had a poor outcome and assuming that all control group patients lost to follow-up had a good outcome. If the recalculated results still demonstrate a treatment benefit, then the loss to follow-up did not cause a falsely positive study result. To avoid recalculations, one short cut is available [26]: only rare studies will still demonstrate a positive treatment effect upon recalculation of study results if more than 15%–20% of patients are lost to follow-up.

Case scenario B – part II

The study comparing NSAID + PPI with NSAID + *H. pylori* eradication in patients with a history of *H. pylori* infection and NSAID-associated peptic ulcer bleeding met all the criteria for a well-designed study: randomization, concealed allocation, equal and minimal use of cointerventions, use of double blinding, use of an intention-to-treat analysis, and minimal number of patients lost to follow-up. Based on this analysis, you decide that the study is likely to produce accurate and unbiased results, and you proceed to review the statistical representations of the results.

Clinically significant results and statistically significant results

Estimating treatment-effect size: relative risk reduction, absolute risk reduction, and number needed to treat

The relative risk reduction (RRR) expresses the decreased risk for an adverse outcome in the treatment group compared with the risk for an adverse outcome in the placebo or control group. For example, in a randomized, double-blind, intention-to-treat trial, patients with endoscopically treated bleeding ulcers received either intravenous PPI or placebo. The study end point was recurrent peptic ulcer bleeding: 22.5% of patients receiving placebo had recurrent bleeding, whereas 7% of patients receiving intravenous PPI had recurrent bleeding [35]. The RRR may be calculated as: (% placebo patients with bleeding – % treatment patients with bleeding) / % placebo patients with bleeding, i.e., (22.5% – 7%) / 22.5%.

This RRR is 69%. Hence, a patient with an endoscopically treated bleeding ulcer is 69% less likely to develop recurrent bleeding from the ulcer when receiving an intravenous PPI compared with a similar patient not receiving an intravenous PPI.

Absolute risk reduction (ARR) is the reduction in adverse outcomes between the placebo group and the treatment group. Although the RRR compares the risk for adverse outcomes between treated and placebo patients, the ARR identifies the actual reduction in adverse outcomes for treated patients. In the study of patients with endoscopically treated bleeding ulcer treated with intravenous PPI, the ARR may be calculated as: % placebo patients with recurrent bleeding ulcer – % patients receiving intravenous PPI with recurrent ulcer bleeding, i.e., 25% – 7% = 15.5%.

Therefore, patients with an endoscopically treated bleeding ulcer who receive intravenous PPI may decrease their individual risk for recurrent ulcer bleeding by 15.5%.

The RRR can be misleadingly large if adverse outcomes are infrequent in patients receiving placebo or no treatment. This concept is best illustrated by comparing the number needed to treat (NNT) and ARR with the RRR. Consider the results from the VIGOR trial [28]. The results from this trial were reported as frequency of serious NSAID-associated GI complications (severe upper GI bleeding, perforation, or obstruction) per 100 patient-years of NSAID use. There were 0.6 complications per 100 patient-years among patients using a COX-2-selective NSAID, rofecoxib, and 1.4 complications per 100 patient-years among patients using naproxen. Based on these data, the RRR is as follows: (% naproxen patients with complications – % rofecoxib patients with complications) / % naproxen patients with complications, i.e., (1.4% – 0.6%) / 1.4% = 60%.

In other words, a patient who uses the COX-2-selective NSAID, rofecoxib, is 60% less likely to have a serious NSAID-associated GI complication compared with a similar patient who uses naproxen. This sounds impressive until you consider the ARR. The ARR is as follows: % naproxen patients with complications – % rofecoxib patients with complications, i.e., 1.4% – 0.6% = 0.8%.

In other words, an average NSAID-using patient who uses a COX-2-selective NSAID, like rofecoxib, reduces his or her individual risk for a serious NSAID-associated GI complication by only about 0.8%. The NNT allows interpretation of study results in terms of patient care, especially when the RRR is large and the incidence of adverse outcomes is small. Specifically, the NNT is the inverse of the ARR, or 1 / ARR, estimating the number of patients who need to be treated to prevent one additional adverse outcome. In the VIGOR trial, the NNT is 1 / ARR, i.e., 1 / 0.8% = 1 / 0.008 = 125.

In other words, for every 125 average patients treated with COX-2-selective NSAIDs instead of naproxen for 1 year, one additional serious GI complication will be prevented. Patients and physicians may be less likely to choose a potentially better, but more expensive, treatment if the study results are presented as the ARR or NNT instead of the RRR [36]. Considering all three statistics (ARR, RRR, NNT) helps both patients and physicians assess the potential benefits of therapy.

Although the ARR and NNT may appear to be more useful than the RRR, the RRR is valuable because of its versatility.

It provides the best estimate of treatment benefit among patients with varying risks of adverse outcomes [37]. Patients using NSAIDs receiving naproxen in the VIGOR trial only had a 1.4% risk for serious NSAID-associated complications per 100 patient-years of use. However, how beneficial would rofecoxib be in a 78-year-old man with a past history of upper GI bleeding? Based on previously published data [33], this patient would have a significantly higher baseline risk for serious NSAID-associated GI complications, approaching 10 per 100 patient-years of use (i.e., 10% risk per year). Given this baseline risk, applying the RRR decreases the risk for serious NSAID-associated GI complications from 10% to 4%. This produces an ARR of about 6% (10% − 4% = 6%) and an NNT of about 17 (1 / 6% = 1 / 0.06 = 17). For this high-risk patient, the added expense of a COX-2 inhibitor is outweighed by the significantly improved safety profile. The value of the RRR is that it can be applied to patient populations with different inherent risks for adverse outcomes [37].

Evaluating the sample size in a non–statistically significant study: were enough patients entered into the study?

Studies that do not demonstrate statistical significance may be interpreted as negative studies (i.e., the treatment is no more likely than placebo to reduce adverse outcomes). However, an adequate number of patients have to enter a trial to demonstrate a statistically significant RRR, regardless of the effectiveness of the treatment. Many trials that do not yield statistically significant results have not entered enough patients into the trial to demonstrate reliably an RRR of 25% or even 50% [38]. When assessing study results, it should be clear if a non-statistically significant result represents a truly ineffective treatment or an inadequate enrollment of patients into a study.

When investigators plan a study, multiple outcomes may be analyzed, but the sample size is calculated based on only one outcome. For example, in a study comparing ligation plus octreotide with ligation alone in the prevention of recurrent bleeding from esophageal varices [39], the investigators estimated that ligation plus octreotide would reduce recurrent bleeding from varices by 70% compared with ligation alone. The study entered enough patients to demonstrate a statistically significant RRR of 70% for recurrent bleeding, and a statistically significant RRR of 76% was measured in the study. Investigators also evaluated 30-day mortality and found that combined treatment reduced 30-day mortality by 52% compared with ligation alone, but this RRR was not statistically significant ($P = 0.09$). However, only enough patients to demonstrate a statistically significant RRR of 70% for recurrent bleeding were enrolled in this study. Because the study demonstrated a strong trend for reduced 30-day mortality with combined treatment, this therapy may truly be efficacious in reducing 30-day mortality, and

this non-statistically significant result is likely the result of inadequate sample size.

What is the precision of the treatment effect: how large are 95% confidence intervals?

Traditionally, a P value of 0.05 or less indicates statistical significance. Studies with P values of 0.05 or less indicate that there is a 5% or less likelihood that the difference between treatment and placebo occurred due to chance. However, P values do not provide data about the accuracy or precision of study results. Confidence intervals do provide information about the precision of study results.

The 95% confidence interval (95% CI) estimates the range within which the true RRR or ARR resides 95% of the time (i.e., if you repeated the same trial 100 times, then the RRR would fall within the 95% CI in 95 of 100 trials). When the lower limit of the confidence interval for RRR is greater than zero, then the treatment is significantly better than placebo. If the upper limit of the confidence interval around the RRR is less than zero, then the treatment is actually harmful or worse than placebo. For example, the RRR in the VIGOR trial for fewer serious NSAID-associated GI complications with rofecoxib is 60% with 95% CI of 20%–80% [28]. Thus, the RRR for serious GI complications with rofecoxib has a 95% likelihood of being between 20% and 80% with the best estimate being 60%.

The magnitude of confidence intervals is determined by the sample size [40]. Studies with large sample sizes have narrower 95% CIs and a more precise estimate of the true RRR. When the upper limit of a confidence interval around an RRR is greater than zero, but the lower limit of the confidence interval is less than zero, it is possible that the treatment could be better, worse, or no different than placebo. If the magnitude of benefit is moderate and the confidence interval is wide and barely crosses zero, then the treatment is probably beneficial and the trial simply did not enter enough patients. For example, one study [41] examined patients with bleeding esophageal varices and compared band ligation with sclerotherapy for reducing rebleeding. The RRR for recurrent variceal bleeding with ligation was 48%, with 95% CI of − 15% to 68%; however, only 77 patients were entered into this study, which was not adequate to demonstrate a statistically significant RRR of 48%. A metaanalysis [42] pooled the results from several studies, allowing the analysis of 547 patients. With this larger sample size, the RRR for recurrent variceal bleeding with ligation was 42% (almost the same RRR as the original randomized trial), but with a statistically significant 95% CI of 16%–60%.

Case scenario B – part III

In the NSAID + PPI vs NSAID + *H. pylori* eradication study [25], patients treated with NSAID + PPI had a 4.4% rate of recurrent bleeding ulcer over 6 months compared with an

18.8% rate of recurrent bleeding ulcer among patients treated with NSAID + *H. pylori* eradication. You assume that the NSAID + *H. pylori* eradication group represents a placebo-type group for your patient. Given these results, you conclude that NSAID + PPI is much better than NSAID + placebo with an RRR = 77%, an ARR = 14.4, and an NNT = 7.

Applying the results of clinical research to your patient

Are the results applicable to your patient?
If your patient meets the inclusion and exclusion criteria of a study, then the results should be applicable to that patient. Even if your patient is a year too old to be included in the study or has a history of a comorbid disease not allowed in the trial, these issues may not prevent the application of study results to your patient. Ultimately, physicians must use their clinical judgment to decide whether a patient differs significantly from study patients, preventing application of study results to that patient.

A study may not identify a statistically significant difference between placebo and treatment for all patients entered in a study, but it may find a significant difference for a subgroup of patients. Often, this subgroup of patients has more severe disease with a higher frequency of adverse outcomes. However, physicians should be cautious before applying subgroup analyses to their patients, even if their patients fit into the subgroups. If investigators evaluate multiple outcomes in many subgroups, eventually one subgroup analysis will be statistically significant simply owing to chance.

The results of subgroup analyses are more likely to be valid if:
- the treatment effect is large
- only a few subgroup analyses were performed
- the subgroup analyses were hypothesized a priori (i.e., before performance of the study)
- it is consistent with current understanding of pathophysiology
- other, independent studies have produced similar findings.

For example, the VIGOR trial demonstrated that rofecoxib decreased clinical upper GI events (i.e., symptomatic ulcers, significant upper GI bleeding, perforation, or obstruction) in the subgroup of patients with a past history of clinical upper GI events. This subgroup analysis was one of only a few subgroup analyses; it was hypothesized a priori. Pathophysiology suggests that selective inhibition of COX-2 isoenzymes reduces the inflammatory response without inhibiting COX-1 isoenzymes in GI mucosal cells and platelets, which should prevent clinical upper GI events.

Are the potential treatment benefits worth the potential side effects, costs, and inconvenience to your patient?
When deciding whether to start a new treatment, both the patient and physician should consider the inconvenience, side effects, and costs associated with the treatment. When balancing the potential benefit of a treatment vs the potential consequences, the NNT is a helpful tool. If the treatment is cheap and convenient and the consequences of the adverse event are potentially severe, then a large NNT may be acceptable. For example, hundreds of health-care providers are vaccinated with hepatitis B vaccine to prevent one case of hepatitis B. If the treatment is expensive and inconvenient and has potentially significant side effects, then the treatment may still be acceptable if the NNT is small and the consequences of an adverse outcome are life-threatening.

Case scenario B – part IV
The NSAID + PPI vs NSAID + *H. pylori* eradication study did not have a true placebo group, although it is likely that some of the patients in the NSAID + *H. pylori* eradication group actually had recurrent ulcers prevented by the *H. pylori* eradication treatment. Therefore, the 18.8% recurrent bleeding peptic ulcer rate is probably an underestimation. Our patient does not have *H. pylori* infection, so we can use the NSAID + *H. pylori* eradication group as a rough estimate of recurrent bleeding peptic ulcer rate in an NSAID + placebo group.

This study was performed in Hong Kong in patients of Asian descent. You are uncertain if you can apply these data to your United States-born patient. There would have to be genetic or environmentally created differences in ulcer pathophysiology or PPI pharmacology between United States-born and Asian patients to prevent you from applying the results of this study to your patient.

Finally, you wonder if you should consider recommending a COX-2-selective NSAID for this patient. COX-2-selective NSAIDs have been associated with increased risks of cardiovascular side effects, which could be detrimental for your patient. Fortunately, your literature search identified a recent study that compared a COX-2-selective NSAID, celecoxib, vs a conventional NSAID, diclofenac, + PPI. This study did not find a statistically significant difference in recurrent ulcer bleeding rates between the two groups: 4.9% vs 6.4% [43]. You also note that the average price of generic PPI + generic NSAID is much less than the cost of branded COX-2-selective NSAIDs. Therefore, you conclude that NSAID + PPI is the most appropriate choice for your patient.

Conclusions

Ultimately, decisions about the use of diagnostic tests and treatments are balanced by possible benefits, harms, costs, patient preferences, and availability of these interventions. In this chapter, principles for the systematic appraisal and application of clinical research have been reviewed. This information will provide a basis to interpret the diagnostic and therapeutic applications of GI technology, which will be discussed in the ensuing chapters.

References

1. Sackett DL, Rosenberg WC, Muir Gray JA, et al. Evidence based medicine: what it is and what it isn't. BMJ 1996;312:71.
2. Straus S, Haynes B, Glasziou P, et al. Misunderstandings, misperceptions, and mistakes. ACP J Club 2007;146:A8.
3. Sharara AI, Aoun E, Abdul-Baki H, et al. A randomized double-blind placebo-controlled trial of rifaximin in patients with abdominal bloating and flatulence. Am J Gastroenterol 2006;101:326.
4. Weiner S. From research evidence to context: the challenge of individualizing care. ACP J Club 2004;141:A11.
5. Haynes RB, Sackett DL, Muir Gray JA, et al. Transferring evidence from research into practice. 1. The role of clinical care research evidence in clinical decisions. ACP J Club 1996;Nov/Dec:A14.
6. Schoenfeld P, Guyatt G, Hamilton F, et al. An evidence-based approach to gastroenterology diagnosis. Gastroenterology 1999;116:1230.
7. Pickhardt PJ, Choi RJ, Hwang I, et al. Computed tomographic virtual colonoscopy to screen for colorectal neoplasia in asymptomatic adults. N Engl J Med 2003;349:2191.
8. Siegel DL, Edelstein PH, Nachamkia I. Inappropriate testing for diarrheal diseases in the hospital. JAMA 1990;263:979.
9. Dolan JG, Bordley DR, Mushlin AI. An evaluation of clinicians' subjective prior probability estimates. Med Decis Making 1986;6:216.
10. Richardson WS, Wilson MW, Guyatt G, Nishikawa J. Users' guides to the medical literature: how to use an article about disease probability for differential diagnosis. JAMA 1999;281:1214.
11. Schoenfeld P, Cash B, Flood A, et al. Colonoscopic screening of average-risk women for colorectal neoplasia. N Engl J Med 2005;352:2061.
12. Winawer S, Fletcher R, Rex D, et al. Colorectal cancer screening and surveillance: clinical guidelines and rationale-update based on new evidence. Gastroenterology 2003;124:544.
13. Chan YL, Chan AC, Lam WW, et al. Choledocholithiasis: comparison of MR cholangiography and ERCP. Radiology 1996;200:85.
14. Barton RJ, Crow HC, Fook SR. Ultrasonographic and radiographic cholecystography. N Engl J Med 1977;296:538.
15. Reid MC, Lachs MS, Feinstein A. Use of methodological standards in diagnostic test research. JAMA 1995;274:6445.
16. Ransohoff D, Feinstein A. Problems of spectrum and bias in evaluating the efficacy of diagnostic tests. N Engl J Med 1978;299:926.
17. Thomson DM, Krupey J, Freedman SO, Gold P. The radioimmunoassay of circulating carcinoembryonic antigen of the human digestive system. Proc Natl Acad Sci U S A 1969;64:161.
18. Bates SE. Clinical applications of serum tumor markers. Ann Intern Med 1991;115:623.
19. Guyatt G, Patterson C, Ali M, et al. Diagnosis of iron deficiency anemia in the elderly. Am J Med 1990;88:205.
20. Fagan TJ. Nomogram for Bayes theorem. N Engl J Med 1975;293:257.
21. Schoenfeld P. Small colonic polyps – do they matter? Clin Gastroenterol Hepatol 2006;4:293.
21. Becker C, Grossholz M, Becker M, et al. Choledocholithiasis and bile duct stenosis: diagnostic accuracy of MRC. Radiology 1997;205:523.
22. Ray Q, Kim C, Scott T, et al. Gastroenterologist interpretation of CTC: Pilot study demonstrating feasibility and similar accuracy compared to radiologists. [abstract] Gastroenterology 2007;132:A6389.
23. Ko CW, Riffle S, Morris C, et al. Complications after screening and surveillance colonoscopy [abstract]. Gastroenterology 2007;132:A994.
24. Zalis ME, Perumpillichira J, Del Frate C, Hahn PF. CT colonography: digital subtraction bowel cleansing with mucosal reconstruction initial observations. Radiology 2003;226:911.
25. Chan FK, Chung SC, Suen BY, et al. Preventing recurrent upper gastrointestinal bleeding in patients with *Helicobacter pylori* infection who are taking low-dose aspirin or naproxen. N Engl J Med 2001;344:967.
26. Schoenfeld P, Cook D, Hamilton F, et al. An evidence-based approach to gastroenterology therapy. Gastroenterology 1998;114:1318.
27. Chalmers TC, Celano P, Sacks HS, Smith H. Bias in treatment assignment in controlled clinical trials. N Engl J Med 1983;309:1358.
28. Bombardier C, Laine L, Reicin A, et al. Comparison of upper gastrointestinal toxicity of rofecoxib and naproxen in patients with rheumatoid arthritis. N Engl J Med 2000;343:1520.
29. Schulz K, Chalmers I, Hayes RJ, Altman DG. Empirical evidence of bias: dimensions of methodological quality with estimates of treatment effects in controlled trials. JAMA 1995;273:408.
30. Drossman DA, Chey W, Panas R, et al. Lubiprostone significantly improves symptom relief rates in adults with irritable bowel syndrome and constipation (IBS-C): data from two, 12-week, randomized, placebo-controlled, double-blind trials [abstract]. Gastroenterology 2007;132:639f.
31. Pascal JP, Cales P. and a Multicenter Study Group. Propranolol in the prevention of first upper gastrointestinal hemorrhage in patients with cirrhosis of the liver and esophageal varices. N Engl J Med 1987;317:856.
32. Angelico M, Carli C, Piat C, et al. Isosorbide-5-mononitrate versus propranolol in the prevention of first bleeding in cirrhosis. Gastroenterology 1993;104:1460.
33. Schoenfeld P, Kimmey M, Scheiman J, et al. Non-steroidal anti-inflammatory drug associated gastrointestinal complications: guidelines for prevention and treatment. Aliment Pharmacol Ther 1999;13:1273.
34. Drossman DA, Toner BB, Whitehead W, et al. Cognitive-behavioral therapy versus education and desipramine versus placebo for moderate to severe functional bowel disorders. Gastroenterology 2003;125:19.
35. Lau JY, Sung JY, Lee KK, et al. Effect of intravenous omeprazole on recurrent bleeding after endoscopic therapy of bleeding peptic ulcers. N Engl J Med 2000;343:310.
36. Forrow L, Taylor WC, Arnold RM. Absolutely relative: how research results are summarized can affect treatment decisions. Ann Intern Med 1992;92:121.
37. Oxman AD, Guyatt G. A consumer's guide to sub-group analysis. Ann Intern Med 1992;116:78.
38. Frieman JA, Chalmers TC, Smith H, et al. The importance of beta, the type II error, and sample size in the design and interpretation of the randomized control trial. Survey of 71 negative trials. N Engl J Med 1978;299:690.
39. Sung JJ, Chung SC, Yung MY, et al. Prospective randomized study of effect of octreotide on re-bleeding from oesophageal varices after endoscopic ligation. Lancet 1995;346:1666.
40. Altman DG. Confidence intervals. In: Sackett DL, Richardson WS, Rosenberg W, Haynes RB (eds). Evidence-based Medicine: How to Practice and Teach EBM. London: Churchill Livingstone, 1997:228.
41. Laine L, El-Newihi HM, Migikovsky B, et al. Endoscopic ligation compared with sclerotherapy for the treatment of bleeding esophageal varices. Ann Intern Med 1993;119:1.
42. Laine L, Cook D. Endoscopic ligation compared with sclerotherapy for treatment of esophageal variceal bleeding. A meta-analysis. Ann Intern Med 1995;123:280.
43. Chan FK, Hung LC, Suen BY, et al. Celecoxib versus diclofenac and omeprazole in reducing the risk of recurrent ulcer bleeding in patients with arthritis. N Engl J Med 2002;347:2104.

Economic analysis in the diagnosis and treatment of gastrointestinal diseases

John M. Inadomi

Forms of economic analysis, 14

Costs, 15

Evidence-based approach to economic studies, 15

Are the results valid? 15

What are the results? 17

Will the results help in caring for my patients? 18

Conclusions, 19

As the costs of providing health care rise in the face of limited available resources, it is more than an academic exercise to identify management strategies that are both effective and cost-effective. There is an increasing requirement to validate one's practice patterns to patients, insurers, and regulatory agencies in a comprehensive fashion that includes demonstration of cost-efficient management. Based on these realities, it is imperative that today's health-care providers possess a solid understanding of economic analysis.

This chapter consists of three sections:
- descriptions of different types of economic analysis
- definitions of the types of costs contained in economic analysis
- essential components of valid economic models.

Forms of economic analysis

Medical decision analysis uses a set of mathematical tools based on probability theory to quantitatively compare the expected outcomes of competing medical management strategies [1–4]. Economic analysis includes a comparison of the costs in competing strategies to identify the optimal management strategies for environments possessing limited economic resources [5]. Guidelines directing the conduct and interpretation of economic analysis in health care have been previously published [6–10].

Principles of Clinical Gastroenterology. Edited by Tadataka Yamada, David H. Alpers, Anthony N. Kalloo, Neil Kaplowitz, Chung Owyang, and Don W. Powell. © 2008 Blackwell Publishing. ISBN 978-1-4051-69103

The simplest form of economic analysis is a *cost-minimization analysis*, also known as a cost-identification analysis. The objective of a cost-minimization analysis is to calculate the least expensive manner in which to treat a specific disorder. For this type of analysis to be valid, the clinical outcomes of competing strategies must be equivalent. The economic resources expended through each strategy are summed, taking into account the costs of the disease and its complications in addition to the costs of treatment. The results of a cost-minimization analysis are expressed in terms of the resources expended through implementation of each strategy.

If the clinical benefits between competing management strategies are expected to differ, then a cost-minimization analysis is an inappropriate tool and more complex analytical methods should be used. A *cost-effectiveness analysis* aims to measure the cost incurred in relationship to the benefit achieved and may be used to compare strategies that are expected to yield different outcomes. The result of a cost-effectiveness analysis is typically reported as the cost required to achieve each unit of benefit, such as the cost per life-year gained, or the cost per symptom-free day achieved. When comparing competing strategies of management, the difference in net costs between strategies can be compared to the difference in net benefits to calculate the incremental cost-effectiveness ratio (ICER). This ratio represents the increase in resource expenditure per unit of benefit achieved with one strategy compared to another, so lower incremental cost-effectiveness ratios are desirable, or more "cost-effective."

For some diseases, time spent in one state of health may not be viewed as equal to time spent in other health states. While a cost-effectiveness analysis assigns the same measure of outcome to all states in which the patient is alive, a *cost–utility analysis* varies the outcome to reflect patient preferences associated with each health state. To incorporate the differences in the quality of life between various states of health, a cost–utility analysis uses a conversion factor or weight that is assigned to each health state. These factors range in value from 1, representing the state of perfect health in which full credit for time spent in this state is accrued, to 0, representing the state of death in which no credit is accrued. These factors, or *utilities*, represent the preferences that patients report for these various health states.

The results of a cost–utility analysis include a unit of measurement that reflects the quality adjustment to the outcome, such as a quality-adjusted life-year (QALY). Comparison between strategies will yield an incremental cost–utility ratio that combines the quantity and quality of the outcome measure in one metric.

A fourth type of economic analysis is the *cost–benefit analysis*. This type of analysis differs from cost-effectiveness and cost–utility analyses in that all outcomes are expressed in monetary terms. While this allows the results of the analysis to be expressed as a single value, it requires assumptions that all benefits can be assigned a specific monetary value. The results of a cost–benefit analysis are calculated by subtracting the costs accrued from implementation of the strategy from the economic benefits gained; if the result is positive, a net gain is perceived to be achieved, while a negative result indicates that the strategy is not cost beneficial [11].

A final form of economic analysis is a *cost–consequence analysis*, in which the components of costs and consequences of competing programs are calculated and presented individually, without an attempt to aggregate the results.

Costs

An important distinction must be made between costs and charges. Costs are defined as the resources required to provide a particular service that represent the foregone opportunity to provide another service. Resources expended for one service cannot be used for another purpose, so this "opportunity cost" is defined by the value of that resource in its next best use to society [5]. Charges may deviate from cost estimates based on inclusion of profit margins, the relative bargaining power of payers and providers, and inaccuracies of accounting systems [12].

Depending on the perspective of the economic analysis, different components of costs are included. Cost components include direct and indirect (productivity) costs. Direct costs are further subdivided into direct health-care costs and direct non-health-care costs [5]. Direct health-care costs are generally borne by *insurers* and *patients* and include the costs of procedures, tests, drugs, supplies, health-care personnel, and medical facilities. Direct non-health-care costs are additional costs accrued by *patients* and include the child-care, elder-care,

and transportation costs required to attend health-care encounters. Indirect or productivity costs represent resources lost by *society* resulting from the inability to work, or engage in leisure activities because of morbidity or death from disease [5].

Evidence-based approach to economic studies

Guidelines outlining the components necessary to produce a valid economic analysis have been previously published [5,6,13]. Table 2.1 describes the criteria by which economic studies should be evaluated. These criteria are based on the Evidence-Based Medicine Working Group series *Users' Guide to the Medical Literature* [7,8]. The three main questions that must be answered affirmatively to accept the conclusions of an economic study include the following.

- Are the results valid?
- What are the results?
- Will the results help in caring for my patients?

Are the results valid?

Did the analysis provide a full economic comparison of health-care strategies?

To answer this question, all clinically relevant strategies must be included in the analysis, and an appropriate perspective of the analysis must be chosen.

Table 2.1 Components essential for economic analysis

Are the results valid?
  Did the analysis provide a full economic comparison of health-care strategies?
    Was a broad enough viewpoint adopted?
    Were all the relevant clinical strategies compared?
  Were the costs and outcomes properly measured and valued?
    Was clinical effectiveness established?
    Were costs measured accurately?
    Were costs and outcomes data appropriately integrated?
  Was appropriate allowance made for uncertainties in the analysis?
  Are estimates of costs and outcomes related to the baseline risk in the treatment population?
What are the results?
  What were the incremental costs and outcomes of each strategy?
  Do incremental costs and outcomes differ between subgroups?
  How much does allowance for uncertainty change the results?
Will the results help in caring for my patients?
  Are the treatment benefits worth the harms and costs?
  Could my patients expect similar health outcomes?
  Could I expect similar costs?

Was a broad enough viewpoint adopted?

When an economic model is constructed, the perspective, or vantage point, from which costs and benefits are observed must be established. A societal perspective is preferred whereby all costs borne by the health-care system, the patient, and society are included; thus direct health-care costs, direct non-health-care costs, and indirect (productivity) costs are included [5,6,13]. Direct non-health-care costs and indirect costs may be difficult to identify, so perspectives that are less comprehensive than the societal perspective are commonly used. These perspectives include a third-party payer or insurer perspective, the perspective of a hospital or clinic, or the patient perspective [5].

In addition to costs, outcomes include the effects examined, such as life-years gained, or the number of cancer cases detected or prevented. If the analysis includes patient preferences for the various health states included in the model (a cost–utility analysis), the outcome will be described in units of QALYs. By examining more global benefits such as life-years or QALYs, an economic analysis may compare resource expenditures among differing disease states; if outcomes are limited to those specific to a disease process, such as the numbers of cancers detected, such comparisons are not possible.

Were all the relevant clinical strategies compared?

All clinically reasonable strategies available to manage a clinical problem should be considered. Moreover, each strategy should be scrutinized to ensure that it conforms to a logical sequence of events. Generally, the investigators will provide a figure summarizing their proposed model to allow readers an opportunity to critique the model's structural and variable assumptions. Although it is beyond the scope of this chapter to discuss the construction of decision models in detail, it should be noted that decision trees are designed to model the temporal flow of clinical events from one initial decision point to subsequent events branching in a tree-like fashion that aims to capture the probabilistic nature of a disease process. In contrast, Markov models allow for movement of hypothetical patients back and forth between various health states in a recursive fashion.

Were the costs and outcomes properly measured and valued?

Was clinical effectiveness established?

The clinical effectiveness of management strategies must be established before any comparison of the cost-effectiveness of these strategies. Results from a single trial, a range of values from multiple trials, or a summary estimate derived from a quantitative analysis of published studies (i.e., a metaanalysis) are generally accepted to approximate effectiveness. It should be noted that *efficacy*, which represents outcomes achieved in research settings using idealized subjects under optimal conditions, may differ from *effectiveness*, which reflects outcomes achieved in "real life" settings using

patients who may not have been represented in clinical trials, under varied management conditions. While published results from randomized clinical trials are considered the best evidence for establishing the efficacy of a therapy, economic studies may be more valid if they are based on effectiveness data that reflect clinical practice in a more generalized manner [7].

Were costs measured accurately?

Depending on the identified perspective of the analysis, different direct and indirect cost components should be included in the economic model. Specifically, a societal perspective that incorporates all direct (health-care and non-health-care) and indirect (productivity) costs is optimally desired. Direct non-health-care costs and indirect costs are generally not available so many economic models are based on the third-party payer or insurer perspectives.

Were costs and outcomes data appropriately integrated?

The most common metric used to integrate the results of a cost-effectiveness analysis is the incremental cost-effectiveness ratio or ICER [7]. The ICER describes the additional cost incurred by providing an alternative strategy to achieve increased effectiveness. In addition to reporting the costs of tested strategies and their associated outcomes, such as life-years or QALYs gained, an economic study should present the ICER between competing strategies. In this manner, the resources required to implement management strategies to improve outcome in one disease may be compared to interventions proposed to manage unrelated disease states.

Economic analyses commonly incorporate discounting or time preferences for outcomes. Discounting reflects people's preference for having money and material goods in the present rather than in the future [6,13]. This concept accounts for the opportunity cost of spending money now to derive benefit at some later time, and is generally based on the financial gain that could have been achieved had the resources required to implement an intervention been invested instead. In a similar manner, health benefits must be adjusted to reflect the time preferences of patients; if not, delaying implementation of an intervention would always appear more cost-effective [6].

Was appropriate allowance made for uncertainties in the analysis?

This is arguably the most important question to answer when critiquing a decision analysis study, including those focusing on health economic questions. Uncertainty in the assumptions of the model may induce variability in the results that may cause the conclusions of the analysis to change. Uncertainty may be present in the parameter estimates (numerical values used for the model variables) as well as in the structural assumptions of the model (i.e., how the model is constructed) [5]. The conventional manner used to examine uncertainty is through sensitivity analysis. Values used as parameter estimates may be tested to observe whether variation within clinically relevant extremes alters the results. The structural assumptions may be tested by changing the relationship between various parts of the model and observing whether differences in conclusions arise. If variations of these factors are associated with substantial changes in conclusions, the model is reported to be sensitive to these factors. One of the major functions of decision analysis is to identify the critical factors necessary to define a clinical problem; the variables to which a model is sensitive identify the areas in which further investigation is necessary.

Uncertainties in parameter estimates may be examined through one-way sensitivity analysis, in which a range of clinically plausible values are assigned to a single variable and the results are examined to determine whether the overall conclusions of the analysis change. In two- or three-way analyses, two or three variables are varied simultaneously to assess their joint influence on the outcome of the model. Multiple (n-way) sensitivity analysis can be accomplished through specialized modeling techniques such as Monte Carlo simulation, in which the values assigned to multiple variables are varied simultaneously [14].

Are estimates of costs and outcomes related to the baseline risk in the treatment population?

It is of great importance to understand the population simulated in an economic model. Specifically, the generalizability of the results of an analysis depend heavily on whether the hypothetical subjects are representative of the population as a whole, or only represent a subpopulation at high or low risk for the outcomes assessed by the model.

What are the results?

If serious methodological flaws are identified through the process outlined above, there is little need to examine the results of the study. It is hoped, however, that published studies are of sufficient quality to achieve favorable responses to the criteria presented thus far and are candidates for examination of the results of the analysis.

What were the incremental costs and outcomes of each strategy?

Results of an economic analysis are best understood by presenting the costs and health outcomes of each strategy, identifying dominated strategies (strategies costing more despite providing less benefit than other strategies), and calculating the incremental cost-effectiveness between successively more effective nondominated strategies [8].

Figure 2.1 illustrates the results of a published cost–utility analysis comparing competing strategies of screening and surveillance to decrease mortality from esophageal adenocarcinoma [15]. In the absence of screening or surveillance, mean per patient costs were $104 over the remaining 16.46 QALYs of the cohort. Screening white men with reflux symptoms at age 50 years and limiting surveillance to those diagnosed with dysplasia associated with Barrett esophagus resulted in mean costs of $1748 and increased the mean QALYs of the cohort to 16.62. The ICER is graphically illustrated as the slope of the line connecting the two strategies and is calculated as $10 440 per additional QALY gained. Most importantly, conducting surveillance in patients with Barrett esophagus in the absence of dysplasia (as is recommended)

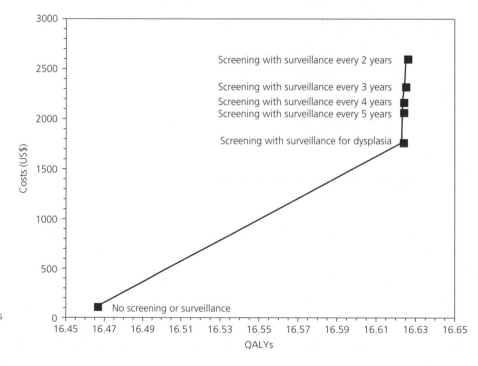

Figure 2.1 Costs and utilities associated with strategies to decrease mortality from esophageal adenocarcinoma. The abscissa denotes the quality-adjusted life-years (QALYs) remaining for the cohort, while the ordinate illustrates the accumulated costs over that period of time. The lines between the strategies illustrate the incremental cost-effectiveness ratio (ICER) between strategies.

increased costs by $300 to $800 per patient while providing a benefit of less than 0.001 QALY compared to the strategy of surveillance limited to patients with Barrett esophagus and dysplasia. The calculated ICER of these strategies was $380 000 to $600 000 per QALY gained.

Do incremental costs and outcomes differ between subgroups?

Much of outcomes research is concerned with identifying populations in whom costs or health outcomes differ substantially from the average results. Subgroup analysis allows the formation of models that can determine whether certain interventions are cost-effective only if limited to populations at high risk for development of poor outcomes, or conversely may be cost-effective for the general population except for those identified at low-risk for poor outcomes.

How much does allowance for uncertainty change the results?

As identified previously, one of the most important functions of a health economic analysis is to identify critical areas of research that must be pursued to establish whether the proposed interventions are cost-effective. A sensitivity analysis illustrates whether variation in the baseline assumptions of a model substantially alter the conclusions of an analysis. Uncertainty exists in the estimates used to populate the variables of all models so it is imperative that the range of clinical plausible values be examined in a systematic fashion. These values are generally obtained through systematic reviews and a metaanalysis of existing literature. Some variables may have insufficient data with which to conduct the analysis; in this case the use of expert opinion may be the only method available to generate values.

If the conclusions of an analysis substantially change with variation in the assumptions of the model, then the model is described as sensitive to these assumptions. If these assumptions are parameter estimates for variables, then clinical research should be directed to more precisely define the value of these variables. If these assumptions are structural assumptions of the model, additional data are required to define the interactions between the variables of the model. The latter generally requires advancements in our understanding of the biology and etiology of a disease process, or of the mechanism by which interventions may provide benefit.

Will the results help in caring for my patients?

An economic analysis will not be useful unless it addresses a clinical question that possesses the potential for improving the treatment of patients. It is of the utmost importance to critically appraise the actual benefits, risks, and costs associated with the implementation of tested strategies, and to determine whether the results of an analysis based on data derived from a research environment can be extrapolated to a general population.

Are the treatment benefits worth the harms and costs?

When comparing competing strategies in terms of their costs and benefits, three outcomes are possible.
• A strategy may be both less costly and provide greater benefit than an alternative strategy, in which case it is defined to be a dominant strategy.
• Conversely, the strategy itself may be dominated by being both more costly and associated with less benefit than the alternative.
• Lastly, one strategy may be more costly but achieve greater benefit than the alternative; in this case the incremental cost-effectiveness or incremental cost–utility may be calculated to determine whether the "bang is worth the buck". Implementation of the more costly strategy depends on the willingness of the health-care system (or whomever the perspective of the analysis was taken from) to commit the required resources to achieve the greater benefit.

Table 2.2 illustrates these possibilities. The difference in cost between strategies is aligned in rows, whereas the difference in effectiveness is listed in columns. The lower left quadrant depicts the case in which strategy A is less expensive than (or the same cost as) strategy B, while achieving greater effectiveness. In this case, strategy A is dominant compared to strategy B. The upper right quadrant examines the converse, in which strategy A is both more expensive and associated with less (or equal) effectiveness compared with strategy B; in this case strategy B dominates strategy A. The remaining two quadrants, upper left and lower right, depict examples where one strategy is associated with greater costs, but also greater effectiveness. In theses cases, the ICER may be calculated, which represents the additional resources required to improve outcome by using one strategy instead of another.

Could my patients expect similar health outcomes?

This question addresses the generalizability of findings from research studies to clinical practice. One must consider the difference between the efficacy of an intervention in a clinical

Table 2.2 Possible outcomes of a cost-effectiveness analysis

Costs	Effectiveness	
	A > B	A ≤ B
A > B	ICER A vs B	B dominant
A ≤ B	A dominant	ICER B vs A[a]

a If costs and effectiveness are equal, strategies are equivalent.
ICER, incremental cost-effectiveness ratio.

trial and the effectiveness of that intervention in a general practice setting. Clinical trials are usually performed in highly selected patient populations at specialized research institutions, so it must be questioned whether patients in one's own health-care population are similar enough to those in clinical trials to warrant extrapolation of the findings. In addition, the infrastructure to successfully implement the intervention must be shown to function as effectively as that available in the clinical trial [20].

Could I expect similar costs?

The perspective of the analysis dictates what types of costs are included in the model. However, even when limiting an economic analysis to direct health-care costs, considerable differences may exist between costs used in a study and the costs inherent in one's own health system. The reasons are varied, but include differences in the resources required to render services that may differ geographically or by the type of health-care system (government, private insurer, health maintenance organization), or because variations in clinical practice may induce cost differences that prevent translation of study costs to one's own practice environment [6].

Conclusions

The topics presented in this chapter construct a framework on which the reader may critically evaluate the information provided by economic analyses published in the literature. For those desiring more detailed information, and for investigators interested in conducting economic studies, several of the listed references provide a more comprehensive review of decision and economic analysis [1,2,4–8,11].

References

1. Petitti DB. Meta-analysis, decision analysis and cost-effectiveness analysis. New York: Oxford University Press, 1994.
2. Pauker SG, Kassirer JP. Decision analysis. N Engl J Med 1987;316: 250.
3. Weinstein M, Fineberg H. Clinical decision analysis. Philadelphia: Saunders, 1980.
4. Sox HC, Blatt MA, Higgins MC, Marton KI. Medical decision making. Stoneham, MA: Butterworth, 1988.
5. Gold MR, Siegel JE, Russell LB, Weinstein MC. Cost-effectiveness in health and medicine. New York: Oxford University Press, 1996.
6. Weinstein MC, Siegel JE, Gold MR, et al. Recommendations of the Panel on Cost-effectiveness in Health and Medicine. JAMA 1996; 276:1253.
7. Drummond MF, Richardson WS, O'Brien BJ, et al. Users' guides to the medical literature. XIII. How to use an article on economic analysis of clinical practice. A. Are the results of the study valid? Evidence-Based Medicine Working Group. JAMA 1997;277:1552.
8. O'Brien BJ, Heyland D, Richardson WS, et al. Users' guides to the medical literature. XIII. How to use an article on economic analysis of clinical practice. B. What are the results and will they help me in caring for my patients? Evidence-Based Medicine Working Group. JAMA 1997;277:1802.
9. Richardson WS, Detsky AS. Users' guides to the medical literature. VII. How to use a clinical decision analysis. B. What are the results and will they help me in caring for my patients? Evidence Based Medicine Working Group. JAMA 1995;273:1610.
10. Richardson WS, Detsky AS. Users' guides to the medical literature. VII. How to use a clinical decision analysis. A. Are the results of the study valid? Evidence-Based Medicine Working Group. JAMA 1995; 273:1292.
11. Provenzale D, Lipscomb J. A reader's guide to economic analysis in the GI literature. Am J Gastroenterol 1996;91:2461.
12. Finkler SA. The distinction between cost and charges. Ann Intern Med 1982;96:102.
13. Siegel JE, Weinstein MC, Russell LB, Gold MR. Recommendations for reporting cost-effectiveness analyses. JAMA 1996;276:1339.
14. Doubilet P, Begg CB, Weinstein MC, et al. Probabilistic sensitivity analysis using Monte Carlo simulation. A practical approach. Med Decis Making 1985;5:157.
15. Inadomi JM, Sampliner R, Lagergren J, et al. Screening and surveillance for Barrett esophagus in high-risk groups: a cost–utility analysis. Ann Intern Med 2003;138:176.
16. Tengs TO, Adams ME, Pliskin JS, et al. Five-hundred life-saving interventions and their cost-effectiveness. Risk Anal 1995;15:369.
17. Laupacis A, Feeny D, Detsky AS, Tugwell PX. Tentative guidelines for using clinical and economic evaluations revisited. CMAJ 1993; 148:927.
18. Laupacis A, Feeny D, Detsky AS, Tugwell PX. How attractive does a new technology have to be to warrant adoption and utilization? CMAJ 1992;146:473.
19. Ell C, May A, Gossner L et al. Endoscopic mucosal resection of early cancer and high-grade dysplasia in Barrett's esophagus. Gastroenterology 2000;118:670.
20. De Ronde T, Martinet JP, Melange M. Endoscopic therapy of Barrett's oesophagus: critical review. Acta Gastroenterol Belg 1999;62:390.

3 Psychosocial factors in the care of patients with functional gastrointestinal disorders

Bruce D. Naliboff, Jeffrey M. Lackner, Emeran A. Mayer

A neurobiological model of functional gastrointestinal disorders and how it relates to symptoms, in particular the psychological and psychiatric aspects of the disorders, 21

Centrally targeted pharmacotherapeutic approaches, 24

Summary of empirically validated psychological treatments, 26

Future development of integrated pharmacological and cognitive–behavioral approaches, 29

Practical advice on how to recognize psychological and psychiatric aspects of patients, with a focus on somatization, anxiety, and depression, 30

Proposed algorithm for management of functional gastrointestinal disorders, 32

Despite the continued uncertainty about the pathophysiology of irritable bowel syndrome (IBS) and related functional gastrointestinal disorders (FGIDs), an extensive body of literature and clinical experience has established clearly the importance of psychosocial factors in symptom expression, and severity and health-related quality of life impairment in patients with FGIDs [1,2]. Traditionally, in disorders that have a well-established organic pathophysiology, psychosocial factors have been considered to be separate, secondary, and less important than biological factors in the overall disease process, as well as in therapeutic approaches. However, in the case of the FGIDs, there is general consensus about:

- the pathophysiogical role of a dysregulated brain–gut axis [3,4]
- the importance of psychosocial stressors in first symptom onset and symptom exacerbation [5]
- the presence of significant psychiatric comorbidity [6].

Therefore, the role of underlying neurobiological and related psychological and psychiatric factors is likely to be of greater pathophysiological importance. The ability to use functional neuroimaging techniques to directly visualize the brain responses in patients with FGID to gut and to psychological stimuli, and to compare these responses to those obtained in patients with frequently comorbid psychiatric and functional pain conditions has provided strong support for this concept [7]. In this chapter, we will briefly review an emerging neurobiological model that is consistent with the key clinical and psychological presentation of FGIDs. We will focus on aspects of this model that are directly relevant for a better understanding and identification of the psychological dimensions of the functional GI syndromes. We will also present a rational approach to treating these dimensions using both pharmacological and nonpharmacological means.

In this chapter, the psychosocial dimensions of FGID are viewed as clinical manifestations of distinct alterations in the neurobiological mechanisms that are engaged in responses to psychosocial stimuli. Psychotherapeutic interventions are viewed as specialized therapies targeted at these distinct neurobiological abnormalities. Within this unifying conceptual framework, both pharmacological and psychological treatments are viewed as biological therapies, the major difference being the respective targets within the central nervous system (CNS) [8,9] (Fig. 3.1).

Principles of Clinical Gastroenterology. Edited by Tadataka Yamada, David H. Alpers, Anthony N. Kalloo, Neil Kaplowitz, Chung Owyang, and Don W. Powell. © 2008 Blackwell Publishing. ISBN 978-1-4051-69103

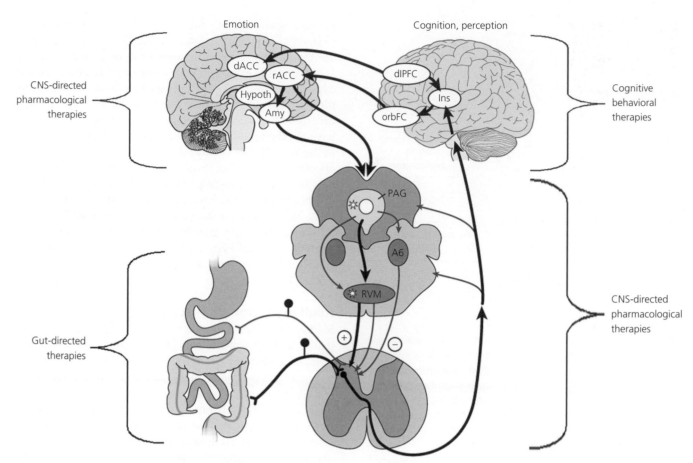

Figure 3.1 General targets within the brain–gut axis for FGID treatments. The principal components of the afferent pathways from the GI tract via spinal afferent pathways to the spinal cord, pontomedullary regions, cortical regions, and limbic and paralimbic regions are shown. While CNS-directed pharmacological therapies generally aim for targets within the spinal cord and subcortical regions, psychological treatments are aimed primarily at processes occurring within the prefrontal cortex. Modified from Mayer et al. [7], with permission from Elsevier.

A neurobiological model of functional gastrointestinal disorders and how it relates to symptoms, in particular the psychological and psychiatric aspects of the disorders

Alterations in the central stress response

The organism's response to stress is generated by a network comprising integrative brain structures that includes cortical, subcortical, and brainstem components (for review, see Mayer, 2000 [4]). The core of the stress system comprises subregions of the hypothalamus, amygdala, and periaqueductal gray. This basic stress circuit receives input from visceral and somatic afferents and from cortical structures. While afferent input from the periphery informs the brain about a wide range of parameters concerning the homeostatic state of the organism (temperature, blood oxygen levels, pH, food intake, and distention and contraction of the GI tract), cortical inputs to the central stress circuits inform the brain about environmental events, including real and perceived threats.

Cortical inputs also play a role in mediating the effects of memories of such environmental events. In turn, the integrative stress circuit provides outputs to the pituitary and to the pontomedullary nuclei, which mediate the neuroendocrine and the autonomic and pain modulatory output to the body, respectively [10–12]. The parallel outputs of this circuit have been referred to as the emotional motor system (EMS), and its principal pathways are summarized in Fig. 3.2 [13]. An important circuit involved in the stress response and in the generation of arousal involves reciprocal interactions between corticotropin-releasing factor (CRF)-positive neurons of the amygdala complex, including the bed nucleus of the stria terminalis (BNST), and catecholaminergic neurons of the locus caeruleus complex [14,15]. Animal studies suggest an important activation of the BNST, and the CRF/CRF subtype 1 receptor signaling system in various anxiety states. Based on neuroimaging studies, an increased responsiveness of this arousal circuit in patients with IBS has been suggested [7], and drugs aimed at reducing the activity within this circuit (including CRF subtype 1 receptor antagonists) are in

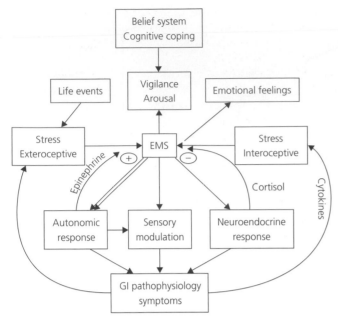

Figure 3.2 Brain–gut interactions and targets for psychological therapies. The schematic illustrates the outputs from the emotional motor system (EMS) to the GI tract and to brain regions involved in the generation of arousal and emotional feelings. While stressors stimulate the outputs of the EMS, cortical influences (mediating the effects of cognitive coping strategies and belief systems) are thought to have primarily an attenuating effect on EMS reactivity. Modified from Mayer [164], with permission from Cambridge University Press.

development as potential novel IBS therapies (see Centrally targeted pharmacotherapeutic approaches).

Adverse early life events and adult stress responsiveness

A series of studies in different patient populations has demonstrated that the quality of the early family environment interacting with genetic factors can serve as a major source of stress vulnerability in later life (Fig. 3.3). Individuals who are the victims of physical, emotional, or sexual abuse are at considerably greater risk for future anxiety disorders and depression [16–20]. Other less dramatic influences in early life, such as cold and distant parent–child relationships, and divorce of the parents or death of the mother before age 10, have also been associated with enhanced vulnerability later in life [21–23]. The enhanced vulnerability is not limited to affective disorders, but extends to a greater risk of chronic illness in general, including a greater risk for the development of IBS [24–26]. It has been suggested that this influence of early life events is mediated in part by parental influences (in conjunction with genetic vulnerabilities) on the development of neural systems that underlie the expression of behavioral, autonomic, and neuroendocrine responses to stress [27–31].

Adult psychosocial stressors

Studies in animals and humans have clearly demonstrated that certain types of stressors can alter the responsiveness of feedback systems by down-regulation of pre- or postsynaptic receptors (adrenergic, serotonergic, glucocorticoid receptors) [32,33]. In the most severe forms, structural changes are evident in certain brain regions [34,35]. Thus, pathological stress can not only activate, but also fundamentally change, the responsiveness and output of the central stress circuits. These alterations could affect the individual output pathways of the general stress response differentially and in different directions (for example, increase or decrease specific sympathetic outputs, increase or decrease certain vagal outputs, up- or down-regulate the hypothalamic–pituitary–adrenal axis, and change pain perception). Some of the best-characterized alterations in this central adaptation to pathological stress are an increase in CRF synthesis and secretion [36–38], an increase in the activity and sensitivity of central noradrenergic systems [39–43], and either a down-regulation or a

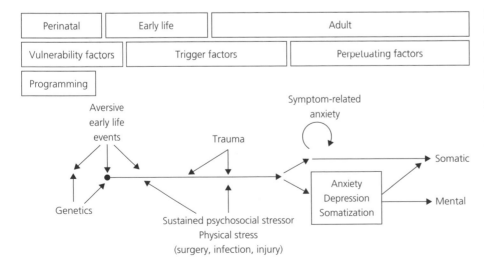

Figure 3.3 The role of stressors in the etiology of FGID and comorbid psychiatric disorders. The schematic illustrates the different effect of stressors on the clinical manifestation of somatic (FGIDs) and mental (psychiatric comorbidities) symptoms and syndromes. While the interaction between genetic factors and aversive early life events plays an important role in determining the vulnerability of an individual for stress-induced (somatic and mental) pathology in adult life, various types of stressors in adulthood play an important role in first onset or in symptom exacerbation. This model emphasizes the close expected relationship between somatic and mental symptoms. Modified from Mayer [164], with permission from Cambridge University Press.

sensitization of glucocorticoid receptors and adrenocorticotropic hormone release [44]. Changes in mood and affect associated with alterations in the stress response have been reported [45,46].

Homeostatic reflex responses and visceral sensitivity

Afferent signals arising from the lumen of the gut are transmitted via various visceral afferent pathways (enteric, spinal, vagal) to the CNS [47–49] (see Fig. 3.1). Homeostatic reflexes, which generate appropriate gut responses to physiological as well as pathological visceral stimuli and are aimed at reestablishing homeostasis, occur at the level of the enteric nervous system, the spinal cord, and the pontomedullary nuclei and limbic regions [48]. The great majority of homeostatic afferent inputs to the CNS from the gut (as well as other viscera) serve as direct input to these reflexes, and are not consciously perceived [50]. However, there are both peripheral and central adaptive mechanisms that can result in the enhanced perception of visceral stimuli ("visceral hypersensitivity"), as well as in the alterations of homeostatic reflex responses, resulting in abdominal pain, discomfort, and altered bowel habits [51]. As illustrated in Fig. 3.1, brain circuits that can down-regulate both enhanced perceptual and reflex responses are plausible targets for both pharmacological and nonpharmacological treatment approaches in FGIDs. Important networks in this context are the corticolimbic pontine circuits, which play a prominent role in the central modulation of emotional, autonomic, and pain responses [7]. Significant cortical components of these circuits are regions within the dorsolateral and ventrolateral prefrontal cortexes. These are thought to be involved in mediating the modulatory effects of beliefs and cognitive coping on the outputs of the EMS to the GI tract, and on associated emotional and arousal responses (see Fig. 3.2).

Central pain amplification

Central pain facilitation mechanisms have been implicated in the enhanced perception of visceral as well as somatic events in patients with chronic functional pain conditions [52]. The characteristic hyperresponsiveness to visceral and emotional stimuli seen in patients with IBS may be related to distinct, but interacting, alterations in central pain modulation systems (reviewed in Mayer et al. [7]). These include enhanced responses in pontine arousal circuits to expected aversive visceral stimuli (resulting in hypervigilance and symptom-related anxiety), ineffective engagement in corticolimbic pontine modulation circuits that normally would attenuate arousal mechanisms, and ineffective engagement of endogenous pain inhibition systems (resulting in compromised pain inhibition) [7]. In turn, these specific alterations can be conceptualized as targets for specific therapeutic interventions. For example, relaxation exercises and anxiolytics are aimed at reducing hyperarousal; cognitive strategies are aimed at

increasing the effectiveness of corticolimbic pontine inhibition circuits; and pharmacological therapies, such as antidepressants, are aimed at normalizing ineffective endogenous pain inhibition systems.

Although not generally discussed in the context of classic stress responses, the modulation of perceptual responses to sensory stimuli originating in the viscera, the musculoskeletal system, or the environment is an integral component of an organism's adaptation to potential or realized perturbations of homeostasis. In general, the anticipation of potentially harmful, but not life-threatening, stimuli are associated with increases in vigilance, attention, and anxiety. This results in an increase in sensitivity in different sensory modalities, including the visual, auditory, and olfactory systems. This increase in sensitivity is also observed in the somatosensory and viscerosensory systems [53]. On the other hand, the actual experience of noxious stimuli or severe stress is sometimes characterized by a decrease in the sensitivity to environmental stimuli, including a powerful inhibition of the pain experience [54,55]. Recent evidence suggests that this stress-induced decrease in somatic pain sensitivity may be accompanied by a stress-induced *increase* in visceral pain sensitivity [56,57]. Certain types of stressor and anxiety states can also be associated with an increase in somatic pain sensitivity [53]. For example, it has been demonstrated that the anticipation of pain in non-human primates can activate the same dorsal horn neurons normally activated by actual pain, providing a possible neurobiological basis for the amplification of pain during an anticipated harmful stimulus [58]. In addition to these phasically responding pain modulation systems, there are tonic pain modulatory influences (including descending serotonergic systems), which bias the system in accordance with the general homeostatic state of the organism [59]. Differences in the activity of these tonic systems may play a role in the altered pain sensitivity frequently seen in disorders of mood and depression, where abnormalities of central serotonergic systems have been demonstrated. As the primary effect of various antidepressants is thought to be mediated by a modulation of these monoaminergic systems, there is good construct validity for beneficial effects of these therapies on chronic abdominal pain and discomfort.

In addition to the activation of descending systems from the brainstem to the spinal cord, there are ascending systems originating in monoaminergic brainstem nuclei. These include the pontine locus caeruleus, which may contribute to stress-induced modulation of perception of visceral and somatic stimuli. Noradrenergic, serotonergic, and cholinergic neurons that project to cortical (prefrontal cortex) and subcortical regions play an important role in emotional arousal, attention, and vigilance towards sensory stimuli.

In summary, patients with IBS present with a pattern of symptoms that is consistent with enhanced responsiveness of the EMS, manifested in altered autonomic and pain modulatory responses. This response pattern is associated with changes in brain activity, characterized by hypervigilance, hyper-arousal, and increased emotional feelings. In patients with FGIDs, abnormal EMS responses are typically observed with the anticipation of and actual experience of aversive visceral stimuli. The fact that the changes are similar to those reported in a variety of other so-called "functional" disorders, suggests a top-down model in which the alterations in the EMS circuits of predisposed individuals can be triggered by psychosocial as well as physical stressors (e.g., gastroenteric infections), resulting in altered EMS outputs to the GI tract, and ultimately the generation of IBS symptoms.

Centrally targeted pharmacotherapeutic approaches

Sedatives and anxiolytics

The rationale for the use of anxiolytic drugs for the treatment of FGIDs likely stems from the clinical observation that the majority of patients also demonstrate comorbid psychological symptoms, particularly anxiety [6, 60]. As reviewed in the preceding paragraph, supportive biological evidence for such an approach comes from studies showing the overlap of brain circuits involved in emotion regulation, autonomic responses, and pain modulation in FDIGs [3,61] (see Figs 3.1 and 3.2). Up to 40% of patients seeking treatment for IBS suffer from anxiety disorders [6,62,63] and also show high scores on measures of symptom-related anxiety [60]. The majority of patients score higher than control subjects on anxiety questionnaires although they may not meet full DSM-IV criteria for an anxiety disorder [6]. Surprisingly, despite the strong theoretical, preclinical, and empirical rationale for the use of sedatives or anxiolytics, there are no well-designed clinical trials of this class of compounds in treating FGID symptoms. For decades, one of the most common treatment strategies for IBS has been the combination of long-acting benzodiazepines (such as Librax) or barbiturates (such as Butibel or Donnata) combined with so-called antispasmodics, which by themselves are probably ineffective. Despite the widespread use of anxiolytics by patients and limited clinical and anecdotal evidence suggesting a possible beneficial effect for benzodiazepines in IBS patients with anxiety disorders [64], there has never been supportive evidence from high-quality clinical trials for their use. Concerns about the side effects of sedation and the potential for addiction have discouraged further investigation of benzodiazepines.

In summary, considerable theoretical, preclinical, epidemiological, and clinical evidence suggests that drugs aimed at central anxiety and arousal circuits may be beneficial in treating patients with functional GI symptoms. However, there is no convincing clinical trial evidence to support the efficacy of these drugs. While the side effect profile of benzodiazepines argues against the use of this class of compounds for chronic treatment, short-term treatment for acute anxiety states in selected patients may be beneficial.

Antidepressants

Multiple central and peripheral mechanisms have been suggested as mediators of the beneficial effect on IBS symptoms of different classes of antidepressant drugs. Proposed central mechanisms include the treatment of comorbid depression, sleep restoration, analgesia, or antihyperalgesia (by strengthening endogenous pain inhibition systems). Proposed peripheral mechanisms include anticholinergic effects, normalization of GI transit, fundic relaxation, and peripheral antineuropathic effects. A detailed review of the relevant studies and a suggested paradigm for their use has been published [65].

Tricyclic antidepressants

Tricyclic antidepressants (TCAs) are prescribed for a number of pain-related disorders, including neuropathic pain, migraine, and fibromyalgia [66–68], as well as FGIDs [64]. The best evidence for their effectiveness is on neuropathic pain [66]. However, a variety of other effects may be important for their therapeutic benefit in FGIDs. For example, TCAs have been shown to slow down orocecal transit and have been shown to alter the duration, but not frequency, of the phase III contractions of the migrating motor complex [69]. Studies of the effect of TCAs on visceral perception as measured by barostat-controlled rectal balloon inflation have been inconclusive [70–72]. Amitriptyline has been shown to alter the activation of limbic brain regions in response to an auditory stressor combined with rectal balloon inflation suggesting a possible benefit for TCAs in stress-related perception of GI symptoms.

Most published studies have shown that TCAs improve symptoms in patients with FGIDs; however the quality and design of these trials have been variable [72–76]. Of the three recent metaanalyses that have evaluated possible beneficial effects of TCAs on functional GI symptoms [77–79], only two concluded that such treatments were beneficial [77,78]. Unfortunately, these metaanalyses are limited by the inclusion of studies with poor study design, including inadequate sample sizes, differences in the functional disorders included, use of different drugs and doses, and choice of outcome measures. In the largest randomized placebo-controlled trial to date, treatment with desipramine was superior to placebo alone in the per-protocol analysis (responder rate 73% vs 49%, number needed to treat = 5.2), but not the intention-to-treat analyses [80]. This is likely the result of the increased side effect profile of TCAs given at higher doses (i.e., dry mouth, drowsiness, constipation, and weight gain) leading to noncompliance and a high drop out rate. In clinical practice, TCAs are typically used at much lower and individually titrated doses (as low as 10 mg/day) and may be better tolerated with sufficient beneficial effect. In the study by

Drossman and colleagues [80], the beneficial effect of desipramine was seen primarily in diarrhea-predominant patients with moderate IBS symptom severity, who reported a history of abuse, but were without depression.

The TCAs have been shown to decrease sensitivity to somatic pain and to improve sleep, thus they might also be particularly beneficial for patients with FGID who have associated extraintestinal symptoms [70,81]. TCAs should not be used primarily to treat psychiatric symptoms in patients with FGID, because the selective serotonin reuptake inhibitors (SSRIs) have a lower side effect profile and greater therapeutic window at effective doses. However, TCAs in low doses may be combined with full therapeutic doses of SSRIs in FGID patients with comorbid depression.

Serotonin reuptake inhibitors

It has long been hypothesized that SSRIs may have beneficial effects in patients with IBS mainly by treating comorbid depression and anxiety. However, preliminary results from several recent clinical trials suggest a possible direct effect on IBS symptoms [82–84]. Other SSRI studies for IBS have shown benefit, but have not differentiated the improvement of psychological symptoms from GI symptoms [85–87].

Newer monoamine reuptake inhibitors, such as the serotonin and norepinephrine reuptake inhibitors (SNRIs) duloxetine and venlafaxine have been proposed as more effective treatments for chronic pain conditions associated with depression [88,89]. It is assumed that the combined effect of these drugs on tonically active descending serotonergic and noradrenergic pain inhibition systems (similar to the effect of TCAs) may be responsible for their effectiveness in the treatment of chronic functional pain conditions. Efficacy has been shown in fibromyalgia [90] and in patients with painful diabetic neuropathy [91,92]. While theoretically there may be an advantage of these newer drugs over TCAs and SSRIs for the treatment of IBS symptoms, clinical trial evidence for such a superiority has not been shown.

Summary

In summary, the theoretical rationales for using centrally acting drugs such as anxiolytics and antidepressants in the treatment of FGIDs are strong. The anxiolytic effect of these drugs on central mechanisms that are thought to play a role in IBS pathophysiology (hypervigilance, symptom-related anxiety, increased stress responsiveness), the potential antihyperalgesic effects of TCAs and SNRIs, and the well-established therapeutic effects on mood suggest their possible mechanism. The use of low-dose TCAs and full-dose SSRIs in selected patients (or patient populations) appears promising, though individualized dosing and patient education may be essential to avoid side effects and to ensure compliance. The reasons for the effectiveness in subgroups of patients are incompletely understood but may be related to differences in underlying pathophysiology, history of early

life trauma, and possibly to differences in genetic polymorphisms. The regular use of benzodiazepine anxiolytics and sedatives is discouraged because of the risk of habituation and the potential for dependency. Novel compounds with anxiolytic or antidepressant activity, such as neurokinin 1 (NK_1) receptor or CRF subtype 1 (CRF_1) receptor antagonists are in development.

Serotonin 5-HT$_3$ receptor antagonists

Serotonin (5-HT) has well-documented effects on gut motility, secretion, and sensation, likely through both central and peripheral pathways, making it a key pharmacological target in the treatment of FGIDs [93,94]. The 5-HT$_3$ receptor antagonists were originally developed as novel anxiolytics [95], followed by a development phase as potential visceral analgesics. The latter approach was based on the rationale of decreasing the responsiveness of spinal afferent neurons innervating the intestine to enterically released 5-HT or to mechanical stimulation [96,97]. More recently, preclinical evidence has implicated 5-HT$_3$ receptors located on central terminals of primary afferent nerves as important components of spinobulbospinal pain facilitation loops [98]. Several large randomized, double-blind, placebo-controlled trials have demonstrated that alosetron 1 mg twice a day for 12 weeks is effective in decreasing stool frequency and bowel urgency, and in providing adequate relief of abdominal pain and discomfort [99–102]. Some trials demonstrated a general global improvement of IBS symptoms and increased health-related quality of life in female [99–101] and male patients with diarrhea-predominant IBS [102]. Despite the unequivocal evidence for clinical effectiveness of this compound, efforts aimed at understanding the mechanism(s) of action of 5-HT$_3$ receptor antagonists have been only partially successful. Clinical [103, 104] and preclinical [105] evidence support the concept that the drug's effect on IBS global symptoms may be mediated in part by central effects. For example, IBS symptom reduction was correlated with reduction in neural activity in central arousal circuits, including the amygdala complex, a brain region involved in the central modulation of gut function and pain [103,106]. The most common adverse effect associated with alosetron use is constipation, which affects 25%–30% of subjects [107]. The occurrence of serious complications from constipation in 1/1000 patients (ileus, bowel obstruction, fecal impaction, and perforation) or ischemic colitis (prevalence 0.1%) has been reported from both clinical trials and postmarketing studies [108, 109]. The adverse event profile of the drug has led to the imposition of restrictions by the Food and Drug Administration of the United States on the prescription of alosetron. Since its reintroduction to the market in November 2002, alosetron is indicated only for women with severe diarrhea-predominant IBS who have experienced chronic IBS symptoms for at least 6 months and for whom conventional IBS therapies have failed.

In summary, 5-HT$_3$ receptor antagonists are highly effective drugs to treat multiple symptoms in male and female patients with diarrhea-predominant IBS. This beneficial effect may in part be related to inhibitory effects on hyperactive arousal circuits. However, because of rare, but potentially serious, side effects, their use is restricted to the most severely ill patients who have failed other therapies.

Summary of empirically validated psychological treatments

The past 20 years has witnessed the development and application of multiple psychosocial therapies for IBS. Their theoretical roots are grounded in the biopsychosocial model [110] and more recently in a more detailed neurobiological model [3,7]. The neurobiological model, described above, holds that individual biology (e.g., genetic predisposition, GI physiology), behavior, and higher order cognitive processes (coping, illness beliefs, abnormal central processing of gut stimuli) influence the development and course of IBS symptoms through their interaction with each other, with early life factors (e.g., trauma, modeling, parenting practices) and the individual's sociocultural environment (e.g., reinforcement contingencies).

Research based on the biopsychosocial model points to three main pathways through which psychological factors influence IBS [111]. The first pathway is directly through biological systems that mediate gut function and sensation [3, 112,113] (see Fig. 3.2). The second pathway is through the adoption of illness behaviors that exacerbate IBS symptoms, obscure symptom profile, and compromise function. Health behaviors are strongly influenced by psychosocial factors [114]. Patients seeking treatment for their IBS show higher levels of psychological distress [115] and higher rates of psychiatric comorbidity [116] than comparison groups (e.g., IBS patients not seeking treatment, IBS patients seen in primary care, patients with organic GI disease). A third pathway is by mediating the risk for development of chronic IBS symptoms [117]. This line of research has focused most extensively on the high rates of early life adversity [118,119] in patients seeking treatment (see also above paragraph and Fig. 3.3).

To the extent that psychological factors influence the expression of IBS, then it is believed that its symptoms are more effectively managed by addressing their presumed underlying psychological processes. By targeting at least one of the pathways linking psychological factors to IBS, psychological treatments presumably effect an improvement in symptoms or other outcome parameters (e.g., function, health-care use, quality of life).

Of psychological treatments, the most widely studied are cognitive–behavior therapies. Their underlying premise is that cognitive and learning processes play an important role in the development and maintenance of FGIDs. These same learning processes can be used to help patients to reduce the pain, distress, and disability associated with IBS. Learning-based or behavioral treatments encompass a number of different techniques, which fall into one of three categories, each reflecting their primary therapeutic focus: respondent techniques, behavioral techniques, cognitive techniques.

Respondent techniques

One type of therapy emphasizes respondent techniques, which are designed to reduce symptoms by teaching patients skills for directly modifying physiological response systems (e.g., decreased muscle tension, autonomic/sympathetic arousal). One may speculate that such techniques will ultimately result in a normalization of hyperresponsive central arousal circuits, a key component of the neurobiological FGID model outlined above. The primary respondent techniques are relaxation strategies, biofeedback, and hypnosis. The outcome literature has featured three types of relaxation training:

- progressive muscle relaxation training
- autogenic therapy
- diaphragmatic breathing retraining.

Progressive muscle relaxation training consists of the systematic tensing and relaxing of selected muscle groups of the whole body. Each muscle group is tensed for 5–10 s followed by approximately 20 s of suggestions to release muscle tension. Tension release cycles are used to deepen relaxation and to sharpen patients' ability to detect tension soon after it develops. The patient first learns to achieve deep relaxation with a relatively lengthy 16 muscle group tension–relaxation exercise. Once the patient masters 16 muscle group exercises, the number of muscle groups is combined (eight muscle groups to five muscle groups) so that the patient achieves a state of deep relaxation within a shorter amount of time before "relaxation by recall" exercises are introduced. In recall relaxation, the patient is taught to elicit a relaxation response without tensing muscles. The final step of relaxation teaches the patient to achieve deep relaxation through the use of counting procedures that require neither tension–relaxation nor a recall procedure. It is believed that unless patients detect tension early and respond to it more adaptively (by applying a more adaptive coping response), physical tension may accumulate to a point that it aggravates or amplifies bodily symptoms. Beyond any beneficial impact on peripheral processes, relaxation training and other somatic control techniques are likely to work by strengthening patients' sense of mastery or self-control over physical symptoms [120].

Biofeedback attempts to teach physiological self-regulation through the use of monitoring instruments that record the activity of physiological signals and displays this to the person being recorded. Biofeedback devices generally measure a specific physiological parameter not ordinarily under voluntary control or conscious awareness. Their activity is recorded by surface sensors, translated into a detectable display (e.g., audio tone or visual display) and "fed back" to the patient in real time as they are being recorded. The patient uses this information, typically in conjunction with the relaxation strategies described above, to regulate the body function being monitored. Biofeedback is typically carried out in a series of 6–10 one-hour-long sessions. Initial sessions are geared toward learning physiological self-regulation in relatively controlled (clinic) settings, while later sessions are designed to generalize this skill in more everyday situations associated with symptom flareups. The most common types of biofeedback modalities are thermal feedback and electromyographic (EMG) feedback. EMG feedback involves measuring the electrical activity of a patient's contracting muscles through the use of visual or auditory modes of feedback, while finger temperature feedback measures peripheral blood flow. The patient's goal is to learn to decrease muscle activity (or increased peripheral blood flow) on demand. Because muscle activity is regarded as an important pathophysiological mechanism underlying IBS, the use of EMG feedback has strong face validity and engages patients in the treatment process. In routine clinical settings where stress management is often the focus of treatment, EMG feedback typically uses the frontalis, masseter, and or trapezius muscles because of their reactivity to stress and ease of measurement. In thermal feedback, peripheral temperature from a finger or from a toe or foot is used to self-regulate autonomic arousal.

Both biofeedback and progressive muscle relaxation are "active" procedures, which require patients to actively attempt to exert control over physiological systems. In progressive muscle relaxation, the control is acquired by tensing and relaxing major muscle groups. In biofeedback, physiological self-control comes about through command of environmental stimuli (audio, video display) via feedback modalities (e.g., EMG, temperature). A second group of relaxation methods are termed passive procedures in that they attempt to elicit relaxation by "allowing sensations to happen" [121]. These methods regard relaxation as an innate physiological state that individuals have difficulty achieving because of competing environmental (noise), cognitive (worrisome thoughts), or emotional (stress, negative emotions) stimuli. Passive relaxation methods teach patients a variety of cognitive skills (deep reflection, attentional focusing, bodily awareness, mental imagery, visualization) to remove these barriers and in the process cultivate states of deep relaxation. Examples of passive relaxation procedures include autogenic training and breathing retraining. Autogenic training requires patients to repeat subvocally a set of verbal commands while attending passively to corresponding bodily sensations (heaviness in the limbs, warmth in the limbs, centering on breathing, warmth in the upper abdomen, and coolness in the forehead) that are suggestive of physiological relaxation. Self-suggestions of heaviness ("My hands, my arms and my shoulders feel heavy, relaxed, and comfort-

able") are theoretically designed to cue skeletal relaxation, while suggestions of warmth ("My hands are warm") are designed to elicit "autonomic relaxation" (peripheral vasodilation). During autogenic training the patient pairs the training phrase ("My hands are heavy and warm") with imagery (e.g., lying on a beach in the sun, holding two hands over a campfire) to evoke the physiological sensations and mental state described in the phrase [122].

In breathing retraining, the patient is taught to take slow, deep, even abdominal/diaphragmatic breaths and attend to relaxing sensations during exhalation. This relaxation procedure is based on the assumption [123,124] that patients with stress-related physical ailments develop abnormalities in breathing patterns (e.g., shallow, chest breathing), which, if chronic, can intensify the physiological arousal that underlies psychosomatic symptoms. By learning to slow down respiration through diaphragmatic respiration, patients presumably reduce the intensity of physical symptoms by normalizing the enhanced responsiveness of circuits of the EMS (see Fig. 3.2). As with all relaxation methods, breathing retraining requires patients to carry out daily practice exercises between sessions to generalize the skills taught in the clinic to the home setting.

In hypnosis [125,126], a therapist typically induces a trance-like state of deep relaxation or concentration using strategically worded verbal suggestions for changes in subjective experience or behavior. While details of hypnotic procedures and suggestion differ depending on the practitioner and clinical problem, sessions have two basic phases. The first is an induction phase during which a trained therapist helps the patient to relax using mental imagery and attention diversion techniques. One common induction method (eye fixation) involves instructing participants to focus on a specific spot or object, to relax more deeply, close his or her eyes to reduce distraction, and follow therapist-delivered suggestions. The provision of hypnotic suggestions is characteristic of the second "application" phase and are directed at achieving specific therapeutic goals such as pain relief, relaxation, restful alertness while the trance persists. Both indirect and direct suggestions may be used during hypnosis. In the context of IBS, hypnotic suggestions are "gut directed" – i.e., the therapists convey suggestions for imaginative experiences incompatible with aversive visceral sensation. Hypnosis for a patient with IBS might include a suggestion that the patient feel a sense of warmth and comfort spreading around the abdominal area. Even though the precise neurobiological mechanisms underlying the beneficial effect of hypnosis on FGID symptoms are not known, several brain-imaging studies have identified distinct changes in brain activity associated with hypnosis, consistent with a down-regulation of affective dimensions of the pain experience [127].

Behavioral techniques

Behavioral interventions focus on changing symptoms by directly altering problem behavior either through skills training exercises [128] or modifying environmental contingencies (e.g., operant behavior therapy) that reinforce symptoms [129]. Operant behavior therapy is based on the operant (or instrumental conditioning) principles set forth by behaviorist B.F. Skinner who emphasized the reinforcing role that the social environment plays in shaping behavior. An operant is an action by an organism that causes an outcome. The outcome of the operant serves to reinforce it, either positively or negatively. If the outcome is favorable to the organism, the probability increases that the operant will reoccur, and the action is regarded as positively reinforced. An outcome is negatively reinforced if the operant is followed by the removal of an aversive stimulus. If the outcome, however, is unfavorable – the probability that the operant will occur again decreases and the action is said to be punished. In clinical settings, the goal of operant techniques is to extinguish or diminish the reinforcing value of illness behaviors and reinforce "well" behaviors. Operant techniques work best for individuals whose illness behaviors (e.g., frequent health-care seeking) are excessive and linked to environmental contingencies such as attention from a solicitous partner, disability payments, and attention from health-care providers. Their responses may unwittingly reinforce illness behaviors that, in the case of functional disorders, have limited, if any, biological value. With repeated occurrence, a vicious cycle of symptoms–illness behaviors–positive reinforcement–symptoms ensues. To the extent that behaviors are shaped by their contingent consequences and the larger environmental context in which they occur, the operant approach focuses mainly on modifying overt illness behaviors through the systematic alteration of environmental consequences (rewards and punishments).

Social skills training is a general term that denotes a set of behavioral strategies aimed at remedying deficits in social behavior and promoting more positive interaction with others. In the context of IBS, these procedures assume that stress reactivity is partly the result of skills deficits that, once remedied, can empower patients to negotiate more effectively the stressors that aggravate IBS symptoms. Examples of social skills techniques include instruction in self-assertion, conflict negotiation, and direct communication (e.g., refusing requests, giving criticism). The therapist provides a rationale for each social skills module, elicits examples of possible scenarios where the skill is required, and role plays sample vignettes highlighting the application of the skill. Social skills training concludes with instruction in effective coping skills, modeling of socially competent behavior, behavioral rehearsal using role play with corrective feedback and coaching, and between-session practice in real-life situations.

Cognitive techniques

Cognitive technique refers to a set of interventions designed to challenge and dispute the negatively skewed thinking patterns characteristic of patients with IBS. These techniques are based on the assumption that cognitive processes, i.e., one's perceptions, attribution, and beliefs, mediate maladaptive responses, reflect errors and biases in information processing of clinical patients, and can be modified in a manner that reduces symptom severity. As outlined in the preceding paragraphs, cognitive techniques are likely to strengthen corticolimbic pontine modulation systems, which aim to attenuate the emotional, autonomic, and pain responses to visceral and expected aversive stimuli. Examples of distortions in thinking include a tendency to catastrophize (overestimate the costs or consequences of negative events), overestimate the likelihood of threat (thinking the worst), and hold unrealistic beliefs regarding the controllability of stressors. For example, an IBS patient may be reluctant to travel on a plane because of worries that she will have an accident mid flight and embarrass herself in front of others. In this case, the patient is overestimating how likely it is that a negative event will occur. To the extent that patients can link catastrophic cognitions to symptom flareups using daily symptom diary records, they would be encouraged to test the validity and usefulness of negative thoughts and their impact on symptoms. Patients are then instructed to challenge and dispute negatively skewed thinking patterns using a variety of techniques. One common strategy requires the patient to learn and apply evidence-based logic ("what is the probability that my worry of having an accident on the plane will definitely occur based on the evidence I have right now") to generate more factual predictions ("I really don't know what's going to happen . . . while I had one accident several years ago, the majority of plane trips have not been a problem") rather than threatening interpretations of life events. By rehearsing structured exercises between clinic visits, patients learn to identify problem beliefs, challenge and dispute their accuracy, and reduce the intensity of behavioral, emotional, and physical responses. Cognitive procedures have been featured as a stand-alone treatment approach [130] and as part of a multicomponent treatment program [80,131–133] that features both cognitive and behavioral techniques (cognitive–behavior therapy).

Psychodynamic–interpersonal treatment

Of non-behaviorally based treatments, brief psychodynamic interpersonal psychotherapy [134,135] has received the most empirical investigation. This approach subordinates the skills training emphasis of cognitive–behavior therapy to a less directive therapeutic stance that encourages the exploration of interpersonal conflicts that are "intertwined with the person's bowel symptoms, resulting in a vicious cycle of pain, distress, and disability" [136; p.153]. Treatment attempts to improve IBS by:
• improving a client's self-awareness and understanding of symptoms and the relationship of those symptoms to emotional difficulties that often arise during interpersonal conflict

- resolving conflict through the vehicle of the patient's relationship with a therapist who imparts insight, encouragement, and reassurance.

In research settings, psychodynamic therapy for IBS is typically scheduled eight times over 3 months (e.g., one 2-h session and seven 45-min sessions) [86]. In routine clinical settings, however, psychodynamic therapy typically involves more than eight sessions (between 16 and 20).

Overview of treatment outcome studies

Evidence for the claim that psychological therapies have therapeutic value comes from a number of systematic reviews. Drossman and colleagues [137] reviewed 15 randomized controlled trials and found evidence for the efficacy of psychological treatments in reducing bowel symptoms post-treatment in 10 of 13 studies. Blanchard and Scharff's [138] review of 21 randomized controlled trials concluded there was "strong" evidence to support the efficacy of hypnotherapy, cognitive therapy, and brief psychodynamic psychotherapy. The Rome III Working Team for Psychosocial Aspects of Functional Gastrointestinal Disorders [139] arrived at a similar conclusion. Appraising essentially the same data against a generic set of criteria for evaluating the quality of both pharmacological and psychological trials, Brandt and colleagues [79] concluded less enthusiastically that only "intermediate-quality" evidence supported the use of psychological treatments for specific IBS symptoms. While narrative reviews have arrived at generally favorable conclusions regarding the efficacy of psychotherapy, they should be interpreted cautiously in light of the subjective and idiosyncratic methodology used for collecting and interpreting information. It is unclear whether statements about treatment efficacy reflect the biases inherent in performing narrative reviews or the true therapeutic value of psychological treatments. For these reasons, Lackner and colleagues [140] conducted a quantitative review (metaanalysis) of 30 randomized controlled trials that compared patients assigned to psychotherapy, treatment as usual, or to control groups who received no treatment (e.g., people on cognitive–behavioral therapy waiting lists). While there were too few studies to establish the relative superiority of any one psychological therapy, psychological treatments as a group appeared to be effective in reducing GI symptoms of IBS (pain, disordered bowel habits), and to a lesser extent psychological distress. The number needed to treat for 50% or greater relief of symptoms in the short term was 2.01. These positive findings should be interpreted somewhat cautiously because the quality of trials is variable, sample sizes are often small, and suffer from other methodological limitations (blinding, vague diagnostic imprecision, inconsistent end points). Larger scale clinical trials have done little to clarify matters. Two studies – one featuring psychodynamic psychotherapy [86] and one a multicomponent cognitive–behavior therapy program [80] – yielded little evidence that either treatment as administered was effective for the set of GI symptoms

for which patients sought therapy. While Creed and colleagues [86] found that neither psychotherapy nor the drug (paroxetine) relieved abdominal pain, psychotherapy and paroxetine were superior to treatment as usual in improving the physical aspects of health-related quality of life, as measured by the SF36 Health Survey. Patients assigned to psychotherapy (but not paroxetine) showed a significant reduction of health-care costs compared with treatment as usual. Psychotherapy was associated with a total cost of $976 (US dollars) compared with paroxetine at a cost of $1252. The trial of cognitive–behavior therapy [80] found that it was associated with improvement on a composite index based largely on patients' ratings of their subjective well-being. No prospective change in specific IBS symptoms was reported. The trial by Creed and colleagues reported that psychodynamic interpersonal therapy was, in comparison with treatment as usual, associated with improvement in physical function but not subjective well-being dimensions of health-related quality of life. A third multicenter study [132] featuring a group-based version of cognitive therapy showed that it was more effective in reducing GI symptoms and quality of life impairment than a waiting list control condition. However, cognitive therapy did not perform consistently better across both treatment sites than an attention placebo condition or as well as the cognitive–behavior therapy featured in previous small-scale randomized controlled trials. These data, coupled with the results of earlier studies, comprise sufficient evidence that psychological treatments are at least moderately effective for reducing GI symptoms and related difficulties among patients with moderate to severe IBS. Unlike most drug treatments, psychological treatments produce changes across the two specific features of IBS, namely pain and irregular bowel habits. Psychological treatments appear more effective than either no treatment or treatment as usual. Few trials have controlled for so-called non-specifics of psychological treatments, such as the therapeutic rationale, adherence and allegiance to the therapeutic protocol, provision of a convincing rationale for the treatment, and time and attention from a warm, supportive clinician. Therefore, it cannot be determined whether psychotherapies are more efficacious than placebo or whether their effect is the result of specific techniques inherent in the featured treatment approach. How long treatment effects persist, what accounts for outcomes, how to abbreviate treatment so that it is more disseminable beyond academic research centers, and what patient is likely to respond are additional questions that remain unanswered.

Future development of integrated pharmacological and cognitive–behavioral approaches

Considerable evidence from treatment and brain-imaging studies in patients with depression suggests that pharmacological and psychotherapeutic approaches may be synergistic, both in terms of outcomes and associated brain activity changes [8,9]. Even though similar evidence is not available for the treatment of patients with FGID, the neurobiological model outlined above provides theoretical evidence supporting such an approach. One may speculate that while psychological therapies improve specifically cognitive coping skills and enhance corticolimbic inhibition, centrally acting drugs are likely to interfere with spinal, pontine, and limbic mechanisms. Both types of approaches are likely to reduce hypervigilance and hyperarousal by decreasing activity in central arousal circuits. On a behavioral basis the combination approach is also appealing because it can emphasize the positive aspects of both the medical model (the problem is real and understandable) and the self-management model.

Practical advice on how to recognize psychological and psychiatric aspects of patients, with a focus on somatization, anxiety, and depression

Assessment of biopsychosocial factors in functional GI disorders

Although the biopsychosocial model presented above has led to a much better understanding of the pathophysiology underlying the interactions between psychosocial factors and the cardinal symptoms of FGIDs, the clinician is still faced with the important task of assessing these issues in each individual patient and putting together a comprehensive, individualized plan. More specifically the clinician needs to make important decisions regarding the following questions.

• Are there non-GI-symptom-related issues that will significantly impact either the choice of treatment or treatment effectiveness?
• Should I consider using psychoactive or pain medications and of what type?
• Is referral to a specialist in psychology, psychiatry, or pain management needed?
• Is there a positive cost–benefit ratio to further GI workup: i.e., does the very low probability of uncovering a new relevant organic finding or the reassurance from another negative workup override the potential negative consequence of reinforcing an unproductive disease/cure model of FGID?
• How best to begin to discuss stress triggers for symptoms and the relevance of psychological and self-management issues.

To answer these and related questions there are some important domains of psychological function that can be assessed. The most common are symptoms of anxiety and depression. Disease-related cognitions and coping ability regarding IBS symptoms, somatization, and presence of past and current stressful life events may also be important areas to assess.

Clinical interview

Indications of how a particular patient might fare on these dimensions can be inferred from the clinical interview – if the patient is comfortable disclosing psychological information and specific questions for these issues are included. A list of specific questions for several domains is included in Table 3.1 [141]. It is important to make sure that patients understand the relevance of such questions and that they are assured of confidentiality. Clinicians should also make sure that there is sufficient time for patients to discuss these sensitive areas and that they are prepared to provide an adequate response

Table 3.1 Psychosocial screening questions

Area of assessment	Sample specific question
Depression	Over the last 2 weeks how often have you been bothered by any of the following problems: (a) little interest in doing things (b) feeling down, depressed or hopeless? Score for each question: not at all = 0, several days = 1, more than half the days = 2, nearly every day = 3 A total of 3 or more indicates an 83% chance of depressive disorder
Anxiety	Have you been anxious or feeling tense recently?
Somatization	In the systems review include questions about headaches, chest pains, palpitations, limb and joint pains, fatigue, tightness of the throat, difficulty with swallowing, difficulty with micturition, dysmenorrhea, dyspareunia
Attribution of symptoms/worry about illness	What do you think causes these symptoms? How worried are you about these symptoms? Have you worried that they might indicate a serious illness, such as cancer?
Illness impact and quality of life	How much do these symptoms interfere with your daily life?

Modified from Creed et al. [140], with permission from Degnon Associates, McLean, VA.

to any significant revelations (such as major depression, suicidal tendencies, domestic violence, etc.) that may occur. A second visit within a week or two may be required to follow up on this area of assessment. Since for many patients discussion of psychosocial issues may be unexpected in a medical interview it is also important to normalize this part of the examination. A good strategy is to open the discussion with questions about how the FGID impacts on the person's life and to use a model of how stress may make symptoms worse in some patients [141].

Screening questionnaires

Empirical studies suggest that medical clinicians often miss psychological problems or underestimate their severity [142]. Fortunately, there are well-validated, brief self-report psychological questionnaires for use with FGIDs. We briefly review some of the important areas for evaluation and example questionnaires most relevant for a FGID screening tool kit in the following sections. A more complete list and detailed descriptions can be found in the ROME III volume [141].

Anxiety and depression

The FGIDs, and especially IBS, have shown significant comorbidity with anxiety disorders and anxiety has been linked to altered pain processing [7,63]. The biopsychosocial model outlined above provides a biological explanation for this comorbidity (see Figs 3.1 to 3.3). The occurrence of depression has also been reported to be higher in patients with FGIDs and may significantly impact the response to treatment [5]. Even in populations of patients with IBS who are without a clear-cut anxiety or depressive disorder, altered mood may be a significant clinical finding that warrants further assessment. Assessment of the severity of anxiety or depression symptoms can be accomplished quite reliably with brief screening questionnaires. Ideally such a questionnaire for use in a population of patients with FGID (or another medical population) will avoid reliance on somatic symptoms to avoid contamination of the mood assessment by the presenting medical complaints. A good example of this type of scale is the Hospital Anxiety and Depression Scale (HADS), which has been specifically developed for medical patient screening. It has been widely used in FGIDs [143,144], and has validated cutoff scores for possible and probable presence of clinically meaningful anxiety and depression.

Gastrointestine-specific anxiety, coping, and cognitions

Chronic and pain-related conditions and certain functional disorders are associated with a variety of unhelpful and sometimes dysfunctional patterns of thinking. Illness-related cognitions and beliefs have an important influence on behavior, well-being, treatment response, and, as illustrated in Figs 3.1 and 3.2, may play an important role in the activity of the corticolimbic pontine circuits, which can modulate

perceptual, emotional, and autonomic responses to actual and anticipated visceral stimuli [6]. Although a variety of cognitive variables have been identified and discussed in the literature, two general categories of particular impact are illness catastrophizing and GI symptom-specific anxiety.

Catastrophizing refers to an exaggerated sense of threat from medical symptoms [145]. Components of illness-related catastrophizing include an overestimation of the negative consequences of symptoms, feelings of helplessness to cope with symptoms, and rumination or inability to distract oneself from symptoms. Catastrophizing has been shown to be an important predictor of poor outcomes in a variety of medical and pain-related disorders, including IBS [146,147]. The *Catastrophizing and Control scales* from the *Coping Strategies Questionnaire* (CSQ) are brief and well-validated measures of coping applicable to patients with FGIDs [148]. A disadvantage of these and other coping questionnaires is the lack of validated cutoffs for determination of mild, moderate, or severe levels of poor coping.

Gastrointestine-specific anxiety is defined as the cognitive, affective, and behavioral response to fear of GI sensations, symptoms, and the context in which these visceral sensations and symptoms occur [60]. Examples of GI symptom-related contexts include situations involving food and eating, like restaurants and parties, or locations in which bathroom facilities are unknown or difficult to reach. As a marker of overresponsiveness to GI sensations, GI-specific anxiety is hypothesized to perpetuate IBS symptoms through alterations in autonomic and pain facilitation, as well as cognitive mechanisms [60]. The GI-specific anxiety may be associated with beliefs of poor symptom control and high illness impact and may, therefore, be a critical element in the severe decrements in quality of life found in IBS patients. GI-specific anxiety has been shown to be significantly associated with IBS severity and impact even after controlling for general anxiety. Recently, the Visceral Sensitivity Index (VSI) was developed as the first instrument to assess GI-specific anxiety. Initial validation efforts indicate that the VSI is an efficient, reliable, and valid measure of GI-specific anxiety in an IBS patient population [149]. The 15-item self-report questionnaire measures fear, anxiety, and hypervigilance that can accompany misappraisals of visceral sensations and discomfort.

Somatization

There are a variety of ways to define somatization. It can refer to the somatoform psychiatric disorders, which have very stringent criteria and therefore do not apply to a significant number of patients with FGID. More commonly, however it is used to describe patients who report a chronic course of multiple functional or pain-related symptoms that are associated with impairment of function and increased demand for health care [150]. Somatization disorder in IBS commonly occurs in the presence of anxiety and depression [151]. Somatization has also been associated with a history of abuse or a rejecting parenting style during childhood, environmental stress, and concurrent anxiety and depression [119] (see also Fig. 3.3). The presence of patients with somatization or what is now sometimes called multiple symptom illness helps explain the frequent extragastrointestinal symptoms of IBS, and the high cooccurrence of other syndromes (e.g., chronic fatigue syndrome, fibromyalgia, multiple chemical sensitivity syndrome) that are defined by unexplained bodily symptoms [63]. As discussed above there is growing evidence that the overlap among functional and psychiatric syndromes reflect certain common CNS processes including affect regulation and pain modulation. There exist well-validated brief screening measures for somatization or breadth of functional symptoms. The Patient Health Questionnaire 15 (PHQ-15) is one such measure with cutoffs for mild, moderate, and severe somatic symptom severity [152].

History of trauma

A history of sexual abuse or physical trauma has been reported to occur in 20%–60% of treatment-seeking patients with IBS and is associated with negative outcomes, including refractory symptoms, greater health-care utilization, and increased receipt of invasive procedures [118,153]. The effects of trauma, especially at an early age, may be related to an increase in somatic vigilance, comorbid psychological disturbances, and poor coping. However, more recent data has pointed to a more complex relationship between negative life experiences and symptom patterns in FGIDs [154]. Many patients report no history of trauma and initial reports of the prevalence of childhood sexual abuse in IBS may have been biased by use of tertiary-care samples. In addition, a variety of factors including parental rejection, household environment, and other non-traumatic but negative events may be significant in vulnerability and later symptom expression for some patients [119] (see also Fig. 3.3).

It is also important not to let the initial speculation about the importance of early sexual abuse in FGIDs overshadow the assessment of current or recent stressors that may be significant for an individual case. For example, domestic violence is a relatively common high-level stressor that is more frequently reported in IBS [155]. Despite these caveats, assessment of early life and recent trauma can be an important part of a comprehensive workup for patients with FGIDs, especially those with multiple symptoms and evidence of more significant psychosocial disturbance. This information should be elicited in a very sensitive fashion and only after establishment of rapport and without undue pressure to reveal information. Encouragement in the form of open-ended questions like "Is there anything else you think might be important such as very painful or difficult experiences," may be used to open this area of discussion. There are also validated instruments for this area that might be considered; however, they should be used with caution and preparation in a clinical setting as most have been developed

for use in research settings. The most frequently used instrument in the literature for clinic-based assessment of abuse is the interview-based measure developed by Leserman and colleagues [156]. The Early Trauma Inventory–Self Report (ETI–SR) is a new brief instrument for the assessment of physical, emotional, and sexual abuse, as well as general traumas, which measures frequency, onset, emotional impact, and other variables [157].

Other variables
Quality of life

Although not often used in a purely clinical setting there are multiple measures for assessing a patient's general quality of life or well-being. The most widely used generic measure is the Medical Outcomes Study Short-Form Health Survey (SF-36) [158]. This and its shortened version, the SF-12, yield scores for physical and mental aspects of quality of life that can be compared across illness groups [159]. Illness-specific quality of life measures for IBS include the well-validated Irritable Bowel Syndrome Quality of Life measurement (IBS-QOL) [160]. There are also quality of life measures for dyspepsia, heartburn, and gastroesophageal reflux disease [141].

Current stress

Events such as divorce, unemployment, financial problems, and other stressful life events can be tallied by instruments such as the Life Experiences Survey [161] while self-perceived stress can be measured by instruments like the Life Stress Scale [162]. While mostly used in research settings, measures like the Life Stress Scale can be used in office screening of a patient's general level of perceived stress.

Recommendations for assessment batteries

If one wishes to use questionnaires for patient screening, a questionnaire for mood (e.g., HADS), a measure of somatization (e.g., PHQ-15), and perhaps a measure of symptom-specific anxiety or coping (e.g., the VSI or Catastrophizing Scale) should be satisfactory; patients with elevated scores on these measures may require further attention and assessment. As an alternative, some clinicians and clinics will choose a multidimensional instrument such as the Symptom Checklist (SCL-90) [163], which includes scales for depression, phobic anxiety, somatization, as well as others. The important point is that both clinical experience and the growing neurobiological evidence suggest that all patients with FGID should at least be minimally screened for psychosocial issues.

Proposed algorithm for management of functional gastrointestinal disorders

The above discussions point to a growing consensus regarding the importance of psychosocial factors in FGIDs, the efficacy of psychological, and to some extent psychopharmacological, treatments, and an emerging neurobiological basis for the biopsychosocial model. This review of the empirical and clinical literature leads to some practical suggestions regarding how to best approach the clinical care of an individual patient with FGID. A first step is to assess the most critical variables that will help determine the level and type of psychosocial intervention that might be warranted.

Severity of FGID symptoms

• Patients with mild or intermittent symptoms and only minimal functional impact should receive clear diagnostic information regarding the nature and expected course of their FGID. They should be encouraged to develop a self-management strategy, which may include symptomatic medications, lifestyle change (such as exercise), and education regarding the appropriate role for further workup.

• As severity of symptoms increases, especially in the presence of significant impact on quality of life and activities, it becomes much more important to include a careful investigation of the psychological issues discussed above and more likely that targeted psychological interventions will become necessary.

Chronicity of symptoms

• Chronicity of symptoms per se is not necessarily a strong predictor of need for psychological intervention. However, longer chronicity in the presence of negative predictors such as poor coping or somatization predicts a complicated treatment course and often a need for behavioral interventions.

Beliefs about the nature and cause of the FGID

• Successful treatment of FGIDs often requires patients to change their focus from looking for a medical cure to developing a self-management approach. The primary clinician can play a significant part in this process by first eliciting the patient's beliefs and then providing the patient with a positive model of FGIDs that is optimistic but realistic.

• For many patients, especially those with poor coping skills, extensive disability, or engrained patient role, referral to a mental health professional familiar with FGIDs will be the most appropriate step for helping the patient develop more advantageous coping skills and behaviors.

Presence of psychological and psychiatric comorbidity

• Indications for comorbid anxiety or depression in patients with FGIDs should signal further inquiry to determine the chronicity and impact of these mood changes and accompanying symptoms of altered sleep, energy level, and social functioning.

• If symptoms have a significant impact on function, a suggestion with explanation for evaluation by a mental health professional is appropriate.

• Use of medications such as antidepressants for mood or sleep should be considered as well.

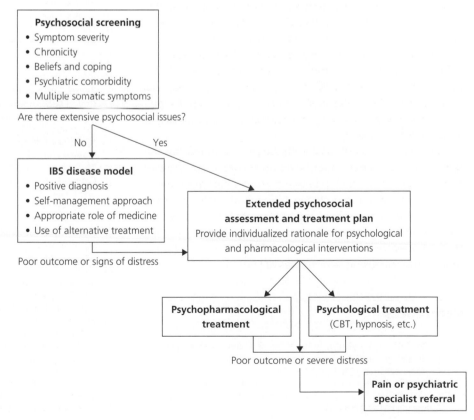

Figure 3.4 FGID biopsychosocial assessment and treatment algorithm. It is recommended that all patients be screened for the presence and severity of the most common psychosocial issues and be given clear and positive information about their disorder. Based on the screening assessment, an individualized plan of pharmacological and nonpharmacological treatments may be instituted with close follow-up (at least in the initial stages). Assessment of progress determines the need for further assessment or referral to a mental health or pain specialist. CBT, cognitive behavioral therapy.

Degree of somatization or comorbid medical problems

- Patients with multiple medical problems and especially multiple pain or functional disorders are likely to have significant psychological or psychiatric comorbidities and poor outcomes from routine medical care for their FGID [150].
- This is a subset of patients with FGID who are likely to benefit most from an integrated plan of care that includes contact with their other providers and inclusion of a mental health provider in the team.

Treatment algorithm

Based on the issues discussed above the decision process regarding the level of psychosocial intervention can be outlined in several steps (see Fig. 3.4).

1 All patients with FGID should at least be screened for the presence and severity of the most common psychosocial issues.

2 All patients should be given a clear and positive explanation of their disorder.

3 Based on the psychosocial screening, the severity of a patient's FGID, and the degree of other comorbid conditions an initial determination is made to either treat specific GI symptoms alone (e.g., diarrhea or constipation), add low-dose TCAs, or include in the plan the use of SSRIs or NSRIs or other psychoactive medications (e.g., short-term anxiolytics), as well as a decision about referral for psychological intervention or other mental health consultation.

4 As discussed above there is good evidence from other subspecialities that the best treatment for functional disorders often involves an individually tailored but interdisciplinary approach that includes combined psychological and psychopharmacological interventions, in addition to GI-specific agents.

5 Even if initially no mental health consultation is included in the plan, a more complete assessment of psychosocial issues and possible referral should be reconsidered if symptoms persist or there is a negative response to symptomatic or antidepressant treatment.

It is important to note that both the process of referral and the likelihood of success may be highly linked to the existence of an ongoing relationship between the primary provider of GI treatment and a knowledgeable mental health provider familiar with the assessment and treatment of FGIDs. Development of one or more of these relationships is an important consideration in being able to provide the best care for the more complicated and severe cases of FGID.

References

1. Spiegel BM, Gralnek IM, Bolus R, et al. Clinical determinants of health-related quality of life in patients with irritable bowel syndrome. Arch Intern Med 2004;164:1773.
2. Mayer EA, Bradesi S, Chang L, et al. Functional GI disorders: from animal models to drug development. Gut 2007; in press. Access online via PMID: 17965064.
3. Mayer EA, Naliboff BD, Chang L, Coutinho SV. Stress and the gastrointestinal tract: V. Stress and irritable bowel syndrome. Am J Physiol Gastrointest Liver Physiol 2001;280:G519.
4. Mayer EA. The neurobiology of stress and gastrointestinal disease. Gut 2000;47:861.
5. Drossman DA, Camilleri M, Mayer EA, Whitehead WE. AGA technical review on irritable bowel syndrome. Gastroenterology 2002;123:2108.
6. Mayer EA, Craske MG, Naliboff BD. Depression, anxiety and the gastrointestinal system. J Clin Psychiatry 2001;62(Suppl. 8):28.
7. Mayer EA, Naliboff BD, Craig AD. Neuroimaging of the brain–gut axis: from basic understanding to treatment of functional GI disorders. Gastroenterology 2006;131:1925.
8. Kennedy SH, Konarski JZ, Segal ZV, et al. Differences in brain glucose metabolism between responders to CBT and venlafaxine in a 16-week randomized controlled trial. Am J Psychiatry 2007;164:778.
9. Goldapple K, Segal Z, Garson C, et al. Modulation of cortical-limbic pathways in major depression: treatment-specific effects of cognitive behavior therapy. Arch Gen Psychiatry 2004;61:34.
10. Sawchenko PE, Li HY, Ericsson A, et al. Circuits and mechanisms governing hypothalamic responses to stress: a tale of two paradigms. In: Mayer EA, Saber CB (eds). The Biological Basis for Mind–Body Interactions. Amsterdam: Elsevier Science, 2000:61.
11. LeDoux JE. The Emotional Brain: The Mysterious Underpinnings of Emotional Life. New York: Simon & Schuster, 1996.
12. Bandler R, Price JL, Keay KA, et al. Brain mediation of active and passive emotional coping. In: Mayer EA, Saber CB (eds). The Biological Basis for Mind–Body Interactions. Amsterdam: Elsevier Science, 2000:333.
13. Mayer EA. Psychological stress and colitis. Gut 2000;46:595.
14. Taché Y, Martinez V, Wang L, Million M. CRF1 receptor signaling pathways are involved in stress-related alterations of colonic function and viscerosensitivity: implications for irritable bowel syndrome. Br J Pharmacol 2004;141:1321.
15. Valentino RJ, Miselis RR, Pavcovich LA. Pontine regulation of pelvic viscera: pharmacological target for pelvic visceral dysfunction. Trends Pharmacol Sci 1999;20:253.
16. Hammen C, Davila J, Brown G, et al. Psychiatric history and stress: predictors of severity of unipolar depression. J Abnormal Psychol 1992;101:45.
17. Wissow LS. Child abuse and neglect. N Engl J Med 1995;332:1425.
18. Bifulco A, Brown GW, Adler Z. Early sexual abuse and clinical depression in adult life. Br J Psychiatry 1991;159:115.
19. Brown GR, Anderson B. Psychiatric morbidity in adult inpatients with childhood histories of sexual and physical abuse. Am J Psychiatry 1993;148:55.
20. McCauley J, Kern DE, Kolodner K, et al. Clinical characteristics of women with a history of childhood abuse: unhealed wounds. J Am Med Assoc 1997;277:1362.
21. Canetti L, Bachar E, Galili-Weisstub E, et al. Parental bonding and mental health in adolescence. Adolescence 1997;32:381.
22. Parker G. Parental representations of patients with anxiety neurosis. Acta Psychiatr Scand 1981;63:33.
23. Russak LG, Schwartz GE. Feelings of parental care predict health status in midlife: A 35 year follow-up of the Harvard Mastery of Stress Study. J Behav Med 1997;20:1.
24. Hislop IG. Childhood deprivation: an antecedent of the irritable bowel syndrome. Med J Austral 1979;1:372.
25. Hill OW, Blendis L. Physical and psychological evaluation of non-organic abdominal pain. Gut 1967;8:221.
26. Lowman BC, Drossman DA, Cramer EM, McKee DC. Recollection of childhood events in adults with irritable bowel syndrome. J Clin Gastroenterol 1987;9:324.
27. Coplan JD, Andrews MW, Rosenblum LA, et al. Persistent elevations of cerebrospinal fluid concentrations of corticotropin-releasing factor in adult nonhuman primates exposed to early-life stressors: implications for the pathophysiology of mood and anxiety disorders. Proc Natl Acad Sci U S A 1996;93:1619.

28. De Bellis M, Chrousos GP, Dorn LD, et al. Hypothalamic–pituitary–adrenal axis dysregulation in sexually abused girls. J Clin Endocrinol Metab 1994;78:249.

29. Francis DD, Meaney MJ. Maternal care and the development of stress responses. Curr Opin Neurobiol 1999;9:128.

30. Heim C, Owens MJ, Plotsky PM, Nemeroff CB. The role of early adverse life events in the etiology of depression and post-traumatic stress disorder. Focus on corticotropin-releasing factor. Ann NY Acad Sci 1997;821:194.

31. Meaney MJ, Diorio J, Francis D, et al. Early environmental regulation of forebrain glucocorticoid receptor gene expression: implications for adrenocortical response to stress. Dev Neurosci 1996;18:49.

32. Fuchs E, Fluegge G. Modulation of binding sites for corticotropin-releasing hormone by chronic psychosocial stress. Psychoneuroendocrinology 1995;20:33.

33. Flügge G. Alterations in the central nervous alpha 2-adrenoceptor system under chronic psychosocial stress. Neuroscience 1996;75:187.

34. Bremner JD, Randall P, Vermetten E, et al. Magnetic resonance imaging-based measurement of hippocampal volume in posttraumatic stress disorders related to childhood physical and emotional abuse – a preliminary report. Biol Psychiatry 1997;41:23.

35. Fuchs E, Uno H, Fluegge G. Chronic psychosocial stress induces morphological alterations in hippocampal pyramidal neurons of the tree shrew. Brain Res 1995;673:275.

36. Bremner JD, Licinio J, Darnell A, et al. Elevated CSF corticotropin releasing factor concentrations in posttraumatic stress disorder. Am J Psychiatry 1997;154:624.

37. Imaki T, Nahan JL, Sawchenko PE, Vale W. Differential regulation of corticotropin-releasing factor mRNA in rat brain regions by glucocorticoids and stress. J Neurosci 1991;11:585.

38. Owens MJ, Nemeroff CB. The role of corticotropin-releasing factor in the pathophysiology of affective and anxiety disorders: laboratory and clinical studies. Presented at the Ciba Foundation Symposium 1993;172:296. Chichester: John Wiley & Sons.

39. Bremner JD, Innis RB, Ng CK, et al. Positron emission tomography measurement of cerebral metabolic correlates of yohimbine administration in combat related posttraumatic stress disorder. Arch Gen Psychiatry 1997;54:246.

40. Reche AJ, Buffington CAT. Increased tyrosine hydroxylase immunoreactivity in the locus coeruleus of cats with interstitial cystitis. J Urol 1998;159:1045.

41. Ladd CO, Huot RL, Thrivikraman KV, et al. Long-term behavioral and neuroendocrine adaptations to adverse early experience. In: Mayer EA, Saber CB (eds). The Biological Basis for Mind–Body Interactions. Amsterdam: Elsevier, 2000:81.

42. Curtis AL, Pavcovich LA, Valentino RJ. Previous stress alters corticotropin-releasing factor neurotransmission in the locus coeruleus. Neuroscience 1995;65:541.

43. Curtis AL, Pavcovich LA, Valentino RJ. Long-term regulation of locus coeruleus sensitivity to corticotropin-releasing factor by swim stress. J Pharmacol Exp Ther 1999;289:1211.

44. Yehuda R, Giller EL, Jr, Levengood RA, et al. Hypothalamic–pituitary–adrenal functioning in post-traumatic stress disorder: expanding the concept of the stress response spectrum. In: Chaney DS, Friedman MJ, Deutch AY (eds). Neurobiological and Clinical Consequences of Stress: From Normal Adaptation to Post-Traumatic Stress Disorder. Philadelphia: Lippincott-Raven Publishers, 1995:351.

45. Gold PW, Goodwin FK, Chrousos GP. Clinical and biochemical manifestations of depression. Relation to the neurobiology of stress (part 2). N Engl J Med 1988;319:348.

46. McEwen BS. Protective and damaging effects of stress mediators. N Engl J Med 1998;338:171.

47. Sengupta JN, Gebhart GF, Johnson LR. Gastrointestinal afferent fibers and sensation. In: Johnson LR (ed.). Physiology of the Gastrointestinal Tract. New York: Raven, 1994:483.

48. Craig AD. How do you feel? Interoception: the sense of the physiological condition of the body. Nat Rev Neurosci 2002;3:655.

49. Bielefeldt K, Christianson JA, Davis BM. Basic and clinical aspects of visceral sensation: transmission in the CNS. Neurogastroenterol Motil 2005;17:488.

50. Ostrowsky K, Isnard J, Ryvlin P, et al. Functional mapping of the insular cortex: clinical implication in temporal lobe epilepsy. Epilepsia 2000;41:681.

51. Mayer EA, Gebhart GF. Basic and clinical aspects of visceral hyperalgesia. Gastroenterology 1994;107:271.

52. Tracey I. Nociceptive processing in the human brain. Curr Opin Neurobiol 2005;15:478.

53. Porreca F, Ossipov MH, Gebhart GF. Chronic pain and medullary descending facilitation. Trends Neurosci 2002;25:319.

54. Basbaum AI, Fields HL. Endogenous pain control mechanisms: review and hypothesis. Ann Neurol 1978;4:451.

55. Fanselow MS. Conditioned fear-induced opiate analgesia: a competing motivational state theory of stress analgesia. Ann N Y Acad Sci 1986;467:40.

56. Coutinho SV, Miller JC, Plotsky PM, Mayer EA. Effect of perinatal stress on responses to colorectal distension in adult rats. Soc Neurosci Abstracts 1999;25:687.

57. Bradesi S, Schwetz I, McRoberts J, et al. Chronic water avoidance stress induces visceral hypersensitivity in male Wistar rats. Gastroenterology 2003;124(Suppl. 1):A671.

58. Duncan GH, Bushnell MC, Bates R, Dubner R. Task related responses of monkey medullary dorsal horn neurons. J Neurophysiol 1987;57:289.

59. Mason P. Ventromedial medulla: pain modulation and beyond. J Comp Neurol 2005 Dec 5;493:2.

60. Labus JS, Mayer EA, Chang L, et al. The central role of gastrointestinal-specific anxiety in irritable bowel syndrome: further validation of the Visceral Sensitivity Index. Psychosom Med 2007;69:89.

61. Taché Y, Martinez V, Million M, Wang L. Stress and the gastrointestinal tract III. Stress-related alterations of gut motor function: role of brain corticotropin-releasing factor receptors. Am J Physiol Gastrointestin Liver Physiol 2001;280:G173.

62. Lydiard RB. Irritable bowel syndrome, anxiety, and depression: What are the links? J Clin Psychiatry 2001;62(Suppl. 8):38.

63. Whitehead WE, Palsson O, Jones KR. Systemic review of the comorbidity of irritable bowel syndrome with other disorders: What are the causes and implications? Gastroenterology 2002;122:1140.

64. Tollefson GD, Luxenberg M, Valentine R, et al. An open label trial of alprazolam in comorbid irritable bowel syndrome and generalized anxiety disorder. J Clin Psychiatry 1991;52:502.

65. Clouse RE, Lustman PJ. Use of psychopharmacological agents for functional gastrointestinal disorders. Gut 2005;54:1332.

66. Saarto T, Wiffen PJ. Antidepressants for neuropathic pain. Cochrane Database of Systematic Rev 2005(3):CD005454.

67. Goldenberg DL, Burckhardt C, Crofford L. Management of fibromyalgia syndrome. J Am Med Assoc 2004;292:2388.

68. Punay NC, Couch JR. Antidepressants in the treatment of migraine headache. Curr Pain Headache Rep 2003;7:51.

69. Gorard DA, Libby GW, Farthing MJ. Effect of a tricyclic antidepressant on small intestinal motility in health and diarrhea-predominant irritable bowel syndrome. Digestive Dis Sci 1995;40:86.

70. Gorelick AB, Koshy SS, Hooper FG, et al. Differential effects of amitriptyline on perception of somatic and visceral stimulation in healthy humans. Am J Physiol 1998;275(3 Pt 1):G460.

71. Poitras P, Riberdy Poitras M, Plourde V, et al. Evolution of visceral sensitivity in patients with irritable bowel syndrome. Dig Dis Sci 2002;47:914.

72. Mertz H, Fass R, Kodner A, et al. Effect of amitryptiline on symptoms, sleep, and visceral perception in patients with functional dyspepsia. Am J Gastroenterol 1998;93:160.

73. Steinhart MJ, Wong PY, Zarr ML. Therapeutic usefulness of amitriptyline in spastic colon syndrome. Int J Psychiatr Med 1981;11:45.

74. Rajagopalan M, Kurian G, John J. Symptom relief with amitriptyline in the irritable bowel syndrome. J Gastroenterol Hepatol 1998;13:738.

75. Myren J, Lovland B, Larssen SE, Larsen S. A double-blind study of the effect of trimipramine in patients with the Irritable Bowel Syndrome. Scand J Gastroenterol 1984;19:835.

76. Greenbaum DS, Mayle JE, Vanegeren LE, et al. Effects of desipramine on irritable bowel syndrome compared with atropine and placebo. Dig Dis Sci 1987;32:257.

77. Jackson JL, O'Malley PG, Tomkins G, et al. Treatment of functional gastrointestinal disorders with antidepressant medications: a meta-analysis. Am J Med 2000;108:65.

78. Lesbros-Pantoflickova D, Michetti P, Fried M, et al. Meta-analysis: the treatment of irritable bowel syndrome. Alim Pharmacol Ther 2004;20:1253.

79. Brandt LJ, Bjorkman D, Fennerty MB, et al. Systematic review on the management of irritable bowel syndrome in North America. Am J Gastroenterol 2002;97(Suppl.):S7.

80. Drossman DA, Toner BB, Whitehead WE, et al. Cognitive-behavioral therapy versus education and desipramine versus placebo for moderate to severe functional bowel disorders. Gastroenterology 2003;125:19.

81. Rodenbeck A, Cohrs S, Jordan W, et al. The sleep-improving effects of doxepin are paralleled by a normalized plasma cortisol secretion in primary insomnia. A placebo-controlled, double-blind, randomized, cross-over study followed by an open treatment over 3 weeks. Psychopharmacology 2003;170:423.

82. Tack J, Muller-Lissner S, Bytzer P, et al. A randomised controlled trial assessing the efficacy and safety of repeated tegaserod therapy in women with irritable bowel syndrome with constipation. Gut 2005;54:1707.

83. Tack J, Broekaert D, Corsetti M, et al. Influence of acute serotonin reuptake inhibition on colonic sensorimotor function in man. Alim Pharmacol Ther 2006;23:265.

84. Broekaert D, Fischler B, Sifrim D, et al. Influence of citalopram, a selective serotonin reuptake inhibitor, on oesophageal hypersensitivity: a double-blind, placebo-controlled study. Alim Pharmacol Ther 2006;23:365.

85. Tabas G, Beaves M, Wang J, et al. Paroxetine to treat irritable bowel syndrome not responding to high-fiber diet: a double-blind, placebo-controlled trial. Am J Gastroenterol 2004;99:914.

86. Creed F, Fernandes L, Guthrie E, et al. The cost-effectiveness of psychotherapy and paroxetine for severe irritable bowel syndrome. Gastroenterology 2003;124:303.

87. Vahedi H, Merat S, Rashidioon A, et al. The effects of fluoxetine in patients with pain and constipation-predominant irritable bowel syndrome: a double-blind randomized-controlled study. Alim Pharmacol Ther 2005;22:381.

88. Barkin RL, Barkin SJ. Antidepressants for the management of pain in geriatric patients. Anesthesia Today 2004;15:23.

89. Bradley RH, Barkin RL, Jerome J, et al. Efficacy of venlafaxine for the long term treatment of chronic pain with associated major depressive disorder. Am J Ther 2003;10:318.

90. Arnold LM, Rosen A, Pritchett YL, et al. A randomized, double-blind, placebo-controlled trial of duloxetine in the treatment of women with fibromyalgia with or without major depressive disorder. Pain 2005;119:5.

91. Raskin J, Pritchett YL, Wang F, et al. A double-blind, randomized multicenter trial comparing duloxetine with placebo in the management of diabetic peripheral neuropathic pain. Pain Med (Malden, MA) 2005;6:346.

92. Westanmo AD, Gayken J, Haight R. Duloxetine: a balanced and selective norepinephrine- and serotonin-reuptake inhibitor. Am J Hlth-Syst Pharm 2005;62:2481.

93. Chial HJ, Camilleri M, Burton D, et al. Selective effects of serotonergic psychoactive agents on gastrointestinal functions in health. Am J Physiol Gastrointestin Liver Physiol 2003;284:G130.

94. Crowell MD. Role of serotonin in the pathophysiology of the irritable bowel syndrome. Br J Pharmacol 2004;141:1285.

95. Gardner CR. Potential use of drugs modulating 5HT activity in the treatment of anxiety. Gen Pharmacol 1988;19:347.

96. Talley NJ. Review article: 5-hydroxytryptamine agonists and antagonists in the modulation of gastrointestinal motility and sensation: clinical implications. Alim Pharmacol Ther 1992;6:273.

97. Humphrey PP, Bountra C, Clayton N, Kozlowski K. Review article: the therapeutic potential of 5-HT 3 receptor antagonists in the treatment of irritable bowel syndrome. Alim Pharmacol Ther 1999; 13(Suppl. 2):31.

98. Suzuki R, Dickenson A. Spinal and supraspinal contributions to central sensitization in peripheral neuropathy. Neurosignals 2005; 14:175.

99. Camilleri M, Chey WY, Mayer EA, et al. A randomized controlled clinical trial of the serotonin type 3 receptor antagonist alosetron in women with diarrhea-predominant irritable bowel syndrome. Arch Intern Med 2001;161:1733.

100. Camilleri M, Northcutt AR, Kong S, et al. Efficacy and safety of alosetron in women with irritable bowel syndrome: a randomised placebo-controlled trial. Lancet 2000;355(9209):1035.

101. Lembo T, Wright RA, Bagby B, et al. Alosetron controls bowel urgency and provides global symptom improvement in women with diarrhea-predominant irritable bowel syndrome. Am J Gastroenterol 2001;96:2662.

102. Chang L, Ameen VZ, Dukes GE, et al. A dose-ranging, phase II study of the efficacy and safety of alosetron in men with diarrhea-predominant IBS. Am J Gastroenterol 2005;100:115.

103. Berman SM, Chang L, Suyenobu B, et al. Condition-specific deactivation of brain regions by 5-HT 3 receptor antagonist alosetron. Gastroenterology 2002;123:969.

104. Mayer EA, Berman S, Derbyshire SW, et al. The effect of the 5-HT3 receptor antagonist, alosetron, on brain responses to visceral stimulation in irritable bowel syndrome patients. Alim Pharmacol Ther 2002;16:1357.

105. Miura M, Lawson DC, Clary EM, et al. Central modulation of rectal distension-induced blood pressure changes by alosetron, a 5-HT3 receptor antagonist. Dig Dis Sci 1999;44:20.

106. Neugebauer V, Li W, Bird GC, et al. Synaptic plasticity in the amygdala in a model of arthritic pain: differential roles of metabotropic glutamate receptors 1 and 5. J Neurosci 2003;23:52.

107. Camilleri M, Mayer EA, Drossman DA, et al. Improvement in pain and bowel function in female irritable bowel patients with alosetron, a 5-HT 3 receptor antagonist. Alim Pharmacol Ther 1999;13:1149.

108. Horton R. Lotronex and the FDA: a fatal erosion of integrity. Lancet 2001;357(9268):1544.

109. Friedel D, Thomas R, Fisher RS. Ischemic colitis during treatment with alosetron. Gastroenterology 2001;120:557.

110. Drossman DA. Presidential address: gastrointestinal illness and the biopsychosocial model. Psychosom Med 1998;60:258.

111. Lackner JM. Irritable bowel syndrome. In: Collins F, Cohen L (eds). Handbook of Health Psychology. Thousand Oaks: Sage, 2003:397.

112. Almy TP, Kern FJ, Tulin M. Alternation in colonic function in man under stress: experimental production of sigmoid spasm in healthy persons'. Gastroenterology 1949;12:425.

113. Naliboff BD, Derbyshire SW, Munakata J, et al. Cerebral activation in patients with irritable bowel syndrome and control subjects during rectosigmoid stimulation. Psychosom Med 2001;63:365.

114. Cohen S, Rodriguez M. Pathways linking affective disturbances and physical disorders. Hlth Psychol 1995;14:374.

115. Whitehead WE, Bosmajian L, Zonderman AB, et al. Symptoms of psychologic distress associated with irritable bowel syndrome: comparison of community and medical clinical samples. Gastroenterology 1988;95:709.

116. Blanchard EB, Scharff L, Schwarz SP, et al. The role of anxiety and depression in the irritable bowel syndrome. Behav Res Ther 1990; 28:401.

117. Drossman DA. Physical and sexual abuse and gastrointestinal illness: what is the link? Am J Med 1994;97:105.

118. Drossman DA, Leserman J, Nachman G, et al. Sexual and physical abuse in women with functional or organic gastrointestinal disorders. Ann Intern Med 1990;113:828.

119. Lackner JM, Gudleski GD, Blanchard EB. Beyond abuse: the association among parenting style, abdominal pain, and somatization in IBS patients. Behav Res Ther 2004;42:41.

120. Rokicki LA, Holroyd KA, France CR, et al. Change mechanisms associated with combined relaxation/EMG biofeedback training for chronic tension headache. Appl Psychophysiol Biofeedback 1997;22:21.

121. Linden W. The autogenic training method of J. H. Schultz. In: Lehrer PM, Woolfolk RL, (eds). Principles and Practice of Stress Management, 2nd edn. New York: Guilford, 1993:205.

122. Schultz JH. Autogenic training: a psychophysiologic approach in psychotherapy. New York: Grune & Stratton, 1959.

123. Fried R. Respiration in stress and stress controll: toward a theorey of stress as a hypoxic phenomenon. In: Lehrer PM, Woolfolk RL, (eds). Principles and Practice of Stress Management, 2nd edn. New York: Guilford, 1993:301.

124. Fried R. The Hyperventilation Syndrome. Baltimore, MD: Johns Hopkins University Press, 1987.

125. Whorwell PJ, Prior A, Faragher EB. Controlled trial of hypnotherapy in the treatment of severe refractory irritable bowel syndrome. Lancet 1984:8414;1232.

126. Galovski TE, Blanchard EB. The treatment of irritable bowel syndrome with hypnotherapy. Appl Psychophysiol Biofeedback 1998;23:219.

127. Rainville P, Duncan GH, Price DD, et al. Pain affect encoded in human anterior cingulate but not somatosensory cortex. Science 1997;277:968.

128. Toner BB, Segal ZV, Emmott S, et al. Cognitive-behavioral group therapy for patients with irritable bowel syndrome. Int J Group Psychother 1998;48:215.

129. Bennett P, Wilkinson S. A comparison of psychological and medical treatment of the Irritable Bowel Syndrome. Br J Clin Psychol 1985;24:215.

130. Payne A, Blanchard EB. A controlled comparison of cognitive therapy and self-help support groups in the treatment of irritable bowel syndrome. J Consult Clin Psychol 1995;63:779.

131. Neff DF, Blanchard EB. A multi-component treatment for irritable bowel syndrome. Behav Ther 1987;18.70.

132. Blanchard EB, Lackner JM, Sanders K, et al. A controlled evaluation of group cognitive therapy in the treatment of irritable bowel syndrome. Behav Res Ther 2007;45:633.

133. Lackner JM, Jaccard J, Krasner SS, et al. How does cognitive behavior therapy for IBS work? A mediational analysis of a randomized clinical trial. Gastroenterology 2007;133:702.

134. Guthrie E, Creed F, Dawson D, Tomenson B. A controlled trial of psychological treatment for the irritable bowel syndrome. Gastroenterology 1991;100:450.

135. Svedlund J, Sjodin I, Ottosson JO, Dotevall G. Controlled study of psychotherapy in irritable bowel syndrome. Lancet 1983;8350:589.

136. Guthrie E, Whorwell PJ. Pscyhotherapy and hypnotherapy in IBS. In: Camilleri M, Spiller RC, (eds). Irritable Bowel Syndrome: Diagnosis and Treatment. London: W. B. Saunders, 2002:157.

137. Drossman DA, Creed FH, Olden KW, et al. Psychosocial aspects of the functional gastrointestinal disorders. Gut 1999;45(Suppl. II):1125.

138. Blanchard EB, Scharff L. Psychosocial aspects of assessment and treatment of irritable bowel syndrome in adults and recurrent abdominal pain in children. J Consult Clin Psychol 2002;70:725.

139. Levy RL, Olden KW, Naliboff BD, et al. Psychosocial aspects of the functional gastrointestinal disorders. Gastroenterology 2006;130:1447.

140. Lackner JM, Morley S, Mesmer C, et al. Psychological treatments for irritable bowel syndrome: a systematic review and meta-analysis. J Consult Clin Psychol 2004;72:1100.

141. Creed F, Levy RL, Bradley LA, et al. Psychosocial aspects of functional gastrointestinal disorders. In: Drossman DA, Corazziari E, Delvaux M, et al., eds. Rome III: The Functional Gastrointestinal Disorders, 3rd edn. McLean, VA: Degnon Associates, Inc. 2006:295.

142. Gelenberg A. Depression is still underrecognized and undertreated. Archiv Intern Med 1999;159:1657.

143. Bjelland I, Dahl AA, Haug TT, Neckelmann D. The validity of the Hospital Anxiety and Depression Scale. An updated literature review. J Psychosom Res 2002;52:69.

144. Zigmond AS, Snaith RP. The hospital anxiety and depression scale. Acta Psychiatr Scand 1983;67:361.

145. Sullivan MJ, Thorn B, Haythornthwaite JA, et al. Theoretical perspectives on the relation between catastrophizing and pain. Clin J Pain 2001;17:52.

146. Lackner JM, Quigley BM, Blanchard EB. Depression and abdominal pain in IBS patients: the mediating role of catastrophizing. Psychosom Med 2004;66:435.

147. Drossman DA, Leserman J, Li Z, et al. Effects of coping on health outcome among women with gastrointestinal disorders. Psychosom Med 2000;62:309.

148. Keefe FJ, Brown GK, Wallston KA, Caldwell DS. Coping with rheumatoid arthritis pain: catastrophizing as a maladaptive strategy. Pain 1989;37:51.

149. Labus J, Bolus R, Chang L, et al. The visceral sensitivity index: development and validation of a gastrointestinal symptom-specific anxiety scale. Alim Pharmacol Ther 2004;20:89.

150. Creed F, Barsky A. A systematic review of the epidemiology of somatisation disorder and hypochondriasis. J Psychosom Res 2004;56:391.

151. North CS, Downs D, Clouse RE, et al. The presentation of irritable bowel syndrome in the context of somatization disorder. Clin Gastroenterol Hepatol 2004;2:787.

152. Kroenke K, Spitzer RL, Williams JB. The PHQ-15: validity of a new measure for evaluating the severity of somatic symptoms. Psychosom Med 2002;64:258.

153. Drossman DA, Talley NJ, Leserman J, et al. Sexual and physical abuse and gastrointestinal illness. Review and recommendations. Ann Intern Med 1995;123:782.

154. Koloski NA, Talley NJ, Boyce PM. A history of abuse in community subjects with irritable bowel syndrome and functional dyspepsia: the role of other psychosocial variables. Digestion 2005;72:86.

155. Perona M, Benasayag R, Perello A, et al. Prevalence of functional gastrointestinal disorders in women who report domestic violence to the police. Clin Gastroenterol Hepatol 2005;3:436.

156. Leserman J, Li Z, Drossman DA, et al. Impact of sexual and physical abuse dimensions on health status: development of an abuse severity measure. Psychosom Med 1997;59:152.

157. Bremner JD, Bolus R, Mayer EA. Psychometric properties of the Early Trauma Inventory-Self Report. J Nerv Ment Dis 2007;195:211.

158. Ware JE, Snow KK, Kosinski M, Gandek B. SF-36 health survey. Manual and interpretation guide. Boston: The Health Institute, New England Medical Center, 1993.

159. Gralnek IM, Hays RD, Kilbourne A, Mayer EA. Impact of irritable bowel syndrome on health-related quality of life (HRQOL). Gastroenterology 1999;116:A1038.

160. Patrick DL, Drossman DA, Frederick IO, et al. Quality of life in persons with irritable bowel syndrome. Development and validation of a new measure. Dig Dis Sci 1998;43:400.

161. Sarason IG, Johnson JH, Siegel JM. Assessing the impact of life changes: development of the Life Experiences Survey. J Consult Clin Psychol 1978;46:932.

162. Cohen S, Kamarck T, Mermelstein R. A global measure of perceived stress. J Hlth Soc Behav 1983;24:385.

163. Derogatis LR, Lazarus L. SCL-90-R, brief symptom inventory, and matching clinical rating scales. Mahwah NJ: Lawrence Erlbaum Associates, Inc. 1994.

164. Mayer EA. Somatic manifestations of traumatic stress. In: Kirmayer LJ, Lemelson R, Barad M (eds) Understanding Trauma: Integrating Biological, Clinical and Cultural Perspectives. Cambridge: Cambridge University Press, 2007:142.

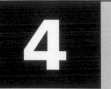

4

Approach to the patient with dyspepsia and related functional gastrointestinal complaints

Nicholas J. Talley, Gerald Holtmann

Clinical presentation of dyspepsia, 38

Dyspepsia in the general population and clinical practice, 41

Causes of dyspepsia, 41

Pathogenesis of functional dyspepsia, 42

Diagnostic approach to the patient with uninvestigated dyspepsia, 46

Management strategies, 47

Prognosis, 54

Dyspepsia is a frequent reason for consultation in primary care and gastrointestinal practice. With the widespread availability and use of endoscopy, it has become evident that a structural explanation is found in only a minority of patients with dyspepsia. The application of appropriate diagnostic and therapeutic strategies in patients with either uninvestigated dyspepsia or documented functional (nonulcer) dyspepsia continues to be a challenge in clinical practice. This chapter aims to summarize the basis for a rational approach to the management of such patients.

Clinical presentation of dyspepsia

Symptoms

The term *dyspepsia* is derived from the Greek roots *dys* ("bad") and *peptein* ("digestion"). Dyspepsia is currently defined as persistent or recurrent epigastric pain or burning, or discomfort from meal-related symptoms (postprandial fullness or early satiation – inability to finish a normal-sized meal) [1,2]; the definition does not exclude those who also have symptoms elsewhere. *Heartburn*, a retrosternal burning discomfort that rises up toward the neck, is often considered distinct from dyspepsia [2] but because of frequent symptom overlap the distinction has been questioned [3,4]. Occasional episodes of dyspepsia often occur in otherwise healthy individuals, but clinically relevant dyspepsia is a relapsing or chronic condition, present for at least 3 months in the previous year [2,5]. Diagnostic tests do not find peptic ulcer disease or another cause for dyspepsia in approximately 60% of patients who are evaluated [1,6,7], and the term *nonulcer dyspepsia* has then been applied [1,8]. However, ulcer disease is decreasing in Western countries, many patients with unexplained dyspepsia do not report typical ulcer-like symptoms, and disturbances of gastroduodenal function have been identified in a subset of patients; hence, the label *functional dyspepsia* is currently most widely applied [9].

Currently, patients with histological gastritis (or duodenitis) are not excluded from the functional dyspepsia category because a link between these abnormalities and symptoms has not been convincingly established [10]. Duodenal eosinophilia has also been observed in a subset of patients with functional dyspepsia, but the pathogenic relevance remains to be established [11–13].

The lack of a structural lesion does not mean that the symptoms are not real. Dyspepsia does negatively impact on quality of life [14]. Moreover, the lack of a clear association between structural lesions and symptoms has been noted in several other gastrointestinal (GI) diseases. For example, endoscopic studies have found that gastric and duodenal ulcer recurrences are frequent in asymptomatic subjects [15,16], and esophagitis and peptic ulcers were found in about 8% and 4% of totally asymptomatic subjects, respectively [6,17].

Principles of Clinical Gastroenterology. Edited by Tadataka Yamada, David H. Alpers, Anthony N. Kalloo, Neil Kaplowitz, Chung Owyang, and Don W. Powell. © 2008 Blackwell Publishing. ISBN 978-1-4051-69103

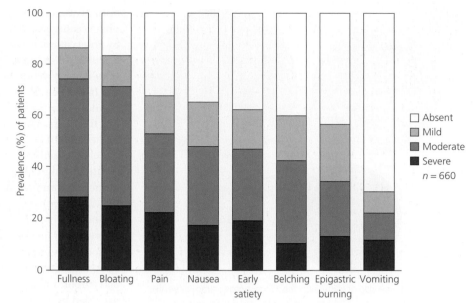

Figure 4.1 Symptom pattern in patients with functional dyspepsia seen at a tertiary referral center. Percentage of dyspeptic symptoms rated as moderate or severe (scores 2 and 3 on a scale 0–3) in 660 patients with functional dyspepsia seen at a tertiary referral center. From Tack et al. [352], with permission from the American Gastroenterological Association.

Subgroups of dyspepsia

The symptom pattern observed in patients with functional dyspepsia seen at tertiary referral centers is summarized in Fig. 4.1. Because multiple symptoms are usual, attempts have been made to categorize patients based on symptom clusters [1,7,18]. In the past, patients with functional dyspepsia were subdivided into ulcer-like and dysmotility-like dyspepsia [1,8,18,19]. The categorization of dyspepsia was introduced for the purposes of better targeting treatment to symptoms; theoretically, for example, patients with dysmotility-like symptoms (e.g., excessive fullness after meals, bloating, nausea) might respond best to prokinetics, whereas patients with ulcer-like symptoms could respond best to antisecretory therapy. However, studies using standardized symptom questionnaires observed considerable overlap (10%–20%) and a lack of stability among the different dyspepsia categories [18–22]. Others have suggested that dividing patients with dyspepsia into those with meal-related and non-meal-related symptoms is most useful [23,24].

The Rome III consensus has redefined functional dyspepsia into two categories for research purposes, namely *postprandial distress syndrome* (PDS, characterized by early satiation or postprandial fullness after most meals) and *epigastric pain syndrome* (EPS, defined by frequent pain or burning in the epigastrium) [2]. Nausea is considered a separate condition, as is bloating. Future studies will need to address the question whether this categorization is important for the targeting of therapy.

Misclassification of gastroesophageal reflux disease as dyspepsia

Whether the symptoms of heartburn or acid regurgitation should be considered a part of the spectrum of functional dyspepsia (or whether symptoms of functional dyspepsia should be thought of as part of gastroesophageal reflux disease) continues to be vigorously debated [1,7]. Despite a lack of endoscopic evidence of esophagitis, pathological acid reflux is detectable in at least 20% of patients with otherwise unexplained epigastric pain or discomfort, but this does not determine whether the epigastric symptoms are truly caused by excess acid in the distal esophagus [25,26].

Classically, heartburn is considered to be of value in identifying true esophageal reflux [27]. The absence of typical heartburn reliably indicates the absence of gastroesophageal reflux disease (GERD) [8,28]; but when present, heartburn is a very insensitive indicator of reflux disease in comparison with 24-h esophageal pH monitoring [8,26,28]. Other data suggest that a subset of patients with functional dyspepsia who respond to acid-lowering therapy have frequent short reflux episodes [29,30]. It is reasonable to conclude that patients who have typical reflux symptoms along with epigastric pain or meal-related symptoms should be considered to have GERD, rather than functional dyspepsia. However, many of these patients do not respond to an adequate trial of acid suppression, and in this situation a diagnosis of functional dyspepsia should be considered. Upper and lower GI symptoms do overlap (e.g., complaints consistent with irritable bowel syndrome, dyspepsia, or heartburn), and this overlap is the norm rather than the exception in patients [31] and in population-based studies (Fig. 4.2) [32,33]. While the term *reflux-like dyspepsia* has been used in the past to describe patients with dyspeptic and reflux symptoms, this has resulted in substantial confusion and should be abandoned [1,7].

Belching, aerophagia, functional vomiting, and rumination

Dyspepsia and reflux are not the only symptom clusters arising from the foregut. Other conditions need to be properly

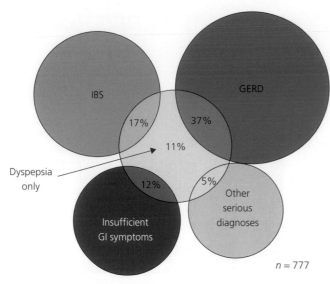

Figure 4.2 The overlap of gastrointestinal (GI) symptoms among female subjects (*n* = 777). About 18% of patients were excluded for reasons unrelated to GI symptoms. Pure dyspepsia represents subjects without predominant gastroesophageal reflux disease (GERD) symptoms or symptoms of irritable bowel syndrome (IBS). From Vakil et al. [33], with permission from Blackwell Publishing.

distinguished. Belching comprises aerophagia (troublesome repetitive belching with observed excessive air swallowing) and unspecified belching (when no evidence of excessive air swallowing is present).

Aerophagia is an excessive unconscious swallowing of air resulting in belching and discomfort. These patients usually report transient improvement of symptoms after belching [1] but often also report dyspeptic symptoms (Fig. 4.3) [34]. Postprandial belching from physiological air swallowing is

normal and occurs up to three to four times per hour. Aerophagia is suggested by a specific history and can be confirmed by observation. Because excessive gas is probably not present, it has been suggested that either disturbed upper GI tract motility or psychopathology accounts for the symptoms, but this has not been carefully studied [1].

Another important category comprises nausea and vomiting disorders, namely chronic idiopathic nausea (frequent bothersome nausea without vomiting), functional vomiting (recurrent vomiting in the absence of self-induced vomiting, or underlying eating disorders, metabolic disorders, drug-induced vomiting, or psychiatric or central nervous system disorders), and cyclic vomiting syndrome (stereotypical episodes of vomiting for days with distinct vomiting-free intervals). Patients with *functional vomiting* have frequent episodes of vomiting, but clinical evaluation does not yield a structural or metabolic cause for the symptoms. Gastroparesis and chronic idiopathic intestinal pseudoobstruction should be excluded by appropriate testing, as should anorexia nervosa, bulimia nervosa, and panic attacks by the clinical assessment.

Rumination in adults without mental retardation or neurological disease is sometimes mislabeled by patients and physicians as vomiting. It is characterized by the regurgitation of recently swallowed food that may be rechewed and expelled or reswallowed. These patients may present with a history of considerable weight loss [35]. Symptoms usually do not occur during sleep [35]. Reflux esophagitis and esophageal motor disorders must be excluded, but the history is virtually diagnostic.

Irritable bowel syndrome

Irritable bowel syndrome (IBS), which affects about one in six persons in the general population, is characterized by recurrent abdominal discomfort or pain and an erratic dis-

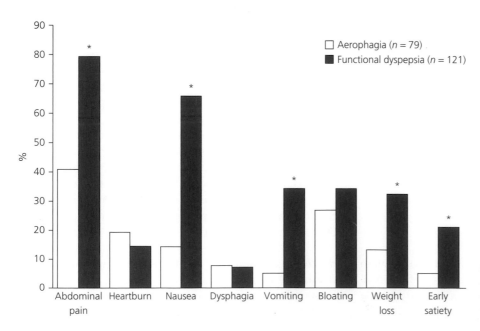

Figure 4.3 Symptoms in patients with aerophagia vs functional dyspepsia. From Chitkara et al. [34], with permission from Blackwell Publishing.

turbance of defecation [5]. A positive diagnosis of IBS can be made based on a careful history in the absence of alarm features such as unexplained weight loss or GI bleeding [5]. Of patients with functional dyspepsia, at least one-third have concurrent symptoms of IBS [18,20,21,31,36,37]. Because many patients do not mention bowel dysfunction unless specifically asked, an explicit inquiry should be made because the presence of concurrent IBS will influence management.

Dyspepsia in the general population and clinical practice

Prevalence and incidence in the population
Population-based studies from around the world have yielded prevalence rates of dyspepsia ranging from 7% to 60% [38–50]. The wide range is unlikely to reflect true variability in prevalence, but is probably explained by methodological differences. Indeed, when two different countries were studied with exactly the same methodology, similar prevalence rates for dyspepsia were observed [18,20].

Although prevalence has been extensively studied, fewer data are available for incidence. One 12- to 20-month population-based study from Olmsted County, Minnesota, identified onset of dyspepsia in approximately 9%, while the same number of subjects who initially reported symptoms became symptom free [51]. In a Swedish study, the calculated 3-month incidence of dyspepsia in previously asymptomatic subjects was under 1% [37]. In subjects enrolled into a 10-year longitudinal study [52], 717 (28%) developed new-onset dyspepsia at 10 years, with an annual incidence of dyspepsia of 2.8%. Lower quality of life at study entry, higher body mass index, presence of IBS at study entry and use of nonsteroidal antiinflammatory drugs or aspirin were significant risk factors for new-onset dyspepsia.

Dyspepsia in clinical practice and health-care-seeking behavior
Fewer than 50% of subjects with dyspepsia and IBS seek medical care, but conservative estimates suggest that these disorders account for 2%–5% of all consultations in family practice [18,20,44,53]. Up to one-third of these patients eventually may be referred to a gastroenterologist [53]. There is an association between the perceived intensity of abdominal (and extraintestinal) symptoms and health-care-seeking behavior in functional dyspepsia [18,20,54]. Psychological distress also may affect the utilization of health-care services [55–57]. Patients with dyspepsia have more concerns about the possible seriousness of their symptoms and are especially worried about cancer [58]. Moreover, patients consulting with dyspepsia have poorer coping capabilities, which may magnify their dyspeptic and psychological symptoms [59]. Gender and symptom type do not appear to influence health-care seeking [54].

Causes of dyspepsia

In patients with dyspepsia presenting for investigation, the four major causes of symptoms are chronic peptic ulcer disease, gastroesophageal reflux (with or without esophagitis), malignancy, and functional dyspepsia [25,60–64].

Structural gastrointestinal disease
The most important structural cause of symptoms to consider is *peptic ulcer disease* because definitive therapy is available [65]. Symptoms discriminate poorly between peptic ulcer disease and functional dyspepsia [49,66]. Indirect evidence for the absence of ulcer disease includes the absence of *Helicobacter pylori* infection on noninvasive testing and no recent nonsteroidal antiinflammatory drug (NSAID) use. However, a normal upper GI endoscopy while the patient is off antisecretory therapy is the definitive diagnostic approach.

In Western countries, the prevalence of *gastric and distal esophageal adenocarcinoma* in previously uninvestigated dyspepsia has been reported to be 1%–2%, but in persons younger than 55 years of age in most Western countries, gastric cancer is a rare cause of dyspepsia [6,67–70]. Nevertheless, the possibility of a neoplasm is often considered because of fear; a delayed diagnosis of early gastric cancer adversely affects patient prognosis, and patient concerns about cancer promote health-care-seeking behavior [58]. However, almost all patients with gastric cancer in Western countries present with advanced (and hence incurable) disease, and there is little evidence that a delay in diagnosis alters the usually very poor outcome [71,72]. In addition, classical alarm symptoms (e.g., weight loss) have a low positive predictive value and thus are not very helpful for identifying patients requiring endoscopic workup [73].

At ultrasonography, *biliary tract disease* (e.g., gallstones) may be found in 1%–3% of patients with dyspepsia but usually this is incidental and not a cause of symptoms [74,75]. Although the prevalence of gallstones increases with age and is three times greater in female patients, there is no clear age-related increase in the prevalence of functional dyspepsia and no gender difference. Cholelithiasis causes biliary pain, which is typically severe, constant pain in the epigastrium or right upper quadrant that persists for hours and occurs episodically [76]. In the absence of characteristic biliary pain, it is unlikely that gallstones are the cause of dyspepsia [77,78]. Obtaining an accurate history is therefore key in differentiating biliary tract disease from functional dyspepsia.

Chronic pancreatitis or *pancreatic carcinoma* may cause symptoms that occasionally are confused with those of functional dyspepsia [79,80]. Patients often have vague symptoms of insidious onset, but postprandial pain is usual that may radiate through to the back; these patients may also have a history of risk factors for pancreatitis, such as excess alcohol use or a family history. Weight loss, nausea, and diarrhea (steatorrhea) are typically late symptoms. Serum amylase and lipase levels are usually normal, but there may be glucose intolerance. In suspected cases, ultrasonography (including endoscopic ultrasonography) or helical computed tomography (including thin sections of the pancreas) will usually aid in the diagnosis.

Endoscopy-negative gastroesophageal reflux

Because 60% of patients with true GERD are endoscopy negative, gastroesophageal reflux should be suspected, despite the absence of esophagitis at endoscopy, in patients with unexplained epigastric burning pain or discomfort, especially if the discomfort has a chest component or radiates up toward the throat, and is relieved by antisecretory therapy [81,82]. The symptomatic response to a short therapeutic trial with a high-dose proton pump inhibitor (PPI) has been advocated as a diagnostic test for GERD, but it has suboptimal sensitivity and specificity [83].

In one center, 20% of dyspeptic patients who were free of peptic ulcer and gallstones had abnormal esophageal acid exposure times [26]. In other studies, between 12% and 40% of patients with otherwise unexplained dyspepsia were found to have pathological gastroesophageal reflux [26,29, 30,85,85]. In clinical practice, there is a substantial group of patients who simultaneously have dyspeptic symptoms and heartburn; most have no esophageal mucosal breaks at endoscopy. It seems likely that at least a large subset of these patients, whether or not they have pathological acid reflux on 24-h pH testing, belong in the spectrum of functional gastrointestinal disorders rather than GERD [86] because only a minority respond to 4 weeks of PPI therapy [87].

Drug-induced dyspepsia

NSAIDs, including the cyclooxygenase-2 (COX-2)-specific NSAIDs, represent the most important cause of drug-induced dyspepsia [88,89]. While many patients will tolerate NSAIDs, clinical experience suggests that patients with functional dyspepsia often develop symptoms when they are treated with NSAIDs. In one experimental study, GI symptoms occurred more frequently in patients with functional dyspepsia compared to healthy controls given aspirin; symptoms were associated with impaired adaptation of visceral thresholds despite mucosal lesions being induced by aspirin in both groups [90].

Other drugs that may produce upper abdominal symptoms include iron or potassium supplements, digitalis, theophylline, and oral antibiotics, especially erythromycin and ampicillin [91]. Reducing the dose or discontinuing drug therapy usually relieves dyspepsia in such cases.

Psychiatric disorders

Patients with constant pain do not have functional dyspepsia; rather, these patients usually have a chronic pain syndrome. Similarly, patients with multisystem complaints plus abdominal symptoms are more likely to have depression or somatoform disorder and should not be mislabeled as having functional dyspepsia; these patients can benefit from formal psychiatric evaluation. Rarely, panic disorder can present with episodic upper abdominal distress or even vomiting. Eating disorders should be considered in any young patient presenting with significant weight loss in addition to dyspepsia [91].

Other disorders

Diabetes mellitus with underlying autonomic neuropathy can cause postprandial fullness, early satiety, nausea, and vomiting, but symptoms correlate poorly with gastroparesis. Poor glycemic control may contribute [92]. Furthermore, diabetic radiculopathy of the thoracic nerve roots can cause upper abdominal pain [91]. Metabolic disturbances (e.g., *hypothyroidism, hypercalcemia*) can produce upper GI distress. *Ischemic heart disease* sometimes presents with just upper abdominal pain that may be induced by exertion. *Intestinal angina* should be considered in older patients, particularly smokers; it typically presents with postprandial pain associated with a fear of eating and significant weight loss [91]. The prevalence of *celiac disease* in patients with dyspepsia may be approximately twice that in the general population in some parts of the world but robust US data are lacking [93,94]; serological screening (e.g., transglutaminase) should be considered to allow diagnosis of an eminently treatable disease.

Malignancies such as colon cancer (e.g., involving the transverse colon), gastric lymphoma or sarcoma, esophageal cancer, pancreatic cancer, and ampullary cancer may cause upper abdominal distress that may initially be confused with functional dyspepsia, although this occurrence is rare [91]. *Infiltrative diseases* of the stomach, including eosinophilic gastritis, Crohn's disease, sarcoidosis, tuberculosis, and syphilis, may also rarely produce dyspepsia [95]. *Ménétrier disease* often presents with upper abdominal symptoms; atrophic gastritis is an asymptomatic condition.

Abdominal wall pain from *muscle strain, nerve entrapment*, or *myositis* can be confused with functional dyspepsia. Characteristically, there is localized tenderness that on palpation reproduces the pain, and the tenderness may be increased by tensing the abdominal muscles [96].

Pathogenesis of functional dyspepsia

Disturbed motor function

Disordered motor function is considered by many to be an important contributor to symptoms. Coordinated phasic and tonic activity of the stomach wall ultimately results in movement, mixture, or storage of lumenal content, but gastric emptying has been the major target of research. Approximately 25%–40% of patients seen with functional dyspepsia at tertiary referral centers have delayed gastric emptying of solids

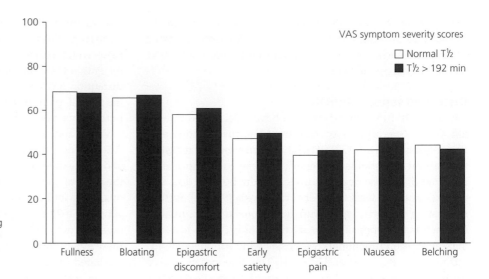

Figure 4.4 Symptom severity scores among patients with functional dyspepsia (*n* = 551), comparing patients with slow gastric emptying vs normal gastric emptying. Note the similarity in symptom severity scores. VAS, visual analog scale. Data derived from Talley et al. [111].

[97–108], and a similar number have antral hypomotility after meals [103,104].

In blood donors with and without dyspepsia, slow gastric emptying was significantly more common in symptomatic cases (with 25% having an abnormality) [109]. In referral patients from Europe, some meal-related symptoms appeared to be associated with slow gastric emptying [105,110] but a link between symptoms and gastric emptying in functional dyspepsia has not been detected by others [9,107,108,111,112] (Fig. 4.4). Accelerated gastric emptying has been observed in up to 10% of tertiary referred patients; this is relevant, because symptoms in such cases might be aggravated by prokinetic therapy [113].

Gastric antral hypomotility, characterized by either a decreased frequency or decreased amplitude of phasic pressure waves, is not a specific finding in functional dyspepsia; such abnormalities have been observed in patients with peptic ulceration and other diseases [103,114,115]. Prolonged ambulatory monitoring of the small intestinal motility of patients with functional dyspepsia has documented symptoms associated with burst activity and retrograde or nonpropagated

phase III activity in some [116]. It is unlikely that this technique will identify specific motility patterns that are closely linked to dyspeptic symptoms [117].

In patients with otherwise unexplained nausea, an elevated slow wave frequency with either a regular (*tachygastria*) or irregular (*tachyarrhythmia*) rhythm has been observed on electrogastrography (EGG) [118,119]. In 72 patients with functional dyspepsia, the EGG findings were abnormal in 50% with delayed gastric emptying and in 22% with normal emptying [119]. Because gastric arrhythmias have also been documented in patients with severe nausea resulting from GERD [120] and other diseases [121], the clinical significance of EGG abnormalities in functional dyspepsia remains in question.

Impaired fundic relaxation has been suggested as a potential mechanism inducing symptoms in functional dyspepsia [122,123]. After a meal, the fundus normally relaxes via a vagal reflex, promoting a pleasant feeling of satiation [124]. A failure of fundic relaxation (or "stiff fundus") occurs in 40% with functional dyspepsia, and has been associated with predominant early satiety and even weight loss (Fig. 4.5) [124]. Others have reported that abnormal fundic accommodation

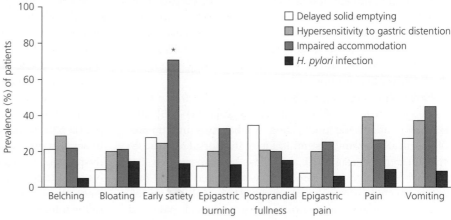

Figure 4.5 Predominant dyspeptic symptom and putative pathophysiological abnormalities. Note that subdividing patients on the basis of symptom predominance does not reliably identify pathophysiological abnormalities aside from early satiety and impaired gastric accommodation. From Karamanolis et al. [353], with permission from the American Gastroenterological Association.

*$P < 0.05$ compared with patients with other predominant symptoms
n = 720: 489 women; mean age 41 years

can overload the antrum, which may also be abnormally sensitive to distention in a subset [125]. However, a lack of symptom association with impaired fundic accommodation has also been reported [122,126].

Disturbed sensory function

Patients with functional dyspepsia have a decreased threshold for the perception of mechanical gastric fundus and antral distention [125,127–131]. It has been shown that gastric mechanical thresholds normally increase (or adapt) after repeated distention or exposure to aspirin, but this does not occur in patients with functional dyspepsia [90,132], further suggesting that sensory dysfunction is one key abnormality in functional dyspepsia. Sensory thresholds can be lowered in patients with functional dyspepsia by intraduodenal lipid, but not glucose, infusion [133,134]. This phenomenon may explain the induction of symptoms after fatty meals reported by some patients with functional dyspepsia. Nevertheless, approximately 60% of patients with functional dyspepsia have normal gastric perception thresholds, and there is considerable overlap between healthy controls and patients, raising questions about the exact relevance of gastric hypersensitivity [135].

Although most studies have observed lowered gastric mechanosensory thresholds, the data regarding small intestinal sensory thresholds in functional dyspepsia are more controversial [136]. Spanish studies [137] found isolated gastric but not intestinal hyperalgesia in functional dyspepsia, and selective jejunal hyperalgesia in patients with IBS [138]. Decreased thresholds for intestinal balloon distention have been observed in patients with functional dyspepsia, although the method used (a latex balloon) may not have produced a well-standardized distention stimulus [139]. Other studies, however, clearly identified lowered duodenal sensory thresholds in a group of patients with functional dyspepsia that were independent of coexisting intestinal dysmotility [130,131].

Lowered sensory thresholds in the stomach and duodenum are not pathognomonic for functional dyspepsia. Both abnormal rectal and esophageal sensory thresholds have been reported in patients with functional dyspepsia [140]. Furthermore, duodenal sensory thresholds did not discriminate patients with functional dyspepsia from those with IBS or those with both conditions [31].

Although there are well-defined experimental animal models for the study of visceral hyperalgesia [141–143], little is known about the underlying mechanisms in humans. Mechanical or chemical stimulation of the dorsal root causes visceral hyperalgesia [144], and it has been speculated that visceral hyperalgesia is associated with altered central projection of central (dorsal horn) neurons [144–146]. The prevalence of extraintestinal complaints, such as back pain and headache, is increased in functional dyspepsia and IBS [147], suggesting that central processing abnormalities may be linked

also to the pathogenesis of symptoms. Positron emission tomography has revealed differences in cerebral blood flow between IBS patients and healthy controls anticipating rectal distention [148]. In functional dyspepsia, proximal stomach distention has now been shown to activate components of the lateral pain system and bilateral frontal inferior gyri, putatively involved in regulation of hunger and satiety [149].

Vagal and spinal afferents mediate visceral sensation. Altered vagal function in patients with functional dyspepsia and IBS has been observed [150, 151], including an increase in the area of the antrum in fasting patients with functional dyspepsia and diabetes mellitus in comparison with healthy subjects [152]. Symptoms of bloating and postprandial fullness are commonly reported by patients after vagotomy, and these symptoms may be linked to an impairment of vagally mediated fundic relaxation [153]. The normal fundic relaxation in response to a meal was significantly diminished in patients with a truncal vagotomy and in patients with functional dyspepsia in comparison with healthy controls [154]. Moreover, other indirect data suggest that the vagus nerve can inhibit the transmission of sensory information, and this inhibition may be impaired in functional dyspepsia [155].

Duodenogastric reflux

Duodenogastric reflux has been postulated to be of importance in the pathogenesis of functional dyspepsia. There is now convincing evidence that duodenogastric reflux is not more common in those with functional dyspepsia than in controls, and it does not appear to be related to either symptoms or antral hypomotility [115,156–158].

Gastric acid

Basal and peak rates of acid output do not differ between patients with functional dyspepsia and controls [159,160]. Acid secretion in response to gastrin-releasing peptide, which simulates the postprandial state, was shown to be significantly increased in *H. pylori*-infected duodenal ulcer patients and *H. pylori*-infected healthy volunteers [161], and gastrin-releasing peptide-stimulated acid secretion was also significantly higher in *H. pylori*-positive patients with functional dyspepsia than in *H. pylori*-positive healthy volunteers [161]. Unfortunately, in the population studied, the background rate of peptic ulcer disease is particularly high, and this may have inadvertently contaminated the functional dyspepsia group [161].

There is increasing evidence that a subset of functional dyspepsia patients have upper GI tract mucosal hypersensitivity to acid. In one study [162], 6 of 18 patients with functional dyspepsia, 15 of whom had histological gastritis, had a positive symptom response to gastric instillation of acid, whereas eight other patients had symptoms during the infusion of saline solution. Pentagastrin injection led to increased reports of pain in patients with functional dyspepsia, although a histamine H_2 antagonist did not significantly reduce the pain

[163]. Because pentagastrin may have other effects in addition to the stimulation of acid secretion, and acid secretion may not be blocked sufficiently by a histamine H_2 antagonist, these data are inconclusive. Esophageal sensory thresholds have been observed to decrease in normal controls during esophageal acid instillation [164], suggesting that physiological esophageal acid reflux may trigger a decrease in sensory thresholds. In fasting dyspeptic patients, the clearance of exogenous acid infused into the duodenal bulb was shown to be impaired and was linked to the induction of nausea [165]. Acid infusion into the duodenum has been observed to increase acid sensitivity [165] and to alter gastric accommodation [166]. Duodenal acid exposure was increased in a subset of patients with functional dyspepsia and prominent nausea, and this was associated with more severe dyspeptic symptoms [167].

Postinfectious dyspepsia

Helicobacter pylori infection is the most common cause of histological gastritis in humans [168,169] and is found in approximately 30%–40% of patients with functional dyspepsia [169–172]. However, it is also common in asymptomatic subjects [173]. There is a lack of convincing evidence to link *H. pylori* with any specific symptom [174–179]. Although chronic gastric inflammation is a potential cause of visceral hyperalgesia [180], two studies failed to find a significant difference in sensory thresholds between *H. pylori*-positive and -negative patients [131,181]. The data do not exclude a role for *H. pylori* infection as an initiating event in functional dyspepsia in a predisposed individual, similar to that proposed for postinfectious IBS [182,183].

A small subgroup of patients with functional dyspepsia characterized by early satiety, nausea, weight loss, and impaired fundic accommodation appeared to develop symptoms following a short episode of infectious gastroenteritis [184]. One study observed that after *Salmonella enteritidis* infection, the relative risks for the new development of dyspepsia was 5.2 and for IBS was 7.8, with significant overlap between dyspepsia and IBS in this population [185].

Duodenitis

The prevalence of histological duodenitis in patients with functional dyspepsia has been reported to be between 14% and 83% [186,187], whereas the prevalence of macroscopic duodenitis in asymptomatic patients may be lower (10%), but an association between duodenitis and functional dyspepsia remains to be established [188]. Duodenal eosinophilia was observed to be associated with functional dyspepsia in an adult population-based endoscopic study performed in northern Sweden [11] and similar findings have been observed in pediatric patients with dyspepsia [12,13] but the clinical implications remain unknown.

It has been claimed that endoscopic irrigation of the duodenum with hydrochloric acid induces symptoms in patients with duodenitis, but unfortunately the results from control subjects have not been evaluated [189]. Based on the available evidence, erosive duodenitis appears to fall more within the spectrum of chronic duodenal ulcer disease and probably should not be considered part of functional dyspepsia.

Psychosocial factors and alterations of the central nervous system

Individuals with functional dyspepsia have been shown to be more psychologically disturbed, in terms of being more anxious and depressed [190–195], and to score higher on measures of neuroticism [196] and somatization [147,197–199] than healthy controls. Other studies suggest that patients with functional dyspepsia are no more psychologically disturbed than patients with organic bowel disease [190,200]. In a case–control study, similar levels of control of anger, anxiety, and unhappiness and of total emotional control over negative reactions in patients with functional dyspepsia and controls, were found [200].

Most of these studies have included only individuals with functional dyspepsia presenting for medical care; they therefore do not rule out the hypothesis that rather than causing symptoms, anxiety and depression simply make patients with functional dyspepsia more likely to present their symptoms to a physician [20], although one Australian study was unable to confirm this concept [201]. In a follow-up study of patients with duodenal ulceration and functional dyspepsia, abnormal personality patterns appeared to normalize after disappearance of the abdominal symptoms [202], suggesting that psychological disturbances in some patients with functional dyspepsia may be a consequence of the symptoms rather than of causal importance. Alternatively, both dyspepsia and psychological disturbances may be caused by another, unknown common environmental or genetic factor.

If psychological factors directly contribute to the development of symptoms in some patients with functional dyspepsia, the precise mechanisms remain to be elucidated. In depressed patients, the hormonal response to a serotonergic challenge is diminished [203]. A similar abnormality of central 5-hydroxytryptaminergic pathways may also exist in the functional GI disorders. The prolactin response to buspirone, an azaperone that stimulates central serotonergic-1A receptors, was found to be significantly greater in patients with functional dyspepsia than in healthy controls, and the difference correlated with the degree of delayed solid-phase gastric emptying assessed scintigraphically [203], but these results require confirmation [204].

The role of stress in the pathogenesis of functional dyspepsia remains controversial. Acute stress may result in decreased gastric contractility that precedes the onset of symptoms [205–207]. It is not known, however, whether chronic dyspeptic symptoms are explained by such mechanisms. The stress of major life events, such as bereavement or divorce, has also been linked to functional dyspepsia [208–210]. On the other hand, patients with functional dyspepsia, with or without antral hypomotility, appear to have normal autonomic and humoral responses to experimental stress [104]. Most studies have not focused on long-term stressors, and it is questionable whether experimental laboratory stressors reflect the stress of real life. Examinations, as an example of a real-life stressor, induced dyspeptic symptoms in medical students that were linked to specific psychological traits, including anxiety [211].

A potential link between childhood or adult sexual, emotional, or verbal abuse and functional GI disorders is based on studies in patients with IBS [212] and population-based surveys [213]. When standard criteria were applied, a surprisingly high prevalence (26%) of abuse in IBS patients (41% in women and 11% in men) was reported by subjects in a US community [213]. Similarly, dyspepsia and heartburn were both significantly associated with abuse [213]. A causal link, however, has not been established, and an Australian study noted that after controlling for other psychosocial factors, abuse was no longer associated with dyspepsia or IBS [214]. People with a history of abuse are more likely to seek medical treatment so it is important to consider exploring this issue in those consulting [213].

Environmental factors

Dyspepsia can be induced by the ingestion of NSAIDs, including low doses of aspirin [19,20] and COX-2 inhibitors [88,215,216]. Most investigations have consistently failed to demonstrate that smoking and alcohol are important risk factors in functional dyspepsia [216–220].

Some patients with functional dyspepsia and IBS report specific food intolerances, but a convincing relationship between diet and chronic dyspepsia remains to be demonstrated [221–223]. In one study, the main difference in eating pattern noted between patients with functional dyspepsia and control subjects was that a significantly lower percentage of patients with functional dyspepsia regularly ate three meals per day. Also, dyspepsia patients in both groups associated certain eating habits and the consumption of specific foods with exacerbations of dyspeptic symptoms, which led to food avoidance in 80% of both groups [223]. In a crosssectional survey from the United Kingdom, 20% of the population reported food intolerance, but food intolerance, as assessed by a double-blind, placebo-controlled food challenge, was confirmed in only one in five [224].

Coffee and decaffeinated coffee stimulate acid secretion [219]. Although the number of cups of coffee ingested has not been linked to functional dyspepsia [217,218], coffee induced symptoms in 53% of patients with functional dyspepsia and in 22% of healthy control subjects [218]. Whether coffee acts as a direct irritant or precipitates gastroesophageal reflux in functional dyspepsia is unknown [225].

Genetics

A specific polymorphism of a G protein (C825T GNβ3) has been associated with functional dyspepsia in two studies from Germany [226]; this was later independently confirmed in a US study [227]. The GNβ3 CC polymorphism leads to reduced signal transduction while the TT polymorphism increases cellular responses; both have been linked to non-meal-related as well as dysmotility-like dyspepsia. It can be speculated that changes in signal transduction may modulate antinociceptive pathways.

Diagnostic approach to the patient with uninvestigated dyspepsia

Identifying patients with structural disease as a cause of dyspepsia

The diagnostic workup of patients with dyspepsia can be time-consuming and costly if undirected. Therefore, attempts have been made to limit diagnostic procedures to patients at higher risk for structural, potentially life-threatening disease. Age, alarm features, symptom patterns, and *H. pylori* status all have been evaluated as predictors of structural disease.

Age

The risk for having a structural cause of symptoms increases with age [6,61,62,228,229]. A cutoff of 45 years has been traditionally applied in dyspepsia management strategies because the risk for gastric cancer in Western countries is extremely low in patients younger than 45 years [61,62]. Indeed, esophagogastroduodenoscopy yielded only three gastric cancers in a sample of more than 7000 dyspeptic patients younger than 45 years without sinister symptoms [67]. However, in the United States upper GI cancer remains rare under the age of 55 years and for this reason current guidelines have endorsed this age cut-off [230]. Patients older than 55 years with new-onset dyspepsia should undergo prompt upper GI endoscopy.

Pattern of symptoms and alarm features

A long duration of symptoms in younger patients makes cancer an unlikely cause of symptoms. Dividing uninvestigated patients into ulcer-like, dysmotility-like, and nonspecific dyspepsia subgroups does not appear to identify subjects at higher risk for a structural lesion [49,66,231–233]. Similarly, individual symptoms are of poor discriminating value [233,234]. In subjects without alarm features, such as weight loss, bleeding, dysphagia, and recurrent vomiting, and who are younger than 55 years, gastric cancer is a rare finding [235]. The positive predictive value of alarm features for cancer, however, is poor (most with an alarm feature do not have cancer) [236,237]. On the other hand, in patients with alarm symptoms where cancer is identified, it is usually advanced and incurable [238].

Helicobacter pylori

Infection with *H. pylori* and traditional NSAID use are strongly associated with peptic ulcer disease [239]. Restricting endoscopy to younger patients who test positive for *H. pylori* (by a ^{13}C- or ^{14}C-urea breath test or stool antigen test), to NSAID users, and to patients older than 55 years reduces the need for endoscopy by 20%–40% without causing a relevant number of peptic ulcers or gastric cancers to be missed [239,240]. This strategy, however, has some limitations; peptic ulcer disease is declining overall in the developed world, and an increasing proportion of patients have *H. pylori*-negative and NSAID-negative ulcer disease [241].

Endoscopy

Peptic ulcer disease, reflux esophagitis, and gastric or esophageal cancer are the most important conditions that must be ruled out to establish a firm diagnosis of functional dyspepsia. Upper GI endoscopy remains the gold standard test and is superior to upper GI radiography [242], but its reassurance value remains poorly established [243,244]. Endoscopy was found to be probably cost effective in patients over 50 years of age compared with usual care [245], but endoscopy in younger patients is not the dominant strategy [246].

Not all structural abnormalities identified at endoscopy are clinically meaningful. In a study from Switzerland, reflux esophagitis or gastric and duodenal ulcers were found in 7% of asymptomatic subjects and in 24% of patients [229]. Asymptomatic esophagitis (usually low grade) occurred in one-third of cases in another population-based endoscopic study from northern Sweden [247,248].

It is notable that some patients with a history of peptic ulceration continue to have dyspepsia even after cure of *H. pylori* infection and in the absence of a persisting ulcer, which suggests that functional dyspepsia has developed [249,250]. If up to 50% of patients with duodenal ulcer have dyspeptic symptoms after apparent cure of their disease [249], it can be speculated that the mechanisms causing ulcer dyspepsia are also linked to the pathophysiology of a subset with functional dyspepsia.

Other diagnostic tests

Abdominal ultrasonography has a low yield [49,91,251]. Whereas endoscopy may yield pathological findings in less than 50% of new patients with dyspepsia, an extended functional workup (including 24-h esophageal pH recording, testing of gastric emptying, biliary scanning, and testing of lactose tolerance) will find abnormalities in only 50% of the remaining patients [25]. The true gain with these additional tests, however, is small. For example, identification of delayed gastric emptying by scintigraphy is unlikely to influence whether or not a prokinetic is prescribed because it has not been established that patients with delayed emptying respond better than those with normal emptying [252]. Similarly, although lactose deficiency may be present, dyspeptic

Table 4.1 Diagnostic studies to be considered in the patient with suspected functional dyspepsia

Useful

A careful history that elicits the symptoms, and a relevant physical examination

Upper gastrointestinal endoscopy during a symptomatic period off acid suppression

Helicobacter pylori testing

Optional

Routine hematological and biochemical tests (full blood count, ESR or CRP, serum glucose measurement, liver function tests, electrolytes and creatinine, calcium, thyroid function)

Ultrasonography of the gallbladder, liver, and pancreas

24-h or 48-h esophageal pH testing

Uncertain clinical value

Gastric-emptying study

Fundus relaxation postprandially (e.g., by SPECT, ultrasound, or MRI)

Water or nutrient load test

Electrogastrography

Gastroduodenal manometry

CRP, C-reactive protein; ESR, erythrocyte sedimentation rate; SPECT, single photon emission computed tomography; MRI, magnetic resonance imaging.

symptoms often fail to respond to lactose withdrawal. The nutrient or water load tests are simple and offer some information on integrated gastric function although their place in clinical practice remains to be defined [123]. A list of recommended tests to establish a diagnosis of dyspepsia is presented in Table 4.1.

Management strategies

Uninvestigated dyspepsia

The initial management options are outlined in Table 4.2. Because only a few patients with dyspepsia have peptic ulcer, and even fewer have cancer, the American College of Physicians recommends empirical medical therapy (e.g., a histamine H_2 blocker) for 4 weeks for younger patients (i.e., younger than 45 years) without alarm features [242]. The use of PPIs has been extended to dyspepsia in clinical practice, and in a metaanalysis of trials in uninvestigated dyspepsia, PPI was superior to H_2 antagonists or antacids for relief of symptoms [253]. The empirical therapy approach has been criticized, however, because it may promote the prolonged use of inappropriate medications, weaken the value of subsequent investigations, cause serious side effects (rarely), mask symptoms of serious disorders, and mask malignancy at subsequent endoscopy [254,255]. Admittedly, while acid suppression can relieve the symptoms of malignancy for a

Table 4.2 Management options for uninvestigated chronic dyspepsia

Exclude symptomatic gastroesophageal reflux, irritable bowel syndrome, and other conditions by
history and examination
Determine whether endoscopy is indicated immediately:
Age > 55 years and new symptoms
Alarm symptoms or signs (e.g., weight loss, recurrent vomiting, bleeding)

If patient is young (< 55 years) and no alarm features:

Option 1
Test for *Helicobacter pylori* status (serology or breath test or stool antigen test)
If *H. pylori*-positive, empirical anti-*H. pylori* treatment; if this fails, go to Option 2
If *H. pylori*-negative, go to Option 3

Option 2
Empirical therapy initially (e.g., antisecretory agent)

Option 3
Prompt endoscopy for all patients
Diagnose ulcer, cancer; treat appropriately
Positively diagnose functional dyspepsia and treat accordingly

period of time, usually the cancer is advanced anyway and incurable so this usually does not change the prognosis [71,72]. If there is a high likelihood of symptom recurrence after the end of treatment, most patients will be investigated anyway, and resources will not be conserved. Lastly, this recommendation also fails to take into account the fact that dyspeptic patients with *H. pylori*-related peptic ulcer usually have a potentially curable disease.

Prompt endoscopy has long been accepted as the gold standard approach. A number of management trials have now shown that empiric *H. pylori* testing and treatment lead to outcomes similar to those observed after prompt endoscopy [246] and is superior to placebo in primary care [256]. The test-and-treat *H. pylori* strategy was associated with a two-thirds reduction in subsequent endoscopies performed within 1 year [257]. In one controlled trial, fewer patients were satisfied with the *H. pylori* test-and-treat strategy [258], but other data suggest that this is not of major clinical concern [257]. In contrast, *H. pylori* testing and referral of positive patients for endoscopy (vs acid suppression) was not cost-effective, and the outcomes were similar [259].

Thus, the *H. pylori* test-and-treat strategy for dyspeptic patients younger than 55 years, appears to be safe and may result in lower costs than initial endoscopy with similar clinical outcomes [257]. For success, the test-and-treat strategy relies on a sufficient background prevalence of *H. pylori* and peptic ulcer disease; the approach will fail if the prevalence of *H. pylori* infection falls below 10%–20% in the population [254]. Furthermore, there may be a potential benefit in terms of reducing the subsequent risk of gastric cancer although this is controversial [260]. The risk of inducing esophagitis after *H. pylori* eradication is very low, and there is no evid-

ence that eradication induces GERD symptoms in Western populations [261, 262]. Other data suggest that if *H. pylori* eradication fails to relieve symptoms, PPI empirical therapy is more cost effective than endoscopy [263].

Therapeutic approach in documented functional dyspepsia

Establishing the diagnosis, and communicating and explaining this diagnosis to the patient are key. In clinical practice, a considerable proportion of patients presenting with dyspeptic symptoms do not need anything else. Establishing a diagnosis on clinical grounds is appropriate in young patients with no alarm features and long-standing symptoms. However, even mild symptoms may trigger the fear that a life-threatening condition is the cause of symptoms in some patients and here ruling out malignancies and other relevant conditions by endoscopy is reasonable.

For the majority of patients, treatment is symptom based [264–266].

Placebo

Several pharmacological treatments are now available for patients with functional dyspepsia (Table 4.3), and most have been compared to placebo in controlled trials. The response to placebo in functional dyspepsia ranges from 30% to 60% [265–267].

In general, placebo response rates in functional bowel disorders (functional dyspepsia, IBS) are considered to be high. However, they are not substantially different from those in nonintestinal diseases (depression, pain disorders, Parkinson disease) or other organic gastrointestinal diseases (duodenal ulcer, inflammatory bowel disease) [268].

Table 4.3 Pharmacological treatment for functional dyspepsia

First-line treatment
Proton pump inhibitor
Anti-*Helicobacter pylori* therapy

Second-line treatment
Histamine H_2-receptor blocker
Tricyclic antidepressants (low dose)
Prokinetic (metoclopramide, domperidone)
$5-HT_1$ agonists (e.g., buspirone, sumatriptan)
Simethicone

Uncertain or unknown efficacy
Gonadotropin-releasing hormone analogues
Somatostatin analogues

Unlikely to be beneficial
Antacids
Prostaglandin analogues
Motilinomimetics
Anticholinergics/antispasmodics
Nitrates

The placebo response may not reflect a nonspecific effect of treatment but rather spontaneous regression of the disease. Indeed, the course of functional dyspepsia typically is characterized by relapsing and remitting symptoms, but during a 1-year period, more than 70% of patients will continue to have symptoms [51,269,270]. A major issue in the treatment of patients with functional dyspepsia is the long-term outcome; unfortunately, most trials have focused on short-term results only. No on-demand (patient-directed) management studies have been conducted.

Very little is known about the predictors of the placebo response. One study suggested that independent predictors of a lower placebo response were lower body mass index and a more consistent predominant symptom pattern, while no association was seen with age, gender, change in gastric emptying, or quality of life [271].

Antacids/simethicone

Randomized controlled studies have failed to show a significant benefit of antacid use over placebo [272–275]. Antacids are probably most effective in those with undiagnosed gastroesophageal reflux [276]. The potential role of gas retention and air swallowing in functional dyspepsia was indirectly examined in one study, which observed a significantly greater improvement in symptoms during treatment with simethicone than with cisapride [277], but more data are needed.

Acid inhibition

Controlled trials testing histamine H_2-receptor antagonists have yielded conflicting results [265,272,274,276,278,279]. These might be explained in part by the relatively small sample sizes, and thus inadequate study power, and the heterogeneity of the study populations. Metaanalysis has suggested a benefit of histamine H_2-receptor antagonists over placebo, but only selected trials could be included, and studies with patients who had GERD symptoms were not specifically excluded [279–282]. The efficacy of the selective muscarinic blocking agent pirenzepine (still available in many countries, but not the United States) is questionable [276,280]. Notably, this drug has a lower acid-inhibitory potency than histamine H_2 blockers and has anticholinergic effects that decrease lower esophageal sphincter pressure.

Reports have described greater relief of symptoms during treatment with a PPI than with placebo or ranitidine in uninvestigated dyspepsia [283] and functional dyspepsia [253, 284]. Several large placebo-controlled studies [285–288] have provided further evidence that inhibition of acid secretion with a PPI relieves symptoms in a subgroup of patients with functional dyspepsia although not all trials agree [289]. However, the therapeutic gain over placebo is modest (number needed to treat = 9), with most patients failing to benefit, and positive results may in part be explained by contamination of the trials with GERD patients. Notably, those with meal-related symptoms probably do not respond better to a PPI than to placebo (Fig. 4.6) [287]. A greater response to PPI than to placebo was observed in *H. pylori*-infected patients in one trial [284], but this was not confirmed by other, methodologically sound trials [287,288].

Cytoprotection

Sucralfate stimulates mucosal prostaglandin synthesis and release of cytokines and has cytoprotective properties in experimental models [290]. One placebo-controlled study [291] reported significant improvement of symptoms in 77% of patients treated with sucralfate, vs 56% of patients in the

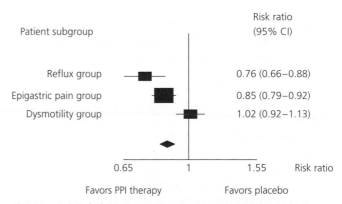

Figure 4.6 Relief of dyspepsia with a proton pump inhibitor vs placebo in functional dyspepsia according to dyspepsia subgroup. Ulcer-like, predominant epigastric pain; dysmotility-like, nonpainful predominant symptom (e.g., fullness, bloating, nausea); reflux-like, symptomatic reflux (heartburn) plus dyspepsia. From Moayyedi et al. [253], with permission from the American Gastroenterological Association.

placebo group. An open study that directly compared sucralfate with ranitidine [292] noted superior symptom improvement in patients treated with sucralfate. Other studies in functional dyspepsia failed to detect a significant effect of sucralfate compared with placebo [292, 293]. Rebamipide, a cytoprotective drug available in the Far East, was not superior to placebo in functional dyspepsia [267]. Misoprostol was also not efficacious in functional dyspepsia [294].

Prokinetic drugs

Few prokinetic drugs are now available to treat functional dyspepsia. The dopaminergic receptor blockers metoclopramide and domperidone may be better than placebo but data are very limited [295]. The safety profiles of some prokinetics limit their use. Metoclopramide can induce side effects through its central antidopaminergic mechanism; these include dystonic reactions, drowsiness, increased prolactin levels, and rarely, particularly in the elderly, tardive dyskinesia. Domperidone, available in Canada, Mexico, and Australia, also increases prolactin levels and may be proarrhythmic. Cisapride, a serotonin $5\text{-}HT_4$ agonist and weak $5\text{-}HT_3$ antagonist, is only available on a compassionate use basis in the United States.

Tegaserod, a $5\text{-}HT_4$ agonist, has been preliminarily evaluated in functional dyspepsia with equivocal results [296]. An increased prevalence of ischemic events led to the drug being suspended in the United States and elsewhere [297]. Erythromycin, a motilin agonist that initiates phase III activity in the antrum and small bowel [298], has not been evaluated in functional dyspepsia, and the drug often induces nausea. Another motilinomimetic, ABT-229, was not superior to placebo in functional dyspepsia patients with or without delayed gastric emptying, and higher doses caused worse outcomes [299]. The dopaminergic prokinetic itopride available in Japan was superior to placebo in a European trial [300]. This study used a modified definition for functional dyspepsia that did not exclude concomitant reflux symptoms. Follow-up studies in Europe and the United States used very rigid entry criteria, excluding reflux, but did not find significant superiority of itopride over placebo [301].

Fundus-relaxing drugs

Fundic relaxation following a meal is impaired in a subset of patients with functional dyspepsia, and this has been linked to early satiety [124]. Hence, drugs that relax the gastric fundus may have therapeutic potential in the syndrome [302, 303]. Administration of the $5\text{-}HT_{1A}$ receptor agonist sumatriptan has been shown in small pilot studies to induce relaxation of the gastric fundus, permitting larger intragastric volumes to accumulate before thresholds for perception or discomfort are reached [302]. Other fundus-relaxing drugs include buspirone (a $5\text{-}HT_{1A}$ agonist), clonidine (an α-adrenergic agonist), and citalopram (a selective serotonin reuptake inhibitor). Randomized controlled trials are needed to confirm

beneficial treatment effects, and while preliminary data are promising [303, 304], there is insufficient information to recommend their use in the routine clinical setting.

Treatment targeting *H. pylori*

Most of the earlier studies of the effects of *H. pylori* eradication in patients with functional dyspepsia had important methodological limitations (i.e., lack of randomization or lack of a placebo control, application of inadequate outcome measures, failure to eradicate infection, lack of adequate follow-up after therapy, or inadequate study power) [170, 305]. More recent studies have assessed the long-term outcome of eradication therapy, but the results have been mixed despite greater methodological rigor [306–318]. Metaanalyses have produced contradictory conclusions [319,320], although the most recent Cochrane metaanalysis suggests that there is a small but clinically relevant benefit (number needed to treat = 15) [321]. Eradication of *H. pylori* should be considered for all infected patients with functional dyspepsia, but despite cure of the infection most will not obtain relief from their dyspepsia.

Visceral analgesic drugs

In recent years, the potential role of serotonin receptors in modulating gut sensation has been recognized [322,323]. The $5\text{-}HT_3$ receptors appear to play a role in the altered nociception that occurs during gastrointestinal inflammation [324], and $5\text{-}HT_3$ antagonists may modulate peripheral gut sensory nerve transmission [325]. One trial with alosetron demonstrated a modest benefit in functional dyspepsia over placebo [326]. However, the development of severe constipation and ischemic colitis limits the use of alosetron.

Leuprolide acetate, a gonadotropin-releasing hormone analogue, has been shown in two randomized placebo-controlled trials to improve symptom scores during a 3-month period in women with poorly defined but severe functional GI complaints [327,328]. The mode of action is unknown, but ovarian hormone release is reduced, and such hormones may modulate GI smooth muscle function. The role of the gonadotropin-releasing hormone analogues remains to be established; moreover, their inconvenient mode of administration as well as their significant side effects resulting from chemical castration substantially restricts their application.

Octreotide in an open label study reduced pain and improved nutritional status in severe functional dyspepsia [329]. Clonidine may reduce pain perception to gastric distention, but any benefit in functional dyspepsia has not been established [330]. Gabapentin or pregabalin may help pain as adjunctive therapy in difficult cases.

Antispasmodic drugs

Because pyloric or antral spasm has not been documented in functional dyspepsia, it is not surprising that neither dicyclomine nor trimebutine was more efficacious than placebo in small cross-over studies [276]. Anticholinergic agents combined with a benzodiazepine have not been tested in functional dyspepsia; such drugs should be used sparingly if at all because of their potential for habituation. On the other hand, a combination of the antispasmodics peppermint oil and caraway oil was superior to placebo in one controlled trial [331].

Antinauseant drugs

Antinausea drugs include the prokinetics and 5-HT$_3$ antagonists (discussed above), and the antihistamines, antimuscarinics (e.g., scopolamine) or phenothiazines (e.g., prochlorperazine, promethazine). Although the therapeutic gain with nonspecific antinauseants has not been formally tested in patients with functional dyspepsia, the histamine H$_1$ antagonists dimenhydrinate and cyclizine decrease gastric dysrhythmias and may be worth a trial [332]. Benzodiazepines (e.g., lorazepam) may also help reduce nausea by their sedative effects. An antinauseant drug combined with a low-dose tricyclic antidepressant may be helpful in difficult cases. Other third-line options of uncertain efficacy include cannabinoids (e.g., dronabinol) that may enhance mood in chronic nausea, or aprepitant (a neurokinin 1 antagonist).

Antidepressant drugs

The data on the efficacy of antidepressants and other psychotropic agents in functional dyspepsia are very limited. However, in one placebo-controlled trial, the antidepressant mianserin (a combined 5-HT$_2$, 5-HT$_3$, and α_2-adrenergic antagonist) was superior to placebo in a heterogeneous group of patients with functional gastrointestinal disorders [333]. Furthermore, the tricyclic antidepressant imipramine at a relatively low dose of 50 mg daily was clearly superior to placebo in patients with noncardiac chest pain [334]. A cross-over study of seven patients with functional dyspepsia reported that their symptoms were significantly less severe after 4 weeks of treatment with amitriptyline, but interestingly, the symptom improvement during treatment was not associated with a normalization of the perceptual responses to gastric distention [335]. In a metaanalysis, tricyclic antidepressants were overall superior to placebo in functional GI disorders [336].

There are as yet no data on the effects of selective serotonin reuptake inhibitors (SSRIs) in patients with functional dyspepsia, and they may aggravate nausea [337]. Mirtazepine or paroxetine may promote weight gain in those who have lost weight because of dyspepsia, while fluoxetine may aggravate weight loss through anorexia. The place of the serotonin and norepinephrine reuptake inhibitors (e.g., duloxetine) is unknown, but may particularly benefit chronic pain.

Regarding the use of antidepressants, it is important to note that tricyclics (but not the SSRIs) appear to be effective at doses well below those currently used for the treatment of depressive disorders, and they may be effective even in patients without obvious psychiatric abnormalities. In pati-

ents with symptoms that are resistant to standard therapy, a trial of a low-dose tricyclic antidepressant (e.g., starting at 10 mg or 25 mg desipramine or imipramine) or an SSRI in full dose is justified.

Complementary and alternative medicine

Major problems of alternative medicines are related to a lack of standardization of the compounds, the inclusion of multiple potentially active extracts, and lack of knowledge about their long-term safety and precise mechanisms of action. Limited placebo-controlled trials have reported improvement of symptoms in functional dyspepsia and IBS during treatment with herbal preparations [338, 339]. For the commercially available preparation Iberogast, there are a few controlled trials supporting its use in patients with functional dyspepsia and IBS [340–342] and the preparation may modulate gastric function [343]. Another readily available herbal remedy that may be promising is artichoke extract [344].

Acupuncture and acupressure can reduce chemotherapy-induced and postoperative nausea and vomiting, but have not been tested in functional dyspepsia [5]. The value of gastric pacing in functional dyspepsia is also unclear but it may improve nausea in those with severe gastroparesis [5].

Patients who fail to respond

If a patient fails to respond to the currently established first-line treatments, a number of questions should be considered.
- Is the diagnosis correct?
- Is the patient properly informed and comfortable with the diagnosis?
- Have realistic goals been set or not?
- Did the patient take the prescribed medication properly?
- Are there other medical or nonmedical treatments available for this patient?

Check the diagnosis

If a diagnostic workup has not been done, the diagnosis should be confirmed utilizing endoscopy and other clinically indicated tests. Other tests may be indicated to rule out atypical GERD (off antisecretory therapy) or a serious motor disorder (e.g., intestinal pseudoobstruction).

Medical therapy

Treatment should be readjusted and other therapeutic avenues should be explored. A trial of high-dose acid suppression, with dose reduction if successful, or changing to a prokinetic if the initial choice was an acid inhibitory agent, can be helpful. Combination therapy (e.g., an antispasmodic plus an antisecretory agent, or simethicone or sucralfate) is not established as being beneficial but may be worth a trial. If early satiety is a prominent symptom a trial of buspirone, sumatriptan, or clonidine can be considered. Another option is to initiate low-dose treatment with a tricyclic antidepressant or an SSRI in full dose.

Psychological therapies

Few controlled trials have evaluated the efficacy of psychological therapies in functional dyspepsia. Haug and colleagues [345] observed significantly greater improvement of symptoms in patients treated with cognitive psychotherapy than in a control group that received no specific treatment. In a randomized trial of patients with functional dyspepsia receiving either psychodynamic interpersonal psychotherapy or supportive therapy, small but significant advantages were observed in the psychotherapy arm compared with the controls in the toal symptom scores of both the gastroenterologists and the patients; 1 year after treatment, the symptom scores were similar [346]. Another trial suggested that hypnotherapy was efficacious in functional dyspepsia compared with an H_2-receptor antagonist or placebo [347,348]. Psychological therapies may specifically address the fear and anxiety of the patients that most likely represent a considerable component of the disease burden [345].

Patients with recurrent or relapsing symptoms

In most patients, symptoms improve after an initial course of treatment. Because functional dyspepsia and related functional disorders are characterized by chronic relapsing symptoms [349], it is highly probable that symptoms will recur after the end of treatment. No long-term strategy has been tested adequately in these patients. If symptoms have responded initially to a specific treatment but recur (usually after weeks or even months), another course of the same treatment is justified. Some patients have frequent symptom relapses that affect their quality of life, and in such cases, intermittent drug treatment can be helpful. Alternatively, consider prescribing on-demand therapy (self-directed therapy only when symptoms develop); this strategy has not been tested in functional dyspepsia but is successful in nonerosive GERD [2]. The patient should also be advised to return for reevaluation if the pattern of symptoms changes or the symptoms do not respond to therapy.

Intractable functional dyspepsia

A small group of patients does not respond to any therapeutic measures, and their quality of life is affected considerably. In these patients – if not already done – rare causes of dyspepsia must be excluded. However, it is equally important that once a comprehensive evaluation has been undertaken, repeated diagnostic testing should be avoided because this undermines patient confidence.

The patient with intractable symptoms can benefit from an ongoing relationship with a physician who demonstrates a commitment to the patient's well-being. The physician should set realistic goals. For example, although improvement in functional status and quality of life is usually possible, complete symptom relief is usually not, and the patient must be made aware of the realities. The patient should be encouraged to become a partner in all management decisions. Regular brief visits will provide useful psychosocial support.

It is important to rule out comorbid major psychiatric disease. Specific behavioral therapy (e.g., psychotherapy or cognitive–behavioral therapy) can reduce anxiety levels and encourage health-promoting behaviors in patients with intractable complaints, giving them greater control over their symptoms. In patients who require continuous therapy, drug holidays should be used to confirm that the therapy is still of value.

Management guidelines

A management algorithm is shown in Fig. 4.7 [350].

Patients with new-onset (uninvestigated) dyspepsia

The medical history is important. If typical reflux symptoms, heartburn, or acid regurgitation is the predominant or most frequent complaint, a diagnosis of gastroesophageal reflux rather than functional dyspepsia should be made and appropriate treatment should be instituted. Similarly, if bowel dysfunction is linked directly to the epigastric pain or discomfort, a diagnosis of IBS should lead to reassurance, explanation, dietary modification, and selective pharmacological therapy or stress management, which constitute the mainstay of treatment for patients with IBS.

Patients older than 55 years with unexplained dyspepsia and those with alarm symptoms should undergo prompt upper GI endoscopy, and management should be based on the findings. In patients without alarm features, management should depend on the degree of uncertainty that both patient and physician are willing to accept.

The use of a noninvasive *H. pylori* test and initiation of anti-*H. pylori* treatment in infected subjects constitute a reasonable initial approach, unless *H. pylori* is very uncommon (< 20%) in the background population [254]. Anti-*H. pylori* therapy should relieve symptoms in most patients with peptic ulcer and substantially eliminate the ulcer diathesis.

No agent has been approved by the Food and Drug Administration for use in functional dyspepsia. If empiric therapy is considered in the uninvestigated patient who is negative for *H. pylori*, the major first-line drug is now a PPI. Patients who fail to respond within 8 weeks or who rapidly relapse should be reassessed; endoscopy in this group, however, has a low yield.

In patients with documented functional dyspepsia after endoscopy, a positive clinical diagnosis and firm reassurance remain the key steps in management, with targeted pharmacological therapy for exacerbations (Table 4.4).

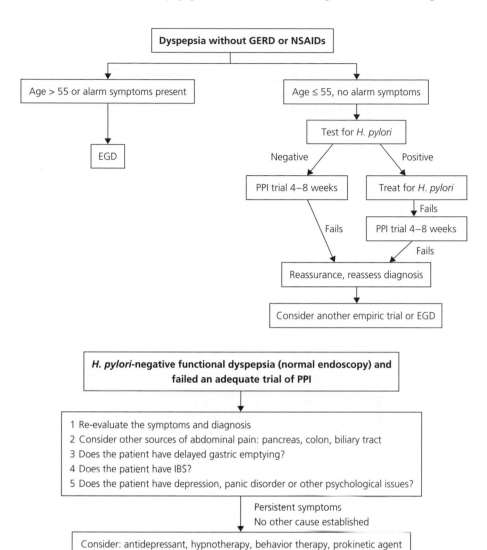

Figure 4.7 Management algorithm for patients presenting with new-onset dyspepsia who have not been previously evaluated. GERD, gastroesophageal reflux disease; IBS, irritable bowel syndrome; NSAID, nonsteroidal antiinflammatory drug; PPI, proton pump inhibitor. Modified from Talley et al. [350], with permission from Blackwell Publishing.

Table 4.4 Management principles in functional dyspepsia

Make a positive clinical diagnosis based on the history and physical examination

Minimize invasive investigations and avoid giving "mixed messages"; do not perform repeated testing (e.g., upper gastrointestinal endoscopy) without substantial indication

Determine the patient's agenda; ask why a patient who has chronic symptoms is presenting now

Provide education about the condition and the benign prognosis

Provide firm reassurance and reinforce this message at subsequent visits

Try dietary modification (e.g., low-fat diet, small meals, split ingestion of solids and liquids, and avoiding foods that precipitate symptoms)

Set realistic treatment goals and center therapy around adjustment to illness and patient-based responsibility for care

Prescribe drugs sparingly, targeting the symptoms of most concern to the patient; remember the placebo response

Consider behavioral treatments or psychotherapy for moderate to severe cases

Organize follow-up care

From Talley et al. [1].

Prognosis

A firm diagnosis of functional dyspepsia after endoscopy is generally safe; few patients are later found to have an ulcer or other structural disease [351]. Population-based studies have demonstrated a considerable turnover of subjects with abdominal symptoms; up to one-third may lose their symptoms for years [349]. Patients with functional dyspepsia seen at tertiary centers represent a subgroup with relatively intractable symptoms, and in this group, evidence that spontaneous remissions occur is only anecdotal. Whereas treatment may relieve symptoms for a limited period, cure cannot be expected.

References

1. Talley NJ, Colin-Jones D, Koch KL. Functional dyspepsia: a classification with guidelines for diagnosis and management. Gastroenterol Int 1991;4:145.
2. Tack J, Talley NJ, Camilleri M, et al. Functional gastroduodenal disorders. Gastroenterology 2006;130:1466.
3. Chiba N. Treat the patients' main dyspepsia complaint, not the ROME criteria. Am J Gastroenterol 2004;99:1059.
4. Thomson A, Barkun A, Armstrong D, et al. The prevalence of clinically significant endoscopic findings in primary care patients with uninvestigated dyspepsia: the Canadian Adult Dyspepsia Empiric treatment-prompt endoscopy (CADET-PE) study. Aliment Pharmacol Ther 2003;17:1481.
5. Drossman DA, Corrazziari E, Talley NJ, et al. Rome II: the functional gastrointestinal disorders. Diagnosis, pathophysiology, and treatment: a multinational consensus. McLean VA: Degnon Associates, 2000.
6. Johnsen R, Bernersen B, Straume B, et al. Prevalences of endoscopic and histological findings in subjects with and without dyspepsia. BMJ 1991;302:749.
7. Colin-Jones DG, Bloom B, Bodemar G, et al. Management of dyspepsia: report of a working party. Lancet 1988;1:576.
8. Talley NJ, Phillips SF. Non-ulcer dyspepsia: potential causes and pathophysiology. Ann Intern Med 1988;108:865.
9. Talley NJ, Locke GRI, Lahr BD, et al. Functional dyspepsia, delayed gastric emptying and impaired quality of life. Gut 2006;55:933.
10. Talley NJ, Vakil N, Delaney B, et al. Management issues in dyspepsia: current consensus and controversies. Scand J Gastroenterol 2004;39:913.
11. Talley NJ, Walker MM, Aro P, et al. Nonulcer dyspepsia and duodenal eosinophilia: an adult endoscopic population-based case–control study. Clin Gastroenterol Hepatol 2007;5:1175.
12. Friesen CA, Sandridge L, Andre L, et al. Mucosal eosinophilia and response to H1/H2 antagonist and cromolyn therapy in pediatric dyspepsia. Clin Pediatr (Phila) 2006;45:143.
13. Friesen CA, Andre L, Garola R, et al. Activated duodenal mucosal eosinophils in children with dyspepsia: a pilot transmission electron microscopic study. J Pediatr Gastroenterol Nutr 2002;35:329.
14. El-Serag HB, Talley NJ. Systematic review: health-related quality of life in functional dyspepsia. Aliment Pharmacol Ther 2003;18:387.
15. Jorde R, Bostad L, Burhol PG. Asytmptomatic gastric ulcer: a follow-up study in patients with previous gastric ulcer disease. Lancet 1986;1:119.
16. Maddern GJ, Vauthey JN, Devitt P, et al. Recurrent peptic ulceration after highly selective vagotomy: long-term outcome. Br J Surg 1991;78:940.
17. Aro P, Ronkainen J, Talley NJ, et al. Body mass index and chronic unexplained gastrointestinal symptoms: an adult endoscopic population-based study. Gut 2005;54:1377.
18. Talley NJ, Zinsmeister AR, Schleck CD, Melton LJ, 3rd. Dyspepsia and dyspepsia subgroups: a population-based study. Gastroenterology 1992;102:1259.
19. Westbrook JI, Talley NJ. Empiric clustering of dyspepsia into symptom subgroups: a population-based study. Scand J Gastroenterol 2002;37:917.
20. Holtmann G, Goebell H, Talley NJ. Dyspepsia in consulters and non-consulters: prevalence, health-care seeking behaviour and risk factors. Eur J Gastroenterol Hepatol 1994;6:917.
21. Agreus L, Svardsudd K, Nyren O, Tibblin G. The epidemiology of abdominal symptoms: prevalence and demographic characteristics in a Swedish adult population. A report from the Abdominal Symptom Study. Scand J Gastroenterol 1994;29:102.
22. Haque M, Wyeth JW, Stace NH, et al. Prevalence, severity and associated features of gastro-oesophageal reflux and dyspepsia: a population-based study. N Z Med J 2000;113:178.
23. Castillo EJ, Camilleri M, Locke GR, et al. A community-based, controlled study of the epidemiology and pathophysiology of dyspepsia. Clin Gastroenterol Hepatol 2004;2:985.
24. Camilleri C, Carlson PJ, Camilleri M, et al. A study of candidate genotypes associated with dyspepsia in a US community. Am J Gastroenterol 2006;101:581.
25. Klauser AG, Voderholzer WA, Knesewitsch PA, et al. What is behind dyspepsia? Dig Dis Sci 1993;38:147.
26. Small PK, Loudon MA, Waldron B, et al. Importance of reflux symptoms in functional dyspepsia. Gut 1995;36:189.
27. Moayyedi P, Duffy J, Delaney B. New approaches to enhance the accuracy of the diagnosis of reflux disease. Gut 2004;53:55.
28. Klauser G, Schindbeck NE, Muller-Lissner SA. Symptoms in gastroesophageal disease. Lancet 1990;335:205.
29. Shi G, Bruley des Varannes S, Scarpignato C, et al. Reflux related symptoms in patients with normal oesophageal exposure to acid. Gut 1995;37:457.
30. Farup PG, Hovde O, Breder O. Are frequent short gastro oesophageal reflux episodes the cause of symptoms in patients with non-ulcer dyspepsia responding to treatment with ranitidine? Scand J Gastroenterol 1995;30:829.
31. Holtmann G, Goebell H, Talley NJ. Functional dyspepsia and irritable bowel syndrome: is there a common pathophysiological basis? Am J Gastroenterol 1997;92:954.
32. Locke GR, 3rd, Zinsmeister AR, Fett SL, et al. Overlap of gastrointestinal symptom complexes in a US community. Neurogastroenterol Motil 2005;17:29.
33. Vakil N, Van Zanten SJ, Chang L, et al. Comprehension and awareness of symptoms in women with dyspepsia. Aliment Pharmacol Ther 2005;22:1147.
34. Chitkara D, Bredenoord AJ, Rucker MJ, Talley NJ. Aerophagia in adults: a comparison with functional dyspepsia. Aliment Pharmacol Ther 2005;22:855.
35. O'Brien MD, Bruce BK, Camilleri M. The rumination syndrome: clinical features rather than manometric diagnosis. Gastroenterology 1995;108:1024.
36. Drossman D, Li Z, Andruzzi E, et al. U.S. householder survey of functional gastrointestinal disorders. Prevalence sociodemography, and health impact. Dig Dis Sci 1993;38:1569.
37. Agreus L, Svardsudd K, Nyren O, Tibblin G. Irritable bowel syndrome and dyspepsia in the general population: overlap and lack of stability over time. Gastroenterology 1995;109:671.
38. Talley NJ, Holtmann G, Agreus L, Jones M. Gastrointestinal symptoms and subjects cluster into distinct upper and lower groupings in the community: a four nations study. Am J Gastroenterol 2000; 95:1439.
39. Talley NJ. Symptom patterns in functional dyspepsia. Eur J Gastroenterol Hepatol 1992;4:597.

40. Weir RD, Backett EM. Studies of the epidemiology of peptic ulcer in a rural community: prevalence and natural history of dyspepsia and peptic ulcer. Gut 1968;9:75.

41. Thompson WG, Heaton KW. Functional bowel disorders in apparently healthy people. Gastroenterology 1980;79:283.

42. Tibblin G. Introduction to the epidemiology of dyspepsia. Scand J Gastroenterol 1985;109:29.

43. Johnsen R, Straume B, Forde OH. Peptic ulcer and non-ulcer dyspepsia – a disease and a disorder. Scand J Prim Health Care 1988;6:239.

44. Jones R, Lydeard S. Prevalence of symptoms of dyspepsia in the community. BMJ 1989;298:30.

45. Jones RH, Lydeard SE, Hobbs FD, et al. Dyspepsia in England and Scotland. Gut 1990;31:401.

46. Penston JG, Pounder RE. A survey of dyspepsia in Great Britain. Aliment Pharmacol Ther 1996;10:83.

47. Bernersen B, Johnsen R, Straume B, et al. Towards a true prevalence of peptic ulcer: the Sorreisa gastrointestinal disorder study. Gut 1990;31:989.

48. Schlemper RJ, van der Werf SD, Vandenbroucke JP, et al. Nonulcer dyspepsia in a Dutch working population and *Helicobacter pylori*. Ulcer history as an explanation of an apparent association. Arch Intern Med 1995;155:82.

49. Bytzer P, Talley NJ. Dyspepsia. Ann Intern Med 2001;134:815.

50. El-Serag HB, Talley NJ. Systematic review: the prevalence and clinical course of functional dyspepsia. Aliment Pharmacol Ther 2004; 19:643.

51. Talley N, Weaver A, Zinsmeister A, Melton LJ, III. Onset and disappearance of gastrointestinal symptoms and functional gastrointestinal disorders. Am J Epidemiol 1992;136:165.

52. Ford AC, Forman D, Bailey AG, et al. Initial poor quality of life and new onset of dyspepsia: results from a longitudinal 10-year follow-up study. Gut 2007;56:321.

53. Knill-Jones RP. Geographical differences in the prevalence of dyspepsia. Scand J Gastroenterol 1991;182:17.

54. Ahlawat SK, Locke GRI, Weaver AL, et al. Dyspepsia consulters and patterns of management: a population-based study. Aliment Pharmacol Ther 2005;22:251.

55. Whitehead WE, Bosmajian L, Zonderman AB, et al. Symptoms of psychologic distress associated with irritable bowel syndrome. Gastroenterology 1988;95:709.

56. Talley NJ, Boyce P, Jones M. Dyspepsia and health care seeking in a community: how important are psychological factors? Dig Dis Sci 1998;43:1016.

57. Koloski NA, Talley NJ, Huskic SS, Boyce PM. Predictors of conventional and alternative health care seeking for irritable bowel syndrome and functional dyspepsia. Aliment Pharmacol Ther 2003; 17:841.

58. Lydeard S, Jones R. Factors affecting the decision to consult with dyspepsia: comparison of consulters and non-consulters. J R Coll Gen Pract 1989;39:495.

59. Cheng C. Seeking medical consultation: perceptual and behavioral characteristics distinguishing consulters and nonconsulters with functional dyspepsia. Psychosom Med 2000;62:844.

60. Davenport PM, Morgan AG, Darnborough A, De Dombal FT. Can preliminary screening of dyspeptic patients allow more effective use of investigational techniques? BMJ 1985;290:217.

61. Forbat LN, Gribble RJ, Baron JH. Gastrointestinal endoscopy in the young. BMJ 1987;295:365.

62. Williams B, Luckas M, Ellingham JH, et al. Do young patients with dyspepsia need investigation? Lancet 1988;2:1349.

63. Mansi C, Mela GS, Pasini D, et al. Patterns of dyspepsia in patients with no clinical evidence of organic diseases. Dig Dis Sci 1990;35:1452.

64. Hansen JM, Bytzer P, Bondesen S, et al. Efficacy and outcome of an open access endoscopy service. Dan Med Bull 1991;38:288.

65. Soll AH. Consensus conference. Medical treatment of peptic ulcer disease: practice guidelines. Practice Parameters of the American College of Gastroenterology. JAMA 1996;275:622.

66. Bytzer P, Schaffalitzky de Muckadell O. Prediction of major pathological conditions in dyspeptic patients referred for endoscopy. A prospective validation study of a scoring system. Scand J Gastroenterol 1992;27:987.

67. Breslin NP, Thomson A, Bailey R, et al. Gastric cancer and other endoscopic diagnoses in patients with benign dyspepsia. Gut 2000;46:93.

68. Christie J, Shepherd NA, Codling BW, Valori RM. Gastric cancer below the age of 55: implications for screening patients with uncomplicated dyspepsia. Gut 1997;41:513.

69. McColl KE, Kidd J, Gillen D. Gastric cancer in patients with benign dyspepsia. Gut 2001;48:581.

70. Crane SJ, Locke GR, III, Harmsen WS, et al. Subsite-specific risk factors for esophageal and gastric adenocarcinoma. Am J Gastroenterol 2007;102:1596.

71. Panter SJ, O'Flanagan H, Bramble MG, Hungin AP. Empirical use of antisecretory drug therapy delays diagnosis of upper gastrointestinal adenocarcinoma but does not effect outcome. Aliment Pharmacol Ther 2004;19:981.

72. Maconi G, Kurihara H, Panizzo V, et al, Cancer IRGfG. Gastric cancer in young patients with no alarm symptoms: focus on delay in diagnosis, stage of neoplasm and survival. Scand J Gastroenterol 2003;38:1249.

73. Veldhuyzen van Zanten S. Review: alarm features in dyspepsia do not have high diagnostic accuracy for predicting upper gastrointestinal cancer. Evid Based Med 2007;12:55.

74. Anonymous. Prevalence of gallstone disease in an Italian adult female population. Rome Group for the Epidemiology and Prevention of Cholelithiasis (GREPCO). Am J Epidemiol 1984;119:796.

75. Bainton D, Davies GT, Evans KT, Gravelle IH. Gallbladder disease. Prevalence in a South Wales industrial town. N Engl J Med 1976; 294:1147.

76. French EB, Robb WA. Biliary and renal colic. BMJ 1963;5350:135.

77. Price WH. Gall-bladder dyspepsia. BMJ 1963;5350:138.

78. Glambek I, Arnesjö B, Soreide O. Correlation between gallstones and abdominal symptoms in a random population. Results from a screening study. Scand J Gastroenterol 1989;24:277.

79. Andersen BN, Scheel J, Rune SJ, Worning H. Exocrine pancreatic function in patients with dyspepsia. Hepatogastroenterology 1982; 29:35.

80. Smith RC, Talley NJ, Dent OF, et al. Exocrine pancreatic function and chronic unexplained dyspepsia. A case–control study. Int J Pancreatol 1991;8:253.

81. Carlsson R, Holloway RH. Endoscopy-negative reflux disease. Baillieres Best Pract Res Clin Gastroenterol 2000;14:827.

82. Dent J, Jones R, Kahrilas P, Talley NJ. Management of gastro-oesophageal reflux disease in general practice. BMJ 2001;322:344.

83. Numans ME, Lau J, de Wit NJ, Bonis PA. Short-term treatment with proton-pump inhibitors as a test for gastroesophageal reflux disease: a meta-analysis of diagnostic test characteristics. Ann Intern Med 2004;140:518.

84. Heikkinen M, Pikkarainen P, Takala J, et al. Etiology of dyspepsia: four unselected consecutive patients in general practice. Scand J Gastroenterol 1995;30:519.

85. Pehl C, Wendl B, Greiner I, et al. Abnormal oesophageal pH-monitoring in patients with functional thoracic and abdominal disorders. Gastroenterol Clin Biol 1995;19:367.

86. Quigley EM. Functional dyspepsia (FD) and non-erosive reflux disease (NERD): overlapping or discrete entities? Best Pract Res Clin Gastroenterol 2004;18:695.

87. Dean BB, Gano ADJ, Knight K, et al. Effectiveness of proton pump inhibitors in nonerosive reflux disease. Clin Gastroenterol Hepatol 2004;2:656.

88. Hawkey CJ. Nonsteroidal anti-inflammatory drug gastropathy. Gastroenterology 2000;119:521.

89. Hawkey CJ, Langman MJ. Non-steroidal anti-inflammatory drugs: overall risks and management. Complementary roles for COX-2 inhibitors and proton pump inhibitors. Gut 2003;52:600.

90. Holtmann G, Gschossmann J, Buenger L, et al. Do changes in visceral sensory function determine the development of dyspepsia during treatment with aspirin? Gastroenterology. 2002;123:1451.

91. Richter JE. Dyspepsia: organic causes and differential characteristics from functional dyspepsia. Scand J Gastroenterol (Suppl.) 1991;182: 11.

92. Bytzer P, Talley NJ, Leemon M, et al. Prevalence of gastrointestinal symptoms associated with diabetes mellitus: a population-based survey of 15,000 adults. Arch Intern Med 2001;161:1989.

93. Locke GR, III, Murray JA, Zinsmeister AR, et al. Celiac disease serology in irritable bowel syndrome and dyspepsia: a population-based case–control study. Mayo Clin Proc 2004;79:476.

94. Bardella MT, Minoli G, Ravizza D, et al. Increased prevalence of celiac disease in patients with dyspepsia. Arch Intern Med 2000;160: 1489.

95. Kalantar SJ, Marks R, Lambert JR, et al. Dyspepsia due to eosinophilic gastroenteritis. Dig Dis Sci 1997;42:2327.

96. Anonymous. Abdominal wall tenderness test. Could Carnett cut costs? Lancet 1991;337:1134.

97. Quartero AO, de Wit NJ, Lodder AC, et al. Disturbed solid-phase gastric emptying in functional dyspepsia: a meta-analysis. Dig Dis Sci 1998;43:2028.

98. Corinaldesi R, Stanghellini V, Raiti C, et al. Effect of chronic administration of cisapride on gastric emptying of a solid meal and on dyspeptic symptoms in patients with idiopathic gastroparesis. Gut 1987;28:300.

99. Wegener M, Borsch G, Schaffstein J, et al. Are dyspeptic symptoms in patients with *Campylobacter pylori*-associated type B gastritis linked to delayed gastric emptying? Am J Gastroenterol 1988;83: 737.

100. Labo G, Bortolotti M, Vezzadini P, et al. Interdigestive gastroduodenal motility and serum motilin levels in patients with idiopathic delay in gastric emptying. Gastroenterology 1986;90:20.

101. Hveem K, Hausken T, Svebak S, Berstad A. Gastric antral motility in functional dyspepsia. Effect of mental stress and cisapride. Scand J Gastroenterol 1996;31:452.

102. Kerlin P. Postprandial antral hypomotility in patients with idiopathic nausea and vomiting. Gut 1989;30:54.

103. Malagelada JR, Stanghellini V. Manometric evaluation of functional upper gut symptoms. Gastroenterology 1985;88:1223.

104. Camilleri M, Malagelada JR, Kao PC, Zinsmeister AR. Gastric and autonomic responses to stress in functional dyspepsia. Dig Dis Sci 1986;31:1169.

105. Waldron B, Cullen PT, Kumar R, et al. Evidence for hypomotility in non-ulcer dyspepsia: a prospective multifactorial study. Gut 1991;32:246.

106. Davis RH, Clench MH, Mathias JR. Effects of domperidone in patients with chronic unexplained upper gastrointestinal symptoms: a double-blind, placebo-controlled study. Dig Dis Sci 1988;33:1505.

107. Stanghellini V, Tosetti C, Paternico A, et al. Risk indicators of delayed gastric emptying of solids in patients with functional dyspepsia. Gastroenterology 1996;110:1036.

108. Talley NJ, Shuter B, McCrudden G, et al. Lack of association between gastric emptying of solids and symptoms in nonulcer dyspepsia. J Clin Gastroenterol 1989;11:625.

109. Haag S, Talley NJ, Holtmann G. Symptom patterns in functional dyspepsia and irritable bowel syndrome: relationship to disturbances in gastric emptying and response to a nutrient challenge in consulters and non-consulters. Gut 2004;53:1445.

110. Sarnelli G, Caenepeel P, Geypens B, et al. Symptoms associated with impaired gastric emptying of solids and liquids in functional dyspepsia. Am J Gastroenterol 2003;98:783.

111. Talley NJ, Verlinden M, Jones M. Can symptoms discriminate among those with delayed or normal gastric emptying in dysmotility-like dyspepsia? Am J Gastroenterol 2001;96:1422.

112. Camilleri M, Talley NJ. Pathophysiology as a basis for understanding symptom complexes and therapeutic targets. Neurogastroenterol Motil 2004;16:135.

113. Delgado-Aros S, Camilleri M, Cremonini F, et al. Contributions of gastric volumes and gastric emptying to meal size and postmeal symptoms in functional dyspepsia. Gastroenterology 2004;127:1685.

114. Stanghellini V, Ghidini C, Maccarini MR, et al. Fasting and postprandial gastrointestinal motility in ulcer and non-ulcer dyspepsia. Gut 1992;33:184.

115. Malagelada JR. Gastrointestinal motor disturbances in functional dyspepsia. Scand J Gastroenterol Suppl.1991;182:29.

116. Jebbink RJ, vanBerge-Henegouwen GP, Akkermans LM, Smout AJ. Antroduodenal manometry: 24-hour ambulatory monitoring versus short-term stationary manometry in patients with functional dyspepsia. Eur J Gastroenterol Hepatol 1995;7:109.

117. Wilmer A, Van Cutsem E, Andrioli A, et al. Ambulatory gastrojejunal manometry in severe motility-like dyspepsia: lack of correlation between dysmotility, symptoms, and gastric emptying. Gut 1998;42: 235.

118. Geldof H, van der Schee EJ, van Blankenstein M, Grashuis JL. Electrogastrographic study of gastric myoelectrical activity in patients with unexplained nausea and vomiting. Gut 1986;27:799.

119. Parkman HP, Miller MA, Trate D, et al. Electrogastrography and gastric emptying scintigraphy are complementary for assessment of dyspepsia. J Clin Gastroenterol 1997;24:214.

120. Brzana RJ, Koch KL. Gastroesophageal reflux disease presenting with intractable nausea. Ann Intern Med 1997;126:704.

121. Verhagen MA, Van Schelven LJ, Samsom M, Smout AJ. Pitfalls in the analysis of electrogastrographic recordings. Gastroenterology 1999;117:453.

122. Boeckxstaens G, Hirsch D, Kuiken S, et al. The proximal stomach and postprandial symptoms in functional dyspeptics. Am J Gastroenterol 2002;97:40.

123. Tack J, Caenepeel P, Piessevaux H, et al. Assessment of meal induced gastric accommodation by a satiety drinking test in health and in severe functional dyspepsia. Gut 2003;52:1271.

124. Tack J, Piessevaux H, Coulie B, et al. Role of impaired gastric accommodation to a meal in functional dyspepsia. Gastroenterology 1998; 115:1346.

125. Caldarella MP, Azpiroz F, Malagelada JR. Antro-fundic dysfunctions in functional dyspepsia. Gastroenterology 2003;124:1220.

126. Bredenoord AJ, Chial HJ, Camilleri M, et al. Gastric accommodation and emptying in evaluation of patients with upper gastrointestinal symptoms. Clin Gastroenterol Hepatol 2003;1:264.

127. Lemann M, Dederding JP, Flourie B, et al. Abnormal perception of visceral pain in response to gastric distension in chronic idiopathic dyspepsia. The irritable stomach syndrome. Dig Dis Sci 1991;36: 1249.

128. Tack J, Caenepeel P, Fischler B, et al. Symptoms associated with hypersensitivity to gastric distention in functional dyspepsia. Gastroenterology 2001;121:526.

129. Moragas G, Azpiroz F, Pavia J, Malagelada JR. Relations among intragastric pressure, postcibal perception, and gastric emptying. Am J Physiol 1993;264:G1112.

130. Holtmann G, Geobell H, Talley NJ. Impaired small intestinal peristaltic reflexes and sensory thresholds are independent functional disturbances in patients with chronic unexplained dyspepsia. Am J Gastroenterol 1996;91:485.

131. Holtmann G, Talley NJ, Goebell H. Association between *H. pylori*, duodenal mechanosensory thresholds, and small intestinal motility in chronic unexplained dyspepsia. Dig Dis Sci 1996;41:1285.

132. Holtmann G, Gschossmann J, Neufang-Huber J, et al. Differences in gastric mechanosensory function after repeated ramp distensions in non-consulters with dyspepsia and healthy controls. Gut 2000;47: 332.

133. Barbera R, Feinle C, Read NW. Nutrient-specific modulation of gastric mechanosensitivity in patients with functional dyspepsia. Dig Dis Sci 1995;40:1636.

134. Feinle C, Grundy D, Read NW. Effects of duodenal nutrients on sensory and motor responses of the human stomach to distension. Am J Physiol 1997;273:G721.

135. Klatt S, Pieramico O, Guethner C, et al. Gastric hypersensitivity in nonulcer dyspepsia: an inconsistent finding. Dig Dis Sci 1997;42:720.

136. Hu WH, Talley NJ. Visceral perception in functional gastrointestinal disorders: disease marker or epiphenomenon? Dig Dis 1996;14:276.

137. Coffin B, Azpiroz F, Guarner F, Malagelada JR. Selective gastric hypersensitivity and reflex hyporeactivity in functional dyspepsia. Gastroenterology 1994;107:1345.

138. Accarino AM, Azpiroz F, Malagelada JR. Selective dysfunction of mechanosensitive intestinal afferents in irritable bowel syndrome. Gastroenterology 1995;108:636.

139. Greydanus MP, Vassallo M, Camilleri M, et al. Neurohormonal factors in functional dyspepsia: insights on pathophysiological mechanisms. Gastroenterology 1991;100:1311.

140. Trimble KC, Farouk R, Pryde A, et al. Heightened visceral sensation in functional gastrointestinal disease is not site-specific. evidence for a generalized disorder of gut sensitivity. Dig Disease Sci 1995;40:1607.

141. Danzebrink RM, Green SA, Gebhart GF. Spinal mu and delta, but not kappa, opioid-receptor agonists attenuate responses to noxious colorectal distension in the rat. Pain 1995;63:39.

142. Grzybicki D, Gebhart GF, Murphy S. Expression of nitric oxide synthase type II in the spinal cord under conditions producing thermal hyperalgesia. J Chem Neuroanat 1996;10:221.

143. Urban MO, Smith DJ, Gebhart GF. Involvement of spinal cholecystokinin B receptors in mediating neurotensin hyperalgesia from the medullary nucleus raphe magnus in the rat. J Pharmacol Exp Ther 1996;278:90.

144. Maves TJ, Pechman PS, Gebhart GF, Meller ST. Possible chemical contribution from chronic gut sutures produces disorders of pain sensation like those seen in man. Pain 1993;54:57.

145. Azpiroz F, Bouin M, Camilleri M, et al. Mechanisms of hypersensitivity in IBS and functional disorders. Neurogastroenterol Motil 2007;19:62.

146. Mayer EA, Gebhart GF. Basic and clinical aspects of visceral hyperalgesia. Gastroenterology 1994;107:271.

147. Talley NJ, Phillips SF, Bruce BK, et al. Multisystem complaints in patients with the irritable bowel syndrome and functional dyspepsia. Eur J Gastroenterol Hepatol 1991;3:71.

148. Silverman DH, Munakata JA, Ennes H, et al. Regional cerebral activity in normal and pathological perception of visceral pain. Gastroenterology 1997;112:64.

149. Vandenberghe J, Dupont P, Van Oudenhove L, et al. Regional cerebral blood flow during gastric balloon distention in functional dyspepsia. Gastroenterology 2007;132:1684.

150. Hausken T, Svebak S, Wilhelmsen I, et al. Low vagal tone and antral dysmotility in patients with functional dyspepsia. Psychosom Med 1993;55:12.

151. Smart HL, Atkinson M. Abnormal vagal function in irritable bowel syndrome. Lancet 1987;2:475.

152. Undeland KA, Hausken T, Svebak S, et al. Wide gastric antrum and low vagal tone in patients with diabetes mellitus type 1 compared to patients with functional dyspepsia and healthy individuals. Dig Dis Sci 1996;41:9.

153. Hartley MN, Mackie CR. Gastric adaptive relaxation and symptoms after vagotomy. Br J Surg 1991;78:24.

154. Troncon LE, Thompson DG, Ahluwalia NK, et al. Relations between upper abdominal symptoms and gastric distension abnormalities in dysmotility like functional dyspepsia and after vagotomy. Gut 1995;37:17.

155. Holtmann G, Goebell H, Jockenhoevel F, Talley NJ. Altered vagal and intestinal mechanosensory function in chronic unexplained dyspepsia. Gut 1998;42:501.

156. Bost R, Hostein J, Valenti M, et al. Is there an abnormal fasting duodenogastric reflux in nonulcer dyspepsia? Dig Dis Sci 1990;35:193.

157. Mearin F, De Ribot X, Balboa A, et al. Duodenogastric bile reflux and gastrointestinal motility in pathogenesis of functional dyspepsia. Role of cholecystectomy. Dig Dis Sci 1995;40:1703.

158. Niemela S. Duodenogastric reflux in patients with upper abdominal complaints or gastric ulcer with particular reference to reflux-associated gastritis. Scand J Gastroenterol (Suppl.) 1985;115:1.

159. Collen MJ, Loebenberg MJ. Basal gastric acid secretion in nonulcer dyspepsia with or without duodenitis. Dig Dis Sci 1989;34:246.

160. Nyren O, Adami HO, Gustavsson S, et al. The "epigastric distress syndrome". A possible disease entity identified by history and endoscopy in patients with nonulcer dyspepsia. J Clin Gastroenterol 1987;9:303.

161. El-Omar E, Penman I, Ardill JE, McColl KE. A substantial proportion of non-ulcer dyspepsia patients have the same abnormality of acid secretion as duodenal ulcer patients. Gut 1995;36:534.

162. George AA, Tsuchiyose M, Dooley CP. Sensitivity of the gastric mucosa to acid and duodenal contents in patients with nonulcer dyspepsia. Gastroenterology 1991;101:3.

163. Bates S, Sjoden PO, Fellenius J, Nyren O. Blocked and nonblocked acid secretion and reported pain in ulcer, nonulcer dyspepsia, and normal subjects. Gastroenterology 1989;97:376.

164. Hu WH, Martin CJ, Talley NJ. Intraesophageal acid perfusion sensitizes the esophagus to mechanical distension: a Barostat study. Am J Gastroenterol 2000;95:2189.

165. Samsom M, Verhagen MA, vanBerge Henegouwen GP, Smout AJ. Abnormal clearance of exogenous acid and increased acid sensitivity of the proximal duodenum in dyspeptic patients. Gastroenterology 1999;116:515.

166. Lee KJ, Vos R, Janssens J, Tack J. Influence of duodenal acidification on the sensorimotor function of the proximal stomach in humans. Am J Physiol Gastrointest Liver Physiol 2004;286:G278.

167. Lee KJ, Demarchi B, Demedts I, et al. A pilot study on duodenal acid exposure and its relationship to symptoms in functional dyspepsia with prominent nausea. Am J Gastroenterol 2004;99:1765.

168. Marshall BJ, Warren JR. Unidentified curved bacilli in the stomach of patients with gastritis and peptic ulceration. Lancet 1984;1:1311.

169. Talley NJ. Helicobacter pylori and dyspepsia. Yale J Biol Med 1999;72:145.

170. Xia HH, Talley NJ. Helicobacter pylori eradication in patients with non-ulcer dyspepsia. Drugs 1999;58:785.

171. Rokkas T, Pursey C, Uzoechina E, et al. Campylobacter pylori and non-ulcer dyspepsia. Am J Gastroenterol 1987;82:1149.

172. Greenberg RE, Bank S. The prevalence of Helicobacter pylori in non-ulcer dyspepsia. Importance of stratification according to age. Arch Intern Med 1990;150:2053.

173. Dooley CP, Cohen H, Fitzgibbons PL, et al. Prevalence of Helicobacter pylori infection and histologic gastritis in asymptomatic persons. N Engl J Med 1989;321:1562.

174. Shallcross TM, Rathbone BJ, Heatley RV. Campylobacter pylori and non-ulcer dyspepsia. In: Rathbone BJ HR, (ed.). Campylobacter pylori and Gastroduodenal Disease, vol. 155, 2nd edn. Oxford: Blackwell Science, 1992.

175. Talley NJ. Is Helicobacter pylori a Cause of Nonulcer Dyspepsia? Berlin: Springer-Verlag, 1990.

176. Caballero-Plasencia AM, Muros-Navarro MC, Martin-Ruiz JL, et al. Dyspeptic symptoms and gastric emptying of solids in patients with functional dyspepsia. Role of Helicobacter pylori infection. Scand J Gastroenterol 1995;30:745.

177. Nandurkar S, Talley NJ, Xia H, et al. Dyspepsia in the community is linked to smoking and aspirin use but not to Helicobacter pylori infection. Arch Intern Med 1998;158:1427.

178. Agreus L, Engstrand L, Svardsudd K, et al. Helicobacter pylori seropositivity among Swedish adults with and without abdominal symptoms. A population-based epidemiologic study. Scand J Gastroenterol 1995;30:752.

179. Danesh J, Lawrence M, Murphy M, et al. Systematic review of the epidemiological evidence on Helicobacter pylori infection and nonulcer or uninvestigated dyspepsia. Arch Intern Med 2000;160:1192.

180. Talley NJ, Hunt RH. What role does Helicobacter pylori play in dyspepsia and nonulcer dyspepsia? Arguments for and against H. pylori

being associated with dyspeptic symptoms. Gastroenterology 1997; 113:S67.

181. Mearin F, de Ribot X, Balboa A, et al. Does *Helicobacter pylori* infection increase gastric sensitivity in functional dyspepsia? Gut. 1995; 37:47.

182. Gwee KA, Leong YL, Graham C, et al. The role of psychological and biological factors in postinfective gut dysfunction. Gut. 1999;44:400.

183. Spiller RC, Jenkins D, Thornley JP, et al. Increased rectal mucosal enteroendocrine cells, T lymphocytes, and increased gut permeability following acute *Campylobacter* enteritis and in post-dysenteric irritable bowel syndrome. Gut. 2000;47:804.

184. Tack J, Demedts I, Dehondt G, et al. Clinical and pathological characteristics of acute-onset functional dyspepsia. Gastroenterology 2002;122:1738.

185. Mearin F, Perez-Oliveras M, Perello A, et al. Dyspepsia and irritable bowel syndrome after a *Salmonella* gastroenteritis outbreak: one-year follow-up cohort study. Gastroenterology 2005;129:98.

186. Jonsson KA, Gotthard R, Bodemar G, Brodin U. The clinical relevance of endoscopic and histologic inflammation of gastroduodenal mucosa in dyspepsia of unknown origin. Scand J Gastroenterol 1989;24:385.

187. Kreuning J, v.d. Wal AM, Kuiper G, Lindeman J. Chronic nonspecific duodenitis. A multiple biopsy study of the duodenal bulb in health and disease. Scand J Gastroenterol Suppl. 1989;167:16.

188. Rypins EB, Sarfeh IJ, Collins-Irby D, et al. Asymptomatic peptic disease in patients undergoing major elective operations: a prospective endoscopic study. Am J Gastroenterol 1988;83:927.

189. Joffe SN, Primrose JN. Pain provocation test in peptic duodenitis. Gastrointest Endosc 1983;29:282.

190. Langeluddecke P, Goulston K, Tennant C. Psychological factors in dyspepsia of unknown cause: a comparison with peptic ulcer disease. J Psychosom Res 1990;34:215.

191. Talley NJ, Fung LH, Gilligan IJ, et al. Association of anxiety, neuroticism, and depression with dyspepsia of unknown cause. A case–control study. Gastroenterology 1986;90:886.

192. Talley NJ, Phillips SF, Bruce B, et al. Relation among personality and symptoms in non-ulcer dyspepsia and the irritable bowel syndrome. Gastroenterology 1990;99:327.

193. Talley NJ, Jones M, Piper DW. Psychosocial and childhood factors in essential dyspepsia. A case–control study. Scand J Gastroenterol 1988;23:341.

194. Drossman DA, Creed FH, Fava GA, et al. Psychosocial aspects of the functional gastrointestinal disorders. Gastroenterol Int 1995;8:47.

195. Walker EA, Gelfand AN, Gelfand MD, Katon WJ. Psychiatric diagnoses, sexual and physical victimization, and disability in patients with irritable bowel syndrome or inflammatory bowel disease. Psychol Med 1995;25:1259.

196. Wilson KC, Whiteoak R, Dewey M, Watson JP. Aspects of personality of soldiers presenting to an endoscopy clinic. J Psychosom Res 1989;33:85.

197. Kutscher SU, Holtmann G, Heuft G, et al. Somatization in Functional Dyspepsia and Irritable Bowel Syndrome: A Short Review. Dordrecht: Kluwer Academic Publishers, 1998.

198. Wilhelmsen I, Haug TT, Ursin H, Berstad A. Discriminant analysis of factors distinguishing patients with functional dyspepsia from patients with duodenal ulcer. Significance of somatization. Dig Dis Sci 1995;40:1105.

199. Jonsson BH, Theorell T, Gotthard R. Symptoms and personality in patients with chronic functional dyspepsia. J Psychosom Res 1995;39:93.

200. Talley NJ, Ellard K, Jones M, et al. Suppression of emotions in essential dyspepsia and chronic duodenal ulcer. A case–control study. Scand J Gastroenterol 1988;23:337.

201. Howell S, Talley NJ. Does fear of serious disease predict consulting behaviour amongst patients with dyspepsia in general practice? Eur J Gastroenterol Hepatol 1999;11:881.

202. Jess P, Eldrup J. The personality patterns in patients with duodenal ulcer and ulcer-like dyspepsia and their relationship to the course of

the diseases. Hvidovre Ulcer Project Group. J Intern Med 1994; 235:589.

203. Chua A, Keating J, Hamilton D, et al. Central serotonin receptors and delayed gastric emptying in non-ulcer dyspepsia. BMJ Clin Res Ed 1992;305:280.

204. Gorard DA, Dewsnap PA, Medbak SH, et al. Central 5-hydroxy-tryptaminergic function in irritable bowel syndrome. Scand J Gastroenterol Suppl. 1995;30:994.

205. Stern RM, Koch KL, Stewart WR, Lindblad IM. Spectral analysis of tachygastria recorded during motion sickness. Gastroenterology 1987;92:92.

206. Thompson DG, Richelson E, Malagelada JR. Perturbation of gastric emptying and duodenal motility through the central nervous system. Gastroenterology 1982;83:1200.

207. Stanghellini V, Malagelada JR, Zinsmeister AR, et al. Stress-induced gastroduodenal motor disturbances in humans: possible humoral mechanisms. Gastroenterology 1983;85:83.

208. Talley NJ, Piper DW. Major life event stress and dyspepsia of unknown cause: a case–control study. Gut 1986;27:127.

209. Hui WM, Shiu LP, Lam SK. The perception of life events and daily stress in nonulcer dyspepsia. Am J Gastroenterol 1991;86:292.

210. Haug TT, Wilhelmsen I, Berstad A, Ursin H. Life events and stress in patients with functional dyspepsia compared with patients with duodenal ulcer and healthy controls. Scand J Gastroenterol 1995;30:524.

211. Erckenbrecht JF, Schäfer R, Köhler G, Enck PJGM. Dyspeptic symptoms in healthy volunteers with stress are related to stress-induced increase of anxiety-results of a prospective study with a long-term "physiological" stress model. J Gastrointest Motil 1993;5:189.

212. Drossman DA, Talley NJ, Leserman J, et al. Sexual and physical abuse and gastrointestinal illness. Review and recommendations. Ann Int Med 1995;123:782.

213. Talley NJ, Fett SL, Zinsmeister AR, Melton LJ. Gastrointestinal tract symptoms and self-reported abuse: a population-based study. Gastroenterology 1994;107:1040.

214. Koloski NA, Talley NJ, Boyce PM. A history of abuse in community subjects with irritable bowel syndrome and functional dyspepsia: the role of other psychosocial variables. Digestion 2005;72:86.

215. Watson DJ, Harper SE, Zhao PL, et al. Gastrointestinal tolerability of the selective cyclooxygenase-2 (COX-2) inhibitor rofecoxib compared with nonselective COX-1 and COX-2 inhibitors in osteoarthritis. Arch Intern Med 2000;160:2998.

216. Talley NJ, Zinsmeister AR, Schleck CD, Melton L, Jr. Smoking, alcohol, and analgesics in dyspepsia and among dyspepsia subgroups: lack of an association in a community. Gut 1994;35:619.

217. Talley NJ, McNeil D, Piper DW. Environmental factors and chronic unexplained dyspepsia. Association with acetaminophen but not other analgesics, alcohol, coffee, tea, or smoking. Dig Dis Sci 1988; 33:641.

218. Elta GH, Behler EM, Colturi TJ. Comparison of coffee intake and coffee-induced symptoms in patients with duodenal ulcer, nonulcer dyspepsia, and normal controls. Am J Gastroenterol 1990;85:1339.

219. Boekema PJ, Samsom M, van Berge Henegouwen GP, Smout AJ. Coffee and gastrointestinal function: facts and fiction. A review. Scand J Gastroenterol Suppl. 1999;230:35.

220. Talley NJ, Weaver AL, Zinsmeister AR, Melton L, Jr. Smoking, alcohol, and nonsteroidal anti-inflammatory drugs in outpatients with functional dyspepsia and among dyspepsia subgroups. Am J Gastroenterol 1994;89:524.

221. Feinle-Bisset C, Vozzo R, Horowitz M, Talley NJ. Diet, food intake, and disturbed physiology in the pathogenesis of symptoms in functional dyspepsia. Am J Gastroenterol 2004;99:170.

222. Kaess H, Kellermann M, Castro A. Food intolerance in duodenal ulcer patients, non ulcer dyspeptic patients and healthy subjects. A prospective study. Klin Wochenschr 1988;66:208.

223. Mullan A, Kavanagh P, O'Mahony P, et al. Food and nutrient intakes and eating patterns in functional and organic dyspepsia. Eur J Clin Nutr 1994;48:97.

224. Young E, Stoneham MD, Petruckevitch A, et al. A population study of food intolerance. Lancet 1994;343:1127.

225. Cohen S. Pathogenesis of coffee-induced gastrointestinal symptoms. N Engl J Med 1980;303:122.

226. Holtmann G, Grote E, Braun-Lang U, et al. G-protein β3 subunit (GNβ3) 825 CC genotype and the manifestation of functional gastrointestinal disorders. Gastroenterology 2004;126(Suppl. 2):A-162.

227. Camilleri CE, Carlson PJ, Camilleri M, et al. A study of candidate genotypes associated with dyspepsia in a U.S. community. Am J Gastroenterol 2006;101:581.

228. Conry BG, McLean AM, Farthing MJ. Diagnostic and therapeutic efficacy of barium meal examination: a prospective evaluation in general practice. BMJ 1989;299:1443.

229. Brignoli R, Merki H, Miazza B, Beglinger C. Endoscopic findings in volunteers and dyspeptic patients. Schweiz Med Wochenschr 1994;124:1240.

230. Talley N, Vakil NB, Moayyedi P. American Gastroenterological Association technical review on the evaluation of dyspepsia. Gastroenterology 2005;129:1756.

231. Boyd EJ. The prevalence of esophagitis in patients with duodenal ulcer or ulcer-like dyspepsia. Am J Gastroenterol 1996;91:1539.

232. Bytzer P, Hansen JM, Havelund T, et al. Predicting endoscopic diagnosis in the dyspeptic patient: the value of clinical judgment. Eur J Gastroenterol Hepatol 1996;8:359.

233. Talley NJ, Weaver AL, Tesmer DL, Zinsmeister AR. Lack of discriminant value of dyspepsia subgroups in patients referred for upper endoscopy. Gastroenterology 1993;105:1378.

234. Kang JY, Ho KY, Yeoh KG, Guan R. Chronic upper abdominal pain due to duodenal ulcer and other structural and functional causes: its localization and nocturnal occurrence. J Gastroenterol Hepatol 1996;11:515.

235. Gillen D, McColl KE. Does concern about missing malignancy justify endoscopy in uncomplicated dyspepsia in patients aged less than 55? Am J Gastroenterol 1999;94:75.

236. Meineche-Schmidt V, Jorgensen T. Alarm symptoms in patients with dyspepsia: a three-year prospective study from general practice. Scand J Gastroenterol 2002;37:999.

237. Hammer J, Eslick G, Howell S, et al. Diagnostic yield of alarm features in irritable bowel syndrome and functional dyspepsia. Gut 2004;53:666.

238. Bowrey DJ, Griffin SM, Wayman J, et al. Use of alarm symptoms to select dyspeptics for endoscopy causes patients with curable esophagogastric cancer to be overlooked. Surg Endosc 2006;20:1725.

239. Sobala GM, Crabtree JE, Pentith JA, et al. Screening dyspepsia by serology to Helicobacter pylori. Lancet 1991;338:94.

240. Patel P, Khulusi S, Mendall MA, et al. Prospective screening of dyspeptic patients by Helicobacter pylori serology. Lancet 1995;346:1315.

241. Xia HH, Phung N, Kalantar JS, Talley NJ. Demographic and endoscopic characteristics of patients with Helicobacter pylori positive and negative peptic ulcer disease. Med J Aust 2000;173:515.

242. Health and Public Policy Committee. Endoscopy in the evaluation of dyspepsia. Ann Intern Med 1985;102:266.

243. Quadri A, Vakil N. Health-related anxiety and the effect of open-access endoscopy in US patients with dyspepsia. Aliment Pharmacol Ther 2003;17:835.

244. Rabeneck L, Wristers K, Souchek J, Ambriz E. Impact of upper endoscopy on satisfaction in patients with previously uninvestigated dyspepsia. Gastrointest Endosc 2003;57:295.

245. Delaney BC, Wilson S, Roalfe A, et al. Cost effectiveness of initial endoscopy for dyspepsia in patients over age 50 years: a randomised controlled trial in primary care. Lancet 2000;356:1965.

246. Delaney B, Moayyedi P, Forman D. Initial management strategies for dyspepsia. Cochrane Database of Systematic Reviews 2003;2.

247. Aro P, Ronkainen J, Storskrubb T, et al. Valid symptom reporting at upper endoscopy in a random sample of the Swedish adult general populaiton. The Kalixanda study. Scand J Gastroenterol 2004;39:1280.

248. Ronkainen J, Aro P, Storskrubb T, et al. High prevalence of gastroesophageal reflux symptoms and esophagitis with or without symptoms in the general adult Swedish population: a Kalixanda study report. Scand J Gastroenterol 2005;40:275.

249. Forbes GM, Glaser ME, Cullen DJ, et al. Duodenal ulcer treated with Helicobacter pylori eradication: Seven-year follow-up. Lancet 1994;343:258.

250. McColl KE, el-Nujumi A, Murray LS, et al. Assessment of symptomatic response as predictor of Helicobacter pylori status following eradication therapy in patients with ulcer. Gut 1998;42:618.

251. Jorgensen T. Abdominal symptoms and gallstone disease: an epidemiological investigation. Hepatology 1989;9:856.

252. Malagelada JR. When and how to investigate the dyspeptic patient. Scand J Gastroenterol (Suppl.) 1991;182:70.

253. Moayyedi P, Delaney B, Vakil N, et al. The efficacy of proton pump inhibitors in non-ulcer dyspepsia: a systematic review and economic analysis. Gastroenterology 2004;127:1329.

254. Talley NJ. Dyspepsia management in the millennium: the death of test and treat? Gastroenterology 2002;122:1521.

255. Bramble MG, Suvakovic Z, Hungin AP. Detection of upper gastrointestinal cancer in patients taking antisecretory therapy prior to gastroscopy. Gut 2000;6:464.

256. Chiba N, Van Zanten SJ, Sinclair P, et al. Treating Helicobacter pylori infection in primary care patients with uninvestigated dyspepsia: the Canadian adult dyspepsia empiric treatment–Helicobacter pylori positive (CADET-Hp) randomised controlled trial. BMJ 2002;324:1012.

257. Delaney BC, Innes MA, Deeks J, et al. Initial management strategies for dyspepsia. Cochrane Database Syst 2000;(2):CD001961.

258. Lassen AT, Pedersen FM, Bytzer P, et al. Helicobacter pylori test-and-eradicate versus prompt endoscopy for management of dyspeptic patients: a randomised trial. Lancet 2000;356:455.

259. Delaney BC, Wilson S, Roalfe A, et al. Randomised controlled trial of Helicobacter pylori testing and endoscopy for dyspepsia in primary care. BMJ 2001;322:898.

260. Wong BC, Lam SK, Wong WM, et al., Group CGCS. Helicobacter pylori eradication to prevent gastric cancer in a high-risk region of China: a randomized controlled trial. JAMA 2004;291:187.

261. Moayyedi P, Talley NJ. Gastro-oesophageal reflux disease. Lancet 2006;367:2086.

262. Raghunath A, Hungin AP, Wooff D, Childs S. Systematic review: the effect of Helicobacter pylori and its eradication on gastro-oesophageal reflux disease in patients with duodenal ulcers or reflux oesophagitis. Aliment Pharmacol Ther 2004;20:733.

263. Spiegel BM, Vakil NB, Ofman JJ. Dyspepsia management in primary care: a decision analysis of competing strategies. Gastroenterology 2002;122:1270.

264. Mason JM, Delaney B, Moayyedi P, et al. Managing dyspepsia without alarm signs in primary care: new national guidance for England and Wales. Alim Pharmacol Ther 2005;21:1135.

265. Veldhuyzen van Zanten SJ, Cleary C, Talley NJ, et al. Drug treatment of functional dyspepsia: a systematic analysis of trial methodology with recommendations for design of future trials. Am J Gastroenterol 1996;91:660.

266. Holtmann G, Talley NJ. Functional dyspepsia. Current treatment recommendations. Drugs 1993;45:918.

267. Talley NJ, Riff DS, Schwartz H, Marcuard SP. Double-blind placebo-controlled multicentre studies of rebamipide, a gastroprotective drug, in the treatment of functional dyspepsia with or without Helicobacter pylori infection. Aliment Pharmacol Ther 2001;15:1603.

268. Enck P, Klosterhalfen S. The placebo response in functional bowel disorders: perspectives and putative mechanisms. Neurogastroenterol Motil 2005;17:325.

269. Morris C, Chapman R, Mayou R. The outcome of unexplained dyspepsia. A questionnaire follow-up study of patients after endoscopy. J Psychosom Res 1992;36:751.

270. Talley NJ, McNeil D, Hayden A, Colreavy C, Piper DW. Prognosis of chronic unexplained dyspepsia. A prospective study of potential predictor variables in patients with endoscopically diagnosed non-ulcer dyspepsia. Gastroenterology 1987;92:1060.

271. Talley NJ, Locke GR, Lahr BD, et al. Predictors of the placebo response in functional dyspepsia. Aliment Pharmacol Ther 2006;23:923.

272. Gotthard R, Bodemar G, Brodin U, Jonsson KA. Treatment with cimetidine, antacid, or placebo in patients with dyspepsia of unknown origin. Scand J Gastroenterol 1988;23:7.

273. Norrelund N, Helles A, Schmiegelow M. [Uncharacteristic dyspepsia in general practice. A controlled trial with an antacid (Alminox)]. Ugeskr Laeger 1980;142:1750.

274. Nyren O, Adami HO, Bates S, et al. Absence of therapeutic benefit from antacids or cimetidine in non-ulcer dyspepsia. N Engl J Med 1986;314:339.

275. Weberg R, Berstad A. Low-dose antacids and pirenzepine in the treatment of patients with non-ulcer dyspepsia and erosive prepyloric changes. A randomized, double-blind, placebo-controlled trial. Scand J Gastroenterol 1988;1988:237.

276. Talley NJ. Drug treatment of functional dyspepsia. Scand J Gastroenterol (Suppl.) 1991;182:47.

277. Holtmann G, Gschossmann J, Mayr P, Talley NJ. A randomised placebo-controlled trial of simethicone and cisapride for the treatment of patients with functional dyspepsia. Aliment Pharmacol Ther 2002;16:1641.

278. Moayyedi P, Soo S, Deeks J, et al. Systematic review: antacids H_2-receptor antagonists, prokinetics, bismuth and sucralfate therapy for non-ulcer dyspepsia. Aliment Pharmacol Ther 2003;17:1215.

279. Talley NJ, McNeil D, Hayden A, Piper DW. Randomized, double-blind, placebo-controlled crossover trial of cimetidine and pirenzepine in nonulcer dyspepsia. Gastroenterology 1986;91:149.

280. Dobrilla G, Comberlato M, Steele A, Vallaperta P. Drug treatment of functional dyspepsia. A meta-analysis of randomized controlled clinical trials. J Clin Gastroenterol 1989;11:169.

281. Finney JS, Kinnersley N, Hughes M, et al. Meta-analysis of antisecretory and gastrokinetic compounds in functional dyspepsia. J Clin Gastroenterol 1998;26:312.

282. Delaney B, Moayyedi P, Deeks J, et al. The management of dyspepsia: a systematic review. Health Technol Assess 2000;4:iii,1.

283. Jones BH, Baxter G. Lansoprazole 30 mg daily versus ranitidine 150 mg b.d. in the treatment of acid-related dyspepsia in general practice. Aliment Pharmacol Ther 1997;11:541.

284. Blum AL, Arnold R, Stolte M, et al. Short course acid suppressive treatment for patients with functional dyspepsia: results depend on *Helicobacter pylori* status. Gut 2000;47:473.

285. Peura DA, Kovacs TOG, Metz DC, et al. Lansoprazole in the treatment of functional dyspepsia: two double blind, randomized, placebo-controlled trials. Am J Med 2004;116:740.

286. Lauritsen K, Aalykke C, Havelund T, et al. Effect of omeprazole in functional dyspepsia: a double-blind, randomized, placebo-controlled study. Gastroenterology 1996;110:A108.

287. Talley NJ, Meineche-Schmidt V, Pare P, et al. Efficacy of omeprazole in functional dyspepsia: double-blind, randomized, placebo-controlled trials (the Bond and Opera studies). Aliment Pharmacol Ther 1998;12:1055.

288. Peura DA, Kovacs TOG, Metz DC, et al. Low-dose lansoprazole: effective for non-ulcer dyspepsia. Gastroenterology 2000;118:A439.

289. Wong WM, Wong BC, Hung WK, et al. Double blind, randomised, placebo controlled study of four weeks of lansoprazole for the treatment of functional dyspepsia in Chinese patients. Gut 2002;51:502.

290. Sheng H, Shah PK, Audus KL. Demonstration of sucralfate-mediated preservation of growth factor bioactivity in the presence of low pH with a human gastric epithelial cell line (AGS). Pharm Res 1996;13:1122.

291. Kairaluoma MI, Hentilae R, Alavaikko M, et al. Sucralfate versus placebo in treatment of non-ulcer dyspepsia. Am J Med 1987;83:51.

292. Misra SP, Dwivedi M, Misra V, Agarwal SK. Sucralfate versus ranitidine in non-ulcer dyspepsia: results of a prospective, randomized, open, controlled trial. Indian J Gastroenterol 1992;11:7.

293. Skoubo-Kristensen E, Funch-Jensen P, Kruse A, et al. Controlled clinical trial with sucralfate in the treatment of macroscopic gastritis. Scand J Gastroenterol 1989;24:716.

294. Hausken T, Stene-Larsen G, Lange O, et al. Misoprostol treatment exacerbates abdominal discomfort in patients with non-ulcer dyspepsia and erosive prepyloric changes. A double-blind, placebo-controlled, multicentre study. Scand J Gastroenterol 1990;25:1028.

295. Hiyama T, Yoshihara M, Matsuo K, et al. Meta-analysis of the effects of prokinetic agents in patients with functional dyspepsia. J Gastroenterol Hepatol 2007;22:304.

296. Zeng J, Zuo XL, Li YQ, et al. Tegaserod for dyspepsia and reflux symptoms in patients with chronic constipation: an exploratory open-label study. Eur J Clin Pharmacol 2007;63:529.

297. Pasricha PJ. Desperately seeking serotonin. A commentary on the withdrawal of tegaserod and the state of drug development for functional and motility disorders. Gastroenterology 2007;132:2287.

298. Peeters TL, Matthijs G, Depoortere I, et al. Erythromycin is a motilin receptor agonist. Am J Physiol 1989;257:G470.

299. Talley NJ, Verlinden M, Snape WJ, et al. Failure of a motilin receptor agonist (ABT-229) to relieve the symptoms of functional dyspepsia in patients with and without delayed gastric emptying: a randomized double-blind placebo-controlled trial. Aliment Pharmacol Ther 2000;14:1653.

300. Holtmann G, Talley NJ, Liebregts T, et al. A placebo-controlled trial of itopride in functional dyspepsia. N Engl J Med 2006;354:832.

301. Talley NJ, Tack J, Ptak T, et al. Efficacy and safety of itopride in functional dyspepsia: results of two phase III multicentre, randomized, double-blind, placebo-controlled trials. Gastroenterology 2007;132:641, A-93.

302. Tack J, Coulie B, Wilmer A, et al. Influence of sumatriptan on gastric fundus tone and on the perception of gastric distension in man. Gut 2000;46:468.

303. Tack J. Functional dyspepsia: impaired fundic accommodation. Curr Treat Options Gastroenterol 2000;3:287.

304. Tack J. Receptors of the enteric nervous system: potential targets for drug therapy. Gut 2000;47 Suppl. 4:iv 20.

305. Talley NJ. A critique of therapeutic trials in *Helicobacter pylori*-positive functional dyspepsia. Gastroenterology 1994;106:1174.

306. Elta GH, Scheiman JM, Barnett JL, et al. Long-term follow-up of *Helicobacter pylori* treatment in non-ulcer dyspepsia patients. Am J Gastroenterol 1995;90:1089.

307. Schutze K HE, Hirschl AM. Clarithromycin or amoxycillin plus high-dose ranitidine in the treatment of *Helicobacter pylori*-positive functional dyspepsia. Eur J Gastroenterol Hepatol 1996;8:41.

308. Veldhuyzen van Zanten S, Malatjialian D, Tanton R, et al. The effect of eradication of *Helicobacter pylori* (Hp) on symptoms in non-ulcer dyspepsia (NUD): a randomized double-blind placebo controlled trial. Gastroenterology 1996;108.

309. McCarthy C, Patchett S, Collins RM, et al. Long-term prospective study of *Helicobacter pylori* in nonulcer dyspepsia. Dig Dis Sci 1995;40:114.

310. Sheu BS, Lin CY, Lin XZ, et al. Long-term outcome of triple therapy in *Helicobacter pylori*-related nonulcer dyspepsia: a prospective controlled assessment. Am J Gastroenterol 1996;91:441.

311. Lazzaroni M, Bargiggia S, Sangaletti O, et al. Eradication of *Helicobacter pylori* and long-term outcome of functional dyspepsia. A clinical endoscopic study. Dig Dis Sci 1996;41:1589.

312. Cucchiara S, Salvia G, Az-Zeqeh N, et al. *Helicobacter pylori* gastritis and non-ulcer dyspepsia in childhood. Efficacy of one-week triple antimicrobial therapy in eradicating the organism. Ital J Gastroenterol 1996;28:430.

313. Greenberg PD, Cello JP. Lack of effect of treatment for *Helicobacter pylori* on symptoms of nonulcer dyspepsia. Arch Intern Med 1999;159:2283.

314. Gilvarry J, Buckley MJ, Beattie S, et al. Eradication of *Helicobacter pylori* affects symptoms in non-ulcer dyspepsia. Scand J Gastroenterol 1997;32:535.

315. Blum AL, Talley NJ, O'Morain C, et al. Lack of effect of treating *Helicobacter pylori* infection in patients with nonulcer dyspepsia. N Engl J Med 1998;339:1875.

316. McColl K, Murray L, El-Omar E, et al. Symptomatic benefit from eradicating *Helicobacter pylori* infection in patients with nonulcer dyspepsia. N Engl J Med 1998;339:1869.

317. Talley NJ, Janssens J, Lauritsen K, et al. Eradication of *Helicobacter pylori* in functional dyspepsia: randomised double blind placebo controlled trial with 12 months' follow up. The Optimal Regimen Cures *Helicobacter* Induced Dyspepsia (ORCHID) Study Group. BMJ 1999;318:833.

318. Talley NJ, Vakil N, Ballard ED, Fennerty MB. Absence of benefit of eradicating *Helicobacter pylori* in patients with nonulcer dyspepsia. N Engl J Med 1999;341:1106.

319. Moayyedi P, Soo S, Deeks J, et al. Systematic review and economic evaluation of *Helicobacter pylori* eradication treatment for non-ulcer dyspepsia. Dyspepsia Review Group. BMJ 2000;321:659.

320. Laine L, Schoenfeld P, Fennerty MB. Therapy for *Helicobacter pylori* in patients with nonulcer dyspepsia. A meta-analysis of randomized, controlled trials. Ann Intern Med 2001;134:361.

321. Moayyedi P, Deeks J, Talley NJ, et al. An update of the Cochrane systematic review of *Helicobacter pylori* eradication therapy in nonulcer dyspepsia: resolving the discrepancy between systematic reviews. Am J Gastroenterol 2003;98:2621.

322. Talley NJ. Review article: 5-hydroxytryptamine agonists and antagonists in the modulation of gastrointestinal motility and sensation: clinical implications. Aliment Pharmacol Ther 1992;6:273.

323. Sanger GJ. 5-Hydroxytryptamine and functional bowel disorders. Neurogastroenterol Motil 1996;8:319.

324. Morteau O, Julia V, Eeckhout C, Bueno L. Influence of 5-HT$_3$ receptor antagonists in visceromotor and nociceptive responses to rectal distension before and during experimental colitis in rats. Fundam Clin Pharmacol 1994;8:553.

325. Blackshaw LA, Grundy D. Effects of 5-hydroxytryptamine (5-HT) on the discharge of vagal mechanoreceptors and motility in the upper gastrointestinal tract of the ferret. J Auton Nerv Syst 1993;45:51.

326. Talley NJ, Van Zanten SV, Saez LR, et al. A dose-ranging, placebo-controlled, randomized trial of alosetron in patients with functional dyspepsia. Aliment Pharmacol Ther 2001;15:525.

327. Mathias JR, Clench MH, Roberts PH, Reeves-Darby VG. Effect of leuprolide acetate in patients with functional bowel disease. Long-term follow-up after double-blind, placebo-controlled study. Dig Dis Sci 1994;39:1163.

328. Mathias JR, Clench MH, Reeves-Darby VG, et al. Effect of leuprolide acetate in patients with moderate to severe functional bowel disease. Double-blind, placebo-controlled study. Dig Dis Sci 1994;39:1155.

329. Ducrotte P, Maillot C, Leroi AM, et al. Octreotide in refractory functional epigastric pain with nutritional impairment – an open study. Aliment Pharmacol Ther 1999;13:696.

330. Kuiken SD, Tytgat GN, Boeckxstaens GE. Review article: drugs interfering with visceral sensitivity for the treatment of functional gastrointestinal disorders-the clinical evidence. Aliment Pharmacol Ther 2005;21:633.

331. Holtmann G, Haag S, Adam B, et al. Effects of a fixed combination of peppermint oil and caraway oil on symptoms and quality of life in patients suffering from functional dyspepsia. Phytomedicine 2003;10 Suppl. 4:56.

332. Quigley EMM, Hasler WL, Parkman HP. AGA technical review on nausea and vomiting. Gastroenterology 2001;120:263.

333. Tanum L, Malt UF. A new pharmacologic treatment of functional gastrointestinal disorder. A double-blind placebo-controlled study with Mianserin. Scand J Gastroenterol 1996;31:318.

334. Cannon RO, 3rd, Quyyumi AA, Mincemoyer R, et al. Imipramine in patients with chest pain despite normal coronary angiograms. N Engl J Med 1994;330:1411.

335. Mertz H, Fass R, Kodner A, et al. Effect of amitriptyline on symptoms, sleep, and visceral perception in patients with functional dyspepsia. Am J Gastroenterol 1998;93:160.

336. Jackson JL, O'Malley PG, Tomkins G, et al. Treatment of functional gastrointestinal disorders with antidepressant medications: a meta-analysis. Am J Med 2000;108:65.

337. Clouse RE, Lustman PJ, Geisman RA, Alpers DH. Antidepressant therapy in 138 patients with irritable bowel syndrome: a five-year clinical experience. Aliment Pharmacol Ther 1994;8:409.

338. Holtmann G, Madisch A, Hotz J, et al. A double-blind, randomized, placebo-controlled trial on the effects of an herbal preparation in patients with functional dyspepsia. Gastroenterology 1999;116: A65.

339. Bensoussan A, Talley NJ, Hing M, et al. Treatment of irritable bowel syndrome with Chinese herbal medicine: a randomized controlled trial. JAMA 1998;280:1585.

340. Rosch W, Liebregts T, Gundermann KJ, et al. Phytotherapy for functional dyspepsia: a review of the clinical evidence for the herbal preparation STW 5. Phytomedicine 2006;13 Suppl. 5:114.

341. Madisch A, Holtmann G, Mayr G, et al. Treatment of functional dyspepsia with a herbal preparation. A double-blind, randomized, placebo-controlled, multicenter trial. Digestion 2004;69:45.

342. Madisch A, Holtmann G, Plein K, Hotz J. Treatment of irritable bowel syndrome with herbal preparations: results of a double-blind, randomized, placebo-controlled, multi-centre trial. Aliment Pharmacol Ther 2004;19:271.

343. Pilichiewicz AN, Horowitz M, Russo A, et al. The herbal medication, Iberogast, relaxes the proximal stomach, stimulates antral motility, but does not affect pyloric and duodenal motility, and slows gastric emptying of liquids in healthy men. Gastroenterology 2007;132:685, A-97.

344. Holtmann G, Adam B, Haag S, et al. Efficacy of artichoke leaf extract in the treatment of patients with functional dyspepsia: a six-week placebo-controlled, double-blind, multicentre trial. Aliment Pharmacol Ther 2003;18.1099.

345. Haug TT, Wilhelmsen I, Svebak S, et al. Psychotherapy in functional dyspepsia. J Psychosom Res 1994;38:735.

346. Hamilton J, Guthrie E, Creed F, et al. A randomized controlled trial of psychotherapy in patients with chronic functional dyspepsia. Gastroenterology 2000,119:661.

347. Calvert EL, Houghton LA, Cooper P, et al. Long-term improvement in functional dyspepsia using hypnotherapy. Gastroenterology 2002; 123.1778.

348. Soo S, Forman D, Delaney B, Moayyedi P. A systematic review of psychological therapies for nonulcer dyspepsia. Am J Gastroenterol 2004;99:1817.

349. Agreus L, Svardsudd K, Talley NJ, et al. Natural history of gastroesophageal reflux disease and functional abdominal disorders: a population-based study. Am J Gastroenterol 2001;96:2905.

350. Talley NJ, Vakil N, Practice Parameters Committee of the American College of Gastroenterology. Guidelines for the management of dyspepsia. Am J Gastroenterol 2005;100:2324.

351. Hsu PI, Lai KH, Lo GH, et al. Risk factors for ulcer development in patients with non-ulcer dyspepsia: a prospective two year follow up study of 209 patients. Gut 2002;51:15.

352. Tack J, Bisschops R, Samelli G. Pathophysiology and treatment of functional dyspepsia. Gastroenterology 2004;127;1239.

353. Karamanolis G, Caenepeel P, Arts J, Tack J. Association of the predominant symptom with clinical characteristics and pathophysiological mechanisms in functional dyspepsia Gastroenterology 2006; 130:296.

5

Approach to the patient with dysphagia, odynophagia, or noncardiac chest pain

Chandra Prakash Gyawali, Ray E. Clouse

Symptom definitions, 62
Approach to the patient with dysphagia, 63
The medical history and physical examination in the patient with dysphagia, 67
Approach to the patient with oropharyngeal dysphagia, 69
Approach to the patient with esophageal dysphagia, 71
Symptomatic treatment of dysphagia, 72
Approach to the patient with odynophagia, 73
Approach to the patient with noncardiac chest pain, 74

Symptom definitions

Dysphagia and odynophagia are common complaints that usually merit prompt investigation and management. Dysphagia, a term derived from Greek roots, literally means to eat badly or with difficulty. In common practice, dysphagia has become an umbrella term encompassing the sensations (short of pain) associated with abnormal bolus transit from mouth to stomach as well as other signs or symptoms accompanying abnormal transit. In a sense, dysphagia has syndromic overtones. Odynophagia, from the Greek "to eat with pain," refers more specifically to pain during any component of the swallowing process. The two terms are not synonymous, they may reflect different underlying disorders, and yet they have overlapping differential diagnoses.

Both dysphagia and odynophagia occur with or shortly after the initiation of a swallow. Pain and discomfort in the neck or retrosternal region that are present between swallows occur through different mechanisms and reflect an expanded differential diagnosis. The *globus sensation*, a sense that something is lodged continuously in the throat, must be differentiated from dysphagia or odynophagia before embarking on an unnecessary investigation [1]. The globus sensation typically is sensed midline at the laryngeal level, but can lateralize in as many as 20% of patients [2]. The sensation classically is

reported as a "lump in the throat," but feeling that a foreign body, sharp object, or food particle is lodged also is a compatible description [1]. Most notably, globus sensation does not interfere with swallowing; although one in five patients with globus sensation notes something abnormal during food swallows, the original symptom abates during the process [3]. Globus may accompany a variety of disorders that cause dysphagia, such as gastroesophageal reflux disease (GERD) and distal esophageal motility disorders. Furthermore, up to 45% of the general population may have intermittent symptoms resembling globus [4]. This symptom most often reflects a functional gastrointestinal disorder [5,6]. A summary of the features differentiating functional globus from oropharyngeal dysphagia is provided in Table 5.1. *Xerostomia*, which means dryness of the mouth, also can be confused with oropharyngeal dysphagia if the medical history is not obtained carefully.

Noncardiac chest pain (NCCP), or *unexplained chest pain*, is a heterogeneous disorder comprising midline chest discomfort with angina-like characteristics, without evident cardiac etiology after comprehensive evaluation [1,7]. The symptom is typically described as burning, gripping, pressing, boring, or stabbing pain in the front of the chest or epigastrium, sometimes radiating to the neck, back, or arms. Since the pain characteristics can resemble cardiac disease, NCCP is the source of much anxiety in patients and physicians alike, leading to repeated office appointments, emergency room visits, and investigative studies. NCCP is reported twice as often by young individuals as by patients over 45 years of age in whom cardiac disease is more prevalent; both genders are equally represented [8]. The first step in the evaluation

Principles of Clinical Gastroenterology. Edited by Tadataka Yamada, David H. Alpers, Anthony N. Kalloo, Neil Kaplowitz, Chung Owyang, and Don W. Powell. © 2008 Blackwell Publishing. ISBN 978-1-4051-69103

Table 5.1 Features distinguishing oropharyngeal dysphagia and functional globus

Characteristic	Oropharyngeal dysphagia	Functional globus
Gender distribution in subjects seeking health care	Not gender dependent	Female predominant
Explanation for symptom persistence	Nature of the underlying structural or neuromuscular diagnosis	Possibly the degree of associated psychological distress
Age at peak incidence	> 50 years	Middle age
Timing of symptom	Occurs immediately (within 1 s) of swallowing	Present between swallows
Effect of swallowing	Induces symptom	Symptom abates
Nasopharyngeal regurgitation	May be present	Always absent
Tracheobronchial aspiration	May be present	Always absent

is the exclusion of cardiac disease. Subsequently, elucidation of a definitive etiology for NCCP may lead to improved symptoms and reduced health-care utilization [9]. GERD is the likely diagnosis when evidence of reflux is present on functional testing or when symptoms respond to antireflux therapy [7]. Esophageal motor disorders, visceral hypersensitivity, and functional chest pain may also contribute to NCCP. Esophageal causes are responsible for NCCP in as many as two-thirds of the cases [10]; other upper gut disorders, pulmonary and mediastinal processes, musculoskeletal syndromes, and neuropsychiatric disorders are other etiologies.

Approach to the patient with dysphagia

Dysphagia is represented by two principal types: oropharyngeal dysphagia and esophageal dysphagia. The differentiation is more than semantic because this segregation reflects differences in pathophysiology, differential diagnosis, investigation and management. For the purposes of this chapter, initiation of swallowing will be considered as occurring at the pharyngeal phase, when velopharyngeal closure, laryngeal elevation and closure, opening of the upper esophageal sphincter, tongue loading and pulsion, and pharyngeal clearance result from highly coordinated central events. Abnormalities preceding the pharyngeal phase, such as bolus preparation and movement, can be detected by bedside evaluation and radiological imaging, if required.

Patients with *oropharyngeal dysphagia* typically complain of food lodging or sticking in the back of the throat or cervical esophageal region and have accurate localization of the site of the swallowing error when it is demonstrated radiologically [11]. The symptom may be perceived as low as the level of the suprasternal notch, but oropharyngeal dysphagia rarely is referred to more distal locations [12]. Hesitation with swallowing, frequent and repeated swallowing attempts, and throat clearing may accompany dysphagia. Not only does the patient sense or demonstrate abnormal pharyngoesophageal transit, but also tracheobronchial aspiration may occur

(with coughing or choking during or after swallows) reflecting discoordination of bolus transit and laryngeal closure. Related symptoms include rough or dysphonic voice after eating; hoarseness may reflect the underlying neuromuscular disorder. Poor neuromuscular coordination or high intrabolus pressure from mechanical obstruction can disrupt protection of the nasopharynx and result in nasopharyngeal regurgitation. Consequently, the spectrum of symptoms associated with oropharyngeal dysphagia can be dramatic and severe. These associated symptoms are often absent, and hence clinical characteristics of the dysphagia are helpful in establishing the cause. Such characteristics, besides location of the symptom, include onset of dysphagia within 1 s of swallowing, inability to swallow any liquids or solids once a food bolus is lodged, and expectoration rather than regurgitation of the bolus [13].

Esophageal dysphagia reflects disorders of the esophageal body and esophagogastric junction as well as anatomical areas abutting these regions, such as the gastric cardia and mediastinum. Obstructing lesions in the proximal esophageal body can produce symptoms that mimic oropharyngeal dysphagia; more distal processes produce esophageal dysphagia with distinctive characteristics. The most telling feature differentiating esophageal from oropharyngeal dysphagia is the sensing of abnormal bolus transit at a retrosternal site. Unfortunately, distal esophageal processes can refer symptoms proximally to the cervical esophageal region and suprasternal notch in nearly 30% of cases [12,14,15]. This fact alone is responsible for the majority of clinical difficulty in segregating types of dysphagia using historical features. In contrast to oropharyngeal dysphagia, esophageal dysphagia is not immediate, typically is not associated with tracheobronchial aspiration, and is more likely to allow further ingestion of liquids to alleviate the dysphagia sensation. Additionally, patients with esophageal dysphagia are more likely to try repeated or forceful swallowing to dislodge or advance food boluses. When bolus impactions occur, patients with esophageal dysphagia regurgitate foamy, bland secretions or ingested liquids that have been retained above the impacted food.

Mechanisms responsible for symptom production

Sensory information from the pharyngeal and proximal esophageal regions is carried by cranial nerves V, X, and XI. Both discomfort and pain can be elicited from the posterior pharynx and hypopharynx by noxious mucosal stimulation. Pressure on pharyngeal surfaces is readily perceived, and minor alterations in bolus pressure dynamics might be sufficient to trigger the reporting of dysphagia in some conditions. Proximal esophageal distention just distal to the upper esophageal sphincter results in upper sphincter hypertonicity, but symptoms have not been linked directly to this motor response [16]. The nasal and tracheobronchial symptoms associated with the oropharyngeal dysphagia syndrome are provoked by noxious stimulation of cranial nerve V innervating nasal passages and activation of the cough reflex, respectively. Little is known about the perception of oropharyngeal dysphagia in patients with normal swallowing dynamics.

Esophageal sensation occurs by way of the vagal and spinal afferent pathways, which also modulate motor activity, although noxious stimuli are carried almost exclusively through spinal afferents [17,18]. At the spinal level, afferents from each esophageal region are widely distributed and overlap with innervation from other organs, such as the heart [19]. This convergence of input contributes to the similarity in the presentations of esophageal and cardiac symptoms [20]. Fine perception of abnormal bolus movement normally is not present in the esophageal body, and retention of a nonobstructing solid bolus in the distal esophagus is poorly recognized [21]. As further evidence, capsule-shaped pH transmitters can be attached to the distal esophageal mucosa and produce few symptoms [22]. Consequently, factors beyond bolus retention are necessary for dysphagia in most cases. Distention of esophageal regions proximal to a lodged bolus may be one important factor. Increased intraesophageal pressure encountered in achalasia before the esophagus becomes markedly dilated may stimulate the sensation of dysphagia [23]. Motility alterations in the esophageal body in response to transient obstruction also may have a sensory counterpart, but it is difficult to attribute dysphagia to specific esophageal body motor patterns alone. Both mild to marked hypomotility and hypermotility are encountered during the routine manometric evaluation of patients who are not reporting dysphagia at the time of the investigation. An exception is the achalasia patient who has increased intraesophageal pressure while being studied [23,24].

In some instances, esophageal dysphagia is produced by mucosal damage. Mucosal inflammation may be partly responsible for the nonobstructive dysphagia seen with GERD [25]. Similarly, mucosal damage overlying strictures or tumors may augment pain sensation through the effects of inflammation on visceral sensitivity [26]. For rings or strictures with little or no associated mucosal injury, dysphagia occurs when food boluses completely and transiently obstruct. Symptoms are corroborated radiographically with brief impaction of radiopaque solid boluses in the narrowed region and are alleviated with dislodgment of the bolus. Dysphagia is not reproduced with liquids or solids that pass freely. Symptoms of dysphagia do not occur until the lumenal diameter is less than 13 mm, a size at which conventional food boluses (e.g., bread, meat) become at least transiently impacted [27]. Persistent obstruction from food bolus impactions produces additional uncomfortable symptoms arising from distention of the proximal esophagus.

Sensitivity to these mechanisms varies considerably from patient to patient. The variation in part may reflect hypersensitivity or hyposensitivity accompanying specific conditions or disease processes [17]. Aging, connective tissue diseases (particularly those overlapping with scleroderma), diabetes, and other conditions associated with esophageal hypomotility are associated with hyposensitivity to experimental stimuli such as acid instillation and balloon distention [17,28–30]. Although not established, such patients may be rather insensitive to transit abnormalities and may underreport dysphagia. Likewise, as the esophagus develops secondary hypomotility and dilates in response to chronic obstruction, there is a resultant decrease of symptoms. In contrast, hypersensitivity to acid and distention stimuli in the functional esophageal syndromes and spastic disorders may help to explain the occurrence of dysphagia in these groups of disorders [31,32]. Many of these patients report a sense of abnormal transit without convincing evidence of an obstructing lesion or mucosal injury [1].

Odynophagia only occasionally accompanies dysphagia and appears to occur through separate mechanisms. With the exception of pain accompanying acute esophageal obstruction, odynophagia requires afferent input not resulting from abnormal bolus transit alone. In the esophageal phase of swallowing, odynophagia may require direct invasion or irritation of intramural nerves, as occurs with malignancies or deep inflammatory processes. Sensory stimulation resulting from some forms of esophagitis also can be responsible for this symptom (e.g., caustic or infectious esophagitis).

Differential diagnoses

Approaching the patient with dysphagia or odynophagia begins with a consideration of the differential diagnoses. Diagnostic possibilities vary markedly between oropharyngeal and esophageal dysphagia, further emphasizing the importance of characterizing dysphagia by type.

Oropharyngeal dysphagia

Symptoms of abnormal transit in any part of the gut can result from disturbed motor function or structural lesions. Oropharyngeal dysphagia can be a manifestation of motor dysfunction or structural disease specific to the oropharynx or its neighboring structures in a ratio of 4 : 1 [33]. Motor dysfunction results from a variety of neurological, striated muscle, and systemic disorders (Table 5.2). Structural lesions are

Table 5.2 Causes of oropharyngeal dysphagia

Neuromuscular diseases
Central nervous system diseases
   Cerebrovascular accident
   Parkinson disease
   Brainstem tumor
   Amyotrophic lateral sclerosis
   Other motor neuron diseases
   Dementia
   Huntington chorea
   Tabes dorsalis
   Poliomyelitis
   Spinocerebellar degeneration
   Syringobulbia
   Progressive bulbar paralysis
   Other congenital or degenerative disorders
Cranial nerve diseases
   Diabetes mellitus
   Recurrent laryngeal nerve palsy (e.g., mediastinal tumor, postsurgical)
   Transection or injury
   Paraneoplastic syndromes
   Diphtheria
   Rabies
   Lead poisoning
   Other neurotoxins (including medications)
Striated muscle disease
   Inflammatory myopathies
   Polymyositis
   Dermatomyositis
   Scleroderma
   Mixed connective tissue disease
   Inclusion body myositis
   Muscular dystrophies
   Oculopharyngeal muscular dystrophy
   Myotonic dystrophy
   Hyperthyroidism
   Myxedema
   Stiff-man syndrome
   Other striated muscle disorders
Primary cricopharyngeal dysfunction (with or without Zenker
   diverticulum)
Other neuromuscular disorders
   Myasthenia gravis
   Amyloidosis
   Botulism

Structural lesions
Intrinsic pharyngoesophageal lesions
   Oropharyngeal carcinoma
   Proximal esophageal carcinoma
   Benign esophageal tumor
   Esophageal web
   High esophageal stricture
   Corrosive damage
   Inflammatory disease (e.g., mucositis, pharyngitis, tonsillar abscess)
   Postsurgical change
   Foreign body
   Postradiation changes
Extrinsic lesions
   Thyroid enlargement or tumor
   Vertebral osteophytes and other skeletal abnormalities
   Cervical lymphadenopathy
   Vascular anomalies

less commonly responsible for oropharyngeal dysphagia, and can be intrinsic or extrinsic to the pharyngoesophageal region. Many of the disorders listed in Table 5.2 have additional manifestations that assist in limiting the differential diagnosis.

Despite the range of diagnostic possibilities, most patients presenting with oropharyngeal dysphagia have suffered a cerebrovascular accident. Parkinson disease is responsible for much of the remainder [34]. Either clinical or videofluoroscopic evidence of swallowing dysfunction can be found in more than 50% of patients following acute stroke, and chest infection (implying tracheobronchial aspiration) occurs in nearly one-third [35–38]. Dysphagia typically improves over the 6 months following the event, but symptoms and signs of oropharyngeal dysfunction persist in 10% to 15% and gradually appear in a small percentage initially free of dysphagia [39]. Laryngopharyngeal sensory deficits accompanying motor dysfunction and thereby impairing the appropriate response to aspiration may contribute to the poor outcome of stroke victims with oropharyngeal dysphagia [40]. Some patients with documented swallowing dysfunction have none of the classic symptoms of oropharyngeal dysphagia, and pulmonary or nutritional complications dominate because of diminished sensation from nerve damage or a reduced level of consciousness.

Laryngopharyngeal cancer surgery is an important structural cause of difficult oropharyngeal dysphagia. Symptoms result from obstruction at the pharyngoesophageal junction or reduced tongue driving force, in the case of resection at the base of the tongue [41]. The importance of the tongue as a pressure generator in the process of swallowing is highlighted in these patients. The esophagus is anchored at the cricoid cartilage, and osteophytes at the fourth through seventh cervical vertebrae can sufficiently impede normal physiology to produce dysphagia [42]. This degree of advanced osteophyte formation is typical of diffuse idiopathic skeletal hyperostosis, or Forestier disease, a disorder that affects 12% of the population and can manifest clinically as dysphagia [43,44]. Careful documentation of the role of the skeletal abnormalities in altering swallowing dynamics and bolus transit using videofluoroscopy is necessary before attributing the symptom to these findings [43,45].

Esophageal dysphagia

In contrast to oropharyngeal dysphagia, wherein motility disorders top the differential diagnosis, esophageal dysphagia is most often caused by structural lesions. As with oropharyngeal dysphagia, the range of possibilities is broad (Table 5.3). Esophageal strictures associated with GERD are common, increase in frequency with age, and are not associated with significant heartburn histories in 25% of patients [46]. Nonobstructive dysphagia is reported to some degree in nearly one-third of patients undergoing preoperative evaluation for antireflux surgery [47]. Distal esophageal rings,

Table 5.3 Causes of esophageal dysphagia

Structural lesions
Intrinsic esophageal lesions
  Peptic stricture
  Reflux esophagitis without stricture
  Esophageal carcinoma and other malignancies
  Benign esophageal tumor
  Esophageal web
  Corrosive damage (e.g., from pills, lye, sclerosants)
  Eosinophilic esophagitis
  Postsurgical change (e.g., following fundoplication)
  Large diverticula
  Foreign body
  Radiation changes
  Amyloidosis and other infiltrative diseases
  Other strictures (congenital, corrugated esophagus)
Extrinsic lesions
  Vascular anomalies or compression (dysphagia lusoria, dysphagia
    aortica)
  Vertebral osteophytes and other skeletal abnormalities
  Mediastinal lymphadenopathy
  Mediastinal tumors
  Other mediastinal disorders
  Gastric volvulus
  Obstructing lesions of the gastric cardia

Neuromuscular diseases (motor disorders)
Hypermotility disorders
  Achalasia
  Achalasia variants (overlap disorders with diffuse esophageal spasm)
  Diffuse esophageal spasm
  Nonspecific spastic disorders
  Lower esophageal dysfunction accompanying epiphrenic diverticula
  Secondary hypermotility disorders (e.g., paraneoplastic syndromes,
    Chagas disease, vagal nerve injury)
Hypomotility disorders
  Idiopathic hypomotility
  Hypomotility associated with systemic disease (e.g., connective tissue
    disease, Raynaud phenomenon, diabetes mellitus, hypothyroidism)
Unclassified motor dysfunction
  Idiopathic food bolus impaction
  Other motor disorders

Esophageal dysmotility can be classified into two predominant categories, hypomotility and hypermotility [17,31] (Fig. 5.1). Hypomotility of either the smooth-muscle esophageal body – also called ineffective esophageal motility [53,54] – or lower esophageal sphincter represents a failure of the contractile mechanisms through neurogenic or myogenic processes. The outcome is feeble or absent esophageal peristalsis and loss of resting tone in the lower esophageal sphincter. Systemic disorders associated with hypomotility have been mentioned previously, but most hypomotility is idiopathic [55,56]. These processes predispose to gastroesophageal reflux disease, and impairment of bolus clearance is often conspicuous. Nevertheless, dysphagia typically is not attributed to hypomotility, even when severe, without careful exclusion of structural explanations that include reflux esophagitis.

In contrast, hypermotility results from deficient inhibitory nerve influence [57]. Nonpropulsive, discoordinated contractions disrupt bolus transit and incomplete lower esophageal sphincter relaxation produces functional obstruction and dysphagia. Consequently, achalasia, diffuse esophageal spasm, and related patterns of severe hypermotility belong in the differential diagnosis [17,31] (Fig. 5.1). A variety of nonspecific spastic disorders, including high-amplitude peristaltic contractions ("nutcracker esophagus"), other vigorous contraction wave abnormalities, and isolated hypermotility features of the lower esophageal sphincter (increased basal pressure or incomplete relaxation), have been found in patients with otherwise unexplained dysphagia [31,58,59]. Transit disruption is less common with these findings, and dysphagia may be related to hypersensitivity that often accompanies the disorders [31]. Spastic disorders typically have no underlying pathological explanation, and their presence does not preclude a functional diagnosis for the presenting complaints nor exclude the possibility that associated psychological factors are contributing to symptoms [1,31,60,61]. Nevertheless, because esophageal dysphagia can represent serious structural explanations, thorough investigation is required before assigning a functional diagnosis. Less classified motor abnormalities also have been reported, e.g., lower esophageal muscular rings [48,62].

Odynophagia
Pain during the oropharyngeal phase of swallowing has been attributed to a variety of processes, particularly malignancies, foreign body ingestion, and mucosal inflammation and ulceration. Oropharyngeal odynophagia may indicate deeper invasion of sensory nerves or extrinsic structures, and a careful evaluation for structural lesions should be undertaken. Odynophagia occurring later in the swallowing process most commonly is caused by specific types of mucosal damage: caustic injury and infection. It also accompanies tumors and other processes associated with deep mural injury, e.g., radiation damage, deep peptic ulceration, and idiopathic ulcer (in immunosuppressed patients)

particularly mucosal rings at the squamocolumnar junction (Schatzki ring), also are common; some indentation of the barium column is detected at this level during radiographic evaluation in as many as 14% of individuals [27,48]. Malignant esophageal neoplasms typically present with dysphagia. Diagnosis of esophageal adenocarcinoma is on a rapid incline, particularly in middle-aged Caucasian males. Other structural explanations listed in the Table are uncommon; vascular anomalies are rare [49–51]. The ability of proximal gastric disorders, e.g., gastric volvulus, to produce this presentation should be considered in the appropriate setting when the cause of esophageal dysphagia is unclear [52].

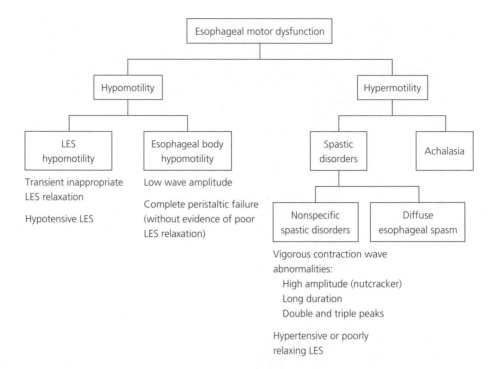

Figure 5.1 A method of categorizing dysmotility in the distal esophagus and lower esophageal sphincter based on the principal type of motor dysfunction. Hypermotility may result from inhibitory nerve deficiency or an imbalance between inhibitory and contractile influences. Some patients have a mixture of hypomotility and hypermotility features and cannot be classified solely into one branch of the scheme. LES, lower esophageal sphincter. From Clouse [31].

– processes more likely to produce chronic or persistent symptoms. Odynophagia rarely results from uncomplicated reflux disease. Chest pain is reported by up to half of patients with achalasia at some period in the course of the illness [63,64]. This pain typically is not directly related to swallowing, runs a course separate from dysphagia, is influenced in a limited fashion by treatment for achalasia, and usually is not confused with purer presentations of odynophagia [64].

The most common causes of acute esophageal odynophagia in immunocompetent subjects are infection with *Candida albicans* or herpes simplex virus and pill-induced injury [65,66]. Other infectious causes for esophagitis can have a similar presentation and include bacteria, fungi, cytomegalovirus, and varicella zoster virus [67]. In fact, the entire range of opportunistic esophageal infections encountered in immunosuppressed individuals may be responsible for this symptom. Whereas herpes simplex virus is the most common viral cause of esophagitis in immunocompetent subjects, cytomegalovirus is a more common offender in the immunosuppressed [68]. In this latter group, however, *Candida* remains the most common cause of infectious esophagitis [67]. Pill-induced caustic injury to the esophagus has been associated with more than 70 medications, including aspirin, potassium supplements, tetracycline, ferrous sulfate, quinidine, alendronate, and nonsteroidal antiinflammatory drugs [66,69,70]. Tissue injury to the esophagus from caustic medications can be deep, and odynophagia reaching severe intensity over 3 to 4 days is a common component of the presentation.

The medical history and physical examination of the patient with dysphagia

Dysphagia is a common clinical problem. Nearly one in five subjects older than 50 years of age describes the symptom in epidemiological surveys [71,72]. Dysphagia is the second most common indication for endoscopy in the United States [73], and a mechanism responsible for the symptom can be found in most cases, even when initially labeled psychogenic [74,75]. Consequently, a systematic approach to the differential diagnosis that results in a well-planned investigation is important. A variety of algorithms have been recommended, but each depends on a carefully obtained medical history at the initial step [76–79]. The physical examination is more likely to provide useful information in patients with oropharyngeal dysphagia.

Establishing the type of dysphagia, either oropharyngeal or esophageal, is of primary importance. Differentiating historical features have been outlined in the opening paragraphs of this chapter. Patients with oropharyngeal dysphagia may have symptoms of oral dysfunction that further support the diagnosis, e.g., poor handling of the food bolus with drooling and spillage, piecemeal swallowing, and dysarthria. When the type of dysphagia remains unclear, discerning the outcome from ingestion of specific foods or liquids can be helpful. Asking for a description of recent meals and resulting symptoms may keep the patient focused on the specific events of swallowing. Additionally, offering the patient a small quantity of water to swallow during the interview may clarify the medical history through firsthand observation.

Certain features in the medical history can help to narrow the differential diagnosis of oropharyngeal dysphagia. Proximal dysphagia for solid foods alone is suggestive of restrictive processes such as strictures, webs, or tumors. Odynophagia in association with oropharyngeal dysphagia also has implications (see p. 69). Sudden onset of symptoms suggests an acute neurological insult; a short but progressive course typifies malignancy; whereas an insidious presentation reflects inflammatory processes, such as myopathies. Delayed expectoration is suggestive of a retaining pharyngeal diverticulum.

Historical evidence and physical findings corroborating a neurological, muscular, or systemic disease should be sought when oropharyngeal dysphagia is suspected, taking into consideration the large differential diagnosis outlined in Table 5.2. Inquiries should be made into past history of cerebrovascular accidents or neurological disability that preceded or accompanied the dysphagia, and a comprehensive neurological examination is essential. The medication history should be reviewed for agents that can either cause or exacerbate dysphagic symptoms, including those with adverse neuromuscular effects (e.g., sedatives, narcotics, muscle relaxants) or that cause xerostomia (e.g., anticholinergics, antihistamines, antidepressants) [80]. Further examination of the neck for masses, thyromegaly, or lymphadenopathy should

be performed. The presence and extent of tracheobronchial aspiration (including history of aspiration pneumonia) should be extracted from the history to determine the severity of the dysphagia syndrome. Likewise, limitations of food intake and their impact on weight should be assessed using the available information. Determining the need and urgency for nonoral feeding is a primary component of the oropharyngeal dysphagia evaluation [81].

If esophageal dysphagia is suspected, the medical history can help to narrow the differential diagnosis and direct the investigative approach [82]. Features or established diagnoses of systemic disorders associated with esophageal dysphagia (Table 5.3), particularly connective tissue diseases and Raynaud phenomenon, should be sought [83,84]. Historical aspects favoring structural diagnoses lead to early endoscopy, biopsy, and dilation. Features favoring a motility disorder may emphasize the importance of barium radiography and manometry, either early in the evaluation or for completion of the work-up. Although presentations of the disorders listed in Table 5.2 are variable from patient to patient, certain features of common diagnoses can be helpful in establishing the initial impression [82] (Fig. 5.2). Structural esophageal lesions typically result in dysphagia following solid food ingestion but not following liquids alone. Bulky foods of larger caliber, such as meats and bread, more

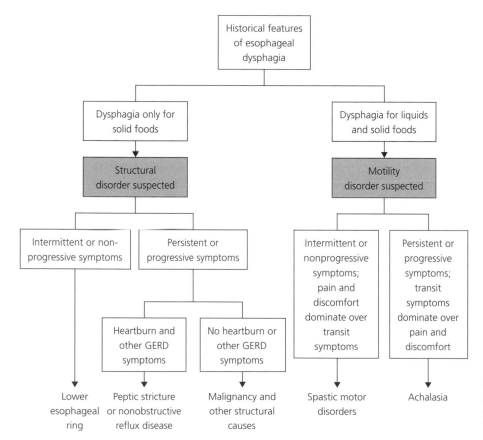

Figure 5.2 Features of the medical history that help focus the differential diagnosis of common causes of esophageal dysphagia. GERD, gastroesophageal reflux disease.

reliably reproduce the symptom. In contrast, precipitants of dysphagia caused by esophageal motility disorders are more variable.

At least 95% of patients with achalasia complain of dysphagia, but the course is frequently nonprogressive [63]. This leaves a large number of patients undiagnosed, an undesirable outcome considering the treatment options available for this disorder. Heartburn also can be reported by achalasia patients so that some are followed for years with a presumptive diagnosis of GERD before the correct diagnosis is established [85,86]. Conventional investigative tests such as endoscopy or barium radiography were not helpful prospectively in as many as one-third of patients with achalasia eventually presenting for manometry, wherein the diagnosis was secured [86]. A careful medical history can enhance the suspicion of achalasia. Dysphagia typically is for liquids as well as solid foods, although one-third of patients may report dysphagia for solid foods alone. Regurgitation of esophageal contents is reported by 60%–90% of subjects, a feature that can be differentiated from gastroesophageal regurgitation by the bland, nonacidic characteristics of the regurgitated material and the ability of the patient to reswallow the bolus without aversion. Maneuvers performed by the patient during meals to increase intraesophageal pressure and enhance esophageal emptying can frequently be elicited (e.g., straightening of the back, raising of the arms above the head, and forceful swallowing) [17,63]. Ability to retain and regurgitate large quantities of ingested food or foamy saliva from a dilated esophagus also characterizes achalasia.

Approach to the patient with oropharyngeal dysphagia

The evaluation of oropharyngeal dysphagia has three important components:
• determination of the structural and physiological abnormalities responsible for symptoms
• discovery of underlying disorders (including neurological and muscular disorders) responsible for these findings
• evaluatation of the safety and practicality of oral feeding [81,87]. The second of these is largely determined from the history and physical findings, as described previously, in conjunction with appropriate laboratory investigations. The other two are most commonly and effectively accomplished by following a protocol for videofluoroscopic swallowing evaluation – referred to as a modified barium swallow [11,77,88]. The examination is structured to detect and analyze functional impairment of the swallowing mechanism and provides evidence for each of the four categories of oropharyngeal swallowing dysfunction:
• inability to initiate or excessive delay in initiation of pharyngeal swallowing
• aspiration of the ingestate

• nasopharyngeal regurgitation
• residue of ingestate within the pharyngeal cavity after swallowing [77].
The modified barium swallow is widely available, well characterizes swallowing dysfunction, and can examine the short-term effects of swallowing interventions (compensatory or corrective swallowing strategies, diet modifications), so it is considered the most applicable initial test in patients with a compatible presentation [75].

Videofluoroscopy also can detect structural abnormalities that are potentially responsible for symptoms, but is less satisfactory than endoscopic evaluation. Transnasal fiberoptic pharyngoscopy/laryngoscopy (nasoendoscopy) is the optimal method for direct inspection of mucosal surfaces in the region, and when combined with a swallowing assessment protocol it provides at least indirect evidence of all categories of swallowing dysfunction except possibly nasopharyngeal regurgitation [89–92]. Nasoendoscopy or indirect laryngoscopy typically is performed early in the evaluation of oropharyngeal dysphagia and is especially important if symptoms suggest a mucosal lesion. Nasoendoscopy also can be used to assess sensory function by applying pulses of air to the mucosa innervated by the superior laryngeal nerve and evoking glottic adduction [92–94]. Thus, in centers where nasoendoscopy combined with a swallowing assessment can be performed, the approach may provide much of the same information as videofluoroscopy and have unique advantages of portability, repeatability without radiation exposure, and technical success in patients with reduced sensorium [91,95,96]. This approach is less effective than videofluoroscopy in determining the cause of swallowing dysfunction, and nasoendoscopy does not obviate the need for videofluoroscopy in all subjects – providing merit to each test in clinical practice. In contrast, manometry has contributed little to the routine evaluation of the patient with oropharyngeal dysphagia despite its capacity to quantify contraction strength [97,98]. It is complementary to videofluoroscopy when the two are performed concurrently, and this approach, or possibly even manometry alone, can be helpful in differentiating obstruction at the level of the upper esophageal sphincter from weak pharyngeal propulsive forces [99,100].

In the systematic assessment of patients with oropharyngeal dysphagia, a specific diagnosis of the underlying cause will be detected in many instances, and the mechanism responsible for the symptom will be detected in nearly all [75]. Important therapeutic recommendations can arise from the evaluation, even when a specific diagnosis is not established. The algorithm shown in Fig. 5.3 demonstrates how these outcomes are accomplished. If local lesions are detected by direct mucosal visualization, further study of swallowing mechanisms may not be required. The videofluoroscopic examination may uncover rings, webs, strictures, posterior pharyngeal diverticula, or tumors that are amenable to specific surgical or endoscopic interventions. However, oropharyngeal

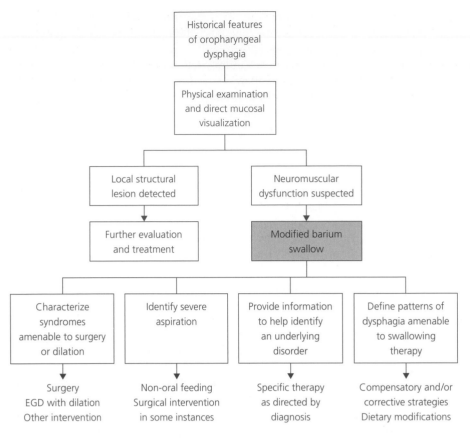

Figure 5.3 Approach to the patient with oropharyngeal dysphagia. The modified barium swallow (videofluoroscopic swallowing evaluation) is a key element in the evaluation of most patients, providing useful information for both diagnosis and management. Nasoendoscopy accompanied by a swallowing protocol is an alternative method to reach similar endpoints. EGD, esophagogastroduodenoscopy. Adapted from the method of Cook & Kahrilas [77].

dysphagia should not be attributed to some common radiological findings without careful consideration of alternative explanations. Such findings include cricopharyngeal bars, prominent vertebral osteophytes, and lateral pharyngeal diverticula. The first of these is found in more than 15% of dysphagic patients evaluated, correlates poorly with the symptomatic state, and would preclude the detection of the true explanation for dysphagia in the vast majority of cases if alternative explanations were not pursued [101,102]. Some authorities believe that dysphagia should not be attributed to a cricopharyngeal bar unless no other explanation is available and coexistent pharyngeal dysfunction is present to accentuate the importance of the bar [74]. The swallowing evaluation also may reveal disorders responsive to cricopharyngeal myotomy or other, less invasive approaches that reduce upper sphincter pressure [103]. The success of myotomy is greatest in situations where the cricopharyngeus opening is limited but pharyngeal function is preserved [104]. Examples include Zenker diverticulum, primary cricopharyngeus dysfunction, and postcricoid stenosis. Success in neurogenic dysphagia can reach 60%, but predictors of response are not readily available [77]. Reviews of this treatment in relation to specific underlying disorders should be consulted [77,105,106].

Detection of aspiration during videofluoroscopy is a predictor of pneumonia risk and future hospitalization, although false negatives also are common with this test in patients with stroke and other forms of neurogenic dysphagia [37,107,108]. Aspiration during nasoendoscopic swallowing assessment has similar predictive value, as does bedside evaluation examining oxygen desaturation with water swallowing [95,109]. As a minimum, compensatory swallowing strategies are required, and oral feeding may be prohibited. If aspiration is demonstrated with all food consistencies despite compensatory maneuvers, nonoral feeding typically is instituted; this approach may not prevent subsequent aspiration pneumonia, however [110–112]. Videofluoroscopic study or nasoendoscopy with swallowing evaluation is also used to direct specific compensatory or corrective swallowing strategies that may reduce the risk of aspiration [95]. Swallowing therapy techniques that have been used are listed in Table 5.4, and, of these, the strongest evidence favors the efficacy of diet modifications in reducing the risk of subsequent aspiration pneumonia [77,113]. Although many of the maneuvers listed in Table 5.4 affect the occurrence of aspiration during a brief swallowing evaluation, such as the modified barium swallow, their actual ability to reduce subsequent morbidity is less established. Nevertheless, the potential benefits at low cost drive recommendation for their use [77,81,114]. After all, the first-year mortality caused by aspiration pneumonia in patients with stroke approaches 20%, and subsequent annual mortality from this complication remains at 10%–15% [34].

Table 5.4 The spectrum of swallowing therapy techniques

Category of technique	Specific example
Swallowing maneuver	Supraglottic swallow
	Supersupraglottic swallow
	Effortful swallow
	Mendelsohn maneuver
Postural adjustment	Head tilt
	Chin tuck
	Head rotation
	Head rotation with extrinsic pressure on thyroid cartilage
	Lying on side, elevation
Facilitatory techniques	Strengthening exercises
	Biofeedback
	Thermal stimulation
	Gustatory stimulation
Dietary modification	Thickening of liquids
	Thinning of liquids

Data from Logemann [11], Logemann [249], Miller & Langmore [250]; table adapted from Cook & Kahrilas [77].

Other interventions for oropharyngeal dysphagia depend on the specific diagnosis that is derived from this initial evaluation, and the reader should refer to discussions of the disorders at other locations in this text. Certain combinations of videofluoroscopic findings can help in determining the correct underlying disorder [34]. Some systemic or neuro-logical disorders that produce oropharyngeal dysphagia can be treated and result in reduction in swallowing symptoms, although this response is not uniform. For example, a reduction of dysphagia in Parkinson disease is inconsistent with levodopa administration, despite improvement in other neurological features of the illness [115,116].

Approach to the patient with esophageal dysphagia

Endoscopy has become the primary tool for investigating esophageal dysphagia, not only for its accuracy but also for its therapeutic potential [117]. In the past, barium radiography was recommended as the initial test in all patients with dysphagia but its popularity is waning. The safety of endoscopy, its high diagnostic yield, and its provision for mucosal biopsy and dilation of commonly encountered structural lesions, favor its use over radiographic screening when esophageal dysphagia is suspected. Likewise, barium radiography is not sufficiently sensitive to the range of tissue damage resulting from GERD, a common cause of esophageal complaints [118]. Barium radiography with fluoroscopy retains a role in the evaluation of esophageal dysphagia (Fig. 5.4); strictures that can be overlooked at endoscopy, particularly those with a lumenal diameter of more than 10 mm, are detectable [119–121]. Barium studies are more sensitive than endoscopy to distal rings and to achalasia and can fully establish the level of dysphagia if symptoms are reproduced

(a) (b) (c) (d) (e) (f)

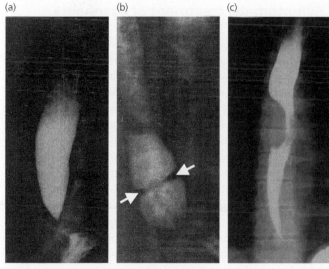
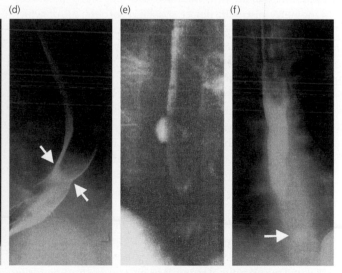

Figure 5.4 Findings on barium radiography can help establish the diagnosis in patients with esophageal dysphagia and unrevealing endoscopy. **(a)** Absent peristalsis and barium retention above a closed lower sphincter suggest achalasia in this patient with minimal esophageal dilation. **(b)** A lower esophageal (Schatzki) ring (arrows) causing intermittent dysphagia was not appreciated at endoscopy. **(c)** Endoscopy was completely normal in this patient with mediastinal adenopathy producing extrinsic compression of the mid-esophagus. **(d)** A stricture with lumenal diameter of 12 mm (arrows) was not appreciated on initial endoscopic evaluation. **(e)** This epiphrenic diverticulum was overlooked at endoscopy yet, once discovered, prompted manometric evaluation and discovery of a severe distal spastic disorder. **(f)** Endoscopy was unrevealing in a patient with a medical history confusing for oropharyngeal vs esophageal dysphagia, but a barium pill (12.5-mm diameter) lodged at the esophagogastric junction (arrow), reproduced symptoms, and led to reevaluation and dilation.

during the study [119,122]. The sensitivity of barium radiography for motor disorders and structural lesions is further enhanced if barium-impregnated solids are employed [123,124]. Although a barium swallow may be required to ultimately establish a diagnosis, its benefits do not overshadow the utility of endoscopy in the typical case, and The American Gastroenterological Association in a practice guideline has recommended endoscopy as the initial investigative test in esophageal dysphagia [117]. Suspicion of achalasia from the outset is an exception [117]. Compatible radiographic findings can be confirmed by manometry, and endoscopy can be reserved until the treatment plan for newly established achalasia is designed.

Once structural explanations for esophageal dysphagia are excluded, the evaluation should proceed with esophageal manometry [125]. Manometry is sensitive to conventional hypermotility and hypomotility disorders but will not establish a conclusive diagnosis or have treatment implications in all patients with otherwise unexplained esophageal dysphagia – even when food bolus impactions have occurred. Nevertheless, manometry is indicated, if only to detect the reasonable proportion of patients with achalasia who would have been overlooked by other investigative tests [86,125]. Manometry occasionally fails to establish the diagnosis of achalasia because of seemingly normal lower esophageal sphincter relaxation, arguably the most important diagnostic criterion; this artifactual error can be reduced if a sleeve sensor is employed, if an averaged value is recorded for lower esophageal sphincter relaxation nadir pressure, or if high-resolution manometric methods are employed [126–128]. Manometry also will detect spastic disorders, all of which may be associated with dysphagia [31]. Although demonstration of a direct relationship between symptoms and these motor disorders is often less convincing, the findings may help direct therapeutic trials [31].

Dysphagia to some degree is the most common complication of antireflux surgery; its occurrence is only predicted with any reliability by preoperative dysphagia [129]. The technical skill of the surgeon is more important than the degree of existent hypomotility in producing this adverse outcome [130]. Early symptoms, even when severe (< 5% of patients), may dissipate within 8 to 12 weeks of the operation with resolution of local inflammatory response [131,132]. Periodic dilation with a 16-mm to 20-mm diameter bougie or balloon may suffice [132]. Persistent dysphagia, occurring to at least mild degree in up to 24% of patients [133], most often is related to suboptimal surgical technique. In cases requiring reoperation, transdiaphragmatic migration of the fundoplication, slipped or misplaced fundoplication, twisted fundoplication, or residual paraesophageal hernia can explain this symptom [134]. Physiological failure of the procedure with persistent reflux is reported following a small percentage of operations, and reflux-related explanations for dysphagia must be excluded.

Multivariate analysis of manometric features in postoperative dysphagia suggests that both the degree of obstruction and the degree of peristaltic competency participate in symptom production, both delaying transit across the lower sphincter [135,136]. The last may be of particular importance [136]. In practice, endoscopy and barium videofluoroscopy are the principal evaluation tools, the emphasis being on detection of an abnormal postoperative appearance and on evaluating the degree of retention [137]. Manometry has a limited role unless used in conjunction with videofluoroscopy or with high-resolution techniques, procedures that remain primarily investigational [23,136]. Dilation for persistent dysphagia is effective in half of subjects when the fundoplication is intact; evidence of slipped fundoplication is predictive of a poor response and reoperation can be avoided with pneumatic dilation in some patients [133,138].

Patients with suspected esophageal dysphagia who remain undiagnosed following endoscopy, barium radiography, and esophageal manometry probably benefit little from additional testing. Ambulatory pH monitoring to define nonobstructive dysphagia from endoscopy-negative reflux disease may have a role that could be obviated with a therapeutic trial of antireflux treatment. When additional evaluation is desired, further efforts at reproducing dysphagia during videofluoroscopy using barium-impregnated liquids or solids could be considered. Reproducing dysphagia in the absence of a transit abnormality helps to establish a functional diagnosis and provides alternative therapeutic approaches.

Symptomatic treatment of dysphagia

Thorough investigation of dysphagia reveals a diagnosis in a majority of cases, and therapy is directed at the specific diagnosis. In some instances, empirical interventions are employed for both diagnosis and treatment. A specific explanation for oropharyngeal dysphagia cannot be found in a reasonable minority of patients with this syndrome, even when abnormalities in swallowing physiology are defined by the modified barium swallow. Compensatory or corrective swallowing strategies and dietary manipulations are the principal empirical interventions (outlined above), aimed at reduced aspiration risk and avoiding nonoral feeding. Empirical use of botulinum toxin or cricopharyngeal myotomy is ill-advised without convincing evidence of restrictive obstruction at the upper sphincter level because of the potential for added morbidity [104,139,140]. Botulinum toxin injection can reduce all indicators of swallowing dysfunction in appropriately selected patients, but the durability of the response is still being evaluated [141]. Balloon catheter or Savary dilation of the cricopharyngeus has been reported for patients with primary cricopharyngeus dysfunction, and the approach has low morbidity [142,143]. There is no evidence that this less invasive approach is effective for oropharyngeal dysphagia unless similar selection criteria are used as for the other techniques. Other empirical therapies are not offered routinely in the management of oropharyngeal dysphagia.

For esophageal dysphagia, empirical strategies include dilation, antireflux therapy, and treatments aimed at sensorimotor dysfunction. The value and safety of dilation with a large caliber (at least 14-mm diameter) bougie or balloon when no abnormality is detected at endoscopy or by videofluoroscopy could be debated, as dilation is not without risk [117,144]. Dysphagia was significantly reduced in a small group of patients with no obstructive lesions who were randomized to dilation with a 16.7-mm Maloney dilator vs those dilated with a small-caliber (8.7-mm) bougie [145]. The benefits were sustained in 80% of initial responders. Empirical use of an 18-mm dilator in an uncontrolled study of patients with esophageal dysphagia for solid foods yet negative endoscopic and radiological evaluations produced immediate response in 95% of subjects and sustained response for nearly 2 years in 68% of the initial responders [146]. By comparison, resolution of dysphagia only occurred in 12% of patients with dysphagia for both solid foods and liquids when managed in the same fashion. Although the risk of perforation or significant bleeding approximates 1% when standard dilation is performed for a variety of benign indications [144], the complication rate is undoubtedly lower when empirical dilation is performed. These findings suggest that dilation with a large caliber dilator is reasonable as a therapeutic trial in patients with significant symptoms from unexplained esophageal dysphagia, especially if the clinical presentation resembles that of a stricture or ring [147].

Antireflux therapy, specifically antisecretory therapy, is offered to many patients with investigation-negative esophageal dysphagia, but a reasonable estimate of its efficacy is unknown. Esophageal prokinetics, such as the serotonin (5-HT$_4$) agonist cisapride, increase midesophageal contraction pressures and could conceivably benefit patients with unexplained esophageal dysphagia [148], but serviceable reports to support this possibility are unavailable. Glucagon inhibits lower esophageal sphincter contraction and has been used acutely in patients with idiopathic food bolus impactions. The limited benefits of this approach may be related to the negative effects of glucagon on esophageal body motility [149]. Smooth-muscle relaxants, such as nitrates, calcium-channel blockers, and peppermint oil, effectively decrease lower esophageal sphincter pressure or reduce distal esophageal contraction amplitudes and improve transit symptoms in achalasia [150–153]. These agents have been tried in patients with spastic disorders with limited benefit. Most trials have studied effects on pain rather than dysphagia, and benefits may be better for transit symptoms. Antidepressants, particularly the tricyclic antidepressants, reduce many unexplained esophageal symptoms, including those associated with spastic esophageal disorders [1,31]. These agents may alter esophageal sensation or the central processing of visceral afferent input [1,154,155]. Although most measured outcomes from antidepressant use have focused on pain, the general cluster of esophageal symptoms, including dysphagia, appears to be responsive when the symptoms represent a functional esophageal disorder [156,157]. Antidepressants typically are reserved for patients without significant transit delay, with no other explanation for dysphagia on thorough investigation, and in whom enhanced tolerance to the symptom would be a suitable outcome.

Approach to the patient with odynophagia

Odynophagia is an uncommon medical problem compared with dysphagia, but its presence usually indicates a significant underlying and definable disorder. The symptom can range from a dull discomfort to a pain of intense severity that interferes with any swallowing attempt.

The medical history and physical examination in the patient with odynophagia

Odynophagia is an important complaint that should be carefully investigated. The most important characteristic is the temporal relationship of pain with swallowing: early pain suggests the oropharyngeal phase, and later pain implicates the esophageal phase. The characteristics used in differentiating types of dysphagia are also helpful in limiting the differential diagnosis. When odynophagia is described accompanying the oropharyngeal phase, malignancy, foreign body, infection, or other causes of inflammation become more likely. Exposure histories that predispose the patient to mucosal irritation, such as prior radiation therapy or corrosive ingestion, should be elicited. A history of tobacco and alcohol use, which are risk factors for head and neck malignancy, should be recorded, and the physical examination should proceed with these diagnostic possibilities in mind. Nasoendoscopy or indirect laryngoscopy is essential when odynophagia is present during the swallowing phase.

When odynophagia originates in esophageal locations, the medical history should focus on factors predisposing the patient to opportunistic infection, including systemic illnesses, immunosuppressive treatment, and antibiotic use. As many as 30%–40% of patients with acquired immunodeficiency syndrome (AIDS) develop symptoms of esophageal disease at some point in the course of their illness [158]. The possibility of foreign body ingestion and use of caustic medications should be carefully explored. Ingestion of pills at bedtime, while reclining, or with little water intake should be determined. The use of caustic medications may not readily be recalled, for example, in young patients using doxycycline for acne management.

Investigation of odynophagia

Whether oropharyngeal or esophageal in location, odynophagia typically requires careful examination of the mucosal surface with direct visualization and biopsy if necessary. This is accomplished with nasoendoscopy, indirect laryngoscopy, or esophagoscopy depending on the nature of the odynophagia. The investigation is altered if a foreign body is the suspected cause of oropharyngeal odynophagia [159–161]. Plain films of the neck with soft tissue technique, including lateral views, are indicated, but many foreign bodies are radiolucent. Sharp or pointed objects lodged at or above the cricopharyngeus should be removed with use of the laryngoscope or by someone experienced in direct laryngoscopy [159,160]. Blunt objects retained in this region, such as coins, mandate protection of the airway during their removal. In some instances, the foreign body may have dislodged, causing residual odynophagia from laceration. Nevertheless, inspection is required and oral contrast studies (that can interfere with direct mucosal inspection) are not indicated in managing oropharyngeal or esophageal foreign bodies [159].

The approach to esophageal odynophagia depends on a combination of the acuity of the presentation, the suspected diagnosis, and the setting (immunocompetent or immunocompromised host). Chronic processes frequently suggest invasion of or extension of mucosa-based processes into deep esophageal layers. Both radiological imaging (chest radiographs, computed tomography, barium radiographs) and endoscopy may be needed to establish the diagnosis and extent of esophageal or mediastinal involvement. In immunocompetent patients with this presentation, initial testing is driven by the suspected diagnosis, and algorithms defining the most expedient or cost-effective approach are not available.

In patients with no history of foreign body ingestion, acute esophageal odynophagia in immunocompetent subjects is most often caused by infectious etiology or pill-induced esophageal damage. Diagnosis can be made by endoscopy or barium radiography [162,163]; endoscopy is more sensitive for the detection of mucosal damage. Management approaches to patients with AIDS with esophageal complaints have been a focus of several studies because of the high incidence of esophageal diseases. *Candida* infection is common, and empirical treatment of patients with AIDS who have oral thrush is recommended [67,164]. Further investigation, including biopsy, may be needed if the patient has a poor response to empirical treatment. In this setting barium radiography is usually not helpful. A randomized trial comparing barium radiography to endoscopy in symptomatic patients with AIDS confirmed the higher sensitivity and utility of the latter technique [165]. In general, cultures taken at the time of endoscopy are less useful than histological study of biopsy specimens because of their inability to differentiate colonization from the pathogen responsible for infection, their

lower sensitivity, and the delay in obtaining results. Treatment for odynophagia in this setting is directed by the specific diagnosis.

Approach to the patient with noncardiac chest pain

Data extracted from cardiac evaluations for chest pain indicate that NCCP is a common disorder, accounting for 2%–5% of all emergency room visits [166], and over one-third of patients admitted for the evaluation of chest pain [167–169]. Population-based studies report an incidence of 25% in the general population (range 14%–33%), accounting for over 69 million diagnoses of NCCP in the United States alone, and annual health-care utilization of over $2 billion [170–174].

Mechanisms and differential diagnosis of noncardiac chest pain

Chemical, mechanical, or thermal irritation of the esophagus, and combinations of sensory and motor abnormalities consequent to central and peripheral neural dysfunction have been invoked as potential mechanisms. The most frequent association is gastroesophageal reflux, which is demonstrated in as many as half of all patients with presumed esophageal etiologies of NCCP [175–177]. Infusing hydrochloric acid can induce chest pain, but for pain to be truly acid related, it must develop promptly when acid is infused and resolve rapidly when acid infusion is discontinued [178,179]. In contrast, many episodes of acid reflux are painless even in NCCP patients with significant chest pain–reflux associations, and correlations between period of exposure to esophageal acid and the severity and frequency of NCCP are poor [180]. Therefore, other factors are thought to contribute to the pathogenesis.

Upon distention of the esophagus with balloon inflation, patients with NCCP perceive sensation, develop discomfort, and experience typical chest pain at much lower inflation pressures compared to controls [181–183]. Patients with other functional disorders (such as irritable bowel syndrome or fibromyalgia) have similar lowered pain thresholds to esophageal balloon distention [179]. Infusion of acid into the esophagus lowers the pain threshold to a greater extent in NCCP patients compared to controls, triggering a state of hypervigilance for esophageal sensation [184,185] that may be reversed with aggressive antireflux therapy [186]. Consequently, subjects with NCCP can be reliably segregated from controls by measuring perception thresholds for pain [182]. This enhanced sensitivity to intralumenal stimuli may be a primary abnormality, but how patients reach this state of heightened awareness is not clear. In susceptible individuals, intermittent stimulation by acid reflux or spontaneous distention events associated with swallowing or belching may be potential triggers. Additionally, alterations in central nervous system processing of afferent signals have been demonstrated; furthermore, increased afferent pathway sensitivity as well as abnormal secondary cortical processing of the afferent signals from the esophagus may also contribute to this disorder [187]. Central processing errors of afferent stimuli are further suggested by heart rate variability and altered vagal reflex responses to esophageal acid instillation in acid-sensitive individuals [188,189].

Esophageal motility testing may identify spastic features in as many as one-third of patients with NCCP, including nutcracker esophagus, nonspecific spastic disorders, diffuse esophageal spasm, hypertensive lower esophageal sphincter, and, rarely, achalasia [190–192]. The role of these disorders in symptom production is not well established, but powerful, prolonged contractions have been reported in NCCP patients, similar to the high-amplitude contractions induced by edrophonium injection. On ambulatory monitoring, however, these abnormal contraction patterns are only rarely associated with pain symptoms, and improvement in chest pain can occur independent of changes in the motor pattern. Sustained increase in esophageal muscle thickness has been identified on high-frequency esophageal intralumenal ultrasound as a correlate of both spontaneous chest pain episodes in patients with NCCP and edrophonium-induced chest pain in normal individuals [193], and the clinical significance of this finding continues to be studied. Additionally, acid reflux episodes have been identified as triggers for chest pain even in spastic disorders such as nutcracker esophagus. Antireflux therapy results in a symptomatic response in a proportion of these patients [176,194].

Psychological factors (somatization) and affective psychiatric disorders (anxiety, depression) appear to be overrepresented in NCCP compared to the general population; panic disorder was diagnosed in up to one-fourth of chest pain sufferers in one study [60,195–197]. Heightened states of awareness of visceral sensation similar to that seen with NCCP have been observed in patients with affective disorders (anxiety, depression), somatization disorders, and panic disorder [179]. Although psychiatric disorders have no direct correlation with physiological findings, they may mediate symptom severity, influence well-being, and impact overall quality of life in patients with NCCP, and specific attention to these disorders can contribute to symptom improvement [60]. Morbidity and utilization of health-care dollars remain high, even though psychiatric disorders as alternative explanations for NCCP are difficult to establish in these patients [198,199].

Cardiac disease is the most important condition to distinguish from other esophageal causes of chest pain because of the potential for significant complications or death if missed. Even with a negative coronary angiogram, microvascular angina manifest as chest pain and a positive stress test (also known as syndrome X) could still exist [200]. Diseases of the upper gut (including peptic ulcer disease), liver, and

biliary tract can potentially present with pain localized to or radiating to the anterior chest wall, as can musculoskeletal pain originating from the chest wall (Table 5.5). Other serious cardiac, pulmonary, and mediastinal conditions to be

Table 5.5 The differential diagnosis of noncardiac chest pain

Esophageal causes
Esophagitis
Esophageal motor disorders
Functional chest pain
Visceral hypersensitivity
Esophageal rupture

Other gastrointestinal causes
Biliary disease
Hepatitis
Pancreatitis
Peptic ulcer disease
Colitis
Irritable bowel syndrome
Functional dyspepsia
Splenic flexure syndrome
Splenomegaly

Cardiac causes
Microvascular angina
Mitral valve prolapse
Myocarditis
Pericarditis
Pulmonary hypertension

Pulmonary causes
Pneumonia
Pleurisy
Pulmonary embolism
Pneumothorax
Lung cancer
Sarcoidosis

Mediastinal causes
Aortic dissection
Mediastinitis
Superior vena cava syndrome
Mediastinal mass lesions

Musculoskeletal causes
Costochondritis
Fibromyalgia
Xiphodynia
Slipping rib syndrome
Herpes zoster
Breast disorders
Sickle cell crisis

Psychiatric causes
Anxiety and depression
Panic disorder
Somatization disorder
Munchausen syndrome

considered include aortic dissection, pulmonary embolism, pericarditis, myocarditis, pneumothorax, and esophageal rupture [201,202].

The medical history and physical examination of the patient with noncardiac chest pain

Esophageal chest pain may be described as pain or discomfort felt retrosternally, in the epigastrium, or even in the front of the neck. Descriptors used by patients can include burning, gripping, pressing, boring or stabbing pain, with radiation to the throat, back or upper arms, features that have considerable overlap in symptom description and location with cardiac pain [179,203]. A history and physical examination does not necessarily help distinguish cardiac from noncardiac sources of chest pain. Presence of any cardiac risk factor therefore warrants consultation with a cardiologist and cardiac investigation before entertaining a noncardiac source as the sole explanation for chest pain. Factors that predict an adverse cardiac event in NCCP patients include male sex, older age, hypercholesterolemia, diabetes mellitus, history of coronary artery disease, and congestive heart failure [204]. However, even patients diagnosed with a noncardiac source on emergency room presentation will have a 3%–4% incidence rate of a cardiac event within the following month [204,205]. Identification of an esophageal cause for chest pain does not exclude a concurrent cardiac source, but if investigation has ruled out cardiac disease, the likelihood of cardiac fatality over 7 years of follow-up has been shown to be negligible [206].

Symptom patterns that suggest an esophageal origin of chest pain include association with meals, prompt relief with antacids, and a history of heartburn or dysphagia. Coexisting esophageal symptoms are reported by almost 90% when GERD is the cause of chest pain, with symptoms at least once a week in over 50% of these patients [172,198,207]. The presence of typical esophageal symptoms, however, does not have a high predictive value in excluding a cardiac source of pain [208] because 50% of patients with coronary artery disease may complain of coexisting esophageal symptoms [209].

The physical examination in patients with esophageal NCCP is typically unremarkable, and therefore serves to exclude other confounding diagnoses. Typical chest pain may be reproduced by chest wall palpation in patients with musculoskeletal chest pain, particularly costochondritis [210,211]. Musculoskeletal etiologies for chest pain may account for 11%–28% of unexplained chest pain [212], but other etiologies could still coexist [213].

Investigation of noncardiac chest pain

The search for evidence of GERD is an important process in the investigation because GERD may be responsible for at least half of NCCP, and GERD symptoms are one of the few predictors of chest pain in community surveys [170,198]. Moreover, 40% of patients with a normal coronary angiogram may have acid-related chest pain [1]. A diagnosis of GERD allows appropriate symptomatic management to be initiated; it prevents unnecessary additional testing for alternative pain explanations and may reduce the functional disability and impaired global well-being seen in patients with undiagnosed chest pain over long periods of time [9,170,214]. If evidence for GERD is inconclusive or absent, further investigations can evaluate for esophageal motor disorders, psychiatric comorbidities, and nonesophageal sources of chest pain.

Therapeutic trial strategies

A brief therapeutic trial with a high-dose antisecretory regimen is a rapid technique for determining clinically relevant reflux–symptom associations and is recommended for its simplicity and cost-effectiveness [175]. The omeprazole test (40 mg in the morning, 20 mg in the afternoon) for 7 days was initially reported to have a sensitivity of 78.3% and a specificity of 85.7% in diagnosing GERD in patients with NCCP [175]. Metaanalysis of studies using the omeprazole test has yielded a sensitivity of 80%, a specificity of 74%, and a summary diagnostic odds ratio of 19.35 [215]. Diagnostic strategies that begin with the omeprazole test have been reported to reduce the use of invasive diagnostic investigation by 43%, resulting in reduced costs and a greater proportion of patients remaining symptom free over 1 year of follow-up (84% vs 73%–74% when invasive tests were initially used) [216]. Despite the enthusiasm for antisecretory therapeutic trials and the acknowledged clinical value of this approach, more than 20% of true reflux-related chest pain may persist despite short-term proton pump inhibitor therapy and therefore render the test falsely negative [217]. In these instances, invasive investigation helps to establish or refute the reflux–chest pain relationship, and evaluates alternative etiologies.

Invasive investigation

Upper endoscopy is frequently performed in patients who have continuing NCCP despite a trial of antisecretory medication. In the absence of alarm symptoms (weight loss, dysphagia, family history of cancer, iron deficiency anemia), the diagnostic utility of endoscopy is low, and endoscopic evidence of esophagitis is found in only 10%–20% of treatment-naïve NCCP patients [192,218,219]; less than 5% have Barrett esophagus or a stricture [218]. Nevertheless, upper endoscopy may have important reassurance value in patients with moderate or high anxiety, and may reduce preoccupation with health and fear of illness or death [220]. A barium esophagogram, on the other hand, has a low utility in the evaluation of NCCP, particularly because of its low sensitivity for detecting evidence of GERD.

Diagnostic tests that establish reflux-related pain are important early tests in the invasive investigation of NCCP. Ambulatory pH monitoring is frequently needed to evaluate for a reflux–chest pain association [22,221]. This is particularly useful when empiric antisecretory medication trials fail [222,223], and may be more useful than endoscopy when alarm features are absent [219]. Since chest pain events may be infrequent and missed during a 24-h pH monitoring study, extended recording with wireless pH monitoring may allow more symptoms to be reported to test for a symptom–reflux association [22,224]. Simple nonstatistical symptom association tests such as the symptom index (a ratio of symptoms associated with reflux events to all symptoms reported during the pH study expressed as a percentage, a value greater than 50% indicating an association) may predict a response to antireflux measures [225]. Statistical assessment of the likelihood of a reflux–pain relationship is provided by the symptom association probability even when the number of symptoms or the proportion of reflux-related symptoms is small, allowing a more robust confidence in the symptom association [226–229]. A probability of cooccurrence by chance of less than 5% (or $P < 0.05$) indicates significant reflux–symptom relationships. Preliminary data suggest that the symptom association probability better predicts successful symptomatic outcome after antireflux therapy, particularly antireflux surgery [229].

Esophageal motility testing is most often performed as part of catheter-based ambulatory pH testing, but can also be considered in patients without GERD evidence after empiric therapeutic trials, upper endoscopy, and ambulatory pH testing. It is useful mainly in excluding achalasia and other advanced spastic processes, including diffuse esophageal spasm, and is not recommended as an initial test for chest pain in the absence of dysphagia or regurgitation [125]. Subtle spastic features may be more readily identified by high-definition manometry as compared to conventional manometry [23]. Advanced techniques, including the acid perfusion test, balloon distention test, impedance planimetry, high-frequency ultrasound, and functional magnetic resonance imaging scans, have been used in the research setting.

As many as 30%–70% of patients with NCCP have evidence of anxiety, panic disorder or other affective disorders, and psychological evaluation may identify individuals who may benefit from formal psychological approaches, including psychiatric medications and cognitive behavioral therapy [230–233]. Psychological evaluation is an option when relief from therapeutic trials for GERD and esophageal motor disorders is inadequate.

Evaluation for nonesophageal causes of NCCP can include radiological imaging to evaluate the hepatobiliary system, lungs, mediastinum, and musculoskeletal system. In certain circumstances, magnetic resonance cholangiopancreatography or even endoscopic retrograde cholangiopancreatography with sphincter of Oddi manometry may be required to exclude a biliary source for upper gut pain.

Long-term approach and outcomes

Ongoing NCCP is associated with impaired functional status and increased health-care utilization. Spontaneous resolution of NCCP is rare, and therefore the long-term management of NCCP hinges on successions of therapeutic trials, starting with treatments geared towards local noxious stimuli, i.e. reflux [213]. When chest pain is suppressed by a therapeutic trial of antisecretory medications, or when GERD is identified on invasive testing, continuation of antireflux measures are of benefit in symptom suppression. Once GERD has been excluded, therapeutic options are limited. Smooth muscle relaxants (anticholinergic agents, nitrates, hydralazine, calcium channel blockers) can be tried when spastic esophageal motor disorders are detected, but controlled trials have failed to demonstrate consistent efficacy in suppressing symptoms [234–237]. Injection of botulinum toxin into the lower esophageal sphincter may be an option for advanced spastic disorders including achalasia and diffuse esophageal spasm, when incomplete or absent lower esophageal sphincter relaxation is found [238,239]. When injected into the esophageal body, there is only limited evidence for efficacy of botulinum toxin in suppressing chest pain in nonachalasia, non-reflux-related spastic motor disorders [240], and this treatment cannot be routinely recommended.

Management options that influence central pain perception or amplification are frequently introduced when success from approaches targeting local irritating influences has proved unsuccessful in suppressing NCCP. Outcomes from antidepressant medication trials are the most encouraging. Benefits do not appear to be dictated by particular physiological or psychological factors, and are probably related to the modulation of central pain perception. Tricyclic antidepressants at low dosages (starting dosage 10 mg to 25 mg, maintenance dosage 50 mg to 125 mg) have documented efficacy in improving symptoms in over three-fourths of patients in the short term, and almost half may maintain their remission over longer-term follow-up [156,157,231,241,242]. Selective serotonin reuptake inhibitors may also be of benefit, and statistically significant improvements in global symptom rating over placebo have been reported in randomized, double blind, placebo-controlled trials using paroxetine and sertaline [243,244]. Theophylline, a nonspecific adenosine receptor antagonist has been demonstrated to reduce frequency, severity, and duration of chest pain episodes [245].

Nonpharmacological interventions including relaxation techniques, cognitive behavioral therapy, and hypnosis are options in refractory NCCP [246–248]. The limited data available suggest sustained benefits, potentially related to improvement in coexistent affective disorders including anxiety and depression.

References

1. Clouse RE, Richter JE, Heading RC, et al. Functional esophageal disorders. In: Drossman DA, Corazziari E, Talley NJ, et al. (eds).

Rome II. The functional gastrointestinal disorders. diagnosis, patho-physiology, and treatment: a multinational consensus, 2nd edn. McClean, VA: Degnon Associates, 2000:569.

2. Batch AJG. Globus pharyngeus (pts I & II). J Laryngol Otol 1988;102:152,227.

3. Wilson JA, Pryde A, Piris J, et al. Pharyngoesophageal dysmotility in globus sensation. Archiv Otolaryngol Head Neck Surg 1989;115:1086.

4. Thompson WG, Heaton KW. Heartburn and globus in apparently healthy people. CMAJ 1982;126:46.

5. Wilson JA, Deary IJ, Maran AG. The persistence of symptoms in patients with globus pharyngis. Clin Otolaryngol Allied Sci 1991;16:202.

6. Rowley H, O'Dwyer TP, Jones AS, Timon CI. The natural history of globus pharyngeus. Laryngoscope 1995;105:1118.

7. Galmiche JP, Clouse RE, Balint A, et al. Functional esophageal disorders. Gastroenterology 2006;130:1459.

8. Drossman DA, Li Z, Andruzzi E, et al. U.S. householders survey of functional gastrointestinal disorders. Prevalence, sociodemography and health impact. Dig Dis Sci 1993;38:1569.

9. Ward BW, Wu C, Richter JE, et al. Long-term follow-up of symptomatic status of patients with noncardiac chest pain. Is diagnosis of esophageal origin helpful? Am J Gastroenterol 1987;82:2156.

10. Vader JP, Larequi-Lauber T, Froehlich F, et al. Appropriateness of gastroscopy: atypical chest pain. Endoscopy 1999;31:611.

11. Logemann JA. Evaluation and treatment of swallowing disorders. San Diego, CA: College Hill, 1983.

12. Wilcox CM, Alexander LN, Clark WS. Localization of an obstructing esophageal lesion. Is the patient accurate? Dig Dis Sci 1995;40:2192.

13. Edwards DA. Discriminative information in the diagnosis of dysphagia. JR Coll Physicians London 1975;9:257.

14. Edwards D. History and symptoms of disease of the esophagus. In: Vantrappen G, Hellemans J (eds). Diseases of the esophagus. New York: Springer Verlag, 1974:103.

15. Smith DF, Ott DJ, Gelfand DW, Chen MY. Lower esophageal mucosal ring: correlation of referred symptoms with radiographic findings using a marshmallow bolus. AJR 1998;171:1361.

16. Cook IJ, Shaker R, Doods WJ, et al. Role of mechanical and chemical stimulation of the esophagus in globus sensation. Gastroenterology 1989;96:A99.

17. Clouse RE, Diamant NE. Esophageal motor and sensory function and motor disorders of the esophagus. In: Feldman M, Scharschmidt BF, Sleisenger MF (eds). Sleisenger and Fordtran's Gastrointestinal disease. Pathophysiology, diagnosis, management, 7th edn. Philadelphia, PA: WB Saunders, 2002:561.

18. Castell JA, Castell DO, Duranceau CA, Topart P. Manometric characteristics of the pharynx, upper esophageal sphincter, esophagus, and lower esophageal sphincter in patients with oculopharyngeal muscular dystrophy. Dysphagia 1995;10:22.

19. Cervero F, Connell LA, Lawson SN. Somatic and visceral primary afferents in the lower thoracic dorsal root ganglia of the cat. J Compar Neurol 1984;228:422.

20. Cervero F, Tattersall JE. Cutaneous receptive fields of somatic and viscerosomatic neurones in the thoracic spinal cord of the cat. J Compar Neurol 1985;237:325.

21. Hey H, Jorgensen F, Sorensen K, et al. Oesophageal transit of six commonly used tablets and capsules. Br Med J (Clin Res Ed) 1982;285(6356):1717.

22. Prakash C, Clouse RE. Value of extended recording time with wireless esophageal pH monitoring in evaluating gastroesophageal reflux disease. Clin Gastroenterol Hepatol 2005;3:329.

23. Clouse RE, Prakash C. Topographic esophageal manometry: an emerging clinical and investigative approach. Dig Dis 2000;18:64.

24. Alrakawi A, Clouse RE. Diagnosing achalasia using a topographic manometric analysis system. Gastroenterology 1997;112:A57.

25. Triadifilopoulos G. Nonobstructive dysphagia in reflux esophagitis. Am J Gastroenterol 1989;84:614.

26. Collins SM. The immunomudulation of enteric neuromuscular function: implications for motility and inflammatory disorders. Gastroenterology 1996;111:1683.

27. Schatzki R. The lower esophageal ring. Am J Radiol 1963;90:805.

28. Fass R, Pulliam G, Johnson C, et al. Symptom severity and oesophageal chemosensitivity to acid in older and young patients with gastro-oesophageal reflux. Age Ageing 2000;29:125.

29. Johnson DA, Winters C, Spurling TJ, et al. Esophageal acid sensitivity in Barrett's esophagus. J Clin Gastroenterol 1987;9:23.

30. Trimble KC, Pryde A, Heading RC. Lowered esophageal sensory thresholds in patients with symptomatic but not excess gastroesophageal reflux: evidence for a spectrum of visceral sensitivity in GORD. Gut 1995;37:7.

31. Clouse RE. Spastic disorders of the esophagus. Gastroenterologist 1997;5:112.

32. Rao SS, Hayek B, Summers RW. Functional chest pain of esophageal origin: hyperalgesia or motor dysfunction. Am J Gastroenterol 2001;96:2584.

33. Staff DM, Shaker R. Oropharyngeal dysphagia and associated disorders. In: Brandt LJ (ed.). Clinical practice of gastroenterology, Vol. 1. Philadelphia, PA: Current Medicine, Inc., 1999:66.

34. Saeian K, Shaker R. Oropharyngeal dysphagia. Clin Perspect Gastroenterol 2000;3:69.

35. Meng NH, Wang TG, Lien IN. Dysphagia in patients with brainstem stroke: incidence and outcome. Am J Phys Med Rehabil 2000; 79:170.

36. Mann G, Hankey GJ, Cameron D. Swallowing disorders following acute stroke: prevalence and diagnostic accuracy. Cerebrovasc Dis 2000;10:380.

37. Perry L, Love CP. Screening for dysphagia and aspiration in acute stroke: a systematic review. Dysphagia 2001;16:7.

38. Sellars C, Campbell AM, Stott DJ, et al. Swallowing abnormalities after acute stroke: a case–control study. Dysphagia 1999;14:212.

39. Smithard DG, O'Neill PA, England RE, Park CL, Wyatt R, Martin DF et al. The natural history of dysphagia following a stroke. Dysphagia 1997;12:188.

40. Aviv JE, Martin JH, Sacco RL, et al. Supraglottic and pharyngeal sensory abnormalities in stroke patients with dysphagia. Ann Otol Rhinol Laryngol 1996;105:92.

41. Walther EK. Dysphagia after pharyngolaryngeal cancer surgery. Part I: Pathophysiology of postsurgical deglutition. Dysphagia 1995; 10:275.

42. Eviatar E, Harell M. Diffuse idiopathic skeletal hyperostosis with dysphagia. J Laryngol Otol 1987;101:627.

43. Akhtar S, O'Flynn PE, Kelly A, Valentine PM. The management of dysphasia in skeletal hyperostosis. J Laryngol Otol 2000;114:154.

44. Ebo D, Goethals L, Bracke P, et al. Dysphagia in a patient with giant osteophytes: case presentation and review of the literature. Clin Rheumatol 2000;19:70.

45. Ladenheim SE, Marlowe FI. Dysphagia secondary to cervical osteophytes. Am J Otolaryngol 1999;20:184.

46. Patterson DJ, Graham DY, Smith JL, et al. Natural history of benign esophageal stricture treated by dilatation. Gastroenterology 1983;85: 346.

47. Patti MG, Feo CV, De Pinto M, et al. Results of laparoscopic antireflux surgery for dysphagia and gastroesophageal reflux disease. Am J Surg 1998;176:564.

48. Bennett JR, Castell DO. Overview and symptom assessment. In: Castell DO, Richter JE (eds). The esophagus. Philadelphia, PA: Lippincott Williams & Wilkins, 1999:33.

49. Storr M, Allescher HD. Esophageal pharmacology and treatment of primary motility disorders. Dis Esophagus 1999;12:241.

50. Janssen M, Baggen MG, Veen HF, et al. Dysphagia lusoria: clinical aspects, manometric findings, diagnosis, and therapy. Am J Gastroenterol 2000;95:1411.

51. Cappell MS. Endoscopic, radiographic, and manometric findings associated with cardiovascular dysphagia. Dig Dis Sci 1995;40:166.

52. Cozart JC, Clouse RE. Gastric volvulus as a cause of intermittent dysphagia. Dig Dis Sci 1998;43:1057.

53. Fouad YM, Katz PO, Hatlebakk JG, Castell DO. Ineffective esophageal motility: the most common motility abnormality in patients

with GERD-associated respiratory symptoms. Am J Gastroenterol 1999;94:1464.

54. Leite LP, Johnston BT, Barrett J, et al. Ineffective esophageal motility (IEM): the primary finding in patients with nonspecific esophageal motility disorder. Dig Dis Sci 1997;42:1859.

55. Schneider HA, Yonker RA, Longley S, et al. Scleroderma esophagus: a nonspecific entity. Ann Intern Med 1984;100:848.

56. Galmiche JP, Janssens J. The pathophysiology of gastro-oesophageal reflux disease: an overview. Scand J Gastroenterol Suppl 1995;211:7.

57. Sifrim D, Janssens J, Vantrappen G. Failing deglutitive inhibition in primary esophageal motility disorders. Gastroenterology 1994;106: 875.

58. Clouse RE, Staiano A. Contraction abnormalities of the esophageal body in patients referred to manometry. A new approach to manometric classification. Dig Dis Sci 1983;28:784.

59. Alrakawi A, Clouse RE. The changing use of esophageal monometry in clinical practice. Am J Gastroenterol 1998;93:2359.

60. Song CW, Lee SJ, Jeen YT, et al. Inconsistent association of esophageal symptoms, psychometric abnormalities and dysmotility. Am J Gastroenterol 2001;96:2312.

61. Shapiro J, Franko DL, Gagne A. Phagophobia: a form of psychogenic dysphagia. A new entity. Ann Otol Rhinol Laryngol 1997;106:286.

62. Hirano I, Gilliam J, Goyal RK. Clinical and manometric features of the lower esophageal muscular ring. Am J Gastroenterol 2000; 95:43.

63. Wong RKH, Johnson LF. Achalasia. In: Castell DO, Johnson LF (eds). Esophageal function in health and disease. New York: Elsevier, 1983:99.

64. Eckardt VF, Stauf B, Bernhard G. Chest pain in achalasia: patient characteristics and clinical course. Gastroenterology 1999;116:1300.

65. Kikendall JW, Friedman AC, Oyewole MA, et al. Pill-induced esophageal injury. Case reports and review of the medical literature. Dig Dis Sci 1983;28:174.

66. Jaspersen D. Drug-induced oesophageal disorders: pathogenesis, incidence, prevention and management. Drug Saf 2000;22:237.

67. Baehr PH, McDonald GB. Esophageal infections: risk factors, presentation, diagnosis, and treatment. Gastroenterology 1994;106:509.

68. Wilcox CM, Diehl DL, Cello JP, et al. Cytomegalovirus esophagitis in patients with AIDS: a clinical, endoscopic, and pathologic correlation. Ann Intern Med 1990;113:589.

69. de Groen PC, Lubbe DF, Hirsch LJ, et al. Esophagitis associated with the use of alendronate. N Engl J Med 1996;335:1016.

70. McCord GS, Clouse RE. Pill-induced esophageal structures: clinical features and risk factors for development. Am J Med 1990;88:512.

71. Bloem BR, Lagaay AM, van Beek W, et al. Prevalence of subjective dysphagia in community residents aged over 87. BMJ 1990; 300(6726):721.

72. Lindgren S, Janzon L. Prevalence of swallowing complaints and clinical findings among 50–79-year-old men and women in an urban population. Dysphagia 1991;6:187.

73. Lieberman DA, De Garmo PL, Fleischer DE, et al. Patterns of endoscopy use in the United States. Gastroenterology 2000;118:619.

74. Ravich WJ, Wilson RS, Jones B, Donner MW. Psychogenic dysphagia and globus: reevaluation of 23 patients. Dysphagia 1989;4:35.

75. Martin-Harris B, Logemann JA, McMahon S, et al. Clinical utility of the modified barium swallow. Dysphagia 2000;15:136.

76. Cook IJ. Investigative techniques in the assessment of oral-pharyngeal dysphagia. Dig Dis 1998;16:125.

77. Cook IJ, Kahrilas PJ. AGA technical review on management of oropharyngeal dysphagia. Gastroenterology 1999;116:455.

78. Rothstein RD. A systematic approach to the patient with dysphagia. Hosp Pract (Off Ed) 1997;32:169.

79. Richter JE. Practical approach to the diagnosis and treatment of esophageal dysphagia. Compr Ther 1998;24:446.

80. Stochus B, Allescher HD. Drug induced dysphagia. Dysphagia 1993;8:154.

81. Logemann JA. Screening, diagnosis, and management of neurogenic dysphagia. Semin Neurol 1996;16:319.

82. Castell DO, Donner MW. Evaluation of dysphagia: a careful history is crucial. Dysphagia 1987;2:65.

83. Lapadula G, Muolo P, Semeraro F, et al. Esophageal motility disorders in the rheumatic diseases: a review of 150 patients. Clin Exp Rheumatol 1994;12:515.

84. Limburg AJ, Beekhuis H, Smit AJ, et al. Esophageal hypomotility in primary and secondary Raynaud's phenomenon: comparison of esophageal scintigraphy with manometry. J Nucl Med 1995;36:451.

85. Spechler SJ, Souza RF, Rosenberg SJ, et al. Heartburn in patients with achalasia. Gut 1995;37:305.

86. Howard PJ, Maher L, Pryde A, et al. Five year prospective study of the incidence, clinical features, and diagnosis of achalasia in Edinburgh. Gut 1992;33:1011.

87. Kahrilas PJ. Current investigation of swallowing disorders. Baill Clin Gastroenterol 1994;8:651.

88. Dodds WJ, Logemann JA, Stewart ET. Radiologic assessment of abnormal oral and pharyngeal phases of swallowing. AJR 1990;154:965.

89. Langmore SE, Schatz K, Olson N. Endoscopic and videofluoroscopic evaluations of swallowing and aspiration. Ann Otol Rhinol Laryngol 1991;100:678.

90. Murray J, Langmore SE, Ginsberg S, Dotsie A. The significance of oropharyngeal secretions and swallowing frequency in predicting aspiration. Dysphagia 1996;11:99.

91. Staff DM, Shaker R. Videoendoscopic evaluation of supraesophageal dysphagia. Curr Gastroenterol Rep 2001;3:200.

92. Aviv JE, Kim T, Sacco RL, et al. FEESST: a new bedside endoscopic test of the motor and sensory components of swallowing. Ann Otol Rhinol Laryngol 1998;107:378.

93. Aviv JE, Martin JH, Keen MS, et al. Air pulse quantification of supraglottic and pharyngeal sensation: a new technique. Ann Otol Rhinol Laryngol, 1993;102:777.

94. Aviv JE, Kaplan ST, Thomson JE, et al. The safety of flexible endoscopic evaluation of swallowing with sensory testing (FEESST): an analysis of 500 consecutive evaluations. Dysphagia 2000;15:39.

95. Aviv JE. Prospective, randomized outcome study of endoscopy versus modified barium swallow in patients with dysphagia. Laryngoscope 2000;110:563.

96. Leder SB. Serial fiberoptic endoscopic swallowing evaluations in the management of patients with dysphagia. Arch Phys Med Rehabil 1998;79:1264.

97. Malhi-Chowla N, Achem SR, Stark ME, DeVault KR. Manometry of the upper esophageal sphincter and pharynx is not useful in unselected patients referred for esophageal testing. Am J Gastroenterol 2000;95:1417.

98. Kelly JH. Use of manometry in the evaluation of dysphagia. Otolaryngol Head Neck Surg 1997;116:355.

99. Jacob P, Kahrilas PJ, Logemann JA, et al. Upper esophageal sphincter opening and modulation during swallowing. Gastroenterology 1989;97:1469.

100. Hila A, Castell JA, Castell DO. Pharyngeal and upper esophageal sphincter manometry in the evaluation of dysphagia. J Clin Gastroenterol 2001;33:355.

101. Jones B, Ravich WJ, Donner MW, et al. Pharyngoesophageal interrelationships: observations and working concepts. Gastroint Radiol 1985;10:225.

102. Curtis DJ, Cruess DF, Berg T. The cricopharyngeal muscle: a videorecording review. AJR 1984;142:497.

103. Mason RJ, Bremner CG. Myotomy for pharyngeal swallowing disorders. Adv Surg 1999;33:375.

104. Mason RJ, Bremner CG, DeMeester TR, et al. Pharyngeal swallowing disorders: selection for and outcome after myotomy. Ann Surg 1998;228:598.

105. Kelly JH. Management of upper esophageal sphincter disorders: indications and complications of myotomy. Am J Med 2000;108 (Suppl. 4a):43S.

106. Ellis FH Jr, Gibb SP, Williamson WA. Current status of cricopharyngeal myotomy for cervical esophageal dysphagia. Eur J Cardio-Thoracic Surg 1996;10:1033.

107. Johnson ER, McKenzie SW, Sievers A. Aspiration pneumonia in stroke. Arch Phys Med Rehab 1993;74:973.
108. Smithard DG, O'Neill PA, Park C, et al. Complications and outcome after acute stroke: does dysphagia matter? Stroke 1996;27:1200.
109. Lim SH, Lieu PK, Phua SY, et al. Accuracy of bedside clinical methods compared with fiberoptic endoscopic examination of swallowing (FEES) in determining the risk of aspiration in acute stroke patients. Dysphagia 2001;16:1.
110. Cogen R, Weinryb J. Aspiration pneumonia in nursing home patients fed via gastrostomy tubes. Am J Gastroenterol 1989;85:1509.
111. Ciocon JO, Silverstone FA, Graver M, Foley CJ. Tube feeding in elderly patients: indications, benefits, and complications. Arch Intern Med 1988;148:429.
112. Hassett JM, Sunby C, Flint LM. No elimination of aspiration pneumonia in neurologically disabled patients with gastrostomy. Surg Gynecol Obstet 1988;167:383.
113. Groher ME. Bolus management and aspiration pneumonia in patients with pseudobulbar dysphagia. Dysphagia 1987;1:215.
114. Martino R, Pron G, Diamant N. Screening for oropharyngeal dysphagia in stroke: insufficient evidence for guidelines. Dysphagia 2000;15:19.
115. Calne DB, Shaw DG, Spiers AS, Stern GM. Swallowing in Parkinsonism. Br J Radiol 1970;43:456.
116. Bushmann M, Dobmeyer SM, Leeker L, Perlmutter JS. Swallowing abnormalities and their response to treatment in Parkinson's disease. Neurology 1989;39:1309.
117. Spechler SJ. AGA technical review on treatment of patients with dysphagia caused by benign disorders of the distal esophagus. Gastroenterology 1999;117:233.
118. Ott DJ. Radiographic techniques and efficacy in evaluating esophageal dysphagia. Dysphagia 1990;5:192.
119. Ott DJ, Chen YM, Wu WC, et al. Radiographic and endoscopic sensitivity in detecting lower esophageal mucosal ring. AJR 1986;147:261.
120. Ott DJ, Gelfand DW, Lane TG, Wu WC. Radiologic detection and spectrum of appearances of peptic esophageal strictures. J Clin Gastroenterol 1982;4:11.
121. Ott DJ, Gelfand DW, Wu WC, Chen YM. Radiological evaluation of dysphagia. JAMA 1986;256:2718.
122. Ott DJ, Richter JE, Chen YM, et al. Esophageal radiography and manometry: correlation in 172 patients with dysphagia. AJR 1987;149:307.
123. Nellemann H, Aksglaede K, Funch-Jensen P, Thommesen P. Bread and barium. Diagnostic value in patients with suspected primary esophageal motility disorders. Acta Radiol 2000;41:145.
124. Ott DJ, Kelley TF, Chen MYM, et al. Use of a marshmallow bolus for evaluating lower esophageal mucosal rings. Am J Gastroenterol 1991;86:817.
125. Kahrilas PJ, Clouse RE, Hogan WJ. American Gastroenterological Association technical review on the clinical use of esophageal manometry. Gastroenterology 1994;107:1865.
126. Mearin F, Malagelada JR. Complete lower esophageal sphincter relaxation observed in some achalasia patients is functionally inadequate. Am J Physiol Gastrointest Liver Physiol 2000;278:G376.
127. Staiano A, Clouse RE. Detection of incomplete lower esophageal sphincter relaxation with conventional point-pressure sensors. Am J Gastroenterol 2001;96:3258.
128. Shi G, Ergun GA, Manka M, Kahrilas PJ. Lower esophageal sphincter relaxation characteristics using a sleeve sensor in clinical manometry. Am J Gastroenterol 1998;93:2373.
129. Herron DM, Swanstrom LL, Ramzi N, Hansen PD. Factors predictive of dysphagia after laparoscopic Nissen fundoplication. Surg Endosc 1999;13:1180.
130. Fibbe C, Layer P, Keller J, et al. Esophageal motility in reflux disease before and after fundoplication: a prospective, randomized, clinical, and manometric study. Gastroenterology 2001;121:5.
131. Pohl D, Eubanks TR, Omelanczuk PE, Pellegrini CA. Management and outcome of complications after laparoscopic antireflux operations. Arch Surg 2001;136:399.
132. Malhi-Chowla N, Gorecki P, Bammer T, et al. Dilation after fundoplication: timing, frequency, indications, and outcome. Gastrointest Endosc 2002;55:219.
133. Wo JM, Trus TL, Richardson WS, et al. Evaluation and management of postfundoplication dysphagia. Am J Gastroenterol 1996;91:2318.
134. Hunter JG, Smith CD, Branum GD, et al. Laparoscopic fundoplication failures: patterns of failure and response to fundoplication revision. Ann Surg 1999;230:595.
135. Prakash C, Soper NJ, Clouse RE. Topographic manometric evaluation following laparoscopic antireflux surgery. Gastroenterology 2001;120 (Suppl. 1):A246.
136. Tatum RP, Shi G, Manka MA, et al. Bolus transit assessed by an esophageal stress test in postfundoplication dysphagia. J Surg Res 2000;91:56.
137. Vaezi MF. Quantitative methods to determine efficacy of treatment in achalasia. Gastrointest Endosc Clin North Am 2001;11:409.
138. Gaudric M, Sabate JM, Artru P, et al. Results of pneumatic dilatation in patients with dysphagia after antireflux surgery. Br J Surg 1999;86:1088.
139. Alberty J, Oelerich M, Ludwig K, et al. Efficacy of botulinum toxin A for treatment of upper esophageal sphincter dysfunction. Laryngoscope 2000;110:1151.
140. Brouillette D, Martel E, Chen LQ, Duranceau A. Pitfalls and complications of cricopharyngeal myotomy. Chest Surg Clin North Am 1997;7:457.
141. Ahsan SF, Meleca RJ, Dworkin JP. Botulinum toxin injection of the cricopharyngeus muscle for the treatment of dysphagia. Otolaryngol Head Neck Surg 2000;122:691.
142. Solt J, Bajor J, Moizs M, et al. Primary cricopharyngeal dysfunction: treatment with balloon catheter dilatation. Gastrointest Endosc 2001;54:767.
143. Hatlebakk JG, Castell JA, Spiegel J, et al. Dilatation therapy for dysphagia in patients with upper esophageal sphincter dysfunction – manometric and symptomatic response. Dis Esophagus 1998;11:254.
144. Clouse RE. Complications of endoscopic gastrointestinal dilation techniques. Gastrointest Endosc Clin North Am 1996;6:323.
145. Colon VJ, Young MA, Ramirez FC. The short- and long-term efficacy of empirical esophageal dilation in patients with nonobstructive dysphagia: a prospective, randomized study. Am J Gastroenterol 2000;95:910.
146. Marshall JB, Chowdhury TA. Does empiric esophageal dilation benefit dysphagia when endoscopy is normal? Dig Dis Sci 1996;41:1099.
147. Gyawali CP, Clouse RE. Do we practice what we preach? Gastrointest Endosc 2007;66:676.
148. Staiano A, Clouse RE. The effects of cisapride on the topography of esophageal peristalsis. Aliment Pharmacol Ther 2002;10:875.
149. Colon V, Grade A, Pulliam G, et al. Effect of doses of glucagon used to treat food impaction on esophageal motor function of normal subjects. Dysphagia 1999;14:27.
150. Bassotti G, Annese V. Review article: pharmacological options in achalasia. Aliment Pharmacol Ther 1999;13:1391.
151. Short TP, Thomas E. An overview of the role of calcium antagonists in the treatment of achalasia and diffuse oesophageal spasm. Drugs 1992;43:177.
152. Bortolotti M. Medical therapy of achalasia: a benefit for few. Digestion 1992;43:177.
153. Pimentel M, Bonorris GG, Chow EJ, Lin HC. Peppermint oil improves the manometric findings in diffuse esophageal spasm. J Clin Gastroenterol 2001;33:27.
154. Clouse RE, Lustman PJ. Antidepressants for irritable bowel syndrome. In: Camilleri M, Spiller RC (eds). Irritable Bowel Syndrome: diagnosis and treatment. London: WB Saunders, 2002:161.
155. Clouse RE. Therapy of functional syndromes. J Functional Syndromes 2001;1:61.
156. Clouse RE, Lustman PJ, Eckert TC, et al. Low-dose trazodone for symptomatic patients with esophageal contraction abnormalities: a double-blind, placebo-controlled trial. Gastroenterology 1987;92:1027.

157. Handa M, Mine K, Yamamoto H, et al. Antidepressant treatment of patients with diffuse esophageal spasm: a psychosomatic approach. J Clin Gastroenterol 1999;28:228.

158. Connolly GM, Hawkins D, Harcourt-Webster JN, et al. Oesophageal symptoms, their causes, treatment, and prognosis in patients with the acquired immunodeficiency syndrome. Gut 1989;30:1033.

159. Webb AA. Management of foreign bodies of the upper gastrointestinal tract: update. Gastrointest Endosc 1995;41:39.

160. Ginsberg GG. Management of ingested foreign objects and food bolus impactions. Gastrointest Endosc 1995;41:33.

161. American Society for Gastrointestinal Endoscopy. Guidelines for the management of ingested foreign bodies. Oak Brook, IL: ASGE Publication, 1995:1026.

162. Levine MS. Radiology of esophagitis: a pattern approach. Radiology 1991;179:1.

163. Yee J. Infectious esophagitis. Radiol Clin North Am 1994;32:1135.

164. Laine L, Dretler RH, Conteas CN, et al. Fluconazole compared with ketoconazole for the treatment of *Candida* esophagitis in AIDS. A randomized trial. Ann Intern Med 1992;117:655.

165. Connolly GM, Forbes A, Gleeson JA, Gazzard BG. Investigation of upper gastrointestinal symptoms in patients with AIDS. AIDS 1989;3:453.

166. Eslick GD, Coulshed DS, Talley NJ. Review article: the burden of illness in non-cardiac chest pain. Aliment Pharmacol Ther 2002; 16:1217.

167. Fruergaard P, Launbjerg J, Hesse B, et al. The diagnosis of patients admitted with acute chest pain but without myocardial infarction. Eur Heart J 1996;17:1028.

168. Spalding L, Reay E, Kelly C. Cause and outcome of atypical chest pain in patients admitted to hospital. J R Soc Med 2003;96:122–125.

169. Imaoka T, Miyaoka Y, Nishi K, et al. Prevalence of noncardiac chest pain in Japanese patients with recurrent chest pain. J Gastroenterol 2005;40:913.

170. Eslick GD, Jones MP, Talley NJ. Non cardiac chest pain: prevalence, risk factors, impact and consulting – a population based study. Aliment Pharmacol Ther 2003;17:1115.

171. Lampe FC, Whincup PH, Wannamethee SG, et al. Chest pain on questionnaire and prediction of major ischemic heart disease events in men. Eur Heart J 1998;19:63.

172. Locke GR 3rd, Talley NJ, Fett SI, . Prevalence and clinical spectrum of gastro-oesophageal reflux: a population based study in Olmsted County, Minnesota. Gastroenterology 1997;112:1448.

173. Tibbling L. Oesophageal dysfunction and angina pectoris in a Swedish population selected at random. Acta Med Scand 1981; 644(Suppl):71.

174. Wong WM, Lam KF, Cheng C, et al. Population based study of non-cardiac chest pain in Southern Chinese: prevalence, psychological factors and health care utilization. World J Gastroenterol 2004;10: 707.

175. Fass R, Fennerty MB, Ofman JJ, et al. The clinical and economic value of a short course of omeprazole in patients with non-cardiac chest pain. Gastroenterology 1998;115:42.

176. Fass R, Winters GF. Evaluation of the patient with noncardiac chest pain: is gastroesophageal reflux disease or an esophageal motility disorder the cause? Medscape Gastroenterol J 2001;3:1.

177. Fass R, Naliboff B, Higa L, et al. Differential effect of long-term esophageal acid exposure on mechanosensitivity and chemosensitivity in humans. Gastroenterology 199;115:1363.

178. Bernstein LM. A clinical test for esophagitis. Gastroenterology 1958;34:760.

179. Bennett J. Oesophagus: Atypical chest pain and motility disorders. BMJ 2001;323:791.

180. Beedassy A, Katz PO, Gruber A, et al. Prior sensitization of esophageal mucosa by acid reflux predisposes to reflux-induced chest pain. J Clin Gastroenterol 2000;31:121.

181. Richter JE, Barish CF, Castell DO. Abnormal sensory perception in patients with esophageal chest pain. Gastroenterology 1986;91:845.

182. Rao SS, Gregersen H, Hayek B, et al. Unexplained chest pain: the hypersensitive, hyperreactive, and poorly compliant esophagus. Ann Intern Med 1996;124:950.

183. Rao SS, Hayek B, Summers RW. Functional chest pain of esophageal origin: hyperalgesia or motor dysfunction. Am J Gastroenterol 2001; 96:2584.

184. Hu WH, Martin CJ, Talley NJ. Intraesophageal acid perfusion sensitizes the esophagus to mechanical distension: a Barostat study. Am J Gastroenterol 2000;95:2189.

185. Sarkar S, Aziz Q, Woolf CJ, . Contribution of central sensitization to the development of non-cardiac chest pain. Lancet 2000;356:1154.

186. Sarkar S, Thompson DG, Woolf CJ, et al. Patients with chest pain and occult gastroesophageal reflux demonstrate visceral pain hypersensitivity which may be partially responsive to acid suppression. Am J Gastroenterol 2004;99:1998.

187. Hobson AR, Furlong PL, Sarkar S, et al. Neurophysiologic assessment of esophageal sensory processing in noncardiac chest pain. Gastroenterology 2006;130:80.

188. Hollerback S, Bulat R, May A, et al. Abnormal cerebral processing of oesophageal stimuli in patients with noncardiac chest pain (NCCP). Neurogastroenterol Motil 2000;12:555.

189. Tougas G, Spaxiani R, Hollerback S, et al. Cardiac autonomic function and oesophageal acid sensitivity in patients with non-cardiac chest pain. Gut 2001;49:706.

190. Katz PO, Dalton CB, Richter JE, et al. Esophageal testing of patients with noncardiac chest pain or dysphagia. Results of three years' experience in 1161 patients. Ann Intern Med 1987;106:593.

191. Dekel R, Pearson T, Wendel C, et al. Assessment of oesophageal motor function in patients with dysphagia or chest pain – the Clinical Outcomes Research Initiative experience. Aliment Pharmacol Ther 2003;18:1083.

192. Battaglia E, Bassotti G, Buonafede G, et al. Noncardiac chest pain of esophageal origin in patients with and without coronary artery disease. Hepatogastroenterology 2005;52:792.

193. Balaban DH, Yamamoto Y, Liu J, et al. Sustained esophageal contraction: a marker of esophageal chest pain identified by intraluminal ultrasonography. Gastroenterology 1999;116:29.

194. Achem SR, Kolts BE, Wears R, et al. Chest pain associated with nutcracker esophagus: a preliminary study of the role of gastroesophageal reflux. Am J Gastroenterol 1993;88:167.

195. Clouse RE, Carney RM. The psychological profile of noncardiac chest pain patients. Eur J Gastroenterol Hepatol 1995;7:1160.

196. Clouse RE, Lustman PJ. Psychiatric illness and contraction abnormalities of the esophagus. N Engl J Med 1983;309:1337.

197. Fleet RP, Dupuis G, Marchand A, et al. Panic disorder in emergency department chest pain patients: prevalence, comorbidity, suicidal ideation, and physician recognition. Am J Med 1996;101:371.

198. Eslick GD. Noncardiac chest pain: epidemiology, natural history, health care seeking, and quality of life. Gastroenterol Clin North Am 2004;33:1.

199. Achem S, DeVault K. Recent developments in chest pain of undetermined origin. Curr Gastroenterol Rep 2000;2:201.

200. Panting JR, Gatehouse PD, Yang GZ, Grothues F, Firmin DN, Collins P, Pennell DJ. Abnormal subendocardial perfusion in cardiac syndrome X detected by cardiovascular magnetic resonance imaging. N Engl J Med 2002;346:1948.

201. Jouriles NJ. Atypical chest pain. Emerg Med Clin North Am 1998; 16:717.

202. Achem SR, DeVault KR. Noncardiac, nonesophageal causes of chest pain. In: Fass R, Eslick GD (eds). Noncardiac chest pain, 1st edn. San Diego: Plural Publishing, 2007:39.

203. Eslick GD. Usefulness of chest pain character and location as diagnostic indicators of an acute coronary syndrome. Am J Cardiol 2005;95:1228.

204. Miller CD, Lindsell CJ, Knandelwal S, et al. Is the initial diagnostic impression of 'noncardiac chest pain' adequate to exclude cardiac disease? Ann Emerg Med 2004;44:565.

205. Hollander JE, Robey JL, Chase MR, et al. Relationship between a clear-cut alternative noncardiac diagnosis and 30-day outcome in

emergency department patients with chest pain. Acad Emerg Med 2007;14:210.

206. Kemp HG, Kronmal RA, Vliestra RE, et al. Seven-year survival of patients with normal or near normal coronary arteriograms. A CASS registry study. J Am Coll Cardiol 1986;7:479.

207. Hewson E, Sinclair J, Dalton C, Richter J. 24-hour esophageal pH monitoring: The most useful test for evaluating noncardiac chest pain. Am J Med 1991;90:576.

208. Voskuil JH, Cramer M, Breumelhof R, et al. Prevalence of eso-phageal disorders in patients with chest pain newly referred to the cardiologist. Chest 1996;109:1210.

209. Alban-Davies H, Jones D, Rhoades J, et al. Angina-like esophageal pain: differentiation from cardiac pain from history. J Clin Gastro-enterol 1985;7:477.

210. Wolf E, Stern S. Costochondral syndrome: its frequency and import-ance in differential diagnosis of coronary heart disease. Arch Intern Med 1976;136:189.

211. Disla E, Rhim HR, Reddy A, et al. Costochondritis, a prospective analysis in an emergency department setting. Arch Intern Med 1994;154:2466.

212. Wise CM, Semble EL, Dalton CB. Musculoskeletal chest wall syndromes in patients with noncardiac chest pain: a study of 100 patients. Arch Phys Med Rehab 1992;73:147.

213. Eslick GD, Coulshed DS, Talley NJ. Diagnosis and treatment of non-cardiac chest pain. Nature Clin Pract 2005;2:463.

214. Bugiardini R, Bairey Merz CN. Angina with "normal" coronary arteries. A changing philosophy. JAMA 2005;293:477.

215. Wang WH, Huang JQ, Zheng GF, et al. Is proton pump inhibitor test-ing an effective approach to diagnose gastroesophageal reflux dis-ease in patients with noncardiac chest pain? A meta-analysis. Arch Intern Med 2005;165:1222.

216. Ofman JJ, Gralnek IM, Udani J, et al. The cost-effectiveness of the omeprazole test in patients with noncardiac chest pain. Am J Med 1999;107:219.

217. Numans ME, Lau J, de Wit NJ, et al. Short-term treatment with proton-pump inhibitors as a test for gastroesophageal reflux dis-ease: a meta-analysis of diagnostic test characteristics. Ann Intern Med 2004;140:518.

218. Dickman R, Mattek N, Holub J, et al. Prevalence of upper gastroin-testinal tract findings in patients with noncardiac chest pain versus those with gastroesophageal reflux disease (GERD)-related symptoms: results from a national endoscopic database. Am J Gastroenterol 2007;102:1173.

219. Kahrilas PJ, Quigley EM. Clinical esophageal pH recording: a tech-nical review for practice guideline development. Gastroenterology 1996;110:1982.

220. Quadri A, Vakil N. Health-related anxiety and the effect of open access endoscopy in US patients with dyspepsia. Aliment Pharmacol Ther 2003;17:835.

221. Wiener GJ, Richter JE, Copper JB, et al. The symptom index: a clin-ically important parameter of ambulatory 24-hour esophageal pH monitoring. Am J Gastroenterol 1988;83:358.

222. Richter JE. Chest pain and gastroesophageal reflux disease. J Clin Gastroenterol 2000;30(suppl.):S39.

223. Hsia PC, Maher KA, Lewis JH, et al. Utility of upper endoscopy in the evaluation of noncardiac chest pain. Gastrointest Endosc 1991; 37:22.

224. Prakash C, Clouse RE. Wireless pH monitoring in patients with non-cardiac chest pain. Am J Gastroenterol 2005;100:1.

225. Patti MG, Molena D, Fisichella PM, et al. Gastroesophageal reflux disease (GERD) and chest pain. Results of laparoscopic anti-reflux surgery. Surg Endosc 2002;16:563.

226. Ghillebert G, Janssens J, Vantrappen G, et al. Ambulatory 24 hour intraoesophageal pH and pressure recordings v provocation tests in the diagnosis of chest pain of oesophageal origin. Gut 1990;31: 738.

227. Weusten BLAM, Roelofs JMM, Akkermans LMA, et al. The symptom-association probability: an improved method for symptom ana-lysis of 24-hour esophageal pH data. Gastroenterology 1994;107: 1741.

228. Snedegar CT, Clouse RE. Comparison of reflux-associated symptom probability (RASP) tests from ambulatory pH monitoring. Gastro-enterology 2004;26(suppl. 2):A-323.

229. Diaz S, Aymerich R, Clouse RE, et al. The symptom association prob-ability is superior to the symptom index for attributing symptoms to gastroesophageal reflux: validation using outcome from laparo-scopic anti-reflux surgery. Gastroenterology 2002;122(suppl.):A75.

230. Carter CS, Servan-Schreiber D, Perlstein WM. Anxiety disorders and the syndrome of chest pain with normal coronary arteries: preval-ence and pathophysiology. J Clin Psychiatry 1997;58:S70.

231. Cannon RO, Quyyumi AA, Mincemoyer R, et al. Imipramine in patients with chest pain despite normal coronary angiograms. N Engl J Med 1994;330:1411.

232. Katon W, Hall ML, Russo J, et al. Chest pain: relationship of psychi-atric illness to coronary arteriographic results. Am J Med 1988;84:1.

233. Kuijpers PM, Denollet J, Lousberg R, et al. Validity of the hospital anxiety and depression scale for use with patients with noncardiac chest pain. Psychosomatics 2003;44:329.

234. Bassoti G, Gaburri M, Imbimbo BP, et al. Manometric evaluation of cimetropium bromide activity in patients with the nutcracker esoph-agus. Scand J Gastroenterol 1988;23:1079.

235. Orlando RC, Bozymski EM. Clinical and manometric effect of nitro-glycerin in diffuse esophageal spasm. N Engl J Med 1973;289:23.

236. Mellow MH. Effect of isosorbide and hydralazine in painful primary esophageal motility disorders. Gastroenterology 1982;83:364.

237. Richter JE, Dalton CB, Bradley LA, et al. Oral nifedipine in the treat-ment of noncardiac chest pain in patients with the nutcracker esoph-agus. Gastroenterology 1987;93:21.

238. D'Onofrio V, Annese V, Miletto P, et al. Long-term follow up of achalasic patients treated with botulinum toxin. Dis Esophagus 2000;13:96.

239. Storr M, Allescher HD, Rosch T, et al. Treatment of symptomatic dif-fuse esophageal spasm by endoscopic injections of botulinum toxin: a prospective study with long-term follow up. Gastrointest Endosc 2001;54:754.

240. Miller LS, Pullela SV, Parkman HP, et al. Treatment of chest pain in patients with noncardiac, nonreflux, nonachalasia spastic esophageal motor disorders using botulinum injection into the gastroesopha-geal junction. Am J Gastroenterol 2002;97:1640.

241. Clouse RE. Antidepressants for functional gastrointestinal syn-dromes. Dig Dis Sci 1994;39:2352.

242. Prakash C, Clouse RE. Long-term outcome from tricyclic antidepres-sant treatment of functional chest pain. Dig Dis Sci 1999;44:2373.

243. Varia I, Logue E, O'Connor C, et al. Randomized trial of sertraline in patients with unexplained chest pain of noncardiac origin. Am Heart J 2000;140:367.

244. Doraiswamy PM, Varia I, Hellegers C, et al. A randomized controlled trial of paroxetine for noncardiac chest pain. Psychopharmacol Bull 2006;39:15.

245. Rao SS, Mudipalli RS, Remes-Troche JM, et al. Theophylline improves esophageal chest pain – a randomized, placebo-controlled study. Am J Gastroenterol 2007;102:930.

246. Hegel MT, Abel GG, Etscheidt M, et al. Behavioral treatment of angina-like chest pain in patients with the hyperventilation syn-drome. J Behav Ther Exp Psychiatry 1989;20:31.

247. Klimes I, Mayou RA, Pearce MJ, et al. Psychological treatments for atypical non-cardiac chest pain. A controlled evaluation. Psychol Med 1990;20:605.

248. Esler JL, Bock BC. Psychological treatments for noncardiac chest pain. Recommendations for a new approach. J Psychosom Res 2004;56:263.

249. Logemann JA. Role of the modified Barium swallow in management of patients with dysphagia. Otolaryngol Head Neck Surg 1997;116: 335.

250. Miller RM, Langmore SE. Treatment efficacy for adults with oropha-ryngeal dysphagia. Arch Phys Med Rehab 1994;75:1256.

6

Approach to the patient with gastroesophageal reflux disease

Joel E. Richter

Clinical manifestations, 83
Diagnostic evaluation, 85
Differential diagnosis, 89
Clinical course, 89
Medical and surgical therapy, 90

Gastroesophageal reflux disease (GERD) results from the failure of the normal antireflux mechanism to protect against frequent and abnormal amounts of gastroesophageal reflux (GER), that is, the effortless movement of gastric contents from the stomach to the esophagus. Gastroesophageal reflux is not itself a disease, but a normal physiological process. It occurs in virtually everyone, multiple times everyday, especially after large meals, without producing either symptoms or signs of mucosal damage. By contrast, GERD is a spectrum of disease usually producing symptoms of heartburn and acid regurgitation. Most patients have no visible mucosal injury at the time of endoscopic examination (nonerosive GERD), whereas others have esophagitis, peptic strictures, Barrett esophagus, or evidence of extraesophageal diseases such as chest pain, pulmonary symptoms, or ear, nose, and throat symptoms. GERD is a multifactorial process and one of the most common human diseases; it is also of economic importance, contributing to the expenditure in the United States of 4 to 5 billion dollars per year for antacid medications. This chapter will review the clinical symptoms associated with GERD and the useful diagnostic tests, and discuss the medical and surgical treatments.

Clinical manifestations

Classical reflux symptoms

Heartburn is the classical symptom of GERD, with patients generally reporting a burning feeling, rising from the stomach or lower chest and radiating toward the neck, throat, and

occasionally the back [1]. Usually, it occurs postprandially, particularly after large meals or the consumption of spicy foods, citrus products, fats, chocolates, or alcohol. Recumbency and bending over may exacerbate heartburn. Nighttime heartburn interferes with restful sleeping and may impair next-day work performance. When heartburn dominates the patient's complaints, it has high specificity (89%), but low sensitivity (38%) for GERD as diagnosed by abnormal 24-h esophageal pH testing [2]. The diagnosis of GERD usually is based on the occurrence of heartburn on two or more days a week, although less frequent symptoms do not preclude the disease [3]. Although this symptom is an aid to diagnosis, the frequency and severity of heartburn do not predict the degree of esophageal damage. Heartburn is caused by acid stimulation of sensory nerve endings in the deeper layers of the esophageal epithelium. These nerve endings are normally protected by a relatively impermeable epithelium, but with epithelial changes caused by reflux, they may be stimulated by H^+ ions or spicy foods [4].

Other common symptoms of GERD are acid regurgitation and dysphagia. The effortless regurgitation of acidic fluid, especially after meals and exacerbated by stooping or recumbency, is highly suggestive of GERD [2]. Among patients with daily regurgitation, the lower esophageal sphincter (LES) pressure usually is low, many have associated gastroparesis, and esophagitis is common. For these reasons, acid regurgitation may be more difficult to control medically then classical heartburn complaints. Dysphagia is reported by more than 30% of patients with GERD [5]. It usually occurs in the setting of long-standing heartburn, with slowly progressive dysphagia primarily for solids. Weight loss is uncommon because patients have good appetites. The most common causes are a peptic stricture or Schatzki ring, but other causes include severe esophageal inflammation alone,

Principles of Clinical Gastroenterology. Edited by Tadataka Yamada, David H. Alpers, Anthony N. Kalloo, Neil Kaplowitz, Chung Owyang, and Don W. Powell. © 2008 Blackwell Publishing. ISBN 978-1-4051-69103

peristaltic dysfunction, and esophageal cancer arising from Barrett esophagus.

Less common reflux-associated symptoms include water brash, odynophagia, burping, hiccups, nausea, and vomiting [6]. *Water brash* is the sudden appearance in the mouth of a slightly sour or salty fluid. It is not regurgitated fluid, but rather secretions from the salivary glands in response to acid reflux [7]. *Odynophagia*, pain on swallowing, can occasionally be seen with severe ulcerative esophagitis. However, its presence should raise the suspicion of an alternative cause of esophagitis, especially infections (candidiasis, herpes) or pills (tetracycline, potassium chloride, quinine, vitamin C, alendronate).

In contrast to the previously described symptomatic presentations, some patients with GERD are asymptomatic. This is particularly true in elderly patients because of decreased acidity of the reflux material or decreased pain perception [8]. Many elderly patients present first with complications of GERD because of long-standing disease with minimal symptoms. For example, up to one-third of patients with Barrett esophagus are insensitive to acid at the time of presentation [9].

Extraesophageal manifestations

It has been suggested that GER may be the cause of a wide spectrum of conditions including noncardiac chest pain, asthma, posterior laryngitis, chronic cough, recurrent pneumonitis, and even dental erosion [10]. Some of these patients have classical reflux symptoms, but many are "silent refluxers," contributing to problems in making the diagnosis. Furthermore, it may be difficult to establish a causal relationship even if GER can be documented by testing (e.g., pH studies), because patients may simply have two common diseases without a cause-and-effect relationship.

Chest pain

GER-related chest pain may mimic angina pectoris. The chest pain is usually described as squeezing or burning, substernal in location, and radiating to the back, neck, jaw, or arm. It often is worse after meals, awakens the patient from sleep, and may worsen during periods of emotional stress. Heavy exercise, even treadmill testing, may provoke GER [11]. Reflux-related chest pain may last minutes to hours, often resolves spontaneously, and may be eased with antacids. Most patients with GERD-induced chest pain have heartburn symptoms [12].

Early studies suggested that spastic motility disorders were the most common esophageal cause of chest pain. However, more recent studies using ambulatory esophageal pH and pressure monitoring suggest that about 25%–50% of patients with noncardiac chest pain have GERD [13]. Overall, these series of reports found that 41% of patients had abnormal 24-h pH test results, whereas 32% had chest pain that was clearly associated with acid reflux. Patients with coronary artery disease commonly have coexisting eso-

phageal diseases, but the evidence that GER causes ischemic pain is controversial [14]. The mechanism for GERD-related chest pain is not clearly understood and probably is multifactorial, related to H^+ ion concentration, volume and duration of acid reflux, and secondary esophageal spasm.

Asthma and other pulmonary diseases

The association of GERD and pulmonary diseases was recognized by Sir William Osler [15], who recommended that asthmatic patients should "learn to take their large daily meal at noon to avoid nighttime asthma which occurred if they ate a full supper." More recent studies suggest the coexistence of the two diseases in up to 80% of asthmatic patients, irrespective of the use of bronchodilators [16,17]. GERD should be considered in asthmatic patients who present in adulthood, those without an intrinsic component, and those not responding to bronchodilators or steroids [18]. Up to 30% of patients with GERD-related asthma have no other esophageal complaints. Other pulmonary diseases associated with GERD include aspiration pneumonia, interstitial pulmonary fibrosis, chronic bronchitis, bronchiectasis, and possibly cystic fibrosis, neonatal bronchopulmonary dysplasia, and sudden infant death syndrome.

Proposed mechanisms of reflux-induced asthma are either aspiration of gastric contents into the lungs with secondary bronchospasm or activation of a vagal reflex from the esophagus to the lungs causing bronchoconstriction. Animal [19] and human [20] studies report bronchoconstriction after esophageal acidification, but the response tends to be mild and unpredictable. In contrast, intratracheal infusion of even small amounts of acid induces profound and reproducible bronchospasm in cats [19]. The reflux of acid into the trachea as compared with the esophagus alone predictably caused marked changes in peak expiratory flow rates in asthmatic patients [21]. Although either mechanism may be responsible for reflux-induced asthma, most patients probably suffer from intermittent microaspiration.

Ear, nose, and throat diseases

GERD may be associated with a variety of laryngeal conditions and symptoms, of which *reflux laryngitis* is perhaps the most common [22,23]. These patients present with hoarseness, globus sensation, frequent throat clearing, recurrent sore throat, and prolonged voice warm-up. Ear, nose, and throat signs attributed to GERD include posterior laryngitis with edema and redness, vocal cord ulcers and granulomas, leukoplakia, and even carcinoma. These changes usually are limited to the posterior third of the vocal cords and interarytenoid areas, both in close proximity to the upper esophageal sphincter. GERD is the third leading cause of chronic cough (after sinus problems and asthma), accounting for 20% of cases [24]. *Dental erosion*, defined as the loss of tooth structure by chemical processes not involving bacteria, can be caused by GER in healthy persons and in patients with bulimia [25].

Despite the association between ear, nose, and throat diseases and GERD, overt esophagitis usually is absent, and most patients have only mild reflux symptoms, if any [22]. Microaspiration of gastric contents is the most likely cause of these complaints. Animal studies find that the combination of acid and pepsin is injurious to the larynx [22]. Human studies report that proximal esophageal acid exposure, especially at night while sleeping, is significantly increased in patients with laryngeal symptoms and signs [26].

Diagnostic evaluation

Many tests are available for evaluating patients with suspected GERD. These tests are often unnecessary because the classical symptoms of heartburn and acid regurgitation are sufficiently specific to identify reflux disease and to begin medical treatment. However, this may not always be the case, and the clinician must decide which test to choose to arrive at a diagnosis in a reliable, timely, and cost-effective manner, depending on the information desired (Table 6.1).

Empirical trial of acid suppression

The simplest and most definitive method for diagnosing GERD and assessing its relation to symptoms (either classical or atypical) is the empirical trial of acid suppression. Unlike other tests that only suggest an association (e.g., esophagitis at endoscopy or positive symptom index on pH testing), the response to antireflux therapy ensures a cause-and-effect

relationship between GERD and symptoms. Therefore, it has become the "first" test used in patients with classical or atypical reflux symptoms without "alarm" complaints. The popularity of this approach was aided by the introduction of the proton pump inhibitors (PPIs), which, unlike the histamine H_2 receptor antagonists (H_2RAs), could drastically reduce the amount of acid reflux into the esophagus. Symptoms usually respond in 7–14 days to a PPI trial. If symptoms disappear with therapy and then return when the medication is stopped, GERD may be assumed.

In the reported empirical trials with heartburn, the initial dose of PPI was high (e.g., omeprazole 40–80 mg/day) and was given for not less than 14 days. A positive response is defined as at least a 50% improvement in heartburn. Using this approach, the PPI empirical trial had a sensitivity of 68%–83% for determining the presence of GERD [27,28]. In non-cardiac chest pain, Fass and colleagues [29] found that a 7-day trial of omeprazole, 40 mg in the morning and 20 mg at night, had a sensitivity of 78% and specificity of 86% for predicting GERD, when compared with traditional tests. Likewise, Ours and colleagues [30] found omeprazole, 40 mg twice a day for 2 weeks, to be a reliable method for identifying acid-related cough. Empirical trials using a 2- to 4-month regimen of PPIs taken twice a day also are commonly used in patients with suspected GERD-associated asthma and GERD complaints related to the ear, nose, and throat.

An empirical trial of PPIs for diagnosing GERD has many advantages. The test is office based, is easily performed, is relatively inexpensive, is available to all physicians, and avoids many needless procedures. For example, Fass and associates [29] showed a saving of more than $570 per average patient because of a 59% reduction in the number of diagnostic tests performed for noncardiac chest pain. Disadvantages are few, but can include a placebo response and uncertain symptomatic end point if symptoms do not resolve totally with extended treatment.

Endoscopy

Upper endoscopy is the standard for documenting the presence and extent of esophagitis, and excluding other etiologies. However, only 40%–60% of patients with abnormal esophageal reflux by pH testing have endoscopic evidence of esophagitis. Thus, the sensitivity of endoscopy for GERD is 60% at best, but it has excellent specificity, at 90%–95% [31].

The earliest endoscopic signs of acid reflux include edema and erythema. Neither finding is specific for GERD, and both are dependent on the quality of endoscopic visual images [31]. More reliable are the findings of friability, granularity, and red streaks. Friability (easy bleeding), occurring with gentle pressure on the mucosa, results from the development of enlarged capillaries near the mucosal surface in response to acid. Red streaks may extend upward from the esophagogastric (EG) junction along the ridges of the esophageal folds. In studies evaluating these stigmata, nearly all patients had

---

Table 6.1 Commonly used tests for assessing the presence, mechanism, and consequences of gastroesophageal reflux disease[a]

Tests for reflux
Intraesophageal pH/impedance monitoring
Ambulatory bilirubin monitoring
Radionuclide ^{99m}Tc scintiscanning
Barium esophagram

Tests to assess symptoms
Empirical trial of acid suppression
Intraesophageal pH/impedance monitoring
Acid perfusion (Bernstein) test

Tests to assess esophageal damage
Endoscopy
Esophageal biopsy
Barium esophagram

Tests to assess pathogenesis
Esophageal manometry
Gastric analysis
Radionuclide ^{99m}Tc scintiscanning

a Order of presentation represents the order of diagnostic usefulness.

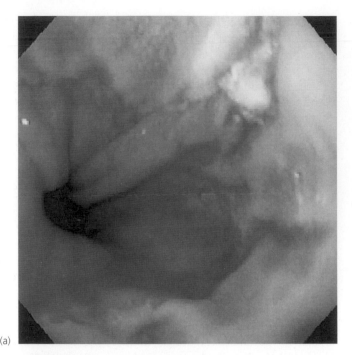

(a)

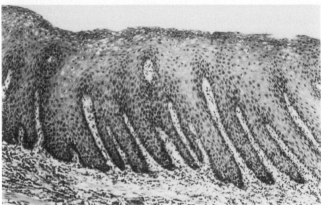

(b)

Figure 6.1 Endoscopic and histological signs of esophagitis. **(a)** Two linear erosions extending proximally from the squamocolumnar junction at the proximal border of a hiatal hernia. This would be classified as grade II esophagitis by the Savary–Miller and Hetzel systems and as grade B by the Los Angeles scale. **(b)** Reparative changes secondary to reflux disease characterized by basal cell hyperplasia (dark cells crowding the papillae) and marked elongation of the rete pegs (pale papillae with finger-like projections).

GERD [32]. With progressive acid injury, erosions develop (Fig. 6.1a) characterized by shallow thinning of the mucosa associated with a white or yellow exudate surrounded by erythema. Commonly located just above the EG junction, erosions may be either single lesions or coalesced regions and occur along the tops of mucosal folds, areas most prone to acid exposure. Erosions may also be caused by nonsteroidal antiinflammatory drugs (NSAIDs), heavy smoking, and infectious esophagitis [32]. Ulcers reflect more severe esophageal damage. They penetrate the mucosa, tend to have either a

white or yellow discolored base, and may be seen either isolated along a fold or surrounding the EG junction.

Multiple classification systems for esophagitis have been proposed; some are confusing and none has worldwide acceptance [33–35] (Table 6.2). In Europe, the most popular scheme is the Savary–Miller classification [33]. In the United States, the Hetzel [34] and Los Angeles [35] systems are most popular, with the latter gaining the most acceptance.

Most patients with GERD are treated initially without endoscopy. The important exception is the patient experiencing alarm symptoms: dysphagia, odynophagia, weight loss, and gastrointestinal bleeding. With such symptoms, endoscopy should be performed early to rule out other entities such as infections, ulcers, cancer, or varices. The role of endoscopy in GERD without alarm symptoms has changed dramatically in the PPI era. Previously, the degree of esophagitis helped direct management, but this is less an issue with PPIs, which effectively heal all grades of esophagitis. The most important reason for performing endoscopy in patients with GERD is to identify peptic strictures or Barrett esophagus. Using this rationale, most patients with chronic GERD need only one endoscopic examination while they are receiving therapy.

Esophageal biopsy

Like endoscopy, the role of esophageal biopsies in evaluating GERD has evolved over the years. Microscopic changes indicative of reflux may occur even when the mucosa appears normal endoscopically [36]. These classic findings are reactive epithelial changes characterized by an increase in the basal cell layer greater than 15% of the epithelium thickness or papilla elongation into the upper third of the epithelium (see Fig. 6.1b), both changes representing increased epithelial turnover of the squamous mucosa. Unfortunately, these changes are also noted in up to 50% of healthy persons when biopsies are taken from the distal 2–3 cm of the esophagus [37]. Hence, the changes are sensitive markers for GERD but have poor specificity.

Acute inflammation characterized by the presence of neutrophils and eosinophils is specific for esophagitis [37]; however, the sensitivity is low, in the range 15%–40% [38]. Eosinophils are found more often on biopsy (19%–63% of subjects) but are less specific, present in up to 33% of healthy adults [39]. Interestingly, the sensitivity and specificity of eosinophils in children are much stronger, reflecting the lack of eosinophils in the juvenile inflammatory response [37,40].

In today's clinical practice, the primary indication for esophageal biopsies is to determine the presence of Barrett epithelium and possible eosinophilic esophagitis. When the former diagnosis is suspected, biopsies are mandatory and should be done when all visual evidence of esophagitis is healed.

Esophageal pH monitoring

Ambulatory intraesophageal pH monitoring is the standard for

Table 6.2 Endoscopic grading systems for esophagitis

Grade	Savary–Miller classification	Hetzel classification
0	Not applicable	Normal-appearing mucosa
I	Single erosive or exudative lesion on one longitudinal fold	Mucosal edema, hyperemia, or friability of mucosa
II	Multiple erosions on more than one longitudinal fold	Superficial erosions involving < 10% of mucosal surface of last 5 cm of distal esophagus
III	Circumferential erosions	Superficial erosions involving 10%–50% of distal esophagus
IV	Ulcer, stricture, or short esophagus isolated or associated with grade I to III lesion	Deep ulceration or confluent erosions > 50% of distal esophagus
V	Barrett esophagus ± grade I to III lesion	Not applicable

	Los Angeles classification
A	One or more mucosal breaks confined to folds, no longer than 5 mm
B	One or more mucosal breaks > 5 mm confined to folds but not continuous between tops of mucosal folds
C	Mucosal breaks continuous between tops of two or more mucosal folds but not circumferential
D	Circumferential mucosal break

establishing pathological reflux (see Chapter 138) [41,42]. The test is performed with a pH probe passed nasally, positioned 5 cm above the manometrically determined LES, and is connected to a battery-powered data logger capable of collecting pH values every 4–6 s. An event marker is activated by the subject in response to symptoms, meals, and body position changes. Patients are encouraged to eat normally and to pursue regular daily activities. Monitoring is carried out usually for 18–24 h. Reflux episodes are detected by a fall to a pH level of less than 4. Commonly measured parameters include the percent of total time that pH is less than 4; the percent of time upright and supine during which the pH is below 4; the total number of reflux episodes; the duration of the longest reflux episode; and the number of episodes longer than 5 min [41]. The total percent of time for which the pH is less than 4 is the most reproducible measurement for GERD, with reported upper limits of normal values ranging from 4%–5.5% [42]. Ambulatory pH testing (using a probe connected to a recording device) can discern positional variations in GER, meals, and sleep-related episodes and helps to relate symptoms to reflux events (Fig. 6.2). As the result of its reliability for measuring GER across normal activities, ambulatory pH testing has replaced other older studies, such as the standard acid reflux (Tuttle) test and radionuclide scintigraphy.

One important problem with esophageal pH monitoring is the lack of an absolute threshold value that reliably identifies pathological GER. Validation studies comparing the presence of esophagitis with abnormal pH findings report sensitivities ranging from 77%–100%, and specificities from 85%–100% [42]. However, these patients with esophagitis rarely need pH testing; rather, the patients with normal endoscopic findings and suspected reflux symptoms should benefit most from ambulatory pH monitoring. Unfortunately, the data are

much less conclusive in this group, with considerable overlap between controls and patients with nonerosive reflux [42]. Other drawbacks of pH testing include possible equipment failure, missed reflux events if the pH probe is buried in a mucosal fold, and false-negative studies resulting from dietary or activity limitations from poor tolerability of the nasal probe.

An important advantage of ambulatory esophageal pH monitoring is its ability to record and correlate symptoms with reflux episodes over extended periods. For this indication, it has essentially replaced the shorter acid perfusion (Bernstein) test. Because only about 10%–20% of reflux episodes are associated with reported symptoms, different statistical analyses have been used in attempting to define a significant association between these two variables, including the symptom index, symptom sensitivity index, and symptom association probability [42]. However, a study found that none of these statistical relationships is superior to a high-dose trial of a PPI in establishing the causal relationship between symptoms and GER [43].

Definite clinical indications for ambulatory pH monitoring have been established [42].
• Before fundoplication – pH testing should be performed in patients with normal endoscopic findings to identify the presence of pathological reflux. If esophagitis is present, pH testing is not necessary because the disease has been established.
• Persistent or recurrent symptoms after antireflux surgery – these warrant repeat pH testing. In these situations, pH monitoring is performed with the patient discontinuing all antireflux medications (PPIs for 1 week, H$_2$RAs for 2 days).
• Reflux symptoms resistant to treatment with normal or equivocal endoscopic findings – esophageal pH testing is particularly helpful in the evaluation of these patients. pH testing is usually done in patients receiving therapy to define

Physiological reflux pattern

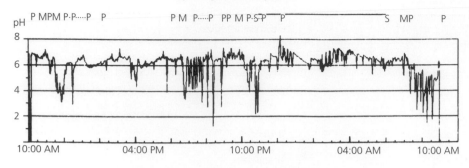

Upright reflux pattern

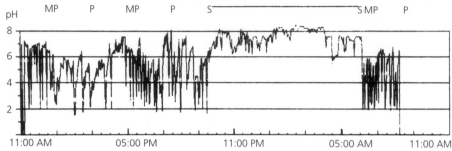

Combined reflux pattern

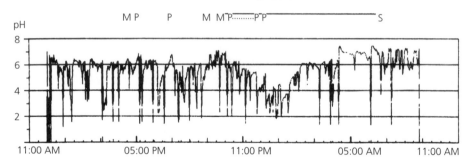

Figure 6.2 Common patterns of 24-h esophageal pH monitoring. **Top:** The physiological pattern of gastroesophageal reflux (GER) in healthy persons. Reflux is noted after meals (M) but not while asleep (S). A reflux episode is defined as a drop in pH to less than 4. **Middle:** Upright reflux pattern with extensive GER during day but not at night. These patients have frequent symptoms, but esophagitis is uncommon. **Bottom:** Combined pattern with GER during day and at night (one episode lasted 3 h). Most of these patients have esophagitis. P, postprandial.

two populations: those with and those without continued abnormal esophageal acid exposure times. The group with persistent GER needs intensification of the medical regimen, whereas those patients with symptoms and adequate acid control have another cause for their complaints.

• Patients with extraesophageal manifestations of GERD – ambulatory pH testing may help in defining this group. In this situation, pH testing is usually done with additional pH probes placed in the proximal esophagus or pharynx [44]. Initially, most of these studies were done when patients were not taking antireflux medications, to confirm the coexistence of GERD; however, this does not guarantee symptom causality. Therefore, the approach is to treat the patients aggressively with PPIs first and to reserve pH testing only for those patients not responding after 4–12 weeks of therapy [45].

Two advances have made pH testing more user-friendly and capable of measuring non-acid reflux. The Bravo pH capsule is a tubeless method of acid monitoring using a radiotelemetry capsule attached directly to the esophageal mucosa. This is more tolerable to the patient, allows 48 h of monitoring, and may improve test accuracy by allowing patients to carry out their usual activities more comfortably [46]. The second improvement combines impedance and pH testing enabling the measurement of both acid and non-acid reflux. This test may be helpful in patients with regurgitation or those with persistent symptoms despite an adequate medical trial of a PPI [47].

Barium esophagram

The barium esophagram is an inexpensive, readily available, and noninvasive esophageal test. It is most useful in demonstrating structural narrowing of the esophagus and in assessing the presence and reducibility of a hiatal hernia. Schatzki rings, webs, or minimally narrowed peptic strictures are often seen only with an esophagram, being missed by endoscopy, which may not adequately distend the esophagus. Administration of a 13-mm radiopaque pill or marshmallow along with the barium liquid can help to identify these subtle narrowings [48]. By giving the patient in the prone oblique position swallows of barium, the barium esophagram also allows good assessment of peristalsis and is helpful preoperatively in identifying a weak esophageal pump [49]. The ability of a barium esophagram to detect esophagitis varies considerably, with sensitivities of 79%–100% for moderate to severe esophagitis, whereas mild esophagitis is usually missed [49]. Barium testing also falls short when addressing the presence of Barrett esophagus. The spontaneous reflux of barium into the proximal esophagus usually suggests reflux, but is infrequent [50]. Provocative maneuvers such as leg lifting, coughing, the Valsalva maneuver, or the water-siphon test can be used to elicit stress reflux. Although these tests can improve the sensitivity of the barium esophagram, some argue that they also decrease its specificity [50,51].

Esophageal manometry

Esophageal manometry allows accurate assessment of LES pressure and relaxation, as well as peristaltic activity including contraction amplitude, duration, and velocity (see Chapter 138). However, esophageal manometry is generally not indicated in the evaluation of the patient with uncomplicated GERD because most of these patients have a normal resting LES pressure [52]. It is an integral component of pH testing to define the LES location accurately, a task poorly performed by endoscopy, fluoroscopy, or the pH pull-through technique. Esophageal manometry is traditionally recommended before antireflux surgery to document adequate esophageal peristalsis [53]. If ineffective peristalsis (low amplitude or frequent failed peristalsis) is identified [54] then a complete fundoplication may be contraindicated. However, several studies have challenged this physiological premise, finding that reflux control was better and dysphagia no more common in patients with weak peristalsis after a complete, compared with a partial, fundoplication [55]. Using impedance combined with traditional manometry, a study found that fewer than 50% of patients with manometric "ineffective" peristalsis have poor esophageal bolus clearance [56]. Thus, this new technology helps to define better a weak esophageal pump and limits the use of the less effective partial fundoplication.

Differential diagnosis

Symptoms associated with GERD may be mimicked by other esophageal and extraesophageal diseases, including achalasia,

Zenker diverticulum, gastroparesis, gallstones, peptic ulcer disease, functional dyspepsia, and angina pectoris. These disorders usually can be identified by failure to respond to aggressive antisecretory therapy and by diagnostic tests such as endoscopy, barium esophagram, esophageal manometry, ultrasound, nuclear emptying studies, and various cardiac tests. Although GERD is the most common cause of esophagitis, other causes (pill-induced esophagitis, infections, or radiation esophagitis) need to be considered in cases that are difficult to manage and in older or immunocompromised patients.

Clinical course

The clinical course of reflux esophagitis depends to a great extent on whether the patient has erosive or nonerosive GERD on initial presentation. Furthermore, patients tend not to cross from one group to another unless they are treated medically or surgically: in follow-up ranging from 6 months to more than 5 years, only 15% of patients with nonerosive disease evolved over time to having esophagitis or complications of GERD [57,58].

Nonerosive reflux disease

Although early studies from tertiary referral centers suggested that nearly half of patients with GERD had esophagitis [59], studies carried out in community practices reveal that up to 70% of patients with GERD had a normal endoscopic examination [60,61]. Furthermore, another community-based study of antacid users found that 53% of patients with GERD had nonerosive disease, and two-thirds of the remainder had only minimal erosive changes at endoscopy [62]. Endoscopy-negative patients with GERD are more likely to be female, younger, thin, and without hiatal hernia. Despite their mild mucosal damage, these patients demonstrate a chronic pattern of symptoms with periods of exacerbation and remission [63]. Studies suggest dilation of intercellular spaces is a histological marker of this disease, irrespective of esophageal acid exposure [64].

Suspicion of *nonerosive GERD* is aroused by the presence of typical reflux symptoms with a normal endoscopic examination, and is confirmed by the patient's response to antisecretory therapy. When performed, 24-h esophageal pH monitoring identifies three distinct subsets of patients with nonerosive disease. First, there are the patients with abnormal acid exposure times who are usually responsive to antisecretory therapy. Second are the patients with normal reflux parameters but a good relationship between acid reflux episodes and symptoms. This group represents 30%–50% of patients with nonerosive GERD and is characterized by "functional heartburn" [63]. These patients probably have heightened esophageal sensitivity to acid and are less likely to respond to antireflux therapy [65]. The third group is characterized by normal acid exposure times and poor symptom correlation. Despite sometimes having classic reflux symptoms, other diseases such as achalasia, gastroparesis, bile reflux, or functional dyspepsia are the cause of their symptoms. Overall, patients with nonerosive GERD do not respond to antireflux treatments as well as do patients with erosive GERD, probably because these three subsets are not carefully defined before treatment [63].

Erosive reflux disease

The clinical course of patients with *erosive esophagitis* is more predictable and is associated with complications of GERD. Controlled studies have shown that in the absence of ongoing maintenance therapy, up to 85% of patients with erosive GERD will have a relapse within 6 months, and the relapse rate is highest in those with the more severe grades of esophagitis [66,67]. This observation, however, should not prevent at least one attempt to withdraw medication, because 20% of patients remain in remission for up to 1 year, especially those with milder esophagitis grades. Although the natural history of untreated erosive GERD is well studied, two European studies suggest that these patients are more prone to reflux complications. In a Finnish study, 20 patients with erosive GERD treated with lifestyle changes, antacids, and prokinetic drugs were followed up for a median of 19 years. Fourteen patients continued to have erosions, and six new cases of Barrett esophagus were detected [68]. Likewise, a large retrospective European study with 6.5 years of follow-up found a high rate of complications (21%), including 13 esophageal ulcers, 15 with strictures, and 45 patients with Barrett epithelium [69]. However, these data must be contrasted with other studies; in one US study, no patients with erosive esophagitis developed Barrett esophagus in a 2-year trial [70]; and in 3800 French patients over a 12-year period, development of stricture was reported in only 0.26% [71].

Medical and surgical therapy

The rationale for GERD therapy depends on a careful definition of specific aims. In patients without esophagitis, the therapeutic goals are simply to relieve the acid-related symptoms and to prevent frequent symptomatic relapses. In patients with esophagitis, the goals are to relieve symptoms and to heal the esophagitis while attempting to prevent further relapses and the development of complications. These goals are set against a complex background: GERD is a chronic disease that may wax and wane in intensity, and relapses are common.

Nonprescription therapy

Although GERD is common in the United States, few persons seek medical care for their complaints, instead choosing to change their lifestyles and self-medicate with over-the-counter (OTC) antacids and low doses of H$_2$RAs. These observations have led to the "iceberg" model of the GERD population. Most heartburn suffers are invisible because they self-medicate and do not seek professional help; only those at the tip of the iceberg, typically patients with severe symptoms or reflux complications, are seen by physicians [72].

Lifestyle modifications

Sensible changes in lifestyle, especially if their rationale is explained to the patient, should be part of the initial management of all subjects. These include head of the bed elevation, avoidance of tight-fitting clothes, weight loss, restriction of alcohol, elimination of smoking, dietary therapy, refraining from lying down after meals, and avoidance of evening snacks before bedtime. Physiological studies show that these maneuvers enhance esophageal acid clearance, minimize acid-reflux-related events, or ease heartburn symptoms, but their therapeutic efficacy in controlled trials usually has not been evaluated [73]. The head of the bed can be elevated either by putting 15- to 20-cm (6- to 8-inch) thick blocks under the legs of the bed or by using a Styrofoam wedge under the mattress to elevate the upper torso. Eating several hours before retiring and avoiding evening snacks keep the stomach empty at bedtime, thereby decreasing the number of nocturnal reflux episodes. These three lifestyle changes are recommended for patients with nocturnal GERD symptoms or laryngeal complaints. One study found that head-of-the-bed elevation was nearly as effective as ranitidine therapy in healing esophagitis [74]. Avoidance of tight-fitting clothes and weight loss are interventions aimed at reducing the incidence of reflux by the abdominal stress mechanism. Although obesity is well established to be a risk factor for GERD, esophagitis, and esophageal adenocarcinoma, the efficacy of weight reduction is controversial [75]. Targeted weight loss may be helpful when discrete periods of weight gain can be associated with exacerbation of reflux symptoms. Cessation of smoking and elimination of alcohol are valuable because both agents reduce LES pressure, reduce acid clearance, and impair intrinsic squamous epithelial protective functions [76,77]. Dietary changes include reducing the size of the meal and intake of fats, carminatives, and chocolate, to reduce the frequency of reflux by decreasing gastric distention and by reducing the episodes of transient low esophageal sphincter relaxations (LESRs), and avoiding foods that lower basal LES pressure [72]. Additionally, some patients complain of heartburn after consuming citrus drinks, spicy foods, tomato-based products, coffee, tea, or cola drinks. Stimulation of gastric acid or esophageal sensitivity to low pH or hyperosmolar liquid solutions may account for these symptoms [78]. However, the indiscriminate prohibition of food products should be avoided, but rather tailored to those foods that bring on individual symptoms, to promote dietary compliance. Finally, patients should avoid, if possible, drugs that lower LES pressure or can promote localized esophagitis.

Over-the-counter medications

Over-the-counter antacids, Gaviscon, and H$_2$RAs are useful in treating mild and infrequent heartburn symptoms, especially when symptoms are brought on by lifestyle indiscretions. Antacids increase LES pressure but work primarily by buffering gastric acid in the esophagus and stomach, albeit for relative short periods. Heartburn symptoms are rapidly relieved, but patients need to take antacids frequently, usually 1–3 h after meals and at bedtime, depending on symptom severity. Gaviscon, containing alginic acid and antacids, mixes with saliva to form a highly viscous solution that floats on the surface of the gastric pool and acts as a mechanical barrier. Both antacids [79] and Gaviscon [80] are more effective than placebo in relieving symptoms induced by a heartburn-promoting meal. However, these agents do not heal esophagitis, and long-term trials suggest effective symptom relief in only 20% of patients using antacids [81]. H$_2$RAs are available in an OTC form at doses that are usually half the standard prescription dose. Although their onset of relief is not as rapid as that of antacids, the OTC H$_2$RAs have a longer duration of action, up to 6–10 h. Therefore, they are particularly useful when taken before a potentially refluxogenic activity, such as a heavy meal or exercise. Like antacids, the OTC H$_2$RAs are ineffective in healing esophagitis [82]. In the summer of 2003, the US Food and Drug Administration (FDA) approved omeprazole (20 mg) as the first OTC PPI. Drug labeling suggested daily use for only 2 weeks and recommended physician follow-up for persistent symptoms. Despite initial fears of patients abusing this drug and not seeing a physician, early consumer data show that individuals accurately self-select if OTC omeprazole is appropriate to use, comply with a 2-week regimen, and seek physician care for long-term management of frequent heartburn [83].

Prescription medication therapy

Patients with frequent heartburn, esophagitis, or complications of GERD usually see a physician and receive prescription medications for their disease. Although prokinetic drugs attempt to correct the motility disorder associated with GERD, the most clinically effective medications for short- and long-term reflux treatment are the acid suppressive drugs.

Prokinetic drugs

Until recently, three prokinetic drugs were available for the treatment of GERD: bethanechol, a cholinergic agonist; metoclopramide, a dopamine antagonist; and cisapride, a serotonin (5-HT$_4$) receptor agonist, which increases acetylcholine release in the myenteric plexus. These drugs improve reflux symptoms by increasing LES pressure, acid clearance, or gastric emptying [84]. However, none alters the frequency of transient LESRs, and their physiological activity decreases as the disease severity worsens [85]. Therefore, prokinetics provide modest benefit in controlling heartburn, but they have little efficacy in healing esophagitis unless they are combined with an acid-inhibiting drug [84].

The use of prokinetic drugs is limited by their side-effect profiles. Bethanechol commonly causes flushing, blurred vision, headaches, abdominal cramps, and urinary frequency. Metoclopramide, which crosses the blood–brain barrier, has a 20%–50% incidence of fatigue, lethargy, anxiety, and restlessness and rarely causes tremor, parkinsonism, or tardive dyskinesia. It is possible to decrease the frequency of these side effects by dose reduction, by increasing the dosing regimen to twice a day, by taking a larger single dose before dinner or at bedtime, or by using a sustained-release tablet. However, the best prokinetic drug for treating GERD, cisapride, was withdrawn from the US market in 2000 because of increased reports of serious cardiac arrhythmias (ventricular tachycardia, ventricular fibrillation, torsades de pointes, and Q–T prolongation) with associated cardiac arrest and deaths related to possible drug interactions [86].

Histamine H$_2$ receptor antagonists

Cimetidine, ranitidine, famotidine, and nizatidine reduce acid secretion by competing with histamine receptors on parietal cells. They are most effective in controlling nocturnal, compared with meal-related, acid secretion because the parietal cells may also be stimulated postprandially by acetylcholine and gastrin [87]. All the H$_2$RAs are equally effective when used in recommended doses, usually twice a day before meals. Clinical GERD trials show that heartburn, both day and night, can be significantly decreased by H$_2$RAs when compared with placebo, although symptoms are rarely abolished (Fig. 6.3a) [88]. Trials and a metaanalysis found that the overall esophagitis healing rates with H$_2$RAs rarely exceeded 60% after up to 12 weeks of treatment, even when higher than standard doses were used (Fig. 6.3b) [88,89]. Healing rates differ in individual trials, depending primarily on the degree of esophagitis being treated: grade I and II esophagitis heals in 60%–90% of patients, whereas grade III and IV heals in 30%–50% of patients despite high-dose regimens [89].

Reflux symptoms associated with nocturnal gastric acid breakthrough during PPI therapy have been recognized [90]. At bedtime, H$_2$RAs successfully eliminated this problem, suggesting a new indication for H$_2$RAs in the PPI era [91]. However, this study used only a single evening dose and did not account for the tolerance to H$_2$RAs that frequently develops over weeks to months [92]. This may impair the ability of chronic long-term nocturnal dosing of H$_2$RAs to eliminate acid breakthrough symptoms [93], but it suggests an important clinical role for H$_2$RAs as medications used on an as-needed basis when lifestyle indiscretions may promote nocturnal symptoms.

The H$_2$RAs are safe, with a side-effect rate (most of which are minor and reversible) of about 4% [87]. Serum concentrations of phenytoin, procainamide, theophylline, and warfarin

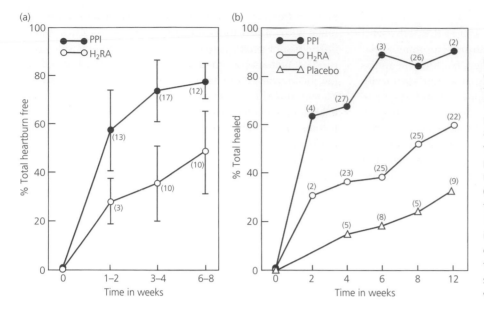

Figure 6.3 **(a)** Symptom relief–time curve expressed as the mean total heartburn relief for proton pump inhibitors (PPIs) or histamine H$_2$ receptor antagonists (H$_2$RAs) corrected for patients free of heartburn at baseline and over 8 weeks. By week 2, more patients treated with PPIs are asymptomatic compared with patients treated with H$_2$RAs even after a much longer duration of treatment (8 weeks). **(b)** Esophagitis healing–time curve as the mean total healing for PPIs, H$_2$RAs, and placebo over 12 weeks. By 4 weeks, PPIs healed esophagitis in more patients than the other two drug classes over 12 weeks, implying a substantial therapeutic gain. The number of studies is shown in parentheses. From Chiba et al. [89], with permission from Elsevier.

are altered after the administration of cimetidine and, to a lesser degree, ranitidine, whereas this interaction is not reported with the other two H$_2$RAs. The former concern that these agents could alter blood ethanol levels has been discounted [87].

Proton pump inhibitors

This class of drugs markedly diminishes gastric acid secretion by inhibiting the final common pathway of acid secretion, the H$^+$,K$^+$-ATPase pump. PPIs inhibit daytime, nocturnal, and meal-stimulated acid secretion to a significantly greater degree than H$_2$RAs [94], but they rarely make patients achlorhydric. Unlike H$_2$RAs, the degree of acid inhibition with PPIs does not correlate with plasma concentration, but it is related to the concentration and duration (area under the curve). After oral ingestion, acid inhibition is delayed because PPIs need to accumulate in the secretory canaliculus of the parietal cell to bind irreversibly to actively secreting proton pumps [95]. Therefore, the more slowly a PPI is cleared from the plasma, the more of it is available for delivery to the proton pumps. PPIs are best taken before the first meal of the day, when most proton pumps are active. Because not all pumps are active at any given time, a single PPI dose does not inhibit all pumps. A second dose, if needed, can be taken before the evening meal.

The five available PPIs are omeprazole, lansoprazole, rabeprazole, pantoprazole, and esomeprazole, the (S)-isomer of the racemic omeprazole. Their superior efficacy compared with H$_2$RAs is based on their ability to maintain an intragastric pH higher than 4 for 15–21 h daily, compared with approximately 8 h daily with the H$_2$RAs [96]. PPIs are superior to H$_2$RAs in completely relieving heartburn symptoms in most patients with severe GERD, usually within 1–2 weeks (Fig. 6.3a) [89]. Symptom relief is better in patients with eros-

ive compared with nonerosive disease [97]. Controlled studies and a large metaanalysis report complete healing of even severe ulcerative esophagitis after 8 weeks in more than 80% of patients taking PPIs, compared with 51% of patients taking H$_2$RAs and 28% receiving placebo (Fig. 6.3b) [98–102]. In those patients not healing initially, prolonged therapy with the same dose or an increased dose usually resulted in 100% healing [103]. Therapeutic efficacy between PPIs was thought to be similar, until large studies found the newest PPI, esomeprazole 40 mg, superior to omeprazole 20 mg and lansoprazole 30 mg in healing esophagitis [104]. The therapeutic advantage is minimal with mild esophagitis (number needed to treat 20–40 patients) and greatest with severe esophagitis (number-to-treat 7–10 patients). This superiority is related to greater systemic bioavailability and less interpatient variability with esomeprazole. Several PPIs are available in the United States for intravenous use.

All the PPIs are well tolerated, with headaches and diarrhea described as the most common side effects in clinical trials. Although increased gastrin levels are reported with all the PPIs, the elevations generally do not exceed the normal range for gastrin and return to normal values within 1 week of stopping the drug. Omeprazole may decrease the clearance of diazepam and warfarin because of competition for the cytochrome P450 isoenzyme P2C19 [105]. The four newer PPIs have minimal or no important drug–drug interactions.

Maintenance therapy

GERD tends to be a chronic relapsing disease, especially in patients with low LES pressure, severe grades of esophagitis, and difficult-to-manage symptoms [96]. Although almost all patients with severe esophagitis can be healed with PPI treatment, recurrence can be anticipated in more than 80% of patients within 6 months of drug discontinuation [66].

The chronicity of less severe forms of GERD is less certain, but relapses probably occur in 15%–30% of patients over 6 months [66,106]. Therefore, maintenance therapy is needed for many patients.

One-year maintenance studies always find the PPIs superior to H2RAs or prokinetics, with remission rates higher than 75% [67,107,108]. Lower overall remission rates (20%–50%) are achieved with H2RAs and prokinetic drugs, and these are most useful in patients with mild or no esophagitis [109]. The US FDA has approved all the PPIs, sometimes at half the short-term dose, for maintenance therapy, but only ranitidine, 150 mg twice daily, has maintenance indications for mild esophagitis. Conversely, clinicians are placing patients with severe erosive esophagitis on long-term PPI therapy indefinitely. The efficacy of this approach is supported by open, compassionate-use data, primarily from The Netherlands and Australia [110,111]. In a study of 230 patients with severe esophagitis healed initially with 40 mg omeprazole, all subjects were kept in remission for up to 11 years. More than 60% were maintained on omeprazole, 20 mg a day, whereas higher doses of 60 mg or more were needed in only 12% of patients, suggesting a lack of tolerance to PPIs. Relapses were rare (1 per 9.4 years of follow-up), strictures did not occur, and Barrett esophagus did not progress [111].

There was concern about the long-term safety of PPIs because of their profound acid suppression. Evidence suggests this fear is unjustified because sufficient gastric acid is produced for normal protein and carbohydrate digestion, iron and calcium absorption, and the prevention of bacterial overgrowth. The clinical effect of omeprazole on vitamin B-12 absorption is controversial [112]. Therefore, it may be prudent to monitor B-12 levels in patients receiving long-term PPI therapy, especially elderly patients or those with poor or unusual diets. The main concern with the long-term safety of PPIs stemmed from reports of that omeprazole produces hypergastrinemia and gastric carcinoid tumors in rats, changes also subsequently demonstrated with long-term ranitidine therapy and subtotal resection of the gastric fundus [113]. However, the rat has a high density of enterochromaffin-like cells and an exaggerated response to achlorhydria; long-term omeprazole therapy in species with lower densities of enterochromaffin-like cells (mice, dogs, humans) has not caused carcinoid tumors. Furthermore, other groups with massive hypergastrinemia (five to ten times the gastrin values on omeprazole), such as patients with pernicious anemia or Zollinger–Ellison syndrome, rarely develop carcinoid tumors [113]. Finally, one study suggested that patients taking long-term omeprazole who are infected with *Helicobacter pylori* develop atrophic gastritis, a precursor to gastric adenocarcinoma, at a more rapid rate than noninfected patients [114]. Nevertheless, a subsequent FDA panel determined that the available data were insufficient for recommending screening and treatment of *H. pylori* infection in patients receiving long-term PPI therapy [115].

Treatment in elderly or pregnant patients

Older patients often complain of less severe reflux symptoms than their younger cohorts, but because of prolonged acid exposure over years, the elderly may have more complicated disease [8]. Treatment of older patients with GERD follows the same principles as in other adults, although they may require more aggressive acid suppression therapy [116]. Pill-induced esophagitis may complicate their treatment. Metoclopramide must be used with caution because of frequent side effects in the elderly. Mental changes in older patients can be associated with H2RAs, and doses need to be decreased in patients with renal insufficiency. Fewer drug interactions are seen with famotidine and nizatidine. Alternative methods of administering PPIs may be necessary in debilitated older patients who cannot swallow intact omeprazole or lansoprazole capsules. Both capsules can be opened and the granules taken with water, a hydrogencarbonate-based suspension, or apple or orange juice, or the granules can be sprinkled on apple sauce or yogurt [117].

Teratogenicity or fetal harm from absorption of medications across the placenta is the foremost consideration in the treatment of GERD during pregnancy [118]. Lifestyle modifications and antacids or Gaviscon remain the cornerstones of treatment, providing adequate relief to the majority of women with mild symptoms. Although rarely used in adults, sucralfate is a nonabsorbable mucosal binder that has been found to be superior to lifestyle changes in a controlled study in pregnant women [119]. Metoclopramide, H2RAs, and most PPIs (except omeprazole) have a category B FDA safety profile for use during pregnancy, based on animal studies showing no risk, and on small case series and anecdotal human reports. Ranitidine is the only one of these drugs shown to be effective during pregnancy [120]. Proton pump inhibitors may be safe for aspiration prophylaxis before anesthesia for elective cesarean sections. Antacids, sucralfate, and most H2RAs (except nizatidine) are safe to use during lactation, although the latter group of drugs is excreted in breast milk. PPIs are not recommended during breast-feeding, based on safety concerns in animal studies [118].

Treatment of extraesophageal presentations

Acid reflux-related chest pain is easily treated by H2RAs or PPIs, with efficacy substantiated by placebo-controlled studies [121]. The efficacy of acid suppression therapy in asthma, cough, and other pulmonary complications of GERD is more mixed [17]. Medical antireflux therapy improves asthma symptoms and reduces the need for asthma medications in more than 60% of patients, but objective improvement of peak expiratory flow rates is observed in only 25% of patients. Best results are found with higher doses of PPIs (usually twice-daily administration) given for 2–3 months. Potential positive predictors of PPI response include asthma that is difficult to control, associated acid regurgitation, proximal reflux on pH testing, and healing of esophagitis with antireflux therapy. Case studies report that 60%–96% of patients with suspected acid-related ear, nose, and throat symptoms and signs improve with acid suppression, but the results of placebo-controlled studies are inconsistent and much less encouraging [45]. Here again, PPIs are more effective than H_2RAs, and extended therapy for up to 3 months may be required. Predictors of response have not been identified, although patients with milder laryngeal signs show better symptom improvement. In all these possible extra-esophageal presentations of GERD, failure to respond to aggressive PPI therapy, confirmed by adequate acid control by pH testing, suggests a cause of these complaints other than acid.

Surgical treatment

Antireflux surgery reduces GER by increasing basal LES pressure, decreasing episodes of transient LESRs, and inhibiting complete LESR [122]. This is accomplished by reducing the hiatal hernia back into the abdomen and thereby restoring an adequate length of intraabdominal sphincter, reconstructing the diaphragmatic hiatus, and reinforcing the LES [123]. Since the advent of minimally invasive surgery, the two most popular operations are the Nissen fundoplication and the Toupet partial fundoplication (Fig. 6.4). The former is a superior operation with more long-term durability, but it has a higher frequency of postoperative dysphagia and gas bloat symptoms [124,125]. Both are routinely performed laparoscopically through the abdomen. The hospital stay is 1–2 days, and many patients return to normal activity in 7–10 days. Patients with more severe disease and a short esophagus manifested by a large nonreducible hernia, a tight stricture, or a long-segment Barrett esophagus require a Collis lengthening procedure creating a 3–5-cm neoesophagus, so the fundoplication can be placed in the abdomen under minimal tension [126].

In the PPI era, the resolution of symptoms on treatment is a good predictor for the success of antireflux surgery for both classical and atypical symptoms [127]. Antireflux surgery is a reasonable option in the following situations:
• healthy patients with GERD that is well controlled on PPIs and who want alternative therapy because of drug expense, poor medication compliance, or a fear of unknown long-term side effects
• patients with atypical GERD symptoms responding to PPIs
• patients with volume regurgitation and aspiration symptoms not controlled on PPIs.
Patients recalcitrant to PPI therapy need to be approached cautiously with surgery because they may have another cause of their disorder (i.e., pill esophagitis, gastroparesis, functional heartburn).

Extensive physiological testing should be done before antireflux surgery is performed. All patients need endoscopy to exclude stricture, Barrett esophagus, and dysplasia. A barium esophagram can help to define a nonreducible hernia,

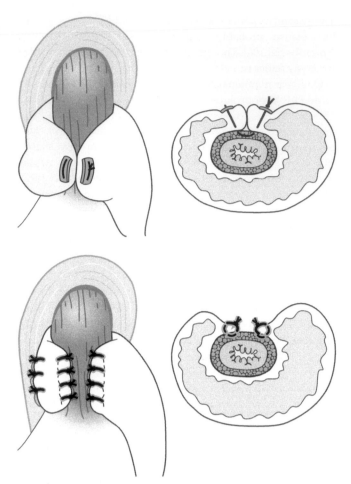

Figure 6.4 Appearance and cross-sectional views of the Nissen fundoplication, a full 360° wrap **(top)**, and the Toupet partial fundoplication **(bottom)**. These are the two most popular fundoplications used in laparoscopic antireflux surgery.

shortened esophagus, and poor esophageal motility. Esophageal manometry combined with impedance will identify ineffective esophageal peristalsis and previously misdiagnosed achalasia or scleroderma. Twenty-four-hour pH testing is needed in all patients with nonerosive GERD or in those with esophagitis not responding to PPI therapy. Gastric analysis and gastric emptying studies may be indicated in selected patients. Careful testing will result in modification of the original operation or an alternative diagnosis in approximately 25% of patients [53].

Antireflux surgery relieves reflux symptoms and reduces the need for stricture dilation in more than 90% of patients [124,125], but Barrett esophagus rarely regresses, and there is insufficient evidence that surgery reduces the risk of esophageal cancer [128]. Comparison studies have found antireflux surgery superior to lifestyle changes, antacids, and H_2RA and prokinetic therapy [70,81], but not PPI therapy, especially when dose titration is permitted [129]. Mortality is rare (< 1%) after antireflux surgery, but new postoperative complaints can occur in up to 25% of patients; these include dysphagia, gas bloat, diarrhea, and increased flatus [130]. Most symptoms improve over 1 year, but persistent complaints suggest too tight a wrap, a displaced fundoplication, or inadvertent damage to the vagus nerve. Successful antireflux surgery, however, does not guarantee a permanent cure. The best surgical results are obtained by experienced surgeons in high-volume centers; these report long-term symptom recurrence in only 10%–15% of patients [124]. However, most operations are performed by community or Veterans Affairs hospital surgeons. Here the results are not as good, with studies finding relapse of symptoms after 2 years in 32%, with 7% requiring repeat surgery [131] and return to regular use of antireflux medications in 62% of patients (one-half on PPIs) 10–15 years after fundoplication [132]. Potential factors contributing to these high relapse rates include inexperienced surgeons, low yearly number of operations per surgeon, and persistence of abdominal stressors (i.e., obesity, heavy isometric exercise or work) that gradually weaken the fundoplication. A suboptimal operation or severe symptom relapse may necessitate a second operation, which has less likelihood of a successful outcome [123]. Because optimal medical therapy is available to all patients with GERD, the risk and benefits of both long-term medical treatment and antireflux surgery must be carefully discussed with patients, so they can take part in this important decision.

New treatments

The future medical treatment of GERD involves drugs that interfere with transient LESRs but do not cause dysphagia. Baclofen, an agonist for γ-aminobutyric acid type B (GABA$_B$) receptors, has been shown to decrease reflux symptoms and to improve pH studies in healthy persons and in patients with GERD [133]. Newer endoscopic treatments of GERD have been approved by the FDA. These techniques include an endoscopic suturing system, radiofrequency energy delivery to the esophagogastric junction, and the injection of non-absorbable polymers into the submucosa surrounding the LES [134–136]. These procedures decrease the frequency of transient LES relaxation, but LES pressure is unchanged and less than 40% of patients have normal pH tests. To date, these techniques have been applied only to patients with small (< 2-cm) or no hernias and mild esophagitis. Results are encouraging, with improvement of symptoms and decreased medication requirements, but the cost-effectiveness and durability of the procedures is suspect (usually > 50% failure by 1–2 years) and reported complications include perforation, hemorrhage, pain, and death. Controlled studies with the radiofrequency and injectable polymer techniques show consistent symptom improvement over the sham procedure, inconsistent reduction in PPIs, and no significant improvement in LES pressure or pH profiles [137,138]. Serious adverse effects with the injectible techniques, including several deaths, led to the voluntary withdrawal of Enteryx

by the manufacturer in September 2005, and suspension of the Gatekeeper clinical program in 2005. A medical position statement by the American Gastroenterological Association (AGA) Institute stated that "current data suggests [sic] that there are no definite indications for endoscopy therapy for GERD at this time" [139].

References

1. Carlsson R, Dent J, Bolling-Sternevold E, et al. The usefulness of a structured questionnaire in the assessment of symptomatic gastro-esophageal reflux disease. Scand J Gastroenterol 1998;33:1023.
2. Klauser AG, Schindlebeck NE, Muller-Lissner SA. Symptoms of gastro-oesophageal reflux disease. Lancet 1990;335:205.
3. Dent J, Brun J, Fendrick AM, et al. An evidence-based appraisal of reflux disease management: the Genval report. Gut 1999;44(Suppl. 2): S1.
4. Powell DW. Barrier function of epithelial. Am J Physiol 1981; 241:G275.
5. Jacob P, Kahrilas PJ, Vanagunos A. Peristaltic dysfunction associated with non-obstructive dysphagia in reflux disease. Dig Dis Sci 1990;35:939.
6. Brzana RJ, Koch KL. Gastroesophageal reflux disease presenting with intractable nausea. Ann Intern Med 1997;126:704.
7. Helm JF, Dodds WJ, Hogan WJ, et al. Acid neutralizing capacity of human saliva. Gastroenterology 1987;83:69.
8. Collen MJ, Abdulian JD, Chen YK. Gastroesophageal disease in the elderly: more severe disease that requires aggressive therapy. Am J Gastroenterol 1995;90:1053.
9. Johnson DA, Winters C, Spurling TJ, et al. Esophageal acid sensitivity in Barrett's esophagus. J Clin Gastroenterol 1987;9:23.
10. Richter JE. Extraesophageal presentations of gastroesophageal reflux disease. Am J Gastroenterol 2000;25(Suppl.):S1.
11. Schofied PM, Bennett DH, Whorewell PJ, et al. Exertional gastro-esophageal reflux: a mechanism for symptoms in patients with angina pectoris and normal coronary angiograms. Br Med J 1987; 294:1459.
12. Hewson EG, Sinclair JW, Dalton CB, et al. Twenty-four hour esophageal pH monitoring: the most useful test for evaluating non-cardiac chest pain. Am J Med 1991;90:576.
13. Richter JE. Approach to the patient with non-cardiac chest pain. In: Yamada T (ed.) Textbook of gastroenterology, 2nd edn. Philadelphia: JB Lippincott, 1995:648.
14. Singh S, Richter JE, Hewson EG, et al. The contribution of gastroesophageal reflux to chest pain in patients with coronary artery disease. Ann Intern Med 1992;117:824.
15. Osler WB. The principles of internal medicine. New York: Appleton, 1892.
16. Sontag SJ, O'Connell S, Khandelwal S, et al. Most asthmatics have gastroesophageal reflux with or without bronchodilator therapy. Gastroenterology 1990;99:613.
17. Harding SM, Sontag SJ. Asthma and gastroesophageal reflux. Am J Gastroenterol 2000;95(Suppl.):S23.
18. Irwin RS, Curley FJ, French CL. Difficult-to-control asthma: contributing factors and outcome of a systematic protocol. Chest 1993; 103:1662.
19. Tuchman DN, Boyle JT, Pack AI, et al. Comparison of airway responses following tracheal or esophageal acidification in the cat. Gastroenterology 1984;87:872.
20. Schan CA, Harding SM, Haile JM, et al. Gastroesophageal reflux-induced bronchoconstriction: an intraesophageal acid infusion study using state-of-the-art technology. Chest 1994;105:731.
21. Jack CIA, Calverley PMA, Donnelly RJ, et al. Simultaneous tracheal and oesophageal pH measurements in asthmatic patients with gastro-oesophageal reflux. Thorax 1995;50:201.

22. Koufman JA. The otolaryngologic manifestations of gastroeso-phageal reflux disease: a clinical investigation of 225 patients using ambulatory 24-hour pH monitoring and an experimental investiga-tion of the role of acid and pepsin in the development of laryngeal injury. Laryngoscope 1978;88:339.

23. Wong RKH, Hanson DG, Waring PJ, Shaw G. ENT manifestations of gastroesophageal reflux. Am J Gastroenterol 2000;95(Suppl.):S15.

24. Irwin RS, Richter JE. Gastroesophageal reflux and cough. Am J Gastroenterol 2000;95(Suppl.):S39.

25. Lazarchik DA, Filler SJ. Dental erosion: predominant oral lesion in gastroesophageal reflux disease. Am J Gastroenterol 2000;95(Suppl.): S33.

26. Jacob P, Kahrilas PH, Herzon G. Proximal esophageal pH: manometry in patients with "reflux laryngitis." Gastroenterology 1991;100:305.

27. Schindlebeck NE, Klauser AG, Voderholzer WA, Mueller-Lissner S. Empiric therapy for gastroesophageal reflux disease. Arch Intern Med 1995;155:1808.

28. Fass R, Ofman JJ, Granelk I, et al. Clinical and economic assessment of the omeprazole test in patients with symptomatic suggestive of gastroesophageal reflux disease. Arch Intern Med 1999;159:2161.

29. Fass R, Fennerty MB, Ofman JJ. The clinical and economic value of a short course of omeprazole in patients with non-cardiac chest pain. Gastroenterology 1998;115:42.

30. Ours TM, Kavuru MS, Schilz R, Richter JE. A prospective evalu-ation of esophageal testing and a double blind, randomized study of omeprazole in a diagnostic and therapeutic algorithm for chronic cough. Am J Gastroenterol 1999;94:3131.

31. Richter JE. Severe reflux esophagitis. Gastrointest Endosc Clin North Am 1994;4:677.

32. Johnson LF, DeMeester, Haggitt RC. Endoscopic signs of gastro-esophageal reflux objectively evaluated. Gastrointest Endosc 1976; 22:151.

33. Ollyo JB, Lang F, Fontolliet C, Monnier P. Savary-Miller's new endoscopic grading of reflux-oesophagitis: a simple, reproducible, logical, complete and useful classification. Gastroenterology 1990;98: A100.

34. Hetzel DJ, Dent J, Reed WD, et al. Healing and relapse of severe pep-tic esophagitis after treatment with omeprazole. Gastroenterology 1988;95:903.

35. Armstrong D, Bennett JR, Blum AL, et al. The endoscopic assess-ment of esophagitis: a progress report of observer agreement. Gastroenterology 1996;111:85.

36. Funch-Jensen P, Kock K, Christensen LA, et al. Microscopic appear-ance of the esophageal mucosa in a consecutive series of patients submitted to endoscopy: correlation with gastroesophageal reflux symptoms and microscopic findings. Scand J Gastroenterol 1986;21:65.

37. Riddell RH. The biopsy diagnosis of gastroesophageal reflux dis-ease, "carditis," and Barrett's esophagus. Am J Surg Pathol 1996;20: 31.

38. Dent J. Microscopic esophageal mucosal injury in non-erosive reflux disease. Clin Gastroenterol Hepatol 2007;5:4.

39. Tunmmala V, Barwick KW, Sontag S, et al. The significance of intraepithelial eosinophils in the histological diagnosis of gastro-esophageal reflux disease. Am J Clin Pathol 1987;87:43.

40. Winters HS, Madara JL, Stafford RJ, et al. Intraepithelial eosinophils: a new diagnostic criterion for reflux esophagitis. Gastroenterology 1982;83:818.

41. DeMeester TR, Johnson LF, Joseph GJ, et al. Pattern of gastro-esophageal reflux in health and disease. Ann Surg 1976;184:459.

42. Hirano I, Richter JE. ACG Practice Guidelines: Esophageal reflux testing. Am J Gastroenterol 2007;102:668.

43. Taghavi SA, Ghasedi M, Firoozi-Saberi M, et al. Symptom associ-ation probability and symptom sensitivity index: preferable but still suboptimal predictors of response of high dose omeprazole. Gut 2005;1067.

44. Shaker R, Milbrath M, Ren J, et al. Esophagopharyngeal distribu-tion of refluxed gastric acid in patients with reflux laryngitis. Gastroenterology 1995;109:1575.

45. Richter JE. Ear nose and throat and respiratory manifestations of GERD; an increasing conundrum. Eur J Gastroenterol Hepatol 2004; 16:1.

46. Pandolfino JE, Richter JE, Ours T, et al. Ambulatory esophageal pH monitoring using a wireless system. Am J Gastroenterol 2003;98:740.

47. Sifrim D, Holloway R, Silny J, et al. Acid, non-acid and gas reflux in patients with gastroesophageal reflux disease during ambulatory 24-hour impedance recordings. Gastroenterology 2001;120:1599.

48. Ott DJ, Kelley TF, Chen MYM, et al. Use of a marshmallow bolus for evaluating lower esophageal mucosal rings. Am J Gastroenterol 1991;86:817.

49. Baker ME, Eistein DM, Hertz BR, et al. Integrating the barium eso-phagram before and after anti-reflux surgery. Radiology 2007;243:329.

50. Thompson JK, Koehler RE, Richter JE. Detection of gastroesophageal reflux: value of the barium studies compared with 24-hour pH monitoring. AJR Am J Roentgenol 1994;162:621.

51. Johnston BT, Troshinsky MB, Castell JA, Castell DO. Comparison of barium radiology with esophageal pH monitoring in the diagnosis of gastroesophageal reflux disease. Am J Gastroenterol 1996;91:1181.

52. Kahrilas PJ, Dodds WJ, Hogan WJ, et al. Esophageal peristaltic dys-function in peptic esophagitis. Gastroenterology 1986;91:897.

53. Waring JP, Hunter JG, Oddsdottir M. The preoperative evaluation of patients considered for laparoscopic antireflux surgery. Am J Gastroenterol 1995;90:35.

54. Leite LP, Johnston BT, Barrett J, et al. Ineffective esophageal motility: the primary finding in patients with non-specific esophageal motil-ity disorder. Dig Dis Sci 1997;42:1853.

55. Oleynikov D, Eubanks TR, Oelschlager BK, Pellegrini CA. Total fun-doplication is the operation of choice for patients with gastro-esophageal reflux and defective peristalsis. Surg Endosc 2002;16:909.

56. Tutian R. Castell DO. Clarification of the esophageal function defect in patients with manometric ineffective esophageal motility: studies using combined impedance-manometry. Gastroenterology 2004;2: 230.

57. Pace F, Santalucia F, Bianchi-Porro G. Natural history of gastro-esophageal reflux disease without esophagitis. Gut 1991;32:845.

58. Labenz J, Nocon M, Lind T, et al. Prospective follow-up from the ProGERD study suggests that GERD is not a categorical disease. Am J Gastroenterol 2006;101:2457.

59. Winters C, Spurling TJ, Chokanian SJ, et al. Barrett's esophagus: a prevalent, occult complication of gastroesophageal reflux disease. Gastroenterology 1987;92:118.

60. Lind T, Havelund T, Carlsson R, et al. Heartburn without oesophag-itis: efficacy of omeprazole therapy and features determining thera-peutic response. Scand J Gastroenterol 1997;32:974.

61. Jones RH, Hungin ADS, Phillips J, et al. Gastroesophageal reflux dis-ease in primary care in Europe: clinical presentation and endoscopic findings. Eur J Gen Pract 1995;1:149.

62. Robinson M, Earnest D, Rodriguez-Stanley S, et al. Heartburn requiring frequent antacid use may indicate significant illness. Arch Intern Med 1998;156:2373.

63. Fass R, Fennerty MB, Vakil N. Nonerosive reflux disease: current concepts and dilemmas. Am J Gastroenterol 2001;96:303.

64. Caviglia R, Ribolsi M, Maggiano N, et al. Dilated intercellular spaces of esophageal epithelium in nonerosive reflux disease patients with physiological esophageal acid exposure. Am J Gastroenterol 2005;100:543.

65. Trimble KC, Douglas S, Pryde A, Heading RC. Clinical character-istics and natural history of symptomatic but not excess gastro-esophageal reflux. Dig Dis Sci 1995;40:1098.

66. Hetzel DJ, Dent J, Reed WD, et al. Healing and relapse of severe pep-tic esophagitis after treatment with omeprazole. Gastroenterology 1988;95:903.

67. Vigneri S, Termini R, Leandro G, et al. A comparison of five main-tenance therapies for reflux esophagitis. N Engl J Med 1995;333:1106.

68. Isolauri J, Luostarinen M, Isolauri E, et al. Natural history of gastro-esophageal reflux disease: 17–22 year follow-up of 60 patients. Am J Gastroenterol 1997;92:37.

69. Brossard E, Monnier JB, Ollyo JB, et al. Serious complications–stenosis, ulcer and Barrett's epithelium – develop in 21.6% of adults with erosive reflux esophagitis. Gastroenterology 1992;100: A36.

70. Spechler SJ. Comparison of medical and surgical therapy for complicated gastroesophageal reflux disease in veterans. N Engl J Med 1992;326:786.

71. Rejeb MB, Bouché O, Zeitoun P. Study of 47 consecutive patients with peptic esophageal stricture compared with 3880 cases of reflux esophagitis. Dig Dis Sci 1992;37:7338.

72. Kaltenback T, Crockett S, Gerson LB. Are lifestyle measures effective in patients with gastroesophageal reflux disease? An evidence based medicine approach. Arch Intern Med 2006;166:965.

73. Meining A, Classen M. The role of diet and lifestyle measures in the pathogenesis and treatment of gastroesophageal reflux disease. Am J Gastroenterol 2000;95:2692.

74. Harvey RF, Gordon PC, Hadley N, et al. Effects of sleeping with the bed-head raised and of ranitidine in patients with severe peptic esophagitis. Lancet 1987;2:1200.

75. Hampel H, Abraham NS, El-Serag HB. Meta-analysis: obesity and the risk of gastroesophageal reflux disease and its complications. Ann Intern Med 2005;143:199.

76. Dennish GW, Castell DO. Inhibiting effect of smoking on the lower esophageal sphincter. N Engl J Med 1971;284:1136.

77. Kaufman SE, Kaye MD. Induction of gastroesophageal reflux by alcohol. Gut 1978;19:336.

78. Feldman M, Barnett C. Relationship between the acidity and osmolality of popular beverages and reported postprandial heartburn. Gastroenterology 195;108:125.

79. Weberg R, Berstad A. Symptomatic effect of a low-dose antacid regimen in reflux oesophagitis. Scand J Gastroenterol 1989;24:401.

80. Buts JP, Barudi C, Otte JB. Double-blind controlled study on the efficacy of sodium alginate (Gaviscon) in reducing gastroesophageal reflux assessed by 24h continuous pH monitoring in infants and children. Eur J Pediatr 1987;146:156.

81. Behar J, Sheahan DG, Biancani P, et al. Medical and surgical management of reflux esophagitis: a 38-month report on a prospective clinical trial. N Engl J Med 1975;293:263.

82. Gonzalez ER, Grillo JA. Over-the-counter histamine₂-blocker therapy. Ann Pharmacother 1994;28:392.

83. Fendrick AM, Shaw M, Schachtel B, et al. Self-selection and use patterns of over-the-counter omeprazole for frequent heartburn. Clin Gastroenterol Hepatol 2004;2:17.

84. Ramirez B, Richter JE. Promotility drugs in the treatment of gastro-oesophageal reflux disease. Aliment Pharmacol Ther 1993;7:5.

85. Dilawari JB, Misiewcz JJ. Action of metoclopramide on the GE junction in man. Gut 1973;14:380.

86. Wysowski DK, Corken A, Gallo-Torres H, et al. Postmarketing reports of QT prolongation and ventricular arrhythmia in association with cisapride and Food and Drug Administration regulatory action. Am J Gastroenterol 2001;96:1698.

87. Lipsy RJ, Fennerty B, Fagan TC. Clinical review of histamine-2 receptor antagonists. Arch Intern Med 1990;150:745.

88. Sontag SJ. Gastroesophageal reflux disease. Brandt LJ. Clinical practice of gastroenterology. Philadelphia: Churchill Livingstone, 1999:21.

89. Chiba N, Gara CJ, Wilkinson JM, Hunt RH. Speed of healing and symptom relief in grade II to IV gastroesophageal reflux disease: a meta-analysis. Gastroenterology 1997;112:1798.

90. Peghini PL, Katz PO, Bracy NA, Castell DO. Nocturnal recovery of gastric acid secretion with twice-daily dosing of proton pump inhibitors. Am J Gastroenterol 1998;93:763.

91. Peghini PL, Katz PO, Castell DO. Ranitidine controls nocturnal gastric acid breakthrough on omeprazole: a controlled study in normal subjects. Gastroenterology 1998;115:1335.

92. Fackler WK, Ours TM, Vaezi MF, Richter JE. Long term effect of H₂RA therapy on nocturnal gastric acid breakthrough. Gastroenterology 2002;112:625.

93. Wilder-Smith CH, Merki HS. Tolerance during dosing with H₂-receptor antagonists: an overview. Scand J Gastroenterol Suppl 1992;27:14.

94. Klinkenberg-Knol EC, Festen HPM, Meuwissen SGM. Pharmacological management of gastro-oesophageal reflux disease. Drugs 1995;49:697.

95. Wolfe MM, Sachs G. Acid suppression: optimizing therapy for gastroduodenal ulcer healing, gastroesophageal reflux disease, and stress-related erosive syndrome. Gastroenterology 2000;118(Suppl.):9.

96. Hunt RH. Importance of pH control in the management of GERD. Arch Intern Med 1999;159:649.

97. Carlson R, Dent J, Watts R, et al. Gastro-oesophageal reflux disease in primary care: an international study of different treatment strategies with omeprazole. Eur J Gastroenterol Hepatol 1998;10:119.

98. Sontag SJ, Hirschowitz BH, Holt S, et al. Two doses of omeprazole versus placebo in symptomatic erosive esophagitis: the US multicenter study. Gastroenterology 1992;102:109.

99. Castell DO, Richter JE, Robinson M, et al. Efficacy and safety of lansoprazole in the treatment of erosive reflux esophagitis. Am J Gastroenterol 1996;91:1749.

100. Cloud ML, Enas N, Humphries TJ, et al. Rabeprazole in treatment of acid peptic diseases. Dig Dis Sci 1998;43:993.

101. Richter JE, Bochenek W. Pantoprazole US GERD Study Group. Oral pantoprazole for erosive esophagitis: a placebo-controlled, randomized clinical trial. Am J Gastroenterol 2000;95:3071.

102. van Pinxteren B, Numan ME, Bonis PA, Lau J. Short-term treatment with proton-pump inhibitors, H₂RAs and prokinetic for gastroesophageal reflux disease-like symptoms and endoscopy negative reflux disease. The Cochrane Database of Systematic Reviews 2004:3: CD002095.

103. Bianchi Porro G, Pace F, Peracchia A, et al. Short-term management of refractory reflux esophagitis with different doses of omeprazole or ranitidine. J Clin Gastroenterol 1992;15:192.

104. Gralnek IM, Dulai GS, Fennerty MB, Spiegel BNR. Esompeprazole vs other proton pump inhibitors in erosive esophagitis: a meta-analysis of randomized clinical trials. Clin Gastroenterol Hepatol 2006;4:1452.

105. Garnett WR. Consideration for long-term use of proton pump inhibitors. Am J Health Syst Pharm 198;55:2269.

106. Toussaint J, Gossuin A, Deruyttere M, et al. Healing and prevention of relapse of reflux esophagitis by cisapride. Gut 1991;35:590.

107. Robinson M, Lanza F, Avener D, Haber M. Effective maintenance treatment of reflux esophagitis with low-dose omeprazole. Ann Intern Med 1996;124:859.

108. Donnellan C, Sharma N, Preston C, Moayyedi P. Medical treatments for the maintenance therapy of reflux esophagitis and endoscopic negative reflux disease. The Cochrane Database of Systematic Reviews 2004;3:CD003245.

109. Vigneri S, Termini R, Leandes G, et al. A comparison of five maintenance therapies for reflex esophagitis. N Engl J Med 1995;333: 1106.

110. Klinkenberg-Knol EC, Feston HPM, Janssen JBM, et al. Long-term treatment with omeprazole for refractory reflux esophagitis: efficacy and safety. Ann Intern Med 1994;121:161.

111. Klinkenberg-Knol EC, Nelis F, Dent J, et al. Long-term omeprazole treatment in resistant gastroesophageal reflux disease: efficacy, safety, and influence on gastric mucosa. Gastroenterology 2000; 118:661.

112. Howden CW. Vitamin B₁₂ levels during prolonged treatment with proton pump inhibitors. J Clin Gastroenterol 2000;30:29.

113. Freston JW. Omeprazole, hypergastrinemia and gastric carcinoid tumors. Ann Intern Med 1994;121:232.

114. Kuipers E, Lundell L, Klinkenberg-Knol EC, et al. Atrophic gastritis and Helicobacter pylori infection in patients with reflux esophagitis treated with omeprazole or fundoplication. N Engl J Med 1996;334: 1018.

115. Food and Drug Administration (FDA). Proton pump inhibitors relabeling for cancer risk not warranted. Washington, DC: FDA, 1996.

116. Richter JE. Gastroesophageal reflux disease in the older patient:

presentation, treatment and complications. Am J Gastroenterol 2000; 95:368.

117. Zimmerman A, Walters JK, Katona B, et al. Alternative methods of proton pump inhibitor administration. Consult Pharm 1997;9:990.

118. Richter JE. Review article: The management of heartburn during pregnancy. Aliment Pharmacol Ther 2005;23:749.

119. Ranchet G, Gangemi O, Petrone M. Sucralfate in the treatment of gravid pyrosis. G Ital Ostet Ginecol 1990;12:1.

120. Larson JP, Patatanian E, Miner PB, et al. Double-blind, placebo controlled study of ranitidine for gastroesophageal reflux disease symptoms during pregnancy. Obstet Gynecol 1997;90:83.

121. Cremmini F, Wise J, Moayyedi P, Talley N. Diagnostic and therapeutic use of proton pump inhibitors in non-cardiac chest pain: a meta-analysis. Am J Gastroenterol 2005;100:1226.

122. Ireland AC, Holloway RH, Toouli J, Dent J. Mechanisms underlying the anti-reflux action of fundoplication. Gut 1993;34:303.

123. Rice TW. Why antireflux surgery fails. Dig Dis 2000;18:43.

124. DeMeester TR, Bonavina L, Albertucci M. Nissen fundoplication for gastroesophageal reflux disease: evaluation of primary repair in 100 consecutive patients. Ann Surg 1986;204:9.

125. Horvath KD, Jobe BA, Herron DM, Swanstrom LL. Laparoscopic Toupet fundoplication is an inadequate procedure for patients with severe reflux disease. J Gastrointest Surg 1999;3:583.

126. Gastal OL, Hagen JA, Peters JH. Short esophagus: analysis of predictors and clinical implications. Arch Surg 1999;134:633.

127. So JBY, Zeitel SM, Rattner DW. Outcomes of atypical symptoms attributed to gastroesophageal reflux treated by laparoscopic fundoplication. Surgery 1998;124:28.

128. Tran T, Spechler SJ, Richardson P, El-Serag HB. Fundoplication and the risk of esophageal cancer in gastroesophageal reflux disease: a Veteran's Affairs cohort study. Am J Gastroenterol 2005;100:1002.

129. Lundell L, Miettinen P, Myrvold HE, et al. Continued (5-year) follow-up of a randomized clinical study comparing antireflux surgery and omeprazole in gastroesophageal reflux disease. J Am Coll Surg 2001;192:172.

130. Perdikis G, Hinder RA, Lund RJ, et al. Laparoscopic Nissen fundoplication: where do we stand? Surg Laparosc Endosc 1997;7:17.

131. Vakil N, Shaw M, Kriby R. Clinical effectiveness of laparoscopic fundoplication in a US community. Am J Med 2003;114:1.

132. Spechler SJ, Lee EL, Ahnen D, et al. Long-term outcome of medical and surgical therapies for gastroesophageal reflux disease: followup of a randomized controlled trial. JAMA 2001;285:23331.

133. Lidums I, Lehmann A, Checklin H, et al. Control of transient lower esophageal sphincter relaxations and reflux by the GABA$_B$ agonist baclofen in normal subjects. Gastroenterology 2000;118:7.

134. Kahrilas PJ. Radiofrequency therapy for the lower esophageal sphincter for the treatment of GERD. Gastrointest Endosc 2003;57: 723.

135. Fennerty MB. Endoscopic suturing for the treatment of GERD. Gastrointest Endosc 2003;57:390.

136. Edmundowicz SA. Injection therapy for the lower esophageal sphincter for the treatment of GERD. Gastrointest Endosc 2004;59:545.

137. Corley DA, Katz P, Wo JM, et al. Improvement of gastroesophageal reflux symptoms after radiofrequency energy: a randomized, shamcontrolled trial. Gastroenterology 2003;125:668.

138. Deviere J, Costamanga G, Neuhas H, et al. Nonresorbable copolymer implantation for gastroesophageal reflux disease: a randomized sham-controlled multicenter trial. Gastroenterology 2005;128:532.

139. Falk GW, Fennerty MB, Rothestein RI. AGA Institute technical review on the use of endoscopic therapy for gastroesophageal reflux disease. Gastroenterology 2006;131:1351.

Approach to the patient with dyspepsia and peptic ulcer disease

Andrew H. Soll, David Y. Graham

Cliinical presentation and diagnosis of peptic ulcer, 99

Natural history of peptic ulcer, 103

Antiulcer pharmacology, 104

Medical treatment of active peptic ulcer disease, 110

Cliinical presentation and diagnosis of peptic ulcer

Peptic ulcer classically presents with symptoms of acid dyspepsia, which appears to reflect gastroduodenal sensitization to H^+ ions. However, it can also present with other symptoms [1–3] (Table 7.1).

"Acid dyspepsia": the classic ulcer symptom

In the era of classic diseases, duodenal ulcer (DU) was thought to be easy to diagnose [4]. Ulcer symptoms are characterized as a burning epigastric "hunger" pain or discomfort that tends to occur when acid is secreted in the absence of food buffer (e.g., 2–3 h after meals) and at night, usually between 23.00 and 02.00, when the circadian stimulation of acid secretion is maximal. Pain rarely occurs before breakfast. Alkali, food, and antisecretory agents produce relief such that "classic" patients tend to "feed" their ulcers. However, the classic presentation proved not to be specific for peptic ulcer disease (PUD), because it occurs in nonulcer dyspepsia, and many ulcer patients have "atypical" symptoms [1–3,5,6]. Despite these qualifications, food relief is more likely to occur with peptic ulcer, whereas food provocation of symptoms (postprandial pain or food intolerance) and nausea have negative predictive value for underlying PUD [7]. Gastric ulcer (GU) is less likely than DU to be relieved by antacids or food and more likely to display food provocation.

The discomfort occurs in the epigastrium in about two-thirds of symptomatic ulcer patients, but may occasionally localize in the right or left upper quadrants or hypochondrium [1]. Radiation of the pain to the back may also occur, but primary back pain is atypical. Clusters of pain lasting a few weeks followed by symptom-free periods of weeks or months is a pattern characteristic of classic DU. However, the classic symptoms of acid dyspepsia with food relief, described above, occur in only about 50% of patients with DU disease (Table 7.1).

Unencumbered by placebo controls, W.L. Palmer demonstrated that aspiration of gastric contents relieved pain and that reinfusion of the acidic (but not neutralized) gastric juice precipitated pain [8], supporting the concept that acid bathing an ulcer crater caused symptoms. In a double-blind protocol, duodenal infusion of acid, but not saline, induced pain in about 40% of patients with active duodenal ulcers [9], whereas infusion of saline produced pain in only 10%. Pain was not produced by infusions in controls. Thus, in at least a portion of patients with DU disease, symptoms are provoked by acid bathing the ulcer.

Data from numerous controlled endoscopic trials, largely in the "pre-*Helicobacter pylori* (Hp) era," have shown that symptoms and mucosal pathology are frequently dissociated such that ulcer healing does not guarantee disappearance of symptoms. Conversely, ulcers may also be present without producing symptoms; 15%–44% of ulcer patients who become symptom-free during therapy still have an ulcer crater at endoscopy. Thus, in a largely Hp-positive group of ulcer patients, resolution of symptoms with antiulcer – but not anti-Hp – therapy does not predict ulcer healing. Complete resolution of dyspeptic symptoms may have different implications when Hp is being treated; complete symptom resolution at 3 months had a 98% positive predictive value for successful eradication of Hp infection [10]. By contrast, persisting symptoms had only a 25% positive predictive value for persisting Hp infection [10]. The presence or

Principles of Clinical Gastroenterology. Edited by Tadataka Yamada, David H. Alpers, Anthony N. Kalloo, Neil Kaplowitz, Chung Owyang, and Don W. Powell. © 2008 Blackwell Publishing. ISBN 978-1-4051-69103

Table 7.1 Symptoms of gastric and duodenal ulcers and nonulcer dyspepsia [1–3]

Symptom	Gastric ulcer (%)	Duodenal ulcer (%)	Nonulcer dyspepsia (%)
Pain/discomfort	100	100	100
Features of the pain:			
Primary pain:			
Epigastric	67	61–86	52–73
Right hypochondrium	6	7–17	4
Left hypochondrium	6	3–5	5
Frequently severe	68	53	37
Within 30 min of food	20	5	32
Gnawing pain	13	16	6
Increased by food	24	10–40	45
Clusters (episodic)	16	56	35
Relieved by alkali	36–87	39–86	26–75
Food relief	2–48	20–63	4–32
Occurs at night	32–43	50–88	24–32
Not related to food or variable	22–53	21–49	22–65
Radiation to back	34	20–31	24–28
Increased appetite		19	
Anorexia	46–57	25–36	26–36
Weight loss	24–61	19–45	18–32
Nausea	54–70	49–59	43–60
Vomiting	38–73	25–57	26–34
Heartburn	19	27–59	28
Nondyspeptic symptoms	2	8	18
Fatty food intolerance		41–72	53
Bloating	55	49	52
Belching	48	59	60

absence of persisting dyspepsia is an inadequate measure of Hp status after therapy and emphasizes the need for testing after Hp eradication (see below).

The dissociation between ulcers and symptoms was also evident in the impact of Hp eradication on the long-term symptomatic outcomes. One to 3 years after successful eradication of Hp, 55% of ulcer patients had resolution of their dyspeptic symptoms compared with only 18% of patients for whom Hp eradication failed [11]. Although Hp cure clearly reduces symptoms in ulcer patients, excluding patients with preexisting gastroesophageal reflux disease (GERD), approximately one-third of Hp-positive ulcer patients can be expected to have persisting symptoms 1 to 3 years after successful cure of the Hp infection. The pathogenesis of these symptoms remains unclear. However, it is clear that the symptoms experienced by ulcer patients reflect factors more complex than simply acid bathing an ulcer crater. Symptoms may relate in part to sensitization of afferent nerves in response to tissue injury (i.e., visceral somatic hypersensitivity) [12,13]. Dyspepsia may result in an exaggerated response to superimposed chemical, mechanical, infectious, or inflammatory insults, and the gastroduodenitis associated with Hp or the inflammatory response to the peptic ulcer itself may produce this sensitization.

Gastroesophageal reflux, duodenal ulcer, *Helicobacter pylori*, and acid secretion

Gastroesophageal reflux disease evident by heartburn, acid reflux, or esophagitis occurs in 20%–60% of DU patients (Table 7.1) [11]. Both GERD and DU are common disorders, and Berkson's fallacy deserves consideration [14] (see Table 7.2). However, the association is strong and has a clear pathophysiological basis. With acid hypersecretion from gastrinoma or idiopathic PUD defined as basal acid output greater than 15 mmol/h, GERD was found in 80% (65% with grade 2 or greater esophagitis and 15% with heartburn only) [15]. Furthermore, patients with esophagitis had a lower median lower esophageal sphincter pressure (LESP) of 15.5 mmHg, compared with 23 mmHg in those without symptoms. Frequent vomiting and obesity were also identified as risk factors for esophagitis, whereas Hp was a strong negative predictor (odds ratio, 0.16) [15]. Therefore, GERD in an ulcer patient should be one clue to an underlying acid hypersecretory disorder.

This association between GERD and PUD has important implications for management. Ulcer patients who are Hp-positive with prominent GERD symptoms are more likely to have persisting symptoms after Hp eradication [11]. In contrast, treatment of Hp in GERD patients either has no effect on requirements for therapy or is associated with an improvement [11,16].

History and physical examination

Clinical evaluation should accomplish three goals. The first is to elicit a history and findings that help discriminate between common and uncommon disorders that overlap with, obscure, or mimic ulcer disease. The second is to evaluate the severity of underlying disease, if present. The third goal is to evaluate the psychosocial dimensions, including patient questions and concerns about the diagnosis, process, and prognosis. Clues to more severe forms of PUD, such as gastrinoma, include the presence of multiple duodenal ulcers, ulcers occurring distal to the duodenal bulb, a strong family history, ulcers that are refractory to medical therapy, and ulcers that recur after surgery. Additional clues to Zollinger–Ellison syndrome (gastrinoma) are peptic ulcers in subjects who are Hp-negative and negative for nonsteroidal antiinflammatory drugs (NSAIDs); an association with diarrhea, steatorrhea, or weight loss; and an association with hypercalcemia and renal stones.

Presentation of ulcer complications

Complications, especially in the absence of NSAID use, are usually associated with chronic peptic ulcers, and are often heralded by the development of ulcer symptoms or a change in symptom pattern. However, in roughly 25% of cases in the absence of NSAIDs, and 50% in the presence of NSAIDs, complications are the presenting symptom of an ulcer that was otherwise clinically silent [17,18]. The difference in symptom reporting between patients presenting with hemorrhage and those with symptoms may reflect the level of visceral sensation [19]. However, in controlled trials the new development of symptoms appears to herald ulcer formation in some patients [20,21]. Classically, penetrating ulcers present with a shift from the typical vague visceral discomfort to a more localized and intense pain that radiates to the back; the expected relief obtained from food or antacids is also diminished. A sudden development of severe, diffuse abdominal pain may indicate perforation. Vomiting is the cardinal feature present in most cases of pyloric outlet obstruction. Hemorrhage may be heralded by nausea, hematemesis, melena, or dizziness.

Unusual complications may also herald the presentation of peptic ulcer. Massive hemorrhage can occur with erosion into a major artery. Posterior perforation is usually characterized by insidious onset of upper abdominal pain caused by a sealed perforation, localized retroperitoneal abscess, or generalized contamination of the lesser sac and peritoneal cavity [22]. Pneumoperitoneum on chest radiography or computed tomography (CT) is a critical diagnostic clue. Valentino syndrome is a DU presenting with retroperitoneal perforation and right lower quadrant pain. The veiled right kidney sign (retroperitoneal air obscuring the right kidney) can be a clue [23]. Penetrating ulcers can also result in fistulae. Gastrocolonic fistulae occur with an anterior GU, and present with halitosis, feculent vomiting, postprandial diarrhea, dyspepsia, and weight loss [24]. An apparent double pylorus has been observed endoscopically to develop as a result of erosion of a GU into the duodenum [25]. Hepatic penetration has been observed with a large DU or GU [26].

Laboratory evaluation

Routine laboratory tests are typically normal. Screening tests should include a complete blood count, liver chemistries, serum creatinine, and serum calcium. A fasting serum gastrin is indicated in ulcers refractory to therapy, in patients with a positive family history, or those requiring surgery. The serum salicylate level can reveal unsuspected aspirin abuse, and determination of this is indicated in refractory and complicated cases. Surreptitious use of aspirin and NSAIDs can also be detected by testing for platelet cyclooxygenase (COX) activity [27].

Acid secretion

Formal gastric analysis has fallen into disfavor exacerbated by the fact that pentagastrin is largely unavailable. However, one can easily assess basal gastric acid secretion using traditional techniques and measure the acid concentration in gastric fluid including that obtained at the time of endoscopy. The presence of an elevated gastrin level should always prompt measurement of gastric acidity to exclude achlorhydria as the cause. A fasting hydrogen ion concentration of approximately 100 mmol/L or greater is highly suggestive of a hypersecretory state.

Testing for *Helicobacter pylori*

Patients with peptic ulcers have high pretest probabilities for the presence of Hp. This high pretest probability means that a positive test, whether it be the presence of anti-Hp IgG antibody, a [13C]urea or [14C]urea breath test (UBT), or a stool antigen test, is strong evidence of the presence of the infection, and treatment can be initiated. By contrast, especially in the setting of ulcer disease, a negative test has a reasonably high probability of being a false negative, and thus negative tests must be confirmed by a second test (e.g., one designed to identify the presence of active infection such as a UBT or stool antigen test). One caveat is that the use of proton pump inhibitors (PPIs), bismuth, or antibiotics reduces the bacterial load and will result in an increased risk of false-negative UBTs, stool antigen tests, histology, rapid urease tests, and culture. Before testing for Hp, administration of a PPI should be stopped for approximately 2 weeks and a histamine H_2 receptor antagonist (H_2RA) substituted, because the latter does not reduce bacterial load. Culture of Hp is generally neither available nor necessary, except for antibiotic susceptibility testing in refractory cases. Another caveat is that whereas experienced pathologists can diagnose Hp using hematoxylin and eosin (H&E) staining, false negatives are frequent, especially when the number of organisms is low. Special stains are recommended, especially when chronic gastritis is present. Because histology is more expensive than biopsy or rapid urease testing, at endoscopy it is reasonable to obtain biopsies from normal-appearing mucosa for both tests and then to discard histology specimens if the urease test is positive. Biopsies for histological testing for Hp should always include sampling of both the antrum and corpus.

Upper gastrointestinal radiography

A definitive radiographic diagnosis of peptic ulcer requires demonstration of barium within an ulcer niche, which is generally round or oval and may be surrounded by a smooth mound of edema [28,29]. Secondary changes include folds radiating to the crater, and deformities in the region secondary to spasm, edema, and scarring. The incisura found encircling a GU reflects secondary spasm of circular muscle. Secondary signs of DU include deformity of the duodenal bulb, which may be evidenced by flattening of the superior or inferior fornices, eccentricity of the pyloric channel, pseudo-diverticulum, or exaggerated outpouching of recesses at the base of the bulb [28]. In the presence of deformity of the duodenal bulb, edema of the folds, or postoperative deformity, ulcer craters become much more difficult to detect. False-positive results occur when barium is trapped between folds. Although endoscopy has replaced radiology as the technique of choice for the evaluation of upper gastrointestinal (GI) complaints in general and detection of cancer in particular, radiology can occasionally be useful. Radiographic signs suggesting gastric malignancy include:

• an ulcer within a definitive mass
• effaced, interrupted, fused, or nodular mucosal folds as they approach the margin of the crater
• negative, irregular filling defects in the ulcer crater.

Endoscopy

Endoscopy provides a sensitive, specific, and safe method for diagnosing peptic ulcers, allowing direct inspection and biopsy. Benign ulcers have smooth, regular, rounded edges, with a flat, smooth ulcer base often filled with exudate. Malignancy [30] is associated with an ulcerated mass that protrudes into the lumen; surrounding folds that are nodular, clubbed, fused, or stop short of the ulcer margin; or margins that are overhanging, irregular, or thickened. The gold standard for determining whether an ulcer is benign or malignant is biopsy. Biopsy should be performed even for gastric lesions with a benign endoscopic appearance; benign-appearing ulcers may harbor malignancy [31]. The proper number of biopsies has been debated and depends upon technique. Four jumbo biopsies of the ulcer margin are equivalent to six or seven adequate, regular-sized biopsies, the number shown to detect nearly all cancers. The description "adequate" biopsy warrants emphasis, because biopsies that do not provide a good sample of the lesion are useless at best and misleading at worst.

In addition to direct endoscopic inspection and biopsy, repeat endoscopy to confirm healing of gastric ulcers may be required for confirmation of benignity. Mandatory follow-up endoscopy for gastric ulcers has been superseded by individualized management based on the clinical situation, endoscopic findings, and the adequacy of initial biopsy. For example, an obviously benign ulcer in a young NSAID user without Hp infection and adequate initial biopsies that were negative would not mandate follow-up endoscopy to rule out malignancy. However, a large, endoscopically indeterminate ulcer in the body of the stomach of an elderly subject generally warrants repeat endoscopy and biopsy.

Computed tomography

Despite limited data, CT is clearly the most valuable test if a penetrating or perforated ulcer is suspected. Furthermore, the much higher resolution of the newer spiral and multislice CT images make them much more valuable for assessing the sometimes subtle findings of complicated ulcers. Advanced CT is clearly more effective than an upright chest radiograph in detecting free air, with positive findings in all 14 consecutive patients with perforation in one surgical series [32]. Ten of these 14 patients also had fluid collections, and five had inflammatory changes in surrounding soft tissues [32]. Extravasation or sinus tracks with intralumenal contrast material, discontinuity of the bowel wall, and mucosal thickening can also be useful findings in localizing the site of perforation or penetration, but these findings only appear to be reliable with the highest-resolution scanning equipment [33,34]. Use of oral contrast is controversial, but also appears to be valuable with higher-resolution equipment [33].

Recommendations regarding evaluation and follow-up

The goal in evaluating a patient with upper gastrointestinal symptoms is to arrive expeditiously at definitive diagnosis without unnecessarily exposing patients to costly and potentially risky diagnostic procedures. These decisions fall within the realm of "good clinical judgment;" there is no gold standard for decisions that are both cost-effective and appropriately cautious. However, decisions must be made and data interpreted in light of specific patient characteristics and diagnosis, such as patient age, socioeconomic background, index event, "ulcer" history, and prior work-up. Decisions would be different for a 25-year-old graduate student with uninvestigated dyspepsia than for a 70-year-old patient with prior documented ulcer complications. Decisions would also be different for patients with a firm, recent endoscopic diagnosis of ulcer, but no Hp testing, compared with a remote "ulcer" diagnosis on clinical grounds.

Complicated gastric ulcer or duodenal ulcer with unknown *H. pylori* status

With all ulcers, the question is "Hp, NSAIDs, neither, or both?" As noted above, testing for Hp is relatively straightforward provided that the caveats for false-negative results are taken

Table 7.2 Etiologies and disease associations for peptic ulcer

Ulcers due to defined mechanisms

Infection
  Helicobacter pylori
  Herpes simplex virus (HSV)
  Cytomegalovirus (CMV)
  Helicobacter heilmanni
  Other rare infections (e.g. tuberculosis, syphilis)
Drug exposure
  NSAIDs and aspirin
  Corticosteroids (when combined with NSAIDs)
  Bisphosphonates
  Clopidogrel
  Mycophenolate mofetil
  Potassium chloride
  Chemotherapy (e.g., hepatic infusion with 5-fluorouracil)
Hormonal or mediator-induced, including acid hypersecretory states
  Gastrinoma (Zollinger–Ellison syndrome)
  Systemic mastocytosis
  Basophilia in myeloproliferative disease
  Antral G cell hyperfunction (existence independent of Hp is
    debatable)
Vascular insufficiency including crack cocaine use
Mechanical: duodenal obstruction (e.g., annular pancreas)
Radiation therapy
Infiltrating disease
  Sarcoidosis
  Crohn's disease

Idiopathic peptic ulcer

Idiopathic hypersecretory (Hp) duodenal ulcer
Non-Hp, non-NSAID familial peptic ulcer
Non-Hp, non-NSAID peptic ulcer

**Comorbid ulcers associated with decompensated chronic disease
or acute multisystem failure**

Stress (ICU) ulcers
Chronic obstructive pulmonary disease
Cirrhosis
Renal failure
Organ transplantation
Other comorbidity, such as cardiovascular disease

Hp, *Helicobacter pylori*; ICU, intensive care unit; NSAIDs, nonsteroidal
antiinflammatory drugs.

into account. The goals include healing the ulcer and preventing its recurrence. If Hp is present it should be treated and at a suitable time (e.g., 4 weeks) after the end of therapy, cure should be confirmed (see "Confirmation of Hp cure" below). Patients with a history of ulcer complications are at a markedly increased risk for future life-threatening events. Hp eradication essentially removes that risk whereas a return to NSAID use is associated with a recurrent risk of a new complication.

H. pylori-negative ulcers

In ulcers that test negative for Hp, alternative etiologies deserve consideration (Table 7.2). However, the most common etiologies for Hp-negative ulcers are false-negative testing for Hp and undiscovered consumption of NSAIDs. Once Hp and NSAID use have been firmly excluded, then alternative etiologies deserve consideration, especially for complicated or troublesome ulcers.

Atypical ulcers
Giant ulcers

Giant ulcers commonly occur in association with NSAID consumption [35]. Giant duodenal or prepyloric ulcers have also been reported in association with end-stage renal failure [36]. Giant GU may also carry an increased risk of harboring carcinoma. Crohn's disease and other disease processes can present with giant ulcers [37].

Atypical duodenal ulcers

Duodenal carcinoma and invading pancreatic carcinoma typically present as masses but may produce benign-appearing ulcers. Because of the low yield, routine DU biopsies cannot be recommended unless the clinical condition warrants it, such as a refractory DU or an atypical endoscopic appearance.

Postbulbar ulcers

Generally, ulcers in the duodenum are located within 2–3 cm of the pylorus. Postbulbar ulcers are uncommon and suggest the presence of gastrinoma and other hypersecretory states. Differential diagnosis should include diverticula, adhesive bands, annular pancreas, and neoplasia of the pancreas and of the duodenum.

Natural history of peptic ulcer

The natural history of Hp-related DU and GU is to recur. Bardhan, following patients for 12 months after documented DU healing, observed that without medical treatment 26% of patients remained symptom-free and 74% relapsed; 33% had one relapse, 24% had two recurrences, and 17% experienced three or more recurrences [38]. The placebo-treated control groups drawn from numerous clinical trials of maintenance therapy indicate a similar 50%–80% recurrence rate during the 6–12 months following initial ulcer healing [39,40]. These recurrences can produce symptoms, but asymptomatic ulcers are frequently found at surveillance endoscopy. A number of factors influence the highly variable rate at which ulcers heal and recur (see "Factors influencing healing" below). Successful eradication of Hp radically changes the natural history and markedly reduces recurrences. However, after Hp eradication erosions may occur in the duodenum that spontaneously heal and do not produce any clinical problems [41,42]. Such posteradication erosions were probably responsible for reports of an unexpectedly high rate of "ulcer" recurrence after successful eradication in a post hoc subgroup analysis of patients participating in a US anti-Hp treatment trial [43].

The natural history of NSAID ulcers has not been formally studied in patients who continue on NSAIDs without ulcer treatment. It is clear that when NSAIDs are stopped, associated ulcers heal unless an independent cause of ulceration exists. Because NSAIDs impair healing, it is possible that such ulcers are more persistent than Hp ulcers.

The limited data that exists for non-HP, non-NSAID ulcers also suggest that they may persist. Persistence of the ulcer diathesis is also expected for hypersecretory, idiopathic PUD [44].

Antiulcer pharmacology

Antisecretory agents
Antisecretory agents accelerate the healing of ulcers regardless of the etiology. They also relieve ulcer-associated dyspepsia. Continued use retards the rate of ulcer recurrence and reduces the risk of complications.

H$_2$-receptor antagonists
Histamine H$_2$-receptor antagonists (H$_2$RAs) are competitive reversible inhibitors of histamine binding at H$_2$-receptors on parietal cells. These drugs are equally efficacious and safe and differ primarily in potency. Available drugs include cimetidine (Tagamet), ranitidine (Zantac), famotidine (Pepcid), and nizatidine (Axid). These drugs are also licensed for sale over the counter at reduced dosages, including Tagamet HB, Zantac 75, Pepcid AC, and Axid. There is no antibacterial activity against Hp from H$_2$RAs.

After oral dosing H$_2$RAs are well absorbed; absorption is inhibited (10%–20%) by concomitant antacids, but not by food. Peak serum concentrations occur 1–3 h after oral dosing. All four drugs cross the blood–brain barrier and placental barrier and are excreted in breast milk [45]. The distribution of cimetidine in cerebrospinal fluid appears to be increased in liver failure [45].

Cimetidine is the least potent of the H$_2$RAs and has the highest incidence of side effects and drug–drug interactions. As such, it has largely fallen into disfavor. For treatment of peptic ulcer disease H$_2$RAs have largely been replaced by PPIs because of the increased potency and lack of tachyphylaxis (tolerance) shown by the latter drugs. The advantages of H$_2$RA are lower cost and avoiding profound acid inhibition, which can have consequences such as impaired calcium absorption, increased fractures, and greater susceptibility to certain GI infections.

Proton pump inhibitors
Proton pump inhibitors (PPIs) block acid secretion at the hydrogen–potassium adenosine triphosphatase (H$^+$,K$^+$-ATPase) pump located on the lumenal border of the gastric parietal cell. This pump exchanges hydrogen for potassium across the parietal cell microvillus membrane, secreting hydrogen ions into the gastric lumen and creating the low-pH environment characteristic of gastric secretions. Proton pump inhibitors bind to and irreversibly inhibit the ATPase. Proton pump inhibitors are the most effective antisecretory agents available, achieving better pH control than provided by H$_2$RAs. Available agents include omeprazole (Prilosec), lansoprazole (Prevacid), pantoprazole (Protonix), rabeprazole (Aciphex), and esomeprazole (Nexium). Although PPIs have some direct antibacterial activity against Hp in vitro, used alone they do not cure the infection. As noted in the section on diagnosis, PPI therapy reduces the Hp load in the stomach and can result in false-negative diagnostic tests.

PPIs are acid-labile and are inactivated if permitted to dissolve in acidic gastric juice. Therefore, enteric coated granules that dissolve at pH 6 or above or sodium bicarbonate are used to protect the drug during transit through the stomach. When given with sodium bicarbonate buffer to fasting patients, PPIs are rapidly absorbed and peak plasma levels are reached in 30 min. With the enteric coated granules the peak concentration occurs 1–3 h after dosing and the drug is detectable in serum for about 6 h (Fig. 7.1a) [46]. The effectiveness of PPIs when given by oral administration relates closely to the AUC (area under the plasma concentration–time curve), rather than to peak plasma drug levels (Fig. 7.1b) [46–51]. The prolonged duration of PPI antisecretory action reflects irreversible inactivation of the parietal cell H$^+$,K$^+$-ATPase, rather than a prolonged serum half-life. Administering PPIs with food delays absorption but does not alter the AUC [52]. Although PPIs differ slightly in metabolism and potency, clinically they are completely interchangeable, and cost should be the primary consideration when choosing which to prescribe. Drug metabolism, as evident by the AUC [53], occurs through cytochrome P450, as considered below, and is prolonged with liver but not renal disease (Fig. 7.1c). Delayed metabolism is also observed with genetic P450 polymorphism and in the elderly. However, in light of the wide safety margin with these drugs and the apparent absence of accumulation, there are no current recommendations to alter dosage in the elderly or in the face of hepatic failure.

The dose- and time-dependency of inhibition of acid secretion by PPIs have the following characteristics.
• *A time lag* in the onset of antisecretory effectiveness is noted over the first 4–7 days of therapy, probably reflecting progressive inhibition of the H$^+$,K$^+$-ATPase and possibly increases in drug bioavailability. This lag period is inversely related to dose.
• *Variability in antisecretory effectiveness* probably is the result of variability in absorption and clearance, as reflected in the AUC. For example, after 7 days of therapy on the 10-mg omeprazole dose, some subjects have minimal inhibition

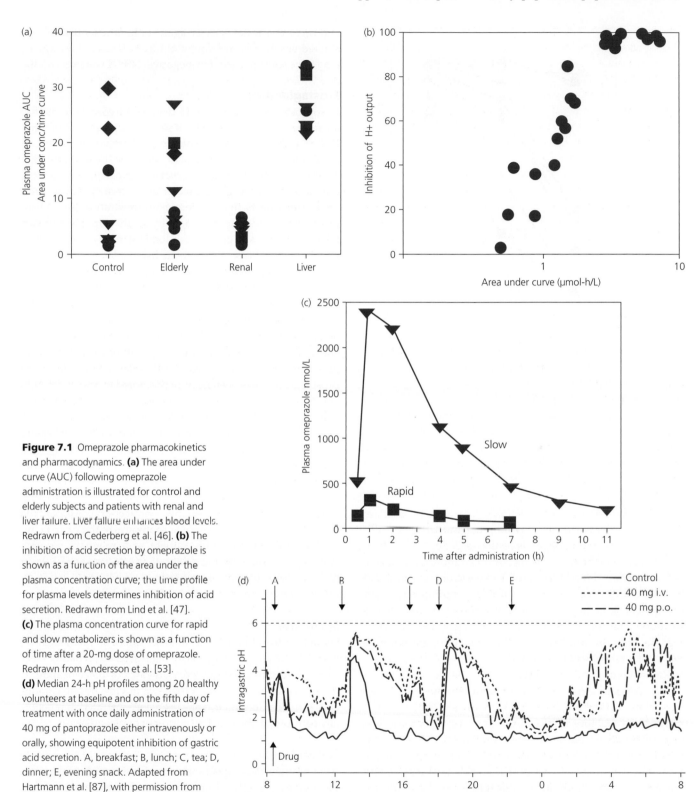

Figure 7.1 Omeprazole pharmacokinetics and pharmacodynamics. **(a)** The area under curve (AUC) following omeprazole administration is illustrated for control and elderly subjects and patients with renal and liver failure. Liver failure enhances blood levels. Redrawn from Cederberg et al. [46]. **(b)** The inhibition of acid secretion by omeprazole is shown as a function of the area under the plasma concentration curve; the time profile for plasma levels determines inhibition of acid secretion. Redrawn from Lind et al. [47]. **(c)** The plasma concentration curve for rapid and slow metabolizers is shown as a function of time after a 20-mg dose of omeprazole. Redrawn from Andersson et al. [53]. **(d)** Median 24-h pH profiles among 20 healthy volunteers at baseline and on the fifth day of treatment with once daily administration of 40 mg of pantoprazole either intravenously or orally, showing equipotent inhibition of gastric acid secretion. A, breakfast; B, lunch; C, tea; D, dinner; E, evening snack. Adapted from Hartmann et al. [87], with permission from Blackwell Publishing.

whereas others have more than 90% inhibition [54]. At 20 mg, inhibition is less variable [55] (Fig. 7.2), with mean inhibition of acidity (H^+ concentration) about 90% [56]. More consistent inhibition of acid secretion is observed at higher doses (Fig. 7.2). A PPI twice daily produces better inhibition of secretion than once daily dosing.

• *PPIs maximally inhibit stimulated parietal cells.* Because PPIs must be concentrated and activated in the acidic compartments

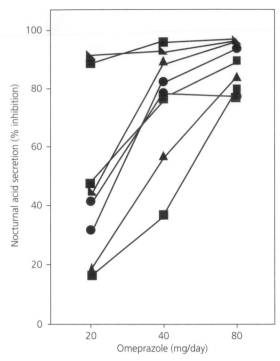

Figure 7.2 Dose response for omeprazole inhibition of nocturnal acid secretion. Acid secretion was determined during four nighttime sessions for seven patients with duodenal ulcer: single doses were given at 08.00 of placebo or omeprazole at 20, 40, or 80 mg. Acid secretion was then determined between 21.00 and 06.00, with the data expressed as a percentage of control secretion. This study illustrates the high variability of inhibition at low, but not high, doses of proton pump inhibitor. Data from Shearman et al. [55].

of the parietal cell, they will only inactivate the H^+,K^+-ATPase present in actively secreting membrane compartments. PPI effectiveness therefore depends on the degree of activation of acid secretion at the time of drug administration. Omeprazole action is reduced if administered while secretion is inhibited by H_2RAs [57], because efficacy varies depending on whether the patient is fasting, has recently taken an H_2RA, or has secretion activated by food, gastrin, or vagal pathways during the time the prodrug is circulating. PPIs are effective when taken shortly before meals.

• Rapid control of acid secretion can be achieved using higher doses of PPIs, or more frequent administration (i.e., 3 or 4 doses of 20 mg of omeprazole in the first 24 h).

• The bioavailability of PPIs administered by nasogastric tube or parenterally is comparable with oral dosing [58,59]. Intravenous formulations of esomeprazole and pantoprazole are available. The pharmacodynamics, duration of action, and effectiveness are essentially identical to the oral administration. In the setting of an intensive care unit (ICU) with fasting patients, intravenous PPI is most effective when given by continuous infusion of 8–10 mg/h after a bolus loading dose [60,61].

Anticholinergics

Anticholinergic medicines have weak antisecretory ability

and no antibacterial activity against Hp and should be considered obsolete for treatment of ulcer disease. These agents may have some place in Hp-negative, NSAID-negative PUD.

Prostaglandins

Misoprostol (Cytotec) is a 15-deoxy-15-hydroxy-16-methyl analogue of prostaglandin E_1; it shares the properties of other E-type prostaglandins, displaying moderate inhibition of basal and food-stimulated acid secretion in humans [62]. Topical activity seems to be crucial in prostaglandin action: oral administration gives greater antisecretory efficacy and fewer side effects than systemic administration [63]. Misoprostol has no antimicrobial activity against Hp. The primary adverse effects are crampy abdominal pain and diarrhea, which are dose-dependent effects [64,65]. Diarrhea occurred in 3%–39% of patients on the 200 µg q.i.d. dose of misoprostol, with the range reflecting trial design and the definition of diarrhea [64,65]. Diarrhea is often mild and transient, and may respond to a temporary reduction in dose. In clinical trials usually less than 20% of subjects drop out because of diarrhea, and the majority can take the drug without problems. The prevalence and significance of side effects associated with prostaglandins has been heavily promoted by manufacturers of other antisecretory drugs competing for the same market (chronic NSAID users). In clinical trials, misoprostol, even when given at half dose, has proven superior to PPIs for healing of endoscopic gastric ulcers and prevention of ulcer relapse among patients without concomitant Hp infections (see below) [66,67]. Prostaglandins of the E group are generally uterotropic and are contraindicated in women of childbearing potential who are not receiving contraception. All patients should be informed of this risk, to minimize the drug being inadvertently given by the patient to a pregnant woman. Although prostaglandins are about as effective as H_2RAs in healing ulcers, they have no role in ulcer healing. Their indication is for the prevention of NSAID-induced ulceration.

Sucralfate

Sucralfate, the aluminum hydroxide salt of sulfated sucrose, is a topical antiulcer drug whose main activity is coating ulcer sites, leading to slightly increased rates of ulcer healing. It does have an effect on Hp adherence in vitro but no convincing anti-Hp effect in vitro has been demonstrated. It is generally considered obsolete for treatment of ulcer disease.

Antacids

Antacids neutralize gastric acid and have a long history in the therapy of peptic ulcer. However, they are inconvenient, requiring multiple doses per day, and are outmoded for peptic ulcer disease.

Antimicrobials

H. pylori occurs as an infection of mucosal surfaces. As with other bacterial infections, the mainstay of therapy is use of antimicrobials to which the bacterium is susceptible. Because the infection is inside the stomach, but outside the body, there may be a place for topical therapy. In fact, because of the hostile acid environment of the stomach, topical therapy may greatly enhance overall effectiveness. It is not clear how much of the effectiveness of current therapies is related to the topical action of the drugs and how much is due to a systemic action, but both are probably important. There is considerable evidence that Hp also invades surface epithelial cells and thus the combination of topical and systemic actions may be best.

Topical agents

Bismuth salts have been used to treat "gastritis" and peptic ulcers for over 200 years. Bismuth is directly bactericidal to Hp and leads to bacterial lysis. Upon ingesting bismuth, there is an immediate and marked reduction in bacterial numbers, thereby reducing the chance that an antimicrobial-resistant subpopulation will survive.

Bismuth has an excellent safety record, with the most problematic side effect being temporary discoloration of the tongue and development of black stools. There is a hypothetical concern for systemic absorption of bismuth leading to bismuth toxicity but this has not proved to be a clinical problem when used for short-duration therapies. Of note, if the common subsalicylate form of bismuth is used, a significant salicylate ingestion will occur. Each tablet of Pepto-Bismol, for example, has 225 mg of salicylate, most of which is absorbed. Patients receiving salicylate therapy should have their doses modified, and patients who should avoid salicylates (e.g., children less than age 16) should consider an alternate form of bismuth. In the United States bismuth is primarily available as bismuth subsalicylate (Pepto-Bismol) although bismuth citrate has become available as part of a combination therapy.

Traditional antimicrobials

H. pylori is susceptible to many different antibiotics, and a variety of antibiotics and antibiotic combinations have been tried. The antibiotics that have proven effective include clarithromycin, amoxicillin, metronidazole/tinidazole, tetracycline, furazolidone, fluoroquinolones, and rifabutin.

Clarithromycin

Clarithromycin (Biaxin) is a macrolide that binds to bacterial ribosomes and disrupts protein synthesis, leading to bacterial cell death. Clarithromycin is the most acid stable of the macrolides and has the lowest minimal inhibitory concentration. The major metabolite of clarithromycin is also active against Hp. Clarithromycin is generally well tolerated. Reported side effects include an altered sense of taste, frequently described as metallic, nausea, vomiting, and headache. Clarithromycin resistance is increasing, and resistance predicts treatment failure.

Amoxicillin

Amoxicillin is an acid-stable semisynthetic penicillin that is bactericidal in vivo. The antimicrobial activity of amoxicillin is pH-dependent with the minimal inhibitory concentration decreasing as the pH increases. Resistance to amoxicillin is rare but has been reported and may be in part responsible for the markedly variable success of the dual combination of a PPI and amoxicillin. Amoxicillin concentrations are highest in the antral mucosa, with lower levels achieved in the corpus mucosa or the mucus layer. Overall, results with combination therapy that includes amoxicillin have been good, suggesting that sufficient levels are achieved and that it is an effective anti-Hp agent when used as part of a combination therapy.

Metronidazole/tinidazole

Metronidazole (Flagyl, Protostat), and the similar tinidazole, are nitroimidazoles that are selectively toxic to microaerophilic microorganisms. A chemically reactive, reduced form of the drug leads to generation of cytotoxic products and destruction of microorganisms. The activity of metronidazole is pH independent, making it theoretically an ideal drug for the gastric environment. Unfortunately, Hp rapidly develops resistance to metronidazole, and the widespread use of this drug has resulted in a high rate of primary resistance. Metronidazole resistance identified in vitro does not always predict resistance in vivo, such that this agent may remain useful despite a high level of resistance in a population or even in an individual (see below).

Tetracyclines

Tetracycline hydrochloride was used in the first effective therapies against Hp and remains an important antibiotic. The activity of tetracycline is independent of gastric acidity making it a potentially useful drug. Tetracycline is also inexpensive and resistance is rare. Success has been reported with tetracycline hydrochloride and with oxytetracycline, whereas doxycycline has produced inferior results. Tetracyclines are contraindicated in children because of the abnormal pigmentation of permanent dentition that occurs when the drug is used while teeth are being calcified.

Fluoroquinolones

Fluoroquinolones have been used increasingly for Hp eradication; they work by blocking DNA gyrase and DNA synthesis of the bacteria. Resistance to fluoroquinolones develops rapidly and prior use of these medications is associated with a high rate of resistance.

Furazolidone

Furazolidone is a monoamine oxidase inhibitor with broad antibacterial activity based on interference of bacterial enzyme activity, and has proven effective as part of triple therapy. Hp is rarely resistant to furazolidone such that it is an underused antimicrobial.

Rifabutin

Rifabutin is a semisynthetic ansamycin antibiotic with a low minimum inhibitory concentration (MIC) for Hp. Rifabutin is being used increasingly, primarily in combination with a PPI and amoxicillin as a rescue therapy.

Drug interactions with antiulcer drugs
Altered absorption

As a result of intralumenal binding, antacids and sucralfate decrease absorption of a number of drugs [68,69] and it is best to advise separation of consumption of antacids and other drugs by an hour before or after (Table 7.3). Bismuth may have the same effect, but data are limited and bismuth is generally given along with the other drugs used in the treatment regimen [70]. Antisecretory agents, by increasing intralumenal pH, can alter drug absorption. For example, the effect of antisecretory agents on reducing absorption of food-bound vitamin B-12 can be dramatic [71,72]. The effect appears to be mediated by the increase in pH and resultant decrease in peptic activity, rather than inhibition of intrinsic factor secretion [73]. The absorption of iron and calcium can also be compromised, and there is increasing evidence of an association of antisecretory drug use, especially PPIs, and the risk of hip fracture [74]. It is not clear whether this is a consequence of the effect on calcium absorption, effects on osteoclast function, or both. There is also evidence that thyroxine absorption is markedly suppressed with either use of PPIs or Hp gastritis, requiring adjustment of a thyroxine dose [75].

Dissolution of some drugs, particularly weak bases, will be decreased with gastric neutralization. The consequences depend on the specific drug and its preparation; for example, decreased dissolution of ketoconazole, a weak base, significantly decreases absorption [45]. Alternatively, the absorption of bismuth from colloidal bismuth subcitrate is increased, presumably because decreased gastric acidity increases free bismuth concentrations [76]. Acid secretory inhibition can decrease the absorption of weak acids from the stomach and increase absorption of weak bases. For example, secretory inhibitors will reduce uptake into gastric mucosa of weak acid NSAIDs, such as aspirin, and decrease superficial damage. However, gastric absorption is usually modest compared with intestinal absorption, and systemic effects override this sparing of gastric mucosa.

Drug interactions involving cytochrome P450

All of the nine PPIs and H$_2$RAs available in the United States that are used for acid inhibition undergo hepatic metabolism to some extent and interact with members of the cytochrome P450 (CYP) superfamily of mixed function oxidases. This topic is inherently complex, reflecting the complexity of the CYP superfamily, which is composed of three major families (CYP1–3), a varying number of subfamilies (e.g., CYP2A–E), and numerous specific members or isoforms in these subfamilies (e.g., CYP2C1–19). For the antisecretory

agents, these interactions with the CYP superfamily generally carry little clinical significance. However, there are specific circumstances where they can become critical and potentially life-threatening (Table 7.3). These serious events are rare and occur in seriously ill subjects with impaired hepatic function and drug metabolism, often confounded by multiple (more than two) interacting drugs and genetic polymorphism of the CYP metabolic pathways. Such factors will not be detected in routine pharmacokinetic studies in young healthy volunteers with usually undefined CYP genetic background; therefore, such studies carry little negative predictive value for excluding uncommon serious interactions encountered in the treatment of complex cases in practice.

Several features of P450 metabolism are important with respect to the antisecretory drugs (this list has been adapted from previous reviews [73,77]).

• *Time and dose dependence.* Drug metabolism and drug interactions undergo dose- and time-dependent changes over the first several days of therapy. Generally, 3 to 5 days are needed to reach maximal inhibition of drug metabolism, although maximal effects can be further delayed in some instances.

• *The therapeutic margin.* Drug interactions are of greatest relevance when the drugs have a narrow therapeutic range. For example, cimetidine may potentially produce significant effects with R-warfarin, theophylline, phenytoin, and nifedipine [45,73].

• *Genetic polymorphism of drug metabolism and interactions.* Genetic polymorphism is particularly important for PPIs, for which the CYP2C19 pathway is a primary metabolic step in degradation. Because of the wide safety margin of PPIs, the major clinical implication is that acid secretory inhibition will be modest in rapid metabolizers and exaggerated in slow metabolizers, because the degree of acid inhibition reflects the AUC. The impact in many situations is modest. For example, in slow metabolizers healing of GU can occur within 2 weeks, compared with 8 weeks in normal metabolizers [78]. In contrast, cure of Hp with omeprazole plus amoxicillin was highly dependent on CYP2C19 metabolism; slow metabolizers had a 100% cure rate, rapid metabolizers a 29% cure rate, and heterozygotes a 60% cure rate [79]. CYP2C19 is also the site of interaction between diazepam and either omeprazole or cimetidine; with the wide therapeutic range for diazepam and marginal effects of the interactions, clinical implications are minimal [52,80]. Omeprazole does not further delay clearance of diazepam or S-mephenytoin in slow metabolizers probably because the point of interaction is defective or absent [77,81]. However, in slow metabolizers, delayed PPI clearance increases the potential for interactions at other CYP sites, such as 3A4 or 2C8. For example, although pharmacokinetic studies indicated that lansoprazole had only minimal P450 drug interactions, in a patient with a CYP2C19 mutation, lansoprazole caused significant increases in tacrolimus levels. These levels returned to normal after replacing lansoprazole with famotidine [82]. Drug interactions may only

Table 7.3 Impact of acid peptic therapy on nutrient absorption and drug interactions

General mechanism	Acid peptic therapeutic agent	Drug or nutrient	Consequences
Intralumenal binding	Sucralfate, antacids, ?bismuth	Potentially binds several drugs in gastric lumen	Prevents absorption, producing lower blood levels
Decreased acid secretion	PPI[a], H$_2$RA	Vitamin B-12	Anemia
		Iron	Anemia
		Calcium	Osteoporosis, pathological fractures
		Thyroxine	Decreased T$_4$ and increased TSH
		Ketoconazole, cefpodoxime, cefuroxime, protease inhibitors (atazanavir and indinavir)	Decreased absorption, particularly of drugs that are weak bases
		Aspirin	Another weak base where gastric absorption is decreased at high pH[b]
		Colloidal bismuth	Increased bismuth absorption
P450 drug interactions	Cimetidine	Alfentanil, amiodarone, nifedipine, carbamazepine, cyclosporine (ciclosporin), citalopram, sulfonylureas, warfarin, and CYP substrates, such as 1A2 (theophylline, trifluoperazine), 2C19 (citalopram, phenytoin, propranolol, sertraline), 3A4[c]	Altered metabolism increases blood levels. Significant consequences may result when the therapeutic margin is small. Consequences are minimal for others, such as diazepam, because of the wide therapeutic margin
	Omeprazole, other PPI[d]	Carbamazepine, CYP2C9 substrates (amiodarone, fluoxetine, phenytoin, sertraline, warfarin), 2C19 substrates (citalopram, propranolol)[e]	
	PPI in slow metabolizers	Antibiotics	Enhanced cure of Hp
	PPI in slow metabolizers or PPI in combination with multiple other drugs that share CYP sites of metabolism, especially 3A4 (e.g., omeprazole plus clarithromycin and carbamazepine)[f]	Any drug metabolized by CYP3A4[c] or possibly other CYP sites	Delayed clearance, with significantly increased levels of drugs metabolized by 3A4

a Effects will be exaggerated in slow metabolizers, because of genetic polymorphism at the CPY2C19 pathway.

b Decreased absorption may decrease superficial mucosal damage, but clinical consequences are minimal because intestinal absorption is so much more important and aspirin and NSAIDs have systemic actions resulting in ulcers.

c Many drugs interact with 3A4, including carbamazepine, cisapride, nifedipine, macrolide antibiotics, azole antifungals, antitumor agents, tacrolimus, psychotropics, diclofenac, doxycycline, imatinib, isoniazid, nefazodone, nicardipine, propofol, protease inhibitors, quinidine, telithromycin, and verapamil.

d Although omeprazole has been implicated for these interactions, in vitro studies suggest that lansoprazole and pantoprazole are potent in vitro inhibitors of CYP2C19 and CYP2C9, respectively [188]. Therefore, caution is appropriate and interactions may become important for other PPIs, especially if combined with other factors, such as in patients who are homozygous slow metabolizers, patients taking a regimen of multiple drugs that amplify interactions, and illness that impairs hepatic metabolism or renal excretion.

e To the extent that these interactions are mediated at CYP2C19, they are NOT more pronounced in slow PPI metabolizers, presumably because the point of interaction is itself defective or absent.

f There may be some differences among PPIs, in that such effects may be less prominent with rabeprazole [189], but data are so limited that no firm conclusions can be reached.

CYP, cytochrome P450; Hp, *Helicobacter pylori*; H$_2$RA, histamine H$_2$-receptor antagonist; PPI, proton pump inhibitor; T$_4$, thyroxine; TSH, thyroid-stimulating hormone.

show up in slow metabolizers, in whom metabolism is shifted to CYP3A4.

- *Variability among individuals.* In addition to genetic polymorphism, other factors can also underlie the variability of drug interactions among individuals. Age can be important at both ends of the spectrum. Elderly subjects are much more likely to have impaired drug metabolism. Infants and young children tend to have rapid metabolism, underlying the use of higher PPI doses in the young [83]. The limited data available suggest that CYPZC19 genetic polymorphism has a similar impact on PPI metabolism in children and adults, with poor metabolizers having 6- to 10-fold higher AUC compared with extensive metabolizers.
- *Multidrug (beyond two-way) interactions.* Three-way drug interactions can produce unexpected results. All of the PPIs are metabolized by CYP3A4 and, therefore, potential interactions with drugs metabolized by this pathway warrant consideration, particularly with drugs having a narrow therapeutic margin. Omeprazole and clarithromycin interact at 3A4 [84], resulting in an increased AUC for omeprazole and clarithromycin. Both drugs have a wide therapeutic window and this interaction may even enhance cure of Hp infection. However, the omeprazole-clarithromycin combination considerably increases carbamazepine (Tegretol) levels [85]. Other drugs metabolized at CYP3A4 should also be used cautiously during combination therapy with a PPI and clarithromycin. Drugs interacting at CPY3A4 include drugs related to cisapride, ketoconazole, macrolide antibiotics, antitumor agents, and several psychotropics.
- Whether interactions produce relevant effects depends upon whether alternate pathways exist for drug metabolism.
- The antisecretory drugs interact with multiple CYP sites. Furthermore, the drugs may act as substrates and thus be metabolized at one or several CYP sites, or the drugs may induce or inhibit the CYP sites.

Medical treatment of active peptic ulcer disease

Factors influencing healing

Several factors potentially affect the rate of ulcer healing and the tendency for recurrence. Reversible factors should be identified and addressed, particularly Hp infection, NSAID use, and cigarette smoking.

Ulcer size influences the time to healing. Large and small GUs heal at the same rate and although effective medical therapy results in more rapid healing, larger ulcers still require more time to heal [86–88].

Conventional ulcer therapy

The superior potency and duration of PPIs have resulted in PPI therapy becoming the therapy of choice with regard to rapid relief of ulcer symptoms and acceleration of ulcer heal-

ing. Numerous marketing studies have attempted to demonstrate differences among the available PPIs. However, when the results are corrected for differences in dose, it becomes clear that the best PPI is the cheapest one (i.e., a PPI is a PPI). It is important to remember that parietal cell hyperplasia and rebound acid hypersecretion follow discontinuation of prolonged PPI therapy [89–92]. Although the rebound acid secretory response is generally small and transient, this hypersecretion may underlie transient exacerbation of acid peptic disease (e.g., the development of duodenal erosions noted above) and GERD symptoms.

Recommendations

Treatment decisions are based on the situation (e.g., presentation, complicating issues, sense of urgency) and etiology of the ulcer disease. Clearly, in the presence of a complicated ulcer (e.g., major upper GI bleeding), diagnosis of the cause can wait until the crisis has passed. For routine symptomatic ulcers diagnosis and treatment can occur concomitantly. Symptomatic ulcers, regardless of cause, typically respond well to antisecretory drug therapy, and most would consider the least expensive PPI as the treatment of choice. There is no place for the routine use of antacids, sucralfate, or prostaglandins for DU, and certainly not for GU. If the ulcer was diagnosed by endoscopy, one would expect that the endoscopist would have obtained samples to diagnose or exclude Hp infection. There is no urgency to diagnose Hp, and diagnosis or confirmation of the diagnosis can certainly be delayed until it is convenient for the patient and physician. However, because antisecretory drug therapy is typically part of anti-Hp therapy, there may be cost savings to do both together. For an uncomplicated small Hp-related DU both treatment of the infection and the ulcer can be done in the same time frame (e.g., 2 weeks) (see below). Treatment of large and complicated ulcers will need to be individualized. The only instance where antiulcer therapy is required beyond the antibiotic treatment period is for larger or complicated ulcers (e.g., bleeding ulcers), or in the setting of sustained NSAID use, as considered below.

H. pylori and ulcer therapy
Drug combinations

Treatment of Hp infection results in acceleration of ulcer healing, prevention of ulcer relapse, and prevention of ulcer complications (Fig. 7.3) [93,94]. Successful eradication of Hp will also reduce the rate of development of gastric cancer in high-risk groups [95,96]. If the infection is cured before significant atrophy develops, it is likely that gastric cancer can be completely prevented [97]. In developed countries, Hp eradication is rarely followed by reinfection. In developing countries where hygiene may be poor, reinfection is common and this remains a major problem for future worldwide eradication programs [98,99].

Although there are a number of drug combinations approved for use, none is ideal and many are outdated. A

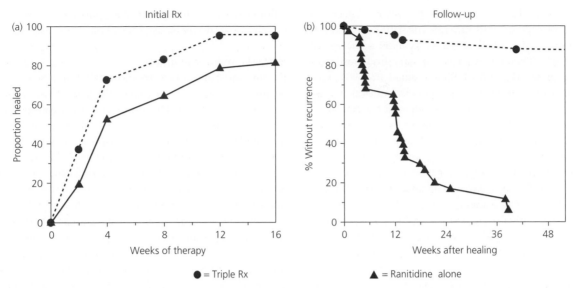

Figure 7.3 **(a)** Patients with duodenal ulcer disease received triple therapy including ranitidine (closed circles) or ranitidine alone (closed triangles) until the ulcer was healed. **(b)** After ulcer healing patients were followed with regular endoscopic evaluation of the ulcer site. Anti-*H. pylori* (Hp) therapy resulted in enhanced ulcer healing and a reduction in ulcer recurrence. All ulcer recurrences in the antibiotic-treated group were related to failed anti-Hp therapy, use of NSAIDs, or both [93,94].

number of studies have shown that subtle changes in protocol, such as changes in drugs, drug formulation, dosing intervals, dosing in relation to meals, and duration of therapy, may have profound effects on outcome [100,101]. There are a number of practical issues to be considered when selecting a regimen for treatment of Hp infection, including cost, simplicity, effectiveness, side effects, the rate of antibiotic resistance in the community, dose, duration, number of administrations per day, whether to administer with meals or when fasting, and whether control of pH is needed [100,101]. None of these issues has been adequately evaluated in a systematic way, and studies with sequential therapy have definitely shown that the outcome of therapy can be improved. The lack of such studies is possibly part of the legacy of Hp infection being a disease studied by gastroenterologists rather than infectious disease specialists, who by their training and experience are less likely to have declared "victory" or "success" at eradication rates considered unacceptable for other serious infectious diseases. The approach for other infectious diseases has been to identify a therapy that is universally effective and then to attempt to simplify it. With Hp, the approach was to simplify only partially effective therapies. To remain competitive the pharmaceutical industry did the minimum required to obtain approval and, in the absence of clear FDA-defined requirements for high eradication rates, attempted to gain marketing advantages by using shorter duration and less frequent administrations instead of attempting to identify regimens with high and reliable cure rates. This has resulted in a number of approved but only partially effective regimens.

An evidence-based choice of the best treatment regimen is nearly impossible because large randomized trials com-

paring the most effective regimens have rarely been done. Metaanalyses have shown that the most commonly used therapies produce cure rates that are typically less than acceptable [102–106]. Although metaanalysis is usually a powerful tool to help understand the overall effectiveness of treatment, it is less helpful in choosing the best therapy because of considerable heterogeneity in the data, including absence of crucial data such as the presence or absence of pretreatment antimicrobial resistance. There are few head-to-head-comparisons of different antibiotic dosages or duration of therapies, leaving the influence of these parameters on treatment success unknown. Finally, and unexpectedly based on the response to treatment of other infectious diseases, the cure rates often differ greatly in different countries despite using the same regime [105,107]. All of the PPIs appear equally effective with the clarithromycin-amoxicillin or metronidazole triple therapies, and they can be used interchangeably depending on local availability and cost [108]. The H$_2$RAs are roughly equally effective, with the only benefit being a slight reduction in cost [109]. However, healing rates and time to pain relief are better with PPIs, and they are generally preferred.

Large population-based trials have also shown that the high rates of success expected on the basis of trials sponsored by the pharmaceutical companies are often unobtainable in clinical practice. Part of this difference is probably attributable to patient selection. Industry-sponsored studies typically studied patients with duodenal ulcer disease, where the cure rates are typically higher than among patients without ulcers [106,110–112].

Fundamentally, *H. pylori* is a serious, chronic transmissible infectious disease that causes damage to gastric structure and function and is a major cause of morbidity and mortality worldwide. As noted above, therapies for bacterial infectious diseases are expected to yield cure rates near 100%. Although Hp proved more difficult than some, by 1989 a successful therapy for Hp had been defined as one that cured more than 80% of the patients [113]. By 1995 it seemed that 90% was achievable [114] and that 95% or greater cure rates were just around the corner. But such cure rates were not achieved, in part because of the failure to learn from the successes of the previous decade. Here, we will use the Maastricht consensus conference definition of a useful therapy as one with an intention to treat (ITT) cure rate of greater than 80% (i.e., therapies with cure rates of 80% or less would be unacceptable) [115].

Legacy-approved triple therapy (e.g., a PPI plus amoxicillin and clarithromycin) yields unacceptably low eradication rates in Europe and the United States, typically below the minimally acceptable 80% success rate (Fig. 7.4a) (Table 7.4) [111,112,116–139].

These results indicate that traditional triple therapy should no longer be considered the initial therapy in Western populations unless pretreatment susceptibility is confirmed, in which case it should be used for 14 days [107,140,141].

Better H. pylori *therapies*

Because most antibiotics are more effective when given with an antisecretory drug, typically a PPI is used along with three or four antimicrobials. The original formulas consisted of a PPI plus two antibiotics chosen from amoxicillin, clarithromycin, metronidazole/tinidazole (i.e., a triple therapy), or four drugs comprising bismuth, tetracycline, metronidazole/tinidazole, and a PPI (i.e., a quadruple therapy). These were administered for 7–14 days, preferably 14 days because longer duration generally provided higher cure rates. Searches for new therapies have followed two basic formulas. One was to start with a PPI plus amoxicillin and add a new drug or drugs. The other was to replace the metronidazole/tinidazole in quadruple therapy with another drug. Whereas triple therapy generally provides unacceptably low cure rates, cure rates with quadruple therapy have largely been maintained.

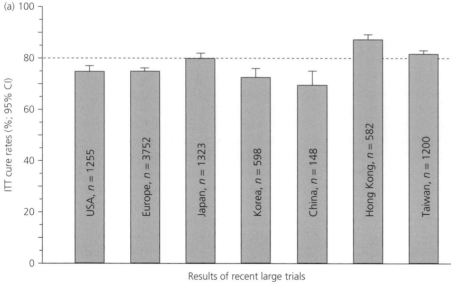

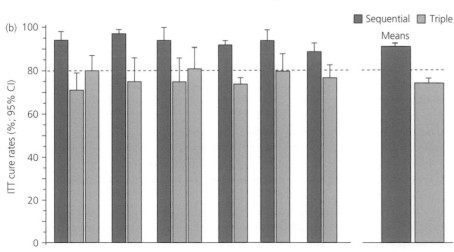

Figure 7.4 (a) The mean pooled results as intention-to-treat (ITT) rates and 95% confidence intervals (CI) of large studies using a proton pump inhibitor (PPI) plus clarithromycin and amoxicillin to treat *H. pylori* infections [111,112,116–121,123,124,126–139]. The 80% or minimally acceptable cure rate is also shown (dotted line). As seen, in the majority of areas the results are unacceptably low, suggesting that this therapy should not be used unless clarithromycin-susceptible strains are definitely present. **(b)** The six direct comparisons of triple therapy consisting of a PPI plus clarithromycin and amoxicillin with sequential therapy. The pooled results of all the comparisons are shown on the right. The mean cure rate (ITT) for sequential therapy was only 90.5% (95% CI 89%–92%), suggesting that additional experiments are needed to further improve the efficacy.

Table 7.4 Regimens for the initial therapy of *Helicobacter pylori* infections

Regimen	Antisecretory adjunct	Antibiotics	Duration	Comments
Quadruple therapy	PPI b.i.d.	Tetracycline hydrochloride, metronidazole, and bismuth	14 days	Higher doses help surmount metronidazole resistance
Sequential therapy	PPI b.i.d.	Amoxicillin Clarithromycin and metronidazole	5 days 5 days	Cure rates low with dual resistance to metronidazole and clarithromycin
Triple therapy	PPI b.i.d.	Clarithromycin plus metronidazole or amoxicillin	7–14 days	Avoid where clarithromycin resistance is high 14-day treatment increased cure by 12%

Note: metronidazole can be replaced by tinidazole.
b.i.d., twice a day; PPI, proton pump inhibitor.

In quadruple therapy the antimicrobials are effective in an acid environment and include either bismuth subcitrate or subsalicylate, tetracycline hydrochloride, metronidazole/tinidazole, and a PPI. Effectiveness requires that the regimen be given at appropriate doses and durations (e.g., a minimum of 1500 mg of tetracycline HCl and 1200 to 1500 mg of metronidazole/tinidazole, and six or eight tablets of a bismuth given in divided doses (e.g., t.i.d. or q.i.d.) for 14 days.

New antibiotic combinations

Quinolones (e.g., ciprofloxacin) were tried in the early phases of searching for effective anti-Hp therapies but were abandoned because of the rapid development of resistance. Fluoroquinolones have seen a renaissance as a replacement for clarithromycin in triple therapy. However, as with legacy triple therapy, 7-day therapy provided an unacceptably low cure rate, which was improved by longer duration [142]. However, the widespread use of these drugs for other indications has led to a rapid increase in fluoroquinolone resistance in many communities such that the usefulness of these drugs will likely be short lived [143]. Furazolidone is an old but effective drug that can be substituted for metronidazole or clarithromycin in either legacy triple or quadruple therapy. Unfortunately, it has become difficult to obtain in the United States because the company that sold it no longer does so. It is, however, easily available in Mexico. Despite the issues about it being a monoamine oxidase inhibitor, it is probably one of the best choices for difficult cases. Rifabutin is also commonly used as a substitution drug, and again longer duration provides better outcomes. None of these approaches is universally satisfactory and, clearly, new drugs are needed.

Sequential therapies

Rather than abandoning triple therapy, Italian investigators decided to provide the drugs sequentially. In this approach a PPI and amoxicillin are given for 5 days followed by the PPI plus clarithromycin (250 or 500 mg) and tinidazole (500 mg) for an additional 5 days [125,129]. This approach has repeat-

edly been proven to be superior to legacy triple therapy in both adults and in children (Fig. 7.4b) [119,122,125,126,144,145]. Sequential administration of antibiotics has traditionally been avoided because of concern that it would promote drug resistance rather than result in increased eradication; however, this sequential therapy starts with drugs against which development of resistance is rare. This approach markedly reduces bacterial load, making it less likely that preexisting resistant organisms remain [100,146]. The addition of the third, or third and fourth, drug would then kill the few remaining organisms. The high rate of success (e.g., reliably ~ 90% ITT) suggests that sequential therapy should supplant triple therapy in regions where the success rates have become unacceptable. However, the success of sequential therapy is reduced in the face of dual resistance (clarithromycin and metronidazole) [126]. Sequential therapy can likely be improved by altering the dose, duration, frequency of administration, or order of administration (e.g., similar effects have been reported when all four drugs are given nonsequentially) [147–149].

Recommendations for therapy

In areas where legacy triple therapy no longer provides adequate cure rates (e.g., the United States, most of Europe, and much of developed Asia), one should use sequential therapy, as described, or add a fourth drug to legacy triple therapy (e.g., metronidazole or tinidazole to the PPI, clarithromycin, and amoxicillin combination). Studies are needed to confirm that sequential therapy can be improved by changes in the dose, duration, or drugs used. The alternative is to use traditional quadruple therapy with a PPI, bismuth, tetracycline, and metronidazole/tinidazole (Table 7.4).

Other approaches for areas with high rates of antimicrobial resistance

Dual therapy with a PPI and amoxicillin was an early attempt at therapy but was soon abandoned because of low and variable eradication rates. However, in Germany this combination is still used clinically, but with a high dose of both PPI and amoxicillin (e.g., 40 mg omeprazole plus 750 mg amoxicillin t.i.d. for 14 days). Reported eradication rates range from 67% to 91% [150–152]. Our experience with the high-dose approach has yielded a cure rate in the range of 70%–75%, and this high-dose dual therapy has formed the basis of our approach to sequential therapy for patients who have proven difficult-to-cure infections. Our approach has been to use 40 mg of omeprazole or esomeprazole and 1 g of amoxicillin t.i.d. for 5 days then on day 6 we add a third antibiotic or third and fourth antibiotic and continue as a triple or quadruple therapy for a total of 12–14 days (e.g., [143]). The choice of the third or fourth antibiotics should be antibiotics that the patient has not used before (such as tetracycline, levofloxacin, furazolidone, or rifabutin). However, therapy is best guided by pretreatment antibiotic susceptibility testing.

Probiotics and nonantibiotic additions

Probiotics are live, nonpathogenic microbial feed or food supplements that can affect the host in a beneficial manner. The best studied probiotics are the lactic acid-producing bacteria, particularly *Lactobacillus* spp. and *Bifidobacterium* spp. Probiotics are thought to play a role in keeping the gut microbial ecosystem stable by restoring resident microflora after antibiotic treatment [153,154]. Some strains of *Lactobacillus* spp. and *Bifidobacterium* spp. have shown in vitro bactericidal effects against Hp, and a protective effect has been confirmed in some animal models [155]. Clinical trials, however, indicate that probiotics generally do not cure Hp infection but may decrease the density of colonization and may decrease the mucosal gastroduodenal inflammation. Metaanalyses have suggested a slight but not dramatic improvement in cure rates by the addition of probiotics [156].

In addition to probiotics, many plant or dairy foodstuffs have been evaluated for gastroprotective and anti-Hp properties [157,158]. Turmeric, cumin, ginger, chili, borage, broccoli sprouts, black caraway, oregano, and liquorices have antimicrobial activities in vitro [159,160]. No data justify therapeutic use of these agents, but further investigation would be of interest. Mucolytics such as *N*-acetylcysteine [161] and the proteolytic enzyme pronase [162] have additive effects to triple therapy, possibly as a result of reducing the mucosal surface gel layer and improving the local antibiotic delivery.

Improving compliance with probiotics

Probiotic cotherapy with antibiotics decreases diarrhea and taste disturbances [163,164]. Additional studies are needed to determine whether such cotherapy improves the poor compliance seen with antibiotic regimens, which is a major reason for ineffective therapy.

Treatment failures

After initial therapy has failed, the best results are obtained when susceptibility testing guides the choice of antibiotics. However, such testing is generally unavailable, and choices must be based on drugs that have not been administered previously [165,166]. Clearly, one should avoid drugs (e.g., clarithromycin) for which resistance eliminates effectiveness during subsequent therapy. Resistance can be expected if fluoroquinolones have been given previously for any other reason. Quadruple therapy is generally recommended after triple therapies have failed [100,101,167] because this combination is effective even with metronidazole resistance [168,169]. Despite the large number of tablets and the frequent drug administrations, drop-out rates and compliance in most clinical trials of quadruple therapy have been comparable with those of twice-daily triple therapy regimens. Furazolidone is often the drug of choice for multiple treatment failures (a salvage therapy).

Explanations for failure of Hp therapy include inappropriate choices of initial therapy (e.g., use of doxycycline instead of tetracycline, or erythromycin instead of clarithromycin), poor compliance with the regimen, and antibiotic resistance. Resistance is the major problem. Compliance can be improved if the patient is counseled regarding the need for continuing the regimen for the prescribed duration although symptoms have disappeared. Compliance is also reduced when side effects occur.

Side effects of therapy

Side effects occur in 20%–30% of patients and are generally mild and transient. Severe side effects are rare. The most common side effect is nausea, which can result from most drugs. Clarithromycin given in doses greater than 1 g/day typically causes a taste disturbance, and patients should be warned to expect it. Patients treated with bismuth salts will have dark stools and they must be warned that this is not blood [170]. Diarrhea is relatively common with antibiotic therapy, and pseudomembranous colitis is rare but can occur. *Candida* vaginitis may occur in women, especially following treatment with tetracycline. Alcoholic beverages should not be consumed during metronidazole therapy and for at least 1 day afterwards because of an Antabuse-like reaction with abdominal cramps, nausea, vomiting, headaches, and flushing.

Antibiotic resistance

Acquired resistance has been demonstrated with all of the antimicrobial agents used to treat Hp infection, especially with nitroimidazoles, macrolides, fluoroquinolones, and rifampicins. Resistance to tetracycline and amoxicillin has been demonstrated but is uncommon. Resistance to metronidazole in the United States is roughly 25%, and rates of metronidazole resistance in excess of 60% have been documented in some developing countries. Increasing the metronidazole dose partially overcomes acquired resistance, but high-dose quadruple therapy is more effective. Hp resistance to clarithromycin has steadily increased, especially in locations where clarithromycin use is high (e.g., Japan and in children in Western countries) [166,171]. Clarithromycin and fluoro-quinolone resistance cannot be overcome by increasing the dosage [103,106,166].

Patient education

Poor compliance is the most controllable factor resulting in treatment failure. An informed, motivated patient is important for success. Patients should be instructed about dose, duration, possible side effects, and the necessity of completing the entire course of therapy, rather than stopping when they feel better [170]. Patients who use tobacco should be educated about the benefits of stopping [106]. Written instructions about how to take the pills are helpful. Gastric distress from the drugs can be reduced by instructing the patient to take them with food. Many pharmacists routinely label tetracycline as "not to be taken with food." We administer all drugs with food, because this greatly simplifies the treatment regimen, is not associated with a reduction in cure rate, reduces nausea, and improves mixing and retention in the stomach. This requires education of both the patient and the pharmacist, who may resist prescribing tetracycline or bismuth with meals.

Confirmation of Hp cure

Confirmation of Hp cure is the standard of care, particularly because poor outcomes accompany persisting infection and because cure rates are often below 80%. Failure to cure the infection in an ulcer patient causes recurrent ulcer disease, continuing risk of ulcer complications, and the need for more testing and treatment. The infected patient also remains a reservoir for transmission to others, especially family members.

Noninvasive, inexpensive, and widely available urea breath tests or stool antigen tests are typically sufficient. Whichever test is used, it is important to wait a sufficient time after stopping antibiotics to ensure that residual Hp have multiplied to detectable levels. The data suggest that a 4-week hiatus is preferable for histology, culture, or urea breath testing. Approximately 8 weeks is required for the stool antigen test. Proton pump inhibitors should be stopped, preferably for 2 weeks, to avoid false-negative results for the tests that require actively growing Hp, including UBT, rapid urease, and stool antigen testing; culture; histology; and culture. A positive test at any time after therapy indicates treatment failure, but a negative test is difficult to interpret as long as prolonged suppression is possible. If confirmation of cure is critical, then endoscopy with biopsy or a UBT should be performed 8–12 weeks post therapy.

Serological testing is not useful for confirming the outcome of therapy, because antibody levels can remain elevated for a long time. A negative test correlates with cure, but is unusual within 2 years after therapy. Recurrent infection is associated with a return of test positivity.

Treatment of NSAID ulcers

There are two critical steps in treating NSAID-associated ulcers. First, whenever possible, discontinue or at least reduce the NSAID dose. Second, search for and cure Hp infection. If NSAIDs can be discontinued, ulcers will generally heal readily with any adequate antisecretory drug therapy, although PPIs are preferred, especially for complicated or large ulcers. Continuing NSAIDs, including COX-2 selective agents, may interfere with ulcer healing, and this should be only done with great caution and with explicit and documented patient consent. The need for and duration of cessation of low-dose aspirin in patients at high cardiac or cerebrovascular risk has been controversial. A controlled trial of patients randomized after endoscopic hemostasis for ulcer bleeding reported that discontinuing low-dose aspirin for 8 weeks led to significantly increased mortality, compared with those randomized to continued aspirin [172]. Both groups were treated with intravenous and then oral PPI; there was no increase in recurrent GI bleeding in the aspirin-treated group. Although preliminary, this study was well done, statistically significant, and indicates that ulcers in high-vascular-risk patients should be treated aggressively with PPI without discontinuing low-dose aspirin.

Proton pump inhibitors are preferred for ulcer healing in patients who continue to take NSAIDs. However, even a double-dose PPI will fail in some patients and recurrences and complications will occur. The data from controlled trials are inadequate to guide treatment decisions in this setting, other than discontinuing NSAIDs. Patient preferences should be included in any decision to continue NSAIDs, and we advise documenting that the patient has elected to continue NSAIDs despite being warned of the consequences.

Misoprostol is generally not a good alternative for the healing of NSAID ulcers; it has only been studied for prevention, as considered below. The H_2RAs, sucralfate, and antacids are inadequate for treatment of NSAID ulcers, especially if NSAIDs will be continued.

Prevention of NSAID ulcers

Early studies on the prevention of NSAID ulcer complications were largely short-term trials on normal subjects or patients free of active ulcer disease and well enough to qualify for study. As noted previously, "endoscopic" ulcers, defined by arbitrary size criteria that may or may not require visible depth, are found at surveillance endoscopy in 5%–25% of subjects taking NSAIDs. In contrast, "clinical" ulcers present with complications at a rate of 0.5%–2% per patient-year of NSAID use. Valid recommendations are those based on preventing complications [173], rather than preventing "endoscopic" ulcers, most of which remain clinically silent.

Determining the most cost-effective means of preventing NSAID ulcer complications is difficult with the available data. Although ulcer complications from NSAIDs are rare, these drugs are widely used, so that the number of patients at risk is high. Several factors impart increased risk for complications; these factors should be taken into account when deciding whether to offer a more costly regimen to reduce ulcer risk. NSAIDs carry a black box warning label regarding ulcer complications; patients should be informed of this risk and if they are in a high-risk category, and this discussion should be documented.

Prostaglandins

Misoprostol (200 µg q.i.d.) is approved for prevention of NSAID-induced GU and DU [65,174]. Diarrhea and abdominal cramps limit patient compliance, but these side effects are often transient and may be reduced by starting therapy with lower doses. The low-dose regimen is less effective in preventing "endoscopic" ulcers, suggesting that the higher dose is preferable, if tolerated [65]. However, in clinical trials with Hp-negative NSAID users, low-dose misoprostol was superior to omeprazole for both endoscopic gastric ulcer healing and ulcer prevention [66]. Data from a randomized clinical trial (RTC) with about 9000 patients indicated that misoprostol (200 µg q.i.d.) reduced NSAID ulcer complications by about 40% [173]. Although patients with active ulcer disease were excluded, misoprostol suppression of complications was evident in the subgroup with history of prior peptic ulcer [173]. Unfortunately, the numbers were small and, most importantly, Hp status was not determined so that it is unknown how well misoprostol works for prevention of clinical complications in Hp-negative subjects compared with Hp-positive subjects.

Antisecretory agents: proton pump inhibitors

There are no approved regimens for the prevention of ulcer complications for patients who cannot tolerate or fail to respond to misoprostol. Data from two RCTs indicate that standard doses of H_2RAs did not prevent NSAID-induced "endoscopic" GU [175,176]. One caveat is that the early studies were done in patients of unknown Hp status. Subsequent studies have shown a marked difference between the outcome of those with and without Hp infections [66]: in the latter, PPIs were remarkably less effective. Interestingly, misoprostol, even at the dose of 400 µg/day, was superior to PPIs for healing of endoscopic gastric ulcers and preventing ulcer relapse, and PPIs were also only marginally superior to low-dose ranitidine [66]. The superiority of misoprostol was confirmed in a separate study of full-dose misoprostol vs full-dose lansoprazole [67]. Epidemiological studies have also shown reduced mortality with the fixed combination of diclofenac and misoprostol (Arthrotec) compared with traditional NSAIDs [177,178]. It is likely that misoprostol us underused.

There are few data regarding H_2RA- or PPI-effected prevention of ulcer complications, particularly in Hp-negative subjects, either naturally or after Hp eradication. However, there are data regarding the highest risk group – namely patients who have experienced an upper gastrointestinal (UGI) bleed and have restarted NSAIDs. In that high-risk group the addition of a PPI to traditional NSAID therapy produced disappointing results, showing rebleeding rates of 12.8% and 13.6% (annualized) with the combination of a PPI and an NSAID [179,180]. The expected rate is between 24% and 36% per year, suggesting that the benefit was probably about 50%–70% protection. In contrast, the combination of a PPI and celecoxib appeared effective in preventing rebleeding whereas the celecoxib alone did not [181].

Overall, the effectiveness of PPIs in preventing clinically important NSAID-associated UGI events is low. As was so elegantly described for gabapentin, medical opinion can be swayed through the use of marketing studies with surrogate end points, opinion leaders' speakers bureaus, and regular consensus conferences despite the lack of data [182]. As noted above, one should probably expect no more than a 50%–80% reduction in serious events with PPI cotherapy. Importantly, there are no data suggesting a dose–response effect (i.e., the lowest PPI doses have proven as effective as higher doses for prevention of endoscopic ulcers) such that the lowest dose of the least expensive PPI would probably suffice. No data support use of sucralfate, antacids, or bismuth for prevention or treatment of NSAID-induced ulceration.

Age alone, and age plus symptoms, markedly influence the baseline risk of NSAID ulcer complications [183]. The issues have become complicated by data suggesting that many traditional NSAIDs have significant cardiovascular risks [184,185] making the choice of therapy among the elderly even more difficult. This has led to rethinking of the role of non-drug therapy [186].

The ulcer risk with different NSAIDs

The choice of agent is dependent on the therapeutic goal. If analgesia is the primary aim, then, in most cases, a trial of full-strength non-NSAID pain relievers should be given first. As with NSAIDs, one should strive for the lowest effective dose. If the patient fails this first-line therapy (e.g., acetaminophen prescribed at regular intervals for the pain of osteoarthritis or other noninflammatory conditions), the cost, safety, and efficacy of individual NSAIDs should be considered prior to prescription of NSAIDs.

In general, one should choose NSAID agents with the shortest half-lives for the temporary treatment of acute painful states. The dental pain model suggests that aspirin and acetaminophen at 650 mg are equally effective as analgesics. The maximum analgesic dose of aspirin or acetaminophen is approximately 650 mg, which is equal to 200 mg of ibuprofen. The maximum analgesic dose of ibuprofen is 400 mg. Thus, there is no reason to give more drug when analgesia is the goal, because it only increases the risk with no additional benefits. As noted above, the issue of cardiovascular risk of selective and nonselective NSAIDs also needs to be taken into account. Deciding which NSAID is suitable for which indication is a continually evolving process.

References

1. Earlam R, Chir M. A computerized questionnaire analysis of duodenal ulcer symptoms. Gastroenterology 1976;71:314.
2. Edwards FC, Coghill NF. Clinical manifestations in patients with chronic atrophic gastritis, gastric ulcer, and duodenal ulcer. Quart J Med 1968;37:337.
3. Horrocks JC, De Dombal FT. Clinical presentation of patients with dyspepsia. Detailed symptomatic study of 360 patients. Gut 1978;19:19.
4. Moynihan BGA, Lond MS. On duodenal ulcer: with notes of 52 operations. Lancet 1905;1:340.
5. Rinaldo JA, Scheinok P, Rupe CE. Symptom diagnosis. A mathematical analysis of epigastric pain. Ann Intern Med 1963;59:145.
6. Sjodin I, Svedlund J, Dotevall G, et al. Symptom profiles in chronic peptic ulcer disease. Scand J Gastroenterol 1985;20:419.
7. Werdmuller BF, van der Putten AB, Loffeld RJ. The clinical presentation of peptic ulcer disease. Neth J Med 1997;50:115.
8. Palmer WL. The "acid test" in gastric and duodenal ulcer. JAMA 1927;88:1778.
9. Kang JY, Yap I, Guan R, et al. Acid perfusion of duodenal ulcer craters and ulcer pain: a controlled double-blind study. Gut 1986;27:942.
10. McColl KE, El-Nujumi A, Murray LS, et al. Assessment of symptomatic response as predictor of Helicobacter pylori status following eradication therapy in patients with ulcer. Gut 1998;42:618.
11. McColl KE, Dickson A, El-Nujumi A, et al. Symptomatic benefit 1–3 years after H. pylori eradication in ulcer patients: impact of gastroesophageal reflux disease. Am J Gastroenterol 2000;95:101.
12. Mayer EA, Gebhart GF. Basic and clinical aspects of visceral hyperalgesia [see comments]. Gastroenterology 1994;107:271 [review].
13. Stanghellini V, Barbara G, de GR, et al. Review article: Helicobacter pylori, mucosal inflammation and symptom perception – new insights into an old hypothesis. Aliment Pharmacol Ther 2001;15(Suppl. 1):28.
14. Donaldson RM, Jr. Factors complicating observed associations between peptic ulcer and other diseases. Gastroenterology 1975;68:1608.
15. Hirschowitz BI, Simmons JL, Johnson LF, et al. Risk factors for esophagitis in extreme acid hypersecretors with and without Zollinger–Ellison syndrome. Clin Gastroenterol Hepatol 2004;2:220.
16. Malfertheiner P, Megraud F, O'Morain C, et al. Current concepts in the management of Helicobacter pylori infection – The Maastricht III Consensus Report. Gut 2007;56:772.
17. Wilcox CM, Alexander LN, Cotsonis GA, et al. Nonsteroidal antiinflammatory drugs are associated with both upper and lower gastrointestinal bleeding. Dig Dis Sci 1997;42:990.
18. Corinaldesi R, Paternico A, Stanghellini V, et al. Patients with duodenitis have gastric secretory and motor functions like those of duodenal ulcer patients: results of a short-term treatment with ranitidine. J Clin Gastroenterol 1991;13:296.
19. Gururatsakul M, Adam B, Liebregts T, et al. Differing clinical manifestations in complicated and uncomplicated peptic ulcer disease: abnormal visceral sensory function may be a key. Gastroenterology 2007;132:A43.
20. Hung LC, Ching JY, Sung JJ, et al. Long-term outcome of Helicobacter pylori-negative idiopathic bleeding ulcers: a prospective cohort study. Gastroenterology 2005;128:1845.
21. Chan FK, Hung LC, Suen BY, et al. Celecoxib versus diclofenac plus omeprazole in high-risk arthritis patients: results of a randomized double-blind trial. Gastroenterology 2004;127:1038.
22. Wong CH, Chow PK, Ong HS, et al. Posterior perforation of peptic ulcers: presentation and outcome of an uncommon surgical emergency. Surgery 2004;135:321.
23. Wang HP, Su WC. Images in clinical medicine. Veiled right kidney sign in a patient with Valentino's syndrome. N Engl J Med 2006;354:e9.
24. Laosebikan AO, Govindasamy V, Chinnery G, et al. Giant gastric ulcer: an endoscopic roller coaster. Gut 2005;54:468.
25. Akazawa Y, Mizuta Y, Osabe M, et al. A case of double pylorus caused by recurrent gastric ulcers: a long-term endoscopic observation. Dig Dis Sci 2005;50:2125.
26. Solomon LK, Vogiatzis I, Craig E, et al. Hepatic penetration of a single large duodenal ulcer. Ulster Med J 2005;74:134.
27. Lanas A, Sekar MC, Hirschowitz BI. Objective evidence of aspirin use in both ulcer and nonulcer upper and lower gastrointestinal bleeding. Gastroenterology 1992;103:862.
28. Glick SN. Duodenal ulcer. Radiol Clin North Am 1994;32:1259.
29. Levine MS. Role of the double-contrast upper gastrointestinal series in the 1990s. Gastroenterol Clin North Am 1995;24:289 [review].
30. Lee JM, Breslin NP, Fallon C, et al. Rapid urease tests lack sensitivity in Helicobacter pylori diagnosis when peptic ulcer disease presents with bleeding. Am J Gastroenterol 2000;95:1166.
31. Graham DY, Schwartz JT, Cain GD, et al. Prospective evaluation of biopsy number in the diagnosis of esophageal and gastric carcinoma. Gastroenterology 1982;82:228.
32. Chen CH, Huang HS, Yang CC, et al. The features of perforated peptic ulcers in conventional computed tomography. Hepatogastroenterology 2001;48:1393.
33. Pun E, Firkin A. Computed tomography and complicated peptic ulcer disease. Australas Radiol 2004;48:516.
34. Yeung KW, Chang MS, Hsiao CP, et al. CT evaluation of gastrointestinal tract perforation. Clin Imaging 2004;28:329.
35. Collen MJ, Santoro MJ, Chen YK. Giant duodenal ulcer. Evaluation of basal acid output, nonsteroidal antiinflammatory drug use, and ulcer complications. Dig Dis Sci 1994;39:1113.
36. Borra S, Gavani S, Kleinfeld M. Giant peptic ulcers in patients with chronic renal failure. Mt Sinai J Med 1990;57:97.
37. Moonka D, Lichtenstein GR, Levine MS, et al. Giant gastric ulcers: an unusual manifestation of Crohn's disease. Am J Gastroenterol 1993;88:297.
38. Bardhan KD. Intermittent treatment of duodenal ulcer for long term medical management. Postgrad Med J 1988;64(Suppl. 1):40.
39. Gudmand-Hoyer F, Jensen KB, Krag E, et al. Prophylactic effect of cimetidine in duodenal ulcer disease. Br Med J 1978;1:1095.
40. Sontag SJ. Current status of maintenance therapy in peptic ulcer disease. Am J Gastroenterol 1988;83:607.
41. Miwa H, Sakaki N, Sugano K, et al. Recurrent peptic ulcers in patients following successful Helicobacter pylori eradication: a multicenter study of 4940 patients. Helicobacter 2004;9:9.
42. Shiotani A, Nishioka S, Iguchi M, et al. Duodenal erosions after eradication of Helicobacter pylori infection. Gastrointest Endosc 2001;54:448.
43. Laine L, Hopkins RJ, Girardi LS. Has the impact of Helicobacter pylori therapy on ulcer recurrence in the United States been overstated? A meta-analysis of rigorously designed trials. Am J Gastroenterol 1998;93:1409.
44. Hirschowitz BI, Simmons J, Mohnen J. Clinical outcome using lansoprazole in acid hypersecretors with and without Zollinger–Ellison syndrome: a 13-year prospective study. Clin Gastroenterol Hepatol 2005;3:39.
45. Feldman M, Burton ME. Histamine2-receptor antagonists. Standard therapy for acid-peptic diseases (first of two parts). N Engl J Med 1990;323:1672.
46. Cederberg C, Andersson T, Skaanberg I. Omeprazole: pharmacokinetics and metabolism in man. Scand J Gastroenterol 1989;24(Suppl. 166):33.
47. Lind T, Cederberg C, Ekenved G, et al. Effect of omeprazole – a gastric proton pump inhibitor – on pentagastrin stimulated acid secretion in man. Gut 1983;24:270.
48. Wilde MI, McTavish D. Omeprazole. An update of its pharmacology and therapeutic use in acid-related disorders. Drugs 1994;48:91.
49. Spencer CM, Faulds D. Lansoprazole. A reappraisal of its pharmacodynamic and pharmacokinetic properties, and its therapeutic efficacy in acid-related disorders. Drugs 1994;48:404 [review].

50. Delhotal Landes BD, Petite JP, Flouvat B. Clinical pharmacokinetics of lansoprazole. Clin Pharmacokinet 1995;28:458.

51. Huber R, Kohl B, Sachs G, et al. Review article: the continuing development of proton pump inhibitors with particular reference to pantoprazole. Aliment Pharmacol Ther 1995;9:363.

52. Andersson T. Pharmacokinetics, metabolism and interactions of acid pump inhibitors. Clin Pharmacokinet 1996;1:9.

53. Andersson T, Cederberg C, Edvardsson G, et al. Effect of omeprazole treatment on diazepam plasma levels in slow versus normal rapid metabolizers of omeprazole. Clin Pharmacol Ther 1990;47:79.

54. Sharma BK, Walt RP, Pounder RE, et al. Optimal dose of oral omeprazole for maximal 24 hour decrease of intragastric acidity. Gut 1984;25:957.

55. Shearman DJC, Buckle PJ, Hetzel DJ. The inhibition of nocturnal gastric acid secretion by omeprazole in patients with duodenal ulcer. Scand J Gastroenterol 1986;21(Suppl. 118):145.

56. Burget DW, Chiverton SG, Hunt RH. Is there an optimal degree of acid suppression for healing of duodenal ulcers? A model of the relationship between ulcer healing and acid suppression. Gastroenterology 1990;99:345.

57. De Graef J, Woussen-Colle M-C. Influence of the stimulation state of the parietal cells on the inhibitory effect of omeprazole on gastric acid secretion in dogs. Gastroenterology 1986;91:333.

58. Larson C, Cavuto NJ, Flockhart DA, et al. Bioavailability and efficacy of omeprazole given orally and by nasogastric tube. Dig Dis Sci 1996;41:475.

59. Han SW, Evans DG, El-Zaatari FAK, et al. The interaction of pH, bile and Helicobacter pylori may explain duodenal ulcer. Am J Gastroenterol 1996;91:1135.

60. Merki HS, Wilder-Smith CH. Do continuous infusions of omeprazole and ranitidine retain their effect with prolonged dosing? Gastroenterology 1994;106:60.

61. Julapalli VR, Graham DY. Appropriate use of intravenous proton pump inhibitors in the management of bleeding peptic ulcer. Dig Dis Sci 2005;50:1185.

62. Monk JP, Clissold SP. Misoprostol – A preliminary review of its pharmacodynamic and pharmacokinetic properties, and therapeutic efficacy in the treatment of peptic ulcer disease. Drugs 1987;33:1.

63. Roszkowski AP, Garay GL, Baker S, et al. Gastric antisecretory and antiulcer properties of enprostil, (+/−)-11alpha, 15alpha-dihydroxy-16-phenoxy-17,18,19,20-tetranor-9-oxoprosta-4,5,13(t)-trienoic acid methyl ester. J Pharmacol Exp Ther 1986;239:382.

64. Bianchi Porro G, Parente F. Side effects of anti-ulcer prostaglandins: an overview of the worldwide clinical experience. Scand J Gastroenterol 1989;24:224.

65. Graham DY, Agrawal NM, Roth SH. Prevention of NSAID-induced gastric ulcer with misoprostol: multicentre, double-blind, placebo-controlled trial. Lancet 1988;2:1277.

66. Graham DY. Critical effect of Helicobacter pylori infection on the effectiveness of omeprazole for prevention of gastric or duodenal ulcers among chronic NSAID users. Helicobacter 2002;7:1.

67. Graham DY, Agrawal NM, Campbell DR, et al. Ulcer prevention in long-term users of nonsteroidal anti-inflammatory drugs: results of a double-blind, randomized, multicenter, active- and placebo-controlled study of misoprostol vs lansoprazole. Arch Intern Med 2002;162:169.

68. Steinberg WM, Lewis, JH, Katz, DM. Antacids inhibit absorption of cimetidine. N Engl J Med 1982;307:400.

69. Hurwitz A. Antacid therapy and drug kinetics. Clin Pharmacokinet 1977;2:269.

70. Wagstaff AJ, Benfield P, Monk JP. Colloidal bismuth subcitrate – A review of its pharmacodynamic and its therapeutic use in peptic ulcer disease. Drugs 1988;36:132.

71. Streeter AM, Goulston KJ, Bathur FA, et al. Cimetidine and malabsorption of cobalamin. Dig Dis Sci 1982;27:13.

72. Belaiche J, Cattan D, Zittoun J, et al. Effect of ranitidine on cobalamin absorption. Dig Dis Sci 1983;28:667.

73. Reynolds JC. The clinical importance of drug interactions with antiulcer therapy. J Clin Gastroenterol 1990;12:S54.

74. Yang YX, Lewis JD, Epstein S, et al. Long-term proton pump inhibitor therapy and risk of hip fracture. JAMA 2006;296:2947.

75. Centanni M, Gargano L, Canettieri G, et al. Thyroxine in goiter, Helicobacter pylori infection, and chronic gastritis. N Engl J Med 2006;354:1787.

76. Nwokolo CU, Prewett EJ, Sawyerr AM, et al. The effect of histamine H2-receptor blockade on bismuth absorption from three ulcer-healing compounds. Gastroenterology 1991;101:889.

77. Petersen KU. Review article: omeprazole and the cytochrome P450 system. Aliment Pharmacol Ther 1995;9:1 [review].

78. Ando T, Minami M, Mizuno T, et al. Long-term follow-up after eradication of Helicobacter pylori with omeprazole, clarithromycin, and tinidazole (OCT regimen) in a Japanese population. Helicobacter 2005;10:379.

79. Furuta T, Ohashi K, Kamata T, et al. Effect of genetic differences in omeprazole metabolism on cure rates for Helicobacter pylori infection and peptic ulcer. Ann Intern Med 1998;129:1027.

80. Smallwood RA, Berlin RG, Castagnoli N, et al. Safety of acid-suppressing drugs. Dig Dis Sci 1995;40:63S.

81. Bertilsson L. Geographical/interracial differences in polymorphic drug oxidation: current state of knowledge of cytochromes P450 (CYP) 2D6 and 2C19. Clin Pharmacokinet 1995;29:192.

82. Takahashi K, Motohashi H, Yonezawa A, et al. Lansoprazole-tacrolimus interaction in Japanese transplant recipient with CYP2C19 polymorphism. Ann Pharmacother 2004;38:791.

83. Litalien C, Theoret Y, Faure C. Pharmacokinetics of proton pump inhibitors in children. Clin Pharmacokinet 2005;44:441.

84. Gustavson LE, Kaiser JF, Edmonds AL, et al. Effect of omeprazole on concentrations of clarithromycin in plasma and gastric tissue at steady state. Antimicrob Agents Chemother 1995;39:2078.

85. Metz DC, Getz HD. Helicobacter pylori gastritis therapy with omeprazole and clarithromycin increases serum carbamazepine levels. Dig Dis Sci 1995;40:912.

86. Walan A, Bader J-P, Classen M, et al. Effect of omeprazole and ranitidine on ulcer healing and relapse rates in patients with benign gastric ulcer. N Engl J Med 1989;320:69.

87. Pace F, Bianchi Porro G, Bode C, et al. Presenting characteristics of benign gastric ulcer and outcome of medical treatment. Eur J Gastroenterol Hepatol 1989;1:175.

88. Reynolds JC, Schoen RE, Maislin G, et al. Risk factors for delayed healing of duodenal ulcers treated with famotidine and ranitidine. Am J Gastroenterol 1994;89:571.

89. el-Omar E, Banerjee S, Wirz A, et al. Marked rebound acid hypersecretion after treatment with ranitidine. Am J Gastroenterol 1996;91:355.

90. Sandvik AK, Brenna E, Waldum HL. Review article: the pharmacological inhibition of gastric acid secretion – tolerance and rebound. Aliment Pharmacol Ther 1997;11:1013.

91. Waldum HL, Brenna E. Personal review: is profound acid inhibition safe? Aliment Pharmacol Ther 2000;14:15.

92. Yeomans ND, Dent J. Personal review: alarmism or legitimate concerns about long-term suppression of gastric acid secretion? Aliment Pharmacol Ther 2000:14:267.

93. Graham DY, Lew GM, Evans DG, et al. Effect of triple therapy (antibiotics plus bismuth) on duodenal ulcer healing. A randomized controlled trial. Ann Intern Med 1991;115:266.

94. Graham DY, Lew GM, Klein PD, et al. Effect of treatment of Helicobacter pylori infection on the long-term recurrence of gastric or duodenal ulcer. A randomized, controlled study. Ann Intern Med 1992;116:705.

95. Uemura N, Okamoto S. Effect of Helicobacter pylori eradication on subsequent development of cancer after endoscopic resection of early gastric cancer in Japan. Gastroenterol Clin North Am 2000;29:819.

96. Uemura N, Okamoto S, Yamamoto S, et al. Helicobacter pylori infection and the development of gastric cancer. N Engl J Med 2001;345:784.

97. Wong BC, Lam SK, Wong WM, et al. Helicobacter pylori eradication to

prevent gastric cancer in a high-risk region of China: a randomized controlled trial. JAMA 2004;291:187.

98. Leal-Herrera Y, Torres J, Monath TP, et al. High rates of recurrence and of transient reinfections of *Helicobacter pylori* in a population with high prevalence of infection. Am J Gastroenterol 2003;98:2395.

99. Soto G, Bautista CT, Roth DE, et al. *Helicobacter pylori* reinfection is common in Peruvian adults after antibiotic eradication therapy. J Infect Dis 2003;188:1263.

100. Graham DY. Antibiotic resistance in *Helicobacter pylori*: implications for therapy. Gastroenterology 1998;115:1272.

101. Graham DY. Therapy of *Helicobacter pylori*: current status and issues. Gastroenterology 2000;118:S2.

102. Chiba N, Rao BV, Rademaker JW, et al. Meta-analysis of the efficacy of antibiotic therapy in eradicating *Helicobacter pylori*. Am J Gastroenterol 1992;87:1716.

103. Dore MP, Leandro G, Realdi G, et al. Effect of pretreatment antibiotic resistance to metronidazole and clarithromycin on outcome of *Helicobacter pylori* therapy: a meta-analytical approach. Dig Dis Sci 2000;45:68.

104. Gisbert JP, Khorrami S, Calvet X, et al. Meta-analysis: proton pump inhibitors vs. H2-receptor antagonists – their efficacy with antibiotics in *Helicobacter pylori* eradication. Aliment Pharmacol Ther 2003;18: 757.

105. Laheij RJ, Rossum LG, Jansen JB, et al. Evaluation of treatment regimens to cure *Helicobacter pylori* infection – a meta-analysis. Aliment Pharmacol Ther 1999;13:857.

106. Broutet N, Tchamgoue S, Pereira E, et al. Risk factors for failure of *Helicobacter pylori* therapy – results of an individual data analysis of 2751 patients. Aliment Pharmacol Ther 2003;17:99.

107. Fischbach LA, Goodman KJ, Feldman M, et al. Sources of variation of *Helicobacter pylori* treatment success in adults worldwide: a meta-analysis. Int J Epidemiol 2002;31:128.

108. Gisbert JP, Khorrami S, Calvet X, et al. Systematic review: Rabeprazole-based therapies in *Helicobacter pylori* eradication. Aliment Pharmacol Ther 2003;17:751.

109. Graham DY, Hammoud F, El-Zimaity HM, et al. Meta-analysis: proton pump inhibitor or H2-receptor antagonist for *Helicobacter pylori* eradication. Aliment Pharmacol Ther 2003;17:1229.

110. Broutet N, Marais A, Lamouliatte H, et al. cagA status and eradication treatment outcome of anti-*Helicobacter pylori* triple therapies in patients with nonulcer dyspepsia. J Clin Microbiol 2001;39:1319.

111. Wong WM, Xiao SD, Hu PJ, et al. Standard treatment for *Helicobacter pylori* infection is suboptimal in non-ulcer dyspepsia compared with duodenal ulcer in Chinese. Aliment Pharmacol Ther 2005;21:73.

112. Calvet X, Ducons J, Bujanda L, et al. Seven versus ten days of rabeprazole triple therapy for *Helicobacter pylori* eradication: a multi-center randomized trial. Am J Gastroenterol 2005;100:1696.

113. Graham DY, Klein PD, Opekun AR, et al. In vivo susceptibility of *Campylobacter pylori*. Am J Gastroenterol 1989;84:233.

114. Graham DY. A reliable cure for *Helicobacter pylori* infection? Gut 1995;37:154.

115. European Helicobacter Pylori Study Group. Current European concepts in the management of *Helicobacter pylori* infection. The Maastricht Consensus Report. Gut 1997;41:8.

116. Della MP, Lavagna A, Masoero G, et al. Effectiveness of *Helicobacter pylori* eradication treatments in a primary care setting in Italy. Aliment Pharmacol Ther 2002;16:1269.

117. Bochenek WJ, Peters S, Fraga PD, et al. Eradication of *Helicobacter pylori* by 7-day triple-therapy regimens combining pantoprazole with clarithromycin, metronidazole, or amoxicillin in patients with peptic ulcer disease: results of two double-blind, randomized studies. Helicobacter 2003;8:626.

118. Boixeda D, Martin dA, Bermejo F, et al. Seven-day proton pump inhibitor, amoxicillin and clarithromycin triple therapy: factors that influence *Helicobacter pylori* eradication success. Rev Esp Enferm Dig 2003;95:206.

119. De Francesco V, Zullo A, Hassan C, et al. The prolongation of triple therapy for *Helicobacter pylori* does not allow reaching therapeutic

outcome of sequential scheme: a prospective, randomised study. Dig Liver Dis 2004;36:322.

120. Fennerty MB, Kovacs TO, Krause R, et al. A comparison of 10 and 14 days of lansoprazole triple therapy for eradication of *Helicobacter pylori*. Arch Intern Med 1998;158:1651.

121. Laine L, Frantz JE, Baker A, et al. A United States multicentre trial of dual and proton pump inhibitor-based triple therapies for *Helicobacter pylori*. Aliment Pharmacol Ther 1997;11:913.

122. Scaccianoce G, Hassan C, Panarese A, et al. *Helicobacter pylori* eradication with either 7-day or 10-day triple therapies, and with a 10-day sequential regimen. Can J Gastroenterol 2006;20:113.

123. Vakil N, Lanza F, Schwartz H, et al. Seven-day therapy for *Helicobacter pylori* in the United States. Aliment Pharmacol Ther 2004;20:99.

124. Zagari RM, Bianchi-Porro G, Fiocca R, et al. Comparison of 1 and 2 weeks of omeprazole, amoxicillin and clarithromycin treatment for *Helicobacter pylori* eradication: the HYPER Study. Gut 2007;56:475.

125. Zullo A, Vaira D, Vakil N, et al. High eradication rates of *Helicobacter pylori* with a new sequential treatment. Aliment Pharmacol Ther 2003;17:719.

126. Vaira D, Zullo A, Vakil N, et al. Sequential therapy versus standard triple-drug therapy for *Helicobacter pylori* eradication: A randomized trial. Ann Intern Med 2007;146:556.

127. De Francesco V, Della VN, Stoppino V, et al. Effectiveness and pharmaceutical cost of sequential treatment for *Helicobacter pylori* in patients with non-ulcer dyspepsia. Aliment Pharmacol Ther 2004;19:993.

128. Paoluzi P, Iacopini F, Crispino P, et al. 2-week triple therapy for *Helicobacter pylori* infection is better than 1-week in clinical practice: a large prospective single-center randomized study. Helicobacter 2006;11:562.

129. Zullo A, Rinaldi V, Winn S, et al. A new highly effective short-term therapy schedule for *Helicobacter pylori* eradication. Aliment Pharmacol Ther 2000;14:715.

130. Furuta T, Shirai N, Xiao F, et al. Polymorphism of interleukin-1beta affects the eradication rates of *Helicobacter pylori* by triple therapy. Clin Gastroenterol Hepatol 2004;2:22.

131. Furuta T, Sagehashi Y, Shirai N, et al. Influence of CYP2C19 polymorphism and *Helicobacter pylori* genotype determined from gastric tissue samples on response to triple therapy for *H. pylori* infection. Clin Gastroenterol Hepatol 2005;3:564.

132. Higuchi K, Maekawa T, Nakagawa K, et al. Efficacy and safety of *Helicobacter pylori* eradication therapy with omeprazole, amoxicillin and high- and low-dose clarithromycin in Japanese patients: a randomised, double-blind, multicentre study. Clin Drug Investig 2006; 26:403.

133. Murakami K, Sato R, Okimoto T, et al. Eradication rates of clarithromycin-resistant *Helicobacter pylori* using either rabeprazole or lansoprazole plus amoxicillin and clarithromycin. Aliment Pharmacol Ther 2002;16:1933.

134. Take S, Mizuno M, Ishiki K, et al. Interleukin-1beta genetic polymorphism influences the effect of cytochrome P 2C19 genotype on the cure rate of 1-week triple therapy for *Helicobacter pylori* infection. Am J Gastroenterol 2003;98:2403.

135. Kim BG, Lee DH, Ye BD, et al. Comparison of 7-day and 14-day proton pump inhibitor-containing triple therapy for *Helicobacter pylori* eradication: neither treatment duration provides acceptable eradication rate in Korea. Helicobacter 2007;12:31.

136. Zhang L, Shen L, Ma JL, et al. Eradication of *H. pylori* infection in a rural population: one-day quadruple therapy versus 7-day triple therapy. World J Gastroenterol 2006;12:3915.

137. Hsu PI, Lai KH, Lin CK, et al. A prospective randomized trial of esomeprazole-versus pantoprazole-based triple therapy for *Helicobacter pylori* eradication. Am J Gastroenterol 2005;100:2387.

138. Lee YC, Wu HM, Chen TH, et al. A community-based study of *Helicobacter pylori* therapy using the strategy of test, treat, retest, and re-treat initial treatment failures. Helicobacter 2006;11:418.

139. Poon SK, Chang CS, Su J, et al. Primary resistance to antibiotics and its clinical impact on the efficacy of *Helicobacter pylori* lansoprazole-based triple therapies. Aliment Pharmacol Ther 2002;16:291.

140. Ford A, Moayyedi P. How can the current strategies for *Helicobacter pylori* eradication therapy be improved? Can J Gastroenterol 2003;17 (Suppl. B):36B.

141. Calvet X, Garcia N, Lopez T, et al. A meta-analysis of short versus long therapy with a proton pump inhibitor, clarithromycin and either metronidazole or amoxicillin for treating *Helicobacter pylori* infection. Aliment Pharmacol Ther 2000;14:603.

142. Saad RJ, Schoenfeld P, Kim HM, et al. Levofloxacin-based triple therapy versus bismuth-based quadruple therapy for persistent *Helicobacter pylori* infection: a meta-analysis. Am J Gastroenterol 2006;101:488.

143. Graham DY, Abudayyeh S, El-Zimaity HM, et al. Sequential therapy using high-dose esomeprazole-amoxicillin followed by gatifloxacin for *Helicobacter pylori* infection. Aliment Pharmacol Ther 2006;24:845.

144. Francavilla R, Lionetti E, Castellaneta SP, et al. Improved efficacy of 10-day sequential treatment for *Helicobacter pylori* eradication in children: a randomized trial. Gastroenterology 2005;129:1414.

145. Zullo A, Gatta L, De Francesco V, et al. High rate of *Helicobacter pylori* eradication with sequential therapy in elderly patients with peptic ulcer: a prospective controlled study. Aliment Pharmacol Ther 2005;21:1419.

146. Wang G, Wilson TJ, Jiang Q, et al. Spontaneous mutations that confer antibiotic resistance in *Helicobacter pylori*. Antimicrob Agents Chemother 2001;45:727.

147. Nagahara A, Miwa H, Ogawa K, et al. Addition of metronidazole to rabeprazole-amoxicillin-clarithromycin regimen for *Helicobacter pylori* infection provides an excellent cure rate with five-day therapy. Helicobacter 2000;5:88.

148. Treiber G, Ammon S, Schneider E, et al. Amoxicillin/metronidazole/omeprazole/clarithromycin: a new, short quadruple therapy for *Helicobacter pylori* eradication. Helicobacter 1998;3:54.

149. Treiber G, Wittig J, Ammon S, et al. Clinical outcome and influencing factors of a new short-term quadruple therapy for *Helicobacter pylori* eradication: a randomized controlled trial (MACLOR study). Arch Intern Med 2002;162:153.

150. Bayerdorffer E, Miehlke S, Mannes GA, et al. Double-blind trial of omeprazole and amoxicillin to cure *Helicobacter pylori* infection in patients with duodenal ulcers. Gastroenterology 1995;108:1412.

151. Miehlke S, Mannes GA, Lehn N, et al. An increasing dose of omeprazole combined with amoxicillin cures *Helicobacter pylori* infection more effectively. Aliment Pharmacol Ther 1997;11:323.

152. Miehlke S, Kirsch C, Schneider-Brachert W, et al. A prospective, randomized study of quadruple therapy and high-dose dual therapy for treatment of *Helicobacter pylori* resistant to both metronidazole and clarithromycin. Helicobacter 2003;8:310.

153. Gotteland M, Brunser O, Cruchet S. Systematic review: are probiotics useful in controlling gastric colonization by *Helicobacter pylori*? Aliment Pharmacol Ther 2006;23:1077.

154. Sheu BS, Wu JJ, Lo CY, et al. Impact of supplement with *Lactobacillus*- and *Bifidobacterium*-containing yogurt on triple therapy for *Helicobacter pylori* eradication. Aliment Pharmacol Ther 2002;16:1669.

155. Aiba Y, Suzuki N, Kabir AM, et al. Lactic acid-mediated suppression of *Helicobacter pylori* by the oral administration of *Lactobacillus salivarius* as a probiotic in a gnotobiotic murine model. Am J Gastroenterol 1998;93:2097.

156. Tong JL, Ran ZH, Shen J, et al. Meta-analysis: the effect of supplementation with probiotics on eradication rates and adverse events during *Helicobacter pylori* eradication therapy. Aliment Pharmacol Ther 2007;25:155.

157. Ali AT, Chowdhury MN, al Humayyd MS. Inhibitory effect of natural honey on *Helicobacter pylori*. Trop Gastroenterol 1991;12:139.

158. Dial EJ, Hall LR, Serna H, et al. Antibiotic properties of bovine lactoferrin on *Helicobacter pylori*. Dig Dis Sci 1998;43:2750.

159. Graham DY, Anderson SY, Lang T. Garlic or jalapeno peppers for treatment of *Helicobacter pylori* infection. Am J Gastroenterol 1999;94:1200.

160. Sato K, Kawakami N, Ohtsu T, et al. Broccoli consumption and chronic atrophic gastritis among Japanese males: an epidemiological investigation. Acta Med Okayama 2004;58:127.

161. Gurbuz AK, Ozel AM, Ozturk R, et al. Effect of N-acetyl cysteine on *Helicobacter pylori*. South Med J 2005;98:1095.

162. Gotoh A, Akamatsu T, Shimizu T, et al. Additive effect of pronase on the efficacy of eradication therapy against *Helicobacter pylori*. Helicobacter 2002;7:183.

163. Armuzzi A, Cremonini F, Bartolozzi F, et al. The effect of oral administration of *Lactobacillus* GG on antibiotic-associated gastrointestinal side-effects during *Helicobacter pylori* eradication therapy. Aliment Pharmacol Ther 2001;15:163.

164. Cremonini F, Di Caro S, Covino M, et al. Effect of different probiotic preparations on anti-*Helicobacter pylori* therapy-related side effects: a parallel group, triple blind, placebo-controlled study. Am J Gastroenterol 2002;97:2744.

165. Miwa H, Nagahara A, Kurosawa A, et al. Is antimicrobial susceptibility testing necessary before second-line treatment for *Helicobacter pylori* infection? Aliment Pharmacol Ther 2003;17:1545.

166. McMahon BJ, Hennessy TW, Bensler JM, et al. The relationship among previous antimicrobial use, antimicrobial resistance, and treatment outcomes for *Helicobacter pylori* infections. Ann Intern Med 2003;139:463.

167. Megraud F, Lamouliatte H. Review article: the treatment of refractory *Helicobacter pylori* infection. Aliment Pharmacol Ther 2003;17:1333.

168. van der Wouden EJ, Thijs JC, van Zwet AA, et al. The influence of in vitro nitroimidazole resistance on the efficacy of nitroimidazole-containing anti-*Helicobacter pylori* regimens: a meta-analysis. Am J Gastroenterol 1999;94:1751.

169. Graham DY, Osato MS, Hoffman J, et al. Metronidazole containing quadruple therapy for infection with metronidazole resistant *Helicobacter pylori*: a prospective study. Aliment Pharmacol Ther 2000;14:745.

170. Buring SM, Winner LH, Hatton RC, et al. Discontinuation rates of *Helicobacter pylori* treatment regimens: a meta-analysis. Pharmacotherapy 1999;19:324.

171. Crone J, Granditsch G, Huber WD, et al. *Helicobacter pylori* in children and adolescents: increase of primary clarithromycin resistance, 1997–2000. J Pediatr Gastroenterol Nutr 2003;36:368.

172. Sung JJ, Lau, JY, Ching, JY, et al. Can aspirin be reintroduced with proton pump inhibitor infusion after endoscopic hemostasis? A double blinded randomized controlled trial. Gastroenterology 2006; 130(Suppl. 2)250.

173. Silverstein FE, Graham DY, Senior JR, et al. Misoprostol reduces serious gastrointestinal complications in patients with rheumatoid arthritis receiving nonsteroidal anti-inflammatory drugs. Ann Intern Med 1995;123:241.

174. Graham DY, White RH, Moreland LW, et al. Duodenal and gastric ulcer prevention with misoprostol in arthritis patients taking NSAIDs. Ann Intern Med 1993;119:257.

175. Robinson MG, Griffin JW, Bowers J, et al. Effect of ranitidine gastroduodenal mucosal damage induced by nonsteroidal antiinflammatory drugs. Dig Dis Sci 1989;34:424.

176. Ehsanullah RSB, Page MC, Tildesley G, et al. Prevention of gastroduodenal damage induced by non-steroidal anti-inflammatory drugs: controlled trial of ranitidine. Br Med J 1988;297:1017.

177. Ashworth NL, Peloso PM, Muhajarine N, et al. A population based historical cohort study of the mortality associated with nabumetone, Arthrotec, diclofenac, and naproxen. J Rheumatol 2004;31:951.

178. Ashworth NL, Peloso PM, Muhajarine N, et al. Risk of hospitalization with peptic ulcer disease or gastrointestinal hemorrhage associated with nabumetone, Arthrotec, diclofenac, and naproxen in a population based cohort study. J Rheumatol 2005;32:2212.

179. Chan FK, Hung LC, Suen BY, et al. Celecoxib versus diclofenac and omeprazole in reducing the risk of recurrent ulcer bleeding in patients with arthritis. N Engl J Med 2002;347:2104.

180. Lai KC, Chu KM, Hui WM, et al. Celecoxib compared with lansoprazole and naproxen to prevent gastrointestinal ulcer complications. Am J Med 2005;118:1271.

181. Chan FK, Wong VW, Suen BY, et al. Combination of a cyclooxygenase-2 inhibitor and a proton-pump inhibitor for prevention

of recurrent ulcer bleeding in patients at very high risk: a double-blind, randomised trial. Lancet 2007;369:1621.

182. Steinman MA, Bero LA, Chren MM, et al. Narrative review: the promotion of gabapentin: an analysis of internal industry documents. Ann Intern Med 2006;145:284.

183. Hernandez-Diaz S, Garcia Rodriguez LA. Cardioprotective aspirin users and their excess risk of upper gastrointestinal complications. BMC Med 2006;4:22.

184. Graham DJ. COX-2 inhibitors, other NSAIDs, and cardiovascular risk: the seduction of common sense. JAMA 2006;296:1653.

185. McGettigan P, Henry D. Cardiovascular risk and inhibition of cyclooxygenase: a systematic review of the observational studies of selective and nonselective inhibitors of cyclooxygenase 2. JAMA 2006;296:1633.

186. Shaughnessy AF, Gordon AE. Life without COX 2 inhibitors. Br Med J 2006;332:1287.

187. Hartmann M, Ehrlich A, Fuder H, et al. Equipotent inhibition of gastric acid secretion by equal doses of oral or intravenous pantoprazole. Aliment Pharmacol Ther 1998;12:1027.

188. Li XQ, Andersson TB, Ahlstrom M, et al. Comparison of inhibitory effects of the proton pump-inhibiting drugs omeprazole, esomeprazole, lansoprazole, pantoprazole, and rabeprazole on human cytochrome P450 activities. Drug Metab Dispos 2004;32:821.

189. Itagaki F, Homma M, Yuzawa K, et al. Effect of lansoprazole and rabeprazole on tacrolimus pharmacokinetics in healthy volunteers with CYP2C19 mutations. J Pharm Pharmacol 2004;56:1055.

8 Approach to the patient with gross gastrointestinal bleeding

Grace H. Elta, Mimi Takami

Clinical presentation, 122
Acute upper gastrointestinal bleeding, 124
Acute lower gastrointestinal bleeding, 137
Obscure gastrointestinal bleeding, 141

Gastrointestinal (GI) bleeding is a common clinical problem requiring more than 300 000 hospitalizations annually in the United States. The annual rate of hospitalization for upper GI bleeding has been estimated at 36 to 102 patients per 100 000 members of the general population and is twice as common in men as in women [1,2]. Lower GI bleeding is less common; the estimate from a large health maintenance organization of cases of acute lower GI bleeding leading to hospitalization was 20 per 100 000 [3]. The rates of acute upper and lower GI bleeding are both increased in patients taking aspirin, and the risk appears to dose related [4,5]. Calcium antagonists and serotonin reuptake inhibitor antidepressants, both of which also inhibit platelet aggregation, may increase GI bleeding [6,7], whereas nitrovasodilator drugs may decrease the risk [8].

Most patients with upper GI bleeding undergo endoscopy within 24 h after admission and one-third of these procedures include endoscopic hemostatic therapy [9]. Several risk scoring systems have been devised for triage of patients with upper GI hemorrhage [10]. The endoscopy-based scoring systems are the most accurate [11], allowing outpatient care of selected patients with significant cost savings [12,13]. Adaptation of clinical care pathways has also been shown to decrease both hospital admissions and length of stay for upper GI bleeding without increasing the number of adverse outcomes [14]. However, shortcomings of both early endoscopic triage [15] and clinical care pathways [16] have been noted because of implementation barriers in actual clinical practice.

Mortality rates from upper GI hemorrhage vary from 3.5% to 7% in the United States [1–3], although a study from the Netherlands in 2000 reported a mortality rate of 13% [17]. The mortality rate for lower GI bleeding has been reported at 3.6%; although similar to upper GI bleeding, mortality is markedly greater in patients who begin bleeding after hospitalization [3]. The early and accurate diagnosis of patients with severe bleeding can facilitate therapeutic maneuvers, leading to lower mortality rates [18]. This trend appears to have developed with the use of therapeutic endoscopic techniques.

Clinical presentation

The overall strategy for management of GI bleeding starts with an assessment of the patient to determine how much blood has been lost and whether the bleeding is ongoing. This is followed by resuscitation because the dire consequences of GI bleeding are those of shock. A brief history and physical examination will often determine whether the source of bleeding is in the upper or lower GI tract and whether the bleeding has ceased, which happens in 80% of patients. The need for urgent vs elective endoscopy can then be determined (although in upper GI bleeding, urgent endoscopy has been proposed for all patients to facilitate triage and decrease resource use). If endoscopy is to be performed electively, empirical medical therapy for the most likely diagnoses can be started to decrease the risk for rebleeding. When a definitive diagnosis is made, specific medical, endoscopic, angiographic, or surgical therapy can be performed.

Patient assessment

The first step in assessing the bleeding patient is to determine the urgency of the situation. Agitation, pallor, hypotension, and tachycardia may indicate shock requiring immediate volume replacement. Patients with severe blood loss may

Principles of Clinical Gastroenterology. Edited by Tadataka Yamada, David H. Alpers, Anthony N. Kalloo, Neil Kaplowitz, Chung Owyang, and Don W. Powell. © 2008 Blackwell Publishing. ISBN 978-1-4051-69103

actually have bradycardia rather than tachycardia secondary to vagal slowing of the heart. Shock occurs when blood loss approaches 40% of the total blood volume. If no evidence of hypotension is found, the orthostatic vital signs can help diagnose lesser degrees of intravascular volume depletion. Postural hypotension with a decrease in systolic blood pressure of 10 mmHg or more usually indicates at least a 20% reduction in blood volume. In the acutely bleeding patient, intravenous access should be established. If the patient has signs of shock or continues to bleed, a large-bore central intravenous line is useful. Blood samples for an assessment of hematocrit, platelets, and coagulation factors and for blood typing and cross-matching should be sent immediately to the laboratory.

The initial hematocrit obtained for a patient with acute bleeding poorly reflects the degree of blood loss. Because the hematocrit is expressed in terms of erythrocyte volume as a percentage of the total blood volume, it does not drop until the blood volume has been restored. This repletion of blood volume from extravascular fluid begins immediately but takes 24–48 h to equilibrate completely. An acutely bleeding patient can be evaluated more effectively by monitoring the blood pressure and pulse and looking for gross evidence of ongoing bleeding than by assessing laboratory tests.

Resuscitation

Patients with severe acute GI bleeding require admission to an intensive care unit (ICU). Fragile patients with a history of cardiopulmonary disease may require measurement of capillary wedge pressure. Rapidly bleeding patients may require endotracheal intubation for airway protection [19]. The intravascular volume should be replenished with normal saline solution to prevent the consequences of shock while blood is being cross-matched for transfusion. This allows adequate circulation of the remaining erythrocytes. The oxygen-carrying capacity of blood can be maximized by administering supplemental oxygen. In rapidly bleeding patients, oxygen availability is markedly decreased during early hemorrhage, reflecting primarily a decreased cardiac output. The decrease in oxygen-carrying capacity of the blood caused by a decrease in hemoglobin is less important. Close attention to vital signs, urine output, and central vascular pressure is mandatory because early intensive resuscitation of patients with upper GI bleeding decreases mortality [20].

The specific criteria that define when a patient requires transfusion vary according to the age of the patient, whether concomitant cardiopulmonary disease is present, and whether the bleeding continues. In general, the hematocrit should be maintained above 30% in elderly patients and above 20% in young, healthy patients. With continued evidence of bleeding, the decision to transfuse cannot be based on the hematocrit alone. Unstable vital signs and gross evidence of active bleeding, such as hematemesis, bright-red blood in the nasogastric aspirate, or hematochezia, are better indicators of the need for transfusion. The hematocrit is a poor index for following the patient's need for additional transfusions. The plasma volume after acute GI bleeding is often overexpanded by intravenous fluids; the immediate posttransfusion hematocrit may underestimate the final value. Overuse of transfusions is probably more common than underuse.

In general, packed erythrocytes are the preferred form of blood transfusion. Whole-blood transfusions should be reserved for the unusual circumstances of massive blood loss and rapid, high-volume replacement, which increases the need for coagulation factor replacement. Preferably, blood volume has already been replenished with saline solution by the time banked blood is available. The use of packed cells also spares components for the blood bank. If the results of coagulation tests are abnormal, as is the case in many patients with cirrhosis, fresh-frozen plasma and platelets may also have to be administered. Even patients with initially normal coagulation factors and platelet counts eventually need plasma and platelet transfusions if they are transfused repeatedly. Patients who require massive transfusions (> 3000 mL) should receive warmed blood to prevent decreases in body temperature. Rarely, in massively transfused patients, calcium supplementation may be necessary to counter the effects of calcium-binding agents in banked blood.

Location of bleeding

In patients with obvious upper GI bleeding who present with hematemesis, a nasogastric tube should be placed to assess further the rate of ongoing blood loss. When upper GI bleeding is suspected, as in the patient with melena or with a history of previous epigastric symptoms or disease, a nasogastric tube aspirate demonstrating blood confirms the upper tract as the source. However, the nasogastric aspirate may be negative in a patient with duodenal bleeding presenting with melena when a competent pylorus prevents duodenogastric reflux. A negative nasogastric aspirate does not preclude the upper gut as the source of bleeding. Melena usually indicates an upper GI source (i.e., above the ligament of Treitz), although bleeding may be from the small bowel or proximal colon. Melena occurs when hemoglobin is converted to hematin or other hemochromes by bacterial degradation. This can be produced experimentally by the ingestion of as little as 100 to 200 mL of blood [21]. If the volume of a lower GI hemorrhage is too small to cause hematochezia but sufficient to supply enough hemoglobin for degradation, and if colonic motility is sufficiently slow, bleeding from the small bowel or proximal colon may cause melena. This is an uncommon occurrence because small bowel bleeding is rare and colonic sources bleed slowly, causing Hemoccult-positive stools, or bleed rapidly enough to cause hematochezia.

Another indication of an upper GI source of bleeding is a mildly elevated level of blood urea nitrogen (BUN) [22]. Some of this azotemia is caused by the absorption of blood, but the experimental ingestion of blood results in lower elevations in BUN of shorter duration, suggesting that part of the azotemia is secondary to hypovolemia [23]. A study has confirmed that the BUN-to-creatinine ratio is higher in upper GI than in lower GI bleeding but is a poor discriminator [24]. Testing for occult blood in nasogastric aspirates is rarely necessary because the blood is often obvious. The one occasion on which occult blood testing is helpful is when a coffee-ground appearance of the aspirate may be produced by some foods. A simple positive test for occult blood may merely indicate nasogastric tube trauma. When occult testing of gastric aspirates is used, it is important not to rely on standard stool kits, which may yield false-negative results in acidic solutions [25].

Hematochezia usually indicates a lower GI source. However, 11% of patients with rapid bleeding from an upper GI source pass bright-red blood rectally because of rapid GI transit [26]. Placement of a nasogastric tube and an endoscopic examination should be considered if there is any question about the location of bleeding in a patient with hematochezia.

Acute upper gastrointestinal bleeding

Upper GI bleeding is a common clinical problem, causing 10 000 to 20 000 deaths each year in the United States. Forty-four percent of hospitalizations for upper GI bleeding are for patients older than 60 years of age [1]. Approximately 80% of upper GI bleeding episodes are self-limited and require only supportive therapy [27]. Patients with continued or recurrent bleeding have mortality rates of 25%–30% [1,27].

Prognostic indicators

Several prognostic indicators in upper GI bleeding have been identified. The most important is the cause of bleeding. Variceal hemorrhages have much higher rebleeding and mortality rates than other conditions. Mortality from variceal hemorrhage during the initial hospitalization has improved over the last 20 years although it is still 14%, with rebleeding rates of 13%–29% [28,29]. A reduction in the mortality rates associated with variceal bleeding would lower the overall mortality of upper GI bleeding because varices account for approximately 10% of all bleeding episodes.

Stigmata of recent bleeding that can be visualized at endoscopy, such as active arterial spurting, oozing of blood, a visible vessel, or a fresh or old blood clot, are important predictors of outcome in peptic ulcer bleeding (Table 8.1). A visible vessel is described endoscopically as an elevated, dark-red, blue, or gray mound that protrudes from the ulcer crater and is resistant to washing. The endoscopic diagnosis of a visible vessel has been validated by pathological correlation in a group of gastric ulcer patients who required surgical resection, although this visible vessel is actually an organizing clot plugging a side hole in the bleeding artery located just below the ulcer base [30]. The evolution of the endoscopic

Table 8.1 Stigmata of hemorrhage and the risk for rebleeding

Stigmata of hemorrhage	Incidence (%)	Rebleeding (%)
Spurting arterial bleeding	8	85–100
Nonbleeding visible vessel	17–50	18–55 (mean 43)
Adherent clot (no visible vessel)	18–26	24–41
Other stigmata	12–18	5–9
No stigmata	10–36	0

Adapted from Johnston [31].

appearance of visible vessels, or sentinel clots, has been described as an initial large, red clot that becomes darker and smaller with time, eventually being replaced with a white plug of fibrin and platelets that finally disappears [31]. Unfortunately, there is considerable disagreement among experts on the endoscopic diagnosis of visible vessels [2,32].

Despite the lack of uniform endoscopic descriptions, the presence of a visible vessel in an ulcer crater at endoscopy predicts an increased risk for required surgical intervention and increased mortality [33]. The incidence of rebleeding in patients who have ulcers with visible vessels is up to 50%, whereas no rebleeding is observed in patients with no stigmata of recent bleeding [34]. When endoscopy is performed within 6–24 h after admission, visible vessels are found in 20%–50% of bleeding ulcers.

The identification of predictors of recurrent hemorrhage directs the need for therapeutic endoscopic techniques, which can lower the mortality rate for patients with ulcers that have stigmata of recent bleeding [35]. Which stigmata indicate a requirement for therapy in patients with bleeding ulcers? Based on numerous randomized trials, there is agreement among experts on the treatment of actively bleeding (i.e., spurting or oozing) visible vessels and nonbleeding visible vessels that are raised and cannot be washed off [36]. Although some controversy still exists on the necessity of endoscopic therapy for adherent clot, several studies and a metaanalysis show superiority for endoscopic therapy over medical therapy alone [37–39].

Other prognostic indicators include the following:
• *Severity of the initial bleed.* Severity is assessed by the transfusion requirement, the presence of bright-red blood in the nasogastric aspirate, or the presence of hypotension (Table 8.2) [40].
• *Age of the patient.* Patients older than 60 years have been shown to have higher mortality rates than their younger counterparts, although this indicator may not be independent from concomitant disease [1].
• *Concomitant disease.* Diseases such as chronic renal failure and severe cardiopulmonary disease affect the ultimate outcome.

Table 8.2 Prognostic value of the severity of upper gastrointestinal bleeding

Nasogastric aspirate	Stool color	Mortality rate (%)
Clear	Red, brown, black	10
Coffee grounds	Brown or black	10
	Red	20
Red blood	Black	10
	Brown	20
	Red	30

Adapted from Silverstein FE, Gilbert DA, Tedesco FJ. The national ASGE survey on upper gastrointestinal bleeding. Gastrointest Endosc 1981;27:73.

- Onset of bleeding during hospitalization. Patients who begin to bleed while hospitalized have a mortality rate of 25%, whereas the rate is only 3.7% for patients who start to bleed before admission [2].

Diagnostic approach

Patients with self-limited minor bleeding and other more serious medical problems may not require endoscopy. However, for most patients, even those with relatively minor bleeding, an accurate diagnosis or localization of the source is desirable to direct further management.

History and physical examination

As initial resuscitative measures are being implemented, a history should be taken and a physical examination performed. Even experienced gastroenterologists can guess the cause of bleeding only 50% of the time after a careful history and physical examination. However, the history may raise specific diagnostic possibilities. A history of peptic ulcer disease (PUD) or dyspeptic symptoms suggests ulcer bleeding. The recent use of nonsteroidal antiinflammatory drugs (NSAIDs) must always be determined, and it is important to obtain a history of ingesting alcohol or a caustic substance. A history of cirrhosis or symptoms of cirrhosis such as ascites may suggest the need for urgent endoscopy to diagnose variceal bleeding. Other medical problems, such as prior aortic graft surgery, coagulopathies, cancer, or recent nosebleeds, may suggest likely diagnoses.

Physical examination of the skin may provide diagnostic clues. Stigmata of cirrhosis, evidence of underlying malignancy (e.g., Kaposi sarcoma), or hereditary vascular anomalies may be revealed. The finding of lymphadenopathy or abdominal masses may suggest malignancy. Abdominal tenderness in the epigastrium is common in peptic disease. Hepatic or splenic enlargement may indicate liver disease or certain malignant disorders. When patients present with upper GI bleeding, a rectal examination may indicate the magnitude of blood loss by demonstrating maroon stool or melena in patients with severe bleeding or normal-colored stool in patients with minimal or recent bleeding.

Endoscopy

The diagnostic accuracy and therapeutic potential of endoscopy makes it the procedure of choice for upper GI bleeding. Diagnostic endoscopy is viewed as a safe and simple procedure by patients and physicians, although morbidity rates of 1.0% and mortality rates of 0.1% have been reported. Endoscopy is contraindicated for an uncooperative patient or a patient with a suspected perforated viscus. Endoscopy can locate precisely the site of bleeding when bleeding continues or the stigmata of bleeding persist. In patients with massive hemorrhage, the source of bleeding occasionally cannot be discerned by endoscopy. In patients whose bleeding has stopped and in whom no stigmata of bleeding remain, a significant lesion seen on endoscopy (e.g., a clean ulcer base) is the presumed source. If more than one lesion or no lesion is identified, a definitive diagnosis cannot be made, and these patients must be restudied if they bleed again. Up to 24% of patients presenting with melena will have a nondiagnostic upper GI endoscopy, with the most common source of bleeding being the right side of the colon [41]. It is important not to mislead those caring for the patient by overstating the certainty of the localization or diagnosis of the bleeding site.

The timing of the diagnostic endoscopy depends on the severity and suspected cause of the hemorrhage. Patients who fail to stop bleeding with simple supportive care require urgent endoscopy to guide further therapeutic techniques. Patients with underlying cirrhosis should undergo endoscopy as close to the bleeding episode as possible because they often have more than one source of potential hemorrhage and the diagnosis of bleeding varices alters future approaches to treatment. For most patients whose bleeding ceases, diagnostic endoscopy can be postponed for 24 h without seriously altering diagnostic accuracy or clinical outcome [42]. A separate reason to perform urgent endoscopy is the use of endoscopic findings as a triage tool, allowing some patients to be discharged from the hospital and managed as outpatients [12].

Angiography

Angiography is used as a diagnostic examination for acute upper GI bleeding only if endoscopy has failed. The bleeding must be arterial and achieve a rate of at least 0.5–0.6 mL/min if extravasation is to be detected. Angiography represents a therapeutic alternative for the delivery of intraarterial vasopressin in stress gastropathy or for embolization of bleeding ulcers or neoplasms in inoperable patients. Angiography may be used to diagnose difficult cases of recurrent GI bleeding from an unknown source. It provides an accurate diagnosis for 50%–75% of patients but is associated with a serious complication rate of about 2%. Complications of angiography

Table 8.3 Final diagnosis of the cause of upper gastrointestinal bleeding in 2225 patients

Diagnosis	Percentage of total diagnoses (%)
Duodenal ulcer	24.3
Gastric erosions	23.4
Gastric ulcer	21.3
Varices	10.3
Mallory–Weiss tear	7.2
Esophagitis	6.3
Erosive duodenitis	5.8
Neoplasm	2.9
Stomal ulcer	1.8
Esophageal ulcer	1.7
Miscellaneous	6.8

Adapted from Silverstein FE, Gilbert DA, Tedesco FJ. The national ASGE survey on upper gastrointestinal bleeding. Gastrointest Endosc 1981;27:73, with permission from Williams & Wilkins.

are related to catheter placement (e.g., dissection, thrombosis, false aneurysm) or to the contrast material (e.g., allergic reactions, renal failure). When embolic occlusion of vessels is used, the complication rate increases because of ischemic necrosis and perforation, although the use of minicoils instead of fluid embolization agents has reduced the risk [43].

Causes and therapy

The three major causes of upper GI bleeding are peptic ulcer disease, gastric erosions, and varices (Table 8.3). Their distribution depends on the patient population studied. In all endoscopic series, no diagnosis is made in 10%–15% of patients, and as many as 20%–30% of patients have more than one diagnosis. The endoscopically examined patients with no diagnosis of disease have an excellent prognosis.

Peptic ulcer bleeding

Duodenal, gastric, and stomal ulcers account for about 50% of upper GI bleeding episodes. Although several effective therapies have been developed for peptic ulcer disease during the past 20 years, these advances have had little or no impact on hospitalization rates for bleeding ulcers. One explanation for this finding may be the widespread use of aspirin and NSAIDs, particularly in the aging population, without adequate proton pump inhibitor (PPI) prophylaxis [17,44]. In addition, ulcers, particularly those that are NSAID-induced, can bleed without a prior history of peptic symptoms.

There is some evidence that ulcers located high on the lesser curvature of the stomach or in the posteroinferior wall of the duodenal bulb are at greater risk for severe bleeding because of their proximity to large vessels [45]. Rebleeding despite endoscopic therapy is more common for ulcers in

these areas [46]. Bleeding tends to occur when an ulcer erodes into the lateral wall of a vessel. The vessel often loops up to the floor of the crater and commonly protrudes with an aneurysmal dilation. A vessel with an eccentric breach is thought to be more likely to be associated with continued or recurrent bleeding than a transected vessel because retraction contraction of a severed vessel is an important mechanism of hemostasis [47].

It has been demonstrated that in patients without stigmata of recent hemorrhage, immediate refeeding and subsequent discharge are as safe as delayed refeeding for 36 h [48]. Patients with continued or recurrent ulcer bleeding have increased mortality rates [49,50]. Therapy is therefore directed at stopping bleeding and preventing recurrent bleeding.

Cessation of bleeding: endoscopic methods

The physician should insert a nasogastric tube (NGT) and perform lavage with tapwater at room temperature for the important task of monitoring the rapidity of bleeding. A study correlated mortality with the color of the fluid from the NGT aspirate and the color of the stool, establishing these parameters as prognostic indicators that might guide medical decision making [51]. A large-bore orogastric tube should replace the diagnostic nasogastric tube when cleaning for subsequent endoscopy is needed. Aliquots of 100 to 500 mL of water are instilled and removed, preferably by gravity drainage to prevent extensive suction trauma. Alternatively, administration of intravenous erythromycin before endoscopy may improve the visual quality of the procedure [52,53]. A spray of 3% hydrogen peroxide has also been suggested as a means of clot dissolution to allow endoscopic visualization [54].

For patients with persistent or recurrent hemorrhage from PUD, endoscopic control of bleeding, which is safer than emergency surgery, should be attempted [55]. In patients with acute nonvariceal upper GI bleeding, early endoscopic hemostatic therapy significantly reduces rates of recurrent bleeding, the need for emergent surgery, and mortality [1,18,56]. Endoscopic methods can be divided into thermal and nonthermal types. Numerous randomized controlled trials have documented the efficacy of injection therapy for bleeding peptic ulcers and for nonbleeding visible vessels [57–61]. Injection agents may be sclerosing, such as alcohol or ethanolamine, vasoconstrictors such as epinephrine (adrenaline), normal saline solution, or clot-producing materials [62,63]. The effect of local compression from injection therapy alone is important because the use of normal saline injection leads to hemostasis. In contrast to thermal therapy, in which precise localization of the bleeding vessel is desirable, injection therapy is feasible even in an actively bleeding patient in whom visualization may be difficult.

Thermal methods include the neodymium:yttrium-aluminum garnet (Nd:YAG) laser, the heater probe, the argon plasma coagulator, and multipolar electrocoagulation.

With electrocautery or heater probe, direct probe pressure is used to tamponade the bleeding vessel, followed by raising the tissue temperature to coagulate and seal the vessel. Controlled trials of multipolar electrocoagulation show efficacy in reducing further bleeding, transfusion requirement, and need for surgery in actively bleeding ulcers and in nonbleeding visible vessels [64,65]. A similar technique that uses pure thermal energy is the heater probe, which has also been efficacious in the treatment of bleeding ulcers and nonbleeding visible vessels [66–68]. The major advantage of these two devices is that they are portable and relatively simple to use. The Nd:YAG laser is as effective as the heater probe and multipolar electrocoagulation, but its immobility, requirement for trained support personnel, and greater equipment expense has markely limited its use [69]. The argon plasma coagulator (APC) is the newest member of the thermal armamentarium. In controlled trials, APC shows results similar to those of the heater probe and electrocautery for primary hemostasis rebleeding, mortality, and need for emergent surgery [70,71]. Although not as well studied, it appears to be as effective as other thermal methods.

Dual endoscopic therapy, combining epinephrine injection and thermal methods, has been shown to be more effective than injection therapy alone. A metaanalysis of randomized trials showed that dual therapy decreased rebleeding rates, the need for surgery, and improved overall survival rates. This is the standard of care for high-risk peptic ulcer hemorrhage [72,73]. Studies have used an endoscopic Doppler ultrasound probe to assess for flow in vessels in addition to traditional endoscopic stigmata to guide endoscopic treatment [74].

Endoscopic clips, which achieve hemostasis mechanically, can also be considered a nonthermal endoscopic therapy for GI bleeding. Mechanical ligation with clips is growing in popularity and is theoretically attractive due to the lack of tissue destruction. This modality compares favorably with standard endoscopic therapies in small clinical trials [75,76].

Although most studies have not shown a reduction in mortality rates with endoscopic therapy [77], a metaanalysis of numerous trials suggested a reduction, although this reached statistical significance only for laser therapy [36].

Prevention of recurrent hemorrhage: pharmacological therapy

Proton pump inhibitors (PPIs)

Most peptic ulcer rebleeding occurs within the first 3 days after presentation. The therapeutic goal is to prevent clot dissolution and allow healing of the underlying lesion. Maintaining gastric pH above 6.0 favors extrinsic and intrinsic coagulation pathways and improves platelet adhesiveness and function [78,79]. The intent of antisecretory therapy in ulcer bleeding is to maintain the gastric pH above 6.0 and increase the likelihood of stable clot formation. In pH studies of healthy volunteers, repeated bolus injections of pantoprazole were compared with continuous infusions at rates of 4 mg/h and 8 mg/h following an 80-mg bolus. The 8 mg/h regimen was noted to be the most efficacious in elevating gastric pH, maintaining a pH greater than 6 for 84% of the day [80]. In a landmark study, a placebo-controlled trial of intravenous omeprazole, administered as an 80-mg bolus followed by 8 mg/h continuous infusion omeprazole after endoscopic treatment of bleeding peptic ulcers, demonstrated a substantial reduction in the risk for rebleeding [81]. A cost-effectiveness analysis of this approach in the United States and Canada revealed that providing high-dose PPI infusions for 3 days following endoscopic therapy was both more effective and less costly than not providing it [82].

Although it is clear that the high-dose PPI infusion is better at suppressing acid and maintaining gastric pH above 6, there is a lack of well-controlled clinical trials comparing high-dose continuous PPI with repeated injections or lower dose infusions in terms of either efficacy or cost effectiveness. One double-blind prospective study randomized patients with bleeding peptic ulcer who had been staged endoscopically and treated when necessary to receive either high-dose intravenous omeprazole (80-mg bolus + 8 mg/h for 3 days) or 20 mg i.v. once a day for 3 days. There was no significant difference in rebleeding rate, need for surgery, or mortality in the two groups, although this study enrolled a high percentage of patients with ulcer lesions at low-risk for rebleeding [83]. A small proportion of patients in this same study group underwent continuous gastric pH monitoring while in the study. Low-dose daily omeprazole resulted in more variability in the gastric pH over a 24-h period, although the mean and median pH values were greater than 4. Continuous infusion of high-dose omeprazole in these patients maintained gastric pH above 6 almost constantly during this period [84]. Similarly, although there have been a few reports suggesting that high-dose oral PPIs after endoscopic treatment do decrease rebleeding rate [85,86], there have been no head-to-head comparison studies of oral vs intravenous PPI in the setting of nonvariceal upper GI bleed. Potent acid suppression with high-dose intravenous or oral proton pump inhibition as an adjunct to endoscopic therapy is the mainstay of medical treatment for peptic ulcer bleeding (see Table 8.4).

Octreotide

Octreotide is a synthetic longer-acting analogue of the inhibitory neuropeptide, somatostatin. It inhibits portal venous blood flow and arterial flow to the stomach and duodenum while preserving renal arterial flow [87]. Its utility for decreasing rebleeding rates of nonvariceal upper GI bleed was initially supported by a metaanalysis of 14 studies, in which it was shown to reduce the risk of continued bleeding and the need for surgery [88]. The favorable effect of somatostatin did not remain statistically significant when the studies were stratified for investigator-blinded trials, however, and the cases were not stratified by severity of bleeding stigmata. Clinical guidelines do not recommend somatostatin in the

Table 8.4 Medical therapy for peptic ulcer bleeding

Decreases rebleeding and need for surgery	High-dose proton pump inhibitors
Efficacy not proven	Somatostatin
	Prostaglandins
	Tranexamic acid
	Intravenous vasopressin
Not effective	Histamine H_2 receptor antagonists

routine treatment of nonvariceal upper GI bleed [89]. This agent may be useful, however, for patients who are bleeding uncontrollably while waiting for upper endoscopy or surgery or for whom surgery and endoscopy are contraindicated [92].

Other agents

Other therapies, such as prostaglandins [91], tranexamic acid (an antifibrinolytic agent) [92], and intravenous vasopressin [93], have been investigated in small trials, although there are no compelling data supporting their utility in bleeding ulcer patients (Table 8.4).

Prevention of rebleeding: endoscopic therapy

The prevention of rebleeding by therapeutic endoscopic methods in high-risk ulcers with stigmata of bleeding is widely accepted [94]. However, some issues remain. The lack of standardized definitions of the various stigmata of recent hemorrhage and sufficient knowledge about each of their natural histories continues to be a problem [95]. Whereas treatment of ulcers with actively bleeding or spurting vessels or with visible nonbleeding vessels is clearly indicated to prevent rebleeding, there has been some disagreement over lower-risk lesions. There continues to be some controversy with regard to the need for endoscopic treatment for ulcers with adherent clot, especially in the era of high-dose PPI therapy [39]. Therapeutic endoscopy does add to the risk of the endoscopic procedure, with a risk for precipitating bleeding as high as 20% and with perforation occurring in as many as 1% of patients. Endoscopy also adds to the cost of treatment, unless it successfully decreases the need for surgery or shortens the hospital stay, and therefore must be applied judiciously.

Cessation of bleeding: when endoscopy and medical therapy fail

Medical and endoscopic treatment to control bleeding from peptic ulcers is followed by recurrence of bleeding in 15% of patients. A randomized controlled trial of repeated endoscopic treatment vs surgery for patients with recurrent ulcer bleeding concluded that endoscopic retreatment is superior to surgery [96]. If hemorrhage is not stopped or if bleeding recurs again, surgery should be considered early because the

risk for death increases as the patient becomes more unstable. Peptic ulcer bleeding is effectively treated with surgery, and this is safer than other therapeutic alternatives, such as angiography.

Unlike bleeding from gastric erosions, bleeding from ulcers is not effectively stopped with intraarterial vasopressin, presumably because of the large size of the bleeding vessel in peptic ulcer disease [97]. Embolization by means of an angiographic catheter with polyvinyl alcohol particles or microcoils can be successful but requires significant expertise and causes complications [98]. This procedure should be reserved for the patient who is too unstable to undergo surgery.

Hemorrhage from gastric erosions

The term *gastritis* should be reserved for the pathologist; *gastric erosions* or *gastropathy* should be used by the endoscopist. Histologically, gastritis is defined by epithelial distortion and inflammatory cell infiltrate, which may be chronic (i.e., predominantly plasma cells) or acute (i.e., polymorphonuclear cells). There may be biopsy evidence of severe histological gastritis with a normal endoscopic appearance [99]. This type of gastritis is not associated with upper GI hemorrhage. Endoscopically, gastropathy is defined by the gross appearance of mucosal hemorrhages, erythema, and erosions. An erosion is technically a break in the mucosa that does not cross the muscularis mucosae. Practically, most endoscopists define an erosion as an area of adherent hemorrhage or a defect in the mucosa with a necrotic base that is less than 3–5 mm in size and without significant depth. This type of gastric erosion may lead to upper GI bleeding and has several different causes [100].

Drug-induced gastropathy

Gastropathy induced by aspirin or other NSAIDs is common. In almost all normal volunteers challenged with aspirin, there is development of mild hemorrhagic gastropathy that involves the proximal or entire stomach within 24 h [101]. The bleeding associated with this acute damage is minimal and only rarely clinically apparent. If the aspirin is continued, adaptation and healing occur. In a smaller percentage of individuals who are continually exposed to NSAIDs, chronic erosive gastropathy, predominantly involving the antrum, develops; symptomatic frank ulcer disease occurs in only 1%–4% of chronic NSAID users [102]. Erosive gastropathy induced by NSAIDs is usually a self-limited disease that heals rapidly after removal of the offending agent.

Interventional treatments, such as therapeutic endoscopy or surgery, are rarely required. Bleeding from NSAID-induced gastric erosions usually resolves spontaneously, and most of the serious upper GI bleeding associated with NSAID intake is the result of NSAID-induced peptic ulcers [103]. Although high-dose PPIs have not been well studied in the treatment of bleeding from NSAID-induced gastric erosions, their use seems reasonable.

A more important issue in the management of NSAID-induced gastropathy is prophylaxis. Prostaglandins have been shown to be effective in preventing acute erosions from NSAIDs and in preventing chronic ulcers although their widespread use has been limited by side effects [104]. A large study of more than 8500 patients did show a 40% reduction in serious NSAID-induced upper GI complications by misoprostol [105]. Prophylactic treatment with histamine H_2-receptor antagonists (H_2RAs) appears effective in duodenal disease but not in the stomach [106], and sucralfate is not effective [104]. Proton pump inhibitors have become the prophylactic drug of choice as a result of their efficacy and tolerability [107,108]. It remains unclear who should receive prophylaxis because significant upper GI bleeding does not develop in most patients on NSAIDs, and routine prophylaxis with PPIs would be extremely expensive. It seems reasonable to recommend additional treatment with PPIs for the patient who has already demonstrated significant upper GI bleeding but requires continued NSAID intake. Additionally, treatment of concomitant *Helicobacter pylori* infection also decreases the risk for recurrent bleeding [109]. Another alternative is to change the NSAID to a less damaging agent, such as the nonacetylated salicylates [110] or etodolac [111]. Much better studied are the specific cyclooxygenase-2 (COX-2) inhibitors, which have been shown to decrease not only gastric erosions but also upper GI tract bleeding [112]. An underrecognized risk by both patients and physicians is that the combination of low-dose aspirin and a COX-2 inhibitor turns the COX-2 inhibitor into a standard NSAID in terms of GI bleeding risk. Unfortunately, low-dose aspirin, whether it is coated or not, significantly increases the risk of upper GI bleeding [44].

An uncommon cause of drug-induced erosive gastropathy is hepatic artery pump chemotherapy. This treatment may cause hemorrhagic gastropathy, duodenitis, and frank ulcer disease [113]. The pathogenesis presumably involves direct tissue injury from the chemotherapeutic agents or from ischemia secondary to catheter placement. Little is known about the management of this entity.

Gastropathy related to alcohol intake

Historically, it was thought that alcohol ingestion caused gastric erosions. In animal models, absolute alcohol does cause severe hemorrhagic gastropathy, although lower doses of intragastric alcohol can produce adaptive cytoprotection [114]. These lower doses are closer to those obtained in human alcohol use. Alcohol consumption is a risk factor for upper GI bleeding only when it is excessive – four or more drinks per day [115]. Perhaps the historical "alcohol-induced gastritis" was actually the result of portal hypertension in patients with alcoholic liver disease. An endoscopic evaluation of GI hemorrhage in alcoholics found the causes to be PUD and disorders related to portal hypertension [116].

Portal gastropathy

Portal gastropathy has been described as a diffuse erythematous, reticular, or mosaic pattern of the gastric mucosa [117]. The endoscopic spectrum of portal gastropathy includes a snakeskin or mosaic appearance, with more severe cases having small areas of intense erythema (e.g., scarlatina rash), frank petechiae, or multiple bleeding spots. Vascular ectasia may be present throughout the stomach or show an antral predilection. A portal gastropathy scoring system has been validated [118]. Hyperdynamic congestion has been the presumed cause [119], with a controversial role suggested for prior variceal obliteration [120,121]. Although mild cases of portal gastropathy have a nonspecific appearance and no clinical consequences, the more severe variants are associated with overt and chronic bleeding [122]. The prevalence of portal gastropathy in patients with cirrhosis is 80%, with acute bleeding occurring in only 2.5% and chronic bleeding in 11% [123]. Portal gastropathy does not respond to treatment with acid suppression, although potent acid suppression has not been studied. Decreasing the portal pressure with propranolol is efficacious in the prevention of rebleeding [124]. Portal systemic shunting in the unusual patient who has continued significant blood loss has been effective [125]. A transjugular intrahepatic portal systemic shunt (TIPS) would likely have similar efficacy.

Stress gastric erosions

Severe illness requiring hospitalization in an ICU is an important cause of gastric erosions causing major hemorrhage, or stress gastropathy. It occurs in patients with respiratory failure, hypotension, sepsis, renal failure, thermal burns, peritonitis, jaundice, or neurological trauma [126]. The risk for bleeding in an individual patient varies with the number of such conditions. Endoscopic evidence of gastropathy is found in almost all ICU patients, although when stress prophylaxis is widely used, clinically important gastrointestinal bleeding occurs in less than 1% of patients [127].

All treatment modalities for significant bleeding from stress erosions are associated with high failure rates and significant morbidity. High-dose PPI and endoscopic therapy are usually the first and safest choices, although neither has been specifically studied in stress gastric erosions. The presence of multiple bleeding sites precludes endoscopic therapy in some patients. Historically, angiographic control of gastric mucosal bleeding reportedly had a good success rate, perhaps because of the small vessel size in these superficial lesions [128]. The operative mortality rate is extremely high for patients bleeding from stress gastric erosions, and rebleeding after surgery is common; surgery is reserved as a last resort [129].

The major emphasis in the management of stress gastric erosions is prophylaxis. Although there has been some controversy about the cost-effectiveness of treating all patients at risk [130], a review of all studies strongly supports routine prophylaxis for all patients ill enough to be in an ICU [131]. The use of high-dose antacids [132], H$_2$RAs [133], or sucralfate [134] in patients at risk has decreased the incidence of bleeding. Their ubiquity of use has made PPIs the most popular agent. Sucralfate administered through the nasogastric tube also seems as effective as high-dose antacids and is cheaper than intravenous H$_2$RAs [135]. However, a large multicenter trial showed a significantly lower rate of clinically important bleeding with ranitidine than with sucralfate [136]. This study also challenged a previous suggestion that agents such as sucralfate, which improve the mucosal defense without altering intragastric pH, may result in lower rates of nosocomial pneumonia in patients on respirators [137]. The validity of the hypothesis that gastric bacterial overgrowth occurs with acid-reducing therapy and that endotracheal intubation establishes a pathway for colonization of the respiratory tract continues to be questioned [136,138].

Esophageal varices

In-hospital mortality rates of patients with cirrhosis and variceal bleeding decreased threefold between 1985 and 2000 (by two-thirds, from 42.6% to 14.5%), although the rate remains as high as 32%–36% in class C patients [28,139]. This high mortality rate attests to the difficulty of managing acute variceal bleeding and preventing further bleeding. It also may explain why so many therapeutic alternatives have been proposed.

Most patients with varices have underlying cirrhosis, and this contributes to the high mortality rate; 40% die of associated medical problems. It has been estimated that one-fourth to one-third of patients with cirrhosis hemorrhage at least once from varices [140]. Despite the increasing array of therapeutic options for variceal hemorrhage, there has been little change in long-term survival.

Determinants of variceal rupture

Portal hypertension must be present, with pressures of 12 mmHg or greater, for varices to develop. However, the degree of pressure elevation does not correlate with the risk for rupture [141]. Portal pressures may be similar in patients with no evidence of varices and in those with large varices. Once a threshold portal pressure develops that permits varices, other factors control their formation and their risk for rupture. It has been suggested that directly measured intravariceal pressure may correlate better with the risk for hemorrhage [142]. The portal pressure measured within 48 h after the bleeding event may also correlate better with bleeding. A higher risk for rebleeding has been demonstrated in patients admitted with variceal hemorrhage who have higher portal pressures [143].

Esophagitis has not been shown to predispose to variceal bleeding, although intuitively it seems reasonable that erosions on top of esophageal varices may cause a vessel to bleed. This remains somewhat controversial [144]. Gastroesophageal reflux as measured by a pH probe is no more common in patients with a history of variceal bleeding than in controls [145]. As in other types of GI bleeding, the recent use of aspirin predisposes to a first episode of variceal bleeding [146].

An important predictor of variceal hemorrhage is the size of the varices. Several studies have shown that large varices are more likely to bleed than small ones [147]. Wall tension is a function of diameter and wall thickness, and it is not surprising that larger varices are more likely to rupture. Another endoscopic finding of value in predicting variceal bleeding is the appearance of the vessel wall. Certain colors of varices are thought to indicate impending hemorrhage. The red color sign is the result of microtelangiectasia of the varix. Variants of this sign are: red wale marks, which look like whip marks; cherry red spots, which are 2 mm in diameter; hemocystic spots, which are round, crimson projections, larger than 4 mm, that look like blood blisters; and diffuse redness. All the red color signs and a blue color are thought to be risk factors for bleeding. Red color signs have been correlated with increased variceal pressure as assessed by direct needle puncture [148]. When examined by endoscopic ultrasonography, hemocystic spots appear as saccular aneurysm projections on the variceal surface [149]. The white nipple sign on a varix, thought to be a platelet–fibrin plug, is considered diagnostic of previous bleeding but not predictive of rebleeding [150]. The presence of cutaneous vascular spiders also correlates with a risk for hemorrhage from esophageal varices [151]. A prognostic index for variceal hemorrhage based on the three variables of variceal size, presence of red wale marks, and a modified Child classification of underlying liver disease could identify subsets of patients with a 1-year incidence of bleeding ranging from 6%–76% [152]. The value of these predictors of variceal rupture depends on the usefulness of prophylactic therapy for variceal bleeding (Table 8.5).

Management of acute variceal hemorrhage

Variceal bleeding is often the most rapid type of upper GI hemorrhage. The emphasis in acute management is on resuscitation. More than 90% of episodes of variceal bleeding cause a drop in the hematocrit to below 30%, so that transfusions are required. However, as in upper GI hemorrhage with other causes, 70%–80% of cases resolve without specific intervention. Urgent endoscopy is indicated for a patient with a suspected variceal source because the methods of treating the acute bleeding episode and preventing recurrent bleeding differ from those for upper GI bleeding with other causes. In more than half to two-thirds of patients with cirrhosis who present with bleeding, the sources are nonvariceal, and many of these patients have more than one lesion [153]. For this reason, early endoscopy is useful to determine the site and cause of bleeding.

In the acutely bleeding patient, intravenous administration of octreotide, a synthetic analogue of somatostatin, is

Table 8.5 Predictors of variceal rupture

Factors correlated with risk for bleeding	Variceal size
	Red marks on varices
	Severity of liver disease
Probably correlated with bleeding	Intravariceal pressure
	Portal pressure during hospitalization for bleeding
	Cutaneous spider angiomas
Not correlated with bleeding	Esophagitis
	Degree of portal pressure elevation over 12 mmHg

often started as soon as the diagnosis is made. This newer agent has replaced vasopressin because of its ease of use, although vasopressin is the historical treatment comparison for octreotide. The efficacy of both agents has been difficult to demonstrate convincingly. Compared with placebo, somatostatin has had conflicting results [154,155], although it has been shown to be equally efficacious with terlipressin and vasopressin [156,157]. There are proponents for using continuous portal pressure monitoring during acute variceal bleeding in the setting of pharmacological therapy [158], although this remains controversial and not widely adapted [159]. The combination of isosorbide 5-mononitrate with somatostatin does not improve therapeutic efficacy and induces more adverse effects so should not be used [160]. Compared with sclerotherapy alone in acute variceal bleeding, vasoactive drugs have similar bleeding outcomes with fewer adverse events [161]. Several studies combining sclerotherapy with octreotide (or vapreotide) vs sclerotherapy alone found less bleeding with combination therapy and no difference in mortality rates [162–165].

An alternative to octreotide or somatostatin for control of variceal hemorrhage is a synthetic analogue of vasopressin, terlipressin, which is reportedly more effective than placebo or vasopressin although not yet available in the United States [166]. When combined with nitroglycerin, it is as effective as balloon tamponade [167] and may be as effective as sclerotherapy [168].

Pharmacological constriction of the lower esophageal sphincter with metoclopramide lowers intravariceal pressure [169], although this is more effective when combined with intravenous nitroglycerin [170]. Only limited data are available regarding metoclopramide in the treatment of bleeding varices [171].

Recombinant coagulation factor VIIa (rFVIIa) acutely normalizes prothrombin time in patients with cirrhosis and variceal bleeding [172] although a randomized placebo-controled trial failed to show an overall benefit despite a decrease in the proportion of patients with advanced cirrhosis who had continued bleeding [173].

After supportive medical therapy and octreotide infusion have been started in the patient with variceal bleeding, the next step in management is urgent band ligation or sclerotherapy. If a skilled endoscopist is not available or, rarely, if the bleeding is too rapid to permit endoscopy, balloon tamponade is indicated.

Variceal band ligation is a superior alternative to sclerotherapy for acutely bleeding patients and for the prevention of rebleeding (Fig. 8.1). Ligation of varices has a significantly lower complication rate than sclerotherapy [174–178], and may further lower the rebleeding rate [174,175,177] and improve survival [174]. Variceal ligation also requires fewer sessions to achieve variceal obliteration. The combination of band ligation and sclerotherapy compared with ligation alone has had conflicting results. Some studies show no benefit for the combined therapy and a higher complication rate than that for ligation alone [179,180]. Other studies suggest that combined therapy may be more effective at variceal eradication [181,182], with a decrease in recurrent bleeding [183]. Another type of "combined therapy" advocated as a way to reduce the rate of variceal recurrence is the use of argon plasma coagulation therapy after eradication of varices [184]. Further confirmatory studies are needed. Although emergent sclerotherapy has a success rate for controlling bleeding of 90% [185], it is relegated to rapidly bleeding patients in whom visualization is insufficient for band ligation or patients with varices too small to ligate. Another ligation technique, in which small detachable snares are used to treat esophageal varices, has been developed [186] and seems comparable with band ligation therapy [187].

Emergency endoscopic therapy in cirrhotics with upper GI hemorrhage is associated with bacteremia, and the administration of prophylactic antibiotics before emergency endoscopy decreases the incidence of clinical infections [188]. In addition, antibiotic prophylaxis in acute variceal hemorrhage appears to decrease rebleeding [189].

When endoscopic and medical therapy fails to control variceal bleeding, balloon tamponade is indicated as a temporizing maneuver. Balloon tamponade with the Sengstaken–Blakemore tube is effective in achieving hemostasis in 70%–90% of patients [190]. Unfortunately, hemostasis is often

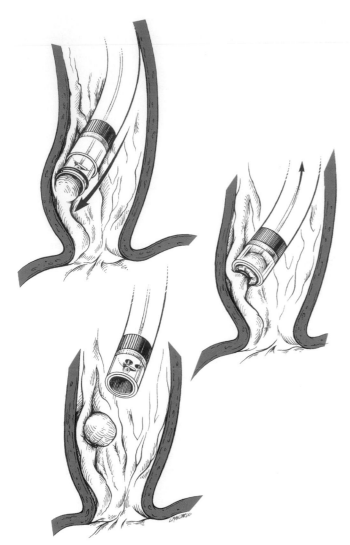

Figure 8.1 Endoscopic band ligation involves the application of a small suction chamber to a standard endoscope tip, which allows the varix to be pulled into the stretched band. A trigger device then releases the band around the varix base, causing subsequent necrosis and scarring.

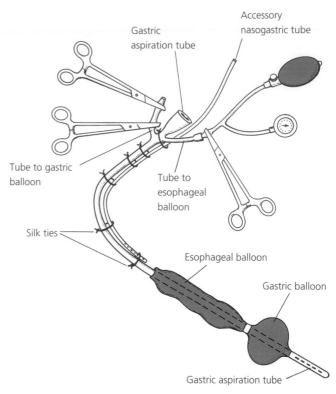

Figure 8.2 Modified Sengstaken–Blakemore tube. Also available is the Minnesota tube, which has a built-in esophageal port.

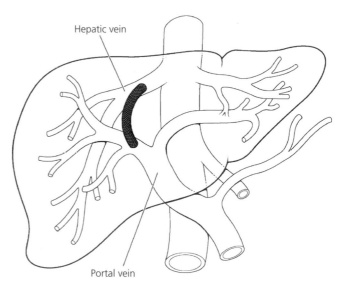

Figure 8.3 The transjugular intrahepatic portosystemic shunt (TIPS) is a metal expandable stent that is placed angiographically between branches of the hepatic and portal veins to create a nonsurgical shunt between the portal and systemic venous systems.

temporary, with rebleeding occurring in 30%–50% of patients after the balloon is deflated. An adapted Sengstaken–Blakemore tube with an esophageal aspiration port, or the Minnesota tube with a built-in esophageal port, are probably the most popular devices (Fig. 8.2) [191]. The complication rate of balloon tamponade is 10%–30%; complications include esophageal perforation, aspiration pneumonia, malfunction requiring replacement, chest pain, gastric erosion, and agitation [192]. Endotracheal intubation before balloon insertion has been recommended to decrease complications [193].

A nonsurgical method of creating portosystemic shunting, used to manage acute variceal hemorrhage and prevent rebleeding, is TIPS. An expandable metallic stent is placed between the hepatic and portal veins within the liver by means of an angiographically guided catheter (Fig. 8.3). Technical success is achieved in 93%–96% of patients, with a 10%–15% procedure complication rate and a 25% incidence of hepatic encephalopathy [194]. In one-third of patients, TIPS stenosis or occlusion develops by 1 year of follow-up, although this is successfully treated by redilation or placement of an additional stent. Some experts advocate the use of hepatic venous pressure gradient measurement 24 h after admission to decide which patients should have early TIPS placement after initial endoscopic and medical stabilization [195]. The TIPS procedure is an effective bridge to liver transplantation because it avoids surgery in patients with advanced liver disease [196].

The surgical shunting of portal blood to the systemic circulation to control ongoing hemorrhage from varices is reserved for patients resistant to other therapies and has become uncommon since the advent of TIPS. The mortality rate for these emergency shunts is as high as 50%–80%, which has dampened enthusiasm for the procedure [197]. This mortality rate is much higher than that of surgery to prevent recurrent variceal bleeding. Although a better survival rate for emergency shunting has been reported, the study may have included patients who would have been controlled with other, simpler techniques at other centers [198]. Staple-gun transection of the esophagus has been advocated as the simplest type of emergency surgery for active variceal bleeding and has been proposed as the salvage procedure of choice after failure of acute sclerotherapy [199]. However, because of lower postsurgical rebleeding rates, portosystemic shunts continue to be favored by many surgeons.

Prevention of recurrent variceal hemorrhage

Up to one-third of patients surviving a variceal hemorrhage rebleed within 6 weeks, and death from bleeding occurs in 40%–60% of these patients. Prevention of recurrent hemorrhage is an important part of therapy. Therapies to prevent rebleeding include endoscopic therapy, medical therapy with propranolol or nitrates, TIPS, and rarely surgical shunts An improvement in the mortality rate is particularly difficult to demonstrate with all these methods, suggesting that the risk for death is more likely correlated to the severity of the underlying liver disease than to rebleeding.

Controversy continues on the choice of medical therapy vs endoscopic therapy for prevention of variceal rebleeding, with patient preference and compliance playing a significant deciding role [200]. Controlled trials of β_1-blockade compared with sclerotherapy showed lower rebleeding rates with sclerotherapy [201], and a metaanalysis confirmed this superiority, although there was no difference in survival [202]. Combination therapy with nadolol and nitrates proved superior to sclerotherapy, with fewer complications and a lower rebleeding rate [203]. Because variceal banding has replaced sclerotherapy at most centers for the prevention of rebleeding, a pivotal trial of the combination of nadolol plus nitrates vs band ligation showed a greater efficacy for the combination medical therapy [204].

The risk for rebleeding is greatest in the first few weeks after the initiation of a endoscopic therapy regimen, before the varices are obliterated. Propranolol has been advocated for the reduction of rebleeding rates during endoscopic sclerotherapy

before variceal obliteration, although the results have been conflicting [205]. A study of variceal ligation vs ligation plus nadolol and sucralfate showed that the combination of ligation and medical therapy decreased both variceal and nonvariceal bleeding [206]. Subcutaneous octreotide has also been combined with endoscopic therapy to prevent rebleeding [207].

Propranolol was proposed more than 25 years ago to prevent rebleeding in patients who had already presented with variceal hemorrhage [208]. Propranolol decreases portal pressures in laboratory animals and humans, although the response is not uniform [209]. Despite early controversy, subsequent studies and several metaanalyses show efficacy with propranolol in doses that reduce the heart rate by 25% [210]. Nadolol is a popular alternative to propranolol because it has to be administered only once daily and is not metabolized by the liver.

Isosorbide mononitrate has been shown to be as effective as propranolol [211] and has been used in patients who either cannot tolerate propranolol or do not respond to it satisfactorily. The combination of propranolol and isosorbide mononitrate enhances portal pressure reduction compared with propranolol alone and has better efficacy in the prevention of rebleeding [212]. Despite some early concerns about the effect of nitrates on renal function and ascites, the combination of nadolol and isosorbide-5-mononitrate appears safe [213].

Comparisons have been made between TIPS and sclerotherapy and band ligation for the prevention of rebleeding [214–217]; TIPS has also been compared with a combination of endoscopic and medical therapy with either sclerotherapy plus propranolol or band ligation plus propranolol [218,219]. Most of these trials showed less rebleeding in the patients receiving TIPS, although survival rates and costs were similar and the incidence of encephalopathy was higher with TIPS treatment. A national guideline recommends use of a combination of nonselective β-blockers plus band ligation as the best option for secondary prophylaxis of variceal hemorrhage [220]. The American College of Gastroenterology guideline recommends reserving TIPS for patients who experience recurrent variceal hemorrhage despite combination pharmacological and endoscopic therapy.

Surgical shunts decompress the portal system by diverting blood into the systemic circulation. Several types of shunts have been used, including end-to-side portacaval, side-to-side portacaval, mesocaval, and splenorenal shunts. Multiple studies have confirmed their efficacy in preventing rebleeding [221]. Unfortunately, encephalopathy developed postoperatively in 10%–40% of patients. This led to the development of the distal splenorenal (i.e., Warren) shunt, which spares portal blood flow to the liver (Fig. 8.4). The proponents of this shunt report lower rates (4%–15%) of encephalopathy [222]. This has been confirmed in some controlled trials [223,224], although other studies comparing nonselective and distal splenorenal shunts have shown similar rates of operative mortality, late mortality, incidence

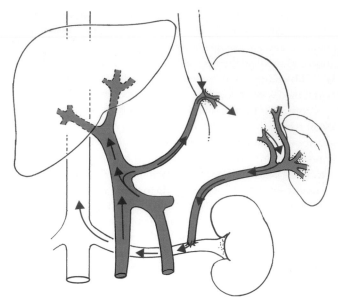

Figure 8.4 The distal splenorenal shunt was designed to prevent diversion of gut venous flow to the liver.

of encephalopathy, and shunt occlusion [225,226]. It appears that the incidence of encephalopathy is related more to the severity of underlying liver disease than to the type of surgery performed. Some surgeons reserve the selective shunt for patients with preserved hepatopetal (i.e., intestine-to-liver) blood flow, although this may be unnecessary. A partial portacaval shunt (i.e., small-diameter or H-graft) has also been advocated as a mechanism to preserve hepatic portal blood flow and decrease postoperative encephalopathy [227,228]. This shunt reportedly does not compromise subsequent liver transplantation, although it may have a higher incidence of occlusion and encephalopathy than the distal splenorenal shunt [229].

Despite the efficacy of all shunts in preventing rebleeding, controlled trials have not shown improved mortality rates [230]. A randomized comparison of surgical shunt and sclerotherapy showed similar survival and efficacy in the prevention of variceal rebleeding, with sclerotherapy having lower costs [231]. Most physicians favor endoscopic therapy as the initial therapy, with surgery reserved for the patients who fail an adequate attempt at variceal obliteration. For patients who are transplantation candidates or have poor hepatic function, TIPS is generally preferred to surgical shunt. For patients with well-preserved hepatic function, controversy continues about the choice between endoscopic treatment or surgery [232,233].

Two other surgical methods of portal decompression have been used. The Sugiura procedure involves esophageal transection with paraesophagogastric devascularization [234]. Many modifications of this esophageal transection and devascularization procedure exist. The results of the Sugiura

procedure in patients with nonalcoholic liver disease have been excellent, but some surgeons have documented high rebleeding rates [235].

A procedure that has not been extensively studied is splenopneumopexy [236]. This can be performed in patients with diffuse splanchnic venous thrombosis when alternative shunts are not technically possible. It involves resection of part of the left diaphragm with apposition of the abraded surfaces of the spleen and left lung to allow decompressive collaterals to form.

Hepatic transplantation is the accepted treatment for otherwise healthy patients with end-stage liver disease. When these patients present with bleeding varices, management of the bleeding should avoid abdominal operations, which makes transplantation more difficult.

Prophylactic treatment of variceal hemorrhage

Because 30% of cirrhotics experience variceal hemorrhage, and the mortality rate associated with even one episode is high, prevention is important. Selection of patients for prophylactic therapy requires endoscopic screening of patients with cirrhosis; prognostic risk scoring primarily relies on varix size [237]. Cirrhotic patients with small or no varices should be followed for the development of varices. The best clinical predictor of the presence of varices is splenomegaly or a platelet count below 88 000/mm^3 [238]. A prospective screening study suggested that patients should undergo endoscopy annually if the initial endoscopy reveals small (grade 1) varices, and that screening every other year is adequate for patients with no varices [239]. Whether screening should be limited to those patients with low platelet counts and more advanced cirrhosis [240], or should be performed with the new esophageal capsule, remain uncertain [241].

Historically, both surgical shunt and sclerotherapy have been used for prophylaxis for the first variceal hemorrhage, although both were abandoned due to their complications [242,243]. Several controlled studies and two metaanalyses concluded that nonselective β-adrenergic antagonists have a beneficial effect in prophylaxis of a first variceal hemorrhage [244–246]. This relatively complication-free treatment can be recommended for patients with large or moderately sized varices. In the 3%–20% of patients who cannot tolerate propranolol, isosorbide-5-mononitrate is an effective alternative [211]. Although combination therapy with propranolol and isosorbide mononitrate is more effective in reducing portal pressure, it causes more side effects and has had controversial benefit compared with propranolol alone for the prevention of a first variceal bleed [247]. Several studies comparing band ligation with medical therapy suggest that endoscopic ligation may be superior [248–250], although in reality the outcomes are similar [251,252], leading many clinicians to reserve endoscopic banding for patients who are intolerant or noncompliant with medical treatment. It is also controversial whether the addition of β-blockade plus band ligation compared with ligation alone is worth the medication side effects [253,254].

Gastric varices

Gastric varices usually accompany esophageal varices, although they may occur alone. In a study of 568 patients with portal hypertension, primary gastric varices were present in 20% of patients, and secondary gastric varices, which developed after treatment of esophageal varices, occurred in 8% of patients [255]. Risk factors for hemorrhage from gastric fundal varices are similar to those for esophageal variceal bleeding: larger variceal size, the presence of red marks, and relatively severe underlying liver disease [256].

Several classification schemes that depend on the variceal location have been suggested [255,257], and it seems that the various subsets have different natural histories and responses to treatment [255,258]. Gastric varices that develop after endoscopic therapy for esophageal varices are referred to as *secondary*. Gastroesophageal varices that cross the gastroesophageal junction along the lesser curvature are most common and often disappear spontaneously with the obliteration of esophageal varices. Gastroesophageal varices that cross the junction along the greater curvature are less common but are associated with a higher incidence of bleeding and are much less likely to disappear after esophageal variceal obliteration. Isolated gastric varices that do not connect with esophageal varices usually occur in the gastric fundus and are the most difficult to treat endoscopically [259]. Isolated gastric varices located elsewhere in the stomach or duodenum (i.e., ectopic varices) are more commonly secondary varices, occur most often in the antrum, and rarely bleed. Isolated gastric varices in the fundus may be the result of splenic vein thrombosis, which can be verified with angiography. These patients are best treated with simple splenectomy, which adequately decompresses their varices. They have an excellent prognosis because they do not have underlying liver disease [260]. Splenic vein thrombosis may occur as a complication of pancreatitis secondary to contiguous inflammation from the body and tail of the pancreas [261].

Bleeding gastric varices commonly are associated with large esophageal varices and are the result of underlying liver disease. When patients with gastroesophageal varices bleed, they are more likely to bleed from their esophageal varices, although bleeding gastric varices are associated with higher transfusion requirements [255]. Acute sclerotherapy to stop bleeding is reportedly effective for all types of gastric varices [262], although sclerotherapy in the stomach may have a higher complication rate. Alternative endoscopic treatments for gastric varices include injection of thrombin [263], snare ligation [264], and a combination of sclerotherapy with percutaneous transhepatic obliteration [265]. Injection of cyanoacrylate glue is effective [266,267], and may be superior to sclerotherapy with alcohol [268] and to band ligation [269]. Shunting with TIPS may be the best treatment for prevent-ing rebleeding from gastric varices, especially from isolated fundal varices, although glue injections may be more cost-effective [270].

Mallory–Weiss tear

Mallory–Weiss tears occur near the gastroesophageal junction in the gastric or esophageal mucosa. They are caused by retching, perhaps with forceful gastric mucosal prolapse as identified at endoscopy [271]. They account for 5%–10% of cases of upper GI hemorrhage [273]. There is usually a history of vomiting food before hematemesis, although bleeding can occur with the first emesis. Many patients with Mallory–Weiss tears have a history of alcohol intake or have portal hypertension [274]. The bleeding usually resolves with conservative management, although endoscopic therapy may be beneficial in patients with high-risk stigmata [274,275]. Rarely, patients with rebleeding or uncontrollable hemorrhage require oversewing of the bleeding mucosa or angiographic treatment.

Esophagitis and esophageal ulcers

Esophagitis and esophageal ulcers account for approximately 8% of cases of upper GI hemorrhage. The primary cause of these lesions is peptic reflux, but other causes include irradiation, infectious esophagitis associated with pathogens such as *Candida* or herpesvirus, pill-induced damage, and endoscopic therapy-induced ulcers. The presentation of bleeding esophageal lesions is similar to that of PUD. Persistent or recurrent bleeding should be treated aggressively with therapeutic endoscopic or angiographic techniques because esophageal lesions are less amenable to surgery than PUD. Proton pump inhibitors may be effective in the treatment of endotherapy-induced ulcers [276,277].

Erosive duodenitis

Hemorrhage resulting from erosive duodenitis is closely related to duodenal ulcer bleeding but is usually less severe because the lesions are shallower and involve smaller vessels. It accounts for approximately 5% of cases of upper GI hemorrhage. The hemorrhage usually occurs in patients with a history of peptic ulcer disease or similar risk factors. Bleeding from duodenitis is almost always self-limited, rarely requiring therapeutic endoscopic intervention.

Neoplasms

Neoplasms of the stomach, esophagus, or duodenum are uncommon causes (2%–5%) of upper GI hemorrhage. Bleeding from these lesions is usually self-limited, and treatment is ultimately in the hands of the oncologist or surgeon. If persistent or recurrent bleeding occurs in a patient unsuitable for surgical resection, endoscopic therapy or angiographic arterial embolization may be used [278]. Intraarterial vasopressin is not usually effective because of the large size of the bleeding vessels.

Angiodysplasia and gastric antral vascular ectasia

Vascular ectasia or angiodysplasia, which occurs less commonly in the stomach or duodenum than in the colon, is the cause of upper GI bleeding in 5%–7% of patients [27,279]. Often found in patients of advanced age, it has been associated with chronic renal failure, hereditary hemorrhagic telangiectasia (Osler–Weber–Rendu syndrome), and prior radiation therapy [280,281]. Angiodysplasia has also been associated with aortic valve disease, although this remains controversial [282]. The diagnosis is usually made endoscopically by visualizing small, punctate, bright-red, vascular mucosal lesions. Controlled studies of therapeutic alternatives are not available, but most clinicians would first attempt endoscopic coagulation techniques [283–285]. These have been successful, although associated with high rebleeding rates in patients with hereditary (Osler–Weber–Rendu) lesions [286]. In cases of vascular ectasia associated with chronic renal failure and its attendant prolonged bleeding time secondary to platelet dysfunction, estrogen–progesterone therapy has been reported as beneficial [287]. Similar efficacy has been reported in patients with normal renal function and chronic GI blood loss from vascular ectasia in a small crossover study [288], although these results were not confirmed in a larger randomized trial [289].

An unusual variant of gastric vascular ectasia is the watermelon stomach [290], also called *gastric antral vascular ectasia* (GAVE). The endoscopic appearance is of a jagged column of vessels that runs along the tops of longitudinal rugal folds, traversing the antrum and converging on the pylorus. This vascular aggregate resembles the stripes on a watermelon. Endoscopic biopsy or resected specimens show dilated mucosal capillaries with focal thrombosis and fibromuscular hyperplasia of vessels in the lamina propria. The condition has been associated clinically with hypochlorhydria, systemic sclerosis, and portal hypertension. In patients with GAVE, ectatic vascular ectasias also commonly occur in the cardia of the stomach [291]. Although GAVE occurs in patients with cirrhosis, it is distinct from portal gastropathy and does not seem to respond to lowering portal pressures [292]. Endoscopic coagulation treatment with Nd:YAG laser, multipolar electrocoagulation, argon plasma coagulator, or the heater probe, is useful in decreasing transfusion requirements [293,294].

Aortoenteric fistulae

Aortoenteric fistulae usually involve the aorta but occasionally arise from branches of the celiac axis. Most aortoenteric fistulae are secondary to prior aortic Dacron graft surgery although they may occur as primary fistulae involving atherosclerotic vessels or more rarely mycotic aneurysms, tuberculosis, or syphilis [295]. Aortoenteric fistulae almost always involve the third portion of the duodenum, although they may rupture into the jejunum, ileum, stomach, and colon. In patients with Dacron grafts, the fistula usually arises from the proximal portion of the graft and may be associated with false aneurysms. The classical clinical presentation is a "herald" bleed that occurs and stops spontaneously hours or occasionally weeks before the exsanguinating hemorrhage.

A high index of suspicion is necessary to make the diagnosis because the fistula is difficult to discern by endoscopy and angiography. Abdominal computed tomography (CT) may demonstrate evidence of the fistula. If there is a history of aortic Dacron graft surgery in a patient presenting with GI hemorrhage, endoscopy should be performed to rule out other causes of bleeding, and the endoscopist should attempt to reach the third portion of the duodenum in an effort to visualize the fistula. If not identified, a fistula should be the presumed source of bleeding.

Hemobilia and hemosuccus pancreaticus

Hemobilia is defined as hemorrhage into the biliary tract from any cause. Hemorrhage traversing the pancreatic duct has been called hemosuccus pancreaticus, although it is often included with hemobilia because it exits through the ampulla. The mortality associated with hemorrhage from both these sites is significant (20%–50%). The most common cause of hemobilia is prior liver or biliary tree trauma, including prior percutaneous liver biopsy or transhepatic cholangiography. Extrahepatic or intrahepatic aneurysms of the hepatic artery or its branches are often caused by the trauma and may communicate with the bile ducts. Angiographic treatment with embolization is usually effective [296]. Less common causes of hemobilia are extrahepatic or intrahepatic tumors, gallstones, and cholecystitis.

Hemosuccus pancreaticus represents bleeding from peripancreatic blood vessels into a pancreatic duct. Blood emanates from digested peripancreatic pseudoaneurysms or veins that rupture into a pseudocyst or from true aneurysms of the peripancreatic vessels that rupture into pancreatic parenchyma and ducts [297]. This usually occurs in patients with a history of chronic pancreatitis and pseudocysts. The diagnosis may be made by endoscopy, with visualization of blood coming from the papilla, although it is easily missed when the bleeding has ceased. Angiography is indicated to define the bleeding site and may be used for treatment by embolizing the vessel [298]. If embolization therapy is not successful, surgery may be required.

Dieulafoy disease

The Dieulafoy lesion is defined as a ruptured, thick-walled artery that is larger than other surrounding submucosal vessels, with little or no associated ulceration. The cause of bleeding is not thought to be a primary ulcerative process but rather pressure erosion of the overlying epithelium by this ectatic vessel [299]. The Dieulafoy vessel usually occurs in the fundus, although up to 34% of the lesions develop outside the stomach [300]. Endoscopically, it appears as a round mucosal defect with a protruding artery at the base. Patients present with hematemesis or melena without any relevant history.

Endoscopic injection therapy, electrocoagulation techniques, band ligation, and hemoclipping have been successful in stopping bleeding in most patients, although surgery is occasionally required [301,302].

Factitious bleeding or bleeding from nongastrointestinal sources

Some patients present with hematemesis or melena that does not originate from a GI source. Usually, it is caused by swallowing blood from epistaxis, hemoptysis, or oral lesions. These diagnoses are best determined by a careful history and physical examination. Endoscopy to rule out GI sources may be required if the diagnosis remains uncertain.

Rarely, patients present with factitious bleeding. They may cause themselves to bleed by venopuncture and then swallow the blood before presentation. A high index of suspicion is necessary to make this diagnosis.

Acute lower gastrointestinal bleeding

Lower GI bleeding is defined as bleeding from a source below the ligament of Treitz. The annual incidence of lower intestinal bleeding is estimated to be 20 to 27 per 100 000 adults at risk [3]. When patients hospitalized for GI bleeding are identified, lower GI sources account for one-fourth to one-third of all bleeding events [303]. Lower GI bleeding is more common in men than in women, and the incidence rate increases with age, with more than a 200-fold increase noted from the third to the ninth decade of life [3]. Overall mortality rates for lower GI bleeding are consistently below 5%, which is lower than mortality rates for upper GI bleeding.

Diagnostic approach

The diagnosis should be sought in all patients with lower GI bleeding unless their overall prognosis is too poor to warrant further tests. In most patients whose bleeding ceases spontaneously, an elective colonoscopy after routine preparation is indicated. Patients with continued bleeding require urgent diagnosis. If a perianal or rectal source is suspected, simple proctoscopy can be performed quickly and may provide the diagnosis. For most colonic bleeding, a more thorough examination is required. Unless the bleeding is massive, rapid intestinal lavage allows adequate preparation for urgent colonoscopy. For patients who are bleeding too rapidly for a cleaning preparation or when urgent colonoscopy is not available, angiography is indicated [304]. As with upper GI bleeding, most angiographers prefer prior radiolabeled nuclide scans to demonstrate active bleeding and direct the examination, although the value of this practice has been questioned [305]. Before angiography or urgent colonoscopy, nasogastric lavage and even upper GI endoscopy should be considered to rule out an upper GI source of bleeding.

History and physical examination

A thorough history and physical examination often point to the correct diagnosis. For example, a prior diagnosis of hemorrhoids or inflammatory bowel disease is important. Symptoms that are associated with bleeding, such as abdominal pain or diarrhea, suggest specific diagnoses. A recent history of anorexia or weight loss or an abdominal mass found during physical examination may indicate an underlying malignancy.

Colonoscopy

Urgent colonoscopy has been defined variably as one performed within 12–48 h of admission. Similar to findings with upper GI bleeding, a retrospective study found that a shorter time to colonoscopy from admission was an independent predictor of hospital length of stay [306]. The longer delay from presentation to endoscopy seen with lower GI bleeding compared with upper GI bleeding reflects the need for oral purge. Rapid purge is best accomplished with polyethylene glycol-based solutions administered by a nasogastric tube or by drinking 1 liter of solution every 30–45 min. A median dose of 5.5 liters (range 4–14 liters) and a time interval of 3–4 h are required to cleanse the colon. For hospitalized patients, about one-third require a nasogastric tube for successful preparation of the colon. Metoclopramide 10 mg i.v. before starting the purge has been recommended to control nausea and promote gastric emptying [26].

Urgent colonoscopy enables a final diagnosis of colonic lesions in 74%–90% of patients. In one series that included prior upper GI endoscopy, upper GI lesions were diagnosed in 11%, presumed small bowel lesions in 9%, and no lesion in 6% of 80 patients with ongoing hematochezia [26]. This diagnostic accuracy is better than that of arteriography.

Radionuclide scans

The site of GI bleeding can be localized by scanning for extravasation of intravascular radioactively labeled blood. Technetium (^{99m}Tc) sulfur colloid scans are obtained shortly after injection. The use of erythrocytes labeled with [^{99m}Tc] pertechnetate allows repeated scanning over 24–36 h after injection to detect intermittent bleeding. These techniques can reveal bleeding even when the rate of blood loss is as low as 0.5 mL/min, and they have no associated morbidity. In comparison with surgical pathology, they have a sensitivity of 88% for correct localization of the bleeding site [307]. The major disadvantage of radionuclide scans is that they localize the bleeding to an area of the abdomen but do not diagnose the specific location or the responsible lesion. For this reason, radionuclide studies are often used to determine which patients have sufficient ongoing bleeding to warrant angiography, although their value as an angiography screen has been questioned [308]. However, they may allow more selective angiographic studies, decreasing the dye load. In the rare situation in which massive hemorrhage makes endoscopy impossible, angiography should be obtained immediately and not be delayed by prior radionuclide scans.

Angiography

In the rapidly bleeding patient, angiography offers accurate diagnosis and therapy. For patients in whom active bleeding cannot be demonstrated, some advocate an aggressive diagnostic angiographic approach based on pharmacological techniques with heparin or streptokinase [309]. When dye extravasation is not demonstrated, angiography can lead to a presumptive diagnosis such as angiodysplasia. Rare small bowel lesions such as arteriovenous malformations or neoplasms may be demonstrated.

Selective arterial embolization with polyvinyl alcohol particles or microcoils has replaced intraarterial vasopressin in the treatment of lower GI hemorrhage [310]. The use of 3F coaxial catheters allows placement of the microcatheter through an outer 5F diagnostic catheter close to the extravasating artery to deliver an embolic agent, thereby lowering the risk for bowel ischemia. Microcoils have become the embolic agent of choice because they are easy to inject and provide reliable arterial occlusion; moreover, flow distal to the coil occlusion can be maintained. Angiographic intervention is reported to be effective in 93% of lower GI hemorrhage patients, with prolonged clinical success in 81% [311]. Angiographic therapy carries the risk of both catheter- and dye-related complications in addition to possible ischemic infarction from embolization. Rebleeding rates are as high as 22%, with ischemia reported in 7%–60% [312,313].

Causes and therapy

Diagnostic certainty for the source of acute colonic bleeding is problematic in much of the literature on lower GI bleeding [314]. A definitive diagnosis is made when there is endoscopic or angiographic evidence of active bleeding, or endoscopic evidence of stigmata of recent bleeding. In the urgent colonoscopy studies, bleeding stigmata providing evidence for a "definitive diagnosis" was present in only 20%–25% of patients. A presumptive diagnosis is made when colonoscopy shows a potential bleeding site such as diverticulosis without bleeding stigmata but no other bleeding lesions. This occurs in up to one-third of patients.

Historically, the two major causes of acute lower GI bleeding were thought to be diverticulosis and angiodysplasia. However, studies using colonoscopy for diagnosis report angiodysplasia much less often [3,303] (Table 8.6). Diverticulosis remains the most frequent cause of gross lower GI bleeding although diverticula are also found incidentally in up to 66% of patients with other bleeding sources. In contrast to patients with upper GI bleeding, patients with lower GI bleeding are less likely to present with shock, and have lower transfusion requirements. Like upper GI bleeding, lower GI bleeding stops spontaneously in approximately 80% of cases.

Table 8.6 Final diagnosis of major lower gastrointestinal bleeding from seven studies

Diagnosis	Percentage of total diagnoses (%)	Mean (%)
Diverticulosis	20–55	33
Angiodysplasia	3–37	8
Cancer/polyp	8–30	19
Colitis[a]	6–22	18
Anorectal	0–9	4
Others[b]	3–14	8
Unknown	1–25	16

a Includes inflammatory bowel disease, infectious colitis, ischemic colitis, radiation colitis, vasculitis, and inflammation of unknown etiology.
b Includes postpolypectomy bleeding, aortocolonic fistula, trauma from fecal impaction, and anastomotic bleeding.
Adapted from Zuckerman & Prakash [314].

Diverticular bleeding

Diverticular bleeding occurs in only 3% of patients with diverticulosis. However, it is the most common cause of major lower GI hemorrhage because of the high prevalence of diverticulosis in the Western world. Despite the left-sided preponderance of diverticula, angiographic studies have demonstrated that 70% of bleeding diverticula occur in the right side of the colon [315]. In contrast, studies in which colonoscopy was used in a limited number of patients suggest that bleeding diverticula are more likely to be left-sided [316,317]. Although most patients with diverticular hemorrhage have always been managed nonoperatively [318], colonoscopic treatment of bleeding further decreases the need for surgical intervention [319].

Diverticula are usually located in the colonic wall at the sites of penetration of nutrient vessels. Bleeding presumably results from a colonic artery that penetrates into the dome of the diverticulum. The artery ruptures into the diverticular sac and causes copious bleeding. Clinical evidence of associated diverticulitis or inflammation is usually not present, and vessel rupture is thought to be the result of pressure erosion.

Diverticular bleeding presents with acute, painless, maroon-to-bright-red hematochezia, although melena may occur. Diverticulosis is not thought to be a cause of Hemoccult-positive stool or slow bleeding [320]. If the initial bout of diverticular bleeding ceases spontaneously, no further therapy is indicated because bleeding does not recur in most patients. Of the 75%–80% of patients in whom bleeding ceases, 65%–75% will not have a recurrence, and 25%–35% will have repeated episodes of diverticular hemorrhage [3,321].

Urgent colonoscopy after purge with endoscopic treatment of diverticular bleeding for patients with active bleeding or stigmata of bleeding has been shown to be highly effective in decreasing the need for surgical intervention compared with historical controls [319]. Endoscopic treatment has not been compared directly with angiographic intervention although it appears to have a higher diagnostic accuracy and a lower complication rate. It is important to remember that despite enthusiasm for therapeutic colonoscopy in acute lower GI bleeding, there are no controlled trials and the number of patients actually reported in case series is small. Also, not all reports are positive [322,323]. Any patient in whom endoscopic or angiographic control of diverticular bleeding fails should undergo urgent surgery to remove the portion of the colon bearing the bleeding site. Additionally, patients with recurrent diverticular bleeding should undergo elective surgery if their general medical condition and anticipated lifespan warrant such aggressive therapy. Accurate preoperative localization of the bleeding site with either angiography or colonoscopy reduces postoperative rebleeding rates by directing the resection to the appropriate segment of colon. Subtotal colon resection is recommended for patients with recurrent bleeding but no demonstration of a bleeding site, and may be associated with lower rebleeding rates than limited colon resection without increasing morbidity or mortality [324]. Surgical mortality rates are between 5% and 10% [325].

Angiodysplasia

Vascular ectasia, or angiodysplasia, is a common cause of acute major lower GI hemorrhage and slow intermittent blood loss. The percentage of cases of acute lower GI bleeding that have been attributed to angiodysplasia varies widely in the literature, from 10% to 40%. Most vascular ectases are degenerative lesions associated with aging. Two-thirds of patients with colonic angiodysplasia are older than 70 years. These lesions are different from the congenital vascular lesions that occur throughout the GI tract in various age groups. Angiodysplastic lesions are usually multiple, less than 5 mm in diameter, and involve primarily the cecum and right side of the colon. A clinical association with aortic valve stenosis is recognized [326], although the validity of the association continues to be controversial [327]. It has been reported that aortic valve replacement decreases bleeding frequency [328]. Acquired von Willebrand disease secondary to aortic stenosis, which is corrected after valve replacement, has been the hypothesized link between bleeding angiodysplasia and aortic valve disease [329]. An abnormal von Willebrand factor has been demonstrated in patients with bleeding angiodysplasia but not in patients with nonbleeding vascular lesions [330].

The pathogenesis of angiodysplasias is unknown, but one theory is that repeated, partial, intermittent obstruction of the submucosal veins where they pierce the muscle layers of the colon leads to dilation and tortuosity of the vessels [331]. Eventually, the entire arteriolar-capillary-venular unit dilates, creating a small arteriovenous communication. The predilection of these degenerative lesions for the right side of the colon may reflect the greater tension in the cecal wall than in the rest of the colon.

The diagnosis of vascular ectasia can be made by colonoscopy or angiography. A sensitivity of 70% for helical CT angiography has been reported in the diagnosis of colonic angiodysplasia by the demonstration of vessel accumulation in the colon wall, an early-filling vein, and an enlarged supplying artery [332]. The diagnostic sensitivity of colonoscopy is 80%–90%, and colonoscopy has the advantage of therapeutic potential [26]. Naloxone may enhance the appearance of both normal colonic vasculature and ectasias [333]. The sensitivity of angiography for angiodysplasia seems to be much lower, although no data based on pathology as the gold standard are available. The earliest angiographic sign is a densely opacified, dilated, tortuous, slowly emptying intramural vein. A vascular tuft represents a more advanced lesion, and an early-filling vein reflects an arteriovenous communication and is a late sign. All diagnostic modalities frequently identify the lesions without demonstrating active bleeding. Because active bleeding is infrequently identified and because these lesions seem to be common in elderly persons without a history of significant blood loss, a definitive diagnosis is difficult. Nevertheless, if no other source of GI bleeding is identified in a patient with recurrent or persistent GI bleeding sufficient to require transfusions or cause significant anemia, the presence of angiodysplasia is an indication for treatment.

Endoscopic techniques of hemostasis and angiographic embolization are both successful for controlling continued gross hemorrhage [334]. Electrocoagulation techniques, including heater probe, hot biopsy with monopolar coagulation, multipolar coagulation, Nd:YAG laser, and the argon plasma coagulator, have all been used successfully for the treatment of bleeding angiodysplasia. Rebleeding rates of 10%–30% have been reported [335]. Options then include further endoscopic therapy or surgery. Complications of endoscopic therapy are uncommon but include induction of bleeding and perforation. A retrospective comparison of medical therapy, coagulation techniques, and surgery showed a significant decrease in transfusion requirements for all three types of management of angiodysplasia [336]. Specimen injection techniques have demonstrated incidental angiodysplastic lesions in as many as 50% of surgically resected colons from autopsy specimens [337]. It seems prudent to reserve endoscopic therapy for lesions causing significant blood loss or anemia. If therapeutic colonoscopy fails to prevent recurrent bleeding, a hemicolectomy or colectomy is indicated, depending on the localization of these lesions.

Neoplasms and postpolypectomy bleeding

Benign and malignant neoplasms of the colon are common and, like diverticula and angiodysplastic lesions, occur predominantly in the elderly. They usually present with small degrees of intermittent bleeding or Hemoccult-positive stools.

However, neoplastic lesions are the cause of acute lower GI bleeding in 2%–26% of cases [338]. The diagnosis is made by colonoscopy, and the treatment is surgical or colonoscopic excision. Small bowel tumors are rare but may be diagnosed by small bowel radiographs, capsule endoscopy, or double balloon enteroscopy. A history of intermittent small bowel obstruction is a clue to a small bowel tumor as the cause of lower GI bleeding.

Postpolypectomy bleeding accounts for 2%–5% of cases of acute lower GI bleeding [3,303]. A review of patients with postpolypectomy hemorrhage noted that half of the patients required transfusions; the presentation time from polypectomy ranged from 0 to 17 days, with a median of 5 days [339]. Antiplatelet agents do not increase the risk of postpolypectomy bleeding although warfarin does [340]. Endoscopic therapy successfully treats more than 95% of patients [339]. In a randomized trial, prophylactic clip application was not shown to decrease the risk of delayed bleeding from polyp excision sites [341].

Perianal disease

Hemorrhoids and anal fissures are the most common causes of minor intermittent lower GI bleeding. Most young and middle-aged persons with rectal bleeding do not even seek medical care [342]. Only rarely is the amount of bleeding severe enough to cause iron deficiency anemia, or acute and severe enough to mandate transfusions. Massive hemorrhage from simple hemorrhoids is rare. Bleeding is usually from internal hemorrhoids and is painless. The characteristic clinical history is the presence of bright-red blood on the toilet tissue or around the stool but not mixed in the stool. Bleeding often occurs with straining or the passage of hard stool. A similar history is common in patients with bleeding from anal fissures, with the exception that anal fissures are often painful. Because rectal polyps and carcinomas may present with a similar bleeding history, patients should be evaluated with flexible sigmoidoscopy, including retroflexion of the flexible sigmoidoscope in the rectum to examine the proximal anal canal. Careful external examination of the external anal canal is also necessary.

Perianal disease is treated with sitz baths, bulk-forming agents, avoidance of straining, and ointments or suppositories. It is unknown whether actual therapeutic benefit is obtained with locally applied medications containing lubricants and hydrocortisone, but many patients report symptomatic relief. When bleeding or other symptoms continue to be troublesome, hemorrhoidal banding, coagulation techniques, or surgery may be indicated [343].

Meckel diverticulum

Meckel diverticulum is the most frequent congenital anomaly of the intestinal tract, with an incidence of 0.3%–3.0% in autopsy reports. It develops from incomplete obliteration of the vitelline duct, leaving an ileal diverticulum. Approxim-
ately 50% of these diverticula contain normal ileal mucosa, and most of the remaining 50% contain gastric mucosa or may occasionally contain duodenal, colonic, or pancreatic ectopic mucosa. The gastric mucosa is capable of acid secretion, which can result in ulceration of adjacent ileal mucosa. Most Meckel diverticula remain asymptomatic and do not require surgical excision when discovered incidentally.

Bleeding, the most common complication, usually occurs in childhood, although bleeding may rarely occur in adults [344]. Patients present with painless bleeding that may be dark or bright red, although its appearance is classically described as "currant jelly." The diagnosis can be made by scanning with radioactively labeled technetium, but false-negative results are not uncommon, and false-positive results have also been reported [345]. Barium filling of the diverticulum may occur, especially with an enteroclysis. Mesenteric angiography may demonstrate the site of bleeding. Surgical excision is the treatment of choice.

Inflammatory bowel disease

Bleeding from inflammatory bowel disease is usually minimal to moderate, although it reportedly accounts for 2%–6% of all cases of acute lower GI bleeding [3,315]. A review of acute major GI hemorrhage in inflammatory bowel disease suggests that it is much more common in Crohn's disease than in ulcerative colitis [346]. However, acute lower GI bleeding accounts for only 1% of hospital admissions for Crohn's disease. Surgery is required for treatment in 20%–35% of cases [347].

Colitis secondary to ischemia, infections, or irradiation

Ischemic colitis is a common entity in the elderly. It is usually caused by "low-flow states" and small vessel disease rather than by large vessel occlusion. Any segment of the colon may be involved, although the most common areas are the splenic flexure, descending colon, and sigmoid colon. The typical presentation is mild, cramping abdominal pain localized to the lower left side, followed within 24 h by rectal bleeding or bloody diarrhea. The blood loss is characteristically minimal, although ischemic colitis causes 3%–9% of all cases of major lower GI bleeding [3,314]. Plain abdominal films may show the classical "thumb-printing" lesion of the colon. The diagnosis is best made by colonoscopy and biopsy. Most cases resolve spontaneously with observation and medical support. Surgery is reserved for the rare circumstance of clinical deterioration with fever and a rising leukocyte count or persistent hemorrhage.

Infectious colitis caused by *Campylobacter jejuni*, *Salmonella* species, *Shigella* species, invasive *Escherichia coli* or *E. coli* 0157:H7, or *Clostridium difficile* often presents with bloody diarrhea. The degree of blood loss is rarely significant. The diagnosis is made by sigmoidoscopy or colonoscopy with biopsy and stool culture. Treatment is either not required or is determined by the specific pathogen.

Radiation-induced colitis is a chronic or recurrent problem that may follow irradiation immediately or several years later. The blood loss is rarely massive but may cause iron deficiency or a need for intermittent blood transfusions. The diagnosis is based on a history of prior irradiation, with endoscopic biopsy confirmation. Medical treatment with bulk-forming agents or sulfasalazine has not been successful. Intrarectal instillation of formalin will stop bleeding in 75%–80% of patients [348]. Endoscopic coagulation treatment with either the argon plasma coagulator, the Nd:YAG, argon, or potassium titanyl phosphate (KTP) laser, bipolar electrocoagulation, or treatment with the heater probe have also been successful in 65%–90% of patients [349–352]. These endoscopic treatment modalities appear safer and technically easier than formalin instillation. Surgical intervention is difficult because of the radiation damage to local tissue, and substantial morbidity has been reported [353].

Intussusception

Intussusception may present with maroon stools and is almost always accompanied by cramping abdominal pain. Uncommon in adults, it usually has a leading point, such as a polyp or malignancy. The diagnosis may be suggested by plain abdominal films or abdominal CT scan and the finding of a sausage-shaped mass during physical examination. Barium enema studies may be useful for diagnosis, and in children may be used for therapeutic reduction. The treatment of intussusception in adults is usually surgical.

Portal hypertension and rectal varices

Ileal or colonic varices, which tend to occur around ostomies [354], may present with massive lower GI bleeding. The diagnosis is often made by angiography, and the treatment is decompression of the portal hypertension by surgery, TIPS, or propranolol and nitrates. Rectal varices may also present with gross lower GI bleeding. Variceal ligation has been used to stop bleeding, although decompression of portal hypertension is probably superior for preventing rebleeding. Multiple colonic vascular ectases in patients with portal hypertension can cause hematochezia or Hemoccult-positive stools; the condition is called *portal colopathy* [355].

Other causes

Several rare causes of lower GI bleeding deserve brief mention. Solitary rectal ulcer, which may be associated with an internally prolapsing rectal mucosa, causes lower GI bleeding, although the bleeding is rarely massive [356]. Idiopathic rectal ulcers, or those caused by rectal impaction or ischemia, may present with major hemorrhage, often displaying peptic-ulcer-type bleeding stigmata [357]. Dieulafoy-like lesions casuing massive lower GI bleeding have been described in the rectum [358]. Aortoenteric fistulae, not associated with prosthetic grafts, can occur in the ileum and colon.

There are two mechanisms by which NSAIDs predispose patients to lower GI bleeding: by causing small bowel or colon ulcers [359,360] and by interfering with platelet function [4,361]. Metronidazole may be effective in decreasing GI blood loss from NSAID-induced enteropathy [362].

Obscure gastrointestinal bleeding

There are always a few unfortunate patients with chronic bleeding (obscure-occult) or recurrent acute bleeding (obscure-overt) in whom a diagnosis cannot be made despite colonoscopy and upper endoscopy. It has been estimated that in as many as 5% of patients a source of bleeding cannot be identified despite extensive examination [363]. The differential diagnosis for the etiology of obscure GI bleeding varies with the age of the patient. Patients younger than 40 are more likely to bleed from mass lesions such as small bowel lymphomas, carcinoids, or adenocarcinomas. Meckel diverticulum, Dieulafoy lesions, polyps from hereditary polyposis syndromes, and Crohn's disease are also more likely in a younger population. Patients older than 40 are more likely to bleed from small bowel intestinal angiodysplasia or NSAID-induced ulcers [364]. Unfortunately, many of these lesions are too small to be detected by angiography and can be missed or not reached by standard endoscopy [365].

Approach to the patient

In young patients with obscure GI bleeding, a radionuclide scan for Meckel diverticulum is indicated. In patients of all ages, the diagnostic yield of repeat upper endoscopy is surprisingly high, ranging from 24%–65% [366–368]. "Push" or small bowel enteroscopy (SBE) can replace this "second look" upper GI endoscopy [369], and has been effective in the evaluation of patients with obscure GI bleeding, with diagnostic yields ranging from 13%–78% [367,370,371]. Unfortunately, SBE, utilizing a pediatric colonoscope or a longer, slimmer "enteroscope," can only examine a short portion of the small bowel, estimated to be between 50 and 150 cm distal to the pylorus. The length of the small intestine (approximately 4.2 m) and its position as a loosely supported and looped structure on the mesentery make conventional endoscopic techniques difficult and inadequate.

Capsule endoscopy

Wireless capsule endoscopy (WCE) allowing imaging of the entire small intestine was developed in the late 1990s [372] and has been available commercially in the United States since 2001. Typically, the capsule is ingested early in the morning after an overnight fast and a minimal bowel preparation. Patients can continue most of their usual activities during the capsule endoscopy, including having a light lunch around 4 h after ingestion of the capsule. Physician presence is not required during the exam and the images are downloaded as a video file that can be reviewed and interpreted at a convenient time. Failure to reach the cecum during the recording period occurs in about 20% of cases [373]. Although capsule endoscopy is a relatively safe procedure, absolute contraindications for its use include GI obstruction or pseudoobstruction due to ileus. In patients with obstructive symptoms, a barium meal with small bowel follow-through (SBFT) may be indicated prior to WCE. The incidence of a retained capsule requiring surgical intervention is about 0.75%, although in many of the reported cases, the retained capsule was considered helpful by identifying the problematic area of small bowel for the surgeon [374,375]. To overcome this problem, a "patency capsule" has been developed. This is a disintegration time-controlled capsule developed to identify patients with strictures that may cause capsule retention. A retained patency capsule is detectable by radiofrequency scanner, with subsequent dissolution after 48 h, enabling passage through tightly strictured areas of small bowel [376]. Although there is concern about the use of capsule endoscopy in patients with pacemakers, evidence suggests that capsule endoscopy may be safely performed in these patients [377].

Wireless capsule endoscopy is the most sensitive modality for seeing the small intestinal mucosa, performing better than SBFT, enteroclysis, push enteroscopy, and CT enterography [378–380]. In a prospective study using intraoperative enteroscopy as the gold standard for diagnosis of obscure GI bleeding lesions, the sensitivity and specificity of WCE proved to be 95% and 75%, respectively, with positive and negative predictive values of 95% and 86% [381]. Far less invasive than intraoperative or double-balloon enteroscopy, WCE has become part of the routine work-up in patients with obscure GI bleeding.

It should be noted, however, that WCE provides images of a portion of the human GI tract not previously studied extensively in vivo. As such, the "normal" appearance of lumenal small bowel in asymptomatic patients is still in the process of being defined. Capsule endoscopy performed in healthy volunteers finds "abnormalities" in 23% of cases [382]. Thus obscure bleed studies that stratify capsule findings into "possible, likely, and definitive" sources of bleeding may reveal somewhat lower sensitivities. In addition, the role of capsule endoscopy in the inpatient setting for patients admitted with brisk or hemodynamically significant GI bleeding has not been well studied. As a result of sedation and lack of ambulation in these patients, the capsule study in this setting may be technically limited. Repeat traditional endoscopy should always be considered before WCE because up to 30% of bleeding lesions noted in the small intestine on WCE lie within the reach of a push enteroscope or colonoscope [383].

Promising as WCE is as a diagnostic tool for obscure gastrointestinal bleeding in the small bowel, the obvious limitation of this modality is the lack of therapeutic ability. Although intraoperative enteroscopy allows definitive treatment of clinically significant small bowel lesions, this is an inherently invasive approach and may not weigh favorably in the risk–benefit analysis for older and more debilitated patients. Balloon enteroscopy serves as an appealing therapeutic corollary for follow-up of lesions noted on capsule endoscopy.

Double-balloon enteroscopy (DBE)

This modality for viewing the small intestine was introduced in Japan in 2001 [384]. Double-balloon enteroscopy (DBE) is unique in that it enables visualization of the entire small intestine without advancing an excessive length of endoscope into the patient. Two inflatable balloons, one at the distal end of a 140-cm long overtube and one at the end of the enteroscope, provide traction against the wall of the small intestine. The overtube is first anchored into position in the duodenum while the enteroscope is advanced through the overtube distally as far as possible. When maximal insertion depth has been reached, the balloon on the tip of the enteroscope is inflated, the balloon at the end of the overtube is deflated and the overtube is advanced over the enteroscope until the ends approximate. At this point the overtube balloon is inflated and the overtube and enteroscope are gently pulled back, causing pleating of the small intestine over the entire apparatus. In this stepwise manner, the length of the small bowel is traversed. The intent is to reach the ileocecal valve, but this goal is often not achieved; however, if it is clinically relevant, a retrograde approach can be used on a separate day. Utilizing DBE, endoscopically directed therapy can be provided throughout the length of the small intestine.

In the largest multicenter report to date, 275 patients with suspected small intestinal disease underwent DBE, 168 of which were referred for obscure bleeding. Of these, the etiology of bleed was determined in 73% and treated in 55%. Panenteroscopy was performed in 42% of patients in whom it was attempted, and the average duration of the procedures was 90 min. Patient tolerance of the procedure was excellent, with a 1% incidence of pancreatitis likely due to duodenal pressure [385]. Jejunal tear, microscopic perforation, aspiration pneumonia, and multiple perforations in a patient with small bowel lymphoma and chemotherapy have also been reported [386]. Therapeutic balloon enteroscopy has a higher complication rate related to the therapy. Single-balloon enteroscopy has been introduced as a competitor to DBE. This technique uses "hooking" of the distal end of the endoscope instead of balloon fixation. Comparative studies of these two techniques are not yet available.

Intraoperative enteroscopy

Intraoperative enteroscopy is still the gold standard of small bowel imaging. The yield of detecting bleeding lesions in the small intestine reaches 83%–100%. This high sensitivity comes at the cost of marked invasiveness, making this a procedure of last resort.

References

1. Yavorski RT, Wong RKH, Maydonovitch C, et al. Analysis of 3294 cases of upper gastrointestinal bleeding in military medical facilities. Am J Gastroenterol 1995;90:568.
2. Longstreth GF. Epidemiology of hospitalization for acute upper gastrointestinal hemorrhage: a population-based study. Am J Gastroenterol 1995;90:206.
3. Longstreth GF. Epidemiology and outcome of patients hospitalized with acute lower gastrointestinal hemorrhage: a population-based study. Am J Gastroenterol 1997;92:419.
4. Lanas A, Sekar C, Hirschowitz BJ. Objective evidence of aspirin use in both ulcer and non-ulcer upper and lower gastrointestinal bleeding. Gastroenterology 1992;103:862.
5. Wilcox CM, Alexander LN, Cotsonis GA, et al. Nonsteroidal antiinflammatory drugs are associated with both upper and lower gastrointestinal bleeding. Dig Dis Sci 1997;42:990.
6. van Walraven C, Mamdani MM, Wells PS, Williams JI. Inhibition of serotonin reuptake by antidepressants and upper gastrointestinal bleeding in elderly patients: retrospective cohort study. Br Med J 2001;323:655.
7. Kaplan RC, Heckbert SR, Koepsell TD, et al. Use of calcium channel blockers and risk of hospitalized gastrointestinal tract bleeding. Arch Intern Med 2000;160:1849.
8. Lanas A, Bajador E, Serrano P, et al. Nitrovasodilators, low-dose aspirin, other nonsteroidal antiinflammatory drugs, and the risk of upper gastrointestinal bleeding. N Engl J Med 2000;343:834.
9. Barkun A, Sabbah S, Enns R, et al. The Canadian Registry on Non-variceal Upper Gastrointestinal Bleeding and Endoscopy (RUGBE): Endoscopic hemostasis and proton pump inhibition are associated with improved outcomes in a real-life setting. Am J Gastroenterol 2004;99:1238.
10. Das A, Wong RCK. Prediction of outcome of acute GI hemorrhage: a review of risk scores and predictive models. Gastrointest Endosc 2004;60:85.
11. Gralnek IM, Dulai GS. Incremental value of upper endoscopy for triage of patients with acute non-variceal upper-GI hemorrhage. Gastrointest Endosc 2004;60:9.
12. Lee JG, Turnipseed S, Romano PS, et al. Endoscopy-based triage significantly reduced hospitalization rates, and costs of treating upper GI bleeding: a randomized controlled trial. Gastrointest Endosc 1999;50:755.
13. Cipolletta L, Bianco MA, Rotondano G, et al. Outpatient management for low-risk nonvariceal upper GI bleeding: a randomized-controlled trial. Gastrointest Endosc 2002;55:1.
14. Podila PV, Ben-Menachem T, Batra SK, et al. Managing patients with acute, nonvariceal gastrointestinal hemorrhage: development and effectiveness of a clinical care pathway. Am J Gastroenterol 2001;96:208.
15. Bjorkman DJ, Zaman A, Fennerty MB, et al. Urgent vs. Elective endoscopy for acute non-variceal upper-GI bleeding: an effectiveness study. Gastrointest Endosc 2004;60:1.
16. Pfau PR, Cooper GS, Carlson MD, et al. Success and shortcomings of a clinical care pathway in the management of acute nonvariceal upper gastrointestinal bleeding. Am J Gastroenterol 2004;99:425.
17. van Leerdam ME, Vreeburg EM, Rauws EA, et al. Acute upper GI bleeding: did anything change? Time trend analysis of incidence and outcome of acute upper GI bleeding between 1993/1994 and 2000. Am J Gastroenterol 2003;98:1494.
18. Chak A, Cooper GS, Lloyd LE, et al. Effectiveness of endoscopy in patients admitted to the intensive care unit with upper GI hemorrhage. Gastrointest Endosc 2001;53:6.
19. Rudolph SJ, Landsverk BK, Freeman ML. Endotracheal intubation for airway protection during endoscopy for severe upper GI hemorrhage. Gastrointest Endosc 2003;57:58.
20. Baradarian R, Ramdhaney S, Chapalamadugu R, et al. Early intensive rescusitation of patients with upper gastrointestinal bleeding decreases mortality. Am J Gastroenterol 2004;99:619.
21. Luke RG, Lees W, Rudick J. Appearances of the stools after the introduction of blood into the caecum. Gut 1964;5:77.
22. Richards RJ, Donica MB, Grayer D. Can the blood urea nitrogen/creatinine ratio distinguish upper from lower gastrointestinal bleeding?. J Clin Gastroenterol 1990;12:500.
23. Stellato T, Rhodes RS, McDougal WS. Azotemia in upper gastrointestinal hemorrhage. Am J Gastroenterol 1980;73:486.
24. Chalasani N, Clark WS, Wilcox CM. Blood urea nitrogen to creatinine concentration in gastrointestinal bleeding. Am J Gastroenterol 1997;92:1796.
25. Layne EA, Mellow MH, Lipman TO. Insensitivity of guaiac slide tests for detection of blood in gastric juice. Ann Intern Med 1981;94:774.
26. Jensen DM, Machicado GA. Diagnosis and treatment of severe hematochezia. The role of urgent colonoscopy after purge. Gastroenterology 1988;95:1569.
27. Fleischer D. Etiology and prevalence of severe persistent upper gastrointestinal bleeding. Gastroenterology 1983;84:538.
28. Carbonell N, Pauwels A, Serfaty L, et al. Improved survival after variceal bleeding in patients with cirrhosis over the past two decades. Hepatology 2004;40:652.
29. Chalasani N, Kahi C, Francois F, et al. Improved patient survival after acute variceal bleeding: a multicenter, cohort study. Am J Gastroenterol 2003;98:653.
30. Swain CP, Storey DW, Bown SG. Nature of the bleeding vessel in recurrently bleeding gastric ulcers. Gastroenterology 1986;90:595.
31. Johnston JH. Endoscopic risk factors for bleeding peptic ulcer. Gastrointest Endosc 1990;36:S16.
32. Lau JYW, Sung JJY, Chan ACW, et al. Stigmata of hemorrhage in bleeding peptic ulcers: an interobserver agreement study among international experts. Gastrointest Endosc 1997;46:33.
33. Griffiths WJ, Neumann DA, Welsh JD. The visible vessel as an indicator of uncontrolled or recurrent gastrointestinal hemorrhage. N Engl J Med 1979;300:1411.
34. Storey DW, Bown SG, Swain CP, et al. Endoscopic prediction of recurrent bleeding in peptic ulcers. N Engl J Med 1981;305:915.
35. Laine L. Multipolar electrocoagulation in the treatment of active upper gastrointestinal tract hemorrhage. N Engl J Med 1987;316:1613.
36. Cook DJ, Salena B, Guyatt GH, Laine L. Endoscopic therapy for acute non-variceal upper gastrointestinal hemorrhage: a meta-analysis. Gastroenterology 1992;102:139.
37. Bleau BL, Sherman KW, Shaw MJ, et al. Recurrent bleeding from peptic ulcer associated with adherent clot: a randomized study comparing endoscopic treatment with medical therapy. Gastrointest Endosc 2002;56:1.
38. Jensen DM, Kovacs TO, Jutabha R, et al. Randomized trial of medical or endoscopic therapy to prevent recurrent ulcer hemorrhage in patients with adherent clots. Gastroenterology 2003;123:407.
39. Kahi CJ, Jensen DM, Sung JJ, et al. Endoscopic therapy versus medical therapy for bleeding peptic ulcer with adherent clot: a meta-analysis. Gastroenterology 2005;129:855.
40. Corley DA, Stefan AM, Wolf M, et al. Early indicators of prgonosis in upper gastrointestinal hemorrhage. Am J Gastroenterol 1998;93:336.
41. Ibach MB, Grier JF, Goldman DE, et al. Diagnostic consideration in evaluation of patients presenting with melena and nondiagnostic esophagogastroduodenoscopy. Dig Dis Sci 1995;40:1459.
42. Leinicke JA, Schaffer RD, Hogan WJ, et al. Emergency endoscopy in acute upper GI bleeding (UGB): does timing affect the significance of diagnostic yield? Gastrointest Endosc 1976;22:228.
43. Kramer SC, Gorich J, Rilinger N, et al. Embolization for gastrointestinal hemorrhages. Eur Radiol 2000;10:802.
44. Sorensen HT, Mellemkjaer L, Blot WJ, et al. Risk of upper gastrointestinal bleeding associated with use of low-dose aspirin. Am J Gastroenterol 2000;95:2218.

45. Swain CP, Salmon PR, Northfield PC. Does ulcer position influence presentation or prognosis of acute gastrointestinal bleeding? Gut 1986;27:A632.

46. Brullet E, Campo R, Bedos G, et al: Site and size of bleeding peptic ulcer: Is there any relation to the efficacy of hemostatic sclerotherapy? Endoscopy 1991;23:73.

47. Swain CP. Pathophysiology of bleeding lesions. Gastrointest Endosc 1990;36:S21.

48. Laine L, Cohen H, Brodhead J, et al. Prospective evaluation of immediate versus delayed refeeding and prognostic value of endoscopy in patients with upper gastrointestinal hemorrhage. Gastroenterology 1992;102:314.

49. Rockall TA, Logan RFA, Devlin HB, Northfield TC. Steering Committee and members of the National Audit of Acute Upper Gastrointestinal Haemorrhage. Incidence of and mortality from acute upper gastrointestinal haemorrhage in the United Kingdom. Br Med J 1995;311:222.

50. Fallah MA, Prakash C, Edmundowicz S. Acute gastrointestinal bleeding. Med Clin N Am 2000;84:1183.

51. Kupfer Y, Cappell MS, Tessler S. Acute gastrointestinal bleeding in the intensive care unit. The intensivist's perspective. Gastroenterol Clin North Am 2000;29:275.

52. Frossard JL, Spahr L, Queneau PE, et al. Erythromycin intravenous bolus infusion in acute upper gastrointestinal bleeding: a randomized, controlled, double-blind trial. Gastroenterology 2002;123:17.

53. Coffin B, Pocard M, Panis Y, et al. Erythromycin improves the quality of EGD in patients with acute upper GI bleeding: a randomized controlled study. Gastrointest Endosc 2002;56:174.

54. Kalloo AN, Canto MI, Wadwa KS, et al. Clinical usefulness of 3% hydrogen peroxide in acute upper GI bleeding: a pilot study. Gastrointest Endosc 1999;49:518.

55. Lin HJ, Lee FY, Chan CY, et al. Heat probe thermocoagulation as a substitute for surgical intervention to arrest massive peptic ulcer hemorrhage: an experience in 153 cases. Surgery 1990;108:18.

56. Cooper GS, Chak A, Way LE, et al. Early endoscopy in upper gastrointestinal hemorrhage: associations with recurrent bleeding, surgery, and length of hospital stay. Gastrointest Endosc 1999;49:145.

57. Rollhauser C, Fleischer DE. Nonvariceal upper gastrointestinal bleeding. Endoscopy 2004;36:52.

58. Lin HJ, Perng CL, Lee FY, et al. Endoscopic injection for the arrest of peptic ulcer hemorrhage: Final results of a prospective, randomized comparative trial. Gastrointest Endosc 1993;39:15.

59. Kubba AK, Palmer KR. Role of endoscopic injection therapy in the treatment of bleeding peptic ulcer. Br J Surg 1996;83:461.

60. Simoens M, Gevers AM, Rutgeerts P. Endoscopic therapy for upper gastrointestinal hemorrhage: A state of the art. Hepatogastroenterology 1999;46:737.

61. Lin HJ, Chan CY, Lee FY, et al. Endoscopic injection to arrest peptic ulcer hemorrhage: a prospective, randomized controlled trial; preliminary results. Hepatogastroenterology 1991;38:291.

62. Chen PC, Wu CS, Liau YU. Hemostatic effect of endoscopic local injection with hypertonic saline-epinephrine solution and pure ethanol for digestive tract bleeding. Gastrointest Endosc 1986;32:319.

63. Pescatore P, John V, Manegold BC, et al. Fibrin sealant in peptic ulcer bleeding: A one year prospective study. Gastrointest Endosc 1996;43:A260.

64. Laine L. Bipolar/multipolar electrocoagulation. Gastrointest Endosc 1990;36:S38.

65. Laine L. Multipolar electrocoagulation in the treatment of peptic ulcers with non-bleeding visible vessels. Ann Intern Med 1989;110:510.

66. Jensen DM. Heat probe for hemostasis of bleeding peptic ulcers: techniques and results of randomized controlled trials. Gastrointest Endosc 1990;36:S42.

67. Lin HJ, Lee FY, Kang WM, et al. A controlled study of therapeutic endoscopy for peptic ulcer with non-bleeding visible vessel. Gastrointest Endosc 1990;36:241.

68. Llach J, Bordas JM, Salmeron JM, et al. A prospective randomized trial of heater probe thermocoagulation versus injection therapy in peptic ulcer hemorrhage. Gastrointest Endosc 1996;43:117.

69. Hui WM, Ng MMT, Lok ASF, et al. A randomized comparative study of laser photocoagulation, heater probe, and bipolar electrocoagulation in the treatment of actively bleeding ulcers. Gastrointest Endosc 1991;37:299.

70. Chau C, Siu W, Law B, et al. Randomized controlled trial comparing epinephrine injection plus heat probe coagulation versus epinephrine injection plus argon plasma coagulation for bleeding peptic ulcers. Gastrointest Endosc 2003;57:455.

71. Cipolletta L, Bianco MA, Rotondano G, et al. Prospective comparison of argon plasma coagulator and heater probe in the endoscopic treatment of major peptic ulcer bleeding. Gastrointest Endosc 1998;48:191.

72. Calvet X, Vergara M, Brullet E, et al. Addition of a second endoscopic treatment following epinephrine injection improves outcome in high-risk bleeding ulcers. Gastroenterology 2004;126:441.

73. Vergara M, Calvet X, Gisbert JP. Epinephrine injection versus epinephrine injection and a second endoscopic method in high risk bleeding ulcers. The Cochrane Database of Systematic Reviews 2007;2:CD005584.

74. Wong RC. Endoscopic Doppler US probe for acute peptic ulcer hemorrhage. Gastrointest Endosc 2004;60:804.

75. Chung IK, Ham JS, Kim HS. Comparison of the hemostatic efficacy of the endoscopic hemoclip method with hypertonic saline± epinephrine injection and a combination of the two for the management of bleeding peptic ulcers. Gastrointest Endosc 1999;49:13.

76. Lin HJ, Hsieh YH, Tseng GY, et al. A prospective, randomized trial of endoscopic hemoclip versus heater probe thermocoagulation for peptic ulcer bleeding. Am J Gastroenterol 2002;97:2250.

77. Matthewson K, Swain CP, Bland M, et al. Randomized comparison of Nd:YAG laser, heater probe, and no endoscopic therapy for bleeding peptic ulcers. Gastroenterology 1990;98:1239.

78. Li Y, Sha W, Nie Y, et al. Effect of intragastric pH on control of peptic ulcer bleeding. J Gastroenterol Hepatol 2000;15:148.

79. Yacyshyn BR, Thomson AB. Critical review of acid suppression in nonvariceal, acute, upper gastrointestinal bleeding. Dig Dis 2000;18:117.

80. Brunner G, Luna P, Hartmann M, Wurst W. Optimizing the intragastric pH as a supportive therapy in upper GI bleeding. Yale J Biol Med 1999;69:225.

81. Lau J, Sung J, Lee K, et al. Effect of intravenous omeprazole on recurrent bleeding after endoscopic treatment of bleeding peptic ulcers. N Engl J Med 2000;343:310.

82. Barkun AN, Herba K, Adam V, et al. High-dose intravenous proton pump inhibition following endoscopic therapy in the acute management of patients with bleeding peptic ulcers in the USA and Canada: A cost-effectiveness analysis. Aliment Pharmacol Ther 2004;19:591.

83. Udd, M, Miettinen P, Palmu A, et al. Regular-dose versus high-dose omeprazole in peptic ulcer bleeding a prospective randomized double-blind study. Scand J Gastroenterol 2001;36:1332.

84. Udd M, Töyry J, Miettinen P, et al. The effect of regular and high doses of omeprazole on the intragastric acidity in patients with bleeding peptic ulcer treated endoscopically: a clinical trial with continuous intragastric pH monitoring. Eur J Gastroenterol Hepatol 2005;17:1351.

85. Javid G, Masoodi I, Zargar SA, et al. Omeprazole as adjuvant therapy to endoscopic combination injection sclerotherapy for treating bleeding peptic ulcer. Am J Med 2001;111:280.

86. Khuroo MS, Yattoo GN, Javid G, et al. A comparison of omeprazole and placebo for bleeding peptic ulcer. N Engl J Med 1997;336:1054.

87. Saruc M, Can M, Kucukmetin N, et al. Somatostatin infusion and hemodynamic changes in patients with non-variceal upper gastrointestinal bleeding: a pilot study. Med Sci Monit 2003;9:PI84.

88. Imperiale TF, Birgisson S. Somatostatin or octreotide compared with

H2 antagonists and placebo in the management of acute nonvariceal upper gastrointestinal hemorrhage: a meta-analysis. Ann Intern Med 1997;127:1062.

89. Adler DG, Leighton JA, Davila RE, et al. ASGE guideline: the role of endoscopy in acute non-variceal upper-GI hemorrhage. Gastrointest Endosc 2004;60:497.

90. Barkun A, Bardou M, Marshall JK. Consensus recommendations for managing patients with nonvariceal upper gastrointestinal bleeding. Ann Int Med 2003;139:843.

91. Yilmaz S, Bayan K, Dursun M, et al. Does adding misoprostol to standard intravenous proton pump inhibitor protocol improve the outcome of aspirin/NSAID-induced upper gastrointestinal bleeding? A randomized prospective study. Dig Dis Sci 2007;52:110.

92. Breckan RK, Wessel-Berg AM, Jorde R. Non-endoscopic first-line treatment of bleeding peptic ulcer with ranitidine and tranexamic acid. Scand J Gastroenterol 2003;38:1000.

93. May G, Musa D. The use of intravenous terlipressin in non-variceal upper GI bleeds. Emerg Med J 2006;23:400.

94. Sacks HS, Chalmers TC, Blum AL, et al. Endoscopic hemostasis: an effective therapy for bleeding peptic ulcers. JAMA 1990;264:494.

95. Benjamin SB. Therapeutic endoscopy and bleeding ulcers: methodology. Gastrointest Endosc 1990;36:S56.

96. Lau J, Sung J, Lam YH, et al. Endoscopic retreatment compared with surgery in patients with recurrent bleeding after initial endoscopic control of bleeding ulcers. N Engl J Med 1999;340:751.

97. Waltman AC, Greenfield AJ, Novelline RA, et al. Pyloroduodenal bleeding and intraarterial vasopressin: clinical results. Am J Roentgenol 1979;133:643.

98. Lieberman DA, Keller FS, Katon RM, et al. Arterial embolization for massive upper gastrointestinal tract bleeding in poor surgical candidates. Gastroenterology 1984;86:876.

99. Elta GH, Appelman HD, Behler EM, et al. A study of the correlation between endoscopic and histologic diagnoses in gastroduodenitis. Am J Gastroenterol 1987;82:749.

100. Borch K, Jansson L, Sjodahl R, et al. Hemorrhagic gastritis. Incidence, etiological factors and prognosis. Acta Chir Scand 1987;154:211.

101. Graham DY, Smith JL. Aspirin and the stomach. Ann Intern Med 1986;104:390.

102. Scheiman JM. NSAIDs, cytoprotection, and gastrointestinal injury. Gastroenterol Clin North Am 1996;25:279.

103. Holvoet J, Terriene L, Van Hee W, et al. Relation of upper gastrointestinal bleeding to non-steroidal anti-inflammatory drugs and aspirin: a case-control study. Gut 1991;32:730.

104. Agrawal NM, Roth S, Graham DY, et al. Misoprostol compared with sucralfate in the prevention of non-steroidal anti-inflammatory drug-induced gastric ulcer. Ann Intern Med 1991;115:195.

105. Silverstein FE, Graham DY, Senior JR, et al. Misoprostol reduces serious gastrointestinal complications in patients with rheumatoid arthritis receiving nonsteroidal anti-inflammatory drugs. Ann Intern Med 1995;123:241.

106. Raskin JB, White RH, Jaszewski R, et al. Misoprostol and ranitidine on the prevention of NSAID-induced ulcers: a prospective, double-blind, multicenter study. Am J Gastroenterol 1996;91:223.

107. Scheiman JM, Yeomans ND, Talley NJ, et al. Prevention of ulcers by esomeprazole in at-risk patients using non-selective NSAIDs and COX-2 inhibitors. Am J Gastroenterol 2006;101:701.

108. Hawkey CJ, Karrasch JA, Szczepanski L, et al. Omeprazole compared with misoprostol for ulcers associated with nonsteroidal anti-inflammatory drugs. N Engl J Med 1998;338:727.

109. Chan F, Chung SC, Suen BY, et al. Preventing recurrent upper gastrointestinal bleeding in patients with Helicobacter pylori infection who are taking low-dose aspirin or naproxen. N Engl J Med 2001;344:967.

110. Scheiman JM, Behler EM, Berardi RR, et al. Salicylsalicylic acid causes less gastroduodenal mucosal damage than enteric-coated aspirin. An endoscopic comparison. Dig Dis Sci 1989;34:229.

111. Laine L, Sloane R, Ferretti M, Cominelli F. A randomized double-blind comparison of placebo, etodolac, and naproxen on gastrointestinal injury and prostaglandin production. Gastrointest Endosc 1995;42:428.

112. Langman MJ, Jensen DM, Watson DJ, et al. Adverse upper gastrointestinal effects of rofecoxib compared with NSAIDS. JAMA 1999;282:1929.

113. Wells JJ, Nostrant TT, Wilson JAP, et al. Gastroduodenal ulcerations in patients receiving selective hepatic artery infusion chemotherapy. Am J Gastroenterol 1985;80:425.

114. Chaudhury TK, Robert A. Prevention by mild irritants of gastric necrosis produced in rats by sodium taurocholate. Dig Dis Sci 1980;25:830.

115. Kelly JP, Kaufman DW, Koff RS, et al. Alcohol consumption and the risk of major upper gastrointestinal bleeding. Am J Gastroenterol 1995;90:1058.

116. Wilcox CM, Alexander LN, Straub RF, et al. A prospective endoscopic evaluation of the causes of upper GI hemorrhage in alcoholics: a focus on alcoholic gastropathy. Am J Gastroenterol 1996;91:134.

117. Vigneri S, Termini R, Piraino A, et al. The stomach in liver cirrhosis. Endoscopic, morphological, and clinical correlations. Gastroenterology 1991;101:472.

118. Stewart CA, Sanyal AJ. Grading portal gastropathy; validation of a gastropathy scoring system. Am J Gastroenterol 2003;98:1758.

119. Sarin SK, Sreenivas DV, Lahoti D, et al. Factors influencing development of portal hypertensive gastropathy in patients with portal hypertension. Gastroenterology 1992;102:994.

120. Lo GH, Lai KH, Cheng JS, et al. The effects of endoscopic variceal ligation and propranolol on portal hypertensive gastropathy: a prospective, controlled trial. Gastrointest Endosc 2001;53:579.

121. Sarin SK, Shahi HM, Jain M, et al. The natural history of portal hypertensive gastropathy; influence of variceal eradication. Am J Gastroenterol 2000;95:2888.

122. Merli M, Nicolini G, Angeloni S, et al. The natural history of portal hypertensive gastropathy in patients with liver cirrhosis and mild portal hypertension. Am J Gastroenterol 2004;99:1959.

123. Primignani M, Carpinelli L, Preatoni P, et al. Natural history of portal hypertensive gastropathy in patients with liver cirrhosis. Gastroenterology 2000;119:181.

124. Perez-Ayuso RM, Pigre JM, Bosch J, et al. Propranolol in prevention of recurrent bleeding from severe portal gastropathy in cirrhosis. Lancet 1991;337:1431.

125. Babb RR, Mitchell RL. Persistent hemorrhagic gastritis in a patient with portal hypertension and esophagogastric varices: the role of portal decompressive surgery. Am J Gastroenterol 1988;83:777.

126. Skillman JJ, Bushnell LS, Goldman H, et al. Respiratory failure, hypotension, sepsis and jaundice – a clinical syndrome associated with lethal hemorrhage from acute stress ulceration of the stomach. Am J Surg 1969;117:523.

127. Pimentel M, Roberts DE, Bernstein CN, et al. Clinically significant gastrointestinal bleeding in critically ill patients in an era of prophylaxis. Am J Gastroenterol 2000;95:2801.

128. Athanasoulis CA, Baum S, Waltman AC, et al. Control of acute mucosal hemorrhage. Intraarterial infusion of posterior pituitary extract. N Engl J Med 1974;290:597.

129. Hubert JP, Kiernan PD, Welch JS, et al. The surgical management of bleeding stress ulcers. Ann Surg 1980;191:672.

130. Ben-Menachem T, Fogel R, Patel RV, et al. Prophylaxis for stress-related gastric hemorrhage in the medical intensive care unit. A randomized, controlled, single-blind study. Ann Intern Med 1994;121:568.

131. Cook DJ, Reeve BK, Guyatt GH, et al. Stress ulcer prophylaxis in critically ill patients. JAMA 1996;275:308.

132. Hastings PR, Skillman JJ, Bushnell LS, et al. Antacid titration in the prevention of acute gastrointestinal bleeding. N Engl J Med 1978;298:1041.

133. Messori A, Trippoli S, Vaiani M, et al. Bleeding and pneumonia in intensive care patients given rantidine and sucralfate for prevention of stress ulcer: meta-analysis of randomised controlled trials. Br Med J 2000;321:1103.

134. Borrero E, Bank S, Margolis I, et al. Comparison of antacid and sucralfate in the prevention of gastrointestinal bleeding in patients who are critically ill. Am J Med 1985;79:62.

135. Tryba M, Zevounov F, Torok M, et al. Prevention of acute stress bleeding with sucralfate, antacids, or cimetidine. Am J Med 1986;79:55.

136. Cook D, Guyatt G, Marshall J, et al. A comparison of sucralfate and ranitidine for the prevention of upper gastrointestinal bleeding in patients requiring mechanical ventilation. N Engl J Med 1998;338:791.

137. Driks MR, Craven DE, Celli BR, et al. Nosocomial pneumonia in intubated patients given sucralfate as compared with antacids or histamine type 2 blockers: the role of gastric colonization. N Engl J Med 1987;317:1376.

138. Simms HH. Gastric alkalinization does not increase the risk of pneumonia in critically ill patients. Semin Respir Infect 1994;9:222.

139. Afessa B, Kubilis PS. Upper gastrointestinal bleeding in patients with hepatic cirrhosis: clinical course and mortality prediction. Am J Gastroenterol 2000;95:484.

140. Snady H, Feinman L. Prediction of variceal hemorrhage: a prospective study. Am J Gastroenterol 1988;83:519.

141. Lebrec D, DeFleury P, Rueff B, et al. Portal hypertension, size of esophageal varices, and risk of gastrointestinal bleeding in alcoholic cirrhosis. Gastroenterology 1980;79:1139.

142. El Atti EA, Nevens F, Bogaerts K, et al. Variceal pressure is a strong predictor of variceal hemorrhage in patients with cirrhosis as well as in patients with non-cirrhotic portal hypertension. Gut 1999;45:618.

143. Moitinho E, Escorsell A, Bandi J, et al. Prognostic value of early measurements of portal pressure in acute variceal bleeding. Gastroenterology 1999;117:626.

144. Beppu K, Inokucki K, Koyanagi N, et al. Prediction of variceal hemorrhage by esophageal endoscopy. Gastrointest Endosc 1981;27:213.

145. Eckardt VF, Grace ND. Gastroesophageal reflux and bleeding esophageal varices. Gastroenterology 1979;76:39.

146. De Ledinghen V, Heresbach D, Fourdan O, et al. Anti-inflammatory drugs and variceal bleeding: a case-control study. Gut 1999;44:270.

147. North Italian Endoscopic Club. Prediction of the first variceal hemorrhage in patients with cirrhosis of the liver and esophageal varices. N Engl J Med 1988;319:983.

148. Kleber G, Sauerbruch T, Fischer G, et al. Pressure of intraesophageal varices assessed by fine needle puncture: its relation to endoscopic signs and severity of liver disease in patients with cirrhosis. Gut 1989;30:228.

149. Schiano TD, Adrain AL, Vega KJ, et al. High-resolution endoluminal sonography assessment of the hematocystic spots of esophageal varices. Gastrointest Endosc 1999;49:424.

150. Siringo S, McCormick PA, Mistry P, et al. Prognostic significance of the white nipple sign in variceal bleeding. Gastrointest Endosc 1991;37:51.

151. Foutch PG, Sullivan JA, Gaines JA, et al. Cutaneous vascular spiders in cirrhotic patients: correlation with hemorrhage from esophageal varices. Am J Gastroenterol 1988;83:723.

152. The North Italian Endoscopic Club. Prediction of the first variceal hemorrhage in patients with cirrhosis of the liver and esophageal varices. A prospective mulitcenter study. New Engl J Med 1989;320:868.

153. Dagradi AE, Mehler R, Tan DTD, et al. Sources of upper gastrointestinal bleeding in patients with liver cirrhosis and large esophagogastric varices. Am J Gastroenterol 1970;54:458.

154. Valenzuela JE, Schubert T, Fogel MR, et al. A multicenter, randomized, double-blind trial of somatostatin in the management of acute hemorrhage from esophageal varices. Hepatology 1989;10:958.

155. Burroughs AK, McCormick PA, Hughes MD, et al. Randomized, double-blind, placebo-controlled trial of somatostatin for variceal bleeding. Gastroenterology 1990;99:1388.

156. Walker S, Kreichgauer HP, Bode JC. Terlipressin vs. somatostatin in bleeding esophageal varices: a controlled, double-blind study. Hepatology 1992;15:1023.

157. Kravetz D, Bosch J, Teres J, et al. Comparison of intravenous somatostatin and vasopressin infusions in the treatment of acute variceal hemorrhage. Hepatology 1984;4:442.

158. Targownik LE, Spiegel BM, Dulai GS, et al. The cost-effectiveness of hepatic venous pressure gradient monitoring in the prevention of recurrent variceal hemorrhage. Am J Gastroenterol 2004;99:1306.

159. Thalheimer U, Mela M, Patch D, Burroughs AK. Targeting portal pressure measurements: a critical reappraisal. Hepatology 2004;39:286.

160. Junquera F, Lopez-Talavera JC, Mearin F, et al. Somatostatin plus isosorbide 5-mononitrate versus somatostatin in the control of acute gastro-oesophageal variceal bleeding: a double-blind, randomised, placebo controlled clinical trial. Gut 2000;46:127.

161. D'Amico G, Pietrosi G, Tarantino I, Pagliaro L. Emergency sclerotherapy versus vasoactive drugs for variceal bleeding in cirrhosis: a Cochrane meta-analysis. Gastroenterology 2003;124:1277.

162. Besson I, Ingrand P, Person B, et al. Sclerotherapy with or without octreotide for acute variceal bleeding. N Engl J Med 1995;333:555.

163. Cales P, Masliah C, Bernard B, et al. Early administration of vapreotide for variceal bleeding in patients with cirrhosis. N Engl J Med 2001;344:23.

164. Avgerinos A, Nevens F, Raptis S, et al. Early administration of somatostatin and efficacy of sclerotherapy in acute oesophageal variceal bleeds: the European Acute Bleeding Oesophageal Variceal Episodes (ABOVE) randomized trial. Gastrointest Endosc 2000;51:372.

165. Banares R, Albillos A, Rincon D, et al. Endoscopic treatment versus endoscopic plus pharmacologic treatment for acute variceal bleeding: a meta-analysis. Hepatology 2002;35:609.

166. Walker S, Stiehl A, Raedsch R, et al. Terlipressin in bleeding esophageal varices: a placebo-controlled, double-blind study. Hepatology 1986;6:112.

167. Fort E, Sautereau D, Silvain C, et al. A randomized trial of terlipressin plus nitroglycerin vs. balloon tamponade in the control of acute variceal hemorrhage. Hepatology 1990;11:678.

168. Escorsell A, Ruiz del Arborl L, Planas R, et al. Multicenter randomized controlled trial of terlipressin versus sclerotherapy in the treatment of acute variceal bleeding: the TEST study. Hepatology 2000;32:471.

169. Saraya A, Sarin SK. Effects of intravenous nitroglycerin and metoclopramide on intravariceal pressure: a double-blind randomized study. Am J Gastroenterol 1993;88:1850.

170. Sarin SK, Saraya A. Effects of intravenous nitroglycerin and nitroglycerin and metoclopramide on intravariceal pressure: a double-blind randomized study. Am J Gastroenterol 1995;90:48.

171. Hosking SW, Doss W, El-Zeiny II, et al. Pharmacological constriction of the lower oesophageal sphincter: a simple method of arresting variceal haemorrhage. Gut 1988;29:1098.

172. Ejlersen E, Melsen T, Ingerslev J, et al. Recombinant activated factor VII (rFVIIa) acutely normalizes prothrombin time in patients with cirrhosis during bleeding from oesophageal varices. Scand J Gastroenterol 2001;36:1081.

173. Bosch J, Thabut D, Bendtsen F, et al. Recombinant factor VIIa for upper gastrointestinal bleeding in patients with cirrhosis: a randomized, double-blind trial. Gastroenterology 2004;127:1123.

174. Stiegmann GV, Goff JS, Michaletz-Onody PA, et al. Endoscopic sclerotherapy as compared with endoscopic ligation for bleeding esophageal varices. N Engl J Med 1992;316:1527.

175. Laine L, El-Newihi HM, Migikovsky B, et al. Endoscopic ligation compared with sclerotherapy for the treatment of bleeding esophageal varices. Ann Intern Med 1993;119:1.

176. Gimson AE, Ramage JK, Panos MZ, et al. Randomized trial of

variceal banding ligation versus injection sclerotherapy for bleeding oesophageal varices. Lancet 1993;342:391.

177. Zargar SAA, JAvid G, Khan BA, et al. Endoscopic ligation vs. sclerotherapy in adults with extrahepatic portal venous obstruction: a prospective randomized study. Gastrointest Endosc 2005;61:58.

178. De La Pena J, Rivero M, Sanchez E, et al. Variceal ligation compared with endoscopic sclerotherapy for variceal hemorrhage: prospective randomized trial. Gastrointest Endosc 1999;49:417.

179. Saeed ZA, Stiegmann GV, Ramirez FC, et al. Endoscopic variceal ligation is superior to combined ligation and sclerotherapy for esophageal varices: a multicenter prospective randomized trial. Hepatology 1997;25:71.

180. Traif IA, Fachartz FS, Jumah AA, et al. Randomized trial of ligation versus combined ligation and sclerotherapy for bleeding esophageal varices. Gastrointest Endosc 1999;50:1.

181. Bhargava DK, Pokharna R. Endoscopic variceal ligation versus endoscopic variceal ligation and endoscopic sclerotherapy: a prospective randomized study. Am J Gastroenterol 1997;92:950.

182. Umehara M, Onda M, Tajiri T, et al. Sclerotherapy plus ligation versus ligation for the treatment of esophageal varices: a prospective randomized study. Gastrointest Endosc 1999;50:7.

183. Garg PK, Joshi YK, Tandon RK. Comparison of endoscopic variceal sclerotherapy with sequential endoscopic band ligation plus low-dose sclerotherapy for secondary prophylaxis of variceal hemorrhage: a prospective randomized study. Gastrointest Endosc 1999;50:369.

184. Cipolletta L, Bianco MA, Rotondano G, et al. Argon plasma coagulation prevents variceal recurrence after band ligation of esophageal varices: preliminary results of a prospective randomized trial. Gastrointest Endosc 2002;56:467.

185. Hartigan PM, Gebhard RL, Gregory PB, et al. Sclerotherapy for actively bleeding esophageal varices in male alcoholics with cirrhosis. Gastrointest Endosc 1997;46:1.

186. Hepworth CC, Burnham WR, Swain P. Development and application of endoloops for the treatment of bleeding esophageal varices. Gastrointest Endosc 1999;50:677.

187. Naga MI, Okasha HH, Foda AR, et al. Detachable endoloop vs. elastic band ligation for bleeding esophageal varices. Gastrointest Endosc 2004;59:804.

188. Hsieh WJ, Lin HC, Hwang SJ, et al. The effect of ciprofloxacin in the prevention of bacterial infection in patients with cirrhosis after upper gastrointestinal bleeding. Am J Gastroenterol 1998;93:962.

189. Hou MC, Lin HC, Liu TT, et al. Antibiotic prophylaxis after endoscopic therapy prevents rebleeding in acute variceal hemorrhage: a randomized trial. Hepatology 2004;39:746.

190. Panes J, Teres J, Bosch J, et al. Efficacy of balloon tamponade in the treatment of bleeding gastric and esophageal varices. Dig Dis Sci 1988;33:454.

191. Boyce MHW. Modification of the Sengstaken-Blakemore balloon tube. N Engl J Med 1962;267:195.

192. Chojkier M, Conn HO. Esophageal tamponade in the treatment of bleeding varices. A decadal progress report. Dig Dis Sci 1980;25:267.

193. Mandelstam P, Zeppa R. Endotracheal intubation should precede esophagogastric balloon tamponade for control of variceal bleeding. J Clin Gastroenterol 1983;5:493.

194. Rossle M, Haag K, Ochs A, et al. The transjugular intrahepatic portosystemic stent-shunt procedure for variceal bleeding. N Engl J Med 1994;330:165.

195. Monescillo A, Martinez-Lagares F, Ruiz-del-Arbol L, et al. Influence of portal hypertension and its early decompression by TIPS placement on the outcome of variceal bleeding. Hepatology 2004;40:793.

196. Ring EJ, Lake JR, Roberts JP, et al. Using transjugular intrahepatic portosystemic shunts to control variceal bleeding before liver transplantation. Ann Intern Med 1992;116:304.

197. Malt RA, Abbolf WM, Warshaw AL, et al. Randomized trial of emergency mesocaval and portacaval shunts for bleeding esophageal varices. Am J Surg 1978;135:584.

198. Orloff MJ, Orloff MS, Rambotti M, et al. Is portal-systemic shunt worthwhile in Child's class C cirrhosis? Ann Surg 1992;216:256.

199. McCormick PA, Kaye GL, Greenslade L, et al. Esophageal staple transection as a salvage procedure after failure of acute injection sclerotherapy. Hepatology 1992;15:403.

200. Rubenstein JH, Eisen GM, Inadomi JM. A cost-utility analysis of secondary prophylaxis for variceal hemorrhage. Am J Gastroenterol 2004;99:1274.

201. Dasarathy S, Dwivedi M, Bhargava DK, et al. A prospective randomized trial comparing repeated endoscopic sclerotherapy and propranolol in decompensated (Child class B and C) cirrhotic patients. Hepatology 1992;16:89.

202. D'Amico G, Pagliaro L, Bosch J. The treatment of portal hypertension: a meta-analytic review. Hepatology 1995;22:332.

203. Villanueva C, Balanzo J, Novella MT, et al. Nadolol plus isosorbide mononitrate compared with sclerotherapy for the prevention of variceal rebleeding. N Engl J Med 1996;334:1624.

204. Villanueva C, Minana J, Ortiz J, et al. Endoscopic ligation compared with combined treatment with nadolol and isosorbide mononitrate to prevent recurrent variceal bleeding. N Engl J Med 2001;345:647.

205. Vinel JP, Lamouliatte H, Cales P, et al. Propranolol reduces the rebleeding rate during endoscopic sclerotherapy before variceal obliteration. Gastroenterology 1992;102:1760.

206. Lo GH, Lai KH, Cheng JS, et al. Endoscopic variceal ligation plus nadolol and sucralfate compared with ligation alone for the prevention of variceal rebleeding: a prospective, randomized trial. Hepatology 2000;32:461.

207. Jenkins SA, Baxter JN, Critchley M, et al. Randomized trial of octreotide for long-term management of cirrhosis after variceal hemorrhage. Gastrointest Endosc 1998;48:328.

208. Lebrec D, Pynard T, Hillon P, et al. Propranolol for the prevention of recurrent gastrointestinal bleeding in patients with cirrhosis: a controlled study. N Engl J Med 1981;305:1371.

209. Garcia-Tsao G, Grace ND, Groszmann RJ, et al. Short-term effects of propranolol on portal venous pressure. Hepatology 1986;6:101.

210. Bernard B, Lebrec D, Maturin P, et al. Beta-adrenergic antagonists in the prevention of gastrointestinal rebleeding in patients with cirrhosis: a meta-analysis review. Hepatology 1995;22:332.

211. Angelico M, Carli L, Piat C, et al. Isosorbide-5-mononitrate versus propranolol in the prevention of first bleeding in cirrhosis. Gastroenterology 1993;104:1460.

212. Gournay J, Masliah C, Martin T, et al. Isosorbide mononitrate and propranolol compared with propranolol alone for the prevention of variceal rebleeding. Hepatology 2000;31:1239.

213. Merkel C, Gatta A, Donada C, et al. Long-term effect of nadolol or nadolol plus isosorbide-5-mononitrate on renal function and ascites formation in patients with cirrhosis. Hepatology 1995;22:808.

214. Pomier-Layrargues G, Villenueve JP, Deschenes M, et al. Transjugular intrahepatic portosystemic shunt (TIPS) versus endoscopic variceal ligation in the prevention of variceal rebleeding in patients with cirrhosis: a randomised trial. Gut 2001;48:390.

215. Cello JP, Olcott EW, Koch J, et al. Endoscopic sclerotherapy compared with percutaneous transjugular intrahepatic portosystemic shunt after initial sclerotherapy in patients with acute variceal hemorrhage. Ann Intern Med 1997;126:858.

216. Cabrera J, Maynar M, Granados R, et al. Transjugular intrahepatic portosystemic shunt versus sclerotherapy in the elective treatment of variceal hemorrhage. Gastroenterology 1996;110:832.

217. Jalan R, Forrest EH, Stanley AJ, et al. A randomized trial comparing transjugular intrahepatic portosystemic stent-shunt with variceal band ligation in the prevention of rebleeding from esophageal varices. Am J Gastroenterol 1999;94:284.

218. Rossle M, Delbert P, Hoag K, et al. Randomized trial of transjugular-intrahepatic-portosystemic shunt versus endoscopy plus propranolol for the prevention of variceal bleeding. Lancet 1997;349:1043.

219. Sauer P, Theilmann L, Stremmel W, et al. Transjugular intrahepatic portosystemic stent shunt versus sclerotherapy plus propranolol for variceal rebleeding. Gastroenterology 1997;113:1623.

220. Garcia-Tsao G, Sanyal AJ, Grace ND, Carey WD. Prevention and management of gastroesophageal varices and variceal hemorrhage in cirrhosis. Am J Gastroenterol 2007;102:2086.

221. Malt RA. Portosystemic venous shunts. N Engl J Med 1976;295:24.

222. Galambos JT, Warren WD, Rudman D, et al. Selective and total shunts in the treatment of bleeding varices. N Engl J Med 1976;295:1089.

223. Langer B, Taylor BR, MacKenzie DR, et al. Further report of a prospective randomized trial comparing distal splenorenal shunt with end-to-side portacaval shunt. Gastroenterology 1985;88:424.

224. Millikan WJ, Jr, Warren WD, Henderson JM, et al. The Emory prospective randomized trial: selective versus non-selective shunt to control variceal bleeding. Ann Surg 1985;201:712.

225. Conn HO, Resnick RH, Grace ND, et al. Comparison of distal and proximal splenorenal shunt vs portal-systemic shunt: current status of a controlled trial. Hepatology 1981;1:151.

226. Harley HAJ, Morgan T, Redker AG, et al. Results of a randomized trial of end-to-side portacaval shunt and distal splenorenal shunt in alcoholic liver disease and variceal bleeding. Gastroenterology 1986;91:802.

227. Johansen K. Prospective comparison of partial versus total portal decompression for bleeding esophageal varices. Surg Gynecol Obstet 1992;175:528.

228. Rosemurgy AS, Zervos EE, Goode SE, et al. Differential effects on portal and effective hepatic blood flow. A comparison between transjugular intrahepatic portasystemic shunt and small-diameter H-graft portacaval shunt. Ann Surg 1997;225:601.

229. Mercado MA, Morales-Linares JC, Granados-Garcia J, et al. Distal splenorenal shunt versus 10-mm low-diameter mesocaval shunt for variceal hemorrhage. Am J Surg 1996;171:591.

230. Reynolds TB, Donovan AJ, Mikkelsen WP, et al. Results of a 12-year randomized trial of portacaval shunt in patients with alcoholic liver disease and bleeding varices. Gastroenterology 1981;80:1005.

231. Cello JP, Grendell JH, Crass RA, et al. Endoscopic sclerotherapy versus portacaval shunt in patients with severe cirrhosis and variceal hemorrhage. N Engl J Med 1984;311:1589.

232. Henderson JM, Boyer TD, Kutner MH, et al. Distal splenorenal shunt versus transjugular intrahepatic portal systemic shunt for variceal bleeding: a randomized trial. Gastroenterology 2006;130:1643.

233. Helton WS, Maves R, Wricks K, Johansen K. Transjugular intrahepatic portasystemic shunt vs. surgical shunt in good-risk cirrhotic patients: a case control comparison. Arch Surg 2001;136:17.

234. Selzner M, Tuttle-Newhall JE, Dahm F, et al. Current indication of a modified Sugiura procedure in the management of variceal bleeding. J Am Coll Surg 2001;193:166.

235. Borganovo G, Gostantini M, Grange D, et al. Comparison of a modified Sugiura procedure with portal systemic shunt for prevention of recurrent variceal bleeding in cirrhosis. Ann Surg 1996;119:214.

236. Ono J, Katsuki T, Kodama Y. Combined therapy for esophageal varices: sclerotherapy, embolization and splenopneumopexy. Surgery 1987;101:535.

237. Merkel C, Zoli M, Siringo S, et al. Prognostic indicators of risk for first variceal bleeding in cirrhosis: a multicenter study in 711 patients to validate and improve the North Italian Endoscopic Club (NIEC) index. Am J Gastroenterol 2000;95:2915.

238. Zaman A, Hapke R, Flora K, et al. Factors predicting the presence of esophageal or gastric varices in patients with advanced liver disease. Am J Gastroenterol 1999;94:3292.

239. Caläs P, Desmorat H, Vinel JP, et al. Incidence of large oesophageal varices in patients with cirrhosis: application to prophylaxis of first bleeding. Gut 1990;31:1298.

240. Zaman A, Becker T, Lapidus J, Benner K. Risk factors for the presence of varices in cirrhotic patients without a history of variceal hemorrhage. Arch Int Med 2001;161:2564.

241. Eisen GM, Eliakim R, Zaman A, et al. A pilot study of the diagnostic accuracy of Given esophageal capsule endoscopy versus conventional upper endoscopy for the diagnosis of esophageal varices. Endoscopy 2006;38:31.

242. Resnick RH, Chalmers TC, Ishihara AM, et al. A controlled study of the prophylactic portacaval shunt. Ann Intern Med 1969;70:675.

243. The Veterans Affairs Cooperative Variceal Sclerotherapy Group. Prophylactic sclerotherapy for esophageal varices in men with alcoholic liver disease. N Engl J Med 1991;324:1179.

244. Conn HO, Grace ND, Bosch J, et al. Propranolol in the prevention of the first hemorrhage from esophagogastric varices: a multicenter, randomized clinical trial. Hepatology 1991;13:902.

245. Pagliaro L, D'Amico G, Sîrensen TIA, et al. Prevention of first bleeding in cirrhosis. A meta-analysis of randomized trials of nonsurgical treatment. Ann Intern Med 1992;117:59.

246. Poynard T, Caläs P, Pasta L, et al. Beta-adrenergic-antagonist drugs in the prevention of gastrointestinal bleeding in patients with cirrhosis and esophageal varices. N Engl J Med 1991;324:1532.

247. Garcia-Pagan JC, Morillas R, Banares R, et al. Spanish Variceal Bleeding Study Group: Propranolol plus placebo versus propranolol plus isosorbide-5-mononitrate in the prevention of a first variceal bleed: a double-blind RCT. Hepatology 2003;37:1260.

248. Sarin SK, Lamba GS, Kumar M, et al. Comparison of endoscopic ligation and propranolol for the primary prevention of variceal bleeding. N Engl J Med 1999;340:988.

249. Jutabha R, Jensen DM, Martin P, et al. Randomized study comparing banding and propranolol to prevent initial variceal hemorrhage in cirrhotics with high-risk esophageal varices. Gastroenterology 2005;128:870.

250. Lo GH, Chen WC, Chen MH, et al. Banding ligation versus nadolol and isosorbide mononitrate for the prevention of esophageal variceal rebleeding. Gastroenterology 2002;123:728.

251. Schepke M, Kleber G, Nurnberg D, et al. Ligation versus propranolol for the primary prophylaxis of variceal bleeding in cirrhosis. Hepatology 2004;40:65.

252. Lui HF, Stanley AJ, Forrest EH, et al. Primary prophylaxis of variceal hemorrhage: a randomized controlled trial comparing banding ligation, propranolol, and isosorbide mononitrate. Gastroenterology 2002;123:735.

253. de la Pena J, Brullet E, Sanchez-Hernandez E, et al. Variceal ligation plus nadolol compared with ligation for prophylaxis of variceal rebleeding: a multicenter trial. Hepatology 2005;41:572.

254. Sarin SK, Wadhawan M, Agarwal SR, et al. Endoscopic variceal ligation plus propranolol versus endoscopic variceal ligation alone in primary prophylaxis of variceal bleeding. Am J Gastroenterol 2005;100:797.

255. Sarin SK, Lahoti D, Saxena SP, et al. Prevalence, classification, and natural history of gastric varices: a long-term follow-up study in 568 portal hypertension patients. Hepatology 1992;16:1343.

256. Kim T, Shijo H, Kokawa H, et al. Risk factors for hemorrhage from gastric fundal varices. Hepatology 1997;25:307.

257. Hashizume M, Kitano S, Yamaga H, et al. Endoscopic classification of gastric varices. Gastrointest Endosc 1990;36:276.

258. Korula J, Chin K, Young K, et al. Demonstration of two distinct subsets of gastric varices. Dig Dis Sci 1991;36:303.

259. Sarin SK. Long-term follow-up of gastric variceal sclerotherapy: an eleven-year experience. Gastrointest Endosc 1997;46:8.

260. Glynn MJ. Isolated splenic vein thrombosis. Arch Surg 1986;121:723.

261. Bernades P, Baetz A, Levy P, et al. Splenic and portal venous obstruction in chronic pancreatitis. Dig Dis Sci 1992;37:340.

262. Sarin SK, Sachdeu G, Nanda R, et al. Endoscopic sclerotherapy in the treatment of gastric varices. Br J Surg 1988;75:747.

263. Heneghan MA, Byrne A, Harrison PM. An open pilot study of the effects of a human fibrin glue for endoscopic treatment of patients with acute bleeding from gastric varices. Gastrointest Endosc 2002;56:422.

264. Lee MS, Cho JY, Cheon YK, et al. Use of detachable snares and elastic bands for endoscopic control of bleeding from large gastric varices. Gastrointest Endosc 2002;56:83.

265. Hashizume M, Tsagawa K, Migos S, et al. Eradication of large gastric varices by sclerotherapy combined with percutaneous transhepatic obliteration. Hepatogastroenterology 1997;44:221.

266. Huang YH, Yeh HZ, Chen GH, et al. Management of gastric varices. Gastroenterology 2001;120:1875.

267. Iwase H, Maeda O, Shimada M, et al. Endoscopic ablation with cyanoacrylate glue for isolated gastric variceal bleeding. Gastrointest Endosc 2001;53:585.

268. Sarin SK, Jain AK, Jain M, Gupta R. A randomized controlled trial of cyanoacrylate versus alcohol injection in patients with isolated fundic varices. Am J Gastroenterol 2002;97:1010.

269. Lo GH, Lai KH, Cheng JS, et al. A prospective, randomized trial of butyl cyanoacrylate injection versus band ligation in the management of bleeding gastric varices. Hepatology 2001;33:1060.

270. Mahadeva S, Bellamy MC, Kessel D, et al. Cost-effectiveness of N-butyl-2-cyanoacrylate (histoacryl) glue injections versus transjugular intrahepatic portosystemic shunt in the management of acute gastric variceal bleeding. Am J Gastroenterol 2003;98:2688.

271. Shepard HA, Harvey J, Jackson A, et al. Recurrent retching with gastric mucosal prolapse. A proposed prolapse gastropathy syndrome. Dig Dis Sci 1984;29:121.

272. Knaver CM. Mallory-Weiss syndrome. Characterization of 75 Mallory-Weiss lacerations in 528 patients with upper gastrointestinal hemorrhage. Gastroenterology 1976;71:5.

273. Paquet KJ, Mercado-Diaz M, Kalk JF. Frequency, significance and therapy of the Mallory-Weiss syndrome in patients with portal hypertension. Hepatology 1990;11:879.

274. Llach J, Elizalde JI, Guevara MC, et al. Endoscopic injection therapy in bleeding Mallory-Weiss syndrome: a randomized controlled trial. Gastrointest Endosc 2001;54:679.

275. Yamaguchi Y, Yamato T, Katsumi N, et al. Endoscopic hemoclipping for upper GI bleeding due to Mallory-Weiss syndrome. Gastrointest Endosc 2001;53:427.

276. Gimson A, Polson R, Westaby D, et al. Omeprazole in the management of intractable esophageal ulceration following injection sclerotherapy. Gastroenterology 1990;99:1829.

277. Shaheen NJ, Stuart E, Schmitz SM, et al. Pantoprazole reduces the size of postbanding ulcers after variceal band ligation: a randomized, controlled trial. Hepatology 2005;41:588.

278. Savides TJ, Jensen DM, Cohen J, et al. Severe upper gastrointestinal tumor bleeding: endoscopic findings, treatments, and outcomes. Endoscopy 1996;28:244.

279. Marwick T, Kerlin P. Angiodysplasia of the upper gastrointestinal tract: clinical spectrum in 41 cases. J Clin Gastroenterol 1986;8:404.

280. Kjeldsen A, Kjeldsen J. Gastrointestinal bleeding in patients with hereditary hemorrhagic telangiectasia. Am J Gastroenterol 2000;95:415.

281. Chalasani N, Cotsonis G, Wilcox CM. Upper gastrointestinal bleeding in patients with chronic renal failure: role of vascular ectasia. Am J Gastroenterol 1996;91:2329.

282. Bhutani MS, Gupta SG, Markert RJ, et al. A prospective controlled evaluation of endoscopic detection of angiodysplasia and its association with aortic valve disease. Gastrointest Endosc 1995;42:398.

283. Olmos JA, Marcolongo M, Pogorelsky V, et al. Argon plasma coagulation for prevention of recurrent bleeding from GI angiodysplasias. Gastrointest Endosc 2004;60:881.

284. Ljubicic N. Endoscopic detachable mini-loop ligation for treatment of gastroduodenal angiodysplasia: case study of 11 patients with long-term follow-up. Gastrointest Endosc 2004;59:420.

285. Kantsevoy SV, Cruz-Correa MR, Vaughn CA, et al. Endoscopic cryotherapy for the treatment of bleeding mucosal vascular lesions of the GI tract: a pilot study. Gastrointest Endosc 2003;57:403.

286. Longacre AV, Gross CP, Gallitelli M, et al. Diagnosis and management of gastrointestinal bleeding in patients with hereditary hemorrhagic telangiectasia. Am J Gastroenterol 2003;98:59.

287. Bronner MH, Pate MB, Cunningham JT, et al. Estrogen-progesterone therapy for bleeding gastrointestinal telangiectasias in chronic renal failure. Ann Intern Med 1986;105:371.

288. Van Cutsen E, Rutgeerts P, Vantrappen G. Treatment of bleeding gastrointestinal vascular malformations with oestrogen-progesterone. Lancet 1990;335:953.

289. Junquera F, Feu F, Papo M, et al. A multicenter, randomized, clinical trial of hormonal therapy in the prevention of rebleeding from gastrointestinal angiodysplasia. Gastroenterology 2001;121:1073.

290. Gretz JE, Achem SR. The watermelon stomach: clinical presentation, diagnosis, and treatment. Am J Gastroenterol 1998;93:890.

291. Stotzer PO, Willen R, Kilander AF. Watermelon stomach: not only antral disease. Gastrointest Endosc 2002;55:897.

292. Spahr L, Villeneuve JP, Dufresne MP, et al. Gastric antral vascular ectasia in cirrhotic patients: absence of relation with portal hypertension. Gut 1999;44:739.

293. Kwan V, Bourke MJ, Williams SJ, et al. Argon plasma coagulation in the management of symptomatic gastrointestinal vascular lesions: experience in 100 consecutive patients with long-term follow-up. Am J Gastroenterol 2006;101:58.

294. Pavey DA, Craig PI. Endoscopic therapy for upper-GI vascular ectasias. Gastrointest Endosc 2004;59:233.

295. Steffes BC, O'Leary JP. Primary aortoduodenal fistulas: a case report and review of the literature. Ann Surg 1980;46:121.

296. Fagan EA, Allison DJ, Chadwick JS, et al. Treatment of haemobilia by selective arterial embolization. Gut 1980;21:541.

297. Risti B, Marincek B, Jost R, et al. Hemosuccus pancreaticus as a source of obscure upper gastrointestinal bleeding: three cases and literature review. Am J Gastroenterol 1995;90:1878.

298. Elton E, Howell DA, Amberson SM, et al. Combined angiographic and endoscopic management of bleeding pancreatic pseudoaneurysms. Gastrointest Endosc 1997;46:544.

299. Juler GL, Labitzke HG, Lamb R, et al. The pathogenesis of Dieulafoy's gastric erosion. Am J Gastroenterol 1984;79:195.

300. Norton ID, Petersen BT, Sorbi D, et al. Management and long-term prognosis of Dieulafoy lesion. Gastrointest Endosc 1999;50:762.

301. Schmulewitz N, Baillie J. Dieulafoy lesions: a review of 6 years of experience at a tertiary referral center. Am J Gastroenterol 2001; 96:1688.

302. Kasapidis P, Georgopoulos P, Delis V, et al. Endoscopic management and long-term follow-up of Dieulafoy's lesions in the upper GI tract. Gastrointest Endosc 2002;55:527.

303. Zuckerman GR, Prakash C. Acute lower intestinal bleeding. Part I: Clinical presentation and diagnosis. Gastrointest Endosc 1998;48:606.

304. Strate LL, Syngal S. Predictors of utilization of early colonoscopy vs. radiography for severe lower intestinal bleeding. Gastrointest Endosc 2005;61:46.

305. Pennoyer WP, Vignati PV, Cohen JL. Mesenteric angiography for lower gastrointestinal hemorrhage: are there predictors for a positive study?. Dis Colon Rectum 1997;40:1014.

306. Schmulewitz N, Fisher DA, Rockey DC. Early colonoscopy for acute lower GI bleeding predicts shorter hospital stay: a retrospective study of experience in a single center. Gastrointest Endosc 2003; 58:841.

307. O'Neill BB, Gosnell JE, Lull RJ, et al. Cinematic nuclear scintigraphy reliably directs surgical intervention for patients with gastrointestinal bleeding. Arch Surg 2000;135:1076.

308. Voeller GR, Bunch G, Britt LG. Use of technetium-labeled red blood cell scintigraphy in the detection and management of gastrointestinal hemorrhage. Surgery 1991;110:799.

309. Koval G, Benner KG, Rosch J, et al. Aggressive angiographic diagnosis in acute lower gastrointestinal hemorrhage. Dig Dis Sci 1987;32:248.

310. DeBarros J, Rosas L, Cohen J, et al. The changing paradigm for the treatment of colonic hemorrhage: superselective angiographic embolization. Dis Col Rectum 2002;45:802.

311. Funaki B, Kostelic JK, Lorenz J, et al. Superselective microcoil embolization of colonic hemorrhage. Am J Roentgenol 2001;177:829.

312. Gordon RL, Ahl KL, Kerlan RK, et al. Selective arterial embolization for the control of lower gastrointestinal bleeding. Am J Surg 1997; 174:24.

313. Silver A, Bendick P, Wasvary H. Safety and efficacy of superselective angioembolization in control of lower gastrointestinal hemorrhage. Am J Surg 2005;189:361.

314. Zuckerman GR, Prakash C. Acute lower intestinal bleeding. Part II: Etiology, therapy, and outcomes. Gastrointest Endosc 1999;49:228.

315. Cassarella WJ, Kanter IE, Seaman WB. Right-sided colonic diverticula as a cause of acute rectal hemorrhage. N Engl J Med 1972;286:450.

316. Foutch PG, Zimmerman K. Diverticular bleeding and the pigmented protuberance (sentinel clot): clinical implications, histopathological correlation, and results of endoscopic intervention. Am J Gastroenterol 1996;91:2589.

317. Foutch PG. Diverticular bleeding: are nonsteroidal anti-inflammatory drugs risk factors for hemorrhage and can colonoscopy predict outcome for patients?. Am J Gastroenterol 1995;90:1779.

318. Bokhari M, Vernava AM, Ure T, et al. Diverticular hemorrhage in the elderly – is it well tolerated? Dis Colon Rectum 1996;39:191.

319. Jensen DM, Machicado GA, Jutabha R, et al. Urgent colonoscopy for the diagnosis and treatment of severe diverticular hemorrhage. N Engl J Med 2000;343:78.

320. Kewenter J, Hellzen-Ingemarsson A, Kewenter G, et al. Diverticular disease and minor rectal bleeding. Scand J Gastroenterol 1985;20:922.

321. McGuire HH. Bleeding colonic diverticula. A reappraisal of natural history and management. Ann Surg 1994;220:653.

322. Bloomfield RS, Jockey DC, Shetzline MA. Endoscopic therapy of acute diverticular hemorrhage. Am J Gastroenterol 2001;96:2367.

323. Angtuaco TL, Reddy SK, Drapkin S, et al. The utility of urgent colonoscopy in the evaluation of acute lower gastrointestinal tract bleeding: a 2-year experience from a single center. Am J Gastroenterol 2001;96:1982.

324. Farner R, Lichliter W, Kuhn J, et al. Total colectomy versus limited colonic resection for acute lower gastrointestinal bleeding. Am J Surg 1999;178:587.

325. Baker R, Senagore A. Abdominal colectomy offers safe management for massive lower GI bleeding. Am Surg 1994;8:578.

326. Greenstein RJ, McElhinney AJ, Reuben D, et al. Colonic vascular ectasias and aortic stenosis: coincidence or causal relationship? Am J Surg 1986;151:347.

327. Imperiale TF, Ransohoff DF. Aortic stenosis, idiopathic gastrointestinal bleeding, and angiodysplasia: is there an association? A methodologic critique of the literature. Gastroenterology 1988;95:1670.

328. Cappell MS, Lebwohl O. Cessation of recurrent bleeding from gastrointestinal angiodysplasias after aortic valve replacement. Ann Intern Med 1986;105:54.

329. Warkentin TE, Moore JC, Morgan DG. Aortic stenosis and bleeding gastrointestinal angiodysplasia: is acquired von Willebrand's disease the link?. Lancet 1992;340:35.

330. Veyradier A, Balian A, Wolf M, et al. Abnormal von Willebrand factor in bleeding angiodysplasias of the digestive tract. Gastroenterology 2001;120:346.

331. Boley SJ, Sammartano R, Adams A, et al. On the nature and etiology of vascular ectasias of the colon. Gastroenterology 1977;72:650.

332. Junquera F, Quiroga S, Saperas E, et al. Accuracy of helical computed tomographic angiography for the diagnosis of colonic angiodysplasia. Gastroenterology 2000;119:293.

333. Brandt LJ, Spinnell MK. Ability of naloxone to enhance the colonoscopic appearance of normal colon vasculature and colon vascular ectasias. Gastrointest Endosc 1999;49:79.

334. Cello JP, Grendell JH. Endoscopic laser treatment for gastrointestinal vascular ectasias. Ann Intern Med 1986;104:352.

335. Santos JCM, Apilli F, Guimaraes AS, et al. Angiodysplasia of the colon: endoscopic diagnosis and treatment. Br J Surg 1988;75:256.

336. Hutcheon DF, Kablin J, Bulkley GB, et al. Effect of therapy on bleeding rates in gastrointestinal angiodysplasia. Am Surg 1987;53:6.

337. Aldabagh SM, Trujillo YP, Taxy JB. Utility of specimen angiography in angiodysplasia of the colon. Gastroenterology 1986;91:725.

338. Peura DA, Lanza FL, Gostout CJ, et al. The American College of Gastroenterology Bleeding Registry: preliminary findings. Am J Gastroenterol 1997;92:924.

339. Sorbi D, Norton I, Conio M, et al. Postpolypectomy lower GI bleeding: descriptive analysis. Gastrointest Endosc 2000;51:690.

340. Hui AJ, Wong RM, Ching JY, et al. Risk of colonoscopic polypectomy

341. Shioji K, Suzuki Y, Kobayashi M, et al. Prophylactic clip application does not decrease delayed bleeding after colonoscopic polypectomy. Gastrointest Endosc 2003;57:691.

342. Talley NJ, Jones M. Self-reported rectal bleeding in a United States community: prevalence, risk factors, and health care seeking. Am J Gastroenterol 1998;93:2179.

343. Randall GM, Jensen DM, Machicado GA, et al. Prospective randomized comparative study of bipolar versus direct current electrocoagulation for treatment of bleeding internal hemorrhoids. Gastrointest Endosc 1994;40:403.

344. Kusumoto H, Yoshida M, Takahashi I, et al. Complications and diagnosis of Meckel's diverticulum in 776 patients. Am J Surg 1992;164:382.

345. Stakianakis GN, Haase GM. Abdominal scintigraphy for ectopic gastric mucosa: a retrospective analysis of 143 studies. Am J Roentgenol 1982;138:7.

346. Pardi DS, Loftus EV, Tremaine WJ, et al. Acute major gastrointestinal hemorrhage in inflammatory bowel disease. Gastrointest Endosc 1999;49:153.

347. Belaiche J, Lousi E, D'Haens G, et al. Acute lower gastrointestinal bleeding in Crohn's disease: characteristics of a unique series of 34 patients. Am J Gastroenterol 1999;94:2177.

348. Saclarides TJ, King DG, Franklin JL, et al. Formalin instillation for refractory radiation-induced hemorrhagic proctitis. Report of 16 patients. Dis Colon Rectum 1996;39:196.

349. Taylor JG, Dijario JA, Buchi KN. Argon laser therapy for hemorrhagic radiation proctitis: long-term results. Gastrointest Endosc 1993;39:641.

350. Jensen DM, Machicado GA, Cheng S, et al. A randomized prospective study of endoscopic bipolar electrocoagulation and heater probe treatment of chronic rectal bleeding from radiation telangiectasia. Gastrointest Endosc 1997;45:20.

351. Taylor JG, DiSario JA, Bjorkman DJ, et al. KTP laser therapy for bleeding from chronic radiation proctopathy. Gastrointest Endosc 2000;52:353.

352. Sebastian S, O'Connor H, O'Morain C, Buckley M. Argon plasma coagulation as first-line treatment for chronic radiation proctopathy. J Gastroenterol Hepatol 2004;19:1169.

353. Pricolo VE, Shellito PC. Surgery for radiation injury to the large intestine. Dis Colon Rectum 1994;37:675.

354. Ricci RL, Lee KR, Greenberger NJ. Chronic gastrointestinal bleeding from ileal varices after total proctocolectomy for ulcerative colitis: correction by mesocaval shunt. Gastroenterology 1980;78:1058.

355. Kozarek RA, Botoman VA, Bredfeldt JE, et al. Portal colopathy: prospective study of colonoscopy in patients with portal hypertension. Gastroenterology 1991;101:1192.

356. Levine DS. "Solitary" rectal ulcer syndrome. Gastroenterology 1987; 92:243.

357. Kanwal F, Dulai G, Jensen GM, et al. Major stigmata of recent hemorrhage on rectal ulcers in patients with severe hematochezia: Endoscopic diagnosis, treatment, and outcomes. Gastrointest Endosc 2003;57:462.

358. Kayali Z, Sangchantr W, Matsumoto B. Lower gastrointestinal bleeding secondary to Dieulafoy-like lesion of the rectum. J Clin Gastroenterol 2000;30:328.

359. Allison MC, Howatson AG, Torrance CJ, et al. Gastrointestinal damage associated with the use of nonsteroidal anti-inflammatory drugs. N Engl J Med 1992;327:749.

360. Lengeling RW, Mitros FA, Brennan JA, Schulze KS. Ulcerative ileitis encountered at ileo-colonoscopy: likely role of nonsteroidal agents. Clin Gastroenterol Hepatol 2003;1:160.

361. Holt S, Rigoglioso V, Sidhu M, et al. Nonsteroidal anti-inflammatory drugs and lower gastrointestinal bleeding. Dig Dis Sci 1993;38:1619.

362. Bjarnason I, Hayllar J, Smethurst P, et al. Metronidazole reduces intestinal inflammation and blood loss in non-steroidal anti-inflammatory drug-induced enteropathy. Gut 1992;33:1204.

363. Thompson JN, Salen RR, Hemingway AP, et al. Specialist investigation of obscure gastrointestinal bleeding. Gut 1987;28:47.

364. Lin S, Rockey DC. Obscure gastrointestinal bleeding. Gastroenterol Clin N Am 2005;34:679.

365. Landi B, Tkoub M, Gaudric M, et al. Diagnostic yield of push-type enteroscopy in relation to indication. Gut 1998;42:421.

366. Chak A, Koehler MK, Sundaram SN, et al. Diagnostic and therapeutic impact of push enteroscopy: analysis of factors associated with positive findings. Gastrointest Endosc 1998;47:18.

367. O'Mahony S, Morris AJ, Straiton M, et al. Push enteroscopy in the investigation of small intestinal disease. Q J Med 1996;89:685.

368. Zaman A, Katon RM. Push enteroscopy for obscure gastrointestinal bleeding yields a high incidence of proximal lesions within reach of a standard endoscope. Gastrointest Endosc 1998;47:372.

369. American Gastroenterological Association. AGA Medical Position Statement: Evaluation and management of occult and obscure gastrointestinal bleeding. Gastroenterology 2000;118:197.

370. Lin S, Branch MS, Shetzline M. The importance of indication in the diagnostic value of push enteroscopy. Endoscopy 2003;35:315.

371. Lewis BS. The history of enteroscopy. Gastrointest Endosc Clin N Am 1999;9:1.

372. Iddan G, Meron G, Glukhovsky A, Swain P. Wireless capsule endoscopy. Nature 2000;405:417.

373. Pennazio M, Santucci R, Rondonotti E, et al. Outcome of patients with obscure gastrointestinal bleeding after capsule endoscopy: report of 100 consecutive cases. Gastroenterology 2004;126:643.

374. Mergener K, Enns R, Brandabur JJ, et al. Complications and problems with capsule endoscopy: results from two referral centers. Gastrointest Endosc 2003;57:AB170.

375. Hutchinson DS, Barawi M, Bermudez F, et al. A prospective study assessing the complication associated with the use of wireless capsule endoscopy (WCE). Am J Gastroenterol 2003;98:S290.

376. Signorelli C, Rondonotti E, Villa F, et al. Use of the Given Patency System for the screening of patients at high risk for capsule retention. Dig Liver Dis 2006;38:326.

377. Leighton JA, Sharma VK, Srivathsan K, et al. Safety of capsule endoscopy in patients with pacemakers. Gastrointest Endosc 2004;59:567.

378. Lewis B, Swain P. Capsule endoscopy in the evaluation of patients with suspected small intestinal bleeding: results of a pilot study. Gastrointest Endosc 2002;56:349.

379. Costamagna G, Shah SK, Riccioni ME, et al. A prospective trial comparing small bowel radiographs and video capsule endoscopy for suspected small bowel disease. Gastroenterology 2002;123:999.

380. Hara AK, Leighton JA, Sharma VK, et al. Small bowel: preliminary comparison of capsule endoscopy with barium study and CT. Radiology 2004;230:260.

381. Hartmann D, Schmidt H, Bolz G, et al. A prospective two-center study comparing wireless capsule endoscopy with intraoperative enteroscopy in patients with obscure GI bleeding. Gastrointest Endosc 2005;61:826.

382. Goldstein J, Eisen G, Lewis B, et al. Abnormal small bowel findings are common in healthy subjects screened for a multi-center, double blind, randomized, placebo-controlled trial using capsule endoscopy. Gastroenterology 2003;124:A37.

383. Rastogi A, Schoen RE, Slivka A. Diagnostic yield and clinical outcomes of capsule endoscopy. Gastrointest Endosc 2004;60:959.

384. Yamamoto H, Sekine Y, Sato Y, et al. Total enteroscopy with a nonsurgical steerable double balloon method. Gastrointest Endosc 2001;53:216.

385. Heine GD, Hadithi M, Groenen MJ, et al. Double-balloon enteroscopy: indications, diagnostic yield, and complications in a series of 275 patients with suspected small-bowel disease. Endoscopy 2006;38:42.

386. Di Caro S, May A, Heine DG, et al. The European experience with double-balloon enteroscopy. Gastrointest Endosc 2005;62:545.

Approach to the patient with occult gastrointestinal bleeding

David A. Ahlquist, Graeme P. Young

Quantifying blood loss, 152

Gastrointestinal hemoglobin metabolism, 152

Iron metabolism and deficiency, 153

Etiology of blood loss, 154

Clinical manifestations of blood loss, 156

Assessment and diagnostic strategies, 156

Fecal blood screening for colorectal neoplasia, 161

Therapeutic considerations, 163

By definition, occult gastrointestinal (GI) bleeding is hidden and not apparent on stool inspection. It occurs commonly, but a test is required for its detection. Elevated fecal blood levels are found in about 1 in 20 adults on prevalence screens [1–4] and probably occur episodically in all persons. Although often trivial, occult GI bleeding may herald a health-threatening lesion arising at any level from mouth to rectum. As such, the clinician is challenged when faced with occult GI bleeding.

The critical metabolic sequela of occult GI bleeding is iron deficiency. Iron deficiency afflicts 20 million people in the United States alone, and global prevalence is estimated at 15% [5,6]. It is the most common cause of anemia and often results from occult GI blood loss [7]. Management of iron deficiency depends on the cause, and GI origin should always be considered.

Fecal occult blood testing is widely used in screening for colorectal cancer and for the evaluation of iron deficiency and anemia. A rational assessment and treatment of occult GI bleeding is based on an appreciation of the pathophysiology of occult blood loss, available diagnostic tools, and therapeutic principles.

Quantifying blood loss

Given a typical daily stool mass of 150 g (150 mL) and a circulating hemoglobin (Hb) of 15 g/dL, the following equival-

ences can be calculated: 2 mL fecal blood loss per day = concentration of 2 mg Hb per gram of stool = total daily Hb loss of 300 mg = daily iron loss of 1 mg.

Depending on the rate and site of GI bleeding, enterocolic transit time, efficiency of lumenal Hb metabolism, and degree of fecal mixing, blood loss may be visually gross or occult. At one extreme, large amounts of blood may be lost into the proximal GI lumen and remain occult. A bolus of more than 150 mL of blood into the stomach or cecum is required to produce melena or hematochezia consistently [8,9]. Fecal Hb concentrations may approach those of circulating blood without being visibly apparent [10]. At the other extreme, a mere drop of blood from anorectal lesions can be visible as a bright-red streak on the stool surface.

Fecal blood is not simply present or absent; the levels range in a continuum from normal to pathologically elevated levels. Fecal blood loss quantified in healthy volunteers averages 0.5–1.5 mL/day (0.5–1.5 mg Hb per gram stool) [11–13], with levels below 2 mL/day found in 95% (Fig. 9.1), using either methods that quantify fecal heme-derived porphyrins or radiolabeled erythrocyte techniques.

Gastrointestinal hemoglobin metabolism

The degree of Hb disassembly during GI transit and fecal storage affects measurement because available fecal blood tests target different components of the Hb molecule (Table 9.1). An appreciation of enterocolic Hb metabolism helps to clarify test limitations and is useful in selecting a test appropriate to the clinical indication.

Principles of Clinical Gastroenterology. Edited by Tadataka Yamada, David H. Alpers, Anthony N. Kalloo, Neil Kaplowitz, Chung Owyang, and Don W. Powell. © 2008 Blackwell Publishing. ISBN 978-1-4051-69103

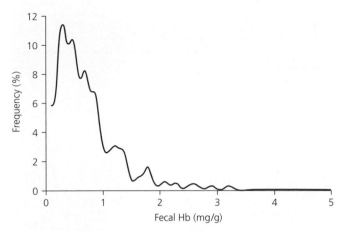

Figure 9.1 Frequency distribution of fecal occult blood levels in 900 asymptomatic subjects undergoing colorectal cancer screening as quantified by the HemoQuant assay. More than 95% of fecal hemoglobin (Hb) levels fall below 2 mg/g, which is considered to be the upper limit of normal.

Heme is cleaved from Hb by enzymes in the upper gut [14]. Some heme, probably less than 15%, is absorbed intact in the proximal small intestine [15–19]. Heme absorption may increase threefold with iron deficiency [20] and decrease after gastrectomy [21]. In the colon, 1%–99% of heme is converted by bacteria to porphyrin [16,22]. Heme-derived porphyrins escape detection by guaiac tests [10,13,18].

The globin chains of Hb are digested by upper gut proteases. Because immunoassays for Hb are directed against globin antigens, they are insensitive for upper GI bleeding [23–25]. Immunoassays fail to detect ingested blood in quantities up to 100 mL [24,26]. Hemoglobin globins are also metabolized by colonic bacteria, and immunoassays are less likely to detect bleeding from the right colon than from the left [27]. Furthermore, immunoreactivity is progressively lost during fecal storage.

Iron metabolism and deficiency

Occult GI bleeding may be compensated by increased iron absorption or mobilization of body iron stores, which, in turn, stimulate erythropoiesis. However, if iron loss from occult bleeding chronically exceeds intestinal iron absorption, iron stores become depleted, and iron deficiency with attendant anemia and other metabolic sequelae ensue. The time required to develop iron deficiency depends on the rate and chronicity of occult bleeding.

Iron absorption

Ordinarily, 1–2 mg iron is absorbed daily, which represents about 10% of that in a typical Western diet [28]. Both heme and elemental forms of iron are absorbed primarily in the duodenum and proximal jejunum. Elemental iron absorption may be increased up to tenfold by iron deficiency, anemia, hypoxia, liver disease, increased erythropoiesis, and elevated lumenal iron concentration [5,28,29]. It is facilitated by reducing substances, bile, pancreatic juice, gastric acid, and a nonacidic gastric modulator [5,30–33]. Iron absorption is impeded by various mucosal diseases of the upper small intestine, such as celiac sprue [34], by duodenal bypass from bariatric surgery [35], and by certain lumenal substances that chelate iron, such as phytates in cereals, tannic acid in tea, and oxalates [28,29]. Selective iron malabsorption occurs rarely due to an inherited defect of transferrin function [36] or to an acquired autoimmunity to the transferrin receptor [37].

Iron loss

A physiological mechanism does not exist for iron excretion. Under normal circumstances, absorption of dietary iron (on average 1–2 mg/day) equals or just exceeds iron loss through normal daily occult GI bleeding (on average 1 mg/day). Trace amounts of iron are also lost through cutaneous desquamation

Table 9.1 Effect of gastrointestinal bleeding site on metabolic fate of intralumenal hemoglobin

Bleeding site	Hb insults during lumenal transit	Hb components in stool[a]		
		Globin	Heme	HDPs
Upper GI tract	Globin completely digested by gastric enteric peptidases Minimal heme absorption to duodenum and jejunum Colonic flora convert heme to HDPs	0	+	+++
Proximal colon	Globin altered by peptidases of colonic flora Colonic flora convert heme to HDPs	+	+	++
Rectosigmoid	Minimal alteration of Hb molecule	+++	+++	0/+

a Immunochemical tests detect globin, guaiac tests react with intact heme, and the heme-porphyrin assay measures both heme and HDPs.
0, absent; 0/+, absent or minor component; +, minor component; ++, moderate component; +++, major component; GI, gastrointestinal; Hb, hemoglobin; HDPs, heme-derived porphyrins.

and intestinal epithelial sloughing. Menorrhagia often contributes to iron deficiency in premenopausal women [38]. Although excessive bleeding can occur from the airway, from the urinary tract, or from multiple phlebotomies, these are uncommon causes of iron deficiency, and, if present, are clinically apparent [5]. Excessive iron loss by occult GI bleeding, the most common cause of iron deficiency, is the most difficult to recognize. As a general rule, daily GI blood losses of at least 5–10 mL are required to overcome compensatory absorptive increases and lead to a negative iron balance.

Iron storage

Most body iron, about 75%, is stored in metabolically active forms, with roughly 70% in Hb and 5% in myoglobin and various tissue enzymes [5]. The remaining 25% of body iron is metabolically inactive and stored in a soluble complex with ferritin or in a particulate state as hemosiderin, especially in hepatocytes and in the reticuloendothelial cells of the liver, bone marrow, and spleen [5]. A small amount of ferritin is present in plasma and correlates well with total body iron stores [39].

Metabolic consequences of iron deficiency

Iron is present in all human cells and is of vital importance for oxygen transport and many metabolic functions. This ubiquitous metal is essential for nearly half of the enzymes of the Krebs tricarboxylic acid cycle, for DNA synthesis, and for many other cellular processes [5,40]. It is not surprising that the clinical and metabolic manifestations of iron deficiency are so generalized.

The fatigue associated with iron deficiency should be recognized as a pancellular phenomenon; it results not only from anemia [41,42] but also from dysfunction in nonhematological tissues [43,44].

Characteristic mucocutaneous findings may be present (see "Clinical manifestations of blood loss"). Gastric atrophy with achlorhydria and a sprue-like small intestinal lesion with malabsorption may occur with iron deficiency and resolve with iron replacement [45–48]. Iron deficiency has also been causally linked to certain behavioral, immunological, and developmental abnormalities [49–54].

Etiology of blood loss

Many of the lesions that cause gross GI bleeding (see Chapter 8) can also cause occult bleeding. The mechanisms of occult GI bleeding necessarily involve a disruption of the epithelium and subepithelial blood vessels, and can be categorized as inflammatory, infectious, vascular, neoplastic, and other (Table 9.2). The prevalence of responsible lesions varies with age and geography. For example, occult bleeding in infants commonly arises from milk-induced enteritis [51], whereas in elderly people peptic ulcer disease or neoplasms are com-

Table 9.2 Disorders that may present as occult gastrointestinal bleeding with or without iron deficiency

Inflammatory causes
Acid peptic disease
Large hiatal hernia (Cameron erosions)
Crohn's disease
Chronic ulcerative colitis
Mild enterocolitis
Whipple disease
Sprue
Eosinophilic gastroenteritis
Meckel diverticulum
Solitary colon ulcer
Anastomotic ulcer
Other

Infectious causes
Hookworm
Strongyloidiasis
Ascariasis
Tuberculous enterocolitis
Amebiasis
Other

Vascular causes
Angiodysplasia and vascular ectasias
Gastroesophageal varices and congestive gastropathy
Hemangiomas
Blue rubber bleb nevus syndrome
Watermelon stomach
Other

Tumors and neoplastic causes
Primary gastrointestinal cancer at any site
Metastases to gastrointestinal tract
Large polyp at any site
Lymphoma
Leiomyoma
Leiomyosarcoma
Lipoma
Other

Drugs
Nonsteroidal antiinflammatory drugs
Other

Miscellaneous causes
Long-distance running
Extra- gastrointestinal bleeding
Benign infiltrative lesions
Factitial causes
Artifact

monplace [7,13,55–57]. Although rare in temperate climes, hookworm infestation is the most common cause of harmful occult bleeding in tropical and subtropical regions [58].

Inflammatory causes

In Western countries, erosions or ulceration of the esophagus, stomach, and duodenum are the most common GI lesions associated with occult bleeding and iron deficiency. Iron deficiency has been attributed to such acid-peptic disease in 30%–70% of adult cases, and is often asymptomatic [7,24,25,55,56]. Acid-peptic disease, particularly reflux esophagitis [59], may also underlie iron deficiency in children. Most peptic disease is caused by drug use (see below) or *Helicobacter pylori* gastritis. In some populations, *H. pylori* disease is pandemic and contributes to widespread iron deficiency [60,61]. Studies suggest that iron deficiency from *H. pylori* disease may occur in the absence of erosions or ulcers and resolves with antibiotic therapy [62,63]; *H. pylori* should be considered in the differential diagnosis of obscure occult GI bleeding [63].

The association between large diaphragmatic hernias and iron deficiency anemia has long been known [64–66]. A large diaphragmatic hernia is found in up to 10% of iron-deficient patients [7,55]. Blood loss is caused by longitudinal mucosal erosions (Cameron erosions) located in the proximal stomach and thought to be secondary to mechanical trauma from breathing [66,67].

Many inflammatory GI conditions of the small bowel may bleed occultly. Bovine milk may produce occult bleeding and iron deficiency in infants as a consequence of inflammation throughout the gut; both resolve after the cow's milk is stopped [68]. Meckel diverticulum may cause occult bleeding in children and young adults [51]. Crohn's disease and chronic ulcerative colitis uncommonly present with occult bleeding alone [7,55]. Occult blood loss may occur with celiac sprue, Whipple disease, eosinophilic gastroenteritis, radiation enteritis, and solitary colon ulcer.

Infectious causes

Whereas occult bleeding may accompany many acute infectious enterocolitides, it may be chronic and lead to iron deficiency in such conditions as GI tuberculosis, amebiasis, ascariasis, and *H. pylori* gastritis (see above). However, the most common infectious cause of harmful occult bleeding worldwide is hookworm.

More than one billion people are infested with hookworm globally, and the prevalence in some tropical countries exceeds 80% [58,69]. The major and often the only manifestation is iron deficiency, which exacts an enormous socioeconomic toll in reduced work-related productivity. Daily occult fecal blood loss averages more than 12 mL from most hosts, and may exceed 100 mL; it correlates with the hookworm burden, and drops sharply after use of a vermifuge [58,70].

Vascular causes

Gastroesophageal varices are occasionally incriminated as the source of occult bleeding and have been reported in up to 3% of patients with iron deficiency [7,13]. The attendant congested mucosa in the gastroduodenum [71] or colon [72] may account for occult blood loss with portal hypertension.

Vascular malformations are found in up to 6% of adults with iron deficiency anemia [7,24,25,55,56] and are common explanations for occult bleeding of obscure origin [73–80]. Gastrointestinal bleeding remains occult in many patients with acquired or hereditary (e.g., hemorrhagic telangiectasia, or Osler–Weber–Rendu syndrome) vascular malformations [81]. An increasingly recognized and endoscopically treatable vascular lesion is watermelon stomach, which characteristically presents with iron deficiency anemia in older women [82,83]. Clinically significant occult bleeding has been described with other vascular lesions, including postradiation telangiectasias [84] and those associated with the blue rubber bleb nevus syndrome [85], scleroderma [86], Turner syndrome [87], and Klippel–Trenaunay syndrome [88].

Tumors and neoplasms

Gastrointestinal tumors are second only to peptic disease as causes for occult bleeding leading to iron deficiency in adults in Western countries [7,24,25,55–57,89–93]. Among adults older than 50 years and with new-onset iron deficiency, a GI malignancy can be found in 15%–30% [57,89–93]. Colorectal cancer is the most common malignant lesion to cause occult bleeding in Western countries, followed by primary cancers in the stomach, esophagus, and ampulla [7,13,24,25,55–57,89–94]. Lymphomas, lipomas, leiomyomas, leiomyosarcomas, hamartomas, juvenile polyps, and metastatic lesions to the gut can also produce occult bleeding.

Iron deficiency may occur in up to 80% of patients with symptomatic colorectal cancer [95]. Because of the importance of fecal occult blood testing in the detection of colorectal neoplasms, these lesions are discussed separately below (see "Fecal blood screening for colorectal neoplasms").

Drugs

Any ingestant that produces direct or indirect injury to the GI tract may cause abnormal occult bleeding. Ethanol can lead to hemorrhagic gastritis only at high concentrations [96,97], and the contribution of social drinking to occult bleeding is probably minor. Anticoagulants appear to unmask bleeding from preexisting lesions rather than produce bleeding per se [98–100]. Certain antibiotics, potassium preparations, antimetabolites, and other drugs may damage the epithelium, but few data on occult bleeding are available.

Aspirin and related nonsteroidal antiinflammatory drugs (NSAIDs) are responsible for most drug-induced occult GI bleeding, owing to their widespread use. In the United States, more than 30 billion NSAID tablets are consumed annually [101]. Except for acetaminophen (paracetamol) and sodium salicylate, all NSAIDs can cause blood loss [102,103]. At therapeutic doses, some NSAIDs induce more bleeding than others [103]. Compared with conventional NSAIDs, cyclooxygenase-2 (COX-2) inhibitors are less mucosotoxic but share cardiovascular risks [104,105]. Most commonly NSAIDs ulcerate the stomach, but they may injure any level of the GI tract and cause bleeding [103,106]. This NSAID gastroenteropathy results from inhibition of epithelial COX and loss of mucoso-protective prostaglandins [107]. The dose of NSAID influences the amount of mucosal injury and blood lost [98,101]. People taking therapeutic amounts of aspirin lose on average 2–5 mL of blood daily, and some more than 30 mL per day [98,101,108]. Fecal blood levels are rarely elevated in those taking low-dose aspirin for cardiovascular prophylaxis [99,109].

Miscellaneous causes

Iron deficiency may develop in long-distance runners and compromise performance [110], and occult GI bleeding appears to be a major cause [111,112]. In elite class runners, both gastric and colonic erosions have been identified and have been shown to resolve with periods of running cessation [113,114]. Occult GI bleeding is less likely to occur with other endurance activities [115,116].

Fecal occult blood levels may be elevated in patients who swallow blood arising from tracheobronchial, dental, oronasopharyngeal, or self-induced sources. Infiltration by benign conditions such as endometriosis [117], amyloidosis [118], and splenosis [119] may become hemorrhagic and result in chronic occult bleeding. Stools sampled from the toilet water may be contaminated if patients have hematuria or menstrual bleeding [120]. Finally, numerous substances other than blood may react with guaiac and other tests to produce false-positive results (see "Fecal blood testing").

Clinical manifestations of blood loss

Symptoms

Occult GI bleeding, in most cases, is clinically silent and unsuspected. However, there may be predominant manifestations of the underlying GI disease responsible for occult bleeding. Also, characteristic symptoms and signs of iron deficiency may occur secondary to chronic occult blood loss from any cause. Fatigue with exercise intolerance is the most frequent symptom occurring with iron deficiency, and can be disabling [40–44]. Rapid palpitations and exertional dyspnea are also common concomitants of advanced iron deficiency. Less common overt sequelae of iron deficiency may be present; for example, iron deficiency may contribute to a restless leg syndrome [121].

Pica, or compulsive eating, may occur in roughly 50% of patients with iron deficiency [122,123]. Pagophagia, or ice eating, is the most frequent form, and some afflicted people have consumed more than 9 kg of ice daily. Other variants of pica include ingestion of soil (geophagia), laundry starch, brittle or crunchy foods (gooberophagia), and chalk. Such bizarre behavior resolves with iron repletion.

Physical findings

Telltale findings may suggest both the presence and cause of iron deficiency. Papilledema, hearing loss, cranial nerve palsies, and retinal hemorrhages occur rarely with severe iron deficiency and may resolve with iron repletion [5,124]. More characteristic of iron deficiency are various epithelial abnormalities. Finger and toe nails may become brittle, longitudinally furrowed, or spooned [125], changes called koilonychia. Glossitis may occur with erythema and loss of lingual papillae [126]. Scaling or fissuring of the lips, called cheilitis, and atrophic rhinitis may also result from iron deficiency. The association of esophageal webs with iron deficiency is known as the Paterson–Kelly syndrome or the Plummer–Vinson syndrome [127,128]. These proximal esophageal webs may cause dysphagia, are more common in women, and may resolve with iron therapy [5,129].

Assessment and diagnostic strategies

Occult GI bleeding may be evidenced either indirectly by laboratory confirmation of iron deficiency or directly by measurement of fecal blood. Neither approach is infallible, and they should be viewed as complementary. Iron deficiency would not be present if enteric blood loss was quantitatively minor or of restricted duration. Fecal blood test results may be negative because of intermittent bleeding or analytical limitations of the tests. It is important to appreciate the strengths, limitations, and complementarity of laboratory techniques used to establish occult bleeding. The subsequent GI evaluation should be tailored to the clinical setting.

Blood and bone marrow tests for iron deficiency

Although a late-stage manifestation, hypochromic microcytic anemia is often the first clue to the presence of iron deficiency [5]. The characteristic erythrocyte morphology on peripheral smear is commonly detected by automated calculations that reveal low mean corpuscular Hb concentration (MCHC) and mean corpuscular volume (MCV). Anisocytosis, or variability in cell size, is also common with iron deficiency anemia and reflected by elevation in the red cell distribution width (RDW). However, these red cell changes are present in fewer than 70% of people with iron deficiency anemia [130], and may occur with anemia of chronic illness, thalassemia, and sideroblastic anemia [5,130,131]. Status of iron stores must be evaluated to determine the cause of microcytic anemia.

Chemical tests

Unlike iron deficiency, other causes of hypochromic microcytic anemia are associated with normal or increased tissue iron stores [5,130,131]. Although typically decreased with iron deficiency, serum iron levels and transferrin saturation correlate rather poorly with marrow iron stores, are influenced by many medical conditions, and are also commonly low with the anemia of chronic illness, the most troublesome differential diagnosis [5,130,131]. By contrast, serum ferritin levels correlate well with tissue iron stores and better discriminate iron deficiency anemia from other anemias [5,131]. Serum ferritin levels fall well before anemia develops, and low serum ferritin is pathognomonic for iron deficiency. Inflammatory, malignant, liver, and renal disease can elevate serum ferritin and uncommonly cause a falsely normal serum level in the face of absent marrow iron stores [5,130,131]. Under such conditions, erythrocyte ferritin [132], serum transferrin receptor [133–135], or erythrocyte protoporphyrin [135–137] levels may more accurately reflect body iron stores. Iron deficiency occasionally presents with normal levels of ferritin or other blood markers, and a bone marrow study is indicated if uncertainty remains. Although the gold standard for iron deficiency is the absence of bone marrow hemosiderin determined by Prussian blue staining, this invasive procedure is seldom required.

Fecal blood testing

A plethora of tests for the detection of fecal occult blood are commercially available. There are four basic approaches, each with advantages and disadvantages.

Guaiac tests

Guaiac preparations have been employed to detect blood for more than a century [138] and remain the most widely used type of fecal blood test. Guaiac-impregnated pad tests, such as Hemoccult, were developed in the 1960s [139]. These pad tests are elegantly simple, inexpensive, highly portable, and require no sophisticated laboratory. Guaiac, a leuco dye, is a colorless compound that becomes colored in the presence of adequate peroxidase-like substances (e.g., Hb) and hydrogen peroxide.

There seems to be no consistent fecal Hb level above which guaiac tests become positive and below which they remain negative [10,13,139–142]. In general, GI blood loss must exceed 10 mL/day before the Hemoccult test is positive at least half the time [10,13,140,141]. Guaiac tests may be positive in stools with less than 1 mg Hb/g [10] or remain negative in those with more than 80 mg/g [10,143]. Hemoccult sensitivity is enhanced by wetting the fecal smear prior to addition of the peroxide catalyst [144] or by hydrating the stool before smearing [10]. Also, the native water content of stools affects Hemoccult reactivity – wetter stools are more likely to be positive than drier stools [10,13].

Another major explanation for variability in guaiac test reactivity is the degradation by fecal flora of heme to porphyrin, which does not possess peroxidase-like activity. This accounts for the relative insensitivity of guaiac tests for occult bleeding arising from the right colon and, especially, more proximal gut [13,16,22,24,145,146]. Conversion of heme to porphyrin continues during fecal storage and causes a corresponding fall in Hemoccult positivity [10,147]. Thus, guaiac tests tend to underestimate enteric blood loss, particularly with bleeding from proximal lesions or when applied to stored wet specimens. If stools are sampled immediately onto collection devices and allowed to dry, heme remains stable for longer.

Several factors besides wet stools can produce chemical false-positive reactions. Certain fruits and vegetables have peroxidase-like activity, and dietary restriction reduces Hemoccult false positives [148]. Whether oral iron causes guaiac false positives is debated [149,150]. Other factors reported to cause a color reaction include sucralfate [151], cimetidine [152], halogens [153], and toilet bowl sanitizers [154]. Factors that inhibit guaiac reactivity, in addition to dry stools and heme degradation, include ascorbic acid [155], antacids [156], heat, acid pH, and defective reagents [157].

Maneuvers to increase guaiac sensitivity, such as hydrating the smeared fecal aliquot before testing or reconfiguring reagent concentrations, often succeed at the expense of specificity [144,158,159].

Immunochemical tests

Immunodetection of fecal hemoglobin, studied for more than a decade, is relatively inexpensive and simple to perform [23–27]. Antihemoglobin or antialbumin antibodies used in these assays do not react with nonhuman blood, diet peroxidases, or medications [160,161], and burdensome dietary preparations are avoided [162]. Metabolism of antigens during transit or storage compromises immunodetection of fecal blood. These tests detect as little as 0.3 mg blood added to a stool, but fail to detect fecal Hb after ingestion of 20–100 mL blood [23,26,146]. It is not surprising that immunochemical tests are less likely to detect upper GI than colorectal bleeding [23–25,146]. Immunochemical tests also seem to be less sensitive for right-sided than left-sided colorectal cancers [163], probably because of bacterial digestion of peptide antigen. Although immunochemical tests promise to improve specificity, some studies have shown that reactions to certain fecal constituents cause false positives at rates comparable with those of guaiac tests [26,164–166]. On the other hand, a study has shown that fecal immunochemical tests achieve improved sensitivity for neoplasia without further loss of specificity [166]. Like guaiac tests, immunochemical tests are often qualitative, variably sensitive, and affected both by the anatomical site of bleeding and by storage.

Immunochemical tests have also been developed to detect blood leukocyte proteins, such as calprotectin [167] and lectoferrin [168]. Although leukocyte proteins may be useful markers for inflammatory diseases, stool assays for these proteins are insensitive for detection of GI bleeding per se and correlate poorly with hemoglobin-directed fecal blood tests [169]. Calprotectin assay from stool appears to offer no advantages over conventional fecal occult blood tests for the detection of colorectal cancer [170,171].

Heme-porphyrin assay

Quantitation of fecal blood provides meaningful diagnostic

information, because the predictive value of an elevated level depends on the degree of elevation [92,172]. A heme-porphyrin-based assay [10,16], called HemoQuant (Mayo Medical Laboratories, Rochester, MN; SmithKline BioSciences, Van Nuys, CA; Nichols Laboratory, Los Angeles, CA), is quantitative, noninvasive, specific for heme, chemically sensitive, and suitable for automation. HemoQuant involves the fluorimetric assay of heme and heme-derived porphyrin. Unlike guaiac and immunochemical tests, the HemoQuant test includes that fraction of heme already degraded to porphyrin during fecal storage [13] or enterocolic transit [10,13,16,22]. Because of this feature, sensitivity for proximal GI bleeding is higher than with guaiac and immunochemical tests [13,24]. The heme-porphyrin test may be affected by red meat, but not by other dietary peroxidases, medications, or fecal contaminants [10,13,16,18].

HemoQuant results are calculated as Hb-equivalents and reported as mg Hb/g stool. Fecal Hb concentrations from 0.01 to 500 mg/g are accurately measured [10–16] and values below 2 mg/g are considered normal [13,92,172]. HemoQuant has been validated by recovery of blood added to stools [10], recovery of ingested blood [16,18,24,146], and close correlation with other quantitative assays [16,17]. HemoQuant is performed for commercial use in reference laboratories only, and the inevitable 2- to 4-day delay in results due to specimen shipment is an inconvenience.

Radiolabeled erythrocyte technique

Fecal recovery of intravenously injected ^{51}Cr-labeled erythrocytes has been used to quantify enteric blood loss for more than three decades [11,12]. After chromium enters the gut lumen, its reabsorption is negligible, and therefore it has proved to be a valid quantitative marker for GI bleeding. However, some have questioned its accuracy at low levels of bleeding because of biliary excretion of free chromium [173]. The test is expensive, requires 3 to 5 days of whole stool collections, and is impractical for large-volume routine use. Slow enterocolic transit may cause falsely low results [174].

Specimen collection and sampling

Accurate fecal blood testing requires control of each step of the testing process. The common practice of sampling stools from the toilet water introduces potential measurement error caused by leaching of blood into the water [154] or by contamination with menstrual or urinary blood [120], urinary reducing substances [153,155], or toilet bowl sanitizers [154]. Use of a collection device prevents these artifacts [154]. Because blood is nonuniformly distributed within the fecal specimen [175], testing of multiple aliquots or multiple stools reduces sampling error [172,176].

Guaiac-based tests have been developed to detect blood in the toilet water or on stool wiped from the perineum, but few published data are available. The historically common practice of fecal blood testing on digital rectal smear leads to substantial artifact [177–180]. Adequate stool is obtained in fewer than half of digital examinations [179], the digital approach may lower test specificity [181], and testing of digital smears may dramatically lower sensitivity [180].

Test selection

No single fecal blood test is appropriate for all applications. Test selection should be guided by judicious consideration of test performance characteristics, availability, and cost relative to the clinical indication (Table 9.3). A simple, inexpensive, qualitative test may be preferred to screen for colorectal bleeding. Immunochemical or guaiac tests are appealing for such screening, as they preferentially detect colorectal bleeding [182]. The heme-porphyrin assay offers no advantage over these simpler tests for screening colorectal lesions [159,183]. However, to evaluate iron deficiency or anemia, the heme-porphyrin assay is most useful because it accurately quantifies lumenal blood loss regardless of the site of bleeding [13,24,146]. The radiolabeled erythrocyte technique yields similar quantitative information [17], but it is time-consuming, much more expensive, and logistically burdensome. Guaiac and immunochemical tests would appear less suitable in the evaluation of anemia because they are insensitive for upper GI bleeding [13,24,92,146]. In a study of anemic patients with hemorrhagic lesions in the proximal gut, the heme-porphyrin test detected 88% compared with 26% by guaiac testing and 2% by immunochemical testing of stools [24].

Patient evaluation

In practice, abnormal occult GI bleeding comes to the attention of clinicians after a positive fecal blood test result in patients undergoing colorectal cancer screening, after iron deficiency anemia is encountered, and, less commonly, after fecal blood tests are applied to investigate those presenting with GI symptoms. The diagnostic strategy should be tailored according to the setting.

Abnormal fecal blood test results in an asymptomatic patient without anemia

This common situation occurs almost exclusively as a result of colorectal cancer screening, because there are few other reasons routinely to check fecal occult blood levels (see "Fecal blood screening for colorectal neoplasia"). The chief aim is to exclude a colorectal cancer, although this finding can be expected in only 2%–10% of test-positive cases [1–4]. Most agree that colonoscopy and other structural approaches are more sensitive and specific for colorectal neoplasia [183,184], but these interventions are also invasive and more expensive.

Because of the relatively low prevalence in most Western countries of malignancies proximal to the colon, physicians could justifiably stop their evaluation after colon studies in the absence of symptoms or anemia [185]. However, a good case can be made for additionally checking the serum ferritin

Table 9.3 Comparative features of fecal occult blood tests

	Guaiac (leuco-dye) tests	Immunoassays	Heme-porphyrin assay	Erythrocyte assay
Quantitative	No	Yes or no	Yes	Yes
Chemical false positives				
Diet peroxidases	Yes	No	No	No
Animal hemoglobin	Yes	No	Yes	No
Halogens	Yes	No	No	No
Toilet sanitizers	Yes	No	No	No
Iron	Yes (?)	No	No	No
Wet stools	Yes	No	No	No
Chemical false negatives				
Ascorbic acid	Yes	No	No	No
Enterocolic Hb metabolism	Yes	Yes	No	No
Fecal storage	Yes	Yes	No	No
Dry stools	Yes	No	No	No
Sensitivity for bleeding				
Upper GI source	Poor	Very poor	Good	Good
Proximal colon	Fair	Fair	Good	Good
Distal colon and rectum	Good	Good	Good	Good
Test performance				
Lab required	No	Yes (small)	Yes	Yes
Assay time	5 min	1–24 h	1–3 h	≥ 72 h
Assay cost	$10–20	~ $30	~ $30	$200–500

level, because this is inexpensive, introduces essentially no morbidity, and, if low, may point to indolent bleeding from a more proximal GI lesion. Documented iron deficiency in the face of a positive fecal blood test suggests chronic occult bleeding and, as with anemia, justifies a careful GI evaluation (see "Occult bleeding in the anemic patient"). Furthermore, in populations with a high prevalence of gastric or esophageal cancer, it may be prudent routinely to extend the evaluation to the upper gut if colorectal studies are negative.

The common practice of fecal occult blood testing on all patients admitted to hospital is of uncertain value. Utilization studies indicate that such testing is inappropriate in most cases because of non-valid valid indications, serious comorbidities, and inadequate patient preparations [186,187].

Occult bleeding in the anemic patient

Unless menorrhagia, gross hematuria, frequent blood donations, or another source of extraintestinal blood loss is clinically apparent, most patients found to have iron deficiency with or without anemia should undergo an aggressive GI evaluation. Because a GI lesion is found in most men and postmenopausal women with new-onset iron deficiency anemia [7,55,56,188], it can be argued that fecal blood testing is superfluous and that GI studies should be done regardless of fecal blood test results. However, nutritional inadequacies,

iron malabsorption, or extraintestinal bleeding may be the crucial etiological factors in some patient groups with iron deficiency anemia. Fecal blood testing may be helpful to assess the contribution of enteric blood loss in selected groups with iron deficiency, including children, menstruating women, postgastrectomy patients, immigrants from less developed countries, strict vegetarians, frequent blood donors, and patients with steatorrhea. For example, premenopausal women with new-onset iron deficiency often demonstrate occult fecal blood loss and, subsequently, are found to harbor hemorrhagic GI lesions [189]. Thus, it should not be assumed that menstrual blood loss alone accounts for iron deficiency in this large subset of patients.

The majority of adults with new-onset iron deficiency anemia are found to have culprit hemorrhagic lesions in the proximal gut (Table 9.4) [24,25,57,89–92,189,190]. However, a small percentage of patients with lesions seen on esophago-gastroduodenoscopy (EGD) also have potential sources of blood loss on colonoscopy [25,89–91,189,190]. Most upper GI lesions in iron-deficient patients are peptic in nature, whereas most colorectal ones are neoplastic [7,24,25,89–91,189–191].

A practical schema for evaluating adults with iron deficiency anemia and occult GI bleeding is shown in Fig. 9.2. The large majority of lesions causing occult bleeding in anemic patients can be demonstrated by routine colonoscopy and EGD and by small intestinal radiography. Some advocate

Table 9.4 Anatomical site of occult gastrointestinal (GI) bleeding in patients with iron deficiency anemia

Series	Number of subjects	Upper GI only	Lower GI only	Both
Zuckerman & Benitez 1992 [89]	53	27	17	9
McIntyre & Long 1993 [90]	63	45	16	2
Gordon et al. 1994 [190]	100	70	30	0
Kepczyk et al. 1995 [189]	50	29	10	11
Rockey et al. 1998 [25]	119	65	48	6
Reyes et al. 1999 [91]	80	37	20	23
Harewood & Ahlquist 2000 [92]	56	39	17	0
Coban et al. 2003 [57]	81	55	26	0
Niv et al. 2005 [93]	33	14	16	3
Combined	635	381 (60%)	200 (31%)	54 (9%)

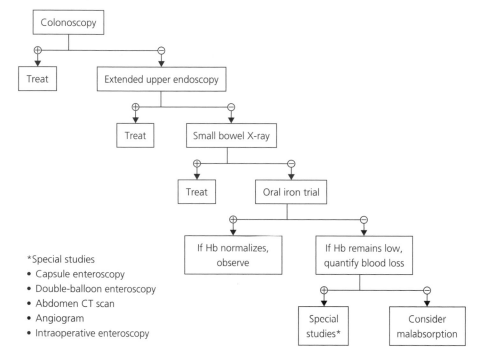

*Special studies
- Capsule enteroscopy
- Double-balloon enteroscopy
- Abdomen CT scan
- Angiogram
- Intraoperative enteroscopy

Figure 9.2 Diagnostic schema for asymptomatic adult patients with iron deficiency anemia and occult gastrointestinal bleeding. CT, computed tomography; Hb, hemoglobin.

extended upper endoscopy rather than conventional EGD for the initial evaluation as a more cost-effective strategy [64,74,192]; and endoscopically treatable lesions, especially vascular ectasias, are not uncommonly discovered in the setting of anemia [73,185,193]. If obvious hemorrhagic lesions are not seen on upper endoscopy, both small bowel and gastric biopsies can appropriately be obtained, as celiac sprue or *H. pylori* gastritis are etiological considerations with obscure iron deficiency and should be excluded [34,194]. In immigrants from tropical or subtropical regions, a stool examination for hookworm or other parasite ova should be considered early in the evaluation of anemia.

Because further studies for obscure bleeding sources are more invasive, expensive, and less revealing of lesions, it is often justifiable to observe a response to iron therapy before embarking on these further studies. Strict avoidance of NSAIDs is necessary during such a trial. Anemia will resolve and no serious pathology will emerge over time in most such patients [194].

In patients who fail to respond to iron therapy, confirmation of GI blood loss with valid fecal blood testing is desirable prior to further evaluation. If GI bleeding is established, special diagnostic studies are indicated. Historically, such studies have included sonde enteroscopy [195], angiography, abdominal computed tomography (CT) scan, and, as last resort, surgical exploration with intraoperative endoscopy [75]. Laparoscopically assisted panenteroscopy has also been explored as an alternative to intraoperative endoscopy [196].

However, many centers recommend use of a swallowed pill-sized videocapsule device (wireless capsule endoscopy) as a minimally invasive procedure to interrogate the small intestine not reachable by conventional endoscopes [76–78,197]. Capsule endoscopy appears to be superior to extended upper endoscopy [76,77,80], and may be comparable with intraoperative endoscopy in finding an obscure bleeding source. In well-selected patients, capsule endoscopy has identified a bleeding lesion in more than 70% of cases [79]. The advent of a double-balloon enteroscope allows operator-controlled inspection of all or most of the small bowel by the oral route or a combination of oral and anal routes [198], and, unlike capsule endoscopy, it has the capacity to obtain biopsies or deliver coagulation therapy [199]. Radioisotope blood loss scans have no role in the evaluation of occult bleeding.

Occult bleeding in the patient with gastrointestinal symptoms

Few data are available on the use of fecal blood testing to evaluate patients with GI symptoms in the absence of iron deficiency or anemia, although some argue that a positive stool result increases the likelihood that organic disease is present [200]. The sequence of diagnostic testing should be initially directed to the anatomical level suggested by symptoms. Site-specific symptoms in patients with iron deficiency are predictive of abnormalities in the corresponding portion of the bowel [64,188]. Clinical judgment is required to determine the extent of evaluation in such instances.

Fecal blood screening for colorectal neoplasia

Fecal blood screening for colorectal cancer is widely practiced, and US surveys suggest that 30%–40% of adults have undergone such screening [201–203]. This section focuses on fecal testing and not on other approaches for the detection of colorectal neoplasia.

Occult bleeding patterns

Fecal blood levels fluctuate widely with colorectal cancer [13,144,172,175,183,204], and vary from markedly elevated to the normal range when individual patients are studied longitudinally (Fig. 9.3). Occult bleeding increases with neoplasm size, surface ulceration, and tumor stage [13,183,205–208].

Although it is well established that symptomatic colorectal polyps may bleed [145], less is known about occult bleeding with asymptomatic polyps. Quantitative studies have shown fecal blood distributions to be comparable in asymptomatic groups with and without adenomas [144,183,204]. Roughly 5% of patients with endoscopically proven polyps are guaiac-positive [183,209], a positivity rate similar to that of the general population. However, larger polyps can become hemorrhagic, and a small proportion of adenomas larger than 1 cm

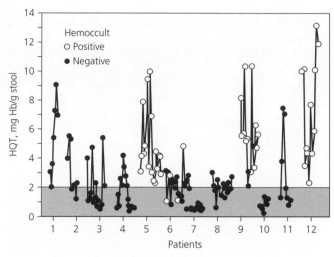

Figure 9.3 Occult blood levels in stools collected for 2 weeks from 12 patients with asymptomatic primary colorectal adenocarcinoma as determined by HemoQuant (HQT) and Hemoccult. The shaded zone below a HemoQuant level of 2 mg Hb/g stool represents the conventional normal range. Hb, hemoglobin. From Ahlquist et al. [172], with permission from Wiley-Liss, a subsidiary of John Wiley and Sons.

are associated with elevated fecal blood levels (Table 9.5). Fecal blood appears to be a poor marker for adenomas, especially small ones.

Test validity

Validity is a function that combines sensitivity, specificity, and predictive value, and it varies with techniques used and populations studied. Validity must be high if a screening test is to perform effectively and efficiently. Sensitivity, or the detection rate, ranges in patients with symptomatic colorectal cancer from 40%–97% [27,160,201,207,210,211]. Based on rigorous prospective studies comparing fecal blood levels against structural gold standards (e.g., colonoscopy) conducted from 1980 to 2005, sensitivity estimates for widely used guaiac tests have averaged about 23% (range 14%–50%) for asymptomatic colorectal cancers (Table 9.5) [163,183,209,212–219]. The newer immunochemical and guaiac tests yield somewhat higher cancer detection rates [158,159,163,220]. However, fecal blood levels from asymptomatic colorectal neoplasms often fall within the normal range (Fig. 9.4), and detection by any fecal blood test is compromised by the intermittency of bleeding.

Screening specificity, the rate of negative tests in those without cancer, ranges from 90% to 98% [1–4,201,218,219], which translates to false-positive rates of 2%–10%. The positive predictive value, or the probability that a positive test will yield a colorectal cancer, is dependent on both test specificity and cancer prevalence. With commonly used guaiac tests in the screening setting, the positive predictive value for colorectal cancer averages 5% (range 2%–18%) [1–4,183,201].

Table 9.5 Hemoccult detection rates for asymptomatic colorectal neoplasms based on comparison against structural gold standards in the screening setting[a]

Series	Number	Gold standard	Hemoccult detection rate % (proportion)	
			Adenoma > 1 cm	Cancer
Ribet et al. 1980 [215]	230	C, CX, S	–	25 (1/4)
Williams et al. 1982 [216]	330	C, CX, S	5 (6/112)[b]	50 (2/4)
Demers et al.1985 [209]	988	S	9 (2/23)	28 (5/18)
Bang et al. 1986 [212]	5715	C	15 (8/53)	43 (3/7)
Rozen 1992 [214]	2255	C, S	–	22 (12/55)
Jahn et al. 1992 [213]	1244	C	24 (10/41)	23 (5/22)
Ahlquist et al. 1993 [183]	2293	C, CX, S	13 (7/56)	26 (12/46)
Robinson et al. 1995 [217]	417	C	18 (3/17)	33 (1/3)
Imperiale et al. 2004 [218]	4404	C	10 (22/214)	14 (10/71)
Ahlquist et al. 2005 [219]	2503	C	7 (9/125)	36 (8/22)
Total	20 379	C, CX, S	10 (67/641)	23 (59/252)

a Only nonrehydrated Hemoccult data included.

b Data represent adenomas ≥ 7 mm.

C, colonoscopy; CX, colon roentgenography; S, proctosigmoidoscopy.

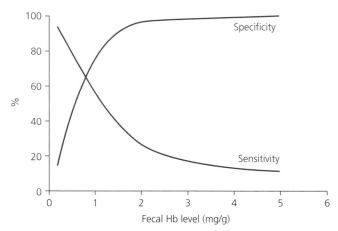

Figure 9.4 Fecal hemoglobin screening for colorectal cancer detection showing inverse relationship between sensitivity and specificity. Quantitative stool testing was performed on 2293 persons who also underwent colorectal evaluation by diagnostic gold standards. From Ahlquist & Gilbert [233], with permission from Karger.

The majority of positive tests yield no pathology and are considered false positives.

A proportion, sometimes the majority, of asymptomatic colorectal cancers can be missed by fecal blood screening tests, and a majority of positive screening tests result from trivial causes other than cancer. Sensitivity can be increased only by reducing specificity, and vice versa (Fig. 9.4).

Test compliance

Screening effectiveness requires not only a good test validity but also a compliant population. Operationally, neoplasm detection rate is the product of test sensitivity and compliance rate in the target population. Compliance rates have been as low as 19% in general populations and as high as 97% in carefully instructed outpatients using a stool collection device [154,201,221], but compliance averages 30%–60% in community-based programs [201,221,222]. Compliance varies with demography, educational effort, and setting [221,223]. Physician compliance in screening programs also varies [201,224,225].

Test effectiveness and cost

Fecal occult blood screening reduces colorectal cancer mortality on an intention-to-screen basis by 15%–30% when regularly applied over 10 years or more (Fig. 9.5) [1–3]. Owing to low detection rates of precursor adenomas, such screening has a lower but nonetheless significant influence on cancer incidence [1–3,226]. The benefit is achieved primarily by detection of early-stage cancer [210] but additionally by adenoma detection [226]. Impact on incidence will be greater if fecal occult blood tests can more effectively detect advanced adenomas; immunochemical tests may be better at detecting these lesions [166]. Screening becomes ineffective when test intervals exceed 2 years [227,228] or when compliance is low [229–231].

Based on mathematical models [229], cost-effectiveness of fecal blood testing is comparable with that of other approaches to colorectal cancer screening. However, the measures of effectiveness are lowest with fecal blood testing, and its comparable cost-effectiveness ratio is due to lower estimated costs [210]. Program costs of fecal blood screening are strongly leveraged by the false-positive rate and the resultant

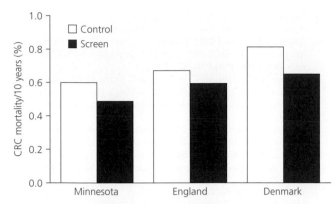

Figure 9.5 Colorectal cancer (CRC) mortality over 10–14 years in controlled trials with Hemoccult screening: screened vs control groups [1–3].

high cost of downstream colonoscopies. Despite their shortcomings, fecal occult blood tests serve to direct colonoscopy to people who are more likely to have neoplasia.

Guidelines for colorectal cancer screening

Because colorectal cancer is so prevalent in the United States, its incidence increases sharply after age 50 years, and its early detection confers a favorable prognosis, the American Cancer Society and other professional organizations recommend annual fecal blood testing for average-risk persons aged 50 years or older. Both guaiac and immunochemical tests performed in standard laboratories have been endorsed for screening [182,232], but the formerly common practice of testing digitally obtained fecal smears is discouraged [180]. If fecal blood testing is to be practiced for cancer detection, clinicians should be aware of test limitations and inform their patients accordingly, understand the common causes of occult GI bleeding, and follow a rational strategy in evaluating elevated test results.

Future approaches to stool screening

Compared with structural screening approaches like colonoscopy, stool testing has several advantages. Stool testing is noninvasive, requires no cathartic preparation, and can be done without a formal health-care visit. Markers with performance characteristics better than occult blood could improve the effectiveness and appeal of stool screening. Exfoliated markers represent rational alternative candidates [180,232–235]. Unlike blood, exfoliated markers enter the colorectal lumen continuously with cell shedding, which enhances sensitivity, and have the potential to be unique to neoplastic tissue, which enhances specificity. Neoplasm-associated DNA alterations are a particularly promising class of exfoliated markers given the known genetic defects in colorectal cancer and the exquisitely sensitive assay techniques available.

Early studies with DNA-based stool testing in selected patient groups suggested high sensitivity and specificity for colorectal cancer [208,235,236] and higher rates of polyp detection than by fecal blood testing [208,235]. Based on the study of a large subject group reflective of the screening setting [218], a first-generation commercial stool DNA test appeared to offer advantages in sensitivity for colorectal cancer detection over the early insensitive guaiac tests at comparable specificity.

Because of its greater unit cost, first-generation stool DNA tests are estimated to be less cost-effective than other approaches to colorectal cancer screening [237]. Future refinements in stool DNA testing and other molecular approaches will likely influence both performance and cost.

Therapeutic considerations

Treatment of abnormal occult GI bleeding is dictated by the clinical setting. The critical first step in management of newly discovered occult bleeding is to exclude a serious underlying lesion. In screening test-positive patients found to have normal structural colorectal studies, it is often appropriate to check whether iron stores are low. If concomitant iron deficiency exists, then an aggressive search for the GI bleeding source is warranted. Specific medical or extirpative therapy of the lesion may not only prevent lesion-associated morbidity but also definitively stop further iron loss (see other chapters for lesion-specific treatments). For those with persistent bleeding from diffuse or inaccessible vascular malformations, some have tried nonspecific medical treatment with systemic estrogen, aminocaproic acid, or somatostatin [238].

Whether the bleeding source is correctable or not, a cornerstone to treatment is the replenishment of iron stores. Some patients with chronically bleeding lesions, such as radiation enteritis or Cameron erosions [66,84], may be appropriately managed with long-term iron replacement alone, because satisfactory medical cures are lacking and surgical approaches may be associated with unwanted morbidity. Uncommonly, blood transfusions are indicated initially in those with severe anemia and cardiovascular compromise.

Oral iron therapy with ferrous sulfate tablets is the preferred approach in most patients with iron deficiency because it is cheap, effective, and usually well tolerated. Other oral preparations include ferrous fumarate, ferrous gluconate, and preparations with added ascorbic acid or other absorption enhancers [5]. Dietary iron replacement is usually inefficient and impractical. For example, it has been calculated that a daily consumption of 5 kg of red meat would be required to provide 60 mg of iron [131], which is the amount contained in one 325-mg tablet of ferrous sulfate. A maximal adult dose of ferrous sulfate is 325 mg t.i.d., as absorption is not appreciably increased with higher doses [5]. With iron replacement, a peak in reticulocytosis occurs after 7 to 10 days, Hb usually normalizes within 2 months, and epithelial abnormalities resolve within months. It should be emphasized that Hb normalizes well before body iron stores are repleted [6]. If blood loss is not ongoing, satisfactory iron replacement usually requires 3–6 months of therapy. Serum ferritin can be used to monitor the adequacy of iron replenishment.

Side effects from oral administration of iron preparations occur in 10%–20% of patients, appear to be dose related, are similar for the different preparations, and result in discontinuation in about 8% of cases [239]. In a large prospective study [239], side effects most commonly reported included constipation (in 13%), diarrhea (6%), heartburn or epigastric pain (5%), and nausea (4%). Side effects from oral iron therapy can often be avoided simply by lowering the dose to one tablet daily or every other day. Low-dose oral iron therapy may be as effective as higher doses but is associated with much fewer side effects [240]. Caution should be taken not to over-replace body iron stores, as excess iron may cause oxidative stress and contribute to long-term risk of inflammatory, cardiovascular, and neoplastic disease [53,241,242]. There is no justification for iron supplementation in iron-replete individuals.

Parenteral iron is indicated in patients who malabsorb iron and in those who do not comply with or tolerate oral iron [243]. Because parenterally administered iron salts are toxic, iron must be injected in a complexed form. Parenteral iron preparations vary in their bioavailability, degradation kinetics, dosimetry, and side effects [5,244,245]. The iron complex is taken up by reticuloendothelial tissues and slowly converted to bioavailable iron. Fatal idiosyncratic reactions occur rarely with parenteral iron dextran [5]. About 10% of patients develop a serum sickness-like illness with fever, myalgias, arthralgias, lymphadenopathy, and urticaria [5]. Some suggest that iron sucrose may be safer and better tolerated than other intravenous preparations [246].

References

1. Mandel JS, Bond JH, Church TR, et al. Reducing mortality from colorectal cancer by screening for fecal occult blood. Minnesota Colon Cancer Control Study. N Engl J Med 1993;328:1365.
2. Hardcastle JD, Chamberlain JO, Robinson MH, et al. Randomised controlled trial of faecal-occult-blood screening for colorectal cancer. Lancet 1996;348:1472.
3. Kronborg O, Fenger C, Olsen J, et al. Randomised study of screening for colorectal cancer with faecal-occult-blood test. Lancet 1996;348:1467.
4. Winawer SJ, Flehinger BJ, Schottenfeld D, Miller DG. Screening for colorectal cancer with fecal occult blood testing and sigmoidoscopy. J Natl Cancer Inst 1993;85:1311.
5. Fairbanks VF. Erythrocyte disorders: anemias related to disturbances of hemoglobin synthesis. In: Williams WJ (ed.). Hematology. New York: McGraw-Hill, 1983:300.
6. DeMaeyer E, Adiels-Tegman M. The prevalence of anaemia in the world. World Health Stat Q 1985;38:302.
7. Kerlin P, Reiner R, Davies M, et al. Iron deficiency anaemia – a prospective study. Aust N Z J Med 1979;9:402.
8. Schiff L, Stevens R, Shapiro N, Goodman S. Observations on the oral administration of citrate blood in man. Am J Med Sci 1942;203:409.
9. Luke RG, Lees W, Rudick J. Appearances of the stools after the introduction of blood into the caecum. Gut 1964;5:77.
10. Ahlquist DA, McGill DB, Schwartz S, et al. HemoQuant, a new quantitative assay for fecal hemoglobin. Comparison with Hemoccult. Ann Intern Med 1984;101:297.
11. Ebaugh FG, Jr, Clemens T, Jr, Rodnan G, Peterson RE. Quantitative measurement of gastrointestinal blood loss. I. The use of radioactive Cr51 in patients with gastrointestinal hemorrhage. Am J Med 1958;25:169.
12. Friedman BI. Radionuclide determination of gastrointestinal blood loss. Semin Nucl Med 1972;2:265.
13. Ahlquist DA, McGill DB, Schwartz S, et al. Fecal blood levels in health and disease. A study using HemoQuant. N Engl J Med 1985;312:1422.
14. Wheby MS, Suttle GE, Ford KT, 3rd. Intestinal absorption of hemoglobin iron. Gastroenterology 1970;58:647.
15. Hallberg L, Bjorn-Rasmussen E, Howard L, Rossander L. Dietary heme iron absorption. A discussion of possible mechanisms for the absorption-promoting effect of meat and for the regulation of iron absorption. Scand J Gastroenterol 1979;14:769.
16. Schwartz S, Dahl J, Ellefson M, Ahlquist D. The "HemoQuant" test: a specific and quantitative determination of heme (hemoglobin) in feces and other materials. Clin Chem 1983;29:2061.
17. Leahy MB, Pippard MJ, Salzmann MB, et al. Quantitative measurement of faecal blood loss: comparison of radioisotopic and chemical analyses. J Clin Pathol 1991;44:391.
18. Schwartz S, Ellefson M. Quantitative fecal recovery of ingested hemoglobin-heme in blood: comparisons by HemoQuant assay with ingested meat and fish. Gastroenterology 1985;89:19.
19. Grasbeck R, Kouvonen I, Lundberg M, Tenhunen R. An intestinal receptor for heme. Scand J Haematol 1979;23:5.
20. Hallberg L, Solvell L. Absorption of hemoglobin iron in man. Acta Med Scand 1967;181:335.
21. Baird IM, Wilson GM. The pathogenesis of anaemia after partial gastrectomy. II. Iron absorption after partial gastrectomy. Q J Med 1959;28:35.
22. Goldschmiedt M, Ahlquist DA, Wieand HS, et al. Measurement of degraded fecal hemoglobin-heme to estimate gastrointestinal site of occult bleeding. Appraisal of its clinical utility. Dig Dis Sci 1988;33:605.
23. Adams EC, Layman KM. Immunochemical confirmation of gastrointestinal bleeding. Ann Clin Lab Sci 1974;4:343.
24. Harewood GC, McConnell JP, Harrington JJ, et al. Detection of occult upper gastrointestinal tract bleeding: performance differences in fecal occult blood tests. Mayo Clin Proc 2002;77:23.
25. Rockey DC, Koch J, Cello JP, et al. Relative frequency of upper gastrointestinal and colonic lesions in patients with positive fecal occult-blood tests. N Engl J Med 1998;339:153.
26. Barrows GH, Burton RM, Jarrett DD, et al. Immunochemical detection of human blood in feces. Am J Clin Pathol 1978;69:342.
27. Songster CL, Barrows GH, Jarrett DD. Immunochemical detection of fecal occult blood – the fecal smear punch-disc test: a new non-invasive screening test for colorectal cancer. Cancer 1980;45:1099.
28. Narasinga BS. Physiology of iron absorption and supplementation. Br Med Bull 1981;37:25.
29. Refsum SB, Schreiner BB. Regulation of iron balance by absorption and excretion. A critical review and a new hypothesis. Scand J Gastroenterol 1984;19:867.
30. Pollack S, Kaufman RM, Crosby WH. Iron absorption: effects of sugars and reducing agents. Blood 1964;24:577.
31. Sorensen EW. Studies on iron absorption. VI. The effect of bile and pancreatin on the absorption of iron. Acta Med Scand 1967;181:707.
32. Jacobs A, Miles PM. Role of gastric secretion in iron absorption. Gut 1969;10:226.
33. Jacobs A, Rhodes J, Eakins J. Gastric factors influencing iron absorption in anemic patients. Scand J Haematol 1967;4:105.
34. Grisolano SW, Oxentenko AS, Murray JA, et al. The usefulness of routine small bowel biopsies in evaluation of iron deficiency anemia. J Clin Gastroenterol 2004;38:756.

35. Alvarez-Leite JI. Nutrient deficiencies secondary to bariatric surgery. Curr Opin Clin Nutr Metab Care 2004;7:569.

36. Goya N, Miyazaki S, Kodate S, Ushio B. A family of congenital atransferrinemia. Blood 1972;40:239.

37. Larrick JW, Hyman ES. Acquired iron-deficiency anemia caused by an antibody against the transferrin receptor. N Engl J Med 1984;311:214.

38. Jacobs A, Butler E. Menstrual blood loss in iron deficiency anemia. Lancet 1965;2:407.

39. Witte DL, Kraemer DF, Johnson GF, et al. Prediction of bone marrow iron findings from tests performed on peripheral blood. Am J Clin Pathol 1986;85:202.

40. Cook JD, Lynch SR. The liabilities of iron deficiency. Blood 1986;68:803.

41. Patterson AJ, Brown WJ, Powers JR, Roberts DC. Iron deficiency, general health and fatigue: results from the Australian Longitudinal Study on Women's Health. Qual Life Res 2000;9:491.

42. Edgerton VR, Gardner GW, Ohira Y, et al. Iron-deficiency anaemia and its effect on worker productivity and activity patterns. Br Med J 1979;2:1546.

43. Schoene RB, Escourrou P, Robertson HT, et al. Iron repletion decreases maximal exercise lactate concentrations in female athletes with minimal iron-deficiency anemia. J Lab Clin Med 1983;102:306.

44. Finch CA, Miller LR, Inamdar AR, et al. Iron deficiency in the rat. Physiological and biochemical studies of muscle dysfunction. J Clin Invest 1976;58:447.

45. Jacobs A, Lawrie JH, Entwistle CC, Campbell H. Gastric acid secretion in chronic iron-deficiency anaemia. Lancet 1966;2:190.

46. Stone WD. Gastric secretory response to iron therapy. Gut 1968;9:99.

47. Guha DK, Walia BN, Tandon BN, et al. Small bowel changes in iron-deficiency anaemia of childhood. Arch Dis Child 1968;43:239.

48. Heldenberg D, Tenenbaum G, Weisman Y. Effect of iron on serum 25-hydroxyvitamin D and 24,25-dihydroxyvitamin D concentrations. Am J Clin Nutr 1992;56:533.

49. Idjradinata P, Pollitt E. Reversal of developmental delays in iron-deficient anaemic infants treated with iron. Lancet 1993;341:1.

50. Scholl TO, Hediger ML, Fischer RL, Shearer JW. Anemia vs iron deficiency: increased risk of preterm delivery in a prospective study. Am J Clin Nutr 1992;55:985.

51. Reeves JD, Vichinsky E, Addiego J, Jr, Lubin BH. Iron deficiency in health and disease. Adv Pediatr 1983;30:281.

52. Sifakis S, Pharmakides G. Anemia in pregnancy. Ann N Y Acad Sci 2000;900:125.

53. Oppenheimer SJ. Iron and its relation to immunity and infectious disease. J Nutr 2001;131:616S; discussion 633S.

54. Ekiz C, Agaoglu L, Karakas Z, et al. The effect of iron deficiency anemia on the function of the immune system. Hematol J 2005;5:579.

55. Cook IJ, Pavli P, Riley JW, et al. Gastrointestinal investigation of iron deficiency anaemia. Br Med J (Clin Res Ed) 1986;292:1380.

56. Calvey HD, Castleden CM. Gastrointestinal investigations for anaemia in the elderly: a prospective study. Age Ageing 1987;16:399.

57. Coban E, Timuragaoglu A, Meric M. Iron deficiency anemia in the elderly: prevalence and endoscopic evaluation of the gastrointestinal tract in outpatients. Acta Haematol 2003;110:25.

58. Roche M, Layrisse M. The nature and causes of "hookworm anemia". Am J Trop Med Hyg 1966;15:1029.

59. Euler AR, Ament ME. Gastroesophageal reflux in children: clinical manifestations, diagnosis, pathophysiology, and therapy. Pediatr Ann 1976;5:678.

60. Yip R, Limburg PJ, Ahlquist DA, et al. Pervasive occult gastrointestinal bleeding in an Alaska native population with prevalent iron deficiency. Role of *Helicobacter pylori* gastritis. JAMA 1997;277:1135.

61. Parkinson AJ, Gold BD, Bulkow L, et al. High prevalence of *Helicobacter pylori* in the Alaska native population and association with low serum ferritin levels in young adults. Clin Diagn Lab Immunol 2000;7:885.

62. Konno M, Muraoka S, Takahashi M, Imai T. Iron-deficiency anemia associated with *Helicobacter pylori* gastritis. J Pediatr Gastroenterol Nutr 2000;31:52.

63. Kurekci AE, Atay AA, Sarici SU, et al. Is there a relationship between childhood *Helicobacter pylori* infection and iron deficiency anemia? J Trop Pediatr 2005;51:166.

64. Rockey DC. Gastrointestinal tract evaluation in patients with iron deficiency anemia. Semin Gastrointest Dis 1999;10:53.

65. Ruhl CE, Everhart JE. Relationship of iron-deficiency anemia with esophagitis and hiatal hernia: hospital findings from a prospective, population-based study. Am J Gastroenterol 2001;96:322.

66. Cameron AJ, Higgins JA. Linear gastric erosion. A lesion associated with large diaphragmatic hernia and chronic blood loss anemia. Gastroenterology 1986;91:338.

67. Moskovitz M, Fadden R, Min T, et al. Large hiatal hernias, anemia, and linear gastric erosion: studies of etiology and medical therapy. Am J Gastroenterol 1992;87:622.

68. Coello-Ramirez P, Larrosa-Haro A. Gastrointestinal occult hemorrhage and gastroduodenitis in cow's milk protein intolerance. J Pediatr Gastroenterol Nutr 1984;3:215.

69. Stoltzfus RJ, Dreyfuss ML, Chwaya HM, Albonico M. Hookworm control as a strategy to prevent iron deficiency. Nutr Rev 1997;55:223.

70. Gilgen D, Mascie-Taylor CG. The effect of anthelmintic treatment on helminth infection and anaemia. Parasitology 2001;122(1):105.

71. Kamath PS, Lacerda M, Ahlquist DA, et al. Gastric mucosal responses to intrahepatic portosystemic shunting in patients with cirrhosis. Gastroenterology 2000;118:905.

72. Kozarek RA, Botoman VA, Bredfeldt JE, et al. Portal colopathy: prospective study of colonoscopy in patients with portal hypertension. Gastroenterology 1991;101:1192.

73. Lewis BS, Waye JD. Chronic gastrointestinal bleeding of obscure origin: role of small bowel enteroscopy. Gastroenterology 1988;94:1117.

74. Descamps C, Schmit A, Van Gossum A. "Missed" upper gastrointestinal tract lesions may explain "occult" bleeding. Endoscopy 1999;31:452.

75. Kendrick ML, Buttar NS, Anderson MA, et al. Contribution of intraoperative enteroscopy in the management of obscure gastrointestinal bleeding. J Gastrointest Surg 2001;5:162.

76. Davis BR, Harris H, Vitale GC. The evolution of endoscopy: wireless capsule cameras for the diagnosis of occult gastrointestinal bleeding and inflammatory bowel disease. Surg Innov 2005;12:129.

77. De Leusse A, Landi B, Edery J, et al. Video capsule endoscopy for investigation of obscure gastrointestinal bleeding: feasibility, results, and interobserver agreement. Endoscopy 2005;37:617.

78. Maieron A, Hubner D, Blaha B, et al. Multicenter retrospective evaluation of capsule endoscopy in clinical routine. Endoscopy 2004;36:864.

79. Fireman Z, Friedman S. Diagnostic yield of capsule endoscopy in obscure gastrointestinal bleeding. Digestion 2004;70:201.

80. Hartmann D, Schilling D, Bolz G, et al. Capsule endoscopy versus push enteroscopy in patients with occult gastrointestinal bleeding. Z Gastroenterol 2003;41:377.

81. Gostout CJ, Bowyer BA, Ahlquist DA, et al. Mucosal vascular malformations of the gastrointestinal tract: clinical observations and results of endoscopic neodymium: yttrium-aluminum-garnet laser therapy. Mayo Clin Proc 1988;63:993.

82. Gostout CJ, Ahlquist DA, Radford CM, et al. Endoscopic laser therapy for watermelon stomach. Gastroenterology 1989;96:1462.

83. Jabbari M, Cherry R, Lough JO, et al. Gastric antral vascular ectasia: the watermelon stomach. Gastroenterology 1984;87:1165.

84. Wellwood JM, Jackson BT. The intestinal complications of radiotherapy. Br J Surg 1973;60:814.

85. Gallo SH, McClave SA. Blue rubber bleb nevus syndrome: gastrointestinal involvement and its endoscopic presentation. Gastrointest Endosc 1992;38:72.

86. Holt JM, Wright R. Anaemia due to blood loss from the telangiectases of scleroderma. Br Med J 1967;3:537.

87. Rosen KM, Sirota DK, Marinoff SC. Gastrointestinal bleeding in Turner's syndrome. Ann Intern Med 1967;67:145.

88. Schmitt B, Posselt HG, Waag KL, et al. Severe hemorrhage from intestinal hemangiomatosis in Klippel-Trenaunay syndrome:

pitfalls in diagnosis and management. J Pediatr Gastroenterol Nutr 1986;5:155.

89. Zuckerman G, Benitez J. A prospective study of bidirectional endoscopy (colonoscopy and upper endoscopy) in the evaluation of patients with occult gastrointestinal bleeding. Am J Gastroenterol 1992;87:62.

90. McIntyre AS, Long RG. Prospective survey of investigations in outpatients referred with iron deficiency anaemia. Gut 1993;34:1102.

91. Reyes Lopez A, Gomez Camacho F, Galvez Calderon C, Mino Fugarolas G. Iron-deficiency anemia due to chronic gastrointestinal bleeding. Rev Esp Enferm Dig 1999;91:345.

92. Harewood GC, Ahlquist DA. Fecal occult blood testing for iron deficiency: a reappraisal. Dig Dis 2000;18:75.

93. Niv E, Elis A, Zissin R, et al. Iron deficiency anemia in patients without gastrointestinal symptoms – a prospective study. Fam Pract 2005;22:58.

94. Croker JR, Beynon G. Gastro-intestinal bleeding – a major cause of iron deficiency in the elderly. Age Ageing 1981;10:40.

95. Beale AL, Penney MD, Allison MC. The prevalence of iron deficiency among patients presenting with colorectal cancer. Colorectal Dis 2005;7:398-402.

96. Lee ER, Dagradi AE. Hemorrhagic erosive gastritis. A clinical study. Am J Gastroenterol 1975;63:201.

97. Fleming JL, Ahlquist DA, McGill DB, et al. Influence of aspirin and ethanol on fecal blood levels as determined by using the HemoQuant assay. Mayo Clin Proc 1987;62:159.

98. Jaffin BW, Bliss CM, LaMont JT. Significance of occult gastrointestinal bleeding during anticoagulation therapy. Am J Med 1987;83:269.

99. Blackshear JL, Baker VS, Holland A, et al. Fecal hemoglobin excretion in elderly patients with atrial fibrillation: combined aspirin and low-dose warfarin vs conventional warfarin therapy. Arch Intern Med 1996;156:658.

100. Bini EJ, Rajapaksa RC, Weinshel EH. Positive predictive value of fecal occult blood testing in persons taking warfarin. Am J Gastroenterol 2005;100:1586.

101. Ivey KJ. Gastrointestinal intolerance and bleeding with non-narcotic analgesics. Drugs 1986;32(Suppl. 4):71.

102. Graham DY, Smith JL. Gastroduodenal complications of chronic NSAID therapy. Am J Gastroenterol 1988;83:1081.

103. Carson JL, Strom BL, Morse ML, et al. The relative gastrointestinal toxicity of the nonsteroidal anti-inflammatory drugs. Arch Intern Med 1987;147:1054.

104. Buttgereit F, Burmester GR, Simon LS. Gastrointestinal toxic side effects of nonsteroidal anti-inflammatory drugs and cyclooxygenase-2-specific inhibitors. Am J Med 2001;110(Suppl. 3A):13S.

105. McGettigan P, Henry D. Cardiovascular risk and inhibition of cyclooxygenase: a systematic review of the observational studies of selective and nonselective inhibitors of cyclooxygenase 2. JAMA 2006;296:1633.

106. Allison MC, Howatson AG, Torrance CJ, et al. Gastrointestinal damage associated with the use of nonsteroidal antiinflammatory drugs. N Engl J Med 1992;327:749.

107. Schoen RT, Vender RJ. Mechanisms of nonsteroidal anti-inflammatory drug-induced gastric damage. Am J Med 1989;86:449.

108. Loeb DS, Talley NJ, Ahlquist DA, et al. Long-term nonsteroidal anti-inflammatory drug use and gastroduodenal injury: the role of *Helicobacter pylori*. Gastroenterology 1992;102:1899.

109. Greenberg PD, Cello JP, Rockey DC. Relationship of low-dose aspirin to GI injury and occult bleeding: a pilot study. Gastrointest Endosc 1999;50:618.

110. Brotherhood J, Brozovic B, Pugh LG. Haematological status of middle- and long-distance runners. Clin Sci Mol Med 1975;48:139.

111. Stewart JG, Ahlquist DA, McGill DB, et al. Gastrointestinal blood loss and anemia in runners. Ann Intern Med 1984;100:843.

112. Fisher RL, McMahon LF, Jr, Ryan MJ, et al. Gastrointestinal bleeding in competitive runners. Dig Dis Sci 1986;31:1226.

113. Cooper BT, Douglas SA, Firth LA, et al. Erosive gastritis and gastrointestinal bleeding in a female runner. Prevention of the bleeding and healing of the gastritis with H2-receptor antagonists. Gastroenterology 1987;92:2019.

114. Moses FM, Brewer TG, Peura DA. Running-associated proximal hemorrhagic colitis. Ann Intern Med 1988;108:385.

115. Robertson JD, Maughan RJ, Davidson RJ. Faecal blood loss in response to exercise. Br Med J (Clin Res Ed) 1987;295:303.

116. Dang CV. Runner's anemia. JAMA 2001;286:714.

117. Miller LS, Barbarevech C, Friedman LS. Less frequent causes of lower gastrointestinal bleeding. Gastroenterol Clin North Am 1994;23:21.

118. Levy DJ, Franklin GO, Rosenthal WS. Gastrointestinal bleeding and amyloidosis. Am J Gastroenterol 1982;77:422.

119. Sikov WM, Schiffman FJ, Weaver M, et al. Splenosis presenting as occult gastrointestinal bleeding. Am J Hematol 2000;65:56.

120. Dardick KR. Hematuria and false-positive tests for stool occult blood. Am Fam Physician 1984;29:201.

121. Earley CJ, Allen RP, Beard JL, Connor JR. Insight into the pathophysiology of restless legs syndrome. J Neurosci Res 2000;62:623.

122. Crosby WH. Pica. JAMA 1976;235:2765.

123. Rector WG, Jr. Pica: its frequency and significance in patients with iron-deficiency anemia due to chronic gastrointestinal blood loss. J Gen Intern Med 1989;4:512.

124. Sun AH, Wang ZM, Xiao SZ, et al. Idiopathic sudden hearing loss and disturbance of iron metabolism. A clinical survey of 426 cases. ORL J Otorhinolaryngol Relat Spec 1992;54:66.

125. Anderson N. Syndrome of spoon nails, anemia, cheilitis, and dysphagia. Arch Dermatol 1938;37:816.

126. Baird IM, Dodge OG, Palmer FJ, Wawman RJ. The tongue and oesophagus in iron-deficiency anaemia and the effect of iron therapy. J Clin Pathol 1961;14:603.

127. Hutton CF. Plummer Vinson syndrome. Br J Radiol 1956;29:81.

128. Jacobs A, Kilpatrick GS. The Paterson-Kelly syndrome. Br Med J 1964;2:79.

129. Khosla SN. Cricoid webs – incidence and follow-up study in Indian patients. Postgrad Med J 1984;60:346.

130. Thompson WG, Meola T, Lipkin M, Jr, Freedman ML. Red cell distribution width, mean corpuscular volume, and transferrin saturation in the diagnosis of iron deficiency. Arch Intern Med 1988;148:2128.

131. Marcus DL, Freedman ML. Clinical disorders of iron metabolism in the elderly. Clin Geriatr Med 1985;1:729.

132. Caravaca F, Vagace JM, Aparicio A, et al. Assessment of iron status by erythrocyte ferritin in uremic patients with or without recombinant human erythropoietin therapy. Am J Kidney Dis 1992;20:249.

133. Ferguson BJ, Skikne BS, Simpson KM, et al. Serum transferrin receptor distinguishes the anemia of chronic disease from iron deficiency anemia. J Lab Clin Med 1992;119:385.

134. Fusaro M, Munaretto G, Spinello M, et al. Soluble transferrin receptors and reticulocyte hemoglobin concentration in the assessment of iron deficiency in hemodialysis patients. J Nephrol 2005;18:72.

135. Metzgeroth G, Adelberger V, Dorn-Beineke A, et al. Soluble transferrin receptor and zinc protoporphyrin – competitors or efficient partners? Eur J Haematol 2005;75:309.

136. Lowenstein W, Cals MJ, De Jaeger C, et al. Free erythrocyte protoporphyrin assay in the diagnosis of iron deficiency in the anemic aged subject. A prospective study of 103 anemic patients. Ann Med Interne (Paris) 1991;142:13.

137. Rettmer RL, Carlson TH, Origenes ML, et al. Zinc protoporphyrin/heme ratio for diagnosis of preanemic iron deficiency. Pediatrics 1999;104:e37.

138. VanDeen J. Tincture gaujaci, und em ozontrague, als reagens auf sehr geringe blutmengen, namentlich in medico-forensischen falen. Arch Holland Beitr Natura Heilk 1864;3:228.

139. Greegor DH. Occult blood testing for detection of asymptomatic colon cancer. Cancer 1971;28:131.

140. Ostrow JD, Mulvaney CA, Hansell JR, Rhodes RS. Sensitivity and reproducibility of chemical tests for fecal occult blood with an emphasis on false-positive reactions. Am J Dig Dis 1973;18:930.

141. Stroehlein JR, Fairbanks VF, McGill DB, Go VL. Hemoccult detection of fecal occult blood quantitated by radioassay. Am J Dig Dis 1976;21:841.

142. Bassett ML, Goulston KJ. False positive and negative hemoccult reactions on a normal diet and effect of diet restriction. Aust N Z J Med 1980;10:1.

143. Heinrich HC. Occult blood tests. Lancet 1980;1:822.

144. Macrae FA, St John DJ. Relationship between patterns of bleeding and Hemoccult sensitivity in patients with colorectal cancers or adenomas. Gastroenterology 1982;82:891.

145. Herzog P, Holtermuller KH, Preiss J, et al. Fecal blood loss in patients with colonic polyps: a comparison of measurements with 51chromium-labeled erythrocytes and with the Haemoccult test. Gastroenterology 1982;83:957.

146. Rockey DC, Auslander A, Greenberg PD. Detection of upper gastrointestinal blood with fecal occult blood tests. Am J Gastroenterol 1999; 94:344–50.

147. Stroehlein JR, Fairbanks VF, Go VL, et al. Hemoccult stool tests: false-negative results due to storage of specimens. Mayo Clin Proc 1976;51:548.

148. Macrae FA, St John DJ, Caligiore P, et al. Optimal dietary conditions for hemoccult testing. Gastroenterology 1982;82:899.

149. Lifton LJ, Kreiser J. False-positive stool occult blood tests caused by iron preparations. A controlled study and review of literature. Gastroenterology 1982;83:860.

150. Coles EF, Starnes EC. Use of HemoQuant assays to assess the effect of oral iron preparations on stool hemoccult tests. Am J Gastroenterol 1991;86:1442.

151. Holman JS, Shwed JA. Influence of sucralfate on the detection of occult blood in simulated gastric fluid by two screening tests. Clin Pharm 1992;11:625.

152. Schentag JJ. False-positive "hemoccult" reaction with cimetidine. N Engl J Med 1980;303:110.

153. Ahlquist DA, Schwartz S. Use of leuco-dyes in the quantitative colorimetric microdetermination of hemoglobin and other heme compounds. Clin Chem 1975;21:362.

154. Ahlquist DA, Schwartz S, Isaacson J, Ellefson M. A stool collection device: the first step in occult blood testing. Ann Intern Med 1988; 108:609.

155. Jaffe RM, Kasten B, Young DS, MacLowry JD. False-negative stool occult blood tests caused by ingestion of ascorbic acid (vitamin C). Ann Intern Med 1975;83:824.

156. Layne EA, Mellow MH, Lipman TO. Insensitivity of guaiac slide tests for detection of blood in gastric juice. Ann Intern Med 1981;94: 774.

157. Markman HD. Errors in the guaiac test for occult blood. JAMA 1967;202:846.

158. Levin B, Hess K, Johnson C. Screening for colorectal cancer. A comparison of three fecal occult blood tests. Arch Intern Med 1997;157:970.

159. Allison JE, Feldman R, Tekawa IS. Hemoccult screening in detecting colorectal neoplasm: sensitivity, specificity, and predictive value. Long-term follow-up in a large group practice setting. Ann Intern Med 1990;112:328.

160. Yoshida Y, Saito H, Tsuchida S. A simple sensitive immunologic fecal occult blood test suitable for mass screening for colorectal cancer. Gastroenterology 1986;90:1699.

161. Nakayama T, Yasuoka H, Kishino T, et al. ELISA for occult faecal albumin. Lancet 1987;1:1368.

162. Federici A, Giorgi Rossi P, Borgia P, et al. The immunochemical faecal occult blood test leads to higher compliance than the guaiac for colorectal cancer screening programmes: a cluster randomized controlled trial. J Med Screen 2005;12:83.

163. Morikawa T, Kato J, Yamaji Y, Wada R, et al. A comparison of the immunochemical fecal occult blood test and total colonoscopy in the asymptomatic population. Gastroenterology 2005;129:422.

164. Castiglione G, Grazzini G, Ciatto S. Guaiac and immunochemical tests for faecal occult blood in colorectal cancer screening. Br J Cancer 1992;65:942.

165. Thomas WM, Hardcastle JD, Jackson J, Pye G. Chemical and immunological testing for faecal occult blood: a comparison of two tests in symptomatic patients. Br J Cancer 1992;65:618.

166. Woo HY, Mok RS, Park YN, et al. A prospective study of a new immunochemical fecal occult blood test in Korean patients referred for colonoscopy. Clin Biochem 2005;38:395.

167. Johne B, Kronborg O, Ton HI, et al. A new fecal calprotectin test for colorectal neoplasia. Clinical results and comparison with previous method. Scand J Gastroenterol 2001;36:291.

168. Roseth A, Kristinsson J, Nygaard K, et al. Faecal lactoferrin: a novel marker of colorectal cancer in rats, a longitudinal in vivo study. Gastroenterology 1995;108:A530.

169. Gilbert JA, Ahlquist DA, Mahoney DW, et al. Fecal marker variability in colorectal cancer: calprotectin versus hemoglobin. Scand J Gastroenterol 1996;31:1001.

170. Limburg PJ, Devens ME, Harrington JJ, et al. Prospective evaluation of fecal calprotectin as a screening biomarker for colorectal neoplasia. Am J Gastroenterol 2003;98:2299.

171. Hoff G, Grotmol T, Thiis-Evensen E, et al. Testing for faecal calprotectin (PhiCal) in the Norwegian Colorectal Cancer Prevention trial on flexible sigmoidoscopy screening: comparison with an immunochemical test for occult blood (FlexSure OBT). Gut 2004;53:1329.

172. Ahlquist DA, McGill DB, Fleming JL, et al. Patterns of occult bleeding in asymptomatic colorectal cancer. Cancer 1989;63:1826.

173. Stephens FO, Lawrenson KB. 51Cr excretion in bile. Lancet 1969;1:158.

174. Chafetz N, Taylor A, Jr., Schleif A, et al. A potential error in the quantitation of fecal blood loss: concise communication. J Nucl Med 1976; 17:1053.

175. Rosenfield RE, Kochwa S, Kaczera Z, Maimon J. Nonuniform distribution of occult blood in feces. Am J Clin Pathol 1979;71:204.

176. Farrands PA, Hardcastle JD. Accuracy of occult blood tests over a six-day period. Clin Oncol 1983;9:217.

177. Hoffman A, Young Q, Bright-Asare P, et al. Early detection of bowel cancer at an urban public hospital: demonstration project. CA Cancer J Clin 1983;33:344.

178. Eisner MS, Lewis JH. Diagnostic yield of a positive fecal occult blood test found on digital rectal examination. Does the finger count? Arch Intern Med 1991;151:2180.

179. Ferreira M, Vanagunas A. Limitations of digital rectal exam for occult blood testing. Gastroenterology 1993;104:A8.

180. Collins JF, Lieberman DA, Durbin TE, Weiss DG. Accuracy of screening for fecal occult blood on a single stool sample obtained by digital rectal examination: a comparison with recommended sampling practice. Ann Intern Med 2005;142:81.

181. Nakama H, Zhang B, Abdul Fattah AS, Kamijo N. Does stool collection method affect outcomes in immunochemical fecal occult blood testing? Dis Colon Rectum 2001;44:871.

182. Allison JE. Colon Cancer Screening Guidelines 2005: the fecal occult blood test option has become a better FIT. Gastroenterology 2005; 129:745.

183. Ahlquist DA, Wieand HS, Moertel CG, et al. Accuracy of fecal occult blood screening for colorectal neoplasia. A prospective study using Hemoccult and HemoQuant tests. JAMA 1993;269:1262.

184. Lieberman DA, Weiss DG. One-time screening for colorectal cancer with combined fecal occult-blood testing and examination of the distal colon. N Engl J Med 2001;345:555.

185. Hsia PC, al-Kawas FH. Yield of upper endoscopy in the evaluation of asymptomatic patients with Hemoccult-positive stool after a negative colonoscopy. Am J Gastroenterol 1992;87:1571.

186. Sharma VK, Komanduri S, Nayyar S, et al. An audit of the utility of in-patient fecal occult blood testing. Am J Gastroenterol 2001;96: 1256.

187. Sharma VK, Corder FA, Raufman JP, et al. Survey of internal medicine residents' use of the fecal occult blood test and their understanding of colorectal cancer screening and surveillance. Am J Gastroenterol 2000;95:2068.

188. Rockey DC, Cello JP. Evaluation of the gastrointestinal tract in patients with iron-deficiency anemia. N Engl J Med 1993;329:1691.

189. Kepczyk T, Cremins JE, Long BD, et al. A prospective, multidisciplinary evaluation of premenopausal women with iron-deficiency anemia. Am J Gastroenterol 1995;94:109.

190. Gordon SR, Smith RE, Power GC. The role of endoscopy in the evaluation of iron deficiency anemia in patients over the age of 50. Am J Gastroenterol 1994;89:1963.

191. Joosten E, Ghesquiere B, Linthoudt H, et al. Upper and lower gastrointestinal evaluation of elderly inpatients who are iron deficient. Am J Med 1999;107:24.

192. Waye JD. Small-bowel endoscopy. Endoscopy 1999;31:56.

193. Hayat M, Axon AT, O'Mahony S. Diagnostic yield and effect on clinical outcomes of push enteroscopy in suspected small-bowel bleeding. Endoscopy 2000;32:369.

194. Schilling D, Grieger G, Weidmann E, et al. Long-term follow-up of patients with iron deficiency anemia after a close endoscopic examination of the upper and lower gastrointestinal tract. Z Gastroenterol 2000;38:827.

195. Gostout CJ. Improving the withdrawal phase of Sonde enteroscopy with the "push-away" method. Gastrointest Endosc 1993;39:69.

196. Bleau BL, Donohue JH, Ahlquist DA, Gostout CJ. Laparoscopically assisted panenteroscopy: a feasibility study in pigs. Gastrointest Endosc 1995;41:154.

197. Appleyard M, Fireman Z, Glukhovsky A, et al. A randomized trial comparing wireless capsule endoscopy with push enteroscopy for the detection of small-bowel lesions. Gastroenterology 2000;119:1431.

198. Di Caro S, May A, Heine DG, et al. The European experience with double-balloon enteroscopy: indications, methodology, safety, and clinical impact. Gastrointest Endosc 2005;62:545.

199. Manabe N, Tanaka S, Fukumoto A, et al. Double-balloon enteroscopy in patients with GI bleeding of obscure origin. Gastrointest Endosc 2006;64:135.

200. Mansson J, Bjorkelund C, Hultborn R. Symptom pattern and diagnostic work-up of malignancy at first symptom presentation as related to level of care. A retrospective study from the primary health care centre area of Kungsbacka, Sweden. Neoplasma 1999;46:93.

201. Simon JB. Occult blood screening for colorectal carcinoma: a critical review. Gastroenterology 1985;88:820.

202. Screening for colorectal cancer – United States, 1997. MMWR Morb Mortal Wkly Rep 1999;48:116.

203. Trends in screening for colorectal cancer – United States, 1997 and 1999. MMWR Morb Mortal Wkly Rep 2001;50:162.

204. Dybdahl JH, Daae LN, Larsen S, Myren J. Occult faecal blood loss determined by a 51Cr method and chemical tests in patients referred for colonoscopy. Scand J Gastroenterol 1984;19:245.

205. Ransohoff DF, Lang CA. Small adenomas detected during fecal occult blood test screening for colorectal cancer. The impact of serendipity. JAMA 1990;264:76.

206. Griffith CD, Turner DJ, Saunders JH. False-negative results of Hemoccult test in colorectal cancer. Br Med J (Clin Res Ed) 1981;283:472.

207. Crowley ML, Freeman LD, Mottet MD, et al. Sensitivity of guaiac-impregnated cards for the detection of colorectal neoplasia. J Clin Gastroenterol 1983;5:127.

208. Ahlquist DA, Skoletsky JE, Boynton KA, et al. Colorectal cancer screening by detection of altered human DNA in stool: feasibility of a multitarget assay panel. Gastroenterology 2000;119:1219.

209. Demers RY, Stawick LE, Demers P. Relative sensitivity of the fecal occult blood test and flexible sigmoidoscopy in detecting polyps. Prev Med 1985;14:55.

210. Ahlquist DA. Fecal occult blood testing for colorectal cancer. Can we afford to do this? Gastroenterol Clin North Am 1997;26:41.

211. Ahlquist DA, Klee GG, McGill DB, Ellesfon RD. Colorectal cancer detection in the practice setting. Impact of fecal blood testing. Arch Intern Med 1990;150:1041.

212. Bang KM, Tillett S, Hoar SK, et al. Sensitivity of fecal hemoccult testing and flexible sigmoidoscopy for colorectal cancer screening. J Occup Med 1986;28:709.

213. Jahn H, Joergensen OD, Kronborg O, Fenger C. Can Hemoccult-II replace colonoscopy in surveillance after radical surgery for colorectal cancer and after polypectomy? Dis Colon Rectum 1992;35:253.

214. Rozen P. Screening for colorectal neoplasia in the Tel Aviv area: cumulative data 1979-89 and initial conclusions. Isr J Med Sci 1992;28:8.

215. Ribet A, Frexinos J, Escourrou J, Delpu J. Occult blood tests and colorectal tumours. Lancet 1980;1:417.

216. Williams CB, Macrae FA, Bartram CI. A prospective study of diagnostic methods in adenoma follow-up. Endoscopy 1982;14:74.

217. Robinson MH, Kronborg O, Williams CB, et al. Faecal occult blood testing and colonoscopy in the surveillance of subjects at high risk of colorectal neoplasia. Br J Surg 1995;82:318.

218. Imperiale TF, Ransohoff DF, Itzkowitz SH, et al. Fecal DNA versus fecal occult blood for colorectal-cancer screening in an average-risk population. N Engl J Med 2004;351:2704.

219. Ahlquist D, Sargent D, Levin T, et al. Stool DNA screening for colorectal cancer; prospective multicenter comparison with Hemoccult. Gastroenterology 2005;128:A-63.

220. Zappa M, Castiglione G, Paci E, et al. Measuring interval cancers in population-based screening using different assays of fecal occult blood testing: the District of Florence experience. Int J Cancer 2001;92:151.

221. Vernon SW. Participation in colorectal cancer screening: a review. J Natl Cancer Inst 1997;89:1406.

222. Kronborg O, Jorgensen OD, Fenger C, Rasmussen M. Randomized study of biennial screening with a faecal occult blood test: results after nine screening rounds. Scand J Gastroenterol 2004;39:846.

223. Hart AR, Eaden J, Barnett S, et al. Colorectal cancer prevention. An approach to increasing compliance in a faecal occult blood test screening programme. J Epidemiol Community Health 1998;52:818.

224. Shields HM, Weiner MS, Henry DR, et al. Factors that influence the decision to do an adequate evaluation of a patient with a positive stool for occult blood. Am J Gastroenterol 2001;96:196.

225. Nadel MR, Shapiro JA, Klabunde CN, et al. A national survey of primary care physicians' methods for screening for fecal occult blood. Ann Intern Med 2005;142:86.

226. Mandel JS, Church TR, Bond JH, et al. The effect of fecal occult-blood screening on the incidence of colorectal cancer. N Engl J Med 2000;343:1603.

227. Mandel JS, Church TR, Ederer F, Bond JH. Colorectal cancer mortality: effectiveness of biennial screening for fecal occult blood. J Natl Cancer Inst 1999;91:434.

228. Selby JV, Friedman GD, Quesenberry CP, Jr, Weiss NS. Effect of fecal occult blood testing on mortality from colorectal cancer. A case-control study. Ann Intern Med 1993;118:1.

229. Khandker RK, Dulski JD, Kilpatrick JB, et al. A decision model and cost-effectiveness analysis of colorectal cancer screening and surveillance guidelines for average-risk adults. Int J Technol Assess Health Care 2000;16:799.

230. Helm JF, Russo MW, Biddle AK, et al. Effectiveness and economic impact of screening for colorectal cancer by mass fecal occult blood testing. Am J Gastroenterol 2000;95:3250.

231. Sonnenberg A, Delco F, Inadomi JM. Cost-effectiveness of colonoscopy in screening for colorectal cancer. Ann Intern Med 2000;133:573.

232. Levin B, Brooks D, Smith RA, Stone A. Emerging technologies in screening for colorectal cancer: CT colonography, immunochemical fecal occult blood tests, and stool screening using molecular markers. CA Cancer J Clin 2003;53:44.

233. Ahlquist DA, Gilbert JA. Stool markers for colorectal cancer screening: future considerations. Dig Dis 1996;14:132.

234. Ahlquist DA. Molecular stool screening for colorectal cancer. Using DNA markers may be beneficial, but large scale evaluation is needed. Br Med J 2000;321:254.

235. Osborn NK, Ahlquist DA. Stool screening for colorectal cancer: molecular approaches. Gastroenterology 2005;128:192.

236. Dong SM, Traverso G, Johnson C, et al. Detecting colorectal cancer in stool with the use of multiple genetic targets. J Natl Cancer Inst 2001;93:858.

237. Song K, Fendrick AM, Ladabaum U. Fecal DNA testing compared

with conventional colorectal cancer screening methods: a decision analysis. Gastroenterology 2004;126:1270.

238. Lewis BS. Medical and hormonal therapy in occult gastrointestinal bleeding. Semin Gastrointest Dis 1999;10:71.

239. Hallberg L, Ryttinger L, Solvell L. Side-effects of oral iron therapy. A double-blind study of different iron compounds in tablet form. Acta Med Scand Suppl 1966;459:3.

240. Rimon E, Kagansky N, Kagansky M, et al. Are we giving too much iron? Low-dose iron therapy is effective in octagenarians. Am J Med 2005;118:1142.

241. Oldenburg B, van Berge Henegouwen GP, et al. Iron supplementation affects the production of pro-inflammatory cytokines in IL-10 deficient mice. Eur J Clin Invest 2000;30:505.

242. Oldenburg B, Koningsberger JC, Van Berge Henegouwen GP, et al. Iron and inflammatory bowel disease. Aliment Pharmacol Ther 2001;15:429.

243. Macdougall IC. Strategies for iron supplementation: oral versus intravenous. Kidney Int Suppl 1999;69:S61.

244. Park L, Uhthoff T, Tierney M, Nadler S. Effect of an intravenous iron dextran regimen on iron stores, hemoglobin, and erythropoietin requirements in hemodialysis patients. Am J Kidney Dis 1998;31:835.

245. Gupta A, Crumbliss AL. Treatment of iron deficiency anemia: are monomeric iron compounds suitable for parenteral administration? J Lab Clin Med 2000;136:371.

246. Schroder O, Mickisch O, Seidler U, et al. Intravenous iron sucrose versus oral iron supplementation for the treatment of iron deficiency anemia in patients with inflammatory bowel disease – a randomized, controlled, open-label, multicenter study. Am J Gastroenterol 2005;100:2503.

10 Approach to screening for colorectal cancer

Graeme P. Young, James E. Allison

Goals of screening, 170
The contexts of screening, 170
The nature of screening, 171
The nature of screening tests, 171
Evidence of effectiveness, 172
Recent developments in screening tests, 178
Other considerations in screening practice, 179
Conclusions, 180

Screening for colorectal cancer can be defined as the testing of asymptomatic people to classify them as likely or unlikely to have the disease [1]. The World Health Organization (WHO) has described the requirements that should be met before it is appropriate to screen [2]. Colorectal cancer meets all these criteria:

- it is a major health problem in many countries
- it has a latent stage
- there are appropriate proven screening tests
- testing is feasible
- treatment can lead to cure.

WHO recommends screening using a simple test. The result of the screening test determines who undergoes a diagnostic test.

Goals of screening

The goal of screening for colorectal cancer is to reduce mortality from or morbidity due to the disease. The natural history and the impact of early detection methods on outcome can be conceptualized as shown in Fig. 10.1. Presymptomatic detection of localized cancer (point S3) reduces morbidity or mortality. If screening detects preinvasive lesions, namely dysplasia or adenoma (points S1 or S2), it will reduce cancer incidence.

Ideally, screening is an ongoing process, which is directed at asymptomatic individuals who are at average risk for developing colorectal cancer [2]. Average risk is defined as age at least 50 years, absence of high-risk factors such as family or

Principles of Clinical Gastroenterology. Edited by Tadataka Yamada, David H. Alpers, Anthony N. Kalloo, Neil Kaplowitz, Chung Owyang, and Don W. Powell. © 2008 Blackwell Publishing. ISBN 978-1-4051-69103

personal history of colorectal neoplasia, resident in a developed or developing country where the lifestyle is changing to that of Western countries, and absence of symptoms suggestive of colorectal cancer [3]. Screening should perhaps be avoided in those individuals where screening is not a health priority, such as when active major illness is present [4]. When high-risk factors are present, an individualized surveillance program is indicated based on specific circumstances.

The most immediate impacts of screening will be adenoma detection, down-staging of the detected cancers and prolonged survival after treatment. The longer-term impacts will be reduction in overall population mortality and incidence.

The contexts of screening

Screening for colorectal cancer is usually undertaken in either personalized or population settings [5]. The health imperatives driving each are different.

In some countries the traditional approach has consisted of a face-to-face meeting between the individual and a physician – sometimes referred to as *case-finding* or *individualistic* screening. It may be initiated by the individual or the physician. Here, the person can be assessed for symptoms and level of risk. What is offered is individualized and done in the context of counseling. Duty of care and doing what is best for the person drive the decision-making – cost-effectiveness tends not to be a consideration, although affordability and access are.

Population or *mass screening* involves an organized and systematic approach aimed at maximum participation in screening within a population. It seeks, through a standardized and often impersonal approach, to engage individuals in at least

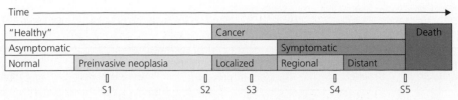

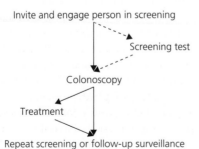

Figure 10.1 Schematic showing stages of colorectal oncogenesis as they relate to different points of early detection as might occur during screening (S1, S2, S3). Relative durations are meant to serve only as a guide. The impact of detection at each point is as follows: S1, detects many adenomas, a proportion of which might not be precursors of cancer but removal should lead to reduced incidence of and mortality from cancer; S2, detects fewer inconsequential adenomas but will remove adenomas and prevent cancer, thereby reducing incidence and mortality; S3, down-stages detected cancers and so will lengthen survival and reduce mortality through increased rate of cure; S4, lesser impact than at S2 but likely to reduce mortality to a degree; S5, probably no impact.

some form of preventive activity – in effect, doing something is better than doing nothing. Outcomes at the population level such as acceptability, feasibility, and low initial cost with proven cost-effectiveness are key issues. Many thousands will be tested in a short time frame, often without ascertainment of presence of symptoms or without profiling risk through a counseling process.

The nature of screening

No matter what the context, screening is by its nature a process that aims to improve the likelihood that affected people, while at a curable and usually unsuspecting stage, receive effective diagnosis and treatment. Screening is, therefore, a process with multiple phases as depicted in Fig. 10.2 [6]. Screening is only beneficial to the individual if the screening test is performed, if diagnosis is accurate, and if treatment is effective.

There are two main choices at the phase where a test is offered (Fig. 10.2).

- *One-step testing* The diagnostic test, colonoscopy, is offered. Selection for colonoscopy is based solely on age and many people will be found to have no neoplasia.
- *Two-step testing* A simpler test is offered first, e.g., a fecal occult blood test (FOBT) or flexible sigmoidoscopy, then those with a positive result proceed to colonoscopy. A simple

screening test calls attention to the likelihood of disease being present and serves to direct resources to those most likely to benefit from diagnostic and therapeutic procedures [6].

Operational phases of the screening process proceed as follows:

- *Invite and encourage* participation in a screening program.
  - Use either a personalized approach within a health-care environment, or
  - Use a mass population approach with wide coverage of the population.
- Where a person is found to have a *high-risk* factor (e.g., colorectal symptoms, family history or personal history of relevant colorectal disease), provide access to an individualized prevention strategy appropriate to that risk.
- Where a person is found to have *symptoms*, offer the appropriate diagnostic test.
- For those who are confirmed *average risk*, provide a safe, effective, acceptable, and affordable screening test in either of two main ways:
  - *two-step testing*: perform a simple test such as a fecal occult blood test (FOBT) to establish risk and select who should proceed to colonoscopy, or
  - *one-step testing*: perform colonoscopy.
- Facilitate *compliance* with any necessary diagnostic and therapeutic follow-up.
- Offer *rescreening* at the appropriate interval, having identified risk status.
- *Monitor* adequacy of participation, quality of tests and clinical procedures, availability of necessary resources, and the outcomes of the program.

Figure 10.2 Diagrammatic representation of the screening process to demonstrate the main phases involved in the screening process and the options of one-step and two-step screening.

The nature of screening tests

The nature of the major screening tests, either established or under study, and their place in the testing phase of the screening process, are summarized in Table 10.1. In general, the efficacy of screening for colorectal cancer is supported by the highest level of evidence, namely randomized controlled trials, at the population level. However, as summarized in Table 10.1, this is not the case for all of the test options. As the

Table 10.1 Overview of available screening tests describing basis for detection of neoplasia, strength of evidence for efficacy, and factors that limit sensitivity and specificity

Detection goal	Technology	Strongest evidence for benefit	Place in screening process	Sensitivity determinants	Specificity determinants
Fecal blood	Guaiac-based FOBT	Population RCT – reduced incidence and mortality	Two-step	Amount of fecal heme	Dietary heme; bleeding nonneoplastic lesions
	Fecal immunochemical test (FIT)	Comparative cohort – better sensitivity or specificity	Two-step	Amount of fecal globin	Bleeding nonneoplastic lesions
Fecal neoplasm-derived DNA	Multitarget fecal DNA test	Comparative cohort – assessing sensitivity and specificity	Two-step	Spectrum of mutations in lesion	Unclear
Visualize lesion	Colonoscopy	Case–control and cohort – reduced incidence and mortality	One-step	Quality of procedure	Histopathology
	Flexible sigmoidoscopy	Case–control – reduced mortality	One- or two-step	Quality of procedure; limited depth of insertion	Histopathology
Imaging of lesion	Barium enema	None	Two-step	Quality of procedure	Lumenal artifact; nonneoplastic pathology
	CT colonography	Comparative cohort – assessing sensitivity and specificity	Two-step	Quality of procedure; precision of technology	Lumenal artifact; nonneoplastic pathology

CT, computed tomography; FOBT, fecal occult blood test, RCT, randomized control trial.

evidence is strongest for tests that detect fecal blood or for those that endoscopically visualize lesions, we will critically evaluate these approaches in detail.

Evidence of effectiveness

As screening is a process where the goal is reduction in population mortality, randomized studies at the population level where mortality has been shown to be reduced even when analyzed on an intention-to-screen basis, i.e., regardless of whether people offered the test actually took it, is the most reliable indicator of effectiveness. We present the evidence available for the best-studied screening tests – namely FOBT, flexible sigmoidoscopy and colonoscopy – with the intention of developing an evidence-based guide for how to undertake screening.

Fecal occult blood tests

The fact that microscopic bleeding may arise from curable cancers and adenomas, provides the basis for screening using an FOBT [7,8]. However, the biology of bleeding is complex and for FOBT screening to be effective, these tests must be used properly in a way that maximizes their ability to detect bleeding from neoplasia.

Types of fecal occult blood test: guaiac and immunochemical tests

Available FOBTs are based on two principal technologies: chemical and immunochemical. The major biological and

technological features of these tests are outlined in Table 10.2 [5,6,8,9].

Chemical fecal occult blood test

The chemical tests (e.g., Hemoccult II) detect the peroxidase activity of heme. The majority use guaiac as the reagent. These guaiac-based FOBT (GFOBT) react to any peroxidase in feces (e.g., plant peroxidases or heme in red meat) and are affected by certain chemicals (e.g., vitamin C). Because heme is relatively stable in the gut (although slow degradation occurs in the colon), GFOBT may detect bleeding from any site in the gastrointestinal tract, including the stomach [11]. Development and interpretation of GFOBT results seem simple but in practice the test is not reliable without training [12]. Most tests employ a wooden spatula for sampling stools, which should ideally be kept clear of the toilet bowl water to avoid leaching of hemoglobin from the stool [13].

Other GFOBT more sensitive than Hemoccult, such as HemoccultSensa, have been developed although at the cost of worsened specificity, especially if red meat has not been excluded from the diet before a sample is collected [9,10]. HemoccultSensa is also more readable [14]. Some studies indicate that if development of GFOBT is delayed 72 h after sampling, the problem of plant peroxidase interference is minimized [14] and dietary restrictions for controlling GFOBT specificity can be simplified such that only red meat and very high-peroxidase foods such as horseradish need be excluded. Unfortunately, unpredictably high positivity rates still occur in several ethnic communities [10,15], resulting in GFOBT not being of practical use.

Table 10.2 Nature, usage, and performance issues for different types of fecal occult blood tests (FOBT) [5, 6]

Type of FOBT	Chemical basis	Diet restrictions	Drug interference	Site of occult bleeding detected	Specificity for neoplasia[d]	Sensitivity for cancer[d]
Chemical (GFOBT)	Guaiac detects peroxidase activity of heme	Required: Red meats Possibly certain raw plant foods[a]	Vitamin C Possibly NSAIDs[b]	Rectum > colon > stomach (in decreasing order of sensitivity)	90%–98% depending on test brand, and usage	35%–67% with one-time testing Over 80% with repeated testing 65%–90% with one-time testing
Immuno-chemical (FIT)	Anti-human hemoglobin antibody detects globin	None required	None	Colon and rectum	Around 95% depending on sensitivity level chosen[c]	Unclear for repeated testing

a Delaying development for 72 h minimizes interference from plant foods and avoids the need for their restriction with standard Hemoccult II. Red meats must be restricted when using a more sensitive GFOBT [9].

b Low-dose aspirin is not a problem, but therapeutic doses, such as those used for rheumatic disorders, may be a problem.

c Tests generally provide a qualitative result, but some newer FIT can be quantifiable.

d Indicative estimates only derived from Tables 10.3 and 10.4 and reference [10].

FIT, fecal immunochemical tests for hemoglobin; GFOBT, guaiac-based FOBT; NSAIDs, nonsteroidal antiinflammatory drugs.

Before the availability of more sensitive GFOBT, rehydration of Hemoccult test cards was applied to increase sensitivity [16], but this has an adverse effect on specificity by activation of plant peroxidases [14]. Guidelines to standardize development have never been established and rehydration is no longer recommended [9,14,17].

To summarize, while of proven efficacy in decreasing colorectal cancer mortality and incidence, chemical FOBT, i.e., GFOBT, has the following shortcomings [8].

• Restrictions of diet and drugs are needed to optimize specificity, especially for the sensitive GFOBT.

• GFOBTs generally use spatula sampling of stools, and stools need to be kept out of contact with toilet bowl water.

• GFOBTs are not selective for colorectal bleeding.

• The end point can be difficult to read and is transient.

• Sensitivity for cancer is suboptimal for less sensitive GFOBT brands.

• More sensitive GFOBTs are subject to unpredictably high false-positive rates.

• GFOBTs are not suitable for automated mass development or reading of the result.

Fecal immunochemical tests

Fecal immunochemical tests for hemoglobin (FIT) use antibodies that are specific for human globin and, therefore, these tests are not affected by diet [11,18,19]. They are subject to less variability in positivity rate than the sensitive GFOBT [15]. Because globin is rapidly degraded by digestive enzymes, these tests are highly selective for occult bleeding of colorectal origin [11].

Depending on the version of FIT and the manufacturer, improvements in fecal sampling have been made; these are discussed elsewhere in detail [8,9,18,20]. The tests may be developed in the office or laboratory and quality assurance of test development is much improved. It is beyond the scope of this chapter to further describe the technological details but laboratory development is preferred in many countries, especially for mass screening when many tests must be performed and quality assurance is vital [5]. Most branded versions of FIT require fewer than three fecal samples, the recommended number for GFOBT.

Several of the latest FIT allow quantification of fecal hemoglobin. The advantage of fecal hemoglobin measurement is that it returns full control of sensitivity and specificity to the end-user [6,8] who can establish the level of fecal hemoglobin that would trigger colonoscopy. At the population level, such an approach allows the test specificity–sensitivity ratio to be maximized, so adapting the colonoscopy rate to the facilities and funds available for screening.

Table 10.2 provides estimates of sensitivity of the different types of the FOBT, i.e., GFOBT and FIT. As a general rule, FITs are at the more sensitive end of the range while GFOBT tests vary widely across the range. A detailed comparison of the different FOBTs has been reported [9] and a recent study has shown a brush-sampling FIT to be more sensitive for cancers and advanced adenomas than even the more sensitive GFOBT [18]. A large-scale study of over 7000 people undergoing screening in California is informative in this respect [10]. It shows that an FIT achieves the same sensitivity as a sensitive GFOBT but with better specificity, i.e., fewer colonoscopies. FITs overcome most of the disadvantages presented by GFOBT and it has been concluded that FIT should replace GFOBT [9,18,20].

Table 10.3 Nature of randomized controlled trials of two-step screening for colorectal cancer by guaiac-based fecal occult blood test

Site	Funen [21–23]	Gothenburg [24,25]	Minnesota [16,26,27]	Nottingham [28–30]	Burgundy [31]
Design					
Status	General population	General population	Volunteers	General population	General population
Age (years)	45–70	60–64	50–80	45–74	45–74
Randomized by:	Individual/household	Individual/household	Individual/household	Individual/household	District
Screen group size	30 967	34 144	15 570 (annual)	76 466	45 642
			15 587 (biennial)		
Control group size	30 966	34 164	15 394	76 384	45 557
GFOBT used	Hemoccult	Hemoccult – rehydrated	Hemoccult (17.5%)	Hemoccult	Hemoccult
			Hemoccult – rehydrated (82.5%)		
Program					
Period	1985–1995	1982–1984	1975–1992	1981–1991	1988–1998
Rounds of screening	5	2	Up to 10	5	6
Frequency	Biennial	18 months	Annual or biennial	Biennial	Biennial
Cumulative endoscopic follow-up[a]	5.3% (after 9 rounds)	6%	Annual – 38% Biennial – 28%	Unclear	3.7%

a Proportion of people undergoing colonoscopy after a positive GFOBT at least once during the trial.
GFOBT, guaiac-based fecal occult blood test.

Screening by fecal occult blood test: evidence of effectiveness

Six controlled trials of screening based on GFOBT have been reported [16,21–32]. The five of these where there was no planned intervention in the control arm [16,21–31] are summarized in Tables 10.3 and 10.4. Follow-up ranged from 8.3 to 18 years for these trials. In all of these trials invitees were asked to sample three separate stools for testing by the GFOBT, as it has been shown that when a cancer is present bleeding may be intermittent [33].

Intermediate outcomes

All studies reported a favorable shift in stage of diagnosed cancers, with more stage A cancers or fewer stage D cancers detected in the screened compared with control groups (Table 10.4).

Test positivity rates, and hence colonoscopy rates, varied greatly between the studies mainly because of the type of test used, but also because of the frequency of testing and the length of the trial (Table 10.3). In the studies where the GFOBT Hemoccult was used without rehydration, positivity rates were low and colonoscopy intervention rates fell in the range 2%–4% [21–23,28–31]. Where the fecal sample was rehydrated before development, the proportion of people undergoing colonoscopy at least once during the trial period was as high as 38% (Table 10.3) [16].

Complication rates for follow-up of positive screening tests are available for several of the trials (Table 10.4). In the

Minnesota trial there were 12 serious complications (perforations or major bleeds) per 10 000 offered screening [16]. No complications were reported in the Burgundy trial [31]. Higher rates were observed in Gothenburg [24]. Bowles and colleagues [34] reported a perforation rate alone of 12 in 9223 colonoscopies examined as part of a prospective audit and six deaths were considered as possibly being a result the procedure.

Behavioral outcomes

In the four true population studies (Funen, Gothenburg, Nottingham, and Burgundy), participation in the first round varied between 53% and 67% (Table 10.4). Participation fell off in the subsequent rounds where only initial participants were reoffered screening but it was maintained when non-participants were reoffered screening (e.g., Burgundy) [31]. When the study groups consisted of volunteers, as in the Minnesota study, initial participation was higher.

Impact on mortality from colorectal cancer

All of the trials offered FOBT on a *repeated* basis. The Gothenburg trial offered screening only twice, i.e., two rounds, and did not see a significant impact on mortality (Table 10.4). All other trials offered more than two rounds of screening and all showed a significant impact on colorectal cancer-related mortality based on an intention-to-screen basis. Analysis on the basis of intention-to-screen takes into account acceptance of screening, not just test performance, and is the public health outcome of greatest impact.

Table 10.4 Outcomes in randomized controlled trials of two-step screening for colorectal cancer by guaiac-based fecal occult blood test

Site	Funen [21–23]	Gothenburg [24,25]	Minnesota [16,26,27]	Nottingham [28–30]	Burgundy [31]
Intermediate measures					
Participation by round	First – 67% All – 46%	First – 63% Any – 68%	Any – 90%	Any – 60%	First – 52.8% Any – 69.5% All – 38.1%
Proportion of cancers at stage 1	Screen[a] – 36% Control – 11%	Screen[a] – 26% Control – 9%	Annual[b] – 33% Biennial[b] –29% Control – 25%	Screen[a] – 21% Control – 12%	Screen[a] – 42% Control – 17%
Sensitivity for cancer	46%	81%	Hemoccult – rehydrated – 92% Hemoccult – 81%	59%	40.1% (computed from screen-detected plus interval cancers)
Main colorectal cancer measures					
Mortality on intention-to-screen basis, OR (CI) (follow-up duration)	0.82 (0.68–0.99) (10 years)	0.88 (0.69–1.12) (8.3 years) [25]	Annual – 0.67 (0.51–0.83) (13 years) Biennial – 0.79 (0.62–0.97) (13 years)	0.86 (0.74–0.99) (7.8 years)	0.84 (0.71–0.99) (11 years)
Participant mortality, OR (CI)	0.66 (0.54–0.81) (7 rounds)	Not stated	Not stated	0.61 (0.50–0.74)	0.67 (0.56–0.81)
Incidence of cancer			Annual – 0.80 (0.70–0.90) (18 years) Biennial – 0.83 (0.78–0.94) (18 years)		1.01 (0.91–1.12) (11 years)
Major complications – colonoscopy		3/2296	15/12 246	"No deaths"	"None"

a Screen-detected lesions not whole screening cohort.
b Whole screening cohort.
CI, confidence interval; OR, odds ratio.

From Table 10.4 it can be seen that biennial screening with Hemoccult (not rehydrated) led to reductions in mortality of 14%–18% (Funen, Nottingham, and Burgundy trials [21,28,31]). A meta-analysis of the early results indicated a reduction in colorectal cancer mortality of 16% [25].

This effect on mortality seems modest but randomized controlled trials tend to underestimate the actual benefit of screening because of nonparticipation in the screened group and uncontrolled access to screening in the control group [35]. A better guide for magnitude of effect comes from the Funen, Nottingham, and Burgundy trials of actual participation in biennial screening with Hemoccult; mortality was reduced by 33%–41% in participants.

The Minnesota trial screened annually and used rehydration of Hemoccult to improve sensitivity [16]; it observed the greatest reduction in mortality on an intention-to-screen basis of 33%. The relative contribution of each is unclear because biennial screening in the Minnesota trial using rehydrated Hemoccult achieved a 21% reduction in mortality compared to the 14%–18% achieved with biennial Hemoccult in

Europe. However, the Minnesota trial is the most informative for the magnitude of benefit because it had the best participation rate and the longest follow-up.

Impact on incidence (Table 10.4)

Cumulative incidence rates for colorectal cancer did not differ between the controls or screened groups in any of the trials by 13 years of follow-up. However, the Minnesota study by 18 years of follow-up (the longest) showed a significant impact on incidence whether screening was annual or biennial [27]. It seems likely that the higher sensitivity of rehydrated Hemoccult and the higher colonoscopy rate have resulted in a better detection (and thus removal) of adenomas.

Doctor's office or home-based fecal sampling?

Performing an in-office GFOBT as part of a digital rectal examination has been common practice [36]. However, usually only one stool sample, rather than the recommended three, is obtained. The patient has not usually undertaken dietary preparation, which increases the risk of falsepositives with

GFOBT [14], and there is always the concern that digital rectal examination will generate minor trauma [37]. FOBT as part of a digital rectal examination was only recently evaluated, in 2005, in a large group of asymptomatic subjects [38]. It was found that sensitivity for neoplasia was much better if 3-day sampling was performed compared to a single in-office test and a negative test did not reduce the odds of cancer being present. Screening based on digital sampling of stool as part of a rectal examination is not recommended.

Endoscopic screening tests: evidence of effectiveness

While the largest population screening trials have been undertaken using FOBT, the use of flexible sigmoidoscopy and colonoscopy for screening is also supported by evidence of impact on mortality of colorectal cancer.

Screening by flexible sigmoidoscopy

The evidence for efficacy of screening sigmoidoscopy comes from case–control studies, the design and outcomes of which are summarized in Table 10.5. In a case–control study of 66 subjects dying from colorectal cancer, the risk of dying was reduced by a single-screening flexible sigmoidoscopy (odds ratio [OR] 0.21; confidence interval [CI] 0.08–0.52) [39]. A similar study involving 261 cases of distal colorectal cancer found an adjusted OR, i.e., risk of death, of 0.41 (CI 0.25–0.69) in those who had had a rigid sigmoidoscopy within 10 years [40]. In both studies, the reduction in risk was limited to rectal and distal colonic lesions, i.e., to lesions within reach. More recent studies of flexible sigmoidoscopy (Table 10.5) continue to support the association [41,42] with similar risk reductions and benefit lasting 10 years or more after the procedure. Mandel [35] provides a critique such case–control studies, pointing out that all such studies are liable to biases that overestimate the effect relative to randomized trials.

Screening sigmoidoscopy is challenged on the grounds that it represents an incomplete examination of the colon, albeit in the region where cancers are more likely [43] and if one is going to the trouble of performing an endoscopic examination, why not perform colonoscopy. Others see it as an efficient way to access a majority of colonic neoplasia at low cost, and include polypectomy as part of the procedure [44].

Table 10.5 Outcomes in case–control and cohort studies addressing impact of endoscopic screening on colorectal cancer

Country	Design	Population	Intervention	Result	Duration of benefit	Reference
USA	Case–control	Dead from CRC, $n = 66$	Single flexible sigmoidoscopy	Dying from distal CRC, OR 0.21 (CI 0.08–0.52)	10 years	[39]
USA	Case–control	Dead from distal CRC, $n = 261$	Rigid sigmoidoscopy	Dying from distal CRC, OR 0.41 (CI 0.25–0.69)	10 years	[40]
USA	Case–control	"Incident CRC"	"Sigmoidoscopy"	Sigmoidoscopy done, OR 0.56 (men, CI 0.44–0.77). Similar in women, minimal impact on proximal CRC		[41]
USA	Case–control	Cases of distal CRC, $n = 1026$	Screening sigmoidoscopy	Sigmoidoscopy done, OR 0.24 (CI 0.17–0.33)	16 years	[42]
Germany	Case–control	Cases of CRC, $n = 320$	Sigmoidoscopy or colonoscopy	Endoscopy done, OR 0.28 (CI 0.16–0.48)	> 10 years	[50]
Israel	Case–control	Cases of CRC, $n = 40$ high-risk surveillance	Colonoscopy	Colonoscopy done, 48.7% of controls compared with 2.5% cases ($P < 0.05$)		[51]
Norway	Cohort	Screened vs not screened, $n = 400$ and $n = 399$, randomized	Flexible sigmoidoscopy initially, subsequent colonoscopy if neoplasia found	Developing CRC, RR 0.20 (CI 0.03–0.95)		[52]
Finland	Cohort	HNPCC complying vs refusing surveillance, $n = 133$ and $n = 119$	Colonoscopy at 3-yearly intervals	Developing CRC, 16% of surveillance vs 6% refusers ($P = 0.014$)		[53]

CI, confidence interval; CRC, colorectal cancer; HNPCC, hereditary nonpolyposis colorectal cancer; OR, odds ratio; RR, relative risk.

There are concerns about feasibility in terms of adequate numbers of proceduralists and inadequacy of reimbursement [45].

Until the randomized population studies underway in UK, Italy, and USA (the PLCO study) [46] are complete and adequate cost-effectiveness studies are undertaken, it is not possible to reach a firm conclusion on the place for flexible sigmoidoscopy in screening.

Screening by colonoscopy

Colonoscopy has long been established as a powerful diagnostic tool for colorectal neoplasia. It is also therapeutic in that successful removal of many adenomas and even early malignant polyps can be undertaken during the procedure. Cohort studies have demonstrated that polypectomy in people prone to develop polyps reduces the risk of cancer [47]. The technology is well established and the reader is referred to other relevant chapters for further discussion on its implementation and practice. Colonoscopy as a screening test is often justified on the basis that it is the most accurate test. Accuracy, however, should not be the sole criterion for choosing a screening test [6,48,49].

The evidence for efficacy of screening colonoscopy for reducing risk of or mortality from colorectal cancer comes from a few case–control studies and small randomized studies [50–53], summarized in Table 10.5. The magnitude of benefit seems large but the studies are small and there are several biases that magnify the effect [35]. The largest, a case–control study of 320 cases, found an OR of 0.28 (0.16–0.48) for diagnosis of colorectal cancer where screening sigmoidoscopy or colonoscopy had been undertaken [50].

Further evidence to support the use of screening colonoscopy comes from the FOBT trials because without colonoscopic follow-up of a positive test, these trials would not have shown benefit. Some argue that further proof of efficacy, in the form of randomized controlled trials, is unnecessary [54] because colonoscopy is more accurate.

Colonoscopic screening has been calculated to be a cost-effective strategy. Several studies have examined effectiveness and incremental cost-effectiveness of multiple screening strategies [48] and two found colonoscopy every 10 years to be the most effective [55,56]. In contrast, a model developed by Lieberman [57] showed that fecal occult blood testing alone was the most cost-effective strategy, but colonoscopy every 10 years became the most cost-effective strategy if the cost for diagnostic colonoscopy was under US$ 750.

How often should endoscopic screening be performed?

For flexible sigmoidoscopy, 5-yearly screening intervals are recommended based on the apparent protection for at least 5 years shown in the case–control studies. Screening flexible sigmoidoscopy may be performed in combination with GFOBT for better detection of proximal lesions although there is little evidence to indicate how much gain is achieved.

For screening colonoscopy, the question of how often to do it in people with average risk remains unanswered. There has been no large prospective study reported that addresses this. If screening colonoscopy is to be a once-only event, then the age at which it is performed is critical [58]. Once-only screening is only sound if we can be confident that most cases destined to develop colorectal cancer in their lifetime will have a "sentinel" lesion at the time the colonoscopy is performed.

When choosing an interval for screening by colonoscopy, there are clues from the few case–control studies where intervals of at least 5 years, and sometimes 10 years, seem justified [50–52]. Some consensus recommendations, e.g., that of the USPSTF [48], recommends 10 years in average risk people. However, cancers may be missed and interval cancers occur in surveillance programs in high-risk individuals [59,60] Without evidence from formal randomized trials, it is not possible to be confident about the appropriate interval.

Is colonoscopy the screening test of first choice?

There are several perspectives to this question and they arise from the two main contexts of screening discussed above.

In the context of individualized screening, differential sensitivity of colonoscopy against FOBT or flexible sigmoidoscopy becomes a consideration in practice, because people often want what is perceived as being best. Colonoscopy is clearly more sensitive [61–63].

On the other hand, some argue that there is a strong case for caution before colonoscopy is accepted as the ideal screening test [48], especially as part of a programmed public-health initiative. Many points must be considered.

• The sensitivity of colonoscopy compared to once-only sigmoidoscopy or FOBT overestimates the benefit. Repeated application of FOBT results in compounding of sensitivity, probably because the dwell time of a curable lesion is longer than the screening interval, meaning that curable lesions may still be detected in a subsequent round of testing. This is borne out in practice: sensitivity of once-only Hemoccult has been shown to be less than 40% [10] yet cumulative sensitivity of unhydrated Hemoccult in the Minnesota trial was 80% (Table 10.4).

• Is the lower sensitivity of the simpler screening tests for advanced neoplasms truly unacceptable? For flexible sigmoidoscopy, the deduced miss rate for advanced proximal neoplasms has been estimated at 24% [61] but the risk of advanced proximal neoplasms progressing to fatal cancer is relatively low, estimated at 1% per year [64–66].

• Colonoscopy is not perfect in practice and lesions are missed [59, 60, 67–69]. Flat lesions in particular are easy to miss during conventional endoscopy [44] and flat or depressed adenomas may progress more rapidly to cancer than polypoid adenomas. If the cancers that are most likely to be fatal are those that develop and grow rapidly [48, 70], there is an advantage to a screening program that allows multiple chances to detect an existing lesion rather than testing just once every 10 years [48,70].

- The serious complication rate with colonoscopic screening is not trivial. One study, where all procedures were carried out by skilled operators, reported a rate of 33 per 10 000 people screened [34]. This is over twice the rate with FOBT screening (Table 10.3).

Colonoscopy may uncover the largest number of neoplasms and minimize the likelihood of missing any colorectal neoplasia but screening policy is not decided by effectiveness alone. If alternative screening strategies can significantly reduce the death rate from colorectal cancer but at an acceptable or lower cost and risk than those associated with colonoscopy, these strategies would be appropriate. The incremental effectiveness of colonoscopy needs to be large enough to justify its disadvantages (considerable manpower and financial resources, bowel preparation, conscious sedation, and serious potential complications). The millions (i.e., almost 95% of the general population) who will undergo colonoscopic screening for no apparent gain are subject to harms that could cumulatively outweigh the benefit to the much smaller number found to have significant colorectal neoplasia [49].

Summary of the effectiveness of available screening tests

Guaiac-based fecal occult blood tests and fecal immunochemical tests

It can be concluded from this evidence that screening of the general population, most of whom will lack high-risk factors, using a GFOBT is justified. The data show that screening should be repeated, with intervals of 1 year possibly giving a better effect than biennial screening. It should be noted that participants in the GFOBT trials were asked to sample three stools in the home environment. There is no evidence that collecting fewer samples by digital rectal examination in the physician's office is effective. Use of a sensitive GFOBT is preferred to rehydration of Hemoccult. Overall, FITs overcome most of the disadvantages presented by GFOBTs. Based on performance, FIT should replace GFOBT in screening for colorectal cancer [18].

Such recommendations are consistent with consensus recommendations from many national or professional groups [17,48]. Most bodies recommend that screening starts in the general population (i.e., undefined or average risk) at age 50 years, because around 90% of colorectal cancer occurs after that age. Cost-effectiveness of screening the general population at a younger age is of questionable value.

Colonoscopy and flexible sigmoidoscopy

On the basis of the studies described above it can be concluded that endoscopic screening will be effective. However, compared to GFOBT, we lack evidence from randomized controlled trials that address acceptability, incremental benefit and complication rates – it is important to understand the balance of risks and benefits. Because case–control studies tend to overestimate benefit, we cannot be certain of the magnitude of incremental benefit provided by endoscopic screening compared with FOBT screening.

Recent developments in screening tests

A recent American Gastroenterological Association Future Trends Committee report on emerging screening and diagnostic technologies for colorectal cancer [19] identified a range of tests and procedures that might be appropriate. These include proteomics or the analysis of broad protein patterns, making it possible to assess small amounts of protein for the presence of identified cancer markers using new protein assessment tools and computerized artificial intelligence analysis. In addition, high-magnification chromoscopic endoscopy [71], spectroscopy, and optical coherence tomography show promise as adjuncts to traditional colonoscopy. Fecal DNA testing also provides new options. The better studied advances, such as stool DNA testing and computed tomography (CT) colonography, will be discussed in some detail.

Fecal DNA tests

Cells shed from cancers and adenomas are detectable in the stools [72]. Detection of molecular or genetic events that either cause cancer or else reflect development of neoplasia could theoretically be useful in selecting who undergoes colonoscopy. Because of the molecular heterogeneity of DNA in neoplasms, selecting the best panel of markers represents a challenge.

The first large-scale evaluation of the value of fecal DNA testing (using a 21-mutation multitarget panel) as a possible first-step test in two-step screening for colorectal cancer has recently been reported [73]. The present version of the stool DNA test is costly (in excess of US$ 400) and requires a cumbersome stool collection that needs to be rapidly delivered to the processing laboratory [74]. The comparators were colonoscopy as the diagnostic reference standard and Hemoccult II (unhydrated) as the proven first-step screening test. A cohort of 4404 subjects completed all three tests and their results were analyzed in a subgroup of 2507, which included all subjects found to have neoplasia. The detection rate of cancer using the fecal DNA panel was 16 of 31 (52%) compared with 4 of 31 (13%, $P = 0.003$) for Hemoccult II. The reported sensitivity of Hemoccult II was substantially lower than that reported in other studies for one-time testing [10] and so it cannot be concluded that Hemoccult, a much cheaper test, is necessarily inferior. The performance of both tests for detecting advanced adenomas was similarly disappointing; 61 of 403 (15.1%) for fecal DNA compared with 43 of 403 (10.7%) for Hemoccult II. In those with negative colonoscopy,

5.6% had tested positive on fecal DNA compared with 4.8% on Hemoccult II (specificities of 94.4% and 95.2%, respectively). Fecal DNA testing did not identify the majority of neoplastic lesions found at colonoscopy and in this format it does not yet represent an advance over the much cheaper FOBT types [74].

It is expected that within the next decade, this innovative technology will eventually lead to more specific and simple tests that will provide an effective first test in a two-step screening process. The newer stool molecular tests might be based on RNA or protein markers that are subject to lesser heterogeneity than DNA tests. A more detailed review is presented by Young [20].

Computed tomography and magnetic resonance imaging colonography

Virtual colonoscopy, also known preferably as computed tomographic colonography (CTC) was first described in 1994. It is an imaging method for detecting pathology in the colon and rectum that is less invasive than colonoscopy [75].

It has been pointed out that CTC avoids some of the drawbacks of colonoscopy, such as the need for intravenous sedation, recovery time, and assistance with transport [76]. The risks of bleeding, perforation, and side effects of sedatives will be much less than with colonoscopy. As the majority of screening colonoscopies identify no clinically significant pathology, CTC, as with other first-step tests such as FOBT, should reduce unnecessary colonoscopies.

With the latest equipment, CTC takes 10–15 min. Advances in software now allow for typical reading times of 10 min or less and final reports can be issued within 2 h. It might eventually prove possible to avoid colonic cleansing using "preparation-less" CTC where an ingested contrast material is used to "tag" lumenal content. Imaging software digitally subtracts tagged material by a process known as electronic cleansing [77].

Performance characteristics of screening CTC have been difficult to assess because CTC is a technology undergoing rapid improvement. In a metaanalysis of 33 studies providing data on 6393 patients [78], sensitivity was 48% for polyps less than 6 mm, 70% for polyps 6–9 mm, and 85% for polyps larger than 9 mm. Specificity also varied according to size: 92% for detection of polyps less than 6 mm, 93% for polyps 6–9 mm and 97% for polyps larger than 9 mm. A weakness of the Mulhall analysis was that only a few studies included in the metaanalysis used the latest technology.

The use of the latest technology including electronic cleansing and multidetector CT scanners which permit faster higher resolution imaging than single detector scanners has been reported on by Pickhardt and colleagues [68]. They prospectively evaluated 1233 average-risk asymptomatic adults who underwent CTC and same-day conventional colonoscopy. The sensitivity of CTC for adenomatous polyps was 93.8% for polyps at least 10 mm in diameter, 93.9% for polyps at least 8 mm in diameter, and 88.7% for polyps at

least 6 mm in diameter. The sensitivities of optical colonoscopy for adenomatous polyps were 87.5%, 91.5%, and 92.3% for the three sizes of polyps, respectively.

While such results are excellent, the practical application of screening CTC requires resolution of the following factors [76,79,80].

- Results in practice are not comparable to those of specialized centers.
- Can some polyps be safely left in place because chance of progression is very low. In other words, which types of lesions require immediate follow-up colonoscopy?
- CTC would ideally be coordinated with follow-up colonoscopy on the same day.
- The workload generated by false-positive CTC, caused by fecal matter, nonadenomatous polyps, or insignificant adenomas, remains unclear.
- Detection rate of flat adenomas by CTC is unclear [81].
- Population acceptance of a procedure that is uncomfortable and that requires time and possibly bowel preparation remains unclear. "Preparation-less" CTC is an unknown at present.
- The impact of finding extracolonic pathology is unclear. One study has undertaken a cost-effectiveness analysis [82]; 118 of 432 subjects (27.3%) had extracolonic lesions. In 7.4% it was felt that findings were clinically relevant and in 2.1% it was felt that subjects may derive a clinical benefit from treatment. Clinical follow-up added just 14.2% to the cost. Such findings suggest that extracolonic lesions might not pose a major problem.
- The cost-effectiveness of population screening with CTC is unclear.

Computed tomographic colonography has the potential to be a valid first-step screening test for colorectal cancer. It can accurately exclude the presence of large polyps and, by inference, cancer with high confidence. Technology improvement is likely to make it more sensitive for target lesions and perhaps more acceptable to those being screened, in the not too distant future. If shown to be cost-effective and applicable to large populations of average risk individuals, it may stand beside other established first-step screening tests such as FOBT, flexible sigmoidoscopy, and colonoscopy.

Other considerations in screening practice

As screening is a process, it is important that each step is feasible, otherwise benefit will not be obtained. Sustainability is also important because screening is unlikely to have a major impact if it is a one-time event in a person's lifetime [74].

Without participation there can be no detection [6]. Removal of dietary restrictions in several populations has been shown to enhance participation in screening with FOBT [83], in one study by 28% [84]. The brush sampling method also simplifies the process and enhances it by 30%. Together, these two advances increase participation by 66% [84]. Obviously, FIT is superior to GFOBT in terms of both participation and performance and should replace GFOBT in two-step screening.

Capacity to undertake colonoscopy, whether as a follow-up assessment of those with a positive FOBT or as a one-step colonoscopic screening test, is critical. Many countries, perhaps all, are unable to comprehensively resource one-step colonoscopic screening. Evidence suggests that the manpower necessary to provide a skilled colonoscopic examination for all age-eligible people in the United States is insufficient [85,86].

Managing risk and duty of care

It is of paramount importance that risks as well as benefits are carefully explained to those being invited to take part. Informed consent must be obtained and the patient must be told that even with colonoscopy, it is possible that polyps or cancers may be missed. As two-step screening is effective and directs colonoscopy to those more likely to have neoplasia [6], there is a duty of care to offer this option. It is important to indicate that better sensitivity of colonoscopy is at the cost of more procedures and higher risk of complication to the screened person.

Conclusions

Screening for colorectal cancer detects unsuspected neoplasia and leads to its removal such that death or suffering from colorectal cancer is avoided. Proof of the value of screening is available even when studies are evaluated at a population level on an intention-to-screen basis where nonparticipating invitees are included in the analysis.

Two-step screening based on FOBT as the initial test is proven to be effective by population randomized controlled trials. FIT has emerged as the FOBT of choice because of a better sensitivity/specificity balance than GFOBT and better population acceptance. Collection of two or three samples for FOBT testing is necessary and there is no evidence that a single fecal sample collected by digital examination in the office is an effective screening strategy. Flexible sigmoidoscopy, while effective as judged from case–control studies, is initially invasive, inconvenient, and uncomfortable compared to FOBT. It will miss proximal lesions although misses can be reduced by coupling with FOBT. The results of the randomized trials of flexible sigmoidoscopic screening are needed before a clear conclusion can be reached on its role.

One-step screening by colonoscopy is likely to provide benefit but incremental cost–benefit and risk–benefit relative to FOBT screening is not clear. Colonoscopy is more likely to be accepted in the context of individual screening where there is face-to-face discussion with a physician. Acceptance at the population level where the offer of screening is more impersonal but also more consistent with the modern lifestyle, is unclear and not likely to be good. Estimates of the workforce required to deliver comprehensive colonoscopic screening raise doubt as to the practicality of using colonoscopy as a public-health initiative.

Fecal DNA tests and CTC are potential additions to FOBT in two-step screening but much more data on their effectiveness, acceptability, and cost–benefit are needed before they can be accepted for routine use. Stool molecular tests hold great promise for the future, especially if they can serve as sensitive and specific tests to identify those who have adenomas.

Screening should not be seen as merely the performance of a one-time test. Repeated testing improves benefit.

On balance, screening of average-risk subjects by the one-step or two-step approach is appropriate practice, starting at age 50 years. An FOBT, preferably of the FIT type, should be undertaken at least as frequently as 2-yearly (biennial), while the maximum safe interval for screening by flexible sigmoidoscopy and colonoscopy remains to be ascertained from prospective studies.

References

1. Morrison AS. Screening. In: Rothman KJ, Greenland S (eds). Modern Epidemiology. Philadelphia PA: Lippincott-Raven, 1998;499.
2. Watson JMG, Junger G. Principles and Practice of Screening for Disease. WHO Public Health Papers No. 34. New York: World Health Organization, 1968.
3. NHMRC. Guidelines for the Prevention, Early Detection and Management of Colorectal Cancer. Canberra: National Health and Medical Research Council, 1999.
4. Goyder E, Barratt A, Irwig LM. Telling people about screening programmes and screening test results: how can we do it better? J Med Screen 2000;7:123.
5. Rozen P, Young GP, Levin B (eds). Colorectal Cancer in Clinical Practice: Prevention and Early Detection, 2nd edn. London: Isis Publications, 2005.
6. Young GP, Macrae FA, St John DJB. Clinical methods of early detection: basis, use and evaluation. In: Young GP, Rozen P, Levin B (eds). Prevention and Early Detection of Colorectal Cancer. London: Saunders, 1996;241.
7. Young GP. Screening for colorectal cancer: an introduction. In: Young GP, Rozen P, Levin B (eds). Prevention and Early Detection of Colorectal Cancer. London: Saunders, 1996;271.
8. Young GP. Fecal immunochemical tests (FIT) vs. office-based guaiac fecal occult blood test (FOBT). Practical Gastroenterol 2004;28:46.
9. Young GP, St John DJB, Winawer SJ, et al. Choice of fecal occult blood tests for colorectal cancer screening: recommendations based on performance characteristics in population studies. Am J Gastroenterol 2002;97:2499.
10. Allison JE, Tekawa IS, Ransom LJ, Adrain AL. A comparison of fecal occult blood tests for colorectal cancer screening. N Engl J Med 1996;334:155.
11. Young GP, St John DJB. Faecal occult blood tests: choice, usage and clinical applications. Clin Biochem Rev 1992;13;161.
12. Selinger RR, Norman S, Dominitz JA. Failure of health care professionals to interpret fecal occult blood tests accurately. Am J Med 2003;114:64.
13. Chin CL, Fox GB, Hradil VP, et al. Pharmacological MRI in awake rats reveals neural activity in area postrema and nucleus tractus solitarius: relevance as a potential biomarker for detecting drug-induced emesis. Neuroimage 2006;33:1152–1160.

14. Sinatra M, St John DJB, Young GP. Interference of plant peroxidases with guaiac-based fecal occult blood tests is avoidable. Clin Chem 1999;45:123.

15. Wong BC, Wong WM, Cheung KL, et al. A sensitive guaiac faecal occult blood test is less useful than an immunochemical test for colorectal cancer screening in a Chinese population. Aliment Pharmacol Ther 2003;18:941.

16. Mandel JS, Bond JH, Church TR, et al. Reducing mortality from colorectal cancer by screening for fecal occult blood. Minnesota Colon Cancer Control Study. N Engl J Med 1993;328:1365.

17. Winawer SJ, Fletcher RH, Rex D, et al. Colorectal cancer screening and surveillance: clinical guidelines and rationale US Multisociety Task Force on Colorectal Cancer. Gastroenterology 2003;124:544.

18. Smith A, Young GP, Cole SR, Bampton P. Comparison of a brush-sampling fecal immunochemical test for hemoglobin with a sensitive guaiac-based fecal occult blood test in detection of colorectal neoplasia. Cancer 2006;107:2152.

19. Regueiro CR AGA Future Trends Committee Report: colorectal cancer: a qualitative review of emerging screening and diagnostic technologies. Gastroenterology 2005;129:1083.

20. Young GP. Molecular approaches to stool screening for colorectal cancer. Curr Colorectal Cancer Rep 2006;2:30.

21. Kronborg O, Fenger C, Olsen J, et al. Randomised study of screening for colorectal cancer with faecal-occult-blood test. Lancet. 1996;348:1467.

22. Jorgensen OD, Kronborg O, Fenger C. A randomised study of screening for colorectal cancer using faecal occult blood testing: results after 13 years and seven biennial screening rounds. Gut 2002;50:29.

23. Kronborg O, Jorgensen OD, Fenger C, et al. Randomized study of biennial screening with a faecal occult blood test: results after nine screening rounds. Scand J Gastroenterol 2004;39:846.

24. Kewenter J, Brevinge H, Engaras B, et al. Results of screening, rescreening, and follow-up in a prospective randomized study for detection of colorectal cancer by fecal occult blood testing. Scand J Gastroenterol 1994;29:468.

25. Towler BP, Irwig L, Glasziou P, et al. Screening for colorectal cancer using the faecal occult blood test, Hemoccult (review). Cochrane Database Syst Rev 2000;(2):CD001216.

26. Mandel JS, Church TR, Ederer F, et al. Colorectal cancer mortality: effectiveness of biennial screening for fecal occult blood. J Natl Cancer Inst 1999;91:434.

27. Mandel JS, Church TR, Bond JH, et al. The effect of fecal occult-blood screening on the incidence of colorectal cancer. N Engl J Med 2000;343:1603.

28. Hardcastle JD, Chamberlain JO, Robinson MH, et al. Randomised controlled trial of faecal-occult-blood screening for colorectal cancer. Lancet 1996;348:1472.

29. Moss SM, Hardcastle JD, Coleman DA, et al. Interval cancers in a randomized controlled trial of screening for colorectal cancer using a faecal occult blood test. Int J Epidemiol 1999;28:386.

30. Robinson MH, Hardcastle JD, Moss SM, et al. The risks of screening: data from the Nottingham randomised controlled trial of faecal occult blood screening for colorectal cancer. Gut 1999;45:588.

31. Faivre J, Dancourt V, Lejeune C, et al. Reduction in colorectal cancer mortality by fecal occult blood screening in a French controlled study. Gastroenterology 2004;126:1674.

32. Screening for colorectal cancer with fecal occult blood testing and sigmoidoscopy. J Natl Cancer Inst 1993;85:1311.

33. Macrae FA, St John DJB, Relationship between patterns of bleeding and Hemoccult sensitivity in patients with colorectal cancers or adenomas. Gastroenterology 1982;82:891.

34. Bowles CJ, Leicester R, Romaya C, et al. A prospective study of colonoscopy practice in the UK today: are we adequately prepared for national colorectal cancer screening tomorrow? Gut 2004;53:277.

35. Mandel JS. Sigmoidoscopy screening probably works, but how well is still unknown. J Natl Cancer Inst 2003;95:571.

36. Bini EJ, Rajapaksa RC, Weinshel EH. The findings and impact of nonrehydrated guaiac examination of the rectum (FINGER) study: a comparison of 2 methods of screening for colorectal cancer in asymptomatic average-risk patients. Arch Intern Med 1999;159:2022.

37. Zhang B, Nakama H, Fattah AS, et al. Lower specificity of occult-blood test on stool collected by digital rectal examination. Hepatogastroenterology 2002;49:165.

38. Collins JF, Lieberman DA, Durbin TE, et al. Accuracy of screening for fecal occult blood on a single stool sample obtained by digital rectal examination: a comparison with recommended sampling practice. Ann Intern Med 2005;142:81.

39. Newcomb PA, Norfleet RG, Storer BE, et al. Screening sigmoidoscopy and colorectal cancer mortality. J Natl Cancer Inst 1992;84:1572.

40. Selby JV, Friedman GD, Quesenberry CP Jr, Weiss NS. A case control study of screening sigmoidoscopy and mortality from colorectal cancer. N Engl J Med 1992;326:653.

41. Slattery ML, Edwards SL, Ma KN, et al. Colon cancer screening, lifestyle, and risk of colon cancer. Cancer Causes Control 2000;11:555.

42. Newcomb PA, Storer BE, Morimoto LM, et al. Long-term efficacy of sigmoidoscopy in the reduction of colorectal cancer incidence. J Natl Cancer Inst 2003;95:622.

43. Podolsky DK. Going the distance – the case for true colorectal-cancer screening. N Engl J Med 2000;343:207.

44. Atkin WS, Saunders BP. Surveillance guidelines after removal of colorectal adenomatous polyps. Gut 2002:51(S5);6.

45. Shaheen NJ, Ransohoff DF. Sigmoidoscopy costs and the limits of altruism. Am J Med 1999;107:286.

46. Lin O, Roy P, Schembre DB, et al. Screening sigmoidoscopy and colonoscopy for reducing colorectal cancer mortality in asymptomatic persons (protocol). Cochrane Database Syst Rev 2005;3.

47. Winawer SJ, Zauber AG, Ho MN, et al. Prevention of colorectal cancer by colonoscopic polypectomy. The National Polyp Study Workgroup. N Engl J Med 1993;329:1977.

48. Pignone M, Saha S, Hoerger T, Mandelblatt J. Cost-effectiveness analyses of colorectal cancer screening: a systematic review for the U.S. Preventive Services Task Force. Ann Intern Med 2002;137:96.

49. Woolf SH. The best screening test for colorectal cancer – a personal choice. Editorial. N Engl J Med 2000;343:1641.

50. Brenner H, Arndt V, Sturmer T, et al. Long-lasting reduction of risk of colorectal cancer following screening endoscopy. Br J Cancer 2001;85:972.

51. Niv Y, Dickman R, Figer A, et al. Case–control study of screening colonoscopy in relatives of patients with colorectal cancer. Am J Gastroenterol 2003;98:486.

52. Thiis-Evensen E, Hoff G S, Sauar J, et al. Population-based surveillance by colonoscopy: effect on the incidence of colorectal cancer. Telemark polyp study I. Scand J Gastroenterol 1999;34:414.

53. Jarvinen HJ, Aarnio M, Mustonen H, et al. Controlled 15-year trial on screening for colorectal cancer in families with hereditary nonpolyposis colorectal cancer. Gastroenterology 2000;118:969.

54. Rex DK, Johnson DA, Lieberman DA, et al. Colorectal cancer prevention 2000: screening recommendations of the American College of Gastroenterology. Am J Gastroenterol 2000;95:868–877.

55. Khandker RK, Dulski JD, Kilpatrick JB, Ellis RP, Mitchell JB, Baine WB. A decision model and cost-effectiveness analysis of colorectal cancer screening and surveillance guidelines for average-risk adults. Int J Technol Assess Health Care 2000;16:799.

56. Sonnenberg A, Delco F, Inadomi JM. Cost-effectiveness of colonoscopy in screening for colorectal cancer. Ann Intern Med 2000;133:573.

57. Lieberman DA. Cost-effectiveness model for colon cancer screening. Gastroenterology 1995;109:1781.

58. Brenner H, Arndt V, Stegmaier C, et al. Reduction of clinically manifest colorectal cancer by endoscopic screening: empirical evaluation and comparison of screening at various ages. Eur J Cancer Prev 2005;14:231.

59. Robertson DJ. Colorectal cancer in patients under close colonoscopic surveillance. Gastroenterology 2005;129:34.

60. Bampton PA, Sandford JJ, Cole SR, et al. Interval faecal occult blood testing in a colonoscopy-based screening programme detects additional pathology. Gut 2005;54:803.

61. Lieberman DA, Weiss DG, Bond JH, et al. Use of colonoscopy to screen asymptomatic adults for colorectal cancer. N Engl J Med 2000;343:162.

62. Imperiale TF, Wagner DR, Lin CY, et al. Risk of advanced proximal neoplasms in asymptomatic adults according to the distal colorectal findings. N Engl J Med 2000;343:169.

63. Schoenfeld P, Cash B, Flood A, et al. Colonoscopic screening of average-risk women for colorectal neoplasia. N Engl J Med 2000;352:2061.

64. Ransohoff DF. Lessons from the UK sigmoidoscopy screening trial. Editorial. Lancet 2002;359:1266.

65. Stryker S, Wolff B, Culp C, et al. Natural history of untreated colonic polyps. Gastroenterology 1987;93:1009.

66. Eide T. Risk of colorectal cancer in adenoma bearing individuals within a defined population. Int J Cancer 1986;38:173.

67. Bressler B, Paszat LE, Vinden C, et al. Colonoscopic miss rates for right-sided colon cancer: a population-based analysis. Gastroenterology 2004;127;452.

68. Pickhardt PJ, Nugent PA, Mysliwiec PA, et al. Location of adenomas missed by colonoscopy. Ann Intern Med 2004;141:352.

69. Lieberman DA. Colonoscopy: as good as gold? Editorial. Ann Intern Med 2004;141:401.

70. Ransohoff DF. Colon cancer screening in 2005: status and challenges. Gastroenterology 2005;128:1685.

71. Lennon VA, Sas DF, Busk MF, et al. Enteric neuronal autoantibodies in pseudoobstruction with small-cell lung carcinoma. Gastroenterology 1991;100:137–142.

72. Osborn NK, Ahlquist DA. Stool screening for colorectal cancer: molecular approaches, Gastroenterology 2005;128:1.

73. Imperiale TF, Ransohoff DF, Itzkowitz SH, et al. Fecal DNA versus fecal occult blood for colorectal-cancer screening in an average-risk population. N Engl J Med 2004;351:2755.

74. Woolf SH. A smarter strategy? Reflections on fecal DNA screening for colorectal cancer. N Engl J Med 2004;351:2755.

75. Vining DJ, Gelfand DW. Non-invasive colonoscopy using helical CT scanning, 3D reconstruction and virtual reality. In: Syllabus: 23rd Annual Meeting, Society of Gastrointestinal Radiologists, Maui, Hawaii, 1994.

76. Morrin MM, LaMont TJ. Screening virtual colonoscopy – ready for prime time? Editorial. N Engl J Med 2003;349:2261.

77. Nicholson FB, Taylor S, Halligan S, Kamm MA. Recent developments in CT colonography. Clin Radiol 2005;60:105.

78. Mulhall BP, Veerappan GR, Jackson JL. Meta-analysis: computed tomographic colonography. Ann Intern Med 2005;142:635.

79. Ransohoff DF. Virtual colonoscopy – what it can do vs what it will do. JAMA 2004;291:1772.

80. Imperiale TF. Editorial. Can computed tomographic colonography become a "good" screening test? Ann Intern Med 2005;142:669.

81. Van Gelder RE, Florie J, Stoker J. Colorectal cancer screening and surveillance with CT colonography: current controversies and obstacles. Abdom Imaging 2005;30:5.

82. Chin MWS, Mendelson RM, Edwards J, Foster NM. Clinical significance of extracolonic findings in a community screening programme. Am J Gastroenterol 2005;100:2771.

83. Cole SR, Young GP. Participation in faecal occult blood test-based screening for colorectal cancer is reduced by dietary restriction, Med J Aust 2001;175:195.

84. Cole SR, Young GP, Esterman A, et al. A randomized trial of the impact of new fecal hemoglobin test technologies on population participation in screening for colorectal cancer. J Med Screening 2003;10:117.

Approach to the patient with unintentional weight loss

Andrew W. DuPont

Etiology, 183

Diagnosis, 188

Treatment and prognosis, 189

Body weight is determined by the balance of caloric intake, activity level, and metabolic rate. Significant alterations in this balance lead to either weight loss or gain. In healthy individuals, body weight typically increases gradually throughout life from early adulthood as a result of an increase in body fat [1]. Overall weight increases, despite a steady decline in lean body mass; therefore substantial weight loss in older individuals should not be dismissed. Weight loss is classified as intentional or unintentional. Unintentional weight loss is most often defined as an involuntary decrease in body weight of at least 5% of the usual body weight in the previous 6–12 months. Unintentional weight loss is usually associated with considerable anxiety for the patient, may be associated with increased mortality and morbidity, and can present a diagnostic challenge to the physician because of multiple potential etiologies.

Involuntary weight loss is not an uncommon entity and has been documented in 1.3%–3% of hospital admissions [2–5]. Unintentional weight loss, which appears more common in the elderly, has been documented in 50%–65% of nursing home residents [6].

Based on available data, approximately 50% of cases of unintentional weight loss are caused by organic diseases including malignancy, and 20%–60% are attributable to psychiatric disorders (Table 11.1) [2–5,7–10]. Results of these studies have demonstrated:
- malignancy is not the most common cause of weight loss
- the etiology is typically established early in the evaluation without extensive testing
- psychiatric disorders are common causes, especially in the elderly.

Principles of Clinical Gastroenterology. Edited by Tadataka Yamada, David H. Alpers, Anthony N. Kalloo, Neil Kaplowitz, Chung Owyang, and Don W. Powell. © 2008 Blackwell Publishing. ISBN 978-1-4051-69103

Mortality in patients with unintentional weight loss has been reported to be as high as 25% during 1-year follow-up [7], and up to 38% when followed for 2 years [3].

Etiology

Although the potential causes of unintentional weight loss are fairly extensive and the mechanism may be multifactorial, the underlying etiology contributes to weight loss by a limited number of physiological processes. These include:
- diminished intake of calories due to anorexia, nausea, or altered smell, taste, or satiety
- loss of calories from the urinary tract in poorly controlled diabetes mellitus or from the gastrointestinal tract in cases of malabsorption
- altered metabolism due to endocrine disorders, increased physical activity, or malignancy.

Although many patients with unintentional weight loss will have loss of appetite, several clinical conditions are associated with weight loss and an increase in appetite; these include hyperthyroidism, pheochromocytoma, significantly increased physical activity, uncontrolled diabetes mellitus, and some cases of malabsorption.

Causes of involuntary weight loss in the geriatric population have been broadly categorized by Morley [11] into social, psychological, medical, or age-related factors (Table 11.2). Robbins [12] has described the "nine Ds" of geriatric weight loss:
- depression
- disease (acute and chronic)
- dementia
- diarrhea
- dysphagia
- dysgeusia
- drugs

Table 11.1 Clinical studies evaluating causes of unintentional weight loss

Etiology (%)[a]	Hernandez et al. [2] (*n* = 276)	Rabinovitz et al. [3] (*n* = 154)	Lankisch et al. [4] (*n* = 158)	Huerta & Viniegra [5] (*n* = 50)	Marton et al. [7] (*n* = 91)	Thompson & Morris [8] (*n* = 45)	Leduc et al. [9] (*n* = 105)	Levine [10] (*n* = 107)	Bilbao-Garay et al. [13] (*n* = 78)
Malignancy	35	36	24	10	19	16	1	6	23
Organic (other than malignancy)	35	30	49	34	50	40	28	36	32
Gastrointestinal disorders	8	17	19		14	11	8	6	6
Other organic disorders	26	13	30		32	18	21	30	26
Psychiatric	24	10	11	42	9	20	60	22	33
Unknown	6	23	16	10	26	24	11	36	11

a Percentages may not equal 100% due to rounding and overlap in diagnostic studies.
n, number of patients in study.

Table 11.2 Causes of weight loss in the geriatric population

Social
Isolation
Poverty
Inadequate education
Lack of transportation
Unavailability of preferred foods
Urban decay

Psychological
Depression
Schizophrenia
Bereavement
Bulimia
Manipulation
Sociopathy
Late-life mania
Dementia
Conversion reaction
Anorexia nervosa
Anxiety
Alcoholism
Late-life paranoia
Excessive burden of life (food refusal)

Medical
Increased metabolism – hyperthyroidism, pheochromocytoma, Parkinson disease
Anorexia – drugs, intestinal ischemia, cancer, hyperparathyroidism
Swallowing problems – dysphagia, cerebrovascular accident
Malabsorption – celiac disease
Increased metabolism and anorexia – COPD, cardiac cachexia

Age-related
Impaired olfactory sensitivity
Appetite suppression
Impaired taste sensitivity

COPD, chronic obstructive pulmonary disease.
From Morley [11], with permission.

- dysfunction
- dentition.

In the majority of cases, the etiology of weight loss is identified; however, in up to one-third of patients the cause remains unknown. In general, those with an undetermined cause have a more favorable mortality rate compared with those having an established diagnosis [4,7,10].

Malignancy

In cases of unexplained weight loss, malignancy is understandably often the most feared underlying cause for patients, and is frequently thought to be the most common etiology by physicians. However, it has been shown not to be the explanation in the majority of patients with involuntary weight loss [2–5,7–10,13].

Weight loss may be the most common manifestation of advanced malignant disease and is present in up to 80% of terminal cases of cancer [14]. At the time of diagnosis, 80% of patients with upper gastrointestinal cancers and 60% with lung cancer have already undergone substantial weight loss [15]. In contrast to the majority of patients with gastric, pancreatic, lung, prostate, and colon cancer [16,17], hematological malignancies and breast cancer are less commonly associated with substantial weight loss [18]. Cachexia, which is defined as weight loss of at least 5% from baseline, is often multifactorial; it is associated with a poor prognosis; and in more than 20% of cases may be the direct cause of death [15]. Mechanisms of weight loss in malignancy include decreased food intake [19], increased adipose tissue lipolysis [20], increased muscle proteolysis [21], and increased resting energy expenditure [22]. Multiple proinflammatory cytokines, including interleukin-6 (IL-6), IL-1β, and tumor necrosis factor-α (TNF-α), are thought to contribute to anorexia and cachexia associated with malignancy [23–25]. Cytokine production in malignancy increases corticotropin-releasing hormone, which is a potent anorectic agent [26]. Increased inflammatory cytokines in malignancy also delay gastric emptying,

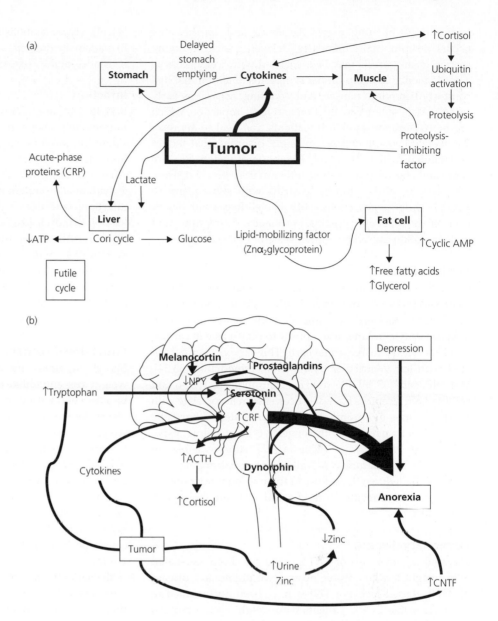

Figure 11.1 The peripheral **(a)** and central **(b)** mechanisms producing anorexia–cachexia syndrome in cancer. ACTH, adrenocorticotropic hormone; AMP, adenosine monophosphate; ATP, adenosine triphosphate; CRF, corticotropin-releasing factor; CNTF, ciliary neurotrophic factor; CRP, C-reactive protein; NPY, neuropeptide Y. Adapted from Morley et al [29], with permission from the American Society for Nutrition.

decrease serum albumin, and enhance lipolysis (Fig. 11.1) [27,28,29].

Gastrointestinal disorders

Weight loss is common in many gastrointestinal disorders, and as with weight loss in malignancy, the mechanism is often multifactorial. Reasons for weight loss in gastrointestinal disease include anorexia, fear of eating (sitophobia), malabsorption, increased energy expenditure due to inflammation, early satiety, compression of abdominal organs as a result of massive splenomegaly or ascites, and intestinal obstruction.

Weight loss can be a consequence of dysphagia, which is seen in achalasia, cerebrovascular accident or other neurological disorders (e.g., amyotrophic lateral sclerosis and Parkinson disease), and esophageal stricture due to gastroesophageal reflux or malignancy.

Benign peptic ulcer disease is a common cause of anorexia and weight loss. Up to 80% of patients with gastric ulcers have been shown to have weight loss of at least 4.5 kg (10 or more pounds) [30], and this may be the result of pain associated with eating, or early satiety and vomiting due to gastric outlet obstruction. Weight loss may also be associated with duodenal ulcers, despite the long-held belief that these patients typically increase their food intake in an effort to ameliorate the pain.

Small intestinal bacterial overgrowth may lead to weight loss because of malabsorption and avoidance of food due to significant bloating, excess flatulence, and diarrhea that occurs postprandially. Similarly, delayed gastric emptying seen in gastroparesis may be associated with weight loss as a consequence of postprandial symptoms of abdominal discomfort, distention, nausea, and vomiting, as well as early satiety. Also, severe constipation and fecal impaction, which are more common in elderly patients, can lead to anorexia and weight loss. Other gastrointestinal disorders that should be included in the differential diagnosis of weight loss are acute and chronic pancreatitis, inflammatory bowel disease, microscopic colitis, atrophic gastritis with subsequent vitamin B-12 deficiency, cholecystitis, cholelithiasis with biliary colic, cirrhosis, acute hepatitis, esophageal dysmotility, and malabsorption caused by celiac disease or other disorders.

Cardiac disease

Congestive heart failure may lead to weight loss through increased metabolic demands, loss of appetite, and dietary restrictions. As seen in patients with malignancy, proinflammatory cytokines also appear to play a role in cardiac cachexia [31,32]. Increased levels of TNF-α have been associated with left ventricular dysfunction, remodeling [33,34], and cell death [35,36]. Elevated concentrations of TNF-α and soluble TNF receptors have also been shown to correlate with low body mass index and abnormalities of steroid hormone metabolism in patients with congestive heart failure, especially those with cardiac cachexia [37]. Atherosclerosis of mesenteric vasculature can lead to intestinal angina as a result of inadequate flood flow to the intestinal tract during digestion, which results in food avoidance and subsequent weight loss.

Pulmonary disease

Elevated serum levels of TNF-α have also been associated with weight loss in chronic obstructive pulmonary disease (COPD). Raised levels of TNF-α have been documented in clinically stable COPD patients with weight loss, compared with COPD patients without weight loss but a similar degree of pulmonary dysfunction [38]. Mechanisms other than proinflammatory cytokines for weight loss in COPD include anorexia (due to underlying disease or medications), increased caloric expenditure due to increased airway resistance, and increased dietary induced thermogenesis and its effect on total energy expenditure [29,39].

Renal disease

Up to 25% of patients with end-stage renal disease have been shown to be severely malnourished [40], and renal insufficiency appears to be an independent risk factor for malnutrition in older adults [41]. Weight loss in chronic renal failure has been attributed to anorexia and hypercatabolism [42,43]. Mechanisms of anorexia associated with renal disease include cytokine excess, medication, gastroparesis, glucose load from dialysate, increased leptin concentrations, and zinc deficiency

[44,45]. Hypercatabolism in renal failure has been ascribed to inadequate dialysis, acidosis, secondary infections, insulin resistance, and increased inflammatory cytokines [46].

Infection

Weight loss and malnutrition are common with human immunodeficiency virus (HIV) infection and should be considered in the differential diagnosis, especially in high-risk individuals. Postulated mechanisms for weight loss in HIV/AIDS include medications, hypermetabolism due to increased activation of proinflammatory cytokines, anorexia, secondary infections, and decreased serum testosterone concentration leading to muscle loss [47,48]. In HIV/AIDS the development of malnutrition may further contribute to clinical immune system dysfunction and progression of the disease. Other infectious causes of weight loss include fungal infections, tuberculosis, parasitic infections, and subacute bacterial endocarditis. Weight loss may be the predominant or only symptom in these patients.

Endocrine disorders

Endocrinopathies are well-known causes of unexplained weight loss, and unlike most other causes of weight loss, may be associated with increased appetite and food intake that is insufficient to fulfill metabolic demand. These entities lead to weight loss by increasing energy expenditure or calorie loss in urine or stool. Unexplained weight loss is commonly seen in undiagnosed or untreated diabetes mellitus, which is the most common cause of weight loss with increased appetite. Weight loss is especially common in new-onset type 1 diabetics as a result of insulin deficiency leading to severe hyperglycemia and glycosuria. Glycosuria, when severe, also causes an osmotic diuresis that leads to extracellular fluid volume depletion and further loss of weight. Noncompliance with insulin therapy has also been reported in young females with type 1 diabetes in an effort to loss weight [49], a finding that may be accompanied by bulimia. Weight loss accompanied by loss of appetite may occur in diabetics with gastroparesis, diabetic diarrhea, malabsorption due to intestinal neuropathy or concomitant celiac disease, or renal disease.

Hyperthyroidism is frequently associated with weight loss despite increased food intake. In a study by Nordyke and colleagues [50], 61% of patients with Graves disease reported weight loss, and 42% had increased appetite. Weight loss in hyperthyroidism is predominantly the result of increased energy expenditure, but may be enhanced by malabsorption due to increased gastrointestinal motility. Anorexia may also occur in hyperthyroidism, particularly in elderly patients with "apathetic" hyperthyroidism [51].

Hypothyroidism typically presents with weight gain, but may lead to weight loss if anorexia is a prominent symptom. Other less common endocrine causes of weight loss include hypercalcemia due to malignancy or hyperparathyroidism, adrenal insufficiency, panhypopituitarism, and pheochro-

Table 11.3 Drug-induced weight loss

Side effect	Drug or supplement
Anorexia	Amantadine, amphetamines, antibiotics (e.g., atovaquone), anticonvulsants, benzodiazepines, decongestants, digoxin, gold, levodopa, metformin, neuroleptics, nicotine, opiates, SSRIs, theophylline
Dry mouth	Anticholinergics, antihistamines, clonidine, loop diuretics
Dysgeusia or dysosmia or both	Acetazolamide, alcohol, allopurinol, amphetamines, ACE inhibitors, antibiotics (e.g., atovaquone, ciprofloxacin, clarithromycin, doxycycline, ethambutol, griseofulvin, metronidazole, ofloxacin, pentamidine, rifabutin, tetracycline), anticholinergics, antihistamines, calcium-channel blockers, carbamazepine, chemotherapy agents, chloral hydrate, cocaine-etidronate, gold, hydralazine, hydrochlorothiazide, iron, levodopa, lithium, methimazole, metformin, nasal vasoconstrictors, nitroglycerin, opiates, penicillamine, pergolide, phenytoin, propranolol, selegiline, sodium cromoglycate, spironolactone, statins, terbinafine, tobacco products, triazolam, tricyclics
Dysphagia	Alendronate, antibiotics (e.g., doxycycline), anticholinergics, bisphosphonates, chemotherapeutic agents, corticosteroids, gold, iron, levodopa, NSAIDs, potassium, quinidine, theophylline
Nausea or vomiting or both	Amantadine, antibiotics, bisphosphonates, digoxin, dopamine agonists, hormone replacement therapy, iron, levodopa, metformin, metronidazole, nitroglycerin, opiates, phenytoin, potassium, SSRIs, statins, theophylline, tricyclics

ACE, angiotensin-converting enzyme; NSAID, nonsteroidal antiinflammatory drug; SSRI, selective serotonin reuptake inhibitor.
From Alibhai et al. [53], with permission from the Canadian Medical Association.

mocytoma due to increased adrenergic activity, which is frequently associated with increased appetite.

Rheumatological disorders

Sixty-seven percent of patients with rheumatoid arthritis (RA) in the United States have significant weight loss [29]. Compared with healthy controls, patients with RA have been shown to have decreased body cell mass, higher resting energy expenditure, decreased physical activity, and increased levels of proinflammatory cytokines (IL-1β and TNF-α), which are associated with altered energy metabolism [52]. Systemic lupus erythematosus is frequently associated with weight loss because of anorexia, nausea, and malaise with decreased oral intake. Scleroderma may lead to weight loss because of swallowing dysfunction and esophageal dysmotility or diffuse intestinal dysmotility, which can lead to diarrhea and malabsorption either alone or in combination with small intestinal bacterial overgrowth.

Medications

Side effects of medications and drug–drug interactions may cause nausea and vomiting, anorexia, dysgeusia, diarrhea, dysphagia, and delayed gastric emptying, and are a frequent cause of weight loss (Table 11.3) [53]. Medication-induced weight loss is especially common in older individuals and has been documented in 9% of ambulatory elderly [8] and 14% of nursing home residents [54].

Age-related factors

Unintentional weight loss in older persons is common and is associated with increased morbidity and mortality and

Table 11.4 "Meals on Wheels:" common treatable causes of unintentional weight loss in the elderly

M	Medication effects
E	Emotional problems, especially depression
A	Anorexia tardive (nervosa), alcoholism
L	Late-life paranoia
S	Swallowing disorders
O	Oral factors (e.g., poorly fitting dentures, cavities)
N	No money
W	Wandering and other dementia-related behaviors
H	Hyperthyroidism, hypothyroidism, hyperparathyroidism, hypoadrenalism
E	Enteric problems (e.g., malabsorption)
E	Eating problems (e.g., inability to feed self)
L	Low-salt, low-cholesterol diets
S	Social problems (e.g., isolation, inability to obtain preferred foods)

From Morley & Silver [56], with permission from the American College of Physicans.

decreased quality of life [55]. Causes of weight loss in the elderly include underlying organic disease, psychiatric disorders, medication, swallowing disorders, delayed gastric emptying, financial and mobility limitations, social isolation, and restrictive diets (Table 11.4; see also Table 11.2) [11,56]. Also, by the age of 65, approximately 50% of individuals will have lost teeth and consequently have difficulty in chewing [57]. Inadequate dentition, poorly fitting dentures, and pain during eating are predictors of significant involuntary weight loss [58].

There seem to be other physiological changes that occur with increasing age, such as elevated levels of the satiating hormone cholecystokinin [59]. Elevated levels of proinflammatory cytokines (TNF-α, IL-1, IL-6) may also contribute to unintentional weight loss in older adults [60]; however, it remains to be firmly established whether cytokine elevation is due to age or other underlying illnesses. Although lean body mass and basal metabolic rate typically decrease with advancing age, body weight typically increases because of an increase in body fat [1]; therefore, weight loss in the elderly should not be considered part of the normal aging process.

Neurological disorders

The incidence of dementia increases with age and has been estimated to occur in 2%–3% of individuals between 65 and 79 years of age [61]. Alzheimer disease has become a recognized cause of weight loss. Weight loss in patients with Alzheimer disease is associated with a more rapid progression of dementia, nursing home placement, and mortality [62]. It has been shown that weight loss may precede the onset of dementia in these patients [63], which suggests that early weight loss in Alzheimer disease is not the result of an inability or unwillingness to eat. Weight loss in institutionalized patients with Alzheimer disease is commonly related to limited assistance and decreased feeding time by staff [11]. Weight loss in demented patients is also related to an inability to recognize the need to eat, difficulty in swallowing, and an increase in energy expenditure in those with habitual wandering.

Weight loss is frequently seen in Parkinson disease, occurring in up to 65% of patients [64]. Weight loss in Parkinson disease is primarily the result of loss of fat from reduced energy intake, increased energy expenditure, or a combination of both, rather than muscle loss from motor impairment [65]. Factors that lead to inadequate food intake in Parkinson disease include loss of appetite, decreased ability to feed oneself, impaired chewing, oropharyngeal dysfunction, dysphagia, and impaired gastrointestinal motility and absorption.

Psychiatric and behavioral causes

Alcoholism frequently leads to weight loss and may be diagnosed at any age. Alcoholism may be associated with depression; however, both are independent risk factors for weight loss. The diagnosis of alcoholism is often difficult to make, as alcohol abuse is not commonly volunteered, and weight loss may be the only obvious physical symptom of the problem.

Apathy and anorexia associated with depression can often lead to weight loss, even without overt evidence of depression. Depression is associated with increased hypothalamic release of corticotropin-releasing hormone, which is a potent anorectic agent [66]. Weight loss as a symptom of depression is more common in the elderly than in the younger population and is the most common cause of weight loss in older individuals [66]. In the elderly population, weight loss due to depression is more common in residents of long-term care facilities. Depression has been reported to occur in 36% of nursing home residents with unintentional weight loss [67]. Overall, psychiatric disorders, including depression, are responsible for 58% of cases of involuntary weight loss in nursing home residents [54]. The loss of a loved one, which is also typically more common in later life, may lead to clinical depression. Reduced food intake associated with the grieving process results in ketosis, and ketone bodies lead to further loss of appetitie, which perpetuates a vicious cycle [11].

Diagnosis

Documentation

Prior to undertaking an extensive evaluation of weight loss, it is imperative that adequate documentation of actual weight loss be done. The perception of weight loss may be influenced by rate of weight loss, initial body weight and size, gender, and underlying medical and psychological disorders [68]. Up to 50% of people who claim to have lost weight will not have evidence of weight loss based on medical records or family questioning [7]. The most accurate way to verify weight loss is by documentation in the patient's medical records; however, if documentation is not available, weight loss may be assessed by inquiring about change in clothing size or corroboration by family or friends.

Evaluation

A directed complete history and physical examination are essential for cost-effective evaluation, diagnosis, and treatment of unintentional weight loss. Marton and colleagues [7] found that in patients with unexplained weight loss, half had a chief complaint that pointed to the specific etiology. The mnemonic "Meals on Wheels" is useful for identifying the etiology in elderly patients (Table 11.4). [56]. It should be determined if the patient feels hungry or has loss of appetite, has difficulty eating or swallowing, or is experiencing functional or social barriers to obtaining food. The history should also include evaluation for psychiatric disorders, which are present in a significant proportion of patients. Information should be obtained regarding medical and surgical history, medications, supplements, cigarette use, and alcohol abuse. A review of symptoms can reveal disease associated with specific organ systems. The adequacy of the patient's diet should be evaluated, and the patient's daily caloric intake should be assessed

The physical examination should initially focus on the patient's mood, affect, and general appearance. Careful assessment of hydration status, including evaluation for orthostatic hypotension, ought to be included. A complete physical examination includes:

- inspection of dentition and the oral cavity
- palpation of the thyroid and lymph nodes of the neck, axillae, and inguinal region
- auscultation of lungs and heart
- abdominal evaluation for the presence of bruits, abnormal bowel sounds, masses, hepatosplenomegaly, tenderness, and distention due to obstruction, ileus, or ascites
- skeletal, breast, genital, and pelvic examination
- prostate and rectal examination, including testing for occult blood
- neurological evaluation and a Mini-Mental Status assessment.

Diagnostic testing should be initially directed at findings identified in the history and physical examination. If no clues are identified in the initial evaluation, simple laboratory testing is indicated including: complete blood cell count, serum chemistries (including renal function and electrolytes), hepatic function tests, urinalysis, chest radiograph, thyroid-stimulating hormone, erythrocyte sedimentation rate or C-reactive protein, and HIV testing if any risk factors are present.

In the absence of localizing symptoms or positive findings on initial laboratory testing, routine screening for malignancy is indicated, as recommended by the American Cancer Society, including:
- fecal occult blood testing (age 40 or older)
- flexible sigmoidoscopy/barium enema or colonoscopy (age 50 or older)
- cervical Papanicolaou smear in women
- mammography (women older than 40 years)
- prostate-specific antigen (men 50 years of age or older).

If the results of these tests are normal and cancer is still suspected, abdominal and pelvic computed tomography (CT) should be considered; however, CT may have a particularly low yield in this patient population. In one series [8] of 45 elderly patients with unintentional weight loss, CT scanning was found unhelpful in the diagnosis beyond merely confirming an already suspected cancer in one patient.

Treatment and prognosis

The treatment of unintentional weight loss is directed at the underlying cause; however, if the etiology is not determined by routine evaluation, management should focus on nutritional support to help prevent further weight loss. Patients may benefit from the elimination of dietary restrictions (e.g., low-cholesterol, low-sodium diets), more frequent smaller meals, unlimited intake of preferred foods, and nutritional supplements. If no cause is found on routine screening, reassurance can be gained from the study by Marton and colleagues [7], who found more than 65% of patients with normal findings on screening tests had a favorable prognosis. In contrast, the patients in this study who had abnormal findings generally had a worse prognosis.

References

1. Wallace JI, Schawartz RS. Epidemiology of weight loss in humans with special reference to wasting in the elderly. Int J Cardiol 2002; 85:15.
2. Hernandez JL, Riancho JA, Matorras P, Gonzales-Macias J. Clinical evaluation for cancer in patients with involuntary weight loss without specific symptoms. Am J Med 2003;114:631.
3. Rabinovitz M, Pitlik SD, Leifer M, et al. Unintentional weight loss. A retrospective analysis of 154 cases. Arch Intern Med 1986;146:186.
4. Lankisch PG, Gerzmann M, Gerzmann JF, Lehnick D. Unintentional weight loss: diagnosis and prognosis. The first prospective follow-up study from a secondary referral center. J Int Med 2001;249:41.
5. Huerta G, Viniegra L. Involuntary weight loss as a clinical problem. Rev Invest Clin (Méx) 1989;41:5.
6. Bouras EP, Lange Sm, Scolapio JS. Rational approach to patients with unintentional weight loss. Mayo Clin Proc 2001;76:923.
7. Marton KI, Sox HC Jr, Krupp JR. Involuntary weight loss: diagnostic and prognostic significance. Ann Intern Med 1981;95:568.
8. Thompson MP, Morris LK. Unexplained weight loss in the ambulatory elderly. J Am Geriatr Soc 1991;39:497.
9. Leduc D, Rouge PE, Rousset H, et al. Clinical study of 105 cases of isolated weight loss in internal medicine. Rev Med Interne 1988;9:480.
10. Levine MA. Unintentional weight loss in the ambulatory setting: etiologies and outcomes. Clin Res 1991;39:580A.
11. Morley JE. Anorexia in older patients: its meaning and management. Geriatrics 1990;45:59.
12. Robbins LJ. Evaluation of weight loss in the elderly. Geriatrics 1989;44:31.
13. Bilbao-Garay J, Barba R, Losa-Garcia JE, et al. Assessing clinical probability of organic disease in patients with involuntary weight loss: a simple score. Eur J Intern Med 2002;13:240.
14. Maltoni M, Nanni O, Pirovano M, et al. Successful validation of the palliative prognostic score in terminally ill cancer patients. Italian Multicenter Study Group on Palliative Care. J Pain Symptom Manage 1999;17:240.
15. Bruera E. Anorexia, cachexia, and nutrition. Br Med J 1997;315:1219.
16. Nixon DW, Heymsfield SB, Cohen AE, et al. Protein-calorie undernutrition in hospitalised cancer patients. Am J Med 1980;68:683.
17. DeWys WD, Begg C, Lavin PT, et al. Prognostic effect of weight loss prior to chemotherapy in cancer patients. Am J Med 1980;69:491.
18. Barber MD, Ross JA, Fearon KC. Cancer cachexia. Surg Oncol 1999;8:133.
19. Levine JA, Morgan MY. Preservation of macronutrient preferences in cancer anorexia. Br J Cancer 1998;78:579.
20. Zuijdgeest-van Leeuwen SD, van den Berg JW, Wattimena JL, et al. Lipolysis and lipid oxidation in weight-losing cancer patients and healthy subjects. Metabolism 2000;49:931.
21. Cohn SH, Gartenhaus W, Sawitsky A, et al. Compartmental body composition of cancer patients by measurement of total body nitrogen, potassium, and water. Metabolism 1981;30:222.
22. Jatoi A, Daly BD, Hughes VA, et al. Do patients with nonmetastatic non-small cell lung cancer demonstrate altered resting energy expenditure? Ann Thorac Surg 2001;72:348.
23. Laviano A, Gleason JR, Meguid MM, et al. Effects of intra-VMN mianserin and IL-1ra on meal number in anorectic tumor-bearing rats. J Investig Med 2000;48:40.
24. Opara EI, Laviano A, Meguid MM, Yang ZJ. Correlation between food intake and CSF IL-1α in anorectic tumor bearing rats. Neuroreport 1995;6:750.
25. Sonti G, Ilyin SE, Plata-Salaman CR. Anorexia induced by cytokine interactions at pathophysiological concentrations. Am J Physiol 1996; 270:R1394.
26. Inui A. Cancer anorexia-cachexia syndrome: current issues in research management. CA Cancer J Clin 2002;52:72.
27. Ramos EJ, Suzuki S, Marks D, et al. Cancer anorexia-cachexia

syndrome: cytokines and neuropeptides. Curr Opin Clin Nutr Metab Care 2004;7:427.

28. Davis MP, Dreicer R, Walsh D, et al. Appetite and cancer-associated anorexia: a review. J Clin Oncol 2004;22:1510.

29. Morley JE, Thomas DR, Wilson MM. Cachexia: pathophysiology and clinical relevance. Am J Clin Nutr 2006;83:735.

30. Palmer ED. Benign chronic gastric ulcer and weight loss. Am Fam Physician 1973;8:109.

31. Anker SD, Ponikowski PP, Clark AL, et al. Cytokines and neurohormones relating to body composition alterations in the wasting syndrome of chronic heart failure. Eur Heart J 1999;20:683.

32. Anker SD, von Haehling S. Inflammatory mediators in chronic heart failure: an overview. Heart 2004;90:464.

33. Bozkurt B, Kribbs S, Clubb FJ, Jr. Pathophysiologically relevant concentrations of tumour necrosis factor-α promote progressive left ventricular dysfunction and remodelling in rats. Circulation 1998;97:1382.

34. Finkel MS, Oddis CV, Jacob TD, et al. Negative inotropic effects of cytokines on the heart mediated by nitric oxide. Science 1992;257:387.

35. Krown KA, Page MT, Nguyen C. Tumour necrosis factor alpha-induced apoptosis in cardiac myocytes; involvement of the sphingolipid signalling cascade in cardiac cell death. J Clin Invest 1996;98:2854.

36. Agnoletti L, Curello S, Bachetti T. Serum from patients with severe heart failure downregulates eNOS and is proapoptotic: role of tumour necrosis factor-alpha. Circulation 1999;100:1983.

37. Anker SD, Clark AL, Kemp M. Tumour necrosis factor and steroid metabolism in chronic heart failure: possible relation to muscle wasting. J Am Coll Cardiol 1997;30:997.

38. Hasegawa Y, Sawada M, Ozaki N, et al. Increased soluble tumor necrosis factor receptor levels in the serum of elderly people. Gerontology 2000;46;185.

39. Farber MO, Mannix ET. Tissue wasting in patients with chronic obstructive pulmonary disease, the acquired immune deficiency syndrome, and congestive heart failure. Neurol Clin 2000;18:245.

40. Cano W. Malnutrition and chronic renal failure. Ann Med Interne (Paris) 2000;151:563.

41. Garg AX, Blake PG, Clark WF, et al. Association between renal insufficiency and malnutrition in older adults: results from the NHAMES III. Kidney Int 2001;60:1867.

42. Guarnieri G, Toigo G, Fiotti N, et al. Mechanisms of malnutrition in uremia. Kidney Int 1997;62(Suppl.):S41.

43. Kalantar-Zadeh K, Stenvinkel P, Bross R, et al. Kidney insufficiency and nutrient-based modulation of inflammation. Curr Opin Clin Nutr Metab Care 2005;8:388.

44. Van Vlem B, Schoonjans R, Vanholder R, et al. Delayed gastric emptying in dyspeptic chronic hemodialysis patients. Am J Kidney Dis 2000;36:962.

45. De Schoenmakere G, Vanholder R, Rottey S, et al. Relationship between gastric emptying and clinical and biochemical factors in chronic hemodialysis patients. Nephrol Dial Transplant 2001;16:1850.

46. Mitch WE, Du J, Bailey JL, Price SR. Mechanisms causing muscle proteolysis in uremia: the influence of insulin and cytokines. Miner Electrolyte Metab 1999;25:216.

47. Dolan S, Wilkie S, Aliabadi N, et al. Effects of testosterone administration in human immunodeficiency virus-infected women with low weight – a randomized placebo-controlled study. Arch Intern Med 2004;164:897.

48. Rietschel P, Corcoran C. Stanley T, et al. Prevalence of hypogonadism among men with weight loss related to human immunodeficiency virus infection who were receiving highly active antiretroviral therapy. Clin Infect Dis 2000;31:1240.

49. Rodin GM, Daneman D. Eating disorders and IDDM: a problematic association. Diabetes Care 1992;15:1402.

50. Nordyke RA, Gilbert FI Jr, Harada ASM. Graves' disease: influence of age on clinical findings. Arch Intern Med 1988;148:626.

51. Trivalle C, Doucet J, Chassagne P, et al. Differences in the signs and symptoms of hyperthyroidism in older and younger patients. J Am Geriatr Soc 1996;44:50.

52. Roubenoff R, Roubenoff RA, Cannon JG, et al. Rheumatoid cachexia: cytokine-driven hypermetabolism accompanying reduced body cell mass in chronic inflammation. J Clin Invest 1994;93:2379.

53. Alibhai SM, Greenwood C, Payette H. An approach to the management of unintentional weight loss in elderly people. CMAJ 2005;172:773.

54. Morley JE, Kraenzle D. Causes of weight loss in a community nursing home. J Am Geriatr Soc 1994;42:583.

55. Fine JT, Colditz GA, Coakley EH, et al. A prospective study of weight change and health-related quality of life in women. JAMA 1999;282:2136.

56. Morley JE, Silver AJ. Nutritional issues in nursing home care. Ann Intern Med 1995;123:850.

57. Fischer J, Johnson MA. Low body weight and weight loss in the aged. J Am Diet Assoc 1990; 90:1697.

58. Sullivan DH, Martin W, Flaxman N, Hagen JE. Oral health problems and involuntary weight loss in a population of frail elderly. J Am Geriatr Soc 1993;41:725.

59. Smith GP, Gibbs J. The satiating effects of cholecystokinin. Curr Concepts Nutr 1988;16:35.

60. Reife CM. Involuntary weight loss. Med Clin North Am 1995;79:299.

61. Morley JE, Silver AJ. Anorexia in the elderly. Neurobiol Aging 1988;9:9.

62. White H, Pieper C, Schmader K. The association of weight change in Alzheimer's disease with severity of disease and mortality: a longitudinal analysis. J Am Geriatr Soc 1998;46:1223.

63. Johnson DK, Wilkins CH, Morris JC. Accelerated weight loss may precede diagnosis in Alzheimer disease. Arch Neurol 2006;63:1312.

64. Moroo I, Yamada T, Hirayama K. Body weight loss in patients with Parkinson's disease. Neurological Med 1994;41:65–67.

65. Markus HS, Tomkins AM, Stern GM. Increased prevalence of under nutrition in Parkinson's disease and its relationship to clinical disease parameters. J Neural Transm 1993;5:117.

66. Rolland Y, Kim MJ, Gammack JK, et al. Office management of weight loss in older persons. Am J Med 2006;119:1019.

67. Morley JE. Anorexia of aging: physiologic and pathologic. Am J Clin Nutr 1997;66:760.

68. Drossman DA. Approach to the patient with unexplained weight loss. In: Yamada T, Alpers DH, Owyand C, et al. (eds). Textbook of Gastroenterology. Philadelphia: JB Lippincott, 1991:634.

Approach to the patient with obesity

Louis A. Chaptini, Steven R. Peikin

Regulation of energy storage, intake, and expenditure, 191
History and physical examination, 194
Gastrointestinal complications of obesity, 194
Systemic complications of obesity, 195
Treatment of obesity, 196
Complications of weight loss, 201
Conclusions, 201

Obesity is defined as an excessive amount of body fat arising from an excess energy intake that exceeds energy expenditure. Accurate measurement of body fat requires expensive and sophisticated techniques not readily available to physicians. The body mass index (BMI) correlates closely with the mass of adipose tissue [1] and therefore constitutes an acceptable estimate of body fat. The BMI represents an index of the relationship between height and weight (calculated as weight in kg divided by height in m^2 or as weight in pounds multiplied by 704 divided by height in inches squared). It is used as a clinical tool to identify overweight (BMI between 25 and 29.9 kg/m^2) and obese (BMI > 30 kg/m^2) patients. This BMI classification is primarily based on several epidemiological studies that assessed the relationship between BMI and mortality and found that men and women with a BMI greater than 30 kg/m^2 are at increased risk of health hazards and mortality [2] (Table 12.1).

According to the most recent National Health and Nutrition Examination Survey (NHANES 2003–2004), the prevalence of obesity among adults in the United States was 32.9% and the prevalence of obesity and overweight was 66.2% (Table 12.2). The number of obese adults has doubled from 1980 to 2000 and the number of morbidly obese (BMI > 40) has quadrupled. More than 300 000 deaths per year are attributed to obesity [3] and poor diet and physical inactivity may soon overtake tobacco as a leading cause of death in the United States [4]. Furthermore, because of the substantial

rise in the prevalence of obesity and its life-threatening complications, we may experience a potential decline in life expectancy in the United States in the 21st century [5].

Obesity has particular relevance to gastroenterologists because of the associated causality with different gastrointestinal diseases. Gastroenterologists should be knowledgeable in the treatment of obesity (dietary interventions and pharmacological treatment) and in the treatment of patients presenting with complications after bariatric surgery. This chapter reviews the complex mechanisms that regulate food intake and body weight, comorbidities in particular those involving gastrointestinal and hepatic complications associated with obesity and the clinical approach to the patient with obesity.

Regulation of energy storage, intake, and expenditure

Concept of energy homeostasis

Fat is the primary form of energy storage. According to the first law of thermodynamics, the amount of stored energy is equal to the difference between energy intake and energy expenditure. This law applies to any biological system, including the human body. Weight gain results from an imbalance in homeostatic mechanisms that, in normal conditions, maintain the difference between intake and expenditure close to zero. A very small imbalance over a long period of time can have a large cumulative effect. To keep a perfect balance between energy intake and expenditure, homeostatic mechanisms rely on neural signals that emanate from adipose tissue, endocrine, neurological, and gastrointestinal systems and are integrated by the central nervous system

Principles of Clinical Gastroenterology. Edited by Tadataka Yamada, David H. Alpers, Anthony N. Kalloo, Neil Kaplowitz, Chung Owyang, and Don W. Powell. © 2008 Blackwell Publishing. ISBN 978-1-4051-69103

Table 12.1 Classification of weight by BMI, waist circumference, and associated disease risk

BMI (kg/m²)	Classification	Disease risk[a] Men ≤ 102 cm (≤ 40″) Women ≤ 88 cm (≤ 35″)	Men > 102 cm (> 40″) Women > 88 cm (> 35″)
< 18.5	Underweight	–	–
18.5–24.9	Normal	–	–
25.0–29.9	Overweight	Increased	High
30.0–34.9	Obese class I	High	Very high
35.0–39.9	Obese class II	Very high	Very high
≥ 40	Obese class III	Extremely high	Extremely high

a Disease risk for type 2 diabetes, hypertension, and cardiovascular disease, relative to normal weight and waist circumference.
BMI, body mass index.
Adapted from World Health Organization [117].

Table 12.2 Age-adjusted prevalence of overweight and obesity among US adults, age 20–74 years

	NHANES II (1976–1980) (n = 11 207)	NHANES III (1988–1994) (n = 14 468)	NHANES (1999–2000) (n = 3603)	NHANES (2001–2002) (n = 3916)	NHANES (2003–2004) (n = 3756)
Percentage of overweight or obese (BMI ≥ 25.0)	47.1	55.9	64.5	65.7	66.2
Percentage of obese (BMI ≥ 30.0)	15.0	23.2	30.9	31.3	32.9

BMI, body mass index; NHANES, National Health and Nutrition Examination Survey.
From Centers for Disease Control and Prevention website accessed on 01/07/2008:
www.cdc.gov/nchs/products/pubs/pubd/hestats/overweight/overwght_adult_03.htm

(CNS) [6, 7] (Fig. 12.1). The CNS subsequently sends signals to multiple organs in the periphery to control energy intake and expenditure and maintain energy homeostasis over long periods of time.

Gastrointestinal hormones and food intake

The gastrointestinal neuroendocrine system plays a substantial role in regulating food intake and maintaining energy homeostasis. Specialized enteroendocrine cells contain chemoreceptors that are sensitive to nutrients present in the chyme as it progresses through the gastrointestinal tract [8]. In response to different classes of nutrients, the enteroendocrine cells secrete peptides that act either as hormones by entering the bloodstream or in a paracrine fashion by diffusing through the extracellular fluid to adjacent cells. Most of these peptides stimulate satiety with the exception of ghrelin, which has an orexigenic effect.

Cholecystokinin

Cholecystokinin (CCK) is the prototypical satiety hormone, produced by I cells in the duodenum and jejunum. It is

secreted in response to the presence of nutrients within the gut lumen, specifically fat and protein [9]. The satiating effect of CCK is mediated by the vagus nerve. The activated vagus in turn stimulates cells in the brainstem (nucleus tractus solitarius) leading to signals to other areas of the brain (paraventricular nucleus and ventromedial hypothalamus) that cause the individual to stop eating [10]. CCK also has endocrine effects on the gastrointestinal system and the CNS, which may be important in stimulating satiety. These include contraction of the pylorus, inhibition of gastric emptying and possibly direct binding to CCK receptors in the area postrema at the base of the fourth ventricle [11].

Peptide tyrosine tyrosine, pancreatic polypeptide

Peptide tyrosine tyrosine (PYY), pancreatic polypeptide (PP), and neuropeptide Y (NPY) are all members of the pancreatic polypeptide family. NPY, a potent short-term stimulus of appetite, is released from NPY neurons in the arcuate nucleus (Fig. 12.1). PYY is secreted by L cells in the distal ileum and colon and is present in two forms, PYY(1–36) and PYY(3–36). PYY release from the gastrointestinal tract is proportional to

Figure 12.1 Pathways of regulation of food intake. Representation of potential action of gut peptides on the hypothalamus. Primary neurons in the arcuate nucleus contain multiple peptide neuromodulators. Appetite-inhibiting neurons (dark purple) contain proopiomelanocortin (POMC) peptides such as α-melanocyte-stimulating hormone (αMSH), which acts on melanocortin receptors (MC3 and MC4) and cocaine- and amphetamine-stimulated transcript peptide (CART), whose receptor is unknown. Appetite-stimulating neurons in the arcuate nucleus (light purple) contain neuropeptide Y (NPY), which acts on Y receptors (Y1 and Y5), and agouti-related peptide (AgRP), which is an antagonist of MC3/4 receptor activity. Integration of peripheral signals within the brain involves interplay between the hypothalamus and hindbrain structures, including the nucleus tractus solitarius (NTS), which receives vagal afferent inputs. Inputs from the cortex, amygdala, and brainstem nuclei are integrated as well, with resultant effects on meal size and frequency, gut handling of ingested food, and energy expenditure. →, direct stimulatory; ⊣, direct inhibitory; PYY, peptide tyrosine tyrosine; PP, pancreatic polypeptide; GLP-1, glucagon-like peptide-1; OXM, oxyntomodulin; CCK, cholecystokinin. Adapted from Badman & Flier [7], with permission from the American Association for the Advancement of Science.

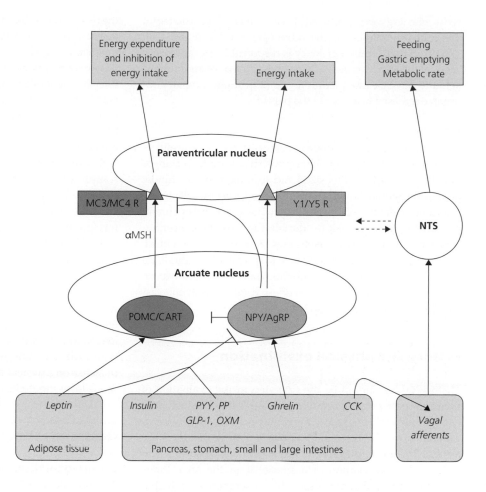

the caloric density of the ingested nutrients, primarily lipids and carbohydrates [12]. When administered peripherally, PYY(3–36) has been shown to reduce food intake in rodents, primates, and in normal weight and obese humans [13,14]. PP is secreted from specific pancreatic islet cells in response to a meal. Several reports have shown a reduction in food intake after peripheral administration of PP [15, 16] (Fig. 12.1).

Glucagon-like peptide-1 and oxyntomodulin

Glucagon-like peptide-1 (GLP-1) is derived from the post-translational modification of proglucagon in the enteroen-docrine L cells in the ileum and colon. The secretion of GLP-1 results from direct nutrient stimulation in the distal small intestine as well as indirect neurohumoral stimulation in proximal regions of the small intestine [17]. A major action of GLP-1 is to help stimulate insulin secretion during a meal. GLP-1 also has an anorectic effect in healthy [18], diabetic [19], and obese [20] human subjects. The peripheral adminis-tration of GLP-1 is thought to elicit satiety by its inhibitory effects on gastrointestinal transit and reduced gastric empty-ing [21].

Oxyntomodulin is another peptide derived from pro-glucagon's posttranslational processing in L cells. It is also an anorectic peptide and reduces caloric intake in humans. Part

of its anorectic effect may result from suppression of plasma ghrelin levels [22].

Amylin

Amylin is a peptide secreted by pancreatic B cells in paral-lel with insulin secretion during meals. The peptide inhibits gastric emptying and gastric acid secretion. Several reports showed a decrease in meal size after systemic administration of amylin [23,24]. Pramlintide, an amylin analogue, has been shown to induce weight loss in diabetic patients [25].

Leptin

Leptin is an adipocyte-derived factor that plays a dominant role in the central regulation of food intake and energy bal-ance by signaling adipose energy reserve to the brain [26]. Leptin is secreted by subcutaneous adipose tissue in response to fat storage or overfeeding. Leptin is also produced in extra-adipose sites such as placenta, skeletal muscle, and stomach. Up to 25% of circulating leptin derives from fundic glands in the stomach [27]. Leptin has the ability to reduce food intake and body weight [28] by suppressing the expression of NPY, a potent appetite stimulatory peptide, and increasing the expression of α-melanocyte-stimulating hormone, which acts to decrease appetite (Fig. 12.1). In contrast, leptin deficiency reduces energy expenditure [7]. The effects of gastric leptin are probably similar to the adipocyte-derived leptin [28]. Although total leptin deficiency is responsible for the obesity seen in the *Ob/Ob* mouse [7], the majority of obese humans actually have elevated leptin levels [29], suggesting an end-organ decreased response to the peptide.

Ghrelin

Unlike the satiety hormones discussed so far, ghrelin is an orexigenic or "appetite" hormone that stimulates hunger [30]. It is primarily synthesized and secreted from the fundic area in the stomach but can also be produced by cells in the duodenum, ileum, cecum, and colon. Plasma levels of ghrelin rise during fasting, peak (to double the baseline concentration) immediately before meals and fall rapidly after a meal, suggesting a role as a meal initiator [31]. The role of ghrelin in obesity in not clear because, unlike what one would expect, ghrelin levels tend to be low in obese humans, only increasing after dietary weight loss [32].

History and physical examination

History taking should be the first step in the evaluation of the obese patient. A review of the patient's lifestyle including eating habits and physical activity may provide helpful information as to why the patient is obese. Eating disorders are a relative contraindication for the treatment of obesity and require the intervention of a specialist in the area. Binge eating is reported more frequently in women with higher BMI [33]. Information about the age at onset of obesity, recent weight changes, previous attempts of weight loss with details of the modalities followed, and family history of obesity is important. A search for drugs that can promote weight gain such as steroid hormones (glucocorticoids, progesterone), neurotropic and psychotropic medications (lithium, antidepressants, phenothiazines), and antidiabetic medications (sulfonylureas, insulin, thiazolidinedione) should be carried out and if possible alternatives should be offered. A review of systems should look for symptoms of secondary causes of obesity such as hypothyroidism, Cushing syndrome and polycystic ovarian syndrome. Attention should be directed to medical conditions associated with obesity like diabetes, hyperlipidemia, hypertension, coronary artery disease, and osteoarthritis. The physician should be aware of symptoms and signs of sleep apnea (loud snoring, daytime fatigue, and morning headaches) and the patient should be referred accordingly. From the gastroenterologist's perspective, a search for symptoms related to gastrointestinal complications of obesity should be undertaken. Those can range from conditions such as gallstones and gastroesophageal reflux disease (GERD) to more serious cases involving cirrhosis or malignancies.

Physical examination should start with the measurement of the height and weight, and calculation of BMI to categorize the risk and severity of obesity. Clinical judgment is necessary in assessing a muscular patient because the BMI may overestimate the degree of fatness. The excess body fat in obese persons may be distributed in an android or gynecoid pattern. Measurement of the patient's waist circumference is important to assess the abdominal distribution of adipose tissue, which by itself is associated with an increased risk of medical complications [34]. Women and men with a waist circumference greater than 88 cm (35 inches) and 102 cm (40 inches), respectively are considered at increased risk for diabetes and other complications of obesity independent of their BMI. Blood pressure should be checked with an appropriately sized cuff. Other key features in the clinical assessment include looking for signs of secondary causes of obesity and conditions that are caused by obesity. Particular attention should be given to the examination of the thyroid gland and the search for signs of hypothyroidism and Cushing syndrome. Hyperinsulinemia, which is typically associated with obesity, can be manifested by acanthosis nigricans around the neck and axilla. Laboratory evaluation should screen for complications of obesity and associated conditions such as nonalcoholic steatohepatitis, type 2 diabetes, and hyperlipidemia that are not necessarily detected on physical examination. Thyroid-stimulating hormone level should be measured to rule out hypothyroidism.

Gastrointestinal complications of obesity

Esophageal disease

The prevalence of GERD and GERD-related complications, particularly erosive esophagitis, Barrett esophagus, and esophageal adenocarcinoma, has been increasing over the past 20 years [35]. Several reports link this increase to the obesity epidemic. The association between reflux symptoms and obesity has been examined in several cross-sectional studies. Most of these studies showed a significant positive association [36–38] with an increased risk ranging from 1.5- to 3-fold in obese subjects, whereas other studies showed no significant link [39,40]. The association between obesity and erosive esophagitis was examined in multiple case–control, cross-sectional, and cohort studies [41–44]: most reports showed a positive association with adjusted odds ratios ranging from 1 to 2.1 in overweight and 1.6 to 14.6 in obese patients.

The incidence of esophageal adenocarcinoma has increased in parallel with that of obesity in the past 15 years, which prompted the performance of several studies looking at an association between them [44–46]. Estimates from pooled studies showed a 2.1-fold increase in the overall risk of esophageal adenocarcinoma in patients with a BMI greater than 25 compared to subjects with a normal BMI [44].

Gallbladder disease

Obesity is an important risk factor for gallbladder disease. Data from the Nurses Health Study demonstrated that the risk for symptomatic gallstones increases linearly with BMI. A twofold and a sevenfold increase in risk for symptomatic gallstones was noted in women with BMI greater than 30 and BMI greater than 45, respectively [47]. Several other epidemiological studies have found the same positive association between BMI and the risk of gallstones [48, 49]. The mechanism of gallstone formation in obese individuals involves an increase in cholesterol saturation index and a decreased response to cholecystokinin [50]. The risk of gallbladder cancer increases with gallstones, hence obesity increases this risk [51].

Pancreatic disease

The increased risk of pancreatitis in obesity is thought to be explained by the increased risk of cholelithiasis. Acute pancreatitis is more severe in overweight and obese subjects [52]. There is an increase in the incidence of infectious complications as well as in the length of hospitalization in obese individuals.

Obesity has also been associated with pancreatic cancer but it has been difficult to determine whether this association is direct or secondary to the association of obesity to diabetes, the latter being an established risk factor for pancreatic cancer. A metaanalysis estimated that obese subjects have a 20% increase in the risk of developing pancreatic cancer when compared to people with a normal body weight [53].

Liver disease

Liver damage can be increased when liver disease occurs in the setting of obesity. This has been shown in chronic hepatitis C, alcoholic liver disease, and toxin-induced liver disease [54,55]. The most common liver abnormality associated with obesity is nonalcoholic fatty liver disease (NAFLD). Several studies have demonstrated a strong link between obesity and NAFLD. There is an increase in prevalence of NAFLD with BMI increase in both genders and in all races. Furthermore, liver biopsies from morbidly obese individuals performed at the time of bariatric surgeries demonstrated NAFLD in over 80% of cases [56]. NAFLD is a spectrum of conditions that range from steatosis at one end to cirrhosis at the most serious end of the spectrum. Nonalcoholic steatohepatitis (NASH) is an intermediate stage in this spectrum, characterized by hepatocyte injury and death accompanied by infiltration of acute and chronic inflammatory cells. NAFLD is the hepatic consequence of insulin resistance and the associated metabolic syndrome that leads to a relative overproduction of proinflammatory mediators [57]. It has also been suggested that hyperleptinemia plays a role in the occurrence of fibrosis by activating hepatic stellate cells (the source of hepatic collagen) [58]. NAFLD is usually diagnosed when patients are referred for further evaluation of abnormal liver enzymes or when fatty infiltration is detected on an abdominal imaging study performed for other reasons. Serum aspartate aminotransferase, alanine aminotransferase, and γ-glutamyl transferase are usually increased less than fourfold and do not correlate with the severity of the condition. The main target in the treatment of NAFLD is the improvement of insulin sensitivity, which can be achieved by dietary modifications and by pharmacological treatment. A gradual weight loss of 10% or more of body weight can correct abnormal liver chemistries and decrease liver size, fat content, and features of steatohepatitis but the impact on the long-term outcome and the progression of the disease remains unknown. Several small clinical trials looking at the efficacy of pharmacological agents such as insulin-sensitizing agents (metformin, troglitazone), lipid-lowering agents (gemfibrozil, atorvastatin), antioxidants (vitamin E), tumor necrosis factor-α-inhibiting agents, and ursodeoxycholic acid showed conflicting results and their impact on the natural progression of the disease remains unknown [59].

Colon disease

Several cohort and case–control studies have looked at the association between obesity and colorectal cancer and a positive association was noted especially in men, with an increased risk of about 1.5-fold to threefold [44,60]. The association was found to be weaker in women, especially older and postmenopausal women [61]. The risk of colon polyps is also increased about twofold in obese individuals [44,62] and appears to be higher in men than in women.

Irritable bowel syndrome

Gastrointestinal motility is regulated by some of the gut peptides involved in feeding behaviors. Hence, the association between irritable bowel syndrome (IBS) and obesity is worth studying. Few studies have examined this association: one demonstrated a significant increase in some IBS symptoms (constipation, diarrhea, straining, and flatus) in obese patients and another showed a threefold increase in the risk of IBS with obesity [63]. Further studies are needed to confirm this association.

Systemic complications of obesity

Since the 1990s, the obesity epidemic has generated a rapid increase in the metabolic syndrome. The metabolic syndrome is defined as the constellation of insulin resistance (manifested by type 2 diabetes or glucose intolerance), visceral adiposity (resulting in abdominal obesity and increased waist circumference), hypertension, and dyslipidemia [64]. One of the direct consequences of metabolic syndrome and obesity is an increase in the prevalence of diabetes, hypertension, and dyslipidemia leading to a two- to threefold increase in cardiovascular disease [64,65] (Fig. 12.2).

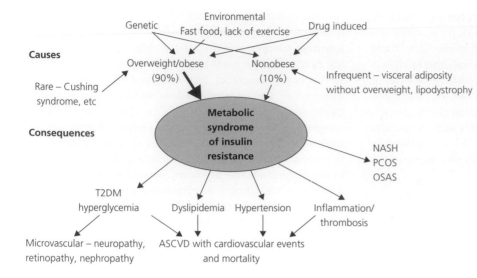

Figure 12.2 Metabolic syndrome. NASH, nonalcoholic steatohepatitis; PCOS, polycystic ovary syndrome; OSAS, obstructive sleep apnea syndrome; ASCVD, atherosclerotic cardiovascular disease; T2DM, type 2 diabetes mellitus. From Richardson & Vinik [64], with permission from Elsevier.

Treatment of obesity

Treatment guidelines

Determination of BMI and waist circumference and the search for comorbid conditions (such as cardiovascular risk factors) help in assessing the degree of overweight and the overall risk status. The next step is to assess how motivated the patient is to lose weight and their degree of understanding of obesity as a disease, its causes, its consequences, and the treatment options, and to discuss any previous unsuccessful treatments and the reasons for failure of those treatments [66] (Table 12.3).

The initial goal of the treatment is a 10% reduction of body weight from baseline. A reasonable time line to achieve this reduction is 6 months of therapy. Further weight loss can be attempted later if indicated [66]. Depending on the degree of overweight and the overall risk status of the patient, different modalities are available to the clinician to achieve the weight loss target. These include lifestyle modifications (dietary interventions and physical activity), pharmacotherapy, and surgical interventions (Table 12.4). Efforts to maintain the achieved weight loss should be put in place through a weight maintenance program involving dietary and behavioral therapy along with physical activity.

Lifestyle modifications
Dietary interventions

To induce weight loss, a calorie deficit must be achieved. Balanced diets should contain a minimum of 1000–1200 kcal per day and provide adequate amounts of all essential nutrients. An average loss of 500 kcal per day should produce a weight loss of about 450 g (1 lb) weekly. There is evidence that weight loss of 5%–15% of initial weight is enough to reduce the risks of dyslipidemia, diabetes, and hypertension associated with obesity [67].

The role of dietary fat in the development of obesity has been studied extensively. Almost all dietary guidelines recommend a reduction in the daily intake of fat to 30% of energy intake or less regardless of weight status. On the other hand, despite a decrease in consumption of fat in the past 30 years, the rate of obesity has risen to an all-time high [68]. This shows that reducing the percentage of fat alone will not produce weight loss unless combined with a reduction of total calories. Furthermore, a metaanalysis of six clinical trials (comparing low-fat to other types of weight-reducing diets) showed that low-fat diets were no better or worse than other weight-reducing diets for achieving sustained weight loss [69]. Despite the controversial role of low-fat diet in the treatment of obesity, the National Institutes of Health (NIH) recommend a low-calorie diet consistent with a step I or II diet (depending on the patient's risk status) in which fat constitutes 30% or less [66].

The popularity of low-carbohydrate diets (Atkins, Sugar Busters, Zone, South Beach) has been increasing since the

Table 12.3 Steps in the assessment and treatment of the overweight and obese patient

Calculate body mass index and measure waist circumference
Look for causes of weight gain, including medications
Assess and treat comorbidities
Assess patient motivation to lose weight and discuss any previous unsuccessful attempt to lose weight:
   If motivated, set reasonable weight loss goal and discuss the options
   If not motivated, urge weight maintenance and manage comorbidities
Develop a treatment plan based on Table 12.4

Table 12.4 Treatment options for the overweight and obese patient

Treatment	BMI 25–26.9	27–29.9	30–34.9	35–39.9	≥ 40
Diet, exercise, behavior therapy	+ (with comorbidities) ± (without comorbidities)[a]	+ (with comorbidities) ± (without comorbidities)[a]	+	+	+
Pharmacotherapy	−	− (without comorbidities) + (with comorbidities)	+	+	+
Surgery	−	−	−	− (without comorbidities) + (with comorbidities)	+

a While weight loss is not necessarily recommended for those with a BMI of 25 to 29.9 kg/m² unless they have two or more comorbidities [66], motivated subjects should be offered lifestyle therapy.
BMI, body mass index.
From NIH [66].

late 1990s. These diets result in a rapid initial weight loss explained by sodium diuresis secondary to ketosis caused by glycogen mobilization in the presence of carbohydrate restriction.

Very-low-calorie diets are diets that provide 500–800 kcal per day. Despite an impressive short-term success, these diets provide no greater weight loss at 1 year than do low-calorie diets (1000–1500 kcal per day) [70].

Portion-controlled, vitamin/mineral-fortified meal replacements have been increasingly used as part of low-calorie diets. These diets using meal replacements are marketed now by several manufacturers and used as components in several large-scale clinical trials. A metaanalysis of trials utilizing these diets showed significant weight loss (7%–8% of body weight) at 3 months and 1 year [71].

Several epidemiological studies looked at the magnitude of weight loss with the different types of diets discussed above. A recent randomized trial comparing four different diets [very-low-carbohydrate (Atkins); macronutrient balance controlling glycemic load (Zone); calorie restriction (Weight Watchers); very-low-fat (Ornish)] with a design intended to simulate their use in a real-world setting [72]. A trend toward higher dropout rates was noted after 1 year with the very low-carbohydrate and very low-fat diets than with the more moderate diets. Average weight loss at 1 year was approximately 4–7 kg (in those who completed the study), and was similar among the four diets. In the intention-to-treat analysis, mean weight loss was similar for all four diets and was more modest (2.1–3.3 kg). Dietary adherence rates were low for all diets and were more important predictors of weight loss. This study illustrates the difficulty of achieving significant weight loss with dietary therapy in a real-world setting.

Physical activity

Physical activity is a key component of any long-term weight loss therapy and weight maintenance program. Physical activity modestly contributes to weight loss in overweight and obese adults. It may also decrease abdominal fat and it increases cardiorespiratory fitness [66]. The combination of a low-calorie diet and increased physical activity produces greater weight loss than diet alone or physical activity alone. Adults should accumulate at least 30 minutes of moderate intensity physical activity on most days of the week.

Behavior therapy

The role of behavior therapy is to alter the eating and activity habits of an obese patient and overcome barriers to compliance with dietary therapy and increased activity [66]. It can be achieved either on an individual basis or in group settings (the latter being less expensive). Behavior therapy can produce a weight loss in the range of 10% of baseline weight over 4 months to 1 year [66,73] but most patients return to baseline weights in the absence of continued intervention. Specific behavioral strategies include self-monitoring, stress management, stimulus control, positive reinforcement, and social support. Self-monitoring consists of recording dietary habits (types, amounts, caloric values, nutrient composition) and physical activity habits (frequency, intensity). Stress management through coping strategies, meditation, and relaxation techniques can defuse situations leading to overeating. Stimulus control includes avoiding stimuli that may encourage eating and situations associated with little amount of exercise. Positive reinforcement through the use of rewards for specific actions encourages behavior change. Social support (family members, friends) can assist in maintaining motivation and providing positive reinforcement [66].

Pharmacotherapy

Antiobesity drugs are indicated as adjuncts to diet and physical activity for patients with BMI of 30 or above in the absence of obesity-related risk factors or diseases, and for patients with BMI of at least 27 in the presence of such conditions [66]. Usually drugs are used after nonpharmacological treatment has been attempted for 6 months with unsatisfactory results of weight loss (less than 450 g per month). Pharmacotherapy for obesity underwent a gigantic turn in the 1990s when Weintraub et al. showed that the combination phentermine-fenfluramine (Phen-fen) induces a sustained weight loss for more than 3 years (74). Fenfluramine was subsequently withdrawn from the market because of an association with valvular heart disease and pulmonary hypertension. Sibutramine and orlistat are the two medications currently approved in the United States for long-term use. Several others, including phentermine, are approved for short-term use but are often used off-label for longer periods of time. Studies are underway regarding new promising antiobesity agents. Other drugs approved for indications other than obesity have been shown to induce some weight loss (Table 12.5).

Sibutramine

Sibutramine (Meridia) is a serotonin and norepinephrine reuptake inhibitor and a weak dopamine reuptake inhibitor. Increasing the availability of these neurotransmitters in the CNS results in appetite suppression. Placebo-controlled trials showed 5%–8% weight reduction after 6 months of sibutramine treatment compared with 2%–4% weight loss in subjects receiving placebo [75,76]. Of note, most of these trials include dietary or exercise interventions for subjects in both the treatment and placebo groups, which likely explains the weight loss in the placebo group. In one study, continued treatment for up to 2 years was associated with some weight regain (approximately 50% of the initial weight loss); however, around 25% of subjects who continued to take sibutramine maintained their reduced weight for the entire 2 years of observation [77]. Side effects of sibutramine include hypertension and tachycardia, therefore routine clinical monitoring of vital signs is recommended. Other less dangerous adverse effects include headache, insomnia, dry mouth, and constipation.

Orlistat

Orlistat (Xenical) alters fat metabolism by inhibiting pancreatic lipase. As a result, ingested fat is not completely digested. Taken with a meal, orlistat can inhibit the absorption of up to 30% of ingested fat [78]. Clinical trials demonstrated that orlistat treatment in conjunction with nutritional counseling results in weight loss of 8%–10% at 1 year, compared to 6% with placebo [79,80]. Extension of the treatment to 2 years results in weight regain of approximately one-third of the initial weight loss (compared with regain of two-thirds with placebo) [79,80]. The use of orlistat is associated with gastrointestinal side effects that include flatulence, steatorrhea, increased stool frequency, fecal incontinence and oily rectal discharge [81]. Malabsorption can be associated with a deficiency in the fat-soluble vitamins A, D, E, and K. Patients on orlistat should receive a daily supplement containing these vitamins given at least 2 hours before or after each dose

Table 12.5 Medications for the treatment of obesity

Medication	Typical dosing	Classification	Common adverse effects
Medications approved by the FDA specifically for weight loss indication			
Phentermine	15–37.5 mg/day	Adrenergic agent	Tachycardia, hypertension
Sibutramine	10–15 mg/day	Serotonergic/adrenergic	Hypertension, tachycardia
Orlistat	120 mg three times/day	Lipase inhibitor	Malabsorption, steatorrhea
Medications approved by the FDA for other indications but shown to have weight loss effect			
Bupropion	150–300 mg/day	Depression	Anticholinergic; agitation
Metformin	500–1000 mg/day	Type 2 diabetes	Hepatic oxidative injury
Topiramate	50–100 mg/day	Seizure disorder	Cognitive impairment
Zonisamide	400–600 mg/day	Seizure disorder	Cognitive impairment

FDA, Food and Drug Administration.
Adapted from Kaplan [81], with permission from Elsevier.

of orlistat [81]. Furthermore, vitamin D levels should be measured before and periodically during orlistat therapy [81]. Few cases of orlistat-induced severe hepatotoxiciy and hepatic failure have been reported [82,83].

Phentermine

Phentermine is an adrenergic reuptake inhibitor that works as an appetite suppressant. It is approved for use over 12 weeks or less. Because phentermine is an adrenergic agonist, it can be associated with tachycardia and hypertension. A weight loss of 1.8 kg (4 lb) over 4 weeks is considered an acceptable therapeutic response [81]. Other noradrenergic agents approved by the Food and Drug Administration (FDA) for short-term use in the treatment of obesity include diethylpropion, phendimetrazine, and benzphetamine [84]. Studies using this class of medications demonstrated up to 10-kg weight loss when compared to placebo [84].

Rimonabant

Rimonabant (Acomplia) is a cannabinoid receptor antagonist. Animal studies have shown that the cannabinoid-1 receptor plays a role in appetite and body weight regulation [85]. Rimonabant has been studied as a potential treatment for both obesity and smoking cessation. In a randomized trial comparing rimonabant to placebo, subjects who took 20 mg rimonabant experienced an average weight loss of 6.6 kg whereas subjects who took placebo lost on average 1.8 kg. Furthermore, improvements in waist circumference, high-density lipoprotein, triglycerides, and insulin resistance were noted with rimonabant [86]. Two other recent randomized controlled trials showed similar effects of rimonabant on weight loss and associated metabolic risk factors [87,88]. In one of the trials, weight regain was noted in subjects who were switched to placebo after 1 year while those who continued on 20 mg rimonabant experienced sustained weight loss at 2 years [88]. Side effects of rimonabant include depression, nausea, headache, dizziness, and diarrhea.

Drugs approved for other indications

Bupropion, a psychotropic agent used in the treatment of depression, is associated with a modest weight loss in the range of 4%–5% when compared to placebo [89]. Similarly, the antidiabetic agent metformin has been associated with weight loss in the range of 4% of the initial body weight over 1–2 years [81]. Topiramate and zonisamide, both anticonvulsant drugs, have been shown to induce some weight loss (up to 6% of the initial body weight with zonisamide) [81].

Over-the-counter products

Over-the-counter dietary supplements are widely used by individuals attempting to lose weight. Such supplements include ephedra (no longer available in the United States to treat obesity), green tea, chromium, chitosan, ginseng, and guar gum. The use of these agents should be discouraged because of the lack of evidence of their efficacy and safety [90].

Surgical therapy

Bariatric surgery is indicated for carefully selected patients with clinically severe obesity (BMI ≥ 40 or BMI ≥ 35 with comorbid conditions) when less invasive methods of weight loss have failed [66]. To be considered effective, a bariatric procedure should result in a sustained excess weight loss of more than 50% and resolution of comorbid conditions. Bariatric surgeries can be divided into two varieties, malabsorptive and restrictive, depending on the mechanism by which weight loss is induced.

Malabsorptive procedures include jejunoileal bypass, biliopancreatic diversion, and biliopancreatic diversion with duodenal switch. These procedures induce weight loss by shortening the length of functional small bowel segment. Profound weight loss can be achieved with these malabsorptive procedures but significant metabolic abnormalities occur, including protein calorie malnutrition and various macronutrient deficiencies [91]. As a result of these dangerous consequences, malabsorptive procedures have been replaced by the restrictive procedures: Roux-en-Y gastric bypass (RYGB), vertical banded gastroplasty (VBG), and laparoscopic adjustable gastric banding (LAGB). RYGB is primarily restrictive but has also some malabsorptive characteristics.

RYGB is accomplished by creating a small, 15–20 mL, gastric pouch and a Roux-en-Y gastrojejunostomy (Fig. 12.3a), hence restricting food intake and at the same time inducing some malabsorption by bypassing the distal stomach, the duodenum, and a variable length of jejunum. RYGB is the most common bariatric procedure performed in the United States. More weight loss is achieved with this procedure than with VBG [92,93]. On average, 50%–75% of excess weight loss is achieved after 1–2 years [94]. Complications of the gastric bypass procedure include stomal stenosis, marginal ulcers, staple line disruption, dilatation of the bypassed stomach, internal hernias, dumping syndrome, and malabsorption of nutrients. RYGB can be performed laparoscopically and results in similar sustained weight loss compared to the open approach [91]. Advantages of the laparoscopic approach include a lower incidence of incisional hernia and wound infection, faster recovery and shorter hospital stay [94,95].

VBG is a purely restrictive procedure that involves creating a gastric pouch by stapling the gastric fundus and placing a circumferential band around the pouch. VBG was the most commonly performed procedure before the advent of gastric bypass (Fig. 12.3b). The average excess weight loss at 3–5 years is around 30%–50% [96]. These more modest long-term results compared with RYGB, along with the significant adverse events associated with VBG (GERD, vomiting, solid food intolerance), explain the decline of popularity of this procedure. Postoperative complications requiring

(a)

(b)

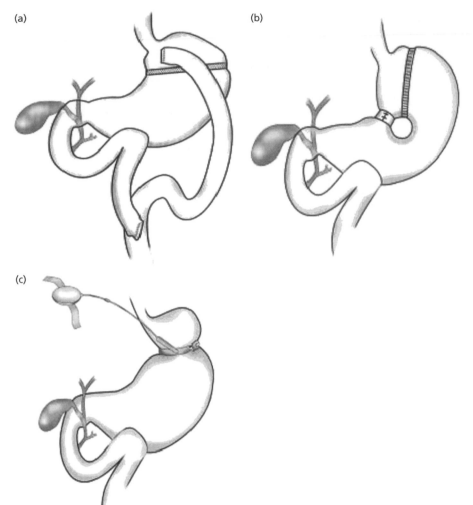

(c)

Figure 12.3 Types of bariatric surgeries: **(a)** Roux-en-Y gastric bypass; **(b)** vertical banded gastroplasty; **(c)** laparoscopic adjustable gastric banding. Redrawn from Brolin [118], with permission from the American Medical Association.

intervention include staple line disruption, stomal stenosis, band erosion, band disruption, and pouch dilatation.

LAGB is another purely restrictive procedure that involves placing a tight, adjustable prosthetic band around the proximal stomach (Fig. 12.3c). The prosthetic band is connected to an infusion port that is placed in the subcutaneous tissue and is accessible with a needle. Injection of saline into the port leads to increased restriction. Advantages of LAGB include technical ease of placement, lack of anastomosis, adjustability (deflation of the port), and reversibility (band removal). Because of its simplicity and lower rate of complications, this procedure has largely replaced VBG, especially in Europe and Australia. Despite initial disappointing data in the United States [97], subsequent studies showed excess weight loss similar to the Australian and European experience, in the range of 45%–75% [98–101].

Patients undergoing bariatric surgery should be followed by a multidisciplinary team including medical, behavioral, and nutritional experts. Gastroenterologists should assess the patient preoperatively and manage any chronic gastro-

intestinal disorders that may complicate the postoperative care. For example, attention should be paid to detecting any gastric, pancreatic, or biliary diseases preoperatively because the alteration of the anatomy with some of the performed surgeries makes parts of the gastrointestinal tract (distal stomach, biliary tree) inaccessible to endoscopic and radiological procedures. Patients should be screened for iron deficiency anemia before surgery and gastrointestinal blood loss should be excluded to avoid confusion after surgery. Fatty liver disease is present in most morbidly obese patients requiring surgery and 3%–7% of these patients have cirrhosis [102]. Portal hypertension and the presence of varices (esophageal and/or gastric) are contraindications to gastric operations and should be excluded before surgery [103].

Gastroenterologists also have a role in the management and follow-up of the bariatric surgery patients postoperatively. Complications of surgery usually present as nausea, vomiting, pain, bleeding, diarrhea, and constipation. Immediately after the surgery, these symptoms are probably directly associated with the operation and are often managed by the surgical team. Later on, the gastroenterologist may get involved to deal with complications indirectly related to the surgery, such as anastomotic ulceration, band erosion, stricture, and fistula, which may require endoscopic therapy. Depending on the type of operation, some nutritional complications may occur. Iron, vitamin B12, and calcium deficiencies can be seen with gastric bypass.

Endoscopic therapy

Minimally invasive endoscopic treatment for obesity is an attractive option, especially in patients who do not respond to lifestyle modifications and pharmacotherapy but are not candidates for bariatric surgery. Various intragastric space-occupying devices have been evaluated for short- and long-term use. In 1985 the FDA approved the Garren–Edwards gastric bubble [104], an air-filled bubble floating in the stomach that is inserted through the esophagus using a gastric tube. Because of a lack of significant weight loss in sham-controlled studies and significant complications such as gastric erosions, gastric ulcers, Mallory–Weiss tear, and esophageal lacerations, this device was abandoned and is no longer commercially available. Several subsequent modifications to the device failed to show improvement in efficacy. More recently, the Bioenterics intragastric balloon (BioEnterics Corp., Carpinteria, CA, USA) has been widely used internationally but not yet in the United States. It consists of a soft, saline-filled balloon placed endoscopically to partially fill the stomach mimicking an intragastric bezoar. Mean excess weight loss with Bioenterics intragastric balloon is reported to be 38%–48% after 4–6 months [105]; however, only a minority of patients has sustained weight reduction after balloon removal [106]. In a recent sham-controlled study, the difference in mean weight loss between patients with Bioenterics intragastric balloons and controls was not significant (10.4% and 9%, respectively) at 3 months [107]. Complications are less frequent with the Bioenterics intragastric balloon than with earlier balloons. They include intolerance to the balloon, vomiting, abdominal pain, esophagitis, and gastric ulcers and erosions [104].

Future endoscopic approaches will aim to duplicate bariatric surgical procedures. Ongoing animal work is directed at attempting gastric partitioning (the equivalent of VBG). Preclinical work is also being undertaken to refine an endoscopic gastrojejunostomy technique [104].

Complications of weight loss

During rapid weight loss, the risk for cholesterol gallstone formation increases [108]. Patients with higher initial BMI and greater absolute rate of weight loss seem to have the highest risk of gallstone formation. The mechanism of this increase in gallstone formation involves an increase in the cholesterol saturation index and in the crystallization pro-

moting proteins (mucin) and a decrease in gallbladder motility with low-calorie low-fat diet [109–111]. Once an individual has lost weight and maintained weight loss, the risk of gallstone formation decreases. Some surgeons recommend the performance of cholecystectomy at the time of gastric bypass surgery because of the high incidence of gallbladder disease in the seriously obese and to avoid postoperative complications as a result of gallstones [112]. More recently, the use of ursodeoxycholic acid has been shown to reduce the risk of gallstone formation in the first 6 months after bariatric surgery [113]. Another complication of rapid and large weight loss is the occurrence of liver disease. Two weight loss studies, one involving patients undergoing gastroplasty and the other involving patients on a very low-calorie diet, showed a decrease in the prevalence of steatosis but an increase in the prevalence of steatohepatitis with the fall of BMI [114,115]. The risk of liver damage may be related to the rapidity of weight loss, which determines the rate of increased delivery to the liver of free fatty acids from lipolysis of adipose triglycerides [116].

Conclusions

Obesity has become a major health problem in most industrialized nations. It has particular relevance to gastroenterologists because of their involvement in managing the associated gastrointestinal disorders, their role in the evaluation and treatment of obese patients before and after bariatric surgery, and their potential future role in the endoscopic therapy for obesity. By becoming actively involved in the management of obesity, gastroenterologists can provide a valuable clinical service to their patients.

References

1. Benn RT. Some mathematical properties of weight-for-height indices used as measures of adiposity. Br J Prev Soc Med 1971;25:42.
2. Troiano RP, Frongillo EA Jr, Sobal J, et al. The relationship between body weight and mortality: a quantitative analysis of combined information from existing studies. Int J Obes Relat Metab Disord 1996;20:63.
3. Fontaine KR, Redden DT, Wang C, et al. Years of life lost due to obesity. JAMA 2003;289:187.
4. Allison DB, Fontaine KR, Manson JE, et al. Annual deaths attributable to obesity in the United States. JAMA 1999;282:1530.
5. Olshansky SJ, Passaro D, Hershow R, et al. A potential decline in life expectancy in the United States in the 21st century. N Engl J Med 2005;352:1138.
6. Strader AD, Woods SC. Gastrointestinal hormones and food intake. Gastroenterology 2005;128:175.
7. Badman MK, Flier JS. The gut and energy balance: visceral allies in the obesity wars. Science 2005;307:1909.
8. Lundgren O. Interface between the intestinal environment and the nervous system. Gut 2004;53(Suppl. 2):16.
9. Douglas BR, Jansen JB, de Jong AJ, et al. Effect of various triglycerides on plasma cholecystokinin levels in rats. J Nutr 1990;120:686.

10. Moran TH, Ladenheim EE, Schwartz GJ. Within-meal gut feedback signaling. Int J Obes Relat Metab Dis 2001;25(Suppl. 5):39.

11. Moran TH, Schwartz GJ. Neurobiology of cholecystokinin. Crit Rev Neurobiol 1994;9:1.

12. Greeley GH Jr, Hashimoto T, Izukura M, et al. A comparison of intraduodenally and intracolonically administered nutrients on the release of peptide-YY in the dog. Endocrinology 1989;125:1761.

13. Batterham RL, Cowley MA, Small CJ, et al. Gut hormone PYY(3-36) physiologically inhibits food intake. Nature 2002;418:650.

14. Batterham RL, Cohen MA, Ellis SM, et al. Inhibition of food intake in obese subjects by peptide YY3-36. N Engl J Med 2003;349:941.

15. Asakawa A, Inui A, Yuzuriha H, et al. Characterization of the effects of pancreatic polypeptide in the regulation of energy balance. Gastroenterology 2003;124:1325.

16. Batterham RL, Le Roux CW, Cohen MA, et al. Pancreatic polypeptide reduces appetite and food intake in humans. J Clin Endocrinol Metab 2003;88:3989.

17. Brubaker PL, Anini Y. Direct and indirect mechanisms regulating secretion of glucagon-like peptide-1 and glucagon-like peptide-2. Can J Physiol Pharmacol 2003;81:1005.

18. Gutzwiller JP, Goke B, Drewe J, et al. Glucagon-like peptide-1: a potent regulator of food intake in humans. Gut 1999;44:81.

19. Gutzwiller JP, Drewe J, Goke B, et al. Glucagon-like peptide-1 promotes satiety and reduces food intake in patients with diabetes mellitus type 2. Am J Physiol 1999;276:1541.

20. Naslund E, Barkeling B, King N, et al. Energy intake and appetite are suppressed by glucagon-like peptide-1 (GLP-1) in obese men. Int J Obes Relat Metab Disord 1999;23:304.

21. Delgado-Aros S, Kim DY, Burton DD, et al. Effect of GLP-1 on gastric volume, emptying, maximum volume ingested, and postprandial symptoms in humans. Am J Physiol 2002;282:424.

22. Cohen MA, Ellis SM, Le Roux CW, et al. Oxyntomodulin suppresses appetite and reduces food intake in humans. J Clin Endocrinol Metab 2003;88:4696.

23. Lutz TA, Del Prete E, Scharrer E. Reduction of food intake in rats by intraperitoneal injection of low doses of amylin. Physiol Behav 1994;55:891.

24. Lutz TA, Geary N, Szabady MM, et al. Amylin decreases meal size in rats. Physiol Behav 1995;58:1197.

25. Schmitz O, Brock B, Rungby J. Amylin agonists: a novel approach in the treatment of diabetes. Diabetes 2004;53(Suppl. 3):233.

26. Flier JS. Obesity wars: molecular progress confronts an expanding epidemic. Cell 2004;116:337.

27. Sobhani I, Bado A, Vissuzaine C, et al. Leptin secretion and leptin receptor in the human stomach. Gut 2000;47:178.

28. Elmquist JK, Elias CF, Saper CB. From lesions to leptin: hypothalamic control of food intake and body weight. Neuron 1999;22:221.

29. Saad MF, Riad-Gabriel MG, Khan A, et al. Diurnal and ultradian rhythmicity of plasma leptin: effects of gender and adiposity. J Clin Endocrinol Metab 1998;83:453.

30. Asakawa A, Inui A, Kaga T, Yuzuriha, et al. Ghrelin is an appetite-stimulatory signal from stomach with structural resemblance to motilin. Gastroenterology 2001;120:337.

31. Cummings DE, Purnell JQ, Frayo RS, et al. A preprandial rise in plasma ghrelin levels suggests a role in meal initiation in humans. Diabetes 2001;50:1714.

32. Cummings DE, Weigle DS, Frayo RS, et al. Plasma ghrelin levels after diet-induced weight loss or gastric bypass surgery. N Engl J Med 2002;346:1623.

33. Spitzer RL, Devlin M, Walsh BT. Binge eating disorder: a multisite field trial of the diagnostic criteria. Int J Eat Disord 1992;11:191.

34. Larsson B, Svardsudd K, Welin L, et al. Abdominal adipose tissue distribution, obesity, and risk of cardiovascular disease and death: 13 year follow up of participants in the study of men born in 1913. BMJ 1984;288:1401.

35. El-Serag HB. The epidemic of esophageal adenocarcinoma. Gastroenterol Clin North Am 2002;31:421.

36. Diaz-Rubio M, Moreno Elola-Olaso C, Rey E, et al. Symptoms of gastro-oesophageal reflux: prevalence, severity, duration and associated factors in a Spanish population. Aliment Pharmacol Ther 2004;19:95.

37. Locke GR III, Talley NJ, Fett SL, et al. Risk factors associated with symptoms of gastroesophageal reflux. Am J Med 1999;106:642.

38. Murray L, Johnston B, Lane A, et al. Relationship between body mass and gastrooesophageal reflux symptoms: the Bristol Helicobacter Project. Int J Epidemiol 2003;32:645.

39. Lagergren J, Bergstrom R, Nyren O. No relation between body mass and gastrooesophageal reflux symptoms in a Swedish population-based study. Gut 2000;47:26.

40. Wu AH, Tseng CC, Bernstein L. Hiatal hernia, reflux symptoms, body size, and risk of esophageal and gastric adenocarcinoma. Cancer 2003;98:940.

41. Nilsson M, Lundegardh G, Carling L, et al. Body mass and reflux oesophagitis: an oestrogen-dependent association? Scand J Gastroenterol 2002;37:626.

42. Stene-Larsen G, Weberg R, Froyshov LI, et al. Relationship of overweight to hiatus hernia and reflux oesophagitis. Scand J Gastroenterol 1988;23:427.

43. Wilson LJ, Ma W, Hirschowitz BI. Association of obesity with hiatal hernia and esophagitis. Am J Gastroenterol 1999;94:2840.

44. El-Serag HB. Obesity and disease of the esophagus and colon. Gastroenterol Clin North Am 2005;34:63.

45. Brown LM, Swanson CA, Gridley G, et al. Adenocarcinoma of the esophagus: role of obesity and diet. J Natl Cancer Inst 1995;87:104.

46. Chow WH, Blot WJ, Vaughan TL, et al. Body mass index and risk of adenocarcinomas of the esophagus and gastric cardia. J Natl Cancer Inst 1998;90:150.

47. Stampfer MJ, Maclure KM, Colditz GA, et al. Risk of symptomatic gallstones in women with severe obesity. Am J Clin Nutr 1992;55:652.

48. Erlinger S. Gallstones in obesity and weight loss. Eur J Gastroenterol Hepatol 2000;12:1347.

49. Kodama H, Kono S, Todoroki I, et al. Gallstone disease risk in relation to body mass index and waist-to-hip ratio in Japanese men. Int J Obes Relat Metab Disord 1999;23:211.

50. Reuben A, Maton PN, Murphy GM, et al. Bile lipid secretion in obese and non-obese individuals with and without gallstones. Clin Sci 1985;69:71.

51. Lowenfels AB, Maisonneuve P, Boyle P, et al. Epidemiology of gallbladder cancer. Hepato-Gastroenterology 1999;46:1529.

52. Martinez J, Sanchez-Paya J, Palazon JM, et al. Obesity: a prognostic factor of severity in acute pancreatitis. Pancreas 1999;19:15.

53. Berrington de Gonzalez A, Sweetland S, Spencer E. A meta-analysis of obesity and the risk of pancreatic cancer. Br J Cancer 2003;89:519.

54. Hodgson M, Van Thiel DH, Goodman-Klein B. Obesity and hepatotoxin risk factors for fatty liver disease. Br J Ind Med 1991;48:690.

55. Giraud NS, Borotto E, Aubert A, et al. Excess weight risk factor for alcoholic liver disease. Hepatology 1997;25:108.

56. Gholam PM, Kotler DP, Flancbaum LJ. Liver pathology in morbidly obese patients undergoing Roux-en-Y gastric bypass surgery. Obes Surg 2002;12:49.

57. Marchesini G, Bugianesi E, Forlani G, et al. Nonalcoholic fatty liver, steatohepatitis, and the metabolic syndrome. Hepatology 2003;37:917.

58. Anania FA. Leptin, liver, and obese mice – fibrosis in the fat lane. Hepatology 2002;36:246.

59. Diehl AM. Hepatic complications of obesity. Gastroenterol Clin North Am 2005;34:45.

60. Moore LL, Bradlee ML, Singer MR, et al. BMI and waist circumference as predictors of lifetime colon cancer risk in Framingham Study adults. Int J Obes Relat Metab Disord 2004;28:559.

61. Giovannucci E. Obesity, gender, and colon cancer. Gut 2002;51:147.

62. Neugut AI, Lee WC, Garbowski GC, et al. Obesity and colorectal adenomatous polyps. J Natl Cancer Inst 1991;83:359.

63. Crowell MD, Cheskin LJ, Musial F. Prevalence of gastrointestinal symptoms in obese and normal weight binge eaters. Am J Gastroenterol 1994;89:387.
64. Richardson DW, Vinik AI. Metabolic implications of obesity: before and after gastric bypass. Gastroenterol Clin North Am 2005;34:9.
65. Isomaa B, Almgren P, Tuomi T, et al. Cardiovascular morbidity and mortality associated with the metabolic syndrome. Diabetes Care 2001;24:683.
66. NIH. The practical guide: identification, evaluation, and treatment of overweight and obesity in adults. Bethesda, MD: National Heart, Lung, and Blood Institute, North American Association for the Study of Obesity, 2000. NIH publication no. 00-4048.
67. Goldstein, DJ. Beneficial health effects of modest weight loss. Int J Obes 1992;16:397.
68. Balart LA. Diet options of obesity: fad or famous. Gastroenterol Clin North Am 2005;34:83.
69. Pirozzo S, Summerbell C, Cameron C, et al. Advice on low-fat diets for obesity. Cochrane Database Syst Rev 2002;CD003640.
70. Wadden TA, Foster GD, Letizia KA. One-year behavioral treatment of obesity: comparison of moderate and severe caloric restriction and the effects of weight maintenance therapy. J Consult Clin Psychol 1994;62:165.
71. Heymsfield SB, van Mierlo CA, van der Knaap HC, et al. Weight management using a meal replacement strategy: meta and pooling analysis from six studies. Int J Obes Relat Metab Disord 2003;27:537.
72. Dansinger ML, Gleason JA, Griffith JL, et al. Comparison of the Atkins, Ornish, Weight Watchers, and Zone diets for weight loss and heart disease risk reduction: a randomized trial. JAMA 2005;293:43.
73. Wing RR. Behavioral approaches to the treatment of obesity. In: Bray GA, Bouchard C (eds). Handbook of Obesity. Clinical applications. New York: Marcel Dekker, Inc., 2004:147.
74. Weintraub M. Long-term weight control study: conclusions. Clin Pharmacol Ther 1992;51:642.
75. Fanghanel G, Cortinas L, Sanchez-Reyes L, et al. A clinical trial of the use of sibutramine for the treatment of patients suffering essential obesity. Int J Obes Relat Metab Disord 2000;24:144.
76. Bray GA, Blackburn GL, Ferguson JM, et al. Sibutramine produces dose-related weight loss. Obes Res 1999;7:189.
77. James WP, Astrup A, Finer N, et al. Effect of sibutramine on weight maintenance after weight loss: a randomised trial. STORM Study Group. Sibutramine Trial of Obesity Reduction and Maintenance. Lancet 2000;356:2119.
78. Ballinger A, Peikin SR. Orlistat: its current status as an anti-obesity drug. Eur J Pharmacol 2002;440:109.
79. Sjostrom L, Rissanen A, Andersen T, et al. Randomised placebo-controlled trial of orlistat for weight loss and prevention of weight regain in obese patients. European Multicentre Orlistat Study Group. Lancet 1998;352:167.
80. Davidson MH, Hauptman J, DiGirolamoM, et al. Weight control and risk factor reduction in obese subjects treated for 2 years with orlistat: a randomized controlled trial. JAMA 1999;281:235.
81. Kaplan LM. Pharmacological therapies for obesity. Gastroenterol Clin North Am 2005;34:91.
82. Thurairajah PH, Syn WK, Neil DA, et al. Orlistat (Xenical)-induced subacute liver failure. Eur J Gastroenterol Hepatol 2005;17:1437.
83. Montero JL, Muntane J, Fraga E, et al. Orlistat associated subacute hepatic failure [Letter]. J Hepatol 2001;34:173.
84. Yanovski SZ, Yanovski JA. Obesity. N Engl J Med 2002;346:591.
85. Kunos G, Batkai S. Novel physiologic functions of endocannabinoids as revealed through the use of mutant mice. Neurochem Res 2001;26:1015.
86. Van Gaal LF, Rissanen AM, Scheen AJ, et al. Effects of the cannabinoid-1 receptor blocker rimonabant on weight reduction and cardiovascular risk factors in overweight patients: 1-year experience from the RIO-Europe study. Lancet 2005;365:1389.
87. Despres JP, Golay A, Sjostrom L. Effects of rimonabant on metabolic risk factors in overweight patients with dyslipidemia. N Engl J Med 2005;353:2121.
88. Pi-Sunyer FX, Aronne LJ, Heshmati HM, et al. RIO-North America Study Group. Effect of rimonabant, a cannabinoid-1 receptor blocker, on weight and cardiometabolic risk factors in overweight or obese patients: RIO-North America: a randomized controlled trial. JAMA 2006;295:761.
89. Jain AK, Kaplan RA, Gadde KM, et al. Bupropion SR vs. placebo for weight loss in obese patients with depressive symptoms. Obes Res 2002;10:1049.
90. Saper RB, Eisenberg DM, Phillips RS. Common dietary supplements for weight loss. Am Fam Physician 2004;70:1731.
91. Demaria EJ, Jamal MK. Surgical options for obesity. Gastroenterol Clin North Am 2005;34:127.
92. Sugerman HJ, Londrey GL, Kellum JM, et al. Weight loss with vertical banded gastroplasty and Roux-Y bypass for morbid obesity with selective versus random assignment. Am J Surg 1989;157:93.
93. Hall JC, Watts JM, O'Brien PE, et al. Gastric surgery for morbid obesity. The Adelaide study. Ann Surg 1990;211:419.
94. Mun EC, Blackburn GL, Matthews JB. Current status of medical and surgical therapy for obesity. Gastroenterology 2001;120:669.
95. Nguyen NT, Goldman C, Rosenquist CJ, et al. Laparoscopic versus open gastric bypass: a randomized study of outcomes, quality of life, and costs. Ann Surg 2001;234:279.
96. MacLean LD, Rhode BM, Forse RA. Late results of vertical banded gastroplasty for morbid and super obesity. Surgery 1990;107:20.
97. US Food and Drug Administration, Centers for Devices and Radiological Health. LAP-BAND Adjustable Gastric Banding (LAGB) System P-000008. Available at: www.fda.gov/cdrh/pdf/p000008.html, accessed 05/08/2007.
98. Ren CJ, Horgan S, Ponce J. US experience with the LAP-BAND system. Am J Surg 2002;184:46.
99. Spivak H, Anwar F, Burton S, et al. The Lap-Band system in the United States: one surgeon's experience with 271 patients. Surg Endosc 2004;18:198.
100. Fox SR, Fox KM, Srikanth MS, et al. The Lap-Band system in a North American population. Obes Surg 2003;13:275.
101. Holloway JA, Forney GA, Gould DE. The Lap-Band is an effective tool for weight loss even in the United States. Am J Surg 2004;188:659.
102. Beymer C, Kowdley KV, Larson A, et al. Prevalence and predictors of asymptomatic liver disease in patients undergoing gastric bypass surgery. Arch Surg 2003;138:1240.
103. Kaplan LM. Gastrointestinal management of the bariatric surgery patient. Gastroenterol Clin North Am 2005;34:105.
104. Huang CS, Farraye FA. Endoscopy in the bariatric surgical patient. Gastroenterol Clin North Am 2005;34:151.
105. Roman S, Napoleon B, Mion F, et al. Intragastric balloon for "nonmorbid" obesity: a retrospective evaluation of tolerance and efficacy. Obes Surg 2004;14:539.
106. Sallet JA, Marchesini JB, Paiva DS, et al. Brazilian multicenter study of the intragastric balloon. Obes Surg 2004;14:991.
107. Mathus-Vliegen E, Tytgat G. Intragastric balloon for treatment-resistant obesity: safety, tolerance, and efficacy of 1-year balloon treatment followed by a 1-year balloon-free follow-up. Gastrointest Endosc 2005;61:19.
108. Shiffman ML, Sugerman HJ, Kellum JM, et al. Gallstone formation after rapid weight loss: a prospective study in patients undergoing gastric bypass surgery for treatment of morbid obesity. Am J Gastroenterol 1991;86:1000.
109. Gebhard RL, Prigge WF, Ansel HJ, et al. The role of gallbladder emptying in gallstone formation during diet induced rapid weight loss. Hepatology 1996;24:544.
110. Shiffman ML, Sugerman HJ, Kellum JM, et al. Changes in gallbladder bile composition following gallstone formation and weight reduction. Gastroenterology 1992;103:214.
111. Gustafsson U, Benthin L, Granstrom L, et al. Changes in gallbladder bile composition and crystal detection time in morbidly obese subjects after bariatric surgery. Hepatology 2005;41:1322.
112. Calhoun R, Willbanks O. Coexistence of gallbladder diseases and morbid obesity. Am J Surg 1987;154:655.

113. Sugerman HJ, Brewer WH, Shiffman ML, et al. A multicenter, placebo-controlled, randomized, double-blind, prospective trial of prophylactic Ursodiol for the prevention of gallstone formation following gastric bypass-induced rapid weight loss. Am J Surg 1995;169:91.

114. Luyckx F, Desaive C, Thiry A, et al. Liver abnormalities in severely obese subjects: effects of drastic weight loss after gastroplasty. Int J Obes 1998;22:222.

115. Andersen T, Gluud C, Franzmann M, et al. Hepatic effects of dietary weight loss in morbidly obese subjects. J Hepatol 1991;12:224.

116. Blackburn G, Mun E. Effects of weight loss surgeries on liver disease. Semin Liver Dis 2004;24:371.

117. World Health Organization. Obesity: preventing and managing the global epidemic. Report of a WHO consultation on obesity. Geneva: World Health Organization, 1997.

118. Brolin RE. Bariatric surgery and long-term control of morbid obesity. JAMA 2002;288:2793.

13

Approach to the patient with nausea and vomiting

William L. Hasler

Definitions, 205
Socioeconomic impacts of nausea and vomiting, 205
Pathophysiology of nausea and vomiting, 206
Causes of nausea and vomiting, 208
History and physical examination, 212
Laboratory studies and diagnostic testing, 213
Principles of management, 216

Definitions

Nausea and vomiting are nonspecific responses to a variety of conditions. *Nausea* is the subjective sensation of an impending urge to vomit and is usually perceived in the throat or epigastrium. *Vomiting* is the forceful ejection of upper gut contents from the mouth. Although usually preceded by nausea, vomiting may occur without nausea. *Retching* may precede vomiting but involves no discharge of gastric contents from the mouth. Nausea and vomiting are distinguished from other symptoms. *Regurgitation* is the effortless return of gut contents into the mouth. *Rumination* is regurgitation with rechewing and reswallowing of food, often occurring multiple times after a meal. In contrast to vomiting, these phenomena can exhibit volitional control. *Anorexia* is a loss of appetite, which may be associated with nausea. *Early satiety* is a sense of gastric fullness before meal completion. Nausea may be part of the general complaint of *indigestion*, which includes abdominal discomfort, heartburn, anorexia, eructation, and bloating.

Socioeconomic impacts of nausea and vomiting

Nausea and vomiting have significant socioeconomic impact. Nausea from acute enteric illness restricts daily activities. Acute

Principles of Clinical Gastroenterology. Edited by Tadataka Yamada, David H. Alpers, Anthony N. Kalloo, Neil Kaplowitz, Chung Owyang, and Don W. Powell. © 2008 Blackwell Publishing. ISBN 978-1-4051-69103

enteric infection increased medical expenses by $1.25 billion and cost $21.8 billion in lost productivity in the United States in 1980 [1]. Pregnant women with nausea and vomiting report fatigue, sleep disturbances, and irritability, which impair interpersonal interactions [2]. It is estimated that 8.5 million working days per year are lost in Britain through the nausea of pregnancy and that severely affected women miss a mean of 62 h of work while pregnant [3]. Twenty-eight percent of all sick-leaves occur because of the nausea of pregnancy in Sweden [4]. A recent Canadian study calculated weekly costs of $132, $355, and $653 for women with mild, moderate, and severe nausea and vomiting of pregnancy, respectively [5]. One percent of pregnant women are hospitalized as a result of nausea and vomiting with an average length of stay of 2.6 days and average charges of nearly US$6000 [4,6]. Chemotherapy-induced nausea and vomiting disrupts normal function in more than 90% of patients [7]. Nausea and vomiting after chemotherapy and after surgery reduce the time spent on leisure and recreation, household tasks, and socializing and cause hardship to family members [8]. Nausea and vomiting after chemotherapy decrease employee productivity and increase health-care costs because of the prolonged hospitalization and home nursing time. Nausea after chemotherapy often restricts functioning to greater degrees than vomiting [7,8]. Postoperative nausea and vomiting costs outpatient surgical centers a mean of $415 per patient [9]. Another British study calculated that nausea and vomiting after surgery prevent the performance of 96–576 surgical procedures per year per center because of increased recovery room stays and extra nursing effort [10]. When queried, 32% of patients scheduled for general anesthesia would pay extra money out of pocket to avoid postoperative nausea and vomiting [11].

Pathophysiology of nausea and vomiting

Vomiting is coordinated by the brainstem and is effected by neuromuscular responses in the gut, pharynx, and thoraco-abdominal wall. The mechanisms underlying nausea are poorly understood but likely involve the cerebral cortex, as nausea requires conscious perception.

Activation of the emetic response

Vomiting is initiated by stimuli acting on the central nervous system (CNS) and peripherally. The area postrema in the dorsal medulla at the caudal aspect of the fourth ventricle is believed to serve as a "chemoreceptor trigger zone" and responds to a range of neurochemical activators. Other CNS and peripheral afferent sites mediate emesis after other stimuli.

Area postrema as a receptor of neurochemical emetic stimuli

Because of its location and its porous blood–brain barrier, the area postrema receives input from the brain and peripheral nerves and samples chemical activators in the bloodstream and cerebrospinal fluid. Several observations confirm the importance of the area postrema. The dopamine agonist apomorphine elicits vomiting when applied directly to the area postrema; conversely, ablation of the structure prevents apomorphine-induced emesis [12]. Magnetic resonance imaging studies show that apomorphine increases blood flow in the area postrema and nucleus tractus solitarius (NTS) reflecting neuronal activation of these structures [13]. Drugs (digoxin, opiates, nicotine, ergot alkaloids, some cancer chemotherapies), metabolic disorders (uremia, diabetic ketoacidosis, hypoxemia, hypercalcemia), radiation therapy, and bacterial toxins induce vomiting by area postrema activation. Neurotransmitters localized to the area postrema include dopamine, serotonin, norepinephrine, enkephalins, γ-aminobutyric acid, and substance P. Receptor subtypes characterized in the structure include dopamine D_2, muscarinic M_1, histamine H_1, serotonin 5-HT_3 and 5-HT_4, vasopressin, N-methyl-D-aspartate, neurokinin NK_1, and μ opioid [14].

Other central nervous system activators of emesis

Different CNS structures mediate emesis in certain settings. Cerebral pathways mediate vomiting from noxious odors, visual stimulation, somatic pain, and unpleasant taste. Brainstem vestibular nuclei activate emesis in motion sickness, Méniére disease, and labyrinthine tumors or infections via area postrema-independent pathways [15]. Motion stimuli and cold caloric irrigation of the ear evoke hypothalamic and brainstem histamine release [16]. Anticholinergic agents binding to neural M_1 receptors are postulated to prevent motion sickness by enhancing habituation responses to rotatory stimuli [16]. Studies report that motion sickness can be attenuated by agonist action at 5-$HT_{1A/7}$ and antagonist action at 5-HT_{2A} receptors, indicating the participation of serotonin pathways in this emetic pathway, whereas another investigation observed no role of serotonin receptors in motion sickness [17,18].

Peripheral afferent neural activation of emesis

Irritants such as copper sulfate, salicylate, staphylococcus toxin, and antral distention activate afferent nerves from the stomach. Nongastric emetic stimuli include distention of the colon, small intestine, and bile ducts, peritoneal inflammation, mesenteric vascular occlusion, and irritation of the pharynx and heart. Emesis evoked by intragastric hypertonic saline or copper sulfate is mediated by activation of gastro-duodenal mucosal afferent fibers, whereas vomiting with gastric distention involves activation of smooth muscle afferents [19]. Vagotomy prevents emesis after intragastric copper sulfate and reduces vomiting provoked by the chemotherapeutic agent cisplatinum and abdominal irradiation [20,21]. Splanchnic afferent pathways modulate emesis after selected stimuli. The threshold for vomiting induced by a 5-HT_3 agonist is increased by acute vagotomy plus splanchnicectomy [22]. However, if vagotomy is performed 14–51 days after splanchnicectomy, the thresholds for induction of emesis are reduced, reflecting recruitment of new pathways. Most afferent vagal fibers project to the NTS, although some project to the area postrema or the dorsal motor nucleus of the vagus (DMNV) [23]. Ablation studies demonstrate that many peripheral stimuli act independently of the area postrema via serotonergic pathways [12]. Serotonin synthesized by enterochromaffin cells or myenteric neurons is believed to act on 5-HT_3 receptors on vagal afferent fibers, in the area postrema, and in the NTS. Antagonists of 5-HT_3 reduce the vomiting evoked by peripheral stimuli such as cisplatinum and copper sulfate [24]. In some species, 5-HT_4 receptors may participate in the emetic response to peripheral stimulation [25].

Central nervous system coordination of the act of vomiting

Multiple brainstem sites coordinate the act of vomiting. Immunohistochemical studies show increased c-fos protein expression after emetic stimulation in the area postrema, NTS, DMNV, phrenic nuclei, medullary nuclei involved with control of respiration, hypothalamus, and amygdala [26]. In addition to activation by vagal stimulation, the NTS receives projections from the area postrema and labyrinths and is postulated to serve as a common focus to initiate the vagally dependent gastrointestinal motor and myoelectric aspects of emesis [23]. The NTS also projects to the Botzinger complex in the medullary retrofacial nucleus, which regulates respiration, the nucleus ambiguous, which supplies the laryngeal and pharyngeal musculature, and the trigeminal, facial, and hypoglossal nuclei, which serve the facial and tongue muscles [27]. Neurons of the medullary reticular formation interact with the nucleus ambiguus, DMNV, and respiratory nuclei. Ablation of the reticular formation prevents emesis in dogs, confirming the importance of this structure [28]. Non-respiratory neurons in the reticular area drive respiratory premotor neurons in the ventral respiratory group [29]. During retching, firing rates in pre-Botzinger complex inspiratory neurons nearly disappear, establishing the interrelation of respiratory and nonrespiratory pathways [30]. These findings are consistent with the postulate that output from the medullary reticular formation with modulatory output from the NTS coordinates neuronal firing in each of these nuclei. Once activated, these brainstem structures stimulate the diaphragm via cervical spinal pathways and the external musculature via the thoracolumbar spinal nerves. The NTS also sends ascending projections into the hypothalamus and limbic regions, suggesting activation of CNS regions regulating the behavioral aspects of emesis [31].

Brainstem tachykinin NK_1 pathways play important roles in mediating emesis. The NK_1 receptors are present in the area postrema, NTS, and other brainstem nuclei [14]. Substance P elicits vomiting when injected into the brainstem, whereas peripheral administration of NK_1 antagonists prevents emesis and retching burst firing patterns in brainstem neurons in response to emetic stimulation [32, 33]. Injections of NK_1 antagonists into the area postrema, medial solitary nucleus, and dorsal vagal complex also prevent vomiting [34]. Studies suggest that the likely site of action of NK_1 antagonists is deeper in the brainstem than the NTS [14]. The NTS and vagal nuclei also are rich in catecholamines, enkephalins, somatostatin, vasopressin, and thyrotropin-releasing hormone

Peripheral responses to the initiation of vomiting
Somatic muscular events associated with vomiting

Emesis results from a coordinated, stereotypic series of somatic muscle actions. During retching, inspiratory thoracic, diaphragmatic, and abdominal muscles contract against a closed glottis producing elevated intraabdominal pressure that forces gastric contents into the esophagus and herniates the gastric cardia into the thorax [35]. A high negative intrathoracic pressure prevents oral expulsion of lumenal contents, even though the upper esophageal sphincter may relax [36]. In contrast, during vomiting, both intraabdominal and intrathoracic pressures are positive because there is no diaphragmatic contraction in the crural region to prevent transmission of the high positive abdominal pressure into the thorax [37]. During emesis, the high positive intrathoracic pressure provides the force for oral expulsion of lumenal contents [35]. Oral propulsion of the vomitus is further facilitated by movement of the hyoid bone and larynx up and forward [38]. Elevation of the soft palate prevents passage of vomitus into the nasal cavities, while glottic closure prevents pulmonary aspiration. Respiration is suppressed except for small inspirations between expulsions [39].

Gastrointestinal events associated with nausea and vomiting

Gastrointestinal contractions are regulated by oscillatory electrical pacemaker activity known as the slow wave, which controls the maximal frequency and direction of contractions. Dominant pacemakers in the stomach and duodenum cycle at 3 and 11–12 cycles/min, respectively. Before emesis, intestinal slow waves are abolished and are followed by bursts of electrical spikes that propagate orally [40]. A retroperistaltic contractile complex (retrograde giant contraction) begins in the mid-small intestine and propagates into the stomach, causing enterogastric reflux [41]. After the retrograde giant contraction has passed, phasic intestinal contractions persist for several minutes and are followed by motor quiescence. Subsequent pyloric closure, antral contraction, and lower esophageal sphincter relaxation facilitate expulsion of intragastric contents. Retroperistaltic contractions of the cervical esophageal body and pharynx have also been described [38]. These motor and myoelectric events are controlled by extrinsic innervation [42]. However, blockade of these phenomena with atropine or vagotomy does not prevent emesis, indicating that they are not strictly needed for vomiting to occur but, rather, enhance evacuation of lumenal contents [41].

Autonomic and endocrine responses to nausea and vomiting

Autonomic disturbances occur because of the proximity of the brainstem nuclei mediating vomiting to those controlling respiratory, vasomotor, cardiac, and salivary activity. Pallor, diaphoresis, hypersalivation, defecation, tachycardia, or hypotension can be experienced with nausea. Elevated parasympathetic vagal activity, as measured by increased beat-to-beat heart rate variability, is observed in women reporting nausea after chemotherapy [43]. Bradycardia and blood pressure variation may occur with retching or vomiting.

Circulating neurohumoral mediators are altered during nausea and vomiting. Vasopressin levels increase during motion sickness, electrical vagal stimulation, and after apomorphine and cisplatinum [44]. Intravenous vasopressin at supraphysiological doses evokes nausea in humans while vasopressin V_1 antagonists prevent motion-induced emesis in monkeys, suggesting that the hormone may contribute to symptoms [45,46]. However, preservation of the emetic capability of apomorphine in patients with central diabetes insipidus indicates that vasopressin is not critical to induce emesis [47]. Highly emetogenic chemotherapies such as cisplatin and carboplatin elicit reductions in cortisol, reflecting disruption of the hypothalamic–pituitary–adrenal axis [48]. Levels of other transmitters such as epinephrine, β-endorphin, growth hormone, and prolactin also change during nausea and vomiting [49].

Pathophysiology of nausea

There is a lack of animal models so the CNS structures that mediate nausea are poorly understood. It has been proposed that nausea is the result of a lower level of activation of the same pathways that produce emesis. Changes in autonomic function or hormone release are proposed to relate to nausea in experimental animals. However, most of these phenomena persist in decerebrate animals that are incapable of perceiving gut sensation. The validity of food avoidance as a marker of nausea is unconfirmed. Activation of the inferior frontal gyrus proportionate to the degree of nausea has been demonstrated by magnetic source imaging in healthy humans exposed to vestibular stimulation or apomorphine [50]. This is similar to observed electroencephalographic changes in temporofrontal regions during motion sickness [51]. These findings suggest possible CNS foci for perception of nausea.

Causes of nausea and vomiting

Nausea and vomiting are caused by a range of pathological and physiological conditions affecting the gut, peritoneal cavity, CNS, and endocrine and metabolic functions (Table 13.1).

Medications

Drug reactions are among the most common causes of nausea and vomiting and usually present soon after the initiation of therapy. Emetogenic drugs may exert their effects by actions on distinct anatomic sites within the CNS and peripheral nervous system. Medications that act on the area postrema include anti-Parkinsonian agents (such as L-dopa, bromocriptine), nicotine, digoxin, and opiate analgesics. Nonsteroidal antiinflammatory drugs and erythromycin activate peripheral afferent pathways, most likely vagal [52]. Other medications that cause nausea and vomiting include cardiac antiarrhythmics, antihypertensives, diuretics, oral antidiabetics, oral contraceptives, and gastrointestinal medications such as sulfasalazine.

Infectious and toxic causes

Infectious illness produces nausea and vomiting that is usually of acute onset. Acute enteric illness occurs most often in children less than 3 years old, but exhibits a second peak incidence in the third decade of life [53]. Viral gastroenteritis may be caused by rotaviruses, reoviruses, adenoviruses, and the Hawaii, Snow Mountain, and Norwalk agents [54–56]. Bacterial infection with *Staphylococcus aureus*, *Salmonella*, *Bacillus cereus*, and *Clostridium perfringens* also produce nausea and vomiting, in many cases via toxins that act on the area postrema [57,58]. The enterotoxin elaborated by *S. aureus* is distinct from enterotoxins A–E and the toxic shock syndrome toxin 1 [59]. *Bacillus cereus* produces one emesis-causing toxin, which can be identified using a polymerase chain reaction assay, and three toxins that induce diarrhea [60,61]. Nausea in immunocompromised patients may result from gastrointestinal infection with cytomegalovirus or herpes simplex [62]. Nongastrointestinal infections that cause nausea include otitis media, meningitis, and hepatitis.

Disorders of the gut and peritoneal cavity

Gut and peritoneal disorders are prevalent causes of nausea and vomiting. Gastric and small intestinal obstructions produce nausea that may be relieved by vomiting. Gastric obstruction is often intermittent, whereas small intestinal obstruction is usually acute and associated with abdominal pain. Superior mesenteric artery syndrome is a rare condition in which the duodenum is compressed by the overlying superior mesenteric artery as it originates from the aorta, causing anatomical obstruction [63]. This syndrome is seen in patients who have experienced profound weight loss, undergone recent surgery, or received prolonged bedrest. Other rare mechanical causes of vomiting include subacute gastric volvulus and antral webs [64].

Gut motor disorders such as gastroparesis and chronic intestinal pseudoobstruction produce nausea through an inability to clear the retained lumenal contents. Systemic diseases that cause gastroparesis include diabetes, scleroderma, systemic lupus erythematosus, polymyositis-dermatomyositis, and amyloidosis. Diabetic gastroparesis commonly results from long-standing poor glycemic control, but is not necessarily associated with a poor prognosis [65]. Delayed gastric emptying of solids is demonstrable in two-thirds of scleroderma patients with abnormal esophageal motility [66]. Gastroparesis develops in fewer than 5% of patients who undergo vagotomy and gastric drainage for ulcer disease. The most common current postsurgical cause of gastroparesis is inadvertent vagal damage during performance of fundoplication for gastroesophageal reflux disease [67]. In patients with acquired immunodeficiency syndrome, human immunodeficiency virus infection may contribute to delays in gastric emptying [68]. Pancreatic adenocarcinoma produces gastroparesis by unknown mechanisms [69]. Gastric ischemia is a rare cause of gastroparesis, especially in women. The median arcuate ligament syndrome produces gastroparesis by compression of the celiac axis [70]. Chronic intestinal pseudoobstruction may be hereditary or result from systemic diseases similar to those that produce gastroparesis. Paraneoplastic intestinal pseudoobstruction is reported with some malignancies, most commonly small cell carcinoma of the lung [71].

One-third of patients with gastroparesis exhibit no underlying systemic disease to explain their symptoms. Some cases of idiopathic gastroparesis are preceded by prodromal symptoms such as diarrhea, fever, headache, or myalgias consistent with a viral etiology. The responsible agent is rarely identified; however, one report in children detected rotavirus in 8 of 11 cases [72]. In general, postviral gastroparesis confers a better prognosis with a shorter duration of illness, less severe symptoms, and better quality of life compared to non-viral idiopathic disease [72,73]. Women with idiopathic

Table 13.1 Causes of nausea and vomiting

Medications

Cancer chemotherapy
  Severe: cisplatinum, dacarbazine, nitrogen mustard
  Moderate: etoposide, methotrexate, cytarabine
  Mild: fluorouracil, vinblastine, tamoxifen
Analgesics
  Aspirin
  Nonsteroidal antiinflammatory drugs
  Auranofin
  Antigout drugs
Cardiovascular medications
  Digoxin
  Antiarrhythmics
  Antihypertensives
  β-Blockers
  Calcium-channel antagonists
Diuretics
Hormonal preparations
  Oral antidiabetics
  Oral contraceptives
Antibiotics
  Macrolides
  Tetracycline
  Sulfonamides
Antituberculous drugs
  Acyclovir
Gastrointestinal medications
  Sulfasalazine
  Azathioprine
Central nervous system activators
  Narcotics
  Antiparkinsonian drugs
  Anticonvulsants
Antiasthmatics
  Theophylline

Disorders of the gastrointestinal tract and peritoneum

Mechanical obstruction
  Gastric outlet obstruction
  Small intestinal obstruction
  Superior mesenteric artery syndrome
  Antral web
  Gastric volvulus
Functional gastroduodenal disorders
  Gastroparesis
  Chronic intestinal pseudoobstruction
  Functional dyspepsia – postprandial distress subset
  Chronic idiopathic nausea
  Functional vomiting
  Gastroesophageal reflux
Radiation therapy
Intraperitoneal inflammation
  Gastroduodenal ulcer
  Cholecystitis
  Pancreatitis
  Hepatitis
  Crohn's disease

Central nervous system causes

Increased intracranial pressure
  Malignant tumor
  Infarction
  Hemorrhage
  Abscess
  Meningitis
  Congenital malformation
Emotional responses
Psychiatric conditions
  Anxiety disorder
  Depression
  Bulimia nervosa
  Anorexia nervosa
Labyrinthine disorders
  Motion sickness
  Labyrinthitis
  Tumor
  Méniére disease

Endocrinological and metabolic causes

Pregnancy
Uremia
Diabetic ketoacidosis
Hyper-, hypoparathyroidism
Hyperthyroidism
Addison disease

Infectious causes

Viral/bacterial gastroenteritis
Otitis media

Postoperative nausea and vomiting

Cyclic vomiting syndrome

Miscellaneous causes

Myocardial infarction
Congestive heart failure
Ethanol abuse
Graft-vs-host disease
Jamaican vomiting sickness
Hypervitaminosis
Starvation

gastroparesis often report physical or sexual abuse, similar to observations in patients with irritable bowel syndrome [74].

It is difficult to distinguish idiopathic gastroparesis from functional dyspepsia in some cases, leading some to speculate that they are variants of the same disorder. As with idiopathic gastroparesis, some functional dyspeptics present after an acute infection. Furthermore, approximately one-third of patients with functional dyspepsia exhibit delayed emptying. The postprandial distress subtype of functional dyspepsia in the current Rome III criteria is characterized by gastroparesis-like symptoms including postprandial fullness and early satiety [75]. Other Rome III diagnoses with symptom overlap with idiopathic gastroparesis include chronic idiopathic nausea and functional vomiting [75]. The prevalence of delayed emptying in these syndromes has not been characterized. From a diagnostic standpoint, a presentation of predominant pain and less nausea is considered to be more typical of functional dyspepsia while dominant nausea with minimal pain is more consistent with idiopathic gastroparesis [76].

Abdominal disorders not involving the gut lumen may produce nausea and vomiting. Inflammatory conditions such as pancreatitis, appendicitis, and cholecystitis activate peritoneal afferent pathways. Biliary colic in the absence of inflammation produces nausea by activating afferents from distention of the biliary tree. Fulminant hepatic failure results in nausea, presumably as the result of retention of unknown emetic toxins and increased intracranial pressure.

Central nervous system causes

Many emetic stimuli produce symptoms by action on the CNS. Increased intracranial pressure from malignancy, infarction, hemorrhage, infection, or congenital causes produces emesis with or without nausea. Maximal emesis occurs at an intracranial pressure of 80 mmHg [77]. Emotional responses to unpleasant smells, tastes, or memories may induce vomiting. Psychiatric conditions (e.g., anxiety, depression) and eating disorders (anorexia nervosa, bulimia nervosa) are often accompanied by nausea and vomiting.

Labyrinthine disorders such as labyrinthitis, tumors, and Ménière's disease produce nausea and vomiting, often with vertigo. Motion sickness is evoked by repetitive movements that activate the vestibular nuclei and is associated with extensive autonomic activation that produces pallor, diaphoresis, and salivation. Space sickness, experienced by most astronauts in zero gravity, is related to motion sickness but may not exhibit the associated autonomic phenomena [78].

Nausea and vomiting in pregnancy

Nausea and vomiting complicate 50%–70% of pregnancies. On average, symptoms begin 39 days after the last menses, peak in the 9th to 11th gestational weeks, and persist for 35–45 days (Fig. 13.1) [3, 79]. Although nausea and vomiting of pregnancy (NVP) is commonly referred to as "morning sickness," only 1.8% of women report symptoms restricted to the morning whereas 80% are symptomatic throughout the day (79). NVP is more common in women who are

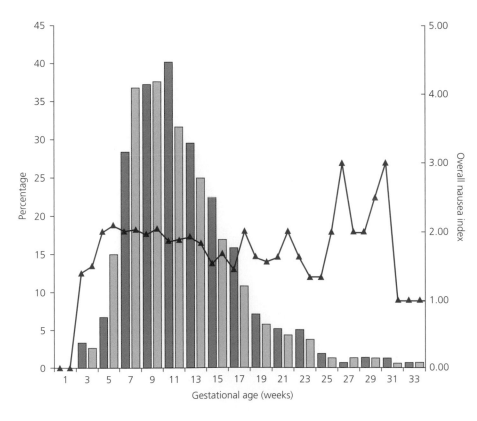

Figure 13.1 The rates and severity of nausea and vomiting of pregnancy (NVP) are plotted as a function of gestation. The filled bars plot the percentage of women who experience NVP each week. The number of women with symptoms is highest in week 11; the number of affected women markedly decreases in the latter half of pregnancy. The line graph plots the nausea severity from 0 to 5. Although many fewer women have nausea later in pregnancy, nausea remains high in these individuals. From Lacroix et al. [79].

primigravid, younger, overweight, less educated, and more economically disadvantaged [80,81]. Twin pregnancies increase the risk of NVP [81]. Factor analysis of dietary constituents has revealed associations of NVP with high intakes of sugars, alcohol, and meats, whereas smoking before pregnancy and use of vitamins during pregnancy decrease the risk [4,82]. Most cases of NVP are not deleterious to either the fetus or mother. Rather, NVP has been associated with longer gestation and reduced incidences of miscarriage, preterm births, congenital heart defects, and fetal demise [83,84]. However, in regions where malnutrition is prevalent, NVP may have nutritional consequences in the later stages of pregnancy that lead to poor outcomes.

Hyperemesis gravidarum, a condition of intractable vomiting, complicates 0.7%–5% of pregnancies and may produce dangerous fluid and electrolyte abnormalities. The risk of hyperemesis is 15% in the second pregnancies of women who had hyperemesis in the first pregnancy, but only 0.7% without prior hyperemesis [85]. Other risk factors for hyperemesis gravidarum requiring hospitalization include hyperthyroidism, psychiatric disease, gastrointestinal disorders, asthma, and preexisting diabetes [86]. Hyperemesis in women with poor weight gain during pregnancy leads to premature birth of infants of low birth weight with low APGAR scores [87].

The cause of NVP is unknown but is believed to relate to altered neurohumoral function. Although symptoms parallel β-human chorionic gonadotropin levels, no pathogenic role has been discerned for this hormone. One group observed an inverse association of prolactin levels with NVP [88]. Leptin levels are elevated in patients with hyperemesis gravidarum [89]. Other studies show associations of nausea severity in pregnancy with maternal androgens such as androstenedione, dehydroepiandrosterone sulfate, and testosterone [90]. Intolerance of oral contraceptives is strongly associated with NVP, suggesting potential roles for estrogen and progesterone [91]. One recent investigation reported an association between elevated maternal serum prostaglandin E_2 levels and NVP [92].

Chemotherapy-induced emesis

Emesis is a common complication of cancer chemotherapy and may be acute, delayed, or anticipatory [93]. Thirty-five per cent of patients develop acute nausea after chemotherapy, while 13% experience acute emesis [94]. Delayed nausea and vomiting are reported by 60% and 50% of patients receiving highly emetogenic chemotherapy and by 52% and 28% of those receiving moderately emetogenic agents [94]. Risk factors for chemotherapy-induced nausea and vomiting include low social functioning, prechemotherapy nausea, female sex, and use of highly emetogenic chemotherapeutic drugs such as cisplatinum, carmustine, high-dose cyclophosphamide, and dacarbazine [95]. These agents elicit acute vomiting within hours of administration with associated increases in plasma serotonin levels, urinary excretion of the serotonin metabolite 5-hydroxyindole acetic acid (5-HIAA), ileal tissue serotonin, and numbers of serotonin immunoreactive cells [93,96]. In contrast, less emetogenic agents evoke little rise in plasma serotonin or urinary 5-HIAA [97]. Cisplatinum-evoked emesis is reduced by vagotomy, suggesting mediation by peripheral afferent pathways [98]. However, the inability of the peripherally active 5-HT$_3$ antagonist zatosetron-QUAT to block cisplatinum-induced emesis when given intravenously, coupled with a significant antiemetic effect when given intracerebroventricularly, indicates an additional site of action in the CNS [99]. Studies quantifying CNS Fos expression observe that cisplatin activates the dorsal vagal complex, central amygdala, and bed nucleus of the stria terminalis [100].

In contrast to acute chemotherapy-evoked emesis, delayed and anticipatory vomiting are mediated by serotonin-independent pathways. Delayed emesis after cisplatinum is not associated with urinary 5-HIAA excretion and is poorly controlled by 5-HT$_3$ antagonists [97]. In dogs, 5-HT$_4$ receptors may participate in delayed chemotherapy-induced emesis [101]. The ability of neurokinin NK$_1$ antagonists to reduce delayed nausea and vomiting after chemotherapy indicates that this phase is mediated by substance P pathways [102]. Another study observed increased norepinephrine production during the delayed phase after cisplatinum [103]. Anticipatory nausea and vomiting occur in 25%–34% of patients by the fourth course of chemotherapy, more often in younger patients [104, 105]. Development of anticipatory symptoms is dependent on anxiety and coping mechanisms. Patient expectations strongly predict the onset of anticipatory nausea but not anticipatory vomiting [106].

Radiation-induced vomiting

Radiation therapy for malignancy produces emesis by effects on both the structure and function of the gut. The incidence of nausea and vomiting is dependent on the region that is irradiated, being as high as 80% when the upper abdomen is included in the radiation field [107]. Involvement of serotonergic pathways is indicated by the ability of 5-HT$_3$ antagonists to reduce the nausea and vomiting that is evoked acutely by abdominal radiation therapy.

Postoperative nausea and vomiting

Nausea and vomiting complicate 17%–37% of surgical operations, more commonly in women [108]. Postoperative nausea and vomiting (PONV) are more frequent after general anesthesia than with regional nerve blocks and correlate with the duration of surgery. PONV occurs more often after abdominal and orthopedic surgery than with laparoscopic or other extraabdominal operations and is exacerbated by the use of opiate agents. Other proven risk factors include non-smoking status, a history of previous PONV or motion sickness, use of volatile anesthetics or nitrous oxide, and high-dose neostigmine [109]. Possible risk factors include a history of migraine, intense preoperative anxiety, decreased perioperative fluids, and administration of perioperative crystalloid solutions instead of colloid [109].

Cyclic vomiting syndrome

Cyclic vomiting syndrome (CVS) is characterized by discrete episodes of intractable emesis with intervening asymptomatic periods. CVS has traditionally been considered a disease of children, who present with a mean age of onset of 5 years old. Affected children typically have eight or nine attacks per year with mean durations of 1–3 days, which may be precipitated by stress or infections [110]. Two-thirds of children with CVS miss more than 10 days of school per year. In children, there are strong associations of CVS with personal or family histories of migraine headaches, motion sickness, gastroesophageal reflux, psychological symptoms, atopy, and forceps delivery [110,111]. CVS is increasingly recognized in adults. The Rome III committee has recently established diagnostic criteria for the disorder that describe stereotypic, self-limited episodes of relentless nausea and vomiting (Fig. 13.2) [75,112]. More than 90% of adults with CVS experience a stereotypic prodrome and many report interepisodic dyspepsia and a history of depression, anxiety, or panic attacks [112,113].

The etiology of CVS is unknown and is likely multifactorial. In children, a migraine-related pathogenesis is suggested by observations that many patients develop migraine headaches in adolescence as the severity of CVS manifestations wane [111]. Children with migraine-associated CVS report milder emetic episodes, more abdominal pain, more headache with photophobia, and increased psychological stress. Some adults report either a personal or a family history of migraines as well [112,113]. In children with CVS, autonomic function testing reveals consistent sympathetic autonomic neuropathic changes, which are postulated to be pathogenic of symptoms [114]. Other proposed causes of CVS in children include food allergy and mitochondrial fatty

acid oxidation disorders such as short-chain and medium-chain acyl-coacetyl A dehydrogenase deficiency and late-onset glutaric acidemia type II [115,116]. Recently, an association of cyclical vomiting patterns in adults with chronic cannabis use was observed [117]. In those individuals who were able to discontinue cannabis abuse, vomiting episodes abated.

Miscellaneous conditions

Endocrinological and metabolic causes of nausea include uremia, diabetic ketoacidosis, hyper- and hypoparathyroidism, hyperthyroidism, and Addison disease. Acute fatty liver of pregnancy, a condition distinct from NVP, produces severe third-trimester vomiting and can be complicated by liver failure, disseminated intravascular coagulation, and fetal or maternal death. Posterior myocardial infarction produces nausea as a result of diaphragmatic irritation. Nausea from acute coronary syndromes is more common in women than men [118]. Nausea occurring with congestive heart failure results from passive congestion of the liver and gut. Excess ethanol intake induces vomiting by local action on the gut and brainstem. Acute graft-vs-host disease is the dominant cause of nausea and vomiting in bone marrow transplant recipients, most commonly occurring within the initial months after transplantation. Jamaican vomiting sickness occurs after eating unripe akee fruit [119]. Excess vitamin intake as well as extended fasting or starvation may also cause nausea.

History and physical examination

Historical features

A detailed history provides useful diagnostic information about the cause of unexplained nausea and emesis. Acute vomiting (for 1 or 2 days) most often results from infection, a medication, or toxin, or accumulation of endogenous toxins

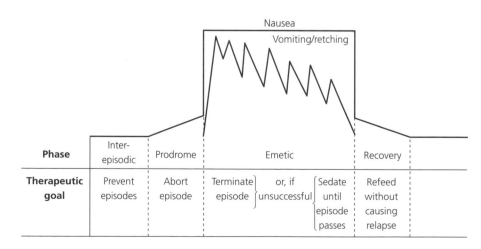

Figure 13.2 The profile of a typical attack of cyclic vomiting syndrome (CVS) in an adult. After a relatively asymptomatic interepisodic interval, a brief prodrome signals the onset of symptoms. This is followed by a period of relentless nausea and vomiting, which terminates in a brief recovery period. Therapeutic goals differ in each phase. Prophylaxis should be offered during the interepisodic period. Antiemetics can be given in the prodrome to attempt to abort the episode. During the attack, if antiemetics are unsuccessful, sedation can shorten symptoms and reduce their impact. Refeeding is attempted during the recovery. From Fleisher et al. [112].

as in uremia or diabetic ketoacidosis. Chronic vomiting (for more than 1 week) usually results from long-standing medical or psychiatric conditions.

Timing of nausea and vomiting

The timing of symptoms provides clues to the underlying disease. Vomiting soon after a meal occurs with mechanical gastric obstruction. However, patients with rumination syndrome also commonly regurgitate undigested food within minutes of consumption – this pattern may be mistaken for early postprandial vomiting. Although patients with gastroparesis may report nausea within 5 min of eating, most vomiting occurs more than 1 h after a meal. Nausea and vomiting from cholecystitis and pancreatitis may present in the first hour. In some cases of esophagitis or ulcer disease, nausea abates with eating. Morning emesis may be reported with pregnancy, uremia, or chronic alcoholism.

Character of the vomitus

Characteristics of the vomitus can assist in diagnosis. Return of undigested food suggests achalasia, rumination, or a Zenker diverticulum. Vomiting of partly digested food hours or days after ingestion suggests gastric obstruction or gastroparesis. Bilious emesis excludes obstruction proximal to the ampulla of Vater, while hematemesis usually results from tissue injury. However, Mallory–Weiss tears may produce bloody vomitus from violent emesis. Gastrinoma patients may vomit voluminous clear acidic liquid, while those with achlorhydria may expel odorless vomitus. Feculent emesis occurs with distal intestinal or colonic obstruction, small intestinal bacterial overgrowth, and gastrocolic fistulae.

Associated symptoms

Abdominal pain is noted with ulcer disease, obstruction, and inflammatory disorders like cholecystitis or pancreatitis. Vomiting may relieve nausea and pain from ulcers and bowel obstruction, but has no effect in inflammatory conditions. Enteric infection may present with associated diarrhea, fever, or myalgias. CNS processes are suggested by headaches, visual changes, altered mentation, and neck stiffness. In these disorders, emesis may be effortless, there may be no nausea, or emesis may be projectile. Labyrinthine diseases present with tinnitus or vertigo. Chest pain, dysphagia, or jaundice suggest cardiac, esophageal, or hepatobiliary disease, respectively. Prolonged vomiting may produce fluid and electrolyte losses, which may cause lightheadedness, rapid heart rate, and mouth dryness.

Complications of nausea and vomiting

Chronic vomiting may promote loss of dental enamel. In addition to Mallory–Weiss tears, violent retching or emesis may cause Boerhaave syndrome, a rupture of the esophagus, which may promote development of mediastinitis or peritonitis. In patients with impaired consciousness, emesis may be complicated by pulmonary aspiration of acidic material leading to chemical pneumonitis.

Physical examination findings

The physical examination provides diagnostic clues and assists in the management of nausea and vomiting. Fever suggests infection or inflammation. Tachycardia, orthostatic hypotension, loss of skin turgor, and dry mucous membranes indicate dehydration. Skin examination may show sclerodactyly in scleroderma or jaundice with hepatobiliary disease. Adenopathy raises concern for neoplasm. Hepatomegaly is found in malignancy as well as benign hepatic infiltration. Absent bowel sounds signify ileus, while high-pitched hyperactive bowel sounds with a distended abdomen are consistent with bowel obstruction. A succession splash on side-to-side movement is found in gastric obstruction or gastroparesis. Ulcers, cholecystitis, pancreatitis, or peritonitis may produce abdominal tenderness or guarding. Gross or occult fecal blood should prompt evaluation for a mucosal injury process. Focal neurological signs, papilledema, and impaired mentation suggest a CNS process while nuchal rigidity is consistent with meningitis. Asterixis is present in metabolic diseases like uremia or hepatic failure. Many gut motor disorders have associated peripheral or autonomic neuropathies.

Laboratory studies and diagnostic testing

For intractable nausea and vomiting or an elusive diagnosis, selected laboratory findings, structural tests, or studies of gut motor function can direct clinical management.

Laboratory testing

Findings of laboratory testing complement the history and physical examination. With long-standing symptoms or dehydration, hypokalemia or an elevated blood urea nitrogen may be detected on electrolyte measurement. Metabolic alkalosis may result from a loss of hydrogen ions in the acidic vomitus and from contraction of the extracellular space from dehydration. A complete blood count can exclude anemia from inflammation or blood loss, leukocytosis from an inflammatory source, or leukopenia from a viral infection. Chronic blood loss also may be suggested by low serum iron saturation or ferritin. Hypoalbuminemia is seen in some chronic diseases and in conditions with gut protein loss. Amylase, lipase, and liver chemistries are obtained for suspected pancreatic or hepatobiliary disease. Endocrinological and metabolic causes can be assessed through pregnancy testing, thyroid chemistry determination, and measurement of blood urea nitrogen, creatinine, glucose, ketones, calcium, and cortisol. Specific serological markers can be obtained for collagen vascular diseases such as lupus. Serological tests in patients with paraneoplastic dysmotility syndromes include type 1 antineuronal nuclear antibody, anti-Purkinje cell cytoplasmic antibody, and ganglionic nicotinic acetylcholine receptor antibody [120]. Such antineuronal antibodies may also be detected in some patients with idiopathic gastroparesis with an autoimmune basis [121]. Meningitis is confirmed by lumbar puncture.

Structural evaluation

Anatomical studies may be indicated if initial testing is nondiagnostic. Flat and upright abdominal radiographs are obtained as a screening test. Small intestinal air–fluid levels with absent colonic air suggest bowel obstruction, while diffuse lumenal distention with absent bowel sounds is consistent with ileus or chronic pseudoobstruction. Subdiaphragmatic free air indicates visceral perforation. Characterization of suspected small intestinal obstruction may be further evaluated by small intestinal contrast radiography. Water contrast agents, such as Gastrografin, provide reasonable degrees of accuracy in excluding obstructions that require surgery [122]. However, barium provides superior visualization of partial obstruction. For those with intermittent symptoms who have a high likelihood of a mechanical process and in whom small bowel contrast radiography is negative, enteroclysis may provide greater discrimination of subtle small intestinal lumenal processes [123]. With this technique, the proximal intestine is intubated under fluoroscopic guidance and barium and methylcellulose are perfused to provide a double-contrast image. If partial colonic obstruction is a consideration, contrast enema radiography should be performed before proceeding with small bowel imaging. Upper endoscopy or contrast radiography may be performed for suspected ulcer disease or outlet narrowing. Endoscopy affords the advantage of providing biopsy capability of abnormal mucosa. Finding retained food on endoscopy in the absence of obstruction suggests gastroparesis. Computed tomography (CT) enterography has been shown to characterize small intestinal inflammation in patients with known or suspected Crohn's disease [124]. Gastric and duodenal dilation on CT scanning with a diminished distance between the superior mesenteric artery and the aorta correlate significantly with symptoms in superior mesenteric artery syndrome [125]. Suspected pancreaticobiliary disease may be evaluated by CT, ultrasound, or biliary scintigraphy. If bowel ischemia is a consideration, mesenteric angiography, CT angiography, or magnetic resonance imaging (MRI) are useful. CT or MRI of the head is indicated if CNS disease is a possibility.

Studies of gastrointestinal motor and myoelectric activity

When lumenal obstruction has been excluded, functional causes of nausea and vomiting such as gastroparesis and pseudoobstruction are entertained. The clinician may elect to treat empirically with a medication designed to stimulate

gut motility. Alternatively, testing of gut motor activity can be performed to characterize the functional defects.

Quantification of gastric emptying

Gastric scintigraphy is the most widely accepted test for diagnosis of gastroparesis and employs a technetium 99m (^{99m}Tc)–sulfur colloid label bound to a solid food. Liquid-phase scans are felt to be less sensitive for detecting the disorder. Solid-phase emptying exhibits a biphasic curve with an initial lag phase, during which the food is mixed in the stomach, followed by a linear emptying phase, which persists until the stomach is emptied. The pattern of solid emptying in gastroparesis may be variable, with some individuals exhibiting prolongation of the lag phase while others show slowed linear emptying after a normal lag phase. A major drawback of gastric scintigraphy has been a lack of standardization of criteria used to diagnose gastroparesis across all medical centers. In a survey of gastric emptying tests performed in academic and community hospitals in Canada, 28% of nuclear medicine departments defined the cutoff for gastroparesis as the degree of gastric retention more than 2 standard deviations above the mean, while 26% used 1 standard deviation, 6.5% employed 1.5 standard deviations, and 40% did not have objective criteria [126]. Among the medical centers surveyed, only 18% validated their results in a population of healthy volunteers. Recently, researchers have advocated acceptance of uniform standards of gastric scintigraphy performance and interpretation. A standardized method using a meal of toast, jam, and EggBeaters labeled with ^{99m}Tc–sulfur colloid was recently validated (Fig. 13.3) [127]. With this technique, gastric retentions over 60% at 2 h and over 10% at 4 h are consistent with gastroparesis. However, even using such a standardized protocol, the diagnosis of gastroparesis may not be clear-cut. In one investigation, 37% of patients

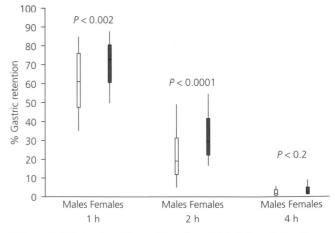

Figure 13.3 Rates of gastric emptying of a radiolabeled low-fat meal are shown for men and women using a standardized scintigraphic method. Normal values for gastric retention are less than 60% at 2 h after meal ingestion and less than 10% after 4 h. From Tougas et al. [127].

with normal emptying at 2 h exhibited delayed emptying at 4 h while 19% with delayed emptying at 2 h showed normalization at 4 h [128]. Although gastric scintigraphy is routinely performed for the diagnosis of gastroparesis, its use has not been rigorously subjected to outcomes analysis. Indeed, one study reported that findings of gastric-emptying scanning did not influence the management of patients undergoing the test [129]. Gastric scintigraphy is also employed to detect rapid gastric emptying, which has been described in adults with CVS and also has been observed in a subset of patients with functional dyspepsia [113,130].

Other techniques for measuring gastric emptying have been promoted. A recently approved method involves ingesting a radiotelemetry capsule that continuously transmits data on lumenal pH and pressure profiles to a receiver worn by the patient. With this test, gastric emptying is determined by measuring the time from ingestion of the capsule to the time a pH reading of near neutrality is recorded, reflecting passage into the proximal duodenum. Correlation coefficients between the capsule technique and gastric scintiscans for detection of gastroparesis exceed 0.8 [131]. This method has potential additional abilities to quantify motility indices in the distal stomach as well as transit, pH, and motor patterns in the small intestine and colon. Performance of breath testing after ingestion of non-radioactive ^{13}C-labeled nutrient substrates such as octanoate, acetate, and *Spirulina platensis* can assess gastric emptying of both solids and liquids. These methods measure liberation of $^{13}CO_2$ in expired breath samples after duodenal assimilation of the ingested compound and are reliable only in persons with normal digestive and absorptive function. Emptying results from the [^{13}C]octanoate and [^{13}C]acetate breath tests show fair to good correlations with scintigraphy [132]. Ultrasonography also can be used to quantify gastric emptying. After ingestion of a liquid, antral scanning is performed in transverse sections and gastric volumes are calculated as a function of time. Solid meals cannot be used because of their echogenic nature. These techniques may be preferred over scintigraphy in selected patients such as pregnant women in whom radioactive tracers are contraindicated. MRI has also been proposed for the assessment of gastric emptying and correlates well with findings of scintigraphy in healthy volunteers. Single photon emission computed tomography (SPECT) employs intravenously administered ^{99m}Tc-pertechnetate that accumulates within the gastric wall rather than the lumen, and thus provides a three-dimensional outline of the stomach [133]. This technique offers the advantage of measuring regional gastric volumes in real time to assess fundic accommodation and intragastric distribution. A potential drawback of SPECT is the need for large radiation doses.

Other tests of gastrointestinal function
Other tests of gastric function performed in academic centers that specialize in the care of patients with disordered gut motor

activity can complement the findings of gastric-emptying testing. A variant of gastric scintigraphy, dynamic antral scintigraphy, is used in research to image nonocclusive antral contractions in real time but this method has not been used clinically [134]. Gastrointestinal manometry involves peroral placement of a catheter to monitor antroduodenojejunal pressures over 6–8 h. The initial 4–5 h records fasting motility, during which one or more fasting motor complexes are usually observed. Motor activity then is measured for 2 h after a solid meal, which should induce a fed pattern. In some centers, manometry is used to test the effects of motor-stimulating drugs or to record motor activity for 24 h in ambulatory fashion. Manometry is considered for patients with unexplained symptoms, who have not responded to treatment, or who are being considered for surgery or enteral vs parenteral nutrition. Gastroparesis is characterized by loss of normal fasting migrating motor complexes and reduced fed antral contractions and, in some cases, spasm of the pylorus [135]. Manometry is most useful in excluding associated small intestinal dysmotilities, including those with myopathic (contractile amplitude < 30 mmHg with normal morphology) and neuropathic (intense, uncoordinated burst contractions) patterns. Small intestinal motor dysfunction is detected in 17%–85% of patients with gastroparesis [136]. Clinical management is influenced in approximately 20% –25% of patients undergoing gastrointestinal manometry [137]. Electrogastrography (EGG) measures gastric slow-wave activity via electrodes affixed to the skin overlying the stomach. Under healthy conditions, EGG recordings exhibit a uniform 3 cycles/min waveform that increases in amplitude with ingestion of water or a nutrient meal. EGG abnormalities include rhythm disruption for more than 30% of the recording time, including tachygastria (frequency > 4 cycles/min) and bradygastria (< 2 cycles/min) and a lack of signal-amplitude increase with eating. EGG abnormalities are prevalent in patients with gastroparesis as well as in patients with nausea from pregnancy, functional dyspepsia, and motion sickness [138]. Impairment of the amplitude response to meals correlates with delayed emptying in patients with gastroparesis. The importance of EGG dysrhythmias in symptom generation is supported by the observation that selected antiemetics normalize slow-wave frequencies [139]. Other electrical techniques, such as epigastric impedance and applied potential tomography, employ cutaneous electrodes to measure changes in resistance afforded by liquid meals that correlate with the rate of emptying. Because gastric myoelectric disturbances have unproven roles in symptom pathogenesis and because no therapies have been characterized to specifically target these abnormalities, EGG, epigastric impedance, and applied potential tomography have not achieved widespread acceptance as useful diagnostic tests. Satiety testing involves the ingestion of water or a liquid nutrient until the patient reports maximal fullness. Volumes consumed in functional dyspeptics with early satiety are reduced compared with healthy volunteers, which is reflective either of impaired relaxation of the proximal stomach or heightened sensitivity of gastric afferent pathways [140].

Principles of management

Care of the patient with nausea and vomiting involves assessing the etiology and severity of the condition, with prompt initiation of therapy to prevent complications. When possible, medical or surgical treatment should be directed at the underlying disease process.

Indications for hospitalization

In some patients, it must be determined if intravenous resuscitation is needed. Poor skin turgor and orthostatic pulse or blood pressure changes indicate that more than 10% of body fluids have been lost and mandate intravenous fluid administration. Potassium supplements are started for hypokalemia if urine output is adequate. Intravenous fluids may be given in the emergency department or outpatient clinic if the patient can resume adequate oral intake at home. If oral replenishment cannot be guaranteed, hospitalization should be considered. Patients with obstruction or ileus may benefit from nasogastric suction. The threshold for hospitalization is lowered for diabetics, patients with concurrent diarrhea, persons with other chronic debilitating disease, and very young or old patients because these patients become rapidly dehydrated.

Dietary and nonmedicinal considerations

Dietary and nonmedicinal measures designed to compensate for gastric motor impairment are advocated for most patients with nausea and vomiting. Ingesting multiple small meals each day, rather than two or three large ones, enhances the efficiency of postprandial intragastric mixing. Liquids empty more rapidly than solids so a reduction of solid food intake is desired. Carbonated liquids are avoided to limit gastric distention. To minimize any inhibition of gastric emptying by lipids, a diet with restricted fat content should be consumed. Inclusion of indigestible fiber in a meal delays its emptying from the stomach and may promote phytobezoar formation [141]. Conversely, reducing the amount of indigestible dietary fiber may decrease symptoms of gastroparesis. Medications that inhibit gastrointestinal motility should be discontinued if possible. In diabetic gastroparesis, maintenance of euglycemia may avoid the inhibitory effects of hyperglycemia on gastric motor function.

Medications for nausea and vomiting

Patients with nausea and vomiting may benefit from medications that suppress emesis (Table 13.2). Others may experience relief from drugs that stimulate gut motor activity (Table 13.3). Such prokinetic agents are commonly given before meals to reduce postprandial gastric stasis with a dose at bedtime to effect gut clearance of undigested residue during sleep.

Antiemetic medications

Antihistamines such as meclizine and dimenhydrinate are useful for vomiting resulting from labyrinthine activation, as with motion sickness or labyrinthitis [142]. They are also effective for nausea in uremia and for PONV. Sedation and dryness of the mouth may limit their use in some settings. Newer, less sedating antihistamines such as astemizole, cetirizine, and fexofenadine have limited antiemetic activity in conditions such as motion sickness [143].

Drugs such as scopolamine that antagonize muscarinic receptors in the vestibular pathways are also effective in motion sickness when given orally or transdermally [144]. Side effects from antimuscarinic agents, such as dryness of the mouth and eyes, sedation, impaired concentration, headaches, constipation, and urinary retention, limit their usefulness in some individuals.

Dopamine antagonists including phenothiazines (prochlorperazine, chlorpromazine) and butyrophenones (droperidol, haloperidol) are the most commonly prescribed antiemetics. Studies employing selective agonists indicate that activation of dopamine D_2 and D_3 receptors, but not D_1 or D_4 receptors, leads to emesis [145]. Thus, most antiemetic antidopaminergics act on the area postrema D_2 receptors to reduce emesis from gastroenteritis, medications, abdominal irradiation, surgery, toxins, and some chemotherapies [146]. Antidopaminergic agents produce many CNS side effects including drowsiness, insomnia, anxiety, mood changes, confusion, dystonic reactions, Parkinsonian symptoms, and irreversible tardive dyskinesia. Through effects on the pituitary, antidopaminergics may induce hyperprolactinemia leading to breast engorgement, galactorrhea, and sexual dysfunction. Other rare side effects include blood dyscrasias and jaundice. Many antidopaminergics bind to other receptors and elicit antihistaminic and antimuscarinic side effects as well.

Serotonin 5-HT$_3$ antagonists are widely used for prophylaxis of acute chemotherapy-induced emesis but are also effective for radiation-induced vomiting and PONV. The antiemetic effects of 5-HT$_3$ antagonists do not show tolerance after multiple courses of chemotherapy [147]. In contrast, 5-HT$_3$ antagonists are less effective against delayed emesis after chemotherapy [97,148]. Other populations who may benefit from 5-HT$_3$ antagonist therapy include those with vomiting refractory to other antiemetics, patients with hepatic or renal impairment, individuals with nausea secondary to human immunodeficiency syndrome, patients with bulimia nervosa, and children with vomiting [149,150]. However, one study reported that patients with nausea and vomiting from causes other than chemotherapy and pregnancy experience no greater relief from intravenous 5-HT$_3$

Table 13.2 Antiemetic medications

Drug class	Medications	Clinical uses	Common side effects
Histamine antagonists	Dimenhydrinate Meclizine Promethazine	Motion sickness Labyrinthitis Uremia Postoperative emesis	Sedation Dry mouth
Muscarinic antagonists	Scopolamine Hyoscine	Motion sickness	Sedation Dry mouth and eyes Impaired concentration Headache Constipation Urinary retention
Dopamine antagonists	Prochlorperazine	Extensive indications including: gastroenteritis, postoperative, toxins, medications, radiation	Sedation Anxiety Mood disturbances Sleep disruption Dystonic reactions Tardive dyskinesia Galactorrhea Sexual dysfunction
Serotonin antagonists	Ondansetron Granisetron	Chemotherapy- and radio-therapy-induced emesis Postoperative emesis Emesis in AIDS	Constipation Headache
Neurokinin antagonists	Aprepitant	Chemotherapy-induced nausea and emesis	Anorexia Diarrhea Constipation
Cannabinoids	Dronabinol	Chemotherapy-induced emesis	Somnolence Ataxia Hallucinations
Antidepressants	Amitriptyline Nortriptyline Mirtazapine	Functional vomiting Diabetic gastropathy Cyclic vomiting syndrome Gastroparesis	Sedation Constipation
Corticosteroids	Dexamethasone	Delayed chemotherapy-induced emesis Postoperative emesis	Anxiety Depression Hyperglycemia Hypertension
Benzodiazepines	Lorazepam	Anticipatory emesis	Sedation

antagonists than from low-dose promethazine [151]. At biologically equivalent doses, the 5-HT$_3$ antagonists ondansetron, granisetron, and dolasetron are equally effective [96]. Newer agents such as palonosetron exhibit longer half-lives and higher binding affinity than older agents and show improved complete response rates as reflected by an absence of emesis and a lack of need for rescue antiemetics after cancer chemotherapy [152,153]. Side effects from 5-HT$_3$ antagonists include constipation, headaches, and rare elevations in liver chemistries. Recent studies suggest that individuals with a single-nucleotide polymorphism (3435C→T) in the gene that codes for the drug efflux transporter adenosine triphosphate-binding cassette subfamily B member 1 (ABCB1) exhibit greater antiemetic responses to 5-HT$_3$ antagonists [154,155]. Other genetic markers may predict responses to selected 5-HT$_3$ antagonists. Patients with duplications of the CPY2D6 allele, which predicts ultrarapid metabolism, exhibit poorer antiemetic responses to dolasetron than granisetron [156].

The neurokinin NK$_1$ antagonist aprepitant is used most often for prevention of acute and delayed chemotherapy-induced

Table 13.3 Prokinetic medications

Medication	Mechanism of action	Common side effects
Commonly used agents for gastroparesis		
Metoclopramide	$5\text{-}HT_4$ receptor facilitation of acetylcholine release from enteric nerves Dopamine receptor antagonist $5\text{-}HT_3$ receptor antagonist (weak)	Sedation Anxiety Mood disturbances Sleep disruption Dystonic reactions Tardive dyskinesia Galactorrhea Sexual dysfunction
Erythromycin	Motilin receptor agonist	Abdominal pain Nausea and vomiting Diarrhea
Agents of limited prescription in gastroparesis		
Domperidone	Peripheral dopamine receptor antagonist	Galactorrhea/gynecomastia Sexual dysfunction
Bethanechol	Muscarinic receptor agonist	Abdominal pain Salivation Nausea Diaphoresis Cardiac dysrhythmias
Physostigmine	Acetylcholinesterase inhibitor	Abdominal pain Salivation Nausea Diaphoresis Cardiac dysrhythmias
Agents for small intestinal dysmotility		
Octreotide	Somatostatin receptor analogue	Diarrhea Altered glycemic control (diabetics) Gallstones Thyroid disease
Leuprolide	Gonadotropin-releasing hormone analogue	Amenorrhea Osteoporosis

emesis, but also exhibits efficacy in PONV and motion sickness [157–159]. Other studies suggest that aprepitant may be less effective than $5\text{-}HT_3$ antagonists in the initial 12 h after chemotherapy [102]. The antiemetic efficacy of aprepitant is preserved after six cycles of chemotherapy [160]. Control of nausea is improved by aprepitant in some studies but not others [161]. Its side effects include anorexia, constipation, diarrhea, nausea, and hiccups [162].

Cannabinoids such as dronabinol exhibit efficacy in chemotherapy-induced emesis prophylaxis comparable to, or slightly better than, the antidopaminergics; however, these drugs produce severe side effects such as somnolence, ataxia, syncope, seizures, and hallucinations, which may be promin-

ent in the elderly [163]. In animal models, the cannabinoid tetrohydrocannabinol suppresses vomiting evoked by lithium via action on CB_1 receptors [164]. Other potential mechanisms of action of the cannabinoids include reduced prostaglandin synthesis and stimulation of endogenous endorphin production [165].

Antidepressant and antipsychotic agents in several classes exhibit antiemetic effects in selected clinical settings. Tricyclic antidepressants are effective in patients with functional vomiting as well as in adults with CVS [113,166]. In one study, tricyclic drugs reduced nausea and vomiting in a mixed group of diabetics with both normal and delayed gastric emptying (Fig. 13.4) [167]. Mirtazepine has shown efficacy

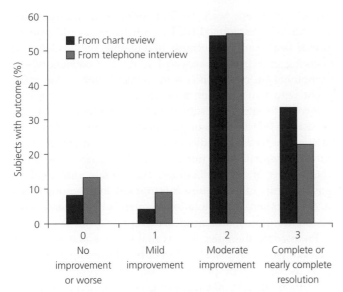

Figure 13.4 The responses of patients with diabetic gastropathy to tricyclic antidepressant treatment. Based on chart review or telephone interview, more than 70% of these patients experienced moderate to complete symptom control while on tricyclic drugs. From Sawhney et al. [167].

in case reports of patients with nausea and vomiting from a variety of causes including gastroparesis [168, 169]. The antipsychotic olanzapine relieves nausea in some patients with drug refractory symptoms [170].

Prokinetic agents

Metoclopramide is a substituted benzamide which acts via 5-HT$_4$ receptor facilitation of gastric cholinergic transmission and dopamine D$_2$ antagonism in the stomach and brainstem. The prokinetic properties of metoclopramide are restricted to the proximal gut, thus the drug is useful for gastroparesis but not small intestinal dysmotility [171]. Antiemetic actions of metoclopramide in the area postrema provide an additional means of symptom control. Because of CNS side effects such as agitation, drowsiness, and dystonias, metoclopramide is poorly tolerated in up to 30% of patients. Irreversible tardive dyskinesia is a catastrophic consequence of metoclopramide therapy which occurs with an incidence of 1%–10% when the drug is taken for longer than 3 months [172]. Because this

condition is disabling and can develop without warning, it should be discussed in detail with the patient before prescription of metoclopramide. This risk should be carefully documented in the patient record. Hyperprolactinemia as a consequence of dopamine antagonism in the pituitary may cause impotence, galactorrhea, and amenorrhea.

Erythromycin induces antroduodenal contractions and accelerates gastric emptying through action on receptors for the hormone motilin, the physiological regulator of fasting gastric motor activity. The abilities of atropine and vagal cooling to block the effects of erythromycin show that vagal cholinergic pathways participate in its prokinetic effects [173]. Patients with gastroparesis and pseudoobstruction may respond to erythromycin, but this agent has a narrow dose range of efficacy thereby limiting its utility [171]. Low doses have no effect whereas high doses induce abdominal pain, nausea, and diarrhea as a result of induction of intense motor spasms. Tolerance to its prokinetic action with chronic oral use has been reported in gastroparesis patients, suggesting that erythromycin may be more useful for short-term administration [174]. Erythromycin also has been associated with an increased risk of sudden cardiac death (Fig. 13.5) [175]. In a large Medicaid cohort, the sudden death rate of current erythromycin users was 2.01 times as high as that of previous erythromycin users or current amoxicillin users. The risk of death was further increased in those who were also on CYP3A inhibitors. Other macrolides including clarithromycin and azithromycin, exhibit prokinetic actions, but their efficacy in gastroparesis has not been investigated.

Domperidone, a benzamidazole derivative, is a dopamine D$_2$ antagonist with prokinetic actions similar to metoclopramide. The drug does not cross the blood–brain barrier so CNS side effects are minimal. As brainstem structures regulating vomiting are outside the blood–brain barrier, domperidone has a potent central antiemetic action. The benefits of domperidone are restricted to the proximal gut, reducing symptoms in patients with gastroparesis and diabetic gastropathy [176]. The drug is approved in most countries except for the United States for oral prescription. Traditionally, domperidone has been obtainable from foreign pharmacies, over the Internet, and from compounding pharmacies in the United States. The Food and Drug Administration (FDA) has discouraged these practices, but has made the drug available in the past under the auspices of a program to academic clinicians who

Figure 13.5 Incidence rate ratios with 95% confidence intervals for sudden cardiac death are plotted for different drug combinations. Erythromycin significantly increased the risk of sudden cardiac death. This risk further increased in patients concurrently taking CYP3A inhibitors. Conversely, those taking amoxicillin or CYP3A inhibitors alone were not at increased risk of sudden cardiac death. From Ray et al. [175].

Study group
Concurrent erythromycin and CYP3A inhibitor use
Erythromycin use
Amoxicillin use
CYP3A inhibitor use alone

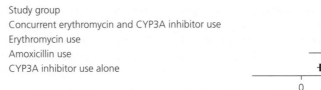

Incidence–rate ratio

submit an Investigational New Drug application to the FDA and who obtain Institutional Review Board approval from the prescribing institution. An intravenous form was withdrawn after case reports of death from cardiac arrhythmias. Hyperprolactinemic side effects may develop because the blood–brain barrier of the anterior pituitary is porous.

Other drugs exhibit motor stimulatory properties and are used in gastroparesis, but clinical trials to document their clinical benefits have not been published. Bethanechol, a muscarinic receptor agonist with direct smooth muscle excitatory effects, is a potent stimulant of gut phasic contractions, but much of this motor activity is not propagative and therefore the drug is a poor prokinetic [177]. Prominent adverse effects include abdominal cramps, skin flushing, diaphoresis, lacrimation, salivation, nausea, vomiting, bronchoconstriction, urinary urgency, and miosis. Dangerous cardiovascular effects include abrupt decreases in blood pressure in hypertensive patients and atrial fibrillation in individuals with hyperthyroidism. Likewise, cholinesterase inhibitors such as physostigmine increase gastric contractions but have limited action to accelerate gastric emptying.

Agents with prokinetic effects on the small intestine may be useful in some patients with intestinal pseudoobstruction. The somatostatin analogue octreotide induces propagative small intestinal motor patterns in patients with pseudoobstruction secondary to scleroderma [178]. Octreotide produces short- and long-term reductions in nausea, vomiting, and abdominal discomfort, and improves measures of intestinal bacterial overgrowth in some patients with pseudoobstruction [178, 179]. The gonadotropin-releasing hormone analogue leuprolide evokes propagative gastric and small intestinal complexes in some patients with intestinal dysmotility and may reduce nausea, bloating, and defecation disturbances in these individuals [180]. Side effects of leuprolide include amenorrhea and osteoporosis.

Management in selected clinical settings
Gastroparesis
To facilitate treatment of patients with gastroparesis, a classification of disease severity has been proposed [76]. Grade 1 or mild gastroparesis is characterized by intermittent, easily controlled symptoms with maintenance of weight and nutrition. In general, patients with grade 1 gastroparesis are asked to modify their diet and avoid medications that can exacerbate the condition. Grade 2 or compensated gastroparesis is characterized by symptoms of moderate severity that are partially controlled with prescription drugs. In general, patients with grade 2 gastroparesis still maintain nutrition and are hospitalized infrequently. These individuals are often given prokinetic and antiemetic agents in combination for symptom control. There have been few direct comparison trials of motor-stimulating drugs in gastroparesis. A metaanalysis reported that erythromycin was most potent at stimulating gastric emptying while erythromycin

and domperidone were both superior to metoclopramide in control of symptoms [181]. This conclusion should be interpreted with caution because of possible publication bias favoring only positive reported trials. For patients whose symptoms are more difficult to control, combination treatment with two prokinetics or administration of drugs by nonenteral routes (e.g., subcutaneous metoclopramide) may be useful [182]. Grade 3 or gastroparesis with gastric failure is characterized by medication-refractory symptoms, inability to maintain oral nutrition, and frequent emergency room visits or hospitalizations. Individuals with grade 3 gastroparesis often require intermittent intravenous fluids and medications, consideration of enteral or parenteral nutrition, and endoscopic or surgical therapy.

Endoscopic therapies are available for some refractory cases of gastroparesis. Injection of botulinum toxin into the pylorus has been proposed as treatment to promote pyloric relaxation, thereby facilitating gastric emptying [76,183]. Several case series have reported symptom reductions and acceleration of emptying which persist for a mean of 5 months after botulinum toxin treatment [184,185]. Likewise, pneumatic dilation of the pylorus has anecdotal benefits. Placing a venting gastrostomy affords the ability to intermittently release retained gas and liquid, thereby relieving fullness, discomfort, and distention-related nausea [186].

Selected patients with medication-unresponsive gastroparesis benefit from surgical intervention. Unpublished case series employing an implantable gastric stimulator that delivers brief, low-energy impulses at a frequency of 12 cycles/min reported impressive reductions in nausea and vomiting in patients with medication-refractory gastroparesis. Because of this apparent benefit, the FDA approved the gastric stimulator as a humanitarian use device and it was granted a humanitarian device exemption to treat refractory diabetic and idiopathic gastroparesis. Implantation of the gastric stimulator is restricted to centers in which Institutional Review Board approval has been granted. Since evaluation by the FDA, the gastric stimulator has shown efficacy in reducing nausea and vomiting, improving nutritional parameters, decreasing the need for supplemental feedings, and improving glycemic control in diabetics in an uncontrolled case series [187]. To date, only one controlled trial has shown modest benefits for the gastric stimulator [188]. Surgical pyloroplasty has shown benefit in an unpublished series of patients with diabetic gastroparesis [189]. Reconstruction of a gastroenteric anastomosis (i.e., conversion of a Billroth I to a Billroth II or vice versa) is rarely effective in gastroparetics. However, performance of completion gastrectomy with preservation of only a small cuff of gastric tissue is an established treatment of postsurgical gastroparesis, providing long-term symptom benefits to 43%–67% of patients [190]. Studies of pancreatic transplantation report no convincing evidence to suggest that this surgery improves gastric function in patients with diabetic gastroparesis. In patients with associated pseudoobstruction, decompression stomas also may reduce symptoms of patients in whom prokinetic drugs are ineffective [191].

Some patients with medication-refractory gastroparesis require enteral or parenteral nutrition on an intermittent basis when symptom flares develop or for permanent caloric and fluid support. In diabetic gastroparesis, surgical jejunostomy placement for enteral feeding improves overall health status with trends to reduced symptoms and hospitalization rates and enhanced nutrition [192]. Total parenteral nutrition (TPN) is less desirable over a prolonged period because of the risks of infectious and hepatobiliary complications and the extreme costs of therapy. Short-term TPN may be offered to reverse rapid weight decline and to ensure adequate fluid delivery. Permanent TPN is usually needed only for gastroparesis patients with superimposed severe intestinal dysmotility who cannot tolerate enteral feeding.

Nausea and vomiting of pregnancy

Several agents have been promoted for treatment of NVP; however, surveys report that pharmacological therapies provide benefits in only 31% of cases [193]. An evidence-based review concluded that antihistamines such as doxylamine, the anticholinergic dicyclomine, and phenothiazines are safe and effective to varying degrees for NVP [194]. Metoclopramide, droperidol, and ondansetron may be effective, but their safety in pregnancy is uncertain. Case reports have observed reductions in intractable hyperemesis gravidarum with intravenous mirtazapine [195]. The benefits of corticosteroids in hyperemesis gravidarum are uncertain with some studies reporting symptom reductions and others showing no effect [196,197]. Because of concerns of the potential toxicity of prescription antiemetics in NVP, complementary and alternative strategies have been employed to treat this condition. In a questionnaire study, 61% of women reported using such therapies during pregnancy with little awareness or supervision by their caregivers [198]. A systematic review of six double-blind, randomized controlled trials of 675 patients reported superiority of ginger over placebo in four studies and equivalence of ginger and pyridoxine in the other two [199]. Another study of 187 women reported no increase in fetal anomalies with ginger [200]. Vitamin B-6 (pyridoxine) may benefit some women with NVP, either given alone or with other agents such as ginger and doxylamine [201, 202]. Acupressure and electrical acustimulation also have reported efficacy in NVP [203, 204].

Chemotherapy-induced emesis

Extensive research has focused on antiemetic regimens to prevent or treat nausea and vomiting that are complicating chemotherapy administration. Most programs include multiple medications, which act on distinct receptor sites. Many regimens include corticosteroids, which exhibit potent antiemetic effects during the delayed period via unknown mech-

anisms [205]. A recent clinical practice guideline advocated a combination of a 5-HT$_3$ antagonist, the corticosteroid dexamethasone, and aprepitant for the acute phase after highly emetogenic chemotherapy regimens with continued use of dexamethasone and aprepitant for the delayed phase [96, 206]. For moderately emetogenic regimens, a 5-HT$_3$ antagonist and dexamethasone with or without aprepitant is recommended for acute prophylaxis, with use of either aprepitant or dexamethasone in the days afterward. Dexamethasone or a dopamine antagonist is advocated for chemotherapy with low emetogenicity. Other consensus documents have concluded that single doses of antiemetic agents are as effective as multiple doses or continuous infusions for the prevention of chemotherapy-induced emesis and that oral agents may be as useful as the intravenous forms of some drugs [207]. Anticipatory emesis is poorly controlled by antiemetic medications and is best managed by relaxation therapy, systematic desensitization techniques, and intravenous anxiolytic medications such as benzodiazepines [208]. Electroacupuncture can reduce acute chemotherapy-induced vomiting whereas acupressure relieves acute nausea [209]. Studies report benefits of ginger and therapeutic massage in reducing nausea after chemotherapy [210,211]. Hypnosis is beneficial in some cases of anticipatory nausea [212].

Radiation-induced vomiting

The 5-HT$_3$ antagonists exhibit proven efficacy in radiotherapy-evoked emesis, but have lesser benefits for nausea after radiation treatments [213]. A consensus document recommended that patients at high risk of radiation-induced emesis receiving total body irradiation should receive prophylaxis with a 5-HT$_3$ antagonist plus dexamethasone [214]. Those with moderate risk from upper abdominal irradiation may receive either prophylaxis or rescue with a 5-HT$_3$ antagonist, whereas those at minimal risk are usually treated with rescue antiemetic therapy.

Postoperative nausea and vomiting

Several antiemetic regimens have been proposed to prevent or control PONV. A systematic review of 737 studies in 103 237 subjects concluded that prophylactic antiemetic therapy provides benefit for 28% of patients whereas 1%–5% experience side effects from the antiemetic regimen [215]. In a factorial trial of six interventions for postoperative nausea and vomiting, antiemetic treatment with ondansetron, dexamethasone, and droperidol each produced similar benefits (Fig. 13.6) [216]. More recently, aprepitant was observed to increase the likelihood of complete prevention of emesis after surgery compared to ondansetron [217]. Consensus guidelines suggest that patients at low risk for PONV should not receive antiemetic prophylaxis while those at moderate risk should be given one or two agents [218]. Double and triple antiemetic drug regimens should be considered for those at high risk. Other consensus guidelines advocate measures to reduce

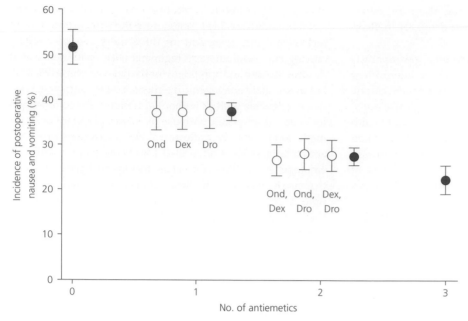

Figure 13.6 The incidence of postoperative nausea and vomiting (PONV) is plotted as a function of prophylactic antiemetic combination. More than 50% of patients developed PONV on no antiemetics. Single antiemetic treatment with ondansetron (Ond), dexamethasone (Dex), and droperidol (Dro) reduced this risk, but no one drug was superior. Dual antiemetic treatment further decreased the risk, but no combination showed an advantage. Triple antiemetic treatment showed minimal additional benefits over dual therapy. From Apfel et al. [216].

risk including use of regional anesthesia, propofol for induction, intraoperative oxygen, and intravenous fluids, avoidance of nitrous oxide and volatile anesthetics, and minimization of opioids and neostigmine [216,219]. Other controlled studies have demonstrated reduced PONV from ginger and acupuncture [220,221].

Cyclic vomiting syndrome

The therapy of CVS represents a major challenge for both pediatric and adult patients. A variety of agents have been proposed for CVS in children including antihistamines, benzodiazepines, 5-HT$_3$ antagonists, prokinetics, nonsteroidal antiinflammatory agents, and L-carnitine [222,223]. Because of its association with migraines, antimigraine therapies including tricyclic antidepressants, β-adrenoceptor antagonists, cyproheptadine, barbiturates, anticonvulsants, and 5-HT$_{1D}$ agonists such as sumatriptan have been employed [222,224]. Management of adult CVS is divided into prophylaxis, attempts to abort the attack, and treatment of the emetic episode (Fig. 13.2) [112]. In one study, 93% of adults with CVS experienced symptom reductions with prophylactic amitriptyline [113]. More recently, the anticonvulsants zonisamide and levetiracetam produced responses that were superior to those to tricyclic agents in prophylaxis of CVS attacks in adult patients, although side effects were observed in 45% of patients [225]. Antiemetic medications are frequently of little benefit in adults with CVS. Thus, a goal of therapy during the attack is to sedate the patient (e.g., parenteral benzodiazepines) to abbreviate the episode and reduce its impact [112].

Miscellaneous settings

Other therapies have shown efficacy in selected emetic disorders in small, often uncontrolled trials. Patients with nausea from opiate withdrawal may respond to opiate antagonists such as naloxone. The α-adrenoceptor agonist clonidine is reported to benefit some patients with gastroparesis [226]. The anticonvulsant agent gabapentin produced symptom benefits in three patients with chemotherapy-induced nausea, whereas the anticonvulsant carbamazepine reduced nausea and vomiting in a patient with meningeal carcinomatosis [227,228]. Ghrelin, a physiological stimulant of food intake with prokinetic properties, exhibits antiemetic activity in ferrets treated with cisplatin; however, its utility in humans with chemotherapy-induced emesis is unknown [229]. Ghrelin is a gastric prokinetic agent in patients with gastroparesis [230]. Motion sickness may respond to ginger, acupressure, and focused regular breathing exercises [231,232]. Transcutaneous electrical nerve stimulation and electrical stimulation of the vestibular system reduce chemotherapy-induced nausea and postoperative nausea, respectively [233,234].

References

1. Garthright WE, Archer DL, Kvenberg JE. Estimates of incidence and costs of intestinal infectious diseases in the United States. Public Health Rep 1988;103:107.
2. O'Brien B, Naber S. Nausea and vomiting during pregnancy: effects on the quality of women's lives. Birth 1992;19:138.
3. Gadsby R, Barnie-Adshead AM, Jagger C. A prospective study of nausea and vomiting during pregnancy. Br J Gen Pract 1993; 43:245–248.
4. Kallen B, Lundberg G, Aberg A. Relationship between vitamin use, smoking, and nausea and vomiting of pregnancy. Acta Obstet Gynecol Scand 2003;82:916.
5. Piwko C, Ungar WJ, Einarson TR, et al. The weekly cost of nausea and vomiting of pregnancy for women calling the Toronto Motherisk Program. Curr Med Res Opin 2007;23:833.
6. Bailit JL. Hyperemesis gravidarum: epidemiologic findings from a large cohort. Am J Obstet Gynecol 2005;193:811.

7. Ballatori E, Roila F, Ruggeri B, et al. The impact of chemotherapy-induced nausea and vomiting on health-related quality of life. Supp Care Cancer 2007;15:179.

8. O'Brien BJ, Rusthoven J, Rocchi A, et al. Impact of chemotherapy-associated nausea and vomiting on patients' functional status and on costs: survey of five Canadian centres. Can Med Assoc J 1993;149:296.

9. Carroll NV, Miederhoff PA, Cox FM, Hirsch JD. Costs incurred by outpatient surgical centers in managing postoperative nausea and vomiting. J Clin Anesth 1994;6:364.

10. Hirsch J. Impact of postoperative nausea and vomiting in the surgical setting. Anaesthesia 1994;49(Suppl.):30.

11. Engoren M, Steffel C. Patient perception of monetary value to avoid unpleasant side effects of anesthesia and surgery. J Clin Anesth 2000;12:388.

12. Borison HL, Wang SC. Physiology and pharmacology of vomiting. Pharmacol Rev 1953;5:193.

13. Chin CL, Fox GB, Hradil VP, et al. Pharmacological MRI in awake rats reveals neural activity in area postrema and nucleus tractus solitarius: relevance as a potential biomarker for detecting drug-induced emesis. Neuroimage 2006;33:1152.

14. Saito R, Takano Y, Kamiya H. Roles of substance P and NK1 receptor in the brainstem development of emesis. J Pharmacol Sci 2003;91:87.

15. Wilpizeski CR, Lowry LD, Goldman WS. Motion-induced sickness following bilateral ablation of area postrema in squirrel monkeys. Laryngoscope 1986;96:1221.

16. Takeda N, Morita M, Hasegawa S, et al. Neuropharmacology of motion sickness and emesis. A review. Acta Otolaryngol Suppl 1993;501:10.

17. Javid FA, Naylor RJ. The effect of serotonin and serotonin receptor antagonists on motion sickness in *Suncus murinus*. Pharmacol Biochem Behav 2002;73:979.

18. Javid FA, Naylor RJ. The effect of the 5-HT$_{1A}$ agonist, 8-OH-DPAT, on motion-induced emesis in *Suncus murinus*. Pharmacol Biochem Behav 2006;85:820.

19. Goldberg SL. The afferent paths of nerves involved in the vomiting reflex induced by distension of the isolated pyloric pouch. Am J Physiol 1931;99:156.

20. Fukui H, Yamamoto M, Sasaki S, Sato S. Involvement of 5-HT$_3$ receptors and vagal afferents in copper sulfate- and cisplatin-induced emesis in monkeys. Eur J Pharmacol 1993;249:13.

21. Makale MT, King GL. Plasticity of autonomic control of emesis in irradiated ferrets. Am J Physiol 1993;265:R1092.

22. Miller AD, Jakus J, Nonaka S. Plasticity of emesis to a 5-HT$_3$ agonist: effect of order of visceral nerve cuts. Neuroreport 1994;5:986.

23. Shapiro RE, Miselis RR. The central organization of the vagus nerve innervating the stomach of the rat. J Comp Neurol 1985;238:473.

24. Read NW, Gwee KA. The importance of 5-hydroxytryptamine receptors in the gut. Pharmacol Ther 1994;62:159.

25. Fukui H, Yamamoto M, Sasaki S, Sato S. Possible involvement of peripheral 5-HT$_4$ receptors in copper sulfate-induced vomiting in dogs. Eur J Pharmacol 1994;257:47.

26. Miller AD, Ruggiero DA. Emetic reflex arc revealed by expression of the immediate-early gene c-fos in the cat. J Neurosci 1994;14:871.

27. Fukuda H, Koga T. Activation of peripheral and/or central chemoreceptors changes retching activities of Botzinger complex neurons and induces expulsion in decerebrate dogs. Neurosci Res 1995;23:171.

28. Koga T, Qu R, Fukuda H. The central pattern generator for vomiting may exist in the reticular area dorsomedial to the retrofacial nucleus in dogs. Exp Brain Res 1998;118:139.

29. Koga T, Fukuda H. Descending pathway from the central pattern generator of vomiting. Neuroreport 1997;8:2587.

30. Fukuda H, Koga T. Most inspiratory neurons in the pre-Botzinger complex are suppressed during vomiting in dogs. Brain Res 1997;763:30.

31. Sawchenko PE. Central connections of the sensory and motor nuclei of the vagus nerve. J Auton Nerve Syst 1983;9:13.

32. Gardner CJ, Twissell DJ, Dale TJ, et al. The broad-spectrum anti-emetic activity of the novel non-peptide tachykinin NK$_1$ receptor antagonist GR203040. Br J Pharmacol 1995;116:3158.

33. Fukuda H, Koga T, Furakawa N, et al. The tachykinin NK$_1$ receptor antagonist GR205171 abolishes the retching activity of neurons comprising the central pattern generator for vomiting in dogs. Neurosci Res 1999;33:25.

34. Ariumi H, Saito R, Nago S, et al. The role of tachykinin NK$_1$ receptors in the area postrema of ferrets in emesis. Neurosci Lett 2000;286:123.

35. McCarthy LE, Borison HL, Spiegel PK, Friedlander RM. Vomiting: radiographic and oscillographic correlates in the decerebrate cat. Gastroenterology 1974;67:1126.

36. Monges H, Salducci J, Naudy B. Dissociation between the electrical activity of the diaphragmatic dome and crura muscular fibres during esophageal distention, vomiting, and eructation. An electromyographic study in the dog. J Physiol 1978;74:541.

37. Tan LK, Miller AD. Innervation of the periesophageal regions of cat's diaphragm: implications for studies of control of vomiting. Neurosci Lett 1986;68:339.

38. Lang IM, Sarna SK, Dodds WJ. Pharyngeal, esophageal, and proximal gastric responses associated with vomiting. Am J Physiol 1993;265:G963.

39. Abe T, Kieser TM, Tomita T, Easton PA. Respiratory muscle function during emesis in awake canines. J Appl Physiol 1994;76:2552.

40. Lang IM, Marvig J, Sarna SK, Condon RE. Gastrointestinal myoelectric correlates of vomiting in the dog. Am J Physiol 1986;251:G830.

41. Lang IM, Sarna SK, Condon RE. Gastrointestinal motor correlates of vomiting in the dog: quantification and characterization as an independent phenomenon. Gastroenterology 1986;90:40.

42. Sha S, Matsushima Y, Habu S, et al. Extrinsic nervous control of retrograde giant contraction during vomiting in conscious dogs. Dig Dis Sci 1996;41:1546.

43. Morrow GR, Andrews PL, Hickok JT, Stern R. Vagal changes following cancer chemotherapy: implications for the development of nausea. Psychophysiology 2000;37:378.

44. Xu LH, Koch KL, Summy-Long J, et al. Hypothalamic and gastric myoelectrical responses during vection-induced nausea in healthy Chinese subjects. Am J Physiol 1993;265:E578.

45. Kim MS, Chey WD, Owyang C, Hasler WL. Role of vasopressin as a mediator of nausea and gastric slow wave dysrhythmias in motion sickness. Am J Physiol 1997;272:G853.

46. Cheung BS, Kohl RL, Money KE, Kinter LB. Etiologic significance of arginine vasopressin in motion sickness. J Clin Pharmacol 1994;34:664.

47. Nussey SS, Hawthorn J, Page SR, et al. Responses of plasma oxytocin and arginine vasopressin to nausea induced by apomorphine and ipecacuanha. Clin Endocrinol 1988;28:297.

48. Morrow GR, Hickok JT, Andrews PL, Stern RM. Reduction in serum cortisol after platinum based chemotherapy for cancer: a role for the HPA axis in treatment-related nausea? Psychophysiology 2002;39:491.

49. Koch KL, Stern RM, Vasey MW, et al. Neuroendocrine and gastric myoelectrical responses to illusory self-motion in humans. Am J Physiol 1990;258:E304.

50. Miller AD, Rowley HA, Roberts TP, Kucharczyk J. Human cortical activity during vestibular- and drug-induced nausea detected using MSI. Ann NY Acad Sci 1996;781:670.

51. Chelen WE, Kabrinsky M, Rogers SK. Spectral analysis of the electroencephalographic response to motion sickness. Aviat Space Environ Med 1993;64:24.

52. Qin XY, Pilot MA, Thompson H, Scott M. Effects of cholinoceptor and 5-hydroxytryptamine$_3$ antagonism on erythromycin-induced canine intestinal motility disruption and emesis. Br J Pharmacol 1993;108:44.

53. Monto AS, Koopman JS. The Tecumseh Study. XI. Occurrence of acute enteric illness in the community. Am J Epidemiol 1980;112:323.

54. Kim KH, Yang JM, Joo SI, et al. Importance of rotavirus and adenovirus types 40 and 41 in acute gastroenteritis in Korean children. J Clin Microbiol 1990;28:2279.

55. Gordon SM, Oshiro LS, Jarvis WR, et al. Foodborne Snow Mountain agent gastroenteritis with secondary person-to-person spread in a retirement community. Am J Epidemiol 1990;131:702.

56. Dolin R, Blacklow NR, DuPont H, et al. Biological properties of Norwalk agent of acute infectious nonbacterial gastroenteritis. Proc Soc Exp Biol Med 1972;140:578.

57. Terranova W, Blake PA. *Bacillus cereus* food poisoning. N Engl J Med 1978;298:143.

58. Loewenstein MS. Epidemiology of *Clostridium perfringens* food poisoning. N Engl J Med 1972;286:1026.

59. Su YC, Wong AC. Identification and purification of a new staphylococcal enterotoxin, H. Appl Environ Microbiol 1995;61:1438.

60. Ehling-Schulz M, Fricker M, Scherer S. *Bacillus cereus*, the causative agent of an emetic type of food-borne illness. Mol Nutr Food Res 2004;48:479.

61. Ehling-Schulz M, Fricker M, Scherer S. Identification of emetic toxin producing *Bacillus cereus* strains by a novel molecular assay. FEMS Microbiol Lett 2004;232:189.

62. Wu D, Hockenberry DM, Brentnall TA, et al. Persistent nausea and anorexia after marrow transplantation: a prospective study of 78 patients. Transplantation 1998;66:1319.

63. Kaiser GC, McKain JM, Shumacher HB. The superior mesenteric artery syndrome. Surgery 1960;110:133.

64. Wadoodi A, MacWalter RS, Dillon JF, Cuschieri A. Subacute gastric volvulus – a rare cause of vomiting in the elderly. Scot Med J 2000;45:54.

65. Kong MF, Horowitz M, Jones KL, et al. Natural history of diabetic gastroparesis. Diabetes Care 1999;22:503.

66. Sridhar KR, Lange RC, Magyar L, et al. Prevalence of impaired gastric emptying of solids in systemic sclerosis: diagnostic and therapeutic implications. J Lab Clin Med 1998;132:541.

67. Hunter RJ, Metz DC, Morris JB, Rothstein RD. Gastroparesis: a potential pitfall of laparoscopic Nissen fundoplication. Am J Gastroenterol 1996;91:2617.

68. Neild PJ, Nijran KS, Yazaki E, et al. Delayed gastric emptying in human immunodeficiency virus infection – correlation with symptoms, autonomic function, and intestinal motility. Dig Dis Sci 2000;45:1491.

69. Barkin JS, Goldberg RJ, Sfakianakis GN, Levi J. Pancreatic carcinoma is associated with delayed gastric emptying. Dig Dis Sci 1986;31:265.

70. Balaban DH, Chen J, Lin Z, et al. Median arcuate ligament syndrome: a possible cause of idiopathic gastroparesis. Am J Gastroenterol 1997;92:519.

71. Lennon VA, Sas DF, Busk MF, et al. Enteric neuronal autoantibodies in pseudoobstruction with small-cell lung carcinoma. Gastroenterology 1991;100:137.

72. Sigurdsson L, Flores A, Putnam PE, et al. Postviral gastroparesis: presentation, treatment, and outcome. J Pediatrics 1997;131:751.

73. Bityutskiy LP, Soykan I, McCallum RW. Viral gastroparesis: a subgroup of idiopathic gastroparesis – clinical characteristics and long-term outcomes. Am J Gastroenterol 1997;92:1501.

74. Soykan I, Sivri B, Sarosiek I, et al. Demography, clinical characteristics, psychological and abuse profiles, treatment, and long-term follow-up of patients with gastroparesis. Dig Dis Sci 1998; 43: 2398–2404.

75. Tack J, Talley NJ, Camilleri M, et al. Functional gastroduodenal disorders. gastroenterology 2006;130:1466–1479.

76. Abell TL, Bernstein RK, Cutts T, et al. Treatment of gastroparesis: a multidisciplinary clinical review. Neurogastroenterol Motil 2006; 18:263.

77. Kacker V, Gupta YK. An experimental model to study intracranial hypertension-induced vomiting in conscious dogs. Methods Find Exp Clin Pharmacol 1996;18:315.

78. Lackner JR, Graybiel A. Sudden emesis following parabolic flight maneuvers: implications for space motion sickness. Aviat Space Environ Med 1986;57:343.

79. Lacroix R, Eason E, Melzack R. Nausea and vomiting during pregnancy: a prospective study of its frequency, intensity, and patterns of change. Am J Obstet Gynecol 2000;182:931.

80. Klebanoff MA, Koslowe PA, Kaslow R, Rhoads GG. Epidemiology of vomiting in early pregnancy. Obstet Gynecol 1985;66:612.

81. Louik C, Hernandez-Diaz S, Werler MM, Mitchell AA. Nausea and vomiting in pregnancy: maternal characteristics and risk factors. Paediatr Perinat Epidemiol 2006;20:270.

82. Pepper GV, Craig Roberts S. Rates of nausea and vomiting in pregnancy and dietary characteristics across populations. Proc Biol Sci 2006;273:2675.

83. Czeizel AE, Puho E. Association between severe nausea and vomiting in pregnancy and lower rate of preterm births. Paediatr Perinat Epidemiol 2004;18:253.

84. Boneva RS, Moore CA, Botto L, et al. Nausea during pregnancy and congenital heart defects: a population-based case–control study. Am J Epidemiol 1999;149:717.

85. Trogstad LI, Stoltenberg C, Magnus P, et al. Recurrence risk in hyperemesis gravidarum. Br J Obstet Gynaecol 2005;112:1641.

86. Fell DB, Dodds L, Joseph KS, et al. Risk factors for hyperemesis gravidarum requiring hospital admission during pregnancy. Obstet Gynecol 2006;107:277.

87. Dodds L, Fell DB, Joseph KS, et al. Outcomes of pregnancies complicated by hyperemesis gravidarum. Obstet Gynecol 2006;107:285.

88. Lagiou P, Tamimi R, Mucci LA, et al. Nausea and vomiting in pregnancy in relation to prolactin, estrogens, and progesterone: a prospective study. Obstet Gynecol 2003;101:639.

89. Aka N, Atalay S, Sayharman S, et al. Leptin and leptin receptor levels in pregnant women with hyperemesis gravidarum. Aust NZ J Obstet Gynaecol 2006;46:274.

90. Carlsen SM, Vanky E, Jacobsen G. Nausea and vomiting associate with increasing maternal androgen levels in otherwise uncomplicated pregnancies. Acta Obstet Gynecol Scand 2003;82:225.

91. Jarnfelt-Samsioe A, Samsioe G, Velinder GM. Nausea and vomiting in pregnancy – a contribution to its epidemiology. Gynecol Obstet Invest 1983;16:221.

92. Gadsby R, Barnie-Adshead A, Grammatoppoulos D, Gadsby P. Nausea and vomiting in pregnancy: an association between symptoms and maternal prostaglandin E_2. Gynecol Obstet Invest 2000; 50:149.

93. Jordan K, Kasper C, Schmoll HJ. Chemotherapy-induced nausea and vomiting: current and new standards in the antiemetic prophylaxis and treatment. Eur J Cancer 2005;41:199.

94. Grunberg SM, Deuson RR, Mavros P, et al. Incidence of chemotherapy-induced nausea and emesis after modern antiemetics. Cancer 2004;100:2261.

95. Osoba D, Zee B, Pater J, et al. Determinants of postchemotherapy nausea and vomiting in patients with cancer. Quality of Life and Symptom Control Committees of the National Cancer Institute of Canada Clinical Trials Group. J Clin Oncol 1997;15:116.

96. Fukui H, Yamamoto M, Ando T, et al. Increase in serotonin levels in the dog ileum and blood by cisplatin as measured by microdialysis. Neuropharmacology 1993;32:959.

97. Cubeddu LX. Serotonin mechanisms in chemotherapy-induced emesis in cancer patients. Oncology 1996;53(Suppl. 1):18.

98. Hawthorn J, Ostler KJ, Andrews PLR. The role of the abdominal visceral innervation and 5-hydroxytryptamine M-receptors in vomiting induced by the cytotoxic drugs cyclophosphamide and cisplatin in the ferret. J Exp Physiol 1988;73:7.

99. Gidda JS, Evans DC, Cohen ML, et al. Antagonism of serotonin$_3$ (5-HT$_3$) receptors within the blood–brain barrier prevents cisplatin-induced emesis in dogs. J Pharmacol Exp Ther 1995;273:695.

100. Horn CC, Ciucci M, Chaudhury A. Brain Fos expression during 48 h after cisplatin treatment: neural pathways for acute and delayed visceral sickness. Auton Neurosci 2007;132:44.

101. Yamakuni H, Sawai H, Maeda Y, et al. Probable involvement of the 5-hydroxytryptamine (4) receptor in methotrexate-induced delayed emesis in dogs. J Pharmacol Exp Ther 2000;292:1002.

102. Hesketh PJ, Van Belle S, Aapro M, et al. Differential involvement of neurotransmitters through the time course of cisplatin-induced emesis as revealed by therapy with specific receptor antagonists. Eur J Cancer 2003;39:1074.

103. Fredrikson M, Hursti TJ, Steineck G, et al. Delayed chemotherapy-induced nausea is augmented by high levels of endogenous noradrenaline. Br J Cancer 1994;70:642.

104. Morrow GR, Rosenthal SN. Models, mechanisms and management of anticipatory nausea and emesis. Oncology 1996;53(Suppl. 1):4.

105. Zachariae R, Paulsen K, Mehlsen M, et al. Anticipatory nausea: the role of individual differences related to sensory perception and autonomic reactivity. Ann Behav Med 2007;33:69.

106. Roscoe JA, Hickok JT, Morrow GR. Patient expectations as predictor of chemotherapy-induced nausea. Ann Behav Med 2000;22:121.

107. Scarantino CW, Ornitz RD, Hoffman LG, Anderson RF. On the mechanism of radiation-induced emesis: the role of serotonin. Int J Radiat Oncol Biol Phys 1994;30:825.

108. Larsson S, Lundberg D. A prospective survey of postoperative nausea and vomiting with special regard to incidence and relations to patient characteristics, anesthetic routines and surgical procedures. Acta Anaesthesiol Scand 1995;39:539.

109. Gan TJ. Risk factors for postoperative nausea and vomiting. Anesth Analg 2006;102:1884.

110. Withers GD, Silburn SR, Forbes DA. Precipitants and aetiology of cyclic vomiting syndrome. Acta Paediat 1998;87:272.

111. Li BU, Murray RD, Heitlinger LA, et al. Is cyclic vomiting syndrome related to migraine? J Pediatr 1999;134:567.

112. Fleisher DR, Gornowicz B, Adams K, et al. Cyclic vomiting syndrome in 41 adults: the illness, the patients, and problems of management. BMC Med 2005;3:20.

113. Namin F, Patel J, Lin Z, et al. Clinical, psychiatric and manometric profile of cyclic vomiting syndrome in adults and response to tricyclic therapy. Neurogastroenterol Motil 2007;19:196.

114. Chelimsky TC, Chelimsky GG. Autonomic abnormalities in cyclic vomiting syndrome. J Pediatr Gastroenterol Nutr 2007;44:326.

115. Lucarelli S, Corrado G, Pelliccia A, et al. Cyclic vomiting syndrome and food allergy/intolerance in seven children: a possible association. Eur J Pediatr 2000;159:360.

116. Seidel J, Streck S, Bellstedt K, et al. Recurrent vomiting and ethylmalonic aciduria associated with rare mutations of the short-chain acyl-CoA dehydrogenase gene. J Inherit Metab Dis 2003;26:37.

117. Allen JH, De Moore GM, Heddle R, Twartz JC. Cannabinoid hyperemesis: cyclical emesis in association with chronic cannabis abuse. Gut 2004;53:1566.

118. Arslanian-Engoren C, Patel A, Fang J, et al. Symptoms of men and women presenting with acute coronary syndromes. Am J Cardiol 2006;98:1177.

119. Tanaka K, Johnson B. Jamaican vomiting sickness. N Engl J Med 1976;295:461.

120. De Giorgio R, Guerrini S, Barbara G, et al. Inflammatory neuropathies of the enteric nervous system. Gastroenterology 2004;126:1872.

121. Pasha SF, Lunsford TN, Lennon VA. Autoimmune gastrointestinal dysmotility treated successfully with pyridostigmine. Gastroenterology 2006;131:1592.

122. Blackmon S, Lucius C, Wilson JP, et al. The use of water-soluble contrast in evaluating clinical equivocal small bowel obstruction. Am Surg 2000;66:238.

123. Maglinte DD, Peterson LA, Vahey TN, et al. Enteroclysis in partial small bowel obstruction. Am J Surg 1984;147:325.

124. Paulsen SR, Huprich JE, Fletcher JG, et al. CT enterography as a diagnostic tool in evaluating small bowel disorders: review of clinical experience with over 700 cases. Radiographics 2006;26:641.

125. Unal B, Akta A, Kemal G, et al. Superior mesenteric artery syndrome: CT and ultrasonography findings. Diag Intervent Radiol 2005;11:90.

126. House A, Champion MC, Chamberlain M. National survey of radionuclide gastric emptying studies. Can J Gastroenterol 1997;11:317.

127. Tougas G, Eaker EY, Abell TL, et al. Assessment of gastric emptying using a low fat meal: establishment of international control values. Am J Gastroenterol 2000;95:1456.

128. Guo JP, Maurer AH, Fisher RS, Parkman HP. Extending gastric emptying scintigraphy from two to four hours detects more patients with gastroparesis. Dig Dis Sci 2001;46:24.

129. Galil MA, Critchley M, Mackie CR. Isotope gastric emptying tests in clinical practice: expectation, outcome, and utility. Gut 1993;34:916.

130. Delgado-Aros S, Camilleri M, Cremonini F, et al. Contributions of gastric volumes and gastric emptying to meal size and postmeal symptoms in functional dyspepsia. Gastroenterology 2004;127:1685.

131. Kuo B, McCallum RW, Koch KL, et al. SmartPill, a novel ambulatory diagnostic test for measuring gastric emptying in health and disease (abstract). Gastroenterology 2006;130:M2205.

132. Braden B, Adams S, Duan LP, et al. The [^{13}C]acetate breath test accurately reflects gastric emptying of liquids in both liquid and semisolid test meals. Gastroenterology 1995;108:1048.

133. Kuiken SD, Samsom M, Camilleri M, et al. Development of a test to measure gastric accommodation in humans. Am J Physiol 1999;277:G1217.

134. Jones K, Edelbroek M, Horowitz M, et al. Evaluation of antral motility in humans using manometry and scintigraphy. Gut 1995;37:643.

135. Mearin F, Camilleri M, Malagelada JR. Pyloric dysfunction in diabetics with recurrent nausea and vomiting. Gastroenterology 1986;90:1919.

136. Camilleri M, Malagelada JR. Abnormal intestinal motility in diabetics with the gastroparesis syndrome. Eur J Clin Invest 1984;14:420.

137. Soffer E, Thongsawat S. Clinical value of duodenojejunal manometry. Its usefulness in diagnosis and management of patients with gastrointestinal symptoms. Dig Dis Sci 1996;41:859.

138. Parkman HP, Hasler WL, Barnett JL, Eaker EY. American Motility Society Clinical GI Motility Testing Task Force. Electrogastrography: a document prepared by the gastric section of the American Motility Society Clinical GI Motility Testing Task Force. Neurogastroenterol Motil 2003;15:89.

139. Koch KL, Stern RM, Stewart WR, Vasey MW. Gastric emptying and gastric myoelectrical activity in patients with diabetic gastroparesis: effect of long-term domperidone treatement. Am J Gastroenterol 1989;84:1069.

140. Tack J, Caenepeel P, Piessevaux H, et al. Assessment of meal induced gastric accommodation by a satiety drinking test in health and in severe functional dyspepsia. Gut 2003;521:1271.

141. Benini L, Castellani G, Brighenti F, et al. Gastric emptying of a solid meal is accelerated by the removal of dietary fibre naturally present in food. Gut 1995;36:825.

142. Wood CD, Kennedy RE, Graybiel A, et al. Clinical effectiveness of anti-motion sickness drugs. JAMA 1966;198:1155.

143. Cheung BS, Heskin R, Hofer KD. Failure of cetirizine and fexofenadine to prevent motion sickness. Ann Pharmacother 2003;37:173.

144. Clissold SP, Heel RC. Transdermal hyoscine (scopolamine). A preliminary review of its pharmacodynamic properties and therapeutic efficacy. Drugs 1985;29:189.

145. Osinski MA, Uchic ME, Seifert T, et al. Dopamine D_2, but not D_4, receptor agonists are emetogenic in ferrets. Pharmacol Biochem Behav 2005;81:211.

146. Wampler G. The pharmacology and clinical effectiveness of phenothiazines and related drugs for managing chemotherapy-induced emesis. Drugs 1983;25(Suppl. 1):35.

147. Markman MR, Peterson G, Kulp B, Markman M. Effectiveness of serotonin-receptor antagonist antiemetic therapy over successive courses of carboplatin-based chemotherapy. Gynecol Oncol 2002;85:435.

148. Cubeddu LX, Hoffmann IS, Fuenmayor NT, Finn AL. Efficacy of ondansetron (GR 38032F) and the role of serotonin in cisplatin-induced nausea and vomiting. N Engl J Med 1990;322:810.

149. Aapro M. Granisetron: an update on its clinical use in the management of nausea and vomiting. Oncologist 2004;9:673.

150. Faris PL, Kim SW, Meller WH, et al. Effect of decreasing afferent vagal activity with ondansetron on symptoms of bulimia nervosa: a randomized, double-blind trial. Lancet 2000;355:792.

151. Moser JD, Caldwell JB, Rhule FJ. No more than necessary: safety and efficacy of low-dose promethazine. Ann Pharmacother 2006;40:45.

152. Oo TH, Hesketh PJ. Drug insight: new antiemetics in the management of chemotherapy-induced nausea and vomiting. Nature Clin Pract Oncol 2005;2:196.

153. Aapro MS, Macciocchi A, Gridelli C. Palonosetron improves prevention of chemotherapy-induced nausea and vomiting in elderly patients. J Supp Oncol 2005;3:369.

154. Babaoglu MO, Bayar B, Aynacioglu AS, et al. Association of the ABCB1 3435C>T polymorphism with antiemetic efficacy of 5-hydroxytryptamine type 3 antagonists. Clin Pharmacol Ther 2005;78:619.

155. Ho KY, Gan TJ. Pharmacology, pharmacogenetics, and clinical efficacy of 5-hydroxytryptamine type 3 receptor antagonists for postoperative nausea and vomiting. Curr Opin Anaesth 2006;19:606.

156. Janicki PK, Schuler HG, Jarzembowski TM, Rossi M. Prevention of postoperative nausea and vomiting with granisetron and dolasetron in relation to CYP2D6 genotype. Anesth Analg 2006;102:1127.

157. Navari RM, Reinhardt RR, Gralla RJ, et al. Reduction of cisplatin-induced emesis by a selective neurokinin-1-receptor antagonist. L-754,030 Antiemetic Trials Group. N Engl J Med 1999;340:190.

158. Gesztesi Z, Scuderi PE, White PF, et al. Substance P (neurokinin-1) antagonist prevents postoperative vomiting after abdominal hysterectomy procedures. Anesthesiology 2000;93:931.

159. Reid K, Palmer JL, Wright RJ, et al. Comparison of the neurokinin-1 antagonist GR205171, alone and in combination with the 5-HT$_3$ antagonist ondansetron, hyoscine and placebo in the prevention of motion-induced nausea in man. Br J Clin Pharmacol 2000;50:61.

160. De Wit R, Herrstedt J, Rapoport B, et al. Addition of the oral NK$_1$ antagonist aprepitant to standard antiemetics provides protection against nausea and vomiting during multiple cycles of cisplatin-based chemotherapy. J Clin Oncol 2003;21:4105.

161. Navari RM. Role of neurokinin-1 receptor antagonists in chemotherapy-induced emesis: summary of clinical trials. Cancer Invest 2004;22:569.

162. Dando TM, Perry CM. Aprepitant: a review of its use in the prevention of chemotherapy-induced nausea and vomiting. Drugs 2004;64:777.

163. Herman TS, Einhorn LH, Jones SE, et al. Superiority of nabilone over prochlorperazine as an antiemetic in patients receiving cancer chemotherapy. N Engl J Med 1979;300:1295.

164. Parker LA, Kwiatkowska M, Burton P, Mechoulam R. Effect of cannabinoids on lithium-induced vomiting in the *Suncus murinus* (house musk shrew). Psychopharmacology 2004;171:156.

165. Wiegant VM, Sweep CG, Nir I. Effect of acute administration of delta 1-tetrahydrocannabinol on beta-endorphin levels in plasma and brain tissue of the rat. Experientia 1987;43:413.

166. Prakash C, Lustman PJ, Freedland KE, Clouse RE. Tricyclic antidepressants for functional nausea and vomiting: clinical outcome in 37 patients. Dig Dis Sci 1998;43:1951.

167. Sawhney MS, Prakash C, Lustman PJ, Clouse RE. Tricyclic antidepressants for chronic vomiting in diabetic patients. Dig Dis Sci 2007;52:418.

168. Pae CU. Low-dose mirtazapine may be successful treatment option for severe nausea and vomiting. Prog Neuropsychopharmacol Biol Psychiatr 2006;30:1143.

169. Teixeira FV, Novaretti TM, Pilon B, et al. Mirtazapine (Remeron) as treatment for non-mechanical vomiting after gastric bypass. Obes Surg 2005;15:707.

170. Srivastava M, Brito-Dellan N, Davis MP, et al. Olanzepine as an antiemetic in refractory nausea and vomiting in advanced cancer. J Pain Sympt Manage 2003;25:578.

171. Parkman HP, Hasler WL, Fisher RS. American Gastroenterological Association technical review on the diagnosis and treatment of gastroparesis. Gastroenterology 2004;127:1592.

172. Ganzini L, Casey DE, Hoffman WF, McCall AL. The prevalence of metoclopramide-induced tardive dyskinesia and acute extrapyramidal movement disorders. Arch Intern Med 1993;153:1469.

173. Mathis C, Malbert CH. Erythromycin gastrokinetic activity is partially vagally mediated. Am J Physiol 1998;274:G80.

174. Richards RD, Davenport K, McCallum RW. The treatment of idiopathic and diabetic gastroparesis with acute intravenous and chronic oral erythromycin. Am J Gastroenterol 1993;88:203.

175. Ray WA, Murray KT, Meredith S, et al. Oral erythromycin and the risk of sudden death from cardiac causes. N Engl J Med 2004;351:1089.

176. Soykan I, Sarosiek I, McCallum RW. The effect of chronic oral domperidone therapy on gastrointestinal symptoms, gastric emptying, and quality of life in patients with gastroparesis. Am J Gastroenterol 1997;92:976.

177. McCallum RW, Fink SM, Lerner E, Berkowitz DM. Effects of metoclopramide and bethanechol on delayed gastric emptying present in gastroesophageal reflux patients. Gastroenterology 1983;84:1573.

178. Soudah HC, Hasler WL, Owyang C. Effect of octreotide on intestinal motility and bacterial overgrowth in scleroderma. N Engl J Med 1991;325:1461.

179. Verne GN, Eaker EY, Hardy E, Sninsky CA. Effect of octreotide and erythromycin on idiopathic and scleroderma-associated intestinal pseudoobstruction. Dig Dis Sci 1995;40:1892.

180. Mathias JR, Clench MH, Reeves-Darby VG, et al. Effect of leuprolide acetate in patients with moderate to severe functional bowel disease. Double-blind, placebo-controlled study. Dig Dis Sci 1994;39:1155.

181. Sturm A, Holtmann G, Goebell H, Gerken G. Prokinetics in patients with gastroparesis: a systematic analysis. Digestion 1999;60:422.

182. McCallum RW, Valenzuela G, Polepalle S, Spyker D. Subcutaneous metoclopramide in the treatment of symptomatic gastroparesis: clinical efficacy and pharmacokinetics. J Pharmacol Exp Ther 1991;258:136.

183. Gupta P, Rao SS. Attenuation of isolated pyloric pressure waves in gastroparesis in response to botulinum toxin injection: a case report. Gastrointest Endo 2002;56:770.

184. Lacy BE, Crowell MD, Schettler-Duncan A, et al. The treatment of diabetic gastroparesis with botulinum toxin injection into the pylorus. Diabetes Care 2004;27:2341.

185. Bromer MQ, Friedenberg F, Miller LS, et al. Endoscopic pyloric injection of botulinum toxin A for the treatment of refractory gastroparesis. Gastrointest Endo 2005;61:833.

186. Kim CH, Nelson DK. Venting percutaneous gastrostomy in the treatment of refractory idiopathic gastroparesis. Gastrointest Endo 1998;47:67.

187. Abell TL, Van Cutsem E, Abrahamsson H, et al. Gastric electrical stimulation in intractable symptomatic gastroparesis. Digestion 2002;66:204.

188. Abell, T, McCallum, R, Hocking, M, et al. Gastric electrical stimulation for medically refractory gastroparesis. Gastroenterology 2003;125:421.

189. Abouezzi ZE, Melvin WS, Ellison EC, Schirmer WJ. Functional and symptomatic improvement in patients with diabetic gastroparesis following pyloroplasty (abstract). Gastroenterology 1998;114:A1374.

190. Eckhauser FE, Conrad M, Knol JA, et al. Safety and long-term durability of completion gastrectomy in 81 patients with postsurgical gastroparesis syndrome. Am Surg 1998;64:711.

191. Heneyke S, Smith VV, Spitz L, Milla PJ. Chronic intestinal pseudo-obstruction: treatment and long term follow up of 44 patients. Arch Dis Child 1999;81:21.

192. Fontana RJ, Barnett JL. Jejunostomy tube placement in refractory diabetic gastroparesis: a retrospective review. Am J Gastroenterol 1996;91:2174.

193. Chandra K, Magee L, Einarson A, Koren G. Nausea and vomiting in pregnancy: results of a survey that identified interventions used by women to alleviate their symptoms. J Psychosom Obstet Gynecol 2003;24:71.

194. Magee LA, Mazzotta P, Koren G. Evidence-based view of safety and effectiveness of pharmacologic therapy for nausea and vomiting of pregnancy (NVP). Am J Obstet Gynecol 2002;186(5 Suppl.):S256.

195. Guclu S, Gol M, Dogan E, Saygili U. Mirtazapine use in resistant hyperemesis gravidarum: report of three cases and review of the literature. Arch Gynecol Obstet 2005;272:298.

196. Bondok RS, El Sharnouby NM, Eid HE, Abd Elmaksoud AM. Pulsed steroid therapy is an effective treatment for intractable hyperemesis gravidarum. Crit Care Med 2006;34:2781.

197. Yost NP, McIntire DD, Wians FH, et al. A randomized, placebo-controlled trial of corticosteroids for hyperemesis due to pregnancy. Obstet Gynecol 2003;102:1250.

198. Hollyer T, Boon H, Georgousis A, et al. The use of CAM by women suffering from nausea and vomiting during pregnancy. BMC Comp Alt Med 2002;2:5.

199. Borrelli F, Capasso R, Aviello G, et al. Effectiveness and safety of ginger in the treatment of pregnancy-induced nausea and vomiting. Obstet Gynecol 2005;105:849.

200. Portnoi G, Chng LA, Karimi-Tabesh L, et al. Prospective comparative study of the safety and effectiveness of ginger for the treatment of nausea and vomiting in pregnancy. Am J Obstet Gynecol 2003; 189:1374.

201. Sripramote M, Lekhyananda N. A randomized comparison of ginger and vitamin B_6 in the treatment of nausea and vomiting of pregnancy. J Med Assoc Thai 2003;86:846.

202. Boskovic R, Einarson A, Maltepe C, et al. Diclectin therapy for nausea and vomiting of pregnancy: effects of optimal dosing. J Obstet Gynaecol Can 2003;25:830.

203. Heazell A, Thorneycroft J, Walton V, Etherington I. Acupressure for the in-patient treatment of nausea and vomiting in early pregnancy: a randomized control trial. Am J Obstet Gynecol 2006;194:815.

204. Rosen T, De Veciana M, Miller HS, et al. A randomized controlled trial of nerve stimulation for relief of nausea and vomiting in pregnancy. Obstet Gynecol 2003;102:129.

205. The Italian Group for Antiemetic Research. Dexamethasone alone or in combination with ondansetron for the prevention of delayed nausea and vomiting induced by chemotherapy. N Engl J Med 2000;342:1554.

206. Aranda Aguilar E, Constenla Figueiras M, Cortes-Funes H, et al. Clinical practice guidelines on antiemetics in oncology. Exp Rev Anticancer Ther 2005;5:963.

207. Kris MG, Hesketh PJ, Herrstedt J, et al. Consensus proposals for the prevention of acute and delayed vomiting and nausea following high-emetic-risk chemotherapy. Supp Care Cancer 2005;13:85.

208. Laszlo J, Clark RA, Hanson DC, et al. Lorazepam in cancer patients treated with cisplatin: a drug having antiemetic, amnesic and anxiolytic effects. J Clin Oncol 1985;3:864.

209. Ezzo J, Vickers A, Richardson MA, et al. Acupuncture-point stimulation for chemotherapy-induced nausea and vomiting. J Clin Oncol 2005;23:7188.

210. Manusirivithaya S, Sripramote M, Tangjitgamol S, et al. Antiemetic effect of ginger in gynecologic oncology patients receiving cisplatin. Int J Gynecol Cancer 2004;14:1063.

211. Billhult A, Bergbom I, Stener-Victorin E. Massage relieves nausea in women with breast cancer who are undergoing chemotherapy. J Alt Comp Med 2007;13:53.

212. Ernst E, Pittler MH. Efficacy of ginger for nausea and vomiting: a systematic review of randomized clinical trials. Br J Anaesthesia 2000;84:367.

213. Tramer MR, Reynolds DJ, Stoner NS, et al. Efficacy of 5-HT_3 receptor antagonists in radiotherapy-induced nausea and vomiting: a quantitative systemic review. Eur J Cancer 1998;34:1836.

214. The Antiemetic Subcommittee of the Multinational Association of Supportive Care in Cancer (MASCC). Prevention of chemotherapy- and radiotherapy-induced emesis: results of the 2004 Perugia International Antiemetic Consensus Conference. Ann Oncol 2006;17:20.

215. Carlisle JB, Stevenson CA. Drugs for preventing postoperative nausea and vomiting. Cochrane Data Sys Rev 2006;3:CD004125.

216. Apfel CC, Korttila K, Abdalla M, et al. A factorial trial of six interventions for the prevention of postoperative nausea and vomiting. N Engl J Med 2004;350:2441.

217. Gan TJ, Apfel CC, Kovac A, et al. A randomized, double-blind comparison of the NK_1 antagonist, aprepitant, versus ondansetron for the prevention of postoperative nausea and vomiting. Anesth Analg 2007;104:1082.

218. Habib AS, Gan TJ. Evidence-based management of postoperative nausea and vomiting: a review. Can J Anaesth 2004;51:326.

219. Gan TJ, Meyer T, Apfel CC, et al. Consensus guidelines for managing postoperative nausea and vomiting. Anesth Analg 2003; 97: 62–71.

220. Chaiyakunapruk N, Kitikannakorn N, Nathisuwan S, et al. The efficacy of ginger for the prevention of postoperative nausea and vomiting: a meta-analysis. Am J Obstet Gynecol 2006;194:95.

221. Streitberger K, Diefenbacher M, Bauer A, et al. Acupuncture compared to placebo-acupuncture for postoperative nausea and vomiting prophylaxis: a randomised placebo-controlled patient and observer blind trial. Anaesthesia 2004;59:142.

222. Li BU. Cyclic vomiting syndrome: age-old syndrome and new insights. Sem Pediatr Neurol 2001;8:13.

223. Van Calcar SC, Harding CO, Wolff JA. L-carnitine administration reduces the number of episodes in cyclic vomiting syndrome. Clin Pediatr 2002;41:171.

224. Benson JM, Zorn SL, Book LS. Sumatriptan in the treatment of cyclic vomiting. Ann Pharmacother 1995;29:997.

225. Clouse RE, Sayuk GC, Lustman PJ, Prakash C. Zonisamide and levetiracetam for adults with cyclic vomiting syndrome: a case series. Clin Gastroenterol Hepatol 2007;5:44.

226. Rosa-e-Silva L, Troncon LE, Oliviera RB, et al. Treatment of diabetic gastroparesis with oral clonidine. Aliment Pharmacol Ther 1995;9: 179.

227. Guttuso T, Roscoe J, Griggs J. Effect of gabapentin on nausea induced by chemotherapy in patients with breast cancer. Lancet 2003;361:1703.

228. Strohscheer I, Borasio GD. Carbamazepine-responsive paroxysmal nausea and vomiting in a patient with meningeal carcinomatosis. Palliat Med 2006;20:549.

229. Rudd JA, Ngan MP, Wai MK, et al. Anti-emetic activity of ghrelin in ferrets exposed to the cytotoxic anti-cancer agent cisplatin. Neurosci Lett 2006;392:79.

230. Murray CD, Martin NM, Patterson M, et al. Ghrelin enhances gastric emptying in diabetic gastroparesis: a double blind, placebo controlled, crossover study. Gut 2005;54:1693.

231. Lien HC, Sun WM, Chen YH, et al. Effects of ginger on motion sickness and gastric slow-wave dysrhythmias induced by circular vection. Am J Physiol – Gastrointest Liver Physiol 2003;284:G481.

232. Yen Pik Sang FD, Golding JF, Gresty MA. Suppression of motion sickness by controlled breathing during mildly nauseogenic motion. Aviat Space Environ Med 2003;74:998.

233. Pearl ML, Fischer M, McCauley DL, et al. Transcutaneous electrical nerve stimulation as an adjunct for controlling chemotherapy-induced nausea and vomiting in gynecologic oncology patients. Cancer Nursing 1999;22:307.

234. Pusch F, Frietag H, Goll V, et al. Electrical stimulation of the vestibular system prevents postoperative nausea and vomiting. Acta Anaesth Scand 2000;44:1145.

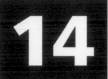

Approach to the patient with abdominal pain

Pankaj Jay Pasricha

Background and importance, 228
The neurobiology of pain, 228
Clinical assessment of the patient with abdominal pain, 238
Approach to the treatment of abdominal pain, 247
Conclusions, 251

We look away from each pain, in the waiting sadness,
Hoping it will pass away. Yet they form our winter's
Bower, darkly filling our senses with green, one
Of our internal seasons, but not merely season,
But place, dwelling, defense, foundation, home.

Rainier Maria Rilke (1875–1926), *The Duino Elegies*

Background and importance

Pain is a paradox, as we are reminded by the haunting words of the Austro-German poet, Rilke. As a sensation, it is an integral component of the normal "defense" system, warning the organism about potentially noxious agents in the internal or external environment; physicians can deal with such acute pain in a relatively straightforward manner in most cases. On the other hand, pain is also unique among sensations in that it can evoke, and to some extent be invoked by, complex alterations in the psychosocial state of human beings. Further, when chronic, it can so dominate the clinical picture that it can no longer be regarded as a sentinel sensation but instead assumes the characteristics of a disease state by itself. It is the purpose of this chapter to provide an overview of the basic neuroscientific tenets of pain, knowledge of which is essential to provide competent and compassionate care.

The gastroenterologist routinely has to deal with abdominal pain, one of the most common symptoms that patients experience. Prevalence rates of more than 20% have been reported and women appear to be disproportionately affected [1]. According to the National Ambulatory Medical Care Survey

in 2002, abdominal pain was the leading gastrointestinal symptom prompting an outpatient visit, with nearly 12 million visits (the next most common symptom was diarrhea, accounting for approximately 4 million visits) [2]. Although abdominal pain is also a major reason for hospitalization, many of these patients do not have a specific diagnosis. Thus, in a consecutive group of 100 patients admitted with lower abdominal pain, 67% were diagnosed as having nonspecific abdominal pain; this represented about 13% of all general surgical admissions [3]. As can be expected, patients with abdominal pain consume significant resources, with mean annual direct health-care costs estimated at US$7646 for abdominal pain [4] (compared with US$5049 for irritable bowel syndrome, US$6140 for diarrhea, and US$7522 for constipation). Although only a small fraction of these persons consult a physician, the symptom is severe enough to impair routine activities in most patients [5]. Furthermore, chronic abdominal pain as an independent predictor of suicidal behavior after adjusting for comorbid psychiatric conditions, shows a risk that is 3- to 11-fold greater than that in controls [6].

The neurobiology of pain

Anatomical pathways
Peripheral pathways

The perception of pain begins in the periphery with the stimulation of spinal sensory neurons (so-called nociceptors), whose cell bodies lie in the dorsal root ganglion (DRG) and whose free nerve endings are located between the smooth muscle layers of hollow organs, on their serosal surface, in the mesentery, and within the mucosa of the gastrointestinal tract (Fig. 14.1). After leaving the viscus that they innervate, these nerve fibers run with the sympathetic fibers (as

Principles of Clinical Gastroenterology. Edited by Tadataka Yamada, David H. Alpers, Anthony N. Kalloo, Neil Kaplowitz, Chung Owyang, and Don W. Powell. © 2008 Blackwell Publishing. ISBN 978-1-4051-69103

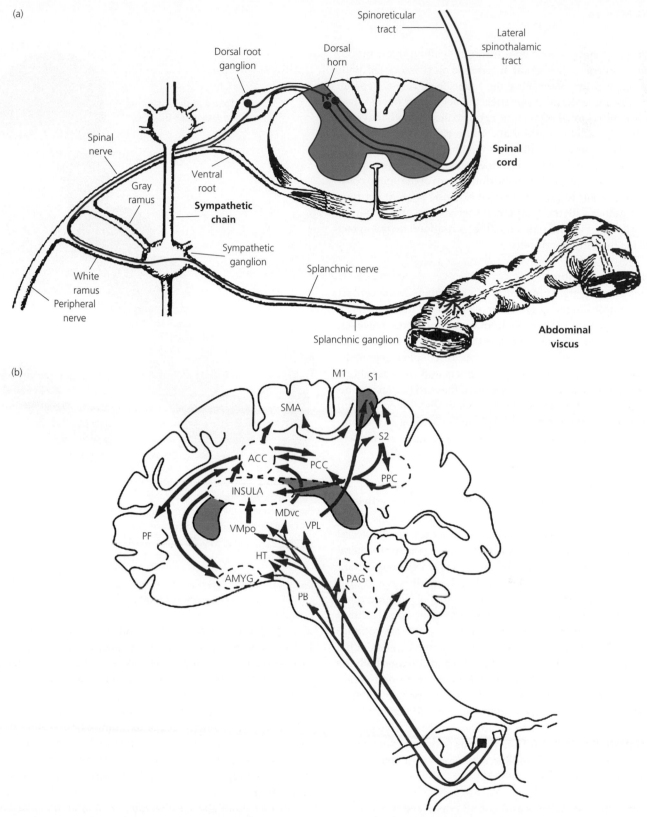

Figure 14.1 Pain pathways. **(a)** Classic neuronal pathways (purple), such as the spinothalamic and spinoreticular tracts, mediating abdominal visceral pain sensation leave the dorsal horn, cross the midline, and ascend to higher centers. Nociceptive information from visceral organs is relayed to cells near the central canal. These postsynaptic dorsal horn cells send their axons in the midline of the dorsal column to synapse in the nucleus gracilis. The pathway then crosses the midline in the lower brainstem to ascend to the ventral posterolateral nucleus of the thalamus. **(b)** Schematic of ascending pathways, subcortical structures, and cerebral cortical structures involved in processing pain. PAG, periaqueductal gray; PB, parabrachial nucleus of the dorsolateral pons; VMpo, ventromedial part of the posterior nuclear complex; MDvc, ventrocaudal part of the medial dorsal nucleus; VPL, ventral posterolateral nucleus; ACC, anterior cingulate cortex; PCC, posterior cingulate cortex; HT, hypothalamus; M1, primary motor cortex; S1 and S2, first and second somatosensory cortical areas; PPC, posterior parietal complex; SMA, supplementary motor area; AMYG, amygdala; PF, prefrontal cortex. This portion of the figure from Price [13], with permission from AAAS.

mesenteric nerves) and pass through, without interruption, one of several prevertebral autonomic plexi associated with the major artery supplying the organ (e.g., celiac, hepatic, superior mesenteric). Thereafter, the nociceptor fibers travel within the regional splanchnic nerve to the sympathetic chain running parallel to the spinal cord on either side. Here they finally part company with the sympathetic nerves, taking the white ramus communicans to the spinal nerve and thence to the eventual termination in the dorsal horn of the spinal cord. It is important to note that while extrinsic afferent neurons run together with the sympathetic nerves for a greater part of their length, visceral pain and other sensations are not in fact carried by sympathetic nerves.

Spinal connections

After entering the spinal cord, afferent fibers make contact with neurons in the gray matter, primarily at the same level. Some innervation, especially from visceral afferents, however, also takes place above and below the level of entry with fibers ascending rostrally and caudally up to six spinal segments. Whereas somatic nociceptor afferents mainly synapse at one level in the most superficial region of the cord (laminae I and II), visceral afferents are more widely distributed in both dorsoventral and craniocaudal planes, providing an anatomical basis for the difficulty in localizing visceral pain precisely [7]. Visceral pain can be difficult to localize clinically.

Ascending pathways

There are two relatively distinct pathways for visceral sensation to ascend cranially from second-order neurons in the spinal cord. The classical one for both somatic and visceral pain involves fibers that cross the midline to the contralateral side, and then travel cephalad in the ventrolateral quadrant of the spinal cord to synapse within the midbrain and thalamic nuclei (see below). The second pathway, which is relatively specific for visceral pain, is relayed in the dorsal column (also known as the dorsal funiculus or posterior column) of the spinal cord (Fig. 14.2) [8]. This column ascends in the midline ipsilaterally in the spinal cord and contains both the central extensions of primary afferent neurons originating in the dorsal root ganglia as well as the postsynaptic dorsal column fibers arising from spinal neurons. Evidence for the functional importance of this pathway is derived from physiological studies as well as from patients with intractable pelvic pain in whom limited midline myelotomy resulted in complete or near-complete relief [9,10].

Supraspinal structures and circuits involved in pain

The spinothalamic tract in the ventrolateral spinal cord relays pain directly to the thalamus whereas the dorsal column pathway is polysynaptic in that there is at least one more relay station in the lower medulla (the gracile or cuneate nuclei) before it reaches the contralateral thalamus. Within the thalamus, the ventral posterior complex, comprising

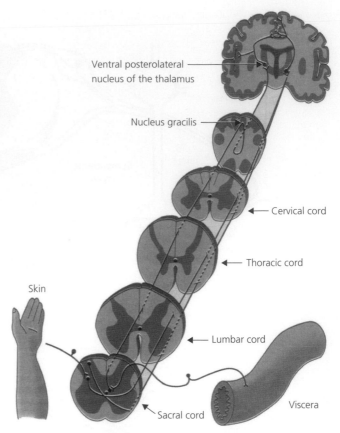

Figure 14.2 "Visceral-specific" pain pathways in the spinal cord. Artist's drawing showing how nociceptive input from the pelvic viscera arrives in the dorsal horn of the spinal cord where it is relayed to higher centers by cells near the central canal. Adapted from Willis & Westlund [15], with permission from Lippincott Williams & Wilkins.

a ventral posterolateral and a ventral posteromedial nucleus, is the main receiving station for nociceptive (as well as mechanosensory) signals. Neurons in these nuclei project to the cerebral cortex where pain is "mapped". Cortical representation of visceral pain is poorly understood but appears to involve both the primary (SI) and secondary (SII) somatosensory cortices. Noxious stimulation from same-segment structures (e.g., esophagus and thoracic skin) in humans reveal some overlaps but also distinct differences in the cortical projection of visceral and superficial nociceptive pathways [11].

Noxious stimulation is also relayed in spinoreticular and other ascending tracts in the anterolateral spinal cord, which are phylogenetically older than the spinothalamic tract but equally important [12]. Spinoreticular fibers make multiple synapses in the reticular formation in the brainstem, which is responsible for arousal and wakefulness. Thus, when these fibers are activated by noxious stimulation, the organism is alerted to the possibility of bodily injury. From the reticular formation, impulses travel to the intralaminar nuclei of the thalamus and are subsequently relayed to the somatosensory cortex as well as the cingulate cortex and prefrontal cortex. Other projections of these nuclei include both the hypothalamus and the limbic system (see below).

In addition to the above major tracts, there are also spinomesencephalic fibers and spinohypothalamic tracts traveling in the anterior spinal cord. The former terminate mainly in the periaqueductal gray matter and the midbrain raphe nuclei (part of the "descending pain-inhibiting system"; see below); some also end in the parabrachial nucleus, which in turn is connected to the limbic system via the amygdala. The spinohypothalamic fibers convey information to neurons in the hypothalamus, which subsequently course to the thalamus; collectively this pathway contributes to the autonomic and reflex responses to painful stimuli.

Integration of noxious stimuli, pain perception, and associated phenomena

Thus it appears that several neural circuits are involved in processing noxious stimuli [12–14]. There is a "sensory-discriminative" circuit, consisting of dorsal column and spinothalamic fibers and their projections, of which the primary function is to characterize the stimuli according to their location and nature. The other circuit is "affective–cognitive" in nature, consisting of the spinoreticular, spinomesencephalic, and other tracts described above, and mediates the accompanying autonomic and emotional responses (arousal, fear, escape). It achieves these functions via its intimate connections to the limbic system, a primitive network in the mammalian brain that is a major center for the interconnected processes of emotion, learning, and memory. It consists of many parts, of which the most important are the cingulate cortex, a long band of cortex that runs from the front of the brain to the back, the parahippocampal gyrus, the dentate gyrus, the hippocampus, and the amygdala. The hippocampus is the main region involved in the generation and storage of memory while the amygdala is responsible for complex emotional processing, including associating various stimuli with specific emotions (emotional memory).

Signals from the somatosensory cortex proceed to the posterior parietal cortex which integrates them with visual and other sensory cues and then relays the information to the insula and the anterior cingulate cortex. The anterior cingulate cortex also receives input from the prefrontal cortex, and they both also receive input from the spinoreticular tracts, as described above. The anterior cingulate cortex thus appears to occupy a critical position in the response to noxious stimuli, integrating information about the immediate environmental threat from the parietal cortex, with behavioral response anticipation and planning originating in the prefrontal cortex, and subsequently initiating the emotional and autonomic responses via the limbic system and hypothalamus.

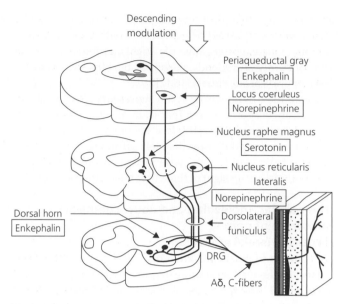

Figure 14.3 Descending pathways involved in modulation of nociception and their principal neuromediators. DRG, dorsal root ganglion. From Russo & Brose [170], with permission from Annual Reviews.

Descending pathways

The functional connections between the spinal cord and higher centers run both ways (Fig. 14.3). Most of the descending pathways are inhibitory and may serve to provide negative feedback to strong painful input; however, excitatory connections also exist. One of the most important centers involved in descending modulation of nociception is the periaqueductal gray (see above), which connects caudally to the spinal cord via the nucleus raphe magnum and raphespinal pathways. It also receives both descending projections from several of the other structures involved in the affective–cognitive aspects of pain, including the limbic system and hypothalamic regions, as well as ascending input from spinomesencephalic fibers (see above). Thus it is in a unique position to coordinate a "dampening" response. Other centers participating in descending inhibition include pontine nuclei such as the locus caeruleus and subcaeruleus [15].

Nociception, suffering, and illness behavior: the biopsychosocial continuum of the pain experience

Finally, it is important to understand that nociception, the detection of tissue damage by specialized cells, is not synonymous with pain. Increased afferent signaling to the central nervous system by itself is not necessarily enough to make a patient with chronic pain seek medical attention. Conversely, pain can be perceived even in the absence of nociception as a result of damage to the peripheral or central nervous system. Illness behavior reflects how pain is acted upon, varies widely among individuals, and is a result of a complex mixture of physiological (e.g., pain intensity/severity or associated features), psychological (mental state, stress, mood, coping style, and memories of or experiences with pain) and social factors (concurrent negative life events, attitudes and behavior of family and friends, perceived benefits such as avoidance of unpleasant duties) [16,17].

The patient with chronic pain represents a dysregulation or dysfunction of a system that is, in effect, a continuum of biopsychosocial factors [18]. In a given patient, the primary disturbance may disproportionately affect one component of the spectrum, and it is the wise physician's task to identify this without losing sight of the whole (see also Chapter 3).

The cellular, molecular, and neurochemical substrate of pain

Types of visceral afferents

By contrast to cutaneous afferents, visceral afferents consist almost exclusively of unmyelinated C-type fibers and small myelinated Aδ-type fibers and can signal both physiological and pathological events. Both Aδ-type and C-type fibers are polymodal and respond to both mechanical and thermal stimuli; the C-type fibers additionally respond to noxious chemical stimuli such as acid and capsaicin, the pungent component in hot chili peppers. From a functional perspective, there are at least three broad types of visceral nociceptors:

• low-threshold afferents that respond faithfully to a broad spectrum of stimulus intensity from the physiological to the noxious

• high-threshold afferents that respond only to stimuli in the noxious range

• "silent" afferents that only become responsive in the presence of tissue injury and inflammation.

These afferents receive input from mucosa, muscle, and serosa [19,20].

Neurobiology of peripheral nociception and key molecules

The nociceptor has to perform three key tasks (Fig. 14.4):

• transduction of noxious stimulus to an electrical signal

• conduction of that electrical signal from the peripheral to the central end of the nociceptor

• encode and relay that signal to second-order neurons in the form of synaptically transmitted chemicals.

In general, nociceptors convert noxious stimuli to an electrical response via specialized receptors. The best example of this is the vanilloid receptor, TRPV1 (transient receptor potential vanilloid 1) [21–23]. It responds to, and appears to integrate, several noxious stimuli produced during tissue injury, including heat, local tissue acidosis, and several proalgesic metabolites. Activation of the receptor results in a cationic, calcium-preferring current that leads to depolarization of the membrane. In addition to TRPV1, nociceptors also possess a variety of other more highly specialized receptors that are capable of interacting only with specific chemical components of the inflammatory "soup" that accompanies tissue injury.

Thermal, mechanical, or chemical stimuli, acting via specific receptors, induce a change in the membrane potential of the nociceptor terminal, called a "receptor" or "generator" potential. Voltage-gated sodium-ion (Nav) and potassium-ion (Kv) channels play a fundamental role in controlling neuronal excitability in response to this relatively small change in membrane potential by setting thresholds for activation of an action potential. Finally, voltage-dependent calcium channels contribute to depolarization but more importantly mediate crucial nociceptor functions such as the release of neurotransmitters and long-term plasticity [24].

Once generated, action potentials are conducted centripetally to the spinal terminals of the nociceptors, where they

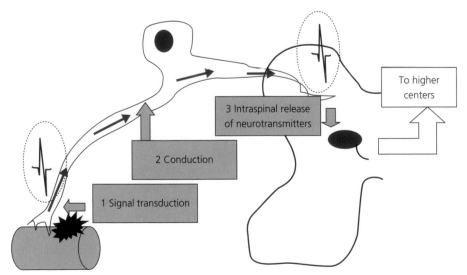

1 Signal transduction

2 Conduction

3 Intraspinal release of neurotransmitters

To higher centers

Figure 14.4 The primary nociceptor and its functions. Sensation from the peripheral organ is carried via fibers whose origin is in cell bodies within the dorsal root ganglia. The central projections of these neurons in turn relay information to second-order neurons in the spinal cord, which transmit this information upwards to the brainstem and higher centers via distinct pathways. This diagram illustrates the three basic components of pain signaling at the level of the first-order neuron in the nociceptive pathway. A painful stimulus is translated into electrical activity, which is conducted centrally and eventually results in the release of neurotransmitters at the central synapses, with stimulation of second-order neurons.

initiate neurotransmitter release (mediated by calcium entry) and thereby relay nociceptive information to second-order neurons. The early response to relatively mild stimuli is transmitted via glutamate acting on the α-amino-3-hydroxy-5-methylisoxazole-4-propionic acid (AMPA) and kainate ligand-gated ion channels [25]. If the stimulus is sustained or intense enough, it causes release of neuropeptides such as substance P, which acts on the neurokinin 1 (NK1) receptor to produce a correspondingly more intense postsynaptic response. This is further boosted by activation of another ionotropic glutamate receptor, the N-methyl-D-aspartate (NMDA) receptor. Calcitonin gene-related peptide, which is coexpressed with substance P, also plays a role in nociceptive transmission, but its role is much less well understood. Several additional neurotransmitters (both inhibitory and excitatory) may also be involved in spinal nociceptive processes including neurokinin A, brain-derived neurotropic factor, vasoactive intestinal peptide, somatostatin, galanin, and nitric oxide.

Inhibitory systems

The dorsal horn cannot be considered a simple way station, but rather as a critical point where peripheral signals may be enhanced or attenuated by caudally directed neural connections from higher centers before they are relayed cranially (Fig. 14.3). Descending inhibitory neurons (see "Descending pathways") counteract the excitation from the periphery via the release of neurotransmitters such as glycine and γ-aminobutyric acid (GABA) [26–28]. While serotonin is also thought to be an important participant in descending inhibition, its effects are not as straightforward, this is the result of the multiplicity of receptors, some of which have conflicting actions on nociception [29]. A closely related inhibitory system involves noradrenaline, whose effects on nociception are largely mediated by α_2-adrenergic presynaptic receptors (the most important of which may be the α_{2A} receptor) [30]. The spinal cord also contains high concentrations of opioid receptors, mainly in the superficial laminae (μ, δ, κ, in order of abundance), activation of which inhibits the release of excitatory neurotransmitters such as substance P and glutamate.

Clinically important physiological characteristics of visceral nociception

With the above knowledge in mind, it is a useful exercise to briefly summarize the differences in the clinically relevant features of pain originating in the viscera as compared with that arising from somatic tissues [31]. First, the visceral afferents are relatively few in number (as compared with somatic structures) and diverge extensively in the central nervous system with the result that the pain tends to be poorly localized. Second, acute visceral pain is often accompanied by autonomic disturbances such as changes in blood pressure and heart rate, pallor and sweating, and visceral motor phenomena such as vomiting and diarrhea. Finally, humans rate

visceral pain as more unpleasant and are more likely to react to it with anxiety and other emotions than cutaneous pain from the same spinal segment and of similar intensity [32].

The above phenomena can be readily explained based on the neuroanatomical principles outlined so far in this chapter. In addition, there are several other clinically important features of visceral pain that need detailed description. These include the phenomena of referred pain, sensitization, and stress-induced exacerbation of pain.

Referred pain

Most clinically significant forms of visceral pain are referred to somatic areas. A patient with "pure" visceral pain is seldom seen in the clinic because this phase usually lasts only a few hours. When it begins, it is felt as a deep and dull discomfort in the midline reflecting the ontogenic origin of the involved organ from the fore-, mid-, or hindgut, respectively (Fig. 14.5). If the underlying insult persists, referred pain sets in. Referred pain is perceived as sharp and readily localized to the overlying or remote superficial somatic structures, such as skin or abdominal wall muscle. Referred pain can occur without hyperalgesia of the somatic structure (simple irradiation) or can be accompanied by sensitization of these structures with resulting hyperalgesia (secondary somatic hyperalgesia) [33]. Examples of both are commonly seen in practice. Thus gallstone induced pain is felt in the right upper quadrant as well as in the back but hyperalgesia (painful to the touch or deeper palpation) is typically experienced at Murphy's point.

The physiological basis of referred pain is incompletely understood and no one theory is completely satisfactory (Fig. 14.6) [34]. In contrast to superficial structure, spinal neurons receiving input from a visceral organ are also connected to afferents from other visceral organs, joints, muscle, and skin. This explains both the lack of precision in being able to localize visceral pain as well as providing a rationale for the "misinterpretation" theory of referred pain. Although central convergence is the most popular paradigm to explain this, it is also possible that somatovisceral convergence occurs in the periphery with dichotomizing primary neurons providing branches to both somatic and visceral structures. Indeed, in animals, both viscerovisceral and somatovisceral dichotomizing afferents have been described [35]. Regardless of the site of convergence, this theory assumes that the brain will consistently assign the origin of the signal to a somatic structure rather than the corresponding visceral organ. This is assumed to be because the brain learns by conditioning and because it experiences sensation from somatic structures far more often than visceral ones, it is more likely to attribute pain from a convergent pathway to the former [34].

Tenderness of overlying regions is a common clinical sign of visceral pain and most experts believe that it results from an "irritative" focus in the spinal cord, representing the site of somatovisceral convergence (Fig. 14.6). A secondary spinal neuron that has been rendered excitable by repeated

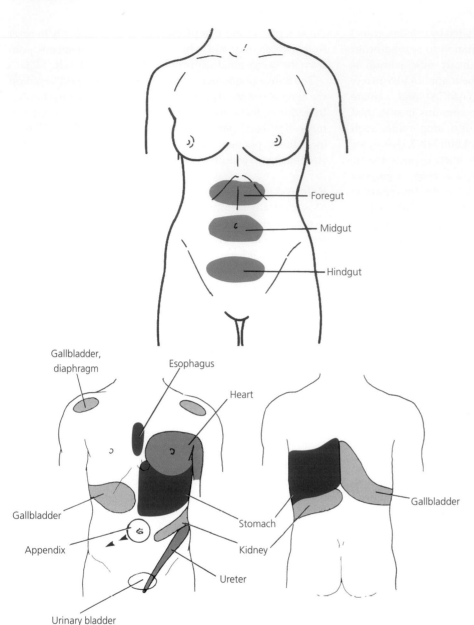

Figure 14.5 True visceral and referred pain patterns. **Top panel**: approximate levels of the abdomen where "true" visceral pain is felt, according to its source. **Lower panel**: important skin areas for referral of visceral pain. From Snell [171], with permission from Lippincott Williams & Wilkins.

stimulation from an injured viscus will therefore now also react in an exaggerated fashion to relatively innocuous input from converging somatic structures, an example of hyperalgesia (see discussion below for greater details). Hyperalgesia of muscle is often accompanied by spasm, which may be secondary to spinal reflexes with their efferent limbs originating in the anterior horn [36,37].

Pain and sensitization

Most clinically important painful conditions occur on a background of a nociceptive system that is operating not at a "normal" level but rather in a potentiated or "sensitized" state [25]. This concept can help to explain many commonly encountered clinical situations. Tissue injury or inflammation results in the local accumulation of several factors that can lead to a sustained and amplified (supranormal) activity of peripheral nociceptors, a phenomenon called peripheral sensitization. In addition, these factors can also result in a change of the responsiveness of previously dormant neurons ("silent nociceptors") such that they now start contributing to nociceptive activity. This increased "afferent barrage" over time leads to changes in second-order neurons within the spinal cord, causing an increase in their responsiveness over time with amplification and persistence of pain [38]: this is an example of central sensitization. The gain of the entire system is therefore reset upwards, with the result that noxious stimuli now elicit a pain response that is much greater when compared with the normal state, a phenomenon

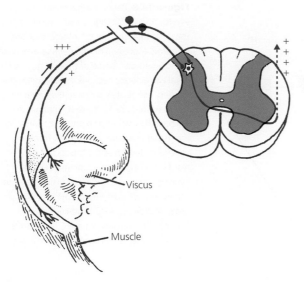

Figure 14.6 Theories of referred pain from a visceral organ, using skeletal muscle as the site of referral. **Left panel**: the convergence-facilitation theory states that painful visceral insults produce an "irritable focus" in the corresponding spinal cord segment, thus facilitating or amplifying signals from somatic structures whose nerves converge on the same spinal neurons. According to this theory, the referred hyperalgesia is mainly central. **Right panel**: the reflex-arc theory states that viscerocutaneous or visceromuscular reflexes traveling through the spinal cord induce neurogenic changes in the muscle or skin that result in a local painful state. According to this theory, referred hyperalgesia can be viewed as peripheral. From Raj [33], with permission from Elsevier.

termed *hyperalgesia*. A further characteristic of the sensitized state is called *allodynia*, a term that refers to the phenomenon in which innocuous or physiological stimuli are perceived as painful. These manifestations of sensitization are graphically illustrated in Fig. 14.7. As an example, one can therefore postulate that patients with painful chronic pancreatitis exhibit pancreatic neuronal sensitization and may experience mechanical allodynia: pain in response to physiological changes in intraductal pressure (which would otherwise have not been perceived). Similarly, subsequent minor flareups of inflammation in such patients could also cause the associated pain to be felt as severe, rather than mild (hyperalgesia).

Pain sensitization results from both early posttranslational changes as well as later transcription-dependent changes in effector genes, with both processes occurring in the peripheral terminals of the nociceptor and in dorsal horn neurons. A variety of factors found in inflamed tissue are capable of producing such sensitization including potassium and hydrogen ions, amines (serotonin [5-HT], histamine), kinins (bradykinin), prostanoids (prostaglandin E_2), purines (adenosine triphosphate), cytokines (tumor necrosis factor, interleukin-1, interleukin-6) and growth factors such as nerve growth factor [39]. In the short-term, several of these agents, acting via specific receptors and/or cellular messengers initiate a chain of events that leads to an increase in the phosphorylated state of critical ion channels (Fig. 14.8), such as TRPV1 and the nociceptor-specific tetrodotoxin-resistant sodium-ion channels, thus enhancing excitability (see above). These early sensitization events are sustained

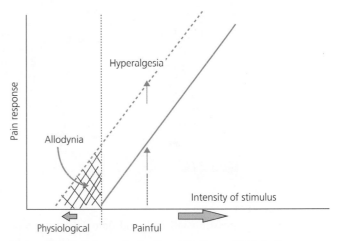

Figure 14.7 Basic concepts of pain sensitization, as illustrated in a theoretical stimulus–response curve. The solid line on the right represents a hypothetical control population while the broken line on the left represents the response in a sensitized population (e.g., patients with pancreatitis). The broken vertical line represents the threshold for painful stimulation in the control population. Note that the sensitized population experiences pain in response to stimulation that is in the nonpainful (physiological range) for the control population, a phenomenon known as allodynia (hatched area). Hyperalgesia refers to a response to painful stimulation that is greater than the control population (arrows).

and further amplified by changes in the expression of several key proteins hours to days after the onset of tissue injury/inflammation. Similar paradigms of sensitization can be used to illustrate the processes underlying central sensitization,

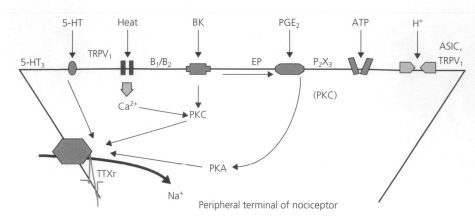

Peripheral terminal of nociceptor

Figure 14.8 Peripheral sensitization: early events. Various biological mediators comprising the inflammatory "soup" interact with specific receptors expressed on the peripheral ends of sensory neurons. Some of these (e.g., noxious heat) can activate neurons directly, while the majority can acutely sensitize the neuron, i.e., make it more excitable by changes in intracellular calcium and phosphorylation states that result in greater activation of critical ion channels such as the tetrodotoxin-resistant (TTXr) sodium channel. 5-HT, 5-hydroxytryptamine; TRPV$_1$, transient receptor potential vanilloid 1; BK, bradykinin; PGE$_2$, prostaglandin E$_2$; ASIC, acid-sensing ion channel; PKC, protein kinase C; PKA, protein kinase A. Adapted from Woolf & Costigan [172].

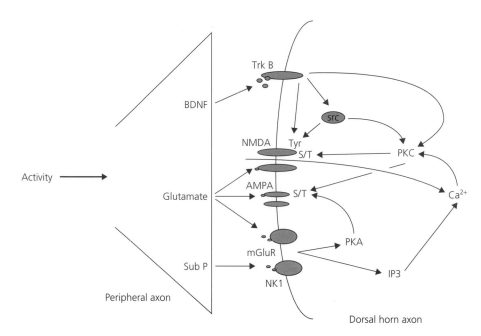

Dorsal horn axon

Figure 14.9 Early sensitization within dorsal horn neurons after release of transmitters from C-type fiber central terminals. These transmitters/neuromodulators act on receptors and ion channels in the dorsal horn to activate protein kinases that phosphorylate membrane-bound *N*-methyl-D-aspartate (NMDA) and α-amino-3-hydroxy-5-methylisoxazole-4-propionic acid (AMPA) receptors and alter their functional properties, increasing membrane excitability and thereby eliciting central sensitization. From Woolf & Costigan [172], with permission from PNAS.

including early posttranslational and late transcriptional events (Fig. 14.9).

These experimental paradigms are beginning to receive confirmation in clinical studies. There is growing evidence that TRPV1 expression is increased in patients with inflammatory bowel disease [40], rectal hypersensitivity [41], and esophagitis [42]. Increased expression of calcitonin gene-related peptide and substance P has been noted in nerve fibers in specimens from patients with chronic pancreatitis [43]. Furthermore, there is a significant correlation between pain and upregulation of pancreatic expression of the NK1 receptor (the principal receptor for substance P, see above) [44], brain-derived neurotropic factor [45], nerve growth factor, and its receptor TrkA [46].

Experimental evidence suggests that both inflammatory and motor events could theoretically set in motion a cascade of events that leads to sensitization even in conditions such as irritable bowel syndrome. Thus, mucosal inflammation accompanying gastrointestinal infections can produce visceral hyperalgesia by both peripheral sensitization and central hyperexcitability [47]. A significant number of patients develop irritable bowel syndrome-like symptoms after a bout of acute infectious gastroenteritis [48,49]. According to this theory, the lack of overt inflammation or disruption of tissue architecture in patients with irritable bowel syndrome is explained by the fact that the initiating event was transient but left persistent changes in its wake that resulted in peripheral and central hyperalgesia. In such a sensitized state even normal contractile events could be perceived as painful (i.e., allodynia).

The relative importance of central and peripheral factors in humans with functional visceral hyperalgesia is not known.

Our present state of knowledge cannot determine if patients with irritable bowel syndrome have increased signaling from a truly "irritable" bowel or if their symptoms arise from changes in the central nervous system response to a relatively normal signal [50]. It is also possible that abnormalities in cognitive–emotional processing of afferent signals, rather than nociception per se, may be important contributors to pain perception in these patients. This is discussed further in the next section.

Stress and visceral pain

Our day-to-day language (e.g., "butterflies in the stomach") attests to the intimate relationship between gut sensation and our mental state. Stress can be classified as either exteroceptive (e.g., psychosocial in origin) or interoceptive (e.g., the result of tissue inflammation or injury) and appears to have opposite effects on somatic and visceral pain, with the former

being suppressed and the latter exacerbated [51]. Clinical experience easily attests to the role of stress in both the onset and modulation of symptoms in patients with irritable bowel syndrome [52].

The biological basis of this is beginning to be explored; a major player appears to be the cortisol release factor/ hormone (CRF or CRH) produced by the hypothalamus in response to stress and exerting a variety of systemic effects via its CRF1 receptor. These include release of adreno-corticotropic hormone as well as changes in gastrointestinal nociception and motility in animals as well as humans [53–55]. These aspects are discussed in greater detail in Chapter 3.

Thus a model emerges in which various components of the biopsychosocial continuum for pain can be seen to interact with each other and produce the final clinical picture (Fig. 14.10) [56].

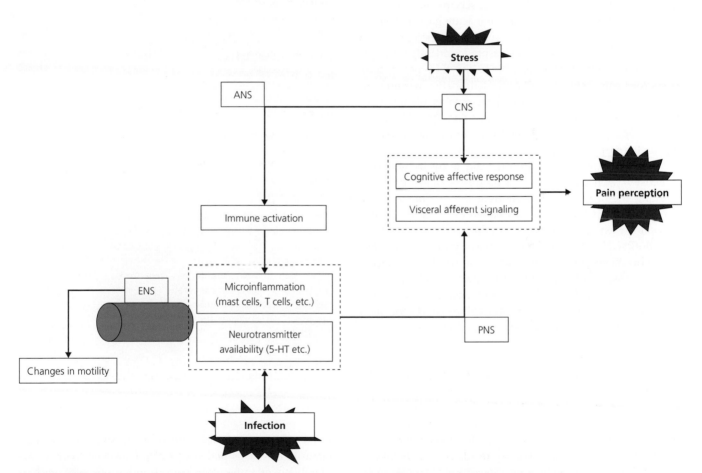

Figure 14.10 Current and emerging pathophysiological concepts of pain in irritable bowel syndrome. The figure assumes a vulnerable background (genetic, developmental phase) that is predisposed to developing a persistent state of activation in response to two major inciting factors, stress and infection, acting initially at central and peripheral sites, respectively. Subgroups of patients with irritable bowel syndrome may differ in the nature of the inciting factor, as well as the activity of the various components that eventually lead to pain perception. Although changes in motility are shown separately, it is possible that in some instances they may also contribute to increased afferent signaling and discomfort. Abbreviations: ANS, autonomic nervous system; CNS, central nervous system; ENS, enteric nervous system; PNS, peripheral nervous system (spinal afferents). From DuPont & Pasricha [56].

Classification of abdominal pain

Pain is a complex syndrome and an attempt to classify it in a comprehensive manner poses a significant challenge. Although some progress has been made in somatic pain syndromes, classification of visceral pain has yet to be undertaken in any systematic fashion. An appealing approach to the classification of pain, used widely in the somatic literature, is based on putative neurophysiological mechanisms. According to this, pain can be either *nociceptive* or *neuropathic* [57]. Nociceptive pain implies an ongoing stimulation of peripheral nociceptors by the persistence of local painful conditions (e.g., injury and/or inflammation). Neuropathic pain, on the other hand, is pain that originates independent of nociceptor stimulation and implies structural or functional changes in the pain pathways (either peripheral or central) that result in persistent but aberrant signaling. Pure nociceptive pain is generally regarded as an experimental concept because clinically relevant pain is almost always accompanied by some changes in the nerves serving the pain pathways. Nevertheless, the pain of some acute gastrointestinal conditions, such as peptic ulcer, colonic ischemia, or acute cholecystitis, can be considered to be predominantly nociceptive in nature. Somatic neuropathic pain syndromes include poststroke pain (central) or diabetic neuropathy (peripheral). Whether there is a visceral counterpart remains unknown but it is possible that certain types of "functional" pain disorders are neuropathic in nature, given the absence of overt pathology in the suspected organ.

Yet another way of classifying pain is by its temporal dimension. Acute pain serves a useful biological function, warning the organism of impending injury. On the other hand, chronic pain, arbitrarily defined as at least a month beyond the expected course of an injury to heal, appears to have outlived its utility and can result in significant secondary morbidity in the form of physical, emotional, or socioeconomic stresses on the patient, family, and society [56] (see discussion above). The challenge for clinicians therefore, is to recognize the various psychosocial attributes of chronic pain without losing track of the underlying problem.

Clinical assessment of the patient with abdominal pain

History

Although patients presenting with acute abdominal pain are dealt with in greater detail in Chapter 16, it is worthwhile to remember that many of the same principles of diagnosis apply to patients in less emergent settings. A carefully taken history often holds the key to an accurate diagnosis of abdominal pain.

Site

Most clinicians find it useful to divide the abdomen into four quadrants (Table 14.1). These general, if crude, inferences are

Table 14.1 Localization of common causes of acute abdominal pain

Right lower quadrant
Appendicitis
Infective terminal ileitis
Crohn's disease
Tuboovarian disorders
Ectopic pregnancy
Ruptured ovarian cyst
Salpingitis
Renal disorders
Right ureteric calculus
Pyelonephritis
Pyogenic sacroiliitis

Right upper quadrant
Acute cholecystitis
Biliary colic
Acute hepatic inflammation or distention

Left upper quadrant
Splenic infarct
Splenic flexure ischemia

Left lower quadrant
Acute diverticulitis
Infectious or inflammatory colitis
Pyogenic sacroiliitis
Tuboovarian disorders

Central abdominal pain
Gastroenteritis, gastritis
Peptic ulcer disease
Small intestinal colic
Acute pancreatitis

Diffuse abdominal pain
Acute infectious peritonitis
Appendicitis
Diverticulitis
Inflammatory bowel disease and toxic megacolon
Perforated ulcer (gastric or duodenal)
Spontaneous peritonitis in cirrhosis
Acute noninfectious peritonitis
Familial Mediterranean fever
Hemorrhagic pancreatitis
Postoperative

supported by studies using balloon insufflation in various organs in conscious patients [58,59]. However, there is considerable overlap between pain from various sites, such as the stomach, bile duct, pancreas, and proximal small intestine. Furthermore, compared to healthy volunteers, patients with chronic painful conditions (including irritable bowel syndrome) often have distorted patterns of pain (as part of the accompanying hyperalgesia) rendering inference about the site of pain even more hazardous [60].

Temporal characteristics

Onset, duration, and the pattern of variation with time are all important features to elicit. Immediate severe pain is suggestive of an acute obstruction of a hollow viscus (e.g., bile duct obstruction by a stone), perforation (e.g., free perforation of a duodenal ulcer), or a catastrophic ischemic condition. The more common situation is a more gradual onset of pain; the transition from a "glowing ember" to a "raging flame" may take hours or days depending upon the underlying condition and is typical of inflammatory conditions such as appendicitis, diverticulitis, pancreatitis, and cholecystitis.

Abrupt cessation of pain can occasionally occur spontaneously and should suggest the relief of an obstructed organ; examples include the intestinal passage of a biliary stone or resolution of a volvulus. In many cases, however, the pain is intermittent in that it wanes for varying intervals of time, only to wax to its original intensity subsequently. Such pain is typical of colic, usually intestinal in origin. Biliary pain, though traditionally labeled as colic also, shows less variability than commonly thought.

In addition to intermittency, another pattern of temporal variation is periodicity, implying a long duration (weeks to months) of pain-free intervals. Such periodicity is seldom regular (unless pain is pelvic and related to the menstrual cycle) and used to be characteristic of conditions such as peptic ulcer disease (in the days before effective therapy was available). Other examples include patients with recurrent urinary stones, patients with irritable bowel syndrome (where the pain often varies with periods of psychosocial stress and associated disturbances in bowel function), and a long list of less common conditions (Table 14.2).

Finally, the duration of the pain should be mentioned as an important factor in that it has a direct bearing on the degree of difficulty in reaching a diagnosis. Many of these patients have already sought medical advice and simple illnesses have generally been excluded by the time they present to a specialist. The clinical picture may further be confounded by the presence of several confounding factors including referred hyperalgesia (see above), secondary psychosocial morbidity, and aberrant illness behaviors.

Character and intensity of pain

These attributes are less useful diagnostically because by their very nature, they are subjective and therefore influenced by the social and educational background of the patient as well as past personal experience. Although patients are often asked to rate pain on simple scales like 1 to 10, often using a previously encountered pain as a reference point, this is seldom useful in distinguishing the cause of the pain or even whether the pain is of the so-called functional type. Similar considerations apply to the description of the nature of the pain. For example, the pain associated with peptic ulcer disease has been described by such apparently contradictory terms as aching, gnawing, sharp, burning, tearing, and squeezing.

Table 14.2 Some causes of intermittent abdominal pain

Physical/obstructive
Ampullary stenosis
Cholelithiasis
Intermittent intestinal obstruction
  Intussusception
  Internal hernia
  Abdominal wall hernia

Metabolic and/or genetic
Acute intermittent porphyria
Familial Mediterannean fever

Neurological
Abdominal epilepsy
Abdominal migraine
Diabetic and other forms of radiculopathy
Nerve entrapment syndromes

Miscellaneous
Endometriosis
Heavy metal (lead) poisoning
Mesenteric ischemia
Acute recurrent pancreatitis

Table 14.3 Common causes of colicky abdominal pain

Biliary colic
Renal colic
Gastrointestinal colic
  Acute gastroenteritis
  Small bowel obstruction
  • Crohn's disease
  • Postsurgical adhesions
  • Pseudoobstruction
  • Intussusception
  Colonic obstruction
  • Carcinoma
  • Diverticulitis

Furthermore, patients often ascribe different meanings to common descriptors. As an example, many patients often associate colic with any diarrheal illness. From a medical perspective, however, the pain of colic refers to a characteristic wave-like build up in intensity culminating in severe pain often associated with other symptoms such a sweating, nausea, and dizziness [61]. The pain of colic is the result of visceral obstruction and peristaltic contractions associated with increased intralumenal pressure and is generally similar in character regardless of the organ involved (Table 14.3).

Relieving and aggravating factors

It is important to elicit the relationship if any between fluctuations in pain and physiological gastrointestinal activity.

Such a relationship may allow the physician to more confidently link the pain to a hollow viscus (rather than musculoskeletal causes) as well as point towards a specific diagnosis. Thus, pain with swallowing (odynophagia) almost invariably points to an esophageal lesion. The pain of duodenal ulcer tends to improve with food or antacid use while gastric ulcer pain may be worsened by food intake. Relief after vomiting suggests a pyloric or proximal small bowel lesion. Colonic pain or distress may be relieved by a bowel movement, particularly in patients with irritable bowel syndrome. On the other hand, anorectal conditions, such as proctitis or fissures, may be aggravated by bowel movements.

Most inflammatory conditions of the bowel or solid organs (such as inflammatory bowel disease or pancreatitis) are associated with varying degrees of systemic reaction including anorexia, malaise, and, perhaps, fever. The exception is duodenal ulcer, which may prompt the patient to increase the food intake because of the perceived association with the lessening of pain. The specific nature of the food that either relieves or aggravates pain is seldom of diagnostic value contrary to popular belief. Thus, the relationship between fatty foods and biliary pain or between spicy foods and peptic ulcer pain is dubious at best [62].

Visceral pain by itself often induces restlessness in the patient but when parietal or somatic structures become involved, aggravation by motion, coughing, or straining is characteristically noted. Retroperitoneal processes, including pancreatitis, tend to be somewhat relieved by maneuvers that increase the volume of this space (sitting up and bending forward).

Physical examination

The patient with acute abdominal pain is best dealt with as an emergency, possibly surgical in nature (see Chapter 16). As with any acute medical condition, the physical examination should first be directed at determining whether the patient is hemodynamically stable and if the patient is in need of emergency surgery. The existence of quantifiable changes in the vital signs of visceral pain (such as bradycardia in response to distention of viscus) has been recognized as far back as the turn of the century [63]. These pseudoaffective responses are objective and reproducible signs of the severity of the patient's condition, and should constitute the first part of clinical assessment of any patient with acute abdominal pain.

In patients with more chronic pain many of the same principles apply but vital signs are less likely to be disturbed. Systemic examination may provide useful clues to the diagnosis, and attention should be paid to skin lesions including purpuric rashes, pallor, jaundice, edema, and other obvious signs of a more generalized disorder (Table 14.4).

Subsequently a careful examination of the abdomen is made. It begins with inspection: note is made of surgical scars and abdominal distention. This is followed by palpation, the success of which depends on the examiner's technique as well on the patient's confidence and cooperation. It can be

Table 14.4 Clues to the etiology of abdominal pain on clinical examination

Physical finding	Related condition
Jaundice	Choledocholithiasis Gallstone pancreatitis Liver congestion or inflammation
Purpura or retinal cytoid bodies	Autoimmune process
Distended abdomen	Bowel obstruction Ascites
Palpable mass	Hernia Neoplasm
Focal neurological finding	Nerve root compression Vertebral body fracture
Anal fissure	Crohn's disease
Dark red "port-wine" urine	Acute intermittent porphyria
Occult blood in stool	Bowel inflammation Peptic ulcer disease Gastrointestinal cancer
Positive Carnett test	Abdominal wall hernia Cutaneous nerve entrapment Myofascial pain syndromes Rectus sheath hematoma Rib tip syndrome

Adapted from Zackowski [173].

very difficult to differentiate guarding and tenderness caused by peritoneal inflammation from voluntary guarding caused by the brusque contact of an examiner's cold hands. Palpation should be performed with warm hands and begin away from the area of maximal tenderness. Abdominal palpation will often identify localized masses, free peritoneal fluid such as ascites, or areas of tenderness. It can also determine if there is localized or diffuse peritoneal inflammation. Eliciting rebound tenderness, a staple of medical school teaching, is generally to be discouraged because it may not only be unreliable [64] but also, because of its painful nature, may compromise the patient's further cooperation. Auscultation of the abdomen is generally limited in utility but does provide broad clues as to the state of the bowels; in this regard it is not necessary or helpful to auscultate all four quadrants. Hypoactive or absent bowel sounds are characteristic in the presence of peritonitis whereas hyperactive sounds throughout the abdomen may be heard with infectious gastroenteritis. Infrequent, prolonged rushes of high-pitched or "tinkling" peristalsis are often heard over the distended loops of bowel seen with intestinal obstruction. Rectal examination in the male and pelvic examination in the female may occasionally reveal signs of local peritonitis in the area. The presence of occult blood in the stools may provide a clue to an intraluminal lesion such as peptic ulcer.

Acute recurrent abdominal pain, characterized by repeated attacks of pain with the patient being entirely well between these episodic bouts, can prove very difficult to diagnose. It is important to try and see the patient during an attack, as it is frequently the only opportunity for making the right diagnosis. When no obvious clinical or laboratory clues to a specific disease process are seen, the Carnett test may help to determine whether chronic intermittent abdominal pain arises from the abdominal wall or has an intraabdominal origin [65, 66]. If a tender spot is identified, the patient is asked to raise his or her head, thus tensing the abdominal musculature. If there is greater tenderness on repeat palpation, the Carnett test is positive and suggests a cause in the abdominal wall (see "Chronic abdominal wall pain"). Diminished tenderness on the other hand may suggest an intraabdominal process.

Differential diagnosis

The differential diagnosis of "abdominal pain" is of course immense. Familiarity with common gastrointestinal diseases and their natural history is a prerequisite for an accurate approach to the patient and clinical suspicion should form the basis for further laboratory and radiological testing. These diseases are dealt with in their entirety in other chapters throughout this textbook. Nevertheless, it is important to point out certain specific clues to such conditions.

Gastroduodenal pain

Gastric pain is usually felt in the midepigastric region but can also be perceived in the left upper quadrant and, occasionally, in the chest [58]. The pain of *peptic ulcer* typifies this kind of pain, which is almost always felt in the epigastric region and unlike other kinds of visceral pain, can often be sharply localized by the patient. Occasional patients with peptic ulcer cannot describe their symptom as a "pain" but rather as "an empty feeling" in the pit of the stomach or other vague descriptions of discomfort. The exact pathogenesis of ulcer pain is still debated: it may reflect direct stimulation of nerves in the ulcer bed by acid, enzymes, or bile or it may be the result of associated spasm of the underlying musculature. It is typically relieved by antacids and food and characteristically, may waken the patient up in the middle of the night.

Peptic ulcers are one cause of *dyspepsia*, which is a syndrome of epigastric pain or discomfort often accompanied by bloating and early satiety as well as other symptoms. Many conditions can cause a similar clinical picture including disorders of the pancreas, biliary tree, gastric malignancy, gastroesophageal reflux, and several medications including antibiotics. When no underlying cause is found, the term nonulcer or functional dyspepsia is used. This is dealt with extensively in Chapter 7.

Biliary pain

Biliary pain, whether arising from the gallbladder or the bile duct, generally follows the same principles of visceral pain and referral (see "Referred pain") as that arising from other organs such as the appendix. Early in its course, the pain is felt as a dull sensation in the midline (epigastrium); with the development of inflammation, or if the pain continues, it is often referred to the right upper quadrant and occasionally to the right infrascapular region. Acute obstruction of the biliary tree is almost always painful although not necessarily "colicky" in the true sense. A gradual dilation of the bile duct, as from a distal ampullary or pancreatic cancer on the other hand may remain painless throughout its course.

Pancreatic pain

Pancreatic pain is usually either the result of inflammation (acute or chronic) or caused by a neoplasm. The pain is typically felt as severe and deep in the midline, and is often associated with referred pain in the left upper quadrant. Because of the proximity of the organ to the underlying vertebral column pain can also radiate to the back. It should also be noted that peripancreatic inflammation in acute pancreatitis can often track to different locations in the abdomen, resulting in pain at sites that are remote from the original insult, such as the lower abdomen or chest.

Liver pain

Most lesions arising deep in the liver parenchyma, including tumors, are typically painless. Liver pain is usually caused by acute stretching or distortion of the liver (Glisson capsule), which can be the result of inflammation, vascular engorgement, or rapidly expanding lesions underneath the surface [58]. Chronic processes such as simple fatty liver or chronic viral hepatitis on the other hand may be entirely painless.

Splenic pain

Similar to the liver, enlargements of the spleen cause pain only when the capsule is stretched. The usual causes of splenomegaly seen in developed countries (hematological disorders and malignancies, portal hypertension) develop slowly and are usually painless. More acute causes including trauma can, however, result in pain that is felt in the left upper quadrant.

Small bowel pain

Small bowel pain is not necessarily associated with disturbances in motility and can be the result of nonobstructing lesions such as inflammation, ulcers, or neoplasms, when it is felt as a dull periumbilical or other midline discomfort that can be aggravated by food intake. Intestinal pain can also be felt occasionally in either flank or in the back [58]. A more dramatic form of small bowel pain is intestinal colic, which reflects intense muscular activity usually proximal to an obstruction but also seen in patients with acute gastro-intestinal infections. Another cause of small intestinal pain is ischemia, acute or chronic. The former type is often cata-strophic in nature but in the latter form, ischemia may give rise to the rare but classic "abdominal angina" with avoid-ance of eating because of the aggravation of pain.

Large bowel, rectal, and pelvic pain

The large bowel has dual nociceptive innervation; pain afferents, via the hypogastric nerves, run with sympathetic nerves to the spinal cord at T10–L2 as well as with the parasympathetic pelvic nerves to spinal cord S2–S4, with the latter being felt to be more important [58]. Inflammatory or neoplastic lesions of the colon can cause pain, which can be similar to small bowel pain, particularly if arising in prox-imal segments. Pain in more distal segments will be felt in the lower abdomen, reflecting its anatomical origin. Again, unless referred pain sets in or the parietal peritoneum is involved, the pain is felt as dull and in the midline. Despite the origin of the word, colic is usually not a typical manifesta-tion of obstructing lesions of the colon, as this organ is rela-tively fixed and capable of dilating significantly. However, inflammatory or infectious lesions of the colon can give rise to a similar syndrome, often described by patients as "spasms," that typically are associated with and usually relieved (at least temporarily) by bowel movements.

Rectal lesions can also cause the symptom of tenesmus, a term that signifies frequent and painful desire to evacuate the bowel that is often unfruitful and/or leaves the patient with a feeling of incomplete evacuation. In this regard it is analogous to the urinary symptom of strangury. It usually signifies proctitis (idiopathic or infectious) but can also be caused by rectal cancers or occasionally thrombosed hemor-rhoids. Another peculiar and incompletely understood rectal syndrome is that of proctalgia fugax which is a transient, but often recurrent and usually severe, ache in the rectal region that typically wakes the patient up at night.

It is important to remember that pain arising in the lower abdomen may be arising in the pelvic organs; such pain is often difficult to distinguish from colonic pain, particularly that seen in functional bowel disorders such as irritable bowel syndrome. Associated clues that should be sought in-clude disturbances in menstruation and dyspspareunia (pain-ful coitus). However, in many instances no obvious cause is found and such patients present as much of a dilemma to gynecologists as they do to gastroenterologists.

Rare and obscure causes of abdominal pain

Epigastric hernias are felt to typically occur in patients lifting heavy weights, possibly resulting in a tear in the linea alba in the midline. They can begin with protrusion of peritoneal fat (epiplocele) or abdominal wall fascia but rarely become large enough to permit entry of a hollow viscus. Although they have been associated with considerable pain, their prevalence and contribution to chronic abdominal wall syn-dromes is unclear. Spigelian hernias, between the external and internal oblique muscles, can also produce a similar pain but this is at the level of the arcuate line. When a careful history and examination and routine laboratory tests fail to reveal a cause of abdominal pain, consideration must be given to even rarer syndromes [67] (Table 14.5). These include disorders that primarily affect visceral nerves rather than the organs themselves, such as acute intermittent por-phyria, chronic poisoning with lead or arsenic, or diabetic radiculopathy. Nerve root disease is relatively common in diabetes and when it affects thoracic segments can present as abdominal pain, which can often be severe and accompanied by weight loss [68–70]. The diagnosis should be suspected in diabetics with unexplained pain that is exacerbated by spinal movement and associated with altered cutaneous sensation and localized muscle weakness. Neural imaging is required and electromyography can confirm the diagnosis. Women on oral contraceptives may experience mysterious attacks of abdominal pain that in some cases can be related to mesen-teric venous thrombosis.

Diagnostic workup

The clinical suspicions generated by a careful history and physical should lead to appropriate laboratory and imaging tests to either confirm or refute the diagnosis. However, despite the fact that acute abdominal pain is traditionally equated with a surgical diagnosis, fewer than 5% of adults presenting with acute abdominal pain will require hospital admission, and even fewer will ever need surgery [71]. Indeed, in a substantial proportion of patients with acute abdominal pain, particularly at the primary-care level and in the emergency room, no definite abdominal pathology will be found to account for the symptoms [72]. The situation with chronic abdominal pain is even worse because many of these patients have already been seen and evaluated by other physicians, with the most straightforward diagnoses having already been excluded. Indeed, in the absence of obvious clinical or laboratory clues, it is relatively unusual to uncover a new pathophysiological basis for all the symptoms in these patients [73]. Tests to exclude other diagnoses must be cau-tiously considered, depending upon the individual presenta-tion and the degree of suspicion for underlying pathology. In recent years, the availability of capsule endoscopy has prompted study of its utility in patients with unexplained abdominal pain. However, the yield is low and the findings likely to be nonspecific [74–78].

In the absence of specific indications, tests such as gastro-intestinal manometry or transit and endoscopic retrograde cholangiopancreatography are rarely helpful in the patient with chronic abdominal pain lasting longer than 6 months. [79,80]. Another example of a relatively invasive diagnostic

Table 14.5 Rare or obscure causes of abdominal pain

Condition	Characteristic features and diagnostic clues	Confirmatory tests
Shingles (varicella-zoster)	Pain may precede rash by 5–7 days Dermatomal distribution	Appearance of rash
Compressive radiculopathy	Dermatomal distribution Tenderness/pain of spinal and paraspinal structures	CT or MRI
Lead poisoning	Crampy intermittent pain Bowel disturbance and nausea Dark blue pigment along gum line Anemia and basophilic stippling	Elevated serum lead levels
Narcotic withdrawal	12–36 h after abrupt cessation Nausea, diarrhea, and cramps Excessive secretion of tears, sweat, rhinorrhea, etc. Hyperdynamic bowel sounds	History of drug intake
Familial Mediterranean fever	Childhood onset Mediterranean ancestry Peritoneal signs and fever Meningitis, pericarditis, pleuritis, and arthritis may occur	Family history Exclusion of other causes
Acute intermittent porphyria	Diffuse "colicky" abdominal pain Associated changes in mental status, muscle weakness, and photosensitivity Port-wine urine False-positive urobilinogen reading on urine dipstick (due to porphobilinogen)	
"Abdominal epilepsy" (temporal lobe seizures)	Pediatric patients Sharp abdominal pain, often periumbilical in nature Accompanied by motor, psychic, or other sensory features	EEG
"Abdominal migraine"	Pediatric patients Associated migraine Nausea and occasional vomiting	Diagnosis of exclusion
Heriditary angioneurotic edema	Submucosal edema with intestinal obstruction Cutaneous manifestations	Measurement of plasma C1 esterase activity
Abdominal vasculitides	Poorly localized pain or tenderness Gastrointestinal bleeding Associated systemic disease (Henoch–Schönlein purpura, lupus, polyarteritis nodosa, etc.)	Angiography Diagnosis of systemic disease

CT, computed tomography; EEG, electroencephalogram; MRI, magnetic resonance imaging.

test that is often contemplated is laparoscopy, particularly if a clinical suspicion of "adhesions" exists. However, the utility of this test and indeed the validity of the diagnosis of adhesions as a cause of unexplained abdominal pain are questionable at best [81]. Laparoscopy for chronic pain seldom leads to a specific diagnosis and even less often to a change in management [82]. Adhesions are very common in women, even in the absence of previous surgery [83] and are found in equal proportion in patients complaining of pelvic pain and those with other complaints [84]. In fact, randomized trials of laparoscopic adhesiolysis vs diagnostic laparoscopy alone

have not shown any benefit from the former and the complication rate is high [85,86].

If enough tests are done, there is a considerable statistical probability of uncovering some abnormalities. However, these abnormalities can be minor and of questionable relevance to the patient's complaints (e.g., minimal changes in the secondary branches of the pancreatic duct). Before acting on these abnormalities, the prudent physician must carefully reevaluate the patient, going through an extensive checklist, such as that in Table 14.6, looking for "red flags." This can often be helpful in making a decision to refer the patient to

Table 14.6 Questions to assess a patient with pain: red flags for referral to specialists in functional bowel disease

Clinical issues

Does the patient:

Have pain that has persisted for 3 months or longer?
- Despite appropriate interventions?
- In the absence of progressive diseases?

Have unrealistic expectations of
- Health-care provider?
- Treatment offered?

Complain about previous health-care providers?

Have a history of substance abuse?

Display pain behaviors?
- Grimacing
- Rigid or guarded movement

Legal and occupational issues

Is litigation pending?

Is the patient receiving disability compensation?

Was the patient employed before the onset of the pain?

Is there a job to which the patient can return?

Does the patient have a history of frequent changes in occupation?

Psychosocial issues

Do other family members also suffer from chronic pain?

Excessive depression or inappropriate moods present?

Major stressful event before onset of pain exacerbation?
- High levels of marital or family conflict?

History of childhood abuse or other sexual trauma?

Activities given up because of pain?
- Plans for renewed or increased activities if pain is reduced?

Adapted from Turk & Okifuji [174].

a more comprehensive center specializing in chronic pain evaluation and treatment.

Despite these efforts, many patients with chronic abdominal pain will be undiagnosed in community practice. There are at least two diagnoses that must then be considered.

Chronic abdominal wall pain

Pain arising primarily in the abdominal wall can result from a heterogeneous and poorly defined group of conditions whose description remains largely anecdotal (Table 14.7) [87]. However, the condition is common and associated with significant health-care costs, largely because it is so often overlooked [88]. In a recent report, chronic abdominal wall pain (CAWP) and irritable bowel syndrome comprised 7.8% and 16.3% of symptomatic referrals, respectively [89]. As with other chronic abdominal pain syndromes, CAWP predominantly affects women and depression and obesity are commonly seen. The prevalence of CAWP has been reported to range from 10% to nearly 40% in referral clinics and to make up to

1% of all general surgical diagnoses [88,90,91]. An accurate diagnosis can result in a marked decrease in physician visits and procedures with overall annual costs decreasing from around $1100 to $500 [89].

The diagnosis is suggested when the pain is superficial, localized to a small area that is usually significantly tender, associated with dysesthesia in the involved region, and when the Carnett sign (see "Physical examination") is positive. If there is an obvious scar from previous surgery or injury, a diagnosis of entrapment neuropathy (with or without a "neuroma") is often entertained. In the absence of a scar, the pain is postulated to arise from so-called "myofascial trigger points" or abdominal cutaneous nerve entrapment as the result of a fibrous ring in the rectus muscle, through which the rectus neurovascular bundle travels [92] (Fig. 14.11).

"Trigger"-point injection with local anesthetics is popularly regarded as a useful method to distinguish abdominal wall pain from that of visceral origin [93]. However, even this may be subject to flawed interpretation. As mentioned above, a characteristic of visceral pain is its referral to somatic structures including the skin and abdominal wall. In some cases, these sites can in turn become sensitized and contribute to the overall pain sensation to varying degrees (Fig. 14.6). It is conceivable that in some patients, this contribution becomes dominant and its interruption by local anesthetics is sufficient to eliminate the pain almost completely, giving rise to a false assumption about the site of pain. This may account for some of the observed inaccuracy in the predictive value of the abdominal wall tenderness test [94]. Nevertheless, clinical experience suggests that the diagnosis of CAWP using a combination of clinical findings and the response to local anesthetic is surprisingly robust and does not change in 90%–97% of patients over the long term [89,95].

Local neural blockade has been reported to be more successful in patients with chronic pain secondary to abdominal wall causes [87,96]. Once a trigger point has been identified by digital examination, the needle is inserted and a small amount of local anesthetic along with a corticosteroid (typically bupivacaine and triamcinolone) is injected at the site of greatest tenderness elicited by the tip of the needle. The response is surprisingly long-lasting and up to two-thirds of patients do not require another injection [88]. For those whose relief is temporary, repeat injections may be necessary. More ablative chemicals, e.g., phenol, are best left to the anesthesiologist to administer.

Functional abdominal pain syndrome

Patients whose chronic abdominal pain remains unexplained despite a careful and detailed evaluation represent a significant clinical challenge to gastroenterologists who often become the de facto caretakers of these patients. In recent years, it has become evident that these patients as a group share enough common features to warrant consideration of a distinct syndrome, the functional abdominal pain syndrome (FAPS) [97]

Table 14.7 Etiology of abdominal wall pain

Etiology	Comments	Diagnosis
Hernia	Protuberance in abdominal wall that usually decreases in size when patient is supine	Abdominal CT scanning, abdominal ultrasonography, herniography
Rectus nerve entrapment	Occurs along lateral edge of rectus sheath; worsening of pain with tensing of muscles	Injection of local anesthetic
Thoracic lateral cutaneous nerve entrapment	Occurs spontaneously, after surgery or during pregnancy	History and physical examination
Ilioinguinal and iliohypogastric nerve entrapment	Lower abdominal pain that occurs after inguinal hernia repair	History and physical examination
Endometriosis	Cyclic abdominal pain	Laparoscopy
Diabetic radiculopathy	Acute, severe truncal pain involving T6–T12 nerve roots	Paraspinal EMG
Abdominal wall tear	Occurs mainly in athletes	History and physical examination
Abdominal wall hematoma	Complication of abdominal laparoscopic procedures	Abdominal CT scanning, abdominal ultrasonography
Spontaneous rectus sheath hematoma	Presents as tender, usually unilateral mass that does not extend beyond midline	Abdominal CT scanning, abdominal ultrasonography
Desmoid tumor	Dysplastic tumor of connective tissue; occurs in young patients (females more often than males)	Surgical excision
Herpes zoster	Pain and hyperesthesia followed by vesicles along a dermatome	History and physical examination
Spinal nerve irritation	Caused by disorders of thoracic spine	CT scanning or MRI studies of thoracic spine
Slipping rib syndrome	Sharp, stabbing pain in upper abdomen caused by luxation of 8th to 10th ribs	Hooking maneuver to pull lower ribs anteriorly, which reproduces the pain and sometimes a click
Idiopathic	Myofascial pain	History and physical examination

CT, computed tomography; EMG, electromyography; MRI, magnetic resonance imaging.
From Suleiman & Johnston [87], with permission from the American Academy of Family Physicians.

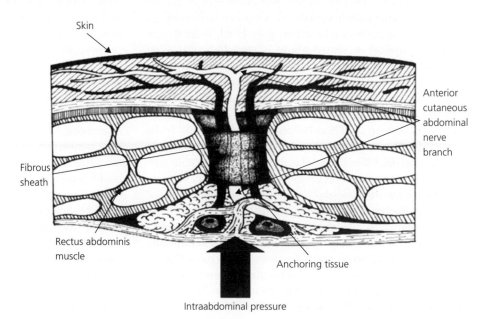

Figure 14.11 Schematized course of the anterior cutaneous nerve in the abdominal wall. Note the theoretical vulnerability to pressure-induced injury and hence generation of neuropathic pain. From Greenbaum [88].

Table 14.8 Diagnostic criteria for functional abdominal pain syndrome

At least 6 months of
- Continuous or nearly continuous abdominal pain
- No or only occasional relationship of pain with physiological events (e.g., eating, defecation, or menses); *and*
- Some loss of daily functioning; *and*
- The pain is not feigned (e.g., malingering); *and*
- Insufficient criteria for other functional gastrointestinal disorders that would explain the abdominal pain

(Table 14.8). It is not synonymous with other functional bowel disorders, which also feature pain, such as irritable bowel syndrome. The distinction is based upon the lack of association with physiological gastrointestinal events such as eating or defecation.

FAPS is relatively uncommon when compared to typical irritable bowel syndrome: in a survey of US householders, it was found in only about 2% of respondents and appeared to increase with age, with women accounting for more than two-thirds of the patients [98]. Nevertheless, patients with FAPS are heavy users of medical resources with a high morbidity [99].

FAPS is a poorly understood and poorly investigated disorder. Theories about its etiopathogenesis are speculative at best. The responsiveness to tricyclic antidepressants has been said to indicate an underlying neuropathic process [97]. On the other hand, patients with FAPS have many psychological disturbances and personality disorders and are often functionally impaired at many levels including work, family, and social settings [100]. They frequently suffer from depression, anxiety, sleep disturbances, withdrawal, decreased activity, fatigue, loss of libido, and morbid preoccupation with the chronic pain [101–103]. Many of these patients have experienced abdominal pain in childhood, and often have relatives with a past or present abdominal pain [100]. A history of previous physical or sexual abuse is very frequent, being reported in as much as one-half of these patients in some series [104]. The onset of pain may also be associated with the demise of a relative, spouse, or other important figure [99].

Based on the Diagnostic and Statistical Manual of Mental Disorders, version IV (DSM-IV) criteria, patients with FAPS qualify for the diagnosis of pain disorder, a subgroup of somatoform disorder (physical complaints for which no adequate medical explanation exists). However, it may be more helpful to view this disorder in terms of the biopsychosocial paradigm discussed previously in this chapter. In this context, the dominant disturbance contributing to the patient's clinical presentation may lie anywhere in this continuum, from heightened nociception to illness behavior. Thus if patients with chronic painful pancreatitis represent an example of a disturbance primarily (but not exclusively) affecting nociceptive signaling, then patients with FAPS can be viewed

as representing a dysfunction of perception, coping or response strategies. Pain may serve many functions in these patients including a means of atonement, derailment of success and a morbid replacement for loss of relationships. Finally, it is possible that because of positive reinforcement, actions that mitigate pain, such as decreasing physical activity or the use of medications, will often continue even after the inciting event (e.g., the acute pain symptom) is resolved. At the same time, other behaviors (e.g., appearing uncomfortable and helpless, not reporting for work) may be reinforced by many of the outcomes that result from the gains the patient may feel he or she is obtaining. These may include increased or renewed attention and empathy from within the family structure, avoidance of the stresses associated with work and family responsibilities, and monetary compensation. Thus, in susceptible individuals, a set of behaviors becomes established that contributes to the maintenance of chronic pain.

FAPS is associated with a characteristic set of behavioral accompaniments. Chronic abdominal pain may occur in bouts lasting from several hours to days or weeks, but even between severe exacerbations, there is residual pain, albeit not as severe or incapacitating. The abdominal pain is often described in vague terms, sometimes through unusual, idiosyncratic or even bizarre language. The pain itself is always or almost always present and is relatively unchanging in character, intensity, and location [99]. Other forms of chronic pain, i.e., those related to a specific pathological diagnosis, usually occur with particular physiological activities (e.g., eating or defecation) and with consistent accompanying gastrointestinal symptoms in addition to pain. Lack of weight loss in the absence of significant depression and lack of fever also suggest FAPS. Although nocturnal pain is often assumed to be "organic", functional pain may also sometimes awaken patients from their sleep [105]. In addition to chronic abdominal pain, pain in locations other than the abdomen is common, as are various somatic complaints [106,107].

Physical examination provides many pointers to this diagnosis but is not by itself conclusive. Suggestive clues include absence of autonomic activation (e.g., tachycardia, diaphoresis), inconsistent tenderness, discrepancy between tenderness elicited with pressure from the stethoscope and that from the examining hand, clutching of the physician's arm during the examination and the "closed eyes sign" (characterized by the patient keeping his or her eyes closed, often with a fixed, beatific smile, during abdominal palpation [108]). Other clues at the time of the interview may provide insight into social impairments contributing to the clinical presentation. These include the constant presence of a spouse or parent who assumes the responsibility as a "go-between" for the physician and the patient, suggesting family "enmeshment" that may be contributing to the illness behavior.

If not established through the initial series of investigations, a gastrointestinal cause for the symptoms is rarely found through subsequent investigations (including surgical exploration) or follow-up visits [107, 109]. Nevertheless, for a variety of reasons, including demands by the patients and their families, physicians often feel compelled to embark on an ever more invasive and expensive series of tests in the hope of uncovering the magical but elusive explanation for the patient's symptoms. Such activity ("furor medicus" [110]) in fact may be counterproductive because it reinforces the patient's conviction that there is something wrong to account for the pain that, if only it were found, could be successfully corrected. Often, when a "cause" is discovered, it is not clear whether it is truly the source of the pain, an incidental finding/epiphenomenonon, or a consequence of the treatment, often surgical, used in an attempt to treat the original complaint [111]. In most of these cases the presumed cause of pain will have been diagnosed and treated, only for the pain to remain, or for a new type of pain to manifest itself elsewhere.

Patients with chronic intractable abdominal pain are rarely substantially pain free after one or more years of follow-up [99], emphasizing the importance of focusing on adaptation to the pain rather than cure. Given our current state of knowledge about this syndrome, it is unrealistic to talk about a cure for FAPS. Palliation is therefore an appropriate goal and in most patients it is achievable. In general, the therapeutic approach to FAPS is similar to the multifactorial approach to other forms of chronic pain described below, with greater emphasis on the psychosocial dimensions.

Approach to the treatment of abdominal pain

Whenever possible, healing of the underlying tissue insult or injury provides the most satisfactory approach to the control of pain. This is discussed in the respective chapters of this book dealing with specific painful conditions. In a significant number of patients with pain of suspected gastrointestinal origin, however, the underlying condition may not be reversible or even identifiable. Pain management then often becomes the primary therapeutic issue and it is critical for the practicing gastroenterologist to become familiar with the general principles of pain management in such patients, as outlined in this section. Although several of these principles also apply to patients with cancer-related pain, physicians in the oncological specialties usually manage these patients and this subject will not be discussed here.

The therapeutic approach to acute severe abdominal pain is reasonably straightforward. Once the need for immediate surgical exploration is ruled out, and a confident working diagnosis is made, attention is quickly turned towards effective pain relief, typically in the form of potent opiate drugs such as morphine (5–10 mg) or the equivalent dose of meperidine. At the same time, specific therapy, if available, is directed towards the suspected underlying cause. Although

analgesics are often withheld in patients with acute abdominal pain for fear of "masking" the diagnosis, this concern has not been validated by any scientific studies and probably dates to the era when high doses of morphine (30 mg or more) were used [112]. When a nonoperative diagnosis is made, arrangements for ongoing pain relief should be made. Although intermittent use of narcotics (either pro re nata or at fixed intervals) is commonly practiced, inadequate dosing or frequency can lead to unnecessary patient discomfort. This is particularly liable to occur when a prolonged duration of recovery (several days to weeks) is expected, such as in patients with severe acute pancreatitis. In such settings, narcotics are best administered using patient-controlled devices.

Patients with chronic abdominal pain present a far greater challenge. For the uninitiated physician, it is tempting to reach for the prescription pad at the conclusion of a visit with such a patient. While pharmacological therapy has a valuable role in these patients, it is also clear that a successful outcome requires taking into consideration several, equally important, factors. As explained previously, chronic pain cannot be viewed as a purely neurophysiological phenomenon and has many other facets, the most important of which is the psychological dimension, consisting of cognitive, emotional, and behavioral processes. The combination of these factors results in functional disability, a third dimension of chronic pain that is often ignored.

The multifactorial and complex nature of chronic pain has made it clear that no single set of skills or techniques can address all the issues that affect the quality of life in most patients. These different dimensions require a multidisciplinary approach, requiring the help of pain-management physicians (internists, anesthesiologists, neurologists, or neurosurgeons), clinical psychologists, nurses, and, often, vocational rehabilitation specialists and nutritionists. The therapeutic interventions available are correspondingly diverse, including exercise programs, cognitive and behavioral therapies, traditional pharmacological agents, alternative therapies, and nerve blocking/ablation techniques, to mention a few. These should be applied either sequentially or in parallel, as part of a pain-management continuum, beginning with the most innocuous and progressing to more invasive strategies. It is important for the gastroenterology physician to broadly understand the entire spectrum of chronic pain management; such an understanding will facilitate appropriate referral to other specialists, promote a more meaningful interaction with them, and maintain a strong and supportive patient–physician relationship instead of leading to feelings of abandonment and other negative attitudes. Since a large number of patients may have chronic abdominal pain or functional bowel syndromes, it is very important for the practicing gastroenterologist to understand the interaction between psychosocial factors and disease in producing gastrointestinal symptoms and illness-related behavior. In this regard, it is necessary to acquire a working knowledge of the concepts and terminology employed by clinical psychologists and psychiatrists. Several of these are discussed in other chapters in this book.

Pharmacological management of chronic pain

Although effective analgesia remains the foremost goal in the pharmacological approach to patients with chronic pain, it must be remembered that there is also a valuable role for drugs in the treatment of concomitant anxiety, depression, and insomnia, a discussion of which can be found in more specialized texts.

Nonsteroidal antiinflammatory drugs and opiates

Gastroenterologists are loath to use traditional nonsteroidal antiinflammatory drugs (NSAIDs), for fear of inducing gastro-intestinal side effects as well as the general feeling that they are less effective in the treatment of chronic abdominal pain than in the relief of acute pain [113]. Indeed, when mild chronic pain necessitates analgesic use, these drugs are often bypassed in favor of the weak opioids propoxyphene or codeine. However, neither of these drugs is very effective compared to NSAIDs; codeine has a number needed to treat (NNT) of around 17, i.e., only an additional 1 in 17 patients experience pain relief after a 60-mg dose, compared to placebo [114]. However, the efficacy may be enhanced to an NNT of 5 by the addition of acetaminophen compared to acetaminophen alone.

The principles of opioid use in patients with visceral pain have recently been reviewed [115]. More severe pain requires stronger analgesics such as morphine, methadone, or trans-dermal fentanyl. Opioids are thought to be more effective in nociceptive pain (see "Classification of abdominal pain") than in neuropathic pain, which may require considerably higher doses. Meperidine is generally felt to be the drug of choice for patients with pancreatitis because of its lesser tendency to cause sphincter of Oddi spasm; however, this has only been shown to be true at subanalgesic doses [116,117]. Because it is more likely to produce other side effects, it is seldom used for chronic pain management. Opioid analgesics share a common adverse-effect profile in general: constipation, nausea, sedation, and respiratory depression. However, the problem most physicians fear with the use of narcotic analgesics is the potential for addiction. This has led to fairly widespread perceptions regarding the patient with chronic pain with suspicion and as among the "most frequently encountered serious user and abuser of psychoactive drugs and opioids" [118]. Coupled with the fact that the efficacy of these drugs in the management of even relatively well-defined chronic somatic pain syndromes is still a matter of controversy, this makes most physicians shy away from their use in these settings. This may be particularly appropriate in patients with functional abdominal pain syndromes. In other cases, such as with chronic painful pancreatitis, these drugs can and should be used judiciously, following fairly

Table 14.9 Guidelines for narcotic use in patients with chronic noncancer pain

1 Clear understanding that opioids are being used for a limited term in the first instance
2 Only one practitioner takes responsibility for opioid prescription
3 Opioid prescription is contingent on certain agreed obligations or goals being met by the patient, e.g., return to work or alteration of inappropriate behaviors. This could take the form of a written contractual arrangement
4 Unauthorized demands for emergency injectable opioids will not be tolerated although some provision can be made for "rescue analgesia" for brief exacerbations of pain
5 The patient understands that opioid dosage compliance will be checked at various random intervals, which may include drug screens and blood samples
6 Physicians must be prepared to terminate the arrangement if the goals are not met or if there is evidence of misuse, even though this may lead to a confrontational meeting with the patient

Derived from Gourlay [175].

rigid guidelines or protocols for narcotic use (Table 14.9). Patient selection remains of paramount importance; the physician must be convinced that there is sufficient evidence for an ongoing nociceptive component and that there is reasonable psychological stability.

Antidepressants

As a class of agents, these are perhaps the most useful drugs for the management of both somatic and gastrointestinal pain syndromes [119]. However, although their usefulness in pain management was first suggested nearly half-a-century ago, these drugs have not been fully embraced by either gastroenterologists or their patients. The latter are often fearful of being stigmatized as having "mental" problems, a misperception that is perpetuated if a clear rationale for their use is not presented by the prescribing physician. The issue if of course confounded by the fact that these patients may also suffer from depression, anxiety, and disturbances of sleep, which are common, but in most patients secondary, accompaniments of any chronic pain syndrome. Effective analgesic doses of these drugs are significantly lower than those required to treat depression and there is reasonable evidence to conclude that the beneficial effects of antidepressants on pain occur independently of changes in mood [120]. In this regard, diminution of anxiety and restoration of mood and sleep patterns should be considered desirable even if they represent primary neuropsychiatric effects of the drug.

From a mechanistic perspective, the common theme shared by these drugs is their ability to modulate central nervous system monoamine (principally serotonin and norepine-phrine) neurotransmitter levels. These are important in mediating central inhibitory pathways (Fig. 14.3); however, peripheral mechanisms may also contribute [121]. Most of these drugs act on the presynaptic pump, inhibiting the uptake of the neurotransmitters and hence increasing their availability in the synaptic cleft. Studies on human volunteers suggest that these drugs affect the threshold for somatic but not visceral pain [122], suggesting perhaps that their target(s) may be peculiar to the sensitized state.

Tricyclic agents ushered in the modern antidepressant era and although they are no longer the preferred agents for depression, they continue to have the most proven track record in the management of chronic pain, both of somatic and visceral origin. A recent meta-analysis of antidepressant treatment for functional gastrointestinal disorders concluded that these agents were quite effective, with an NNT of 3.2 (i.e., three patients needing treatment for one patient to experience symptom improvement) and a relatively large improvement in pain (about 0.9 standard deviations) [123]. Gastroenterologists therefore should become familiar with the pharmacology and therapeutic use of one or more of these agents. They are well absorbed after oral administration, undergo extensive first-pass hepatic metabolism with long elimination half-lives (measured in days and weeks) and have active metabolites, some of which are also marketed as drugs. In addition to the putative analgesic effects on monoamine uptake, several of the older agents have anticholinergic (muscarinic) and antihistaminic (both H_1 and H_2) properties that contribute to their side effect profile. Other serious side effects include cardiac conduction problems including a prolonged QT interval and dysrhythmia.

Selective serotonin reuptake inhibitors (SSRIs), such as paroxetine, sertraline, and fluoxetine, which are currently the mainstay in the treatment of depression, have fewer side effects and have been advocated particularly for patients with functional constipation because they can increase bowel movements and even cause diarrhea. However, they have been less well evaluated in the management of pain than tricyclic antidepressants; the somatic pain literature suggests that the efficacy of these agents for chronic pain is equivocal at best [124]. A randomized trial of paroxetine in patients with irritable bowel syndrome showed no effect on abdominal pain, although overall wellbeing was improved [125]. Similarly, fluoexitine does not appear to affect colorectal sensitivity [126]. However, recent studies suggest that citalopram may be effective in relieving pain in patients with irritable bowel syndrome as well as have acute effects on esophageal sensitivity [127,128]. Newer antidepressants may also have promise in this regard [124]. These include the serotonin/norepinephrine reuptake inhibitors (SNRIs) such as venlafaxine, which inhibits the uptake of both norepinephrine and serotonin almost equally and also has additional inhibitory effects on dopamine and the $5-HT_2$ receptor.

It has been shown to attenuate the pain response to colorectal distention in healthy volunteers [129]. Initial reports from the somatic pain literature also suggest a possible analgesic role for tetracyclic compounds such as maprotiline and mirtazepine with a greater effect on the uptake of norepinephrine compared with serotonin (mirtazepine also has several postsynaptic effects including $5-HT_2$, $5-HT_3$, α_2, and H_1). Other agents being evaluated include the triazolopyridines such as nefazadone, which not only selectively inhibits serotonin uptake but also has significant postsynaptic effects on the $5-HT_{2A}$ receptor and perhaps the α_1 receptor [130–133]. An older agent in the same class, trazadone, has been used with good effect in patients with noncardiac chest pain [134]; although it does not have the usual side effects of the tricyclic antidepressants, it is more sedating and can cause priapism in males.

Before beginning antidepressants it is important to assess the psychological profile of the patient, as this may be important in determining the choice of therapy. If the patient is depressed then it may be more appropriate to use full antidepressant doses of a drug that also has analgesic properties. This could be either a tricyclic antidepressant with a low side effect profile or perhaps one of the newer agents discussed above (not an SSRI). If the patient is already on an antidepressant but this does not have proven analgesic activity (such as an SSRI), consideration should be given to switching to one that does.

If the patient is not depressed, it is critical to spend some time explaining the scientific rationale for the use of antidepressants, with an attempt to clearly separate the analgesic effects from the antidepressant ones. The most appropriate agent to start with in this setting is one of the tricyclic anti depressants. A typical regimen would start with 25 mg amitryptyline or nortryptyline (an even lower dose such as 10 mg may be considered in the elderly patient). This is given at night and will almost immediately begin helping the disturbed sleep patterns that often accompany chronic pain. Daytime sedation may occur but tolerance develops rapidly. Tolerance to the antimuscarinic effects may take longer and it is important to advise the patients about this. In the absence of significant side effects, the dose of the antidepressant is gradually increased until adequate benefit is achieved or the upper limit of the recommended dose is reached. It is also important to tell the patient that the analgesic effect may take several days to weeks to develop and that unlike conventional analgesics, the drug is not to be taken on a pro re nata basis but on a fixed schedule. A trial of at least 4–6 weeks at a stable maximum dose is recommended before discontinuation. If a particular tricyclic antidepressant is clearly not found to be effective under these circumstances, one may consider switching to another class of antidepressants such as nefazadone, mirtazepine, or venlafaxine. Venflaxine may also be substituted for a tricyclic antidepressant if excessive sedation is observed with the latter.

Other neuropsychiatric drugs

Unlike the antidepressants, the use of neuroleptics in chronic pain management is controversial, with equivocal evidence of efficacy and the lack of a clear biological rationale [118]. Their use is further tempered by the risk of significant adverse extrapyramidal effects related to nigrostriatal dopamine blockade. The most experience with these drugs, particularly fluphenazine and haloperidol, has been in neuropathic pain syndromes and there is little if any literature on which to base their use in patients with chronic abdominal pain. Because of the risk of side effects, these drugs should only be considered if antidepressants have failed; they should be begun at low dosages (e.g., 1 mg fluphenazine) with careful monitoring for neurological effects. A variety of antiepileptic drugs with neuronal stabilizing properties (phenytoin, carmazepine, gabapentin, pregabalin), or γ-aminobutyric acid-enhancing properties (clonazepam, valproic acid) have found some utility in somatic pain syndromes, particularly of the neuropathic variety [135,136]. In this regard the N-type calcium-ion channel blockers, gabapentin and pregabalin show particular promise and early studies suggest a specific effect on hypersensitivity in both animal studies and patients with irritable bowel syndrome [137–141].

Finally, mention must be made of the use of benzodiazepines, which are frequently used by patients with chronic pain including insomnia, anxiety, and muscle spasm. While useful in these settings for short-term use, there is a significant risk for dependence on these drugs and there is little if any evidence that they have any real analgesic effect.

The somatostatin analogue octreotide has been reported to attenuate visceral sensitivity but is probably not very practical to use because of costs and need for multiple injections [142–145]. Other drugs that have shown reasonable efficacy in patients with neuropathic pain include clonidine, an α_2-adrenergic agonist with some efficacy in diarrhea-predominant irritable bowel syndrome [146], baclofen (a γ-aminobutyric acid B receptor agonist) and the NMDA receptor antagonists, ketamine and dextromethorphan [147–152]. Although the rationale for the use of these drugs is appealing (see discussion earlier in this chapter), their use in gastrointestinal pain disorders is limited by gastroenterologists' lack of familiarity, inadequate or no controlled studies, and side effects.

Neural blockade and neuorolytic therapy

Theoretically, interruption of the pain pathways should provide relief of pain that is peripheral in origin. This has led to the development of various techniques, both for diagnostic and therapeutic purposes. The rationale for the diagnostic use of neural blockade in a given patient is based on several assumptions [153], the most important of which are:

• that pain impulses arise from injury in a peripheral location and subsequently travel along well-defined nerves

• that interruption of this pathway (either temporarily or permanently) completely abolishes the sensory function of these nerves.

However, these assumptions have several limitations, leading to difficulty in the universal endorsement of such techniques in patients with chronic abdominal pain. Thus, functional or anatomical interruption of the peripheral ends of the nociceptive nerves may not relieve pain if impulses continue to be generated at the proximal end including the dorsal root ganglia. Furthermore, the relative contribution of central (i.e., spinal and higher centers) vs peripheral sensitization in chronic visceral pain syndromes, particularly of the "functional" type, is not known. Conceivably, central sensitization could lead to continuous pain signaling in the absence of peripheral input. Alternatively, if interruption of peripheral input is incomplete, altered spinal processing of nonnociceptive fiber input will continue to cause allodynic pain. Variability in these biological factors, combined with inconsistencies in blockade techniques may be one explanation why for instance, celiac plexus blocks may work for pain arising from pancreatic cancer but are generally ineffective in patients with chronic pancreatitis.

Despite these limitations, it is clear that neurolytic techniques are valuable for certain subsets of patients, particularly with cancer where celiac neurolysis may be effective for up to 85% of patients with pancreatic cancer pain and in about 70% of patients with pain from nonpancreatic cancers [154]. By contrast, pain relief in nonneoplastic pain such as chronic pancreatitis is not routinely recommended because of low efficacy (50% or less) and the short duration of relief (around 2 months) even in those patients that initially respond [155].

Nonconventional methods of treating chronic abdominal pain

Indwelling epidural and intrathecal access systems have been effectively used for some patients with intractable chronic pain and have been used to deliver opiates and other drugs such as clonidine and baclofen [156]. A variety of electrical stimulation techniques, including peripheral (transcutaneous electrical nerve stimulation or TENS), spinal, and cerebral stimulations, have been used for various somatic pain conditions as well as for angina pectoris with encouraging results [157]. This has also been shown to decrease esophageal pain sensitivity [158]. Spinal cord electrical stimulation via implantable electrodes is a recent technique with some promise in refractory visceral pain syndromes including chronic pancreatitis [159–162]. The underlying rationale for these techniques is based on the original "gate theory" of Melzack and Wall. According to this, the pain gate in the spinal cord is closed in the presence of large afferent fiber activity invoked by electrical stimulation of the nerve, root, or cord. Although γ-aminobutyric acid and serotonin may be involved as neuromediators, the effects of electrical stimulation do not rely on endogenous opioids [163]. Much more clinical experience in visceral pain is required before these techniques can be generally endorsed.

Acupressure and acupuncture (electrical or conventional) are alternative medicine techniques that have been widely used for somatic pain, with results that are mixed. It has been postulated that these techniques invoke supraspinal mechanisms of inhibition [164–166]. There is limited clinical information on this technique in patients with irritable bowel syndrome and other functional gastrointestinal disorders [167–169].

Conclusions

The diagnosis and management of abdominal pain, particularly when chronic, is one of the most challenging clinical problems faced by gastroenterologists. Significant progress has been made in our understanding of the pathogenesis of somatic sensitization and it is hoped that this will lead to similar advances in visceral pain. While there is a clear role for pharmacotherapy, the successful management of pain requires an intensely engaged physician who can interpret this symptom along with the psychosocial context of the patient.

References

1. Sandler RS, Stewart WF, Liberman JN, et al. Abdominal pain, bloating, and diarrhea in the United States: prevalence and impact. Dig Dis Sci 2000;45:1166.
2. Shaheen NJ, Hansen RA, Morgan DR, et al. The burden of gastrointestinal and liver diseases, 2006. Am J Gastroenterol 2006;101:2128.
3. Sheridan WG, White AT, Havard T, Crosby DL. Non-specific abdominal pain: the resource implications. Ann R Coll Surg Engl 1992;74:181.
4. Nyrop KA, Palsson OS, Levy RL, et al. Costs of health care for irritable bowel syndrome, chronic constipation, functional diarrhoea and functional abdominal pain. Aliment Pharmacol Ther 2007;26:237.
5. Halder SLS, Locke III GR. Epidemiology and socioeconomic impact of visceral and abdominal pain syndromes. In: Pasricha PJ, Willis WD, Gebhart GF (eds). Chronic Abdominal and Visceral Pain: Theory and Practice, 1st edn. New York: Informa 2007:11.
6. Spiegel B, Schoenfeld P, Naliboff B. Systematic review: the prevalence of suicidal behaviour in patients with chronic abdominal pain and irritable bowel syndrome. Aliment Pharmacol Ther 2007;26:183.
7. Willis WJ. Visceral inputs to sensory pathways in the spinal cord. In: Cervero F, JFB M, eds. Visceral Sensation. Amsterdam: Elsevier 1986:207.
8. Willis W, Al-Chaer E, Quast M, Westlund K. A visceral pain pathway in the dorsal column of the spinal cord. Proc Natl Acad Sci USA 1999;96:7675.
9. Palecek J. The role of dorsal columns pathway in visceral pain. Physiol Res 2004;53(Suppl. 1):S125.
10. Al-Chaer ED, Feng Y, Willis WD. A role for the dorsal column in nociceptive visceral input into the thalamus of primates. J Neurophysiol 1998;79:3143.
11. Strigo IA, Duncan GH, Bushnell MC, et al. The effects of racemic ketamine on painful stimulation of skin and viscera in human subjects. Pain 2005;113:255.
12. Craig AD. Pain mechanisms: labeled lines versus convergence in central processing. Annu Rev Neurosci 2003;26:1.
13. Price D. Psychological and neural mechanisms of the affective dimension of pain. Science 2000;288:1769.
14. Mayer EA, Naliboff BD, Craig AD. Neuroimaging of the brain–gut axis: from basic understanding to treatment of functional GI disorders. Gastroenterology 2006;131:1925.
15. Willis W, Westlund K. Neuroanatomy of the pain system and the pathways that modulate pain. J Clin Neurophysiol 1997;14:2.
16. Loeser JD. Pain and suffering. Clin J Pain 2000;16(2 Suppl.):S2.
17. Turk DC, Okifuji A. Does sex make a difference in the prescription of treatments and the adaptation to chronic pain by cancer and non-cancer patients? Pain 1999;82:139.
18. Levy RL, Olden KW, Naliboff BD, et al. Psychosocial aspects of the functional gastrointestinal disorders. Gastroenterology 2006;130:1447.
19. Al-Chaer ED, Willis WD. Neuroanatomy of visceral pain: pathways and processes. In: Pasricha PJ, Willis WD, Gebhart GF (eds). Chronic Abdominal and Visceral Pain: Theory and Practice, 1st edn. New York: Informa, 2007:33.
20. Brierly SM, Blackshaw LA. The neurobiology of visceral nociceptors. In: Pasricha PJ, Willis WD, Gebhart GF (eds). Chronic Abdominal and Visceral Pain: Theory and Practice, 1st edn. New York and London: Informa healthcare 2007:45.
21. Ma W, Quirion R. Inflammatory mediators modulating the transient receptor potential vanilloid 1 receptor: therapeutic targets to treat inflammatory and neuropathic pain. Expert Opin Ther Targets 2007;11:307.
22. Pingle SC, Matta JA, Ahern GP. Capsaicin receptor: TRPV1 a promiscuous TRP channel. Handb Exp Pharmacol 2007;179:155.
23. Szallasi A, Cortright DN, Blum CA, Eid SR. The vanilloid receptor TRPV1: 10 years from channel cloning to antagonist proof-of-concept. Nat Rev Drug Discov 2007;6:357.
24. Bielefeldt K. Neurochemical and molecular basis of peripheral sensitization. In: Pasricha PJ, Willis WD, Gebhart GF (eds). Chronic Abdominal and Visceral Pain: Theory and Practice, 1st edn. New York: Informa 2007:67.
25. Woolf CJ, Salter MW. Neuronal plasticity: increasing the gain in pain. Science 2000;288:1765.
26. Zeilhofer HU. The glycinergic control of spinal pain processing. Cell Mol Life Sci 2005;62:2027.
27. Enna SJ, McCarson KE. The role of GABA in the mediation and perception of pain. Adv Pharmacol 2006;54:1.
28. Kirsch J. Glycinergic transmission. Cell Tissue Res 2006;326:535.
29. Sommer C. Is serotonin hyperalgesic or analgesic? Curr Pain Headache Rep 2006;10:101.
30. Pertovaara A. Noradrenergic pain modulation. Prog Neurobiol 2006;80:53.
31. Ness TJ. Distinctive clinical and biological characteristics of visceral pain. In: Pasricha PJ, Willis WD, Gebhart GF (eds). Chronic Abdominal and Visceral Pain: Theory and Practice, 1st edn. New York: Informa 2007:1.
32. Strigo IA, Bushnell MC, Boivin M, Duncan GH. Psychophysical analysis of visceral and cutaneous pain in human subjects. Pain 2002;97:235.
33. Raj P. Visceral pain. In: Raj P (ed.). Practical Management of Pain. St Louis: Mosby 2000:145.
34. Giamberardino MA, Cervero F. The neural basis of referred visceral pain. In: Pasricha PJ, Willis WD, Gebhart GF (eds). Chronic Abdominal and Visceral Pain: Theory and Practice, 1st edn. New York: Informa 2007:177.
35. Christianson JA, Liang R, Ustinova EE, et al. Convergence of bladder and colon sensory innervation occurs at the primary afferent level. Pain 2007;128:235–43.
36. Giamberardino MA, Affaitati G, Lerza R, et al. Evaluation of indices of skeletal muscle contraction in areas of referred hyperalgesia from an artificial ureteric stone in rats. Neurosci Lett 2003;338:213.
37. Giamberardino MA, Dalal A, Valente R, Vecchiet L. Changes in activity of spinal cells with muscular input in rats with referred

muscular hyperalgesia from ureteral calculosis. Neurosci Lett 1996; 203:89.

38. Cervero F, Laird JM. Visceral pain. Lancet 1999;353(9190):2145.

39. Dray A. Inflammatory mediators of pain. Br J Anaesth 1995;75: 125.

40. Yiangou Y, Facer P, Dyer NH, et al. Vanilloid receptor 1 immunoreactivity in inflamed human bowel. Lancet 2001;357:1338.

41. Chan CL, Facer P, Davis JB, et al. Sensory fibres expressing capsaicin receptor TRPV1 in patients with rectal hypersensitivity and faecal urgency. Lancet 2003;361:385.

42. Matthews PJ, Aziz Q, Facer P, et al. Increased capsaicin receptor TRPV1 nerve fibres in the inflamed human oesophagus. Eur J Gastroenterol Hepatol 2004;16:897.

43. Buchler M, Weihe E, Friess H, et al. Changes in peptidergic innervation in chronic pancreatitis. Pancreas 1992;7:183.

44. Shrikhande SV, Friess H, di Mola FF, et al. NK-1 receptor gene expression is related to pain in chronic pancreatitis. Pain 2001; 91:209.

45. Chung N, Cho SY, Choi DH, et al. STATT: a titrate-to-goal study of simvastatin in Asian patients with coronary heart disease. Simvastatin treats Asians to target. Clin Ther 2001;23:858.

46. Friess H, Zhu Z, di Mola F, et al. Nerve growth factor and its high-affinity receptor in chronic pancreatitis. Ann Surg 1999;230:215.

47. Cervero F. Visceral pain: mechanisms of peripheral and central sensitization. Ann Med 1995;27:235.

48. Camilleri M, Ford MJ. Review article: colonic sensorimotor physiology in health, and its alteration in constipation and diarrhoeal disorders. Aliment Pharmacol Ther 1998;12:287.

49. Rhodes DY, Wallace M. Post-infectious irritable bowel syndrome. Curr Gastroenterol Rep 2006;8:327.

50. Naliboff BD, Mayer EA. Brain imaging in IBS: drawing the line between cognitive and non-cognitive processes. Gastroenterology 2006;130:267.

51. Coutinho SV, Plotsky PM, Sablad M, et al. Neonatal maternal separation alters stress-induced responses to viscerosomatic nociceptive stimuli in rat. Am J Physiol Gastrointest Liver Physiol 2002;282:G307.

52. Mayer EA, Naliboff BD, Chang L, Coutinho SV. V. Stress and irritable bowel syndrome. Am J Physiol Gastrointest Liver Physiol 2001;280:G519.

53. Tache Y, Perdue MH. Role of peripheral CRF signalling pathways in stress-related alterations of gut motility and mucosal function. Neurogastroenterol Motil 2004;16 Suppl. 1:137.

54. Fukudo S, Saito K, Sagami Y, Kanazawa M. Can modulating corticotropin releasing hormone receptors alter visceral sensitivity? Gut 2006;55:146.

55. Tache Y, Million M. Stress, visceral pain and the brain–gut connections. In: Pasricha PJ, Willis WD, Gebhart GF (eds). Chronic Abdominal and Visceral Pain: Theory and Practice, 1st edn. New York: Informa, 2007:205.

56. Dupont AW, Pasricha PJ. Irritable bowel syndrome and functional abdominal pain syndromes: pathophysiology. In: Pasricha PJ, Willis WD, Gebhart GF (eds). Chronic Abdominal and Visceral Pain: Theory and Practice, 1st edn. New York: Informa, 2007:33.

57. Derasari M. Taxonomy of pain syndromes: classification of chronic pain syndromes. In: Raj PP (ed.). Practical Management of Pain, 3rd edn. St Louis: CV Mosby, 2000:10.

58. Cervero F. Sensory innervation of the viscera: peripheral basis of visceral pain. Physiol Rev 1994;74:95.

59. Ness TJ, Gebhart GF. Visceral pain: a review of experimental studies. Pain 1990;41:167.

60. Ness T, Metcalf A, Gebhart G. A psychophysiological study in humans using phasic colonic distension as a noxious visceral stimulus. Pain 1990;43:377.

61. French E, Robb W. Biliary and renal colic. BMJ 1963;2:135.

62. Horrocks J, De Dombal F. Clinical presentation of patients with "dyspepsia. Detailed symptomatic study of 360 patients. Gut 1978; 19:19.

63. Beaumont PR, Glauberg AF. Necrotizing lymphadenitis as a cause of acute abdominal distress in a dog. Mod Vet Pract 1979;60:890.

64. Liddington MI, Thomson WH. Rebound tenderness test. Br J Surg 1991;78:795.

65. Thomson H, Francis DM. Abdominal-wall tenderness: A useful sign in the acute abdomen. Lancet 1977;2:1053.

66. Thomson WH, Dawes RF, Carter SS. Abdominal wall tenderness: a useful sign in chronic abdominal pain. Br J Surg 1991;78:223–5.

67. Roy S, Weimersheimer P. Nonoperative causes of abdominal pain. Surg Clin N Am 1997;77:1433.

68. Longstreth GF, Newcomer AD. Abdominal pain caused by diabetic radiculopathy. Ann Intern Med 1977;86:166.

69. Longstreth GF. Diabetic thoracic polyradiculopathy: ten patients with abdominal pain. Am J Gastroenterol 1997;92:502.

70. Longstreth GF. Diabetic thoracic polyradiculopathy. Best Pract Res Clin Gastroenterol 2005;19:275.

71. Stevenson RJ. Abdominal pain unrelated to trauma. Surg Clin North Am. 1985;65:1181.

72. Blendis L. Abdominal pain. In: Wall P, Melzack R (eds). Textbook of Pain. London: Churchill Livingstone, 1994:583.

73. Drossman DA. The patient with chronic undiagnosed abdominal pain. Hosp Pract (Off Ed) 1986;21:22, 4–5, 9.

74. Bardan E, Nadler M, Chowers Y, et al. Capsule endoscopy for the evaluation of patients with chronic abdominal pain. Endoscopy 2003;35:688.

75. Fry LC, Carey EJ, Shiff AD, et al. The yield of capsule endoscopy in patients with abdominal pain or diarrhea. Endoscopy 2006;38:498.

76. May A, Manner H, Schneider M, et al. Prospective multicenter trial of capsule endoscopy in patients with chronic abdominal pain, diarrhea and other signs and symptoms (CEDAP-Plus Study). Endoscopy 2007;39:606.

77. Pasha SF, Fleischer DE. Capsule endoscopy for abdominal pain – is it of value or just another test for doctors to do? Endoscopy 2007;39: 650.

78. Spada C, Pirozzi GA, Riccioni ME, Iacopini F, Marchese M, Costamagna G. Capsule endoscopy in patients with chronic abdominal pain. Dig Liver Dis 2006;38:696.

79. Camilleri M. Management of the patient wtih chronic abdominal pain and clinical pharmacology of nonopioid drugs. In: Pasricha PJ, Willis WD, Gebhart GF (eds). Chronic Abdominal and Visceral Pain: Theory and Practice, 1st edn. New York: Informa 2007:271.

80. Ruddell WS, Lintott DJ, Axon AT. The diagnostic yield of ERCP in the investigation of unexplained abdominal pain. Br J Surg 1983;70:74.

81. Olden KW. Rational management of chronic abdominal pain. Comprehensive Ther 1998;24:180.

82. Easter DW, Cuschieri A, Nathanson LK, Lavelle-Jones M. The utility of diagnostic laparoscopy for abdominal disorders. Audit of 120 patients. Arch Surg 1992;127:379.

83. Weibel M. Peritoneal adhesions and their relation to abdominal surgery. Am J Surg 1973;126:345.

84. Rapkin A. Adhesions and pelvic pain: a retrospective study. Obstet Gynecol 1986;68:13.

85. Swank DJ, Swank-Bordewijk SC, Hop WC, et al. Laparoscopic adhesiolysis in patients with chronic abdominal pain: a blinded randomised controlled multi-centre trial. Lancet 2003;361(9365):1247.

86. Swank DJ, Van Erp WF, Repelaer Van Driel OJ, et al. A prospective analysis of predictive factors on the results of laparoscopic adhesiolysis in patients with chronic abdominal pain. Surg Laparosc Endosc Percutan Tech 2003;13:88.

87. Suleiman S, Johnston DE. The abdominal wall: an overlooked source of pain. Am Fam Physician 2001;64:431.

88. Greenbaum DS. Abdominal wall pain. In: Pasricha PJ, Willis WD, Gebhart GF (eds). Chronic Abdominal and Visceral Pain: Theory and Practice, 1st edn. New York: Informa, 2007:427.

89. Costanza CD, Longstreth GF, Liu AL. Chronic abdominal wall pain: clinical features, health care costs, and long-term outcome. Clin Gastroenterol Hepatol 2004;2:395.

90. Srinivasan R, Greenbaum DS. Chronic abdominal wall pain: a frequently overlooked problem. Practical approach to diagnosis and management. Am J Gastroenterol 2002;97:824.

91. Thomson WH, Dawes RF, Carter SS. Abdominal wall tenderness: a useful sign in chronic abdominal pain. Br J Surg 1991;78:223.

92. Applegate WV, Buckwalter NR. Microanatomy of the structures contributing to abdominal cutaneous nerve entrapment syndrome. J Am Board Fam Pract 1997;10:329.

93. Gallegos N, Hobsley M. Abdominal pain: parietal or visceral? J R Soc Med 1992;85:379.

94. Gray DW, Dixon JM, Seabrook G, Collin J. Is abdominal wall tenderness a useful sign in the diagnosis of non-specific abdominal pain? Ann R Coll Surg Engl 1988;70:233.

95. Greenbaum DS, Greenbaum RB, Joseph JG, Natale JE. Chronic abdominal wall pain. Diagnostic validity and costs. Dig Dis Sci 1994;39:1935.

96. Gallegos NC, Hobsley M. Abdominal wall pain: an alternative diagnosis. Br J Surg 1990;77:1167.

97. Clouse RE, Mayer EA, Aziz Q, et al. Functional abdominal pain syndrome. Gastroenterology. 2006;130:1492.

98. Drossman DA, Li Z, Andruzzi E, et al. U.S. householder survey of functional gastrointestinal disorders. Prevalence, sociodemography, and health impact. Dig Dis Sci 1993;38:1569.

99. Drossman DA. Chronic functional abdominal pain. Am J Gastroenterol 1996;91:2270.

100. Hill OW, Blendis L. Physical and psychological evaluation of "non-organic" abdominal pain. Gut 1967;8:221.

101. Rose JD, Troughton AH, Harvey JS, Smith PM. Depression and functional bowel disorders in gastrointestinal outpatients. Gut 1986;27:1025.

102. Magni G, Rossi MR, Rigatti-Luchini S, Merskey H. Chronic abdominal pain and depression. Epidemiologic findings in the United States. Hispanic Health and Nutrition Examination Survey. Pain 1992;49:77.

103. Gomez J, Dally P. Psychologically mediated abdominal pain in surgical and medical outpatients clinics. BMJ 1977;1:1451.

104. Drossman DA, Leserman J, Nachman G, et al. Sexual and physical abuse in women with functional or organic gastrointestinal disorders. Ann Intern Med 1990;113:828.

105. Lawson MJ, Grant AK, Paull A, Read TR. Significance of nocturnal abdominal pain: a prospective study. BMJ 1980;280:1302.

106. Drossman DA. Patients with psychogenic abdominal pain: six years' observation in the medical setting. Am J Psychiatry 1982;139:1549.

107. Sloth H, Jorgensen LS. Chronic non-organic upper abdominal pain: diagnostic safety and prognosis of gastrointestinal and non-intestinal symptoms. A 5- to 7-year follow-up study. Scand J Gastroenterol 1988;23:1275.

108. Gray DW, Dixon JM, Collin J. The closed eyes sign: an aid to diagnosing non-specific abdominal pain. BMJ 1988;297:837.

109. Devor D, Knauft RD. Exploratory laparotomy for abdominal pain of unknown etiology. Diagnosis, management, and follow-up of 40 cases. Arch Surg 1968;96:836.

110. DeVaul RA, Faillace LA. Persistent pain and illness insistence: a medical profile of proneness to surgery. Am J Surg 1978;135:828.

111. Sarfeh IJ. Abdominal pain of unknown etiology. Am J Surg 1976;132:22.

112. LoVecchio F, Oster N, Sturmann K, et al. The use of analgesics in patients with acute abdominal pain. J Emerg Med 1997;15:775.

113. Brooks P, Day R. Drug therapy: nonsteroidal antiinflammatory drugs – differences and similarities. N Engl J Med 1991;324:1716.

114. Wiffen PJ. An evidence base for WHO "essential analgesics". Pain Clin Updates 2000:1.

115. Ballantyne JC. Pharmacology and practice of opioid drugs for visceral pain. In: Pasricha PJ, Willis WD, Gebhart GF (eds). Chronic Abdominal and Visceral Pain: Theory and Practice, 1st edn. New York: Informa, 2007:287.

116. Thompson D. Narcotic analgesic effects on the Sphincter of Oddi: a review of the data and therapeutic implications in treating pancreatitis. Am J Gastroenterol 2001;96:1266.

117. Ruskis A. Effects of narcotics on gastrointestinal tract, liver and kidneys. In: Kitahata L, Collins J (eds). Narcotic Analgesics in Anesthesiology. Baltimore: Williams and Wilkins 1982:143.

118. Hendler N. Pharmacological management of pain. In: Raj PP (ed.). Practical Management of Pain. St Louis: Mosby, 2000:145.

119. Olden KW. The use of antidepressants in functional gastrointestinal disorders: new uses for old drugs. CNS Spectr 2005;10:891.

120. Drossman DA, Toner BB, Whitehead WE, et al. Cognitive-behavioral therapy versus education and desipramine versus placebo for moderate to severe functional bowel disorders. Gastroenterology 2003;125:19.

121. Su X, Gebhart GF. Effects of tricyclic antidepressants on mechanosensitive pelvic nerve afferent fibers innervating the rat colon. Pain 1998;76:105.

122. Gorelick AB, Koshy SS, Hooper FG, et al. Differential effects of amitriptyline on perception of somatic and visceral stimulation in healthy humans. Am J Physiol 1998;275:G460.

123. Jackson JL, O'Malley PG, Tomkins G, et al. Treatment of functional gastrointestinal disorders with antidepressant medications: a meta-analysis. Am J Med 2000;108:65.

124. Mays TA. Antidepressants in the management of cancer pain. Curr Pain Headache Rep 2001;5:227.

125. Tabas G, Beaves M, Wang J, et al. Paroxetine to treat irritable bowel syndrome not responding to high-fiber diet: a double-blind, placebo-controlled trial. Am J Gastroenterol 2004;99:914.

126. Kuiken SD, Tytgat GN, Boeckxstaens GE. The selective serotonin reuptake inhibitor fluoxetine does not change rectal sensitivity and symptoms in patients with irritable bowel syndrome: a double blind, randomized, placebo-controlled study. Clin Gastroenterol Hepatol 2003;1:219.

127. Broekaert D, Fischler B, Sifrim D, et al. Influence of citalopram, a selective serotonin reuptake inhibitor, on oesophageal hypersensitivity: a double-blind, placebo-controlled study. Aliment Pharmacol Ther 2006;23:365.

128. Tack J, Broekaert D, Fischler B, et al. A controlled crossover study of the selective serotonin reuptake inhibitor citalopram in irritable bowel syndrome. Gut 2006;55:1095.

129. Chial HJ, Camilleri M, Ferber I, et al. Effects of venlafaxine, buspirone, and placebo on colonic sensorimotor functions in healthy humans. Clin Gastroenterol Hepatol 2003;1:211.

130. Coluzzi F, Mattia C. Mechanism-based treatment in chronic neuropathic pain: the role of antidepressants. Curr Pharm Des 2005;11:2945.

131. Mico JA, Ardid D, Berrocoso E, Eschalier A. Antidepressants and pain. Trends Pharmacol Sci 2006;27:348.

132. Saarto T, Wiffen PJ. Antidepressants for neuropathic pain. Cochrane Database Syst Rev 2005:CD005454.

133. Sindrup SH, Otto M, Finnerup NB, Jensen TS. Antidepressants in the treatment of neuropathic pain. Basic Clin Pharmacol Toxicol 2005;96:399.

134. Clouse RE, Lustman PJ, Eckert TC, et al. Low-dose trazodone for symptomatic patients with esophageal contraction abnormalities. A double-blind, placebo-controlled trial. Gastroenterology 1987;92:1027.

135. Tremont-Lukats IW, Megeff C, Backonja MM. Anticonvulsants for neuropathic pain syndromes: mechanisms of action and place in therapy. Drugs 2000;60:1029.

136. Magnus L. Nonepileptic uses of gabapentin. Epilepsia 1999;40 Suppl. 6:S66; discussion S3.

137. Houghton LA, Fell C, Whorwell PJ, et al. Effect of a second-generation Alpha2Delta ligand, Pregabalin on visceral sensation in hypersensitive patients with irritable bowel syndrome. Gut 2007;56:1218.

138. Diop L, Raymond F, Fargeau H, et al. Pregabalin (CI-1008) inhibits the trinitrobenzene sulfonic acid-induced chronic colonic allodynia in the rat. J Pharmacol Exp Ther 2002;302:1013.

139. Feng Y, Cui M, Willis WD. Gabapentin markedly reduces acetic acid-induced visceral nociception. Anesthesiology 2003;98:729.

140. Lee KJ, Kim JH, Cho SW. Gabapentin reduces rectal mechanosensitivity and increases rectal compliance in patients with diarrhoea-predominant irritable bowel syndrome. Aliment Pharmacol Ther 2005;22:981.

141. Smiley MM, Lu Y, Vera-Portocarrero LP, et al. Intrathecal gabapentin enhances the analgesic effects of subtherapeutic dose morphine in a rat experimental pancreatitis model. Anesthesiology 2004;101:759.

142. Chey WD, Beydoun A, Roberts DJ, et al. Octreotide reduces perception of rectal electrical stimulation by spinal afferent pathway inhibition. Am J Physiol 1995;269:G821.

143. Bradette M, Delvaux M, Staumont G, et al. Octreotide increases thresholds of colonic visceral perception in IBS patients without modifying muscle tone. Dig Dis Sci 1994;39:1171.

144. Hasler WL, Soudah HC, Owyang C. A somatostatin analogue inhibits afferent pathways mediating perception of rectal distention. Gastroenterology 1993;104:1390.

145. Hasler WL, Soudah HC, Owyang C. Somatostatin analog inhibits afferent response to rectal distention in diarrhea-predominant irritable bowel patients. J Pharmacol Exp Ther 1994;268:1206.

146. Camilleri M, Kim DY, McKinzie S, et al. A randomized, controlled exploratory study of clonidine in diarrhea-predominant irritable bowel syndrome. Clin Gastroenterol Hepatol 2003;1:111.

147. Kuiken SD, Lei A, Tytgat GN, et al. Effect of the low-affinity, noncompetitive N-methyl-D-aspartate receptor antagonist dextromethorphan on visceral perception in healthy volunteers. Aliment Pharmacol Ther 2002;16:1955.

148. Fisher K, Coderre TJ, Hagen NA. Targeting the N-methyl-D-aspartate receptor for chronic pain management. Preclinical animal studies, recent clinical experience and future research directions. J Pain Symptom Manage 2000;20:358.

149. Ben-Ari A, Lewis MC, Davidson E. Chronic administration of ketamine for analgesia. J Pain Palliat Care Pharmacother 2007;21:7.

150. Chizh BA. Low dose ketamine: a therapeutic and research tool to explore N-methyl-D-aspartate (NMDA) receptor-mediated plasticity in pain pathways. J Psychopharmacol 2007;21:259.

151. Miller MA, Harrison BP. Ketamine: it is not just for kids anymore. Am J Emerg Med 2007;25:725.

152. Okon T. Ketamine: an introduction for the pain and palliative medicine physician. Pain Physician 2007;10:493.

153. Hogan QH, Abram SE. Neural blockade for diagnosis and prognosis. A review. Anesthesiology 1997;86:216.

154. Mercadante S, Nicosia F. Celiac plexus block: a reappraisal. Reg Anest Pain Med 1998;23:37.

155. Patt R. Outcomes, efficacy, complications, and sequelae of visceral pain management. In: Raj PP (ed.). Practical Pain Management. St Louis: Mosby, 2000:904.

156. Bennett AT, Collins KA. Pathologic quiz case: abdominal pain. Arch Pathol Lab Med 2000;124:1089.

157. Gadsby JG, Flowerdew MW. Transcutaneous electrical nerve stimulation and acupuncture-like transcutaneous electrical nerve stimulation for chronic low back pain. Cochrane Database Syst Rev 2000:CD000210.

158. Borjesson M, Pilhall M, Eliasson T, et al. Esophageal visceral pain sensitivity: effects of TENS and correlation with manometric findings. Dig Dis Sci 1998;43:1621.

159. Kapur S, Mutagi H, Raphael J. Spinal cord stimulation for relief of abdominal pain in two patients with familial Mediterranean fever. Br J Anaesth 2006;97:866.

160. Kapural L, Narouze SN, Janicki TI, Mekhail N. Spinal cord stimulation is an effective treatment for the chronic intractable visceral pelvic pain. Pain Med 2006;7:440.

161. Patrizi F, Freedman SD, Pascual-Leone A, Fregni F. Novel therapeutic approaches to the treatment of chronic abdominal visceral pain. ScientificWorldJournal 2006;6:472.

162. Tiede JM, Ghazi SM, Lamer TJ, Obray JB. The use of spinal cord stimulation in refractory abdominal visceral pain: case reports and literature review. Pain Pract 2006;6:197.

163. Brooker CD, Cousins MJ. Neuromodulation techniques for visceral pain from benign disorders. In: Pasricha PJ, Willis WD, Gebhart GF (eds). Chronic Abdominal and Visceral Pain: Theory and Practice, 1st edn. New York: Informa, 2007:311.

164. Du HJ, Chao YF. Localization of central structures involved in descending inhibitory effect of acupuncture on viscero-somatic reflex discharges. Sci Sin 1976;19:137.

165. Shu J, Li KY, Huang DK. The central effect of electro-acupuncture analgesia on visceral pain of rats: a study using the [3H]2-deoxyglucose method. Acupunct Electrother Res 1994;19:107.

166. Rong PJ, Zhu B, Huang QF, et al. Acupuncture inhibition on neuronal activity of spinal dorsal horn induced by noxious colorectal distention in rat. World J Gastroenterol 2005;11:1011.

167. Lim B, Manheimer E, Lao L, et al. Acupuncture for treatment of irritable bowel syndrome. Cochrane Database Syst Rev 2006:CD005111.

168. Takahashi T. Acupuncture for functional gastrointestinal disorders. J Gastroenterol 2006;41:408.

169. Sierpina VS, Kuncharapu I. Complementary and integrative medicine approaches to visceral pain. In: Pasricha PJ, Willis WD, Gebhart GF (eds). Chronic Abdominal and Visceral Pain: Theory and Practice, 1st edn. New York: Informa, 2007:33.

170. Russo CM, Brose WG. Chronic pain. Annu Rev Med 1998;49:123.

171. Snell, RS. Clinical Anatomy for Medical Students, 6th edn. Philadelphia: Lippincott, Williams & Wilkins, 2000.

172. Woolf CJ, Costigan M. Transcriptional and posttranslational plasticity and the generation of inflammatory pain. Proc Natl Acad Sci USA 1999;96:7723.

173. Zackowski SW. Chronic recurrent abdominal pain. Emerg Med Clin N Am 1998;16:877.

174. Turk DC, Okifuji A. Pain: assessment of patients' reporting of pain: an integrated perspective. Lancet 1999;353:1784.

175. Gourlay GK. Clinical pharmacology of the treatment of chronic non-cancer pain. In: Committee IASP (ed.). Pain 1999 – an Updated Review. Seattle: IASP Press, 1999:433.

15

Approach to the patient with gas and bloating

William L. Hasler

Normal physiology, 255
Clinical syndromes, 256
Pathogenesis of gas and bloating, 257
Evaluation of the patient with gas and bloating, 261
Principles of management, 263

Normal physiology

Gas production

The gastrointestinal tract contains less than 200 mL gas; daily gas expulsion averages 600–700 mL after consumption of a standardized diet plus 200 g baked beans [1]. On average, healthy men pass flatus 14 times per day, especially after meals. Daily flatus numbers up to 25 are normal. Ingestion of a nonabsorbable carbohydrate such as lactulose nearly doubles flatus frequency [2]. The major gases in flatus are nitrogen, oxygen, carbon dioxide, hydrogen, and methane [3] (Fig. 15.1). Gases produced by colonic bacterial fermentation of ingested nutrients and endogenous glycoproteins (hydrogen, methane, and carbon dioxide) represent 74% of flatus. Flatus odor correlates with hydrogen sulfide concentrations; other sulfur-containing gases in flatus include methanethiol and dimethyl sulfide [4]. Age, gender, and the methane-producing capabilities of a given individual's flora do not significantly affect flatus frequency although men produce more aromatic flatus than women [5]. Major shifts in production of methane or reduction of sulfates occur spontaneously, indicating the inconstancy of bacterial flora populations. Variability in bacterial hydrogen production reflects changes in methane production or mixing of the stool within the colon [6]. Daily lactose feedings to patients with lactase deficiency lead to reductions in hydrogen production, indicating dietary modulation of gut flora metabolic pathways [7].

Gas transit

Insight into normal patterns of intestinal gas transit has been provided by experiments in which physiological gas mixtures containing nitrogen, oxygen, and carbon dioxide are perfused into the jejunum. In healthy volunteers, gas perfusion produces steady-state flow with little distention and few symptoms [8]. Gas collected from the rectum in such studies is expelled in pulsatile fashion indicating that flow is regulated by intrinsic motor patterns in the distal gut (Fig. 15.2) [9]. Gas transit is accelerated by caloric liquid or solid meals whereas non-caloric liquids have no stimulatory effects, providing an experimental correlate to the observation that gas passage and gaseous symptoms increase postprandially [10]. Conversely, intestinal lipid perfusion retards the propulsion of gas perfused into the jejunum, demonstrating nutrient-induced reflex modulation of gas transit [11]. Retardation of gas flow by lipid is more pronounced with ileal perfusion than with duodenal perfusion, which is indicative of region-specific activation of this reflex [12]. Other factors regulate physiological gas flow. Assuming an upright posture expedites gas flow compared with studies performed when supine [13]. Likewise, mild physical activity accelerates gas transit and reduces gas retention in healthy individuals [14].

Recent studies detail some of the motor events that regulate gastrointestinal gas flow in healthy humans. Using combined colonic manometry with concurrent jejunal gas perfusion and rectal gas collection, one group has shown increases in propagative distal colonic pressure waves that temporally correlate with pulsatile gas expulsions [15]. Furthermore, there is some correlation between fasting duodenojejunal motility and gas expulsion, indicating the participation of phasic motor activity throughout the gut in the transit of lumenal gas. In addition, employing barostat

Principles of Clinical Gastroenterology. Edited by Tadataka Yamada, David H. Alpers, Anthony N. Kalloo, Neil Kaplowitz, Chung Owyang, and Don W. Powell. © 2008 Blackwell Publishing. ISBN 978-1-4051-69103

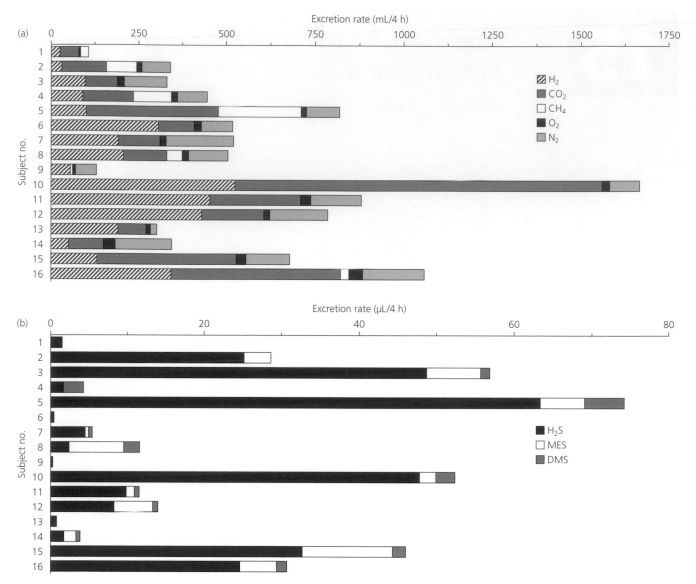

Figure 15.1 The volume of each gas passed from the rectum over a 4-h period is shown for 16 healthy volunteers. The major gases **(a)** are hydrogen (H$_2$), carbon dioxide (CO$_2$), methane (CH$_4$), oxygen (O$_2$), and nitrogen (N$_2$). Sulfur-containing gases **(b)** are passed in much smaller quantities and include hydrogen sulfide (H$_2$S), methanethiol (MES), and dimethylsulfide (DMS). From Suarez et al. [3].

methods, increases in duodenal tone with reductions in gut capacitance are observed during jejunal gas perfusion [16].

Disruption of normal gas transit by different stimuli produces variable perception of bloating, indicating stimulus-specific activation of gut sensory pathways. Retardation of gas flow with intravenous glucagon produces significant distention but little symptomatic bloating, whereas similar degrees of distention occurring with voluntary anal contraction cause significant gaseous symptomatology [17]. Jejunal and rectal gas perfusion produces similar degrees of gas retention in healthy volunteers; however, significant symptoms are elicited only with jejunal gas loading [18]. Retardation of gas flow by intestinal lipid perfusion is prevented by concurrent rectal or duodenal distention; however, symptomatic bloating is reported only during duodenal distention [19].

Clinical syndromes

Gas in the gastrointestinal tract is responsible for several clinical phenomena. Eructation, or belching, is the retrograde expulsion of esophageal or gastric gas from the mouth. Involuntary belching after eating is caused by release of swallowed air after gastric distention, and may be exacerbated by foods that reduce lower esophageal sphincter tone. The Magenblase syndrome is defined as epigastric fullness and bloating relieved by belching. Manometric studies of eructation show decreases in lower esophageal sphincter tone followed by upper esophageal sphincter relaxation [20]. Flatulence is the volitional or involuntary release of gas from the anus. Manometric studies performed during flatulence

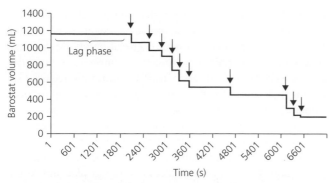

Figure 15.2 A sample rectal gas evacuation profile from a healthy volunteer during jejunal perfusion of a physiological gas mixture is shown. Before gas perfusion, the barostat cylinder was emptied (starting volume 1170 mL). After initiation of gas perfusion, there was a lag period of approximately 1900 s during which no gas was evacuated at the level of the rectum. Thereafter, gas evacuation into the barostat cylinder was pulsatile with passage of discrete boluses (arrows) with a total expulsion of approximately 900 mL over a 2-h period. From Gonlachanvit et al. [9].

demonstrate propagated colon contractions with increased rectal pressure coupled with early anal sphincter relaxation [21]. Bloating is the perception of retained excess gas within the gut lumen. Bloating is experienced monthly by 15.9% of individuals in the United States compared with the 21.8% who experience abdominal pain or discomfort [22]. Bloating was more common in women (19.2%) than men (10.5%) in one study, but was reported less often by women in another large survey [22,23]. Other symptoms experienced by patients with complaints of excess gas include abdominal pain, halitosis, anorexia, early satiety, nausea, belching, loud borborygmi, and constipation.

Pathogenesis of gas and bloating

Gas and bloating are reported in a number of disorders. These gaseous symptoms may result from excess gas production, abnormal gas transit with generation of retarding motor patterns, abnormal perception of normal amounts of gas within the gut, and abnormal somatic muscular activity in the abdominal wall.

Carbohydrate maldigestion
Maldigestion and malabsorption of carbohydrates are commonly associated with intestinal gas production. Substances that cause gaseous symptoms include simple and complex carbohydrates and dietary fiber. Unabsorbed carbohydrates are propelled to the colon where they serve as nutrient substrates for enteric bacteria. Unlike their handling by mammalian tissues, carbohydrates subjected to bacterial metabolism liberate hydrogen gas and short-chain fatty acids. Flatulence is the initial symptom reported, with borborygmi and bloating occurring with greater degrees of malabsorption, and

abdominal pain and diarrhea occurring with the highest levels. Carbohydrate maldigestion and malabsorption may result from loss of enterocyte enzymes in normal intestinal mucosa, inability to transport a poorly absorbed sugar in an otherwise healthy individual, or an organic disorder of the intestinal mucosa such as celiac disease.

Maldigestion and malabsorption of simple sugars
The most common carbohydrate maldigestion syndrome, lactose intolerance, results from insufficient levels of enterocyte lactase, which hydrolyzes ingested lactose into glucose and galactose. Lactase deficiency is present in 21% of white Americans but is more prevalent in individuals of African (75%), Hispanic (51%), and Native American (79%) background [24]. Absence of intestinal lactase is rare, so most individuals can tolerate small amounts of milk products. In individuals who consider themselves severely lactose intolerant, symptoms attributable to lactase deficiency are uncommon unless more than 240 mL milk is ingested per day [25]. However, most lactase-deficient individuals develop symptoms after ingesting at least 1 liter of milk.

Other simple sugars may lead to gas and bloating as well. Furthermore, nonabsorbable sugars such as lactulose accelerate small intestinal transit, further increasing gastrointestinal symptoms [26]. Increased gas production is recognized as resulting from consumption of fruits or juices. Only 60% of fructose, a sugar in fruits and soft drinks, is absorbed in the normal human intestine. As little as 37.5 g fructose can produce significant symptoms in some individuals [27]. Patients with fructose-intolerance pass flatus more frequently and produce more hydrogen for given amounts of fructose vs asymptomatic individuals. Sorbitol, a natural substance in fruits and an artificial sweetener in diet foods, is malabsorbed by 43% of white subjects and 55% of non-white subjects [28]. Severe sorbitol intolerance is reported in 32% of non-whites vs 4% of whites. Some subjects are susceptible to as little as 5 g sorbitol, while nearly all develop severe symptoms with 20 g [29]. Consumption of chocolate containing isomalt produces greater increases in breath hydrogen than chocolate with sucrose, while xylitol is also malabsorbed to variable degrees [30]. In fact, 2%–4% of sucrose is malabsorbed by healthy individuals, although most of this is salvaged in the colon [31].

Finally, hereditary syndromes of intolerance of specific sugars are described. Sucrase-isomaltase deficiency is a rare condition presenting with symptoms of carbohydrate malabsorption after sucrose ingestion. Symptoms typically, but not always, begin in infancy. The disorder is inherited in autosomal recessive fashion and results from one of several defects in the sucrase-isomaltase gene [32].

Maldigestion of complex carbohydrates and fiber
Ingested complex carbohydrates may also be poorly assimilated. The average amounts malabsorbed out of 100-g meals

are 20 g for baked beans, 7–10 g for wheat, oats, potatoes, and corn, and 0.9 g for rice [33]. Comparisons of pH and concentrations of lactic and volatile fatty acids in cecal fluid and expelled feces indicate that most unabsorbed starch is metabolized in the colon. Whole grains produce five times more hydrogen than refined flours. There is no evidence that significant adaptation develops with respect to the volumes of gas expelled in persons habitually ingesting a diet rich in beans. Nondigestible oligosaccharides, such as stachyose, raffinose, and verbascose, are abundant in beans and legumes. Flour derived from soy beans that are low in these oligosaccharides produces less gas than that from standard soybeans [34].

Fiber intake correlates with flatus production in many individuals, although some studies have found no association of gas and bloating with ingestion of psyllium or methylcellulose [5]. In one investigation, fiber-free diets reduced daily gas expulsion from 700 mL to 200 mL [1]. The intrinsic flora may contribute to bloating after fiber ingestion, as individuals who produce low levels of methane experience greater symptoms than high methane producers [35]. However, fecal gas production from incubation with bran produces only 10% as much hydrogen and carbon dioxide as with lactulose, supporting the observations that fiber supplements elicit feelings of bloating but do not increase flatus frequency, while lactulose causes elevations in both [36]. In a recent study in healthy humans, ingesting 30 g of psyllium daily retarded transit of a jejunally perfused gas mixture, providing a possible mechanism for increased gaseous symptoms after fiber supplementation [9].

Abnormal gut flora

The human colon contains up to 10^{14} bacteria [37]. Colonic bacteria serve several roles, including fermentation of food residue, modulation of gut immune function, synthesis of essential vitamins, and protection against pathogens [38–41]. Normal jejunal and ileal bacterial counts are 10^3–10^4 and 10^7–10^9 colony-forming units (CFU) per mL, respectively, whereas densities in the colon approach 10^{12} CFU/mL. Small intestinal bacterial overgrowth is defined by the presence of more than 10^5 CFU/mL in proximal intestinal fluid. The main organisms cultured are *Streptococcus*, *Escherichia coli*, *Lactobacillus*, and *Bacteroides*. Gaseous symptoms with bacterial overgrowth are thought to result from microbial metabolism of consumed and endogenous carbohydrates. In addition to producing gas, bloating, diarrhea, abdominal discomfort, and nausea, bacterial overgrowth leads to nutrient malabsorption and weight loss. Other complications include the development of metabolic bone disease as well as an increased risk of spontaneous bacterial peritonitis in patients with cirrhosis [42].

There are several reported organic causes of bacterial overgrowth. The condition complicates small intestinal obstruction from a variety of causes. Stasis within small intestinal diverticula predisposes to bacterial overgrowth, while vagotomy increases intestinal microbial colonization because of hypochlorhydria. Small intestinal bacterial counts are increased by proton-pump inhibitors; however, symptoms are not usually observed [43]. Common variable immunodeficiency syndrome may present with bacterial overgrowth from reduced lumenal immune surveillance. Forty-three percent of cases of diabetic diarrhea are attributed to bacterial overgrowth, mostly from altered motor function [44]. Patients with intestinal pseudoobstruction develop overgrowth from impaired gut clearance. Cologastric and coloenteric fistulae and coprophagia increase bacterial delivery to the upper gut, overwhelming defenses against infection. Bacterial overgrowth is a recognized cause of gaseous symptoms in the elderly and is probably the result of altered motility, acid production, and immune function.

Dysmotility syndromes

Conditions that alter gut motor function may produce prominent gas and bloating. Bloating and fullness are commonly reported by individuals with gastroparesis and are postulated to stem from gastric retention of solids, liquids, and gases. Recently, an increased prevalence of bacterial overgrowth was reported in patients with gastroparesis, providing another potential cause of gaseous symptoms in these individuals [45]. Patients with fat intolerance and rapid gastric emptying also complain of bloating [46]. Fundoplications for gastroesophageal reflux involve wrapping the gastric fundus around the lower esophagus, thus reducing the ability to belch or vomit. In the early postoperative period, up to 73% of patients experience bloating [47]. Two years later, this gas-bloat syndrome has improved in 71% of individuals. Preoperative delay in gastric emptying is a risk factor for gas-bloat syndrome. Patients with chronic intestinal pseudoobstruction experience gas and bloating and exhibit small intestinal dilation as a result of delayed gas transit and small intestinal bacterial overgrowth. Causes of gastroparesis and intestinal pseudoobstruction include diabetes mellitus, scleroderma, amyloidosis, familial conditions, paraneoplastic syndromes, and endocrinological disease. Many cases are idiopathic in nature. Bloating is also reported by patients with chronic constipation.

Acute processes producing adynamic ileus also produce prominent gas and bloating. Ileus may involve the entire gut or may be localized as in acute colonic pseudoobstruction. Causes of acute ileus include systemic infection or inflammation, the postoperative state, medications, generalized or localized gut hypotension, metabolic disturbances, and cardiovascular disease.

Functional bowel disorders

Gas and bloating are prevalent complaints of patients with functional bowel disorders such as irritable bowel syndrome (IBS) and functional dyspepsia. In one investigation, bloating

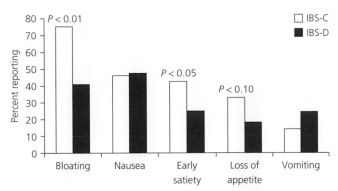

Figure 15.3 The percentages of constipation-predominant (IBS-C) and diarrhea-predominant (IBS-D) irritable bowel syndrome (IBS) patients reporting selected upper gastrointestinal symptoms. More IBS-C patients experienced bloating as well as early satiety and loss of appetite compared with IBS-D patients. From Talley et al. [55].

was rated the most bothersome symptom by 60% of IBS patients, whereas 29% considered pain to be most intrusive [48]. Bloating was experienced on 28% of days in another study, while pain was reported on 33% of days [49]. Abdominal distention and bloating are more often reported by women with IBS than men, with symptom increases noted in relation to menstruation [50]. In premenopausal women with IBS, bloating is strongly associated with uterine cramping and breast tenderness, suggesting that gastrointestinal complaints may be confounded by menses-associated symptoms [51]. Bloating in IBS may be worsened by stress and relieved by relaxation [52,53]. Most studies show more prominent bloating with constipation-predominant IBS than those with diarrhea, although some investigations report no relation of bloating to a particular defecation profile (Fig. 15.3) [54–56]. Recent investigations distinguish the sensation of bloating from objective measures of abdominal distention. In one study, constipated patients reported bloating and exhibited abdominal distention whereas those with diarrhea noted bloating without distention [52]. Objective distention shows diurnal variability in IBS patients, being higher later in the day [57].

The pathogenesis of gas and bloating in IBS is not well defined and is likely multifactorial in nature. Five published studies on IBS report increases in abdominal distention while two report no change [58–60]. Likewise, two studies report increased gas production while two do not and three investigations observe more gas within the gut lumen whereas four reports show no change [58]. It is likely that only some of these pathogenic factors contribute to symptoms in any given IBS patient.

Carbohydrate intolerance in irritable bowel syndrome

Lactose intolerance is common in patients with IBS [61]. However, the symptom responses of patients with IBS are not clearly improved by lactose restriction or lactase supplementation; this questions the pathogenic relevance of lactase deficiency in these individuals [62,63]. Most investigations show no increase in the prevalence of fructose or sorbitol intolerance in IBS, although some studies do report a response to dietary restriction of these sugars [64,65]. Several studies report increases in bloating with dietary bran supplementation in patients with IBS [66]. Conversely, dietary fiber restriction may lead to symptom reduction in some individuals [67].

Abnormal colonic flora in irritable bowel syndrome

Extensive investigation suggests that alterations in the enteric flora of patients with IBS may relate to symptom development. Cumulative 3-h breath hydrogen excretion from colonic fermentation of ingested lactulose is reportedly greater in patients with IBS than in healthy controls [68]. However, other studies report no increase in breath hydrogen excretion in IBS patients with bloating [69]. In an older study, patients with IBS exhibited fewer fecal coliforms, lactobacilli, and bifidobacteria compared with controls [70]. More recently, *Bifidobacterium* and *Lactobacillus* densities were observed to be lower in patients with constipation, and concentrations of potentially pathogenic bacteria and fungi were higher [71]. A variety of immune alterations were observed in these individuals, including increases in CD3[+], CD4[+], and CD25[+] lymphocytes, reduced CD72[+] B lymphocytes, diminished neutrophil and monocyte phagocytosis, and elevated antibody titers to *Escherichia coli* and *Staphylococcus aureus*, indicating prominent interactions of the gut flora with the host immune system [71]. Recent studies employing polymerase chain reaction methods have characterized differences in fecal flora in different IBS subtypes. Using these methods, diarrhea-predominant patients exhibited decreases in lactobacilli and trends to reduced *Desulfovibrio* and *Bifidobacterium* [72]. Counts of *Veillonella* were higher in constipated IBS patients compared with healthy volunteers. *Clostridium coccoides* and *Bifidobacterium catenulatum* counts were reduced in all IBS subsets compared with controls.

Small intestinal bacterial overgrowth in irritable bowel syndrome

Small intestinal bacterial overgrowth has been promoted as a cause of symptoms in IBS. Recent studies have reported positive lactulose breath tests in large subsets (78%) of patients with IBS, which have been attributed to bacterial overgrowth in the small intestine [73]. Furthermore, those with positive breath tests exhibit reductions in fasting small intestinal motor complexes, thereby predisposing to bacterial colonization of the small intestine [74]. Patients with diarrhea-predominance tend to produce increases in breath hydrogen after lactulose or glucose, whereas those with constipation generate excess methane (Fig. 15.4) [75–77]. This

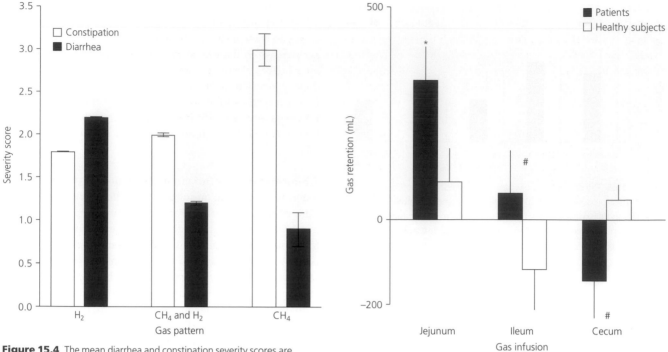

Figure 15.4 The mean diarrhea and constipation severity scores are shown for patients with purported small intestinal bacterial overgrowth as a function of the gas pattern [hydrogen (H_2), methane (CH_4), or both ($CH_4 + H_2$)] on lactulose breath testing. Constipation scores were significantly greater for individuals with methane production. From Pimentel et al. [75].

Figure 15.5 Responses to proximal vs distal gas perfusion are shown for patients with irritable bowel syndrome (IBS) and healthy volunteers. Compared with healthy subjects, patients with IBS developed significant gas retention with jejunal ($*P < 0.05$) but not ileal (#, not significant) or cecal (#, not significant) gas perfusion. From Salvioli et al. [84].

differential gas production may have pathogenic relevance. Constipated IBS patients with excess methane production exhibit reduced blood serotonin release after a glucose meal compared with hydrogen-producers [78]. In dogs, small intestinal methane perfusion delays transit while in isolated guinea pig ileum, methane augments contractile responsiveness to mechanical stimulation [76]. However, other groups using other diagnostic methods report much lower rates of overgrowth (10%–31%) in IBS and show no response to antibiotics [79, 80]. This is an area of active investigation.

Altered gas transit/perception in irritable bowel syndrome

Abnormal gut motor and sensory functions probably contribute to the pathogenesis of bloating in many cases of IBS [58]. Early studies referred to a splenic flexure syndrome with localized air trapping, which was suggestive of altered transit of lumenal gas. Small intestinal transit, measured scintigraphically, is accelerated in IBS patients with bloating compared with healthy volunteers [81]. In an argon washout study, patients with functional abdominal pain retained normal amounts of infused gas [82]. However, half of patients exhibited prolonged gas transit and many showed abnormal retrograde gas reflux into the stomach. In jejunal gas perfusion investigations, many patients with IBS exhibit abnormal gas

retention, which correlates with increased distention and symptoms of bloating [83]. In a recent study combining gas perfusion with radiolabeled xenon gas transit, patients with bloating exhibited selective retardation of gas flow in the small intestine, suggesting that this region is responsible for the generation of abdominal distention (Fig. 15.5) [84]. In these subjects, gas retention was observed only when gas was perfused into the jejunum whereas transit of gas perfused into the ileum or colon was normal. Lipid perfusion of the duodenum and jejunum but not ileum retards transit of jejunally perfused gas with associated increases in bloating and abdominal distention in patients with IBS [85, 86]. Indeed, the changes in gas retention observed during proximal intestinal lipid perfusion distinguish patients with IBS from healthy controls with more than 90% sensitivity and specificity [85]. Furthermore, reflex inhibition of nutrient-modulated gas flow is impaired in IBS. Rectal distention prevents retardation of gas flow during duodenal lipid perfusion in healthy subjects but has no effect in IBS, leading to gas retention in affected patients [87].

Other investigators report no alterations in retention and postulate that bloating results from visceral hypersensitivity. In one study, patients with IBS reported more pain with duodenal nitrogen perfusion and with sham gas perfusion compared with healthy volunteers [88]. Duodenojejunal motility indices were unaffected by true or sham gas perfusion in either subject group, suggesting that gaseous symptoms result from heightened perception rather than from alterations in gut transit. Recent studies suggest that perceptual hypersensitivity may be greater in those who complain of bloating without distention than in those with bloating and associated distention [89].

Abdominal wall factors in irritable bowel syndrome

In addition to gut neuromuscular factors, some cases of bloating may stem from dysfunctional somatic muscular activity within the abdominal wall [58]. Older studies postulated roles for weak abdominal muscles, a low diaphragm, or exaggerated lumbar lordosis [54]. Computed tomography (CT) scans of patients with IBS show increased lateral abdominal profiles, which may relate to changes in gut or abdominal wall muscle tone [90]. In a 2005 CT study in patients with bloating, severe episodes of abdominal distention were associated with exaggerated diaphragmatic descent [91]. Measurements of abdominal girth in healthy humans with inductance plethysmography demonstrate increases while sitting or standing compared with lying supine [92]. Likewise, girth increases after meal ingestion and decreases during sleep [92,93]. Using this method, bloated IBS patients with constipation exhibited significantly greater distention compared with bloated IBS patients with diarrhea [94]. However, in electromyographic studies of patients with IBS compared with healthy controls, no differences in abdominal wall activity were seen [95]. More recently, rectal gas perfusion studies reported increases in perception in IBS and functional bloating that were associated with changes in external and internal oblique muscle contraction, indicating an interaction of visceral and somatic musculature in the production of gaseous symptomatology [96].

Miscellaneous causes of gas and bloating

Most upper gut air in healthy individuals results from aerophagia, which occurs when intrathoracic pressure is negative. Aerophagia may be worsened by gum chewing, smoking, or oral irritation. Patients who have undergone laryngectomy experience gaseous complaints as a consequence of their air swallowing to facilitate esophageal speech. Patients with ulcer disease, gastroesophageal reflux, or biliary colic exhibit aerophagia and chronically belch in an effort to reduce their symptoms. Celiac disease may produce gaseous symptoms, including bloating and flatulence. Population-based studies observe increases in the prevalence of celiac disease in patients with presumed IBS compared with healthy controls [97]. Food allergy has been proposed to contribute to bloating in IBS; however, its importance remains to be defined. Selected immunoglobulin G4 antibodies to food antigens are reportedly elevated in some IBS patients with bloating [98,99]. Medications (anticholinergics, opiates, calcium blockers, antidepressants) produce gas by

their effects on gut motility. Psychological factors may play a role in the genesis of bloating in some patients with IBS. One-third of patients relate symptoms of bloating to stress or anxiety [52,53]. However, other studies observe no relation of bloating severity with degree of anxiety [100].

Evaluation of the patient with gas and bloating

The diagnostic approach to the patient with unexplained gas and bloating relies on a careful history and physical examination complemented by directed laboratory, structural, and functional testing.

History and physical examination

Patients with complaints of excess gas may report symptoms that are consistent with functional disease but which also could result from a structural abnormality. The clinician must search for clues that suggest an organic cause. Relief of symptoms with defecation or flatus is consistent with IBS, as is the absence of symptoms that awaken the patient from deep sleep. In contrast, vomiting, fever, weight loss, nocturnal diarrhea, rectal bleeding, or steatorrhea indicates probable organic disease. Conditions that predispose to small intestinal bacterial overgrowth should be determined by history. The use of medications that delay gut transit should be questioned. Assessment of ethnic background and family history can determine the risks for lactase deficiency or celiac disease. Finally, a history of anxiety or other psychiatric disease raises the possibility of aerophagia or a functional bowel disorder.

A dietary history may correlate symptoms with specific foods. Ingestion of legumes, fruits, unrefined starches, and lactose-containing foodstuffs should be addressed. The clinician should ascertain if soft drinks containing fructose or diet foods and gums containing sorbitol are being consumed. Activities that involve excess swallowing, such as gum chewing, smoking, and chewing tobacco, predispose to aerophagia.

The results of the physical examination are usually normal in patients with excess gas, but anxiety, hyperventilation, and air swallowing may be evident as an initial impression. Findings suggestive of organic disease include sclerodactyly with scleroderma, dermatitis herpetiformis in celiac disease, peripheral or autonomic neuropathy with dysmotility syndromes, and cachexia, jaundice, or palpable masses with malignant obstruction. Abdominal inspection may reveal scars from previous fundoplication, vagotomy, or other operations, which might cause adhesions. Auscultation assesses for absent bowel sounds with ileus or myopathic dysmotility, high-pitched bowel sounds with intestinal obstruction, or a succussion splash in gastric obstruction or gastroparesis. Abdominal percussion and palpation may reveal tympany and distention in the patient with mechanical obstruction or intestinal dysmotility. The presence of shifting dullness or a fluid wave indicates ascites rather than excess intestinal gas. Rectal examination is performed to exclude occult fecal blood, which would suggest lumenal inflammation or neoplasm.

In general, patients with gas and bloating do not experience serious sequelae as a consequence of their condition. However, some patients with complete mechanical intestinal obstruction or toxic megacolon secondary to inflammatory colitis may develop lumenal perforation, which can be life threatening. Patients with acute colonic pseudoobstruction are at risk of perforation because of thinning of the cecal wall. Rarely, patients with excess hydrogen-producing bacteria in the small intestine develop pneumatosis cystoides intestinalis [101]. Other complications from organic disease occur rarely and are generally manifestations of the underlying disease rather than of the gas itself. There have been case reports of explosions resulting from the ignition by tobacco smoking of feculent gas expelled by eructation in patients with gastrointestinal obstruction with bacterial overgrowth [102]. Colonic explosions have been reported infrequently in patients undergoing colonoscopy with mucosal cautery. These rare complications result from inadequate bowel cleansing or use of mannitol or sorbitol purging solutions, which generate hydrogen and methane to concentrations approaching 30%–45% [103].

Laboratory and structural testing

Laboratory tests facilitate the exclusion of organic disease. However, those individuals who satisfy the Rome criteria for IBS without evidence of alarm features may need only limited testing. In addition to standard hematology and chemistry determinations to screen for inflammatory or mucosal processes, thyroid chemistries or fasting cortisol levels are indicated in some individuals. Serological testing for celiac disease (tissue transglutaminase or endomysial antibodies) is performed in patients from appropriate ethnic backgrounds with IBS-like symptoms because of the increased prevalence of celiac sprue in these populations [104–106]. Other serologies of value in rare cases include antinuclear antibodies and scleroderma antibodies to evaluate for collagen vascular disease and antinuclear neuronal antibodies to screen for paraneoplastic visceral neuropathy [107]. Stool analysis for *Giardia* may be indicated in some patients with diarrhea.

Imaging tests may be performed in selected cases to distinguish mechanical obstruction from functional gas retention. Flat and upright abdominal radiographs may reveal diffuse distention consistent with ileus or pseudoobstruction, diffuse haziness in ascites, or air–fluid levels in the patient with intestinal obstruction. Distinguishing ileus from obstruction may not be accomplished by plain radiography alone. Contrast enema radiography can detect colonic or distal small intestinal obstruction. Small intestinal contrast radiography can evaluate for partial gastric outlet or small intestinal obstruction. Upper or lower endoscopy facilitates the identification

and biopsy of lesions producing partial blockage. Small bowel barium studies can also crudely quantify intestinal transit and assess motor patterns in patients with possible chronic intestinal pseudoobstruction. If suspicion for partial obstruction is high, enteroclysis may provide more detailed assessment of small intestinal lumenal processes [108]. With this technique, the proximal intestine is intubated under fluoroscopic guidance and barium and methylcellulose are perfused to provide a double-contrast image. Ultrasonography or CT scanning may provide useful information regarding the causes of gaseous distention and can exclude processes such as ascites, which may be misinterpreted as abdominal gas.

Functional testing

When results from structural tests are negative, methods to assess carbohydrate absorption, quantify gut transit and motor function, or measure flatus production can provide insight into the cause of symptoms.

Breath testing

Hydrogen breath testing can be used to confirm carbohydrate intolerance as a cause of gaseous symptoms. These methods quantify the hydrogen produced by lumenal bacteria during the metabolism of ingested test substrates. Conversely, carbohydrate metabolism by human tissues does not elicit hydrogen production. Expired breath samples are obtained before and for 2 h after ingesting a solution of the sugar, which is presumed to be maldigested or malabsorbed. Proper breath holding followed by immediate exhalation reduces the variability in hydrogen levels from 28% to 10% [109]. An increase in hydrogen of more than 20 parts per million within 120 min of lactose ingestion distinguishes biopsy-proven lactase deficiency from lactase-sufficiency with 90% sensitivity [110]. Hydrogen excretion after lactose ingestion correlates well with symptoms of carbohydrate maldigestion, while lactose tolerance testing with measurement of plasma glucose concentrations shows a poor correlation [111]. Hydrogen breath testing has also been used to detect fructose or sorbitol malabsorption; however, normal values for these tests are less well defined [112]. Hydrogen measurement may be extended to 10 h to test for maldigestion of complex carbohydrates. Even for lactose, some have proposed extending hydrogen measurements to 5–7 h to increase the sensitivity and specificity of the test [113]. Children with sucrose intolerance may be tested for sucrase-isomaltase deficiency with sucrose hydrogen breath testing. Some patients may be tested for fructose or sorbitol malabsorption using hydrogen breath testing, although normal values for these tests are less well defined.

Breath testing is also used to test for small intestinal bacterial overgrowth. Elevated fasting hydrogen or early rises within 30 min of substrate ingestion suggest overgrowth. Breath testing after glucose consumption provides sensitivities and specificities of 60%–90% for the diagnosis of bacterial overgrowth [114]. Lactulose and rice have been used as substrates; however, the sensitivities of these methods are as low as 17%–33% for detecting overgrowth [115]. False-negative results occur in patients without hydrogen-producing bacteria, while false-positive tests occur with rapid small intestinal transit. As a consequence, lactulose breath testing has not been universally accepted as a reliable test for bacterial overgrowth. Other centers rely on ^{14}C-labeled or ^{13}C-labeled substrates, with measurement $^{14}CO_2$ or $^{13}CO_2$ in the breath, although special facilities are necessary for these analyses. If the diagnosis is uncertain, diagnosis of bacterial overgrowth is made by documentation of bacterial counts greater than 10^5 CFU/mL on quantitative culture of duodenal or jejunal secretions [114].

Finally, hydrogen breath testing using lactulose is able to quantify orocecal transit in suspected intestinal pseudoobstruction. The transit time is measured from the time of ingestion until an increase in breath hydrogen is observed, reflecting colonic bacterial metabolism of the substrate. This method has significant limitations. Lactulose accelerates small intestinal transit [116]. Furthermore, erroneous values are obtained with superimposed bacterial overgrowth.

Tests of gut motor function

Gastric emptying tests or gastrointestinal manometry are sometimes performed for suspected gastrointestinal dysmotility as a cause of bloating. Scintigraphic measures of the emptying of radiolabeled solid meals (technetium 99m sulfur colloid in eggs) are used to exclude gastroparesis or rapid emptying. Other methods of quantifying gastric emptying include isotopic breath tests (e.g., ^{13}C-labeled octanoate) and ingested capsule techniques. In some centers, scintigraphy is used to the assess rates of small intestinal or colonic transit in suspected pseudoobstruction and constipation [117]. More often, radioopaque marker techniques are ordered to diagnose slow transit constipation [118]. In some cases, full thickness biopsy may be required to document degeneration of nerve or muscle layers.

Flatus analysis

In some research institutions, flatus analysis is performed to gain insight into the cause of excess flatulence [119]. Flatus passages are counted and expelled gas is analyzed. Excess release of nitrogen indicates probable aerophagia, whereas increases in carbon dioxide, hydrogen, and methane suggest increased colonic metabolism of ingested food residue.

Principles of management

Gaseous symptoms may respond to dietary measures, enzyme preparations that facilitate digestion, adsorbents and agents that decrease surface tension, treatments that alter gut flora, or drugs that modify gut transit. Evidence favoring any individual therapy is limited because few controlled investigations have been performed to compare the various treatments of gaseous symptoms.

Dietary and nonmedication therapy

Dietary measures may reduce gaseous symptoms in selected patients. Most lactase-deficient persons have residual enzyme activity and tolerate small amounts of lactose [120]. When consumed in yogurt with active cultures, lactose may be better tolerated because of bacterial β-galactosidase activity [121]. Breath hydrogen concentrations are 39% higher after consumption of pasteurized yogurt compared with unpasteurized samples because of the loss of intrinsic lactase activity. However, pasteurized yogurt containing up to 20 g lactose is tolerated by lactase-deficient individuals, suggesting that some of the benefits of yogurt stem from factors other than its enzymatic capabilities. Dairy products containing lactase-producing *Lactobacillus acidophilus*, *Bifidobacterium*, and *Lactobacillus bulgofilus* reduce bloating in some patients with lactose intolerance [122]. Children with sucrase-isomaltase deficiency also benefit from dietary modifications with elimination of sucrose. In some individuals, sucrose can slowly be reintroduced into the diet because the colon possesses some capacity for fermentation of the sugar. In some instances, the foods themselves may be modified to decrease their propensity to produce gas. Soaking cowpeas and yam beans for 12 h and cooking for 30 min eliminates most malabsorbed oligosaccharides, reducing raffinose from 0.71%–6.86% to 0.04%–0.40% and stachyose from 2.38%–4.14% to 0.12%–0.72% [123]. Gamma irradiation to levels used for insect disinfestation (0.25–0.75 kGy) also reduces raffinose in mung beans [124].

Studies of carbohydrate exclusion diets in patients with IBS do not show convincing benefits. Only a small fraction of patients with IBS who have documented lactase deficiency respond to lactose restriction. Similarly, in an older study, less than 40% experience symptom improvement on exclusion of fructose and sorbitol [64]. However, some newer studies report more impressive responses to dietary restriction of these compounds. In a recent investigation of patients with functional causes of bloating, 72% exhibited evidence of malabsorption of lactose, fructose plus sorbitol, or both [125]. Two-thirds of these individuals reported symptom improvements on diets that restricted sugars that were malabsorbed. In another investigation of 62 IBS patients with fructose intolerance demonstrated by hydrogen breath testing, dietary fructose exclusion led to symptom improvement in 85% [126]. Low gas diets that exclude many complex carbohydrates reduce flatus frequency by up to 50% in some individuals (Table 15.1) [127]. Patients with IBS who have evidence of celiac disease may respond to dietary gluten exclusion [128]. In IBS patients with food allergy documented by elevated immunoglobulin G4 antibodies to

Table 15.1 Foods that promote significant gas production

Dairy products
Vegetables
    Onions
    Beans
    Celery
    Carrots
    Brussels sprouts
Fruits
    Raisins
    Bananas
    Apricots
    Prune juice
Complex carbohydrates
    Pretzels
    Bagels
    Wheat germ

Adapted from Levitt [127].

food antigens, exclusion diets have been reported to be beneficial [98,99,129].

Lifestyle changes are useful for selected patients. Aerophagia may be reduced by stopping gum chewing and smoking. Chronic belchers may better understand the role of aerophagia by observing their swallowing mechanics in a mirror. Initiation of mild exercise has been shown to enhance clearance of jejunal gas loads in patients with IBS [130]. Gas-trapping undergarments are available for those with excess malodorous flatus [4].

Enzymes, adsorbents, and agents to reduce surface tension

Exogenous enzymes facilitate the breakdown of undigested food residue (Table 15.2). Preparations of β-galactosidase (lactase) are marketed to treat lactase deficiency. In adults, lactase supplements reduce hydrogen excretion and bloating, cramps, and flatulence after ingestion of lactose [131]. Similarly, in lactose-intolerant children, lactase tablets reduce hydrogen levels after a lactose challenge from 60 to 7 parts per million with reductions in pain, bloating, diarrhea, and flatulence [132]. Small studies have reported differential efficacy of different lactase preparations, but this finding must be confirmed in larger trials [133]. Bacterial α-galactosidase derived from *Aspergillus niger* (Beano) reduces flatulence in healthy volunteers who consume meatless chili [134]. However, most indigestible fiber does not contain galactose so this agent is unlikely to produce benefit when diets that are not legume-rich are consumed. Pancreatic enzymes reduce bloating, gas, and fullness after high-calorie, high-fat meals in healthy individuals; however, their utility in patients with excess gas and bloating is unexplored [135]. Hydrogen production and bloating and cramping decrease when children with sucrase-isomaltase deficiency are given sacrosidase, a liquid from *Saccharomyces cerevisiae* that contains 6000 IU sucrase activity per mg of protein [136].

Agents that reduce the surface tension of gas bubbles and adsorbents are commonly used for gaseous symptoms (Table 15.2). Simethicone promotes the rupture of thick foam films. Effects of simethicone on hydrogen production are inconsistent; however, benefits have been reported in some patients with functional dyspepsia and with gas-related discomfort from chronic diarrhea [137,138]. Activated charcoal

Table 15.2 Medication therapies for gas and bloating

Medication class	Examples	Comments
Enzyme preparations	β-Galactosidase (lactase)	For lactose intolerance; variable effectiveness in lactose-intolerant IBS patients
	α-Galactosidase	Effective for legume-rich meals in healthy volunteers
	Pancreatic enzymes	Uncertain efficacy for gas and bloating of any cause
Adsorbents and agents that reduce surface tension	Simethicone in IBS	Possible benefits in functional dyspepsia and gas with diarrhea; uncertain benefits in IBS
	Activated charcoal	Possible benefits in gas production and malodorous flatus; charcoal-lined undergarments are available
	Bismuth subsalicylate	Possible benefits in reducing malodorous flatus
Treatments to modify gut flora	Antibiotics	Useful for bacterial overgrowth secondary to organic disease; possible benefits in IBS
	Probiotics (*Lactobacillus*, *Bifidobacterium*)	Possible benefits in IBS
	Prebiotics	Uncertain benefits in IBS
Prokinetic medications	Tegaserod	Reduces bloating in IBS; recently withdrawn from US market
	Neostigmine	Reduces lumenal distention in acute colonic pseudoobstruction; uncertain benefits in bloating

IBS, irritable bowel syndrome.

reduced flatulence and hydrogen production after consumption of carbohydrate-rich meals in two studies; however, another investigation showed no reductions from charcoal after eating baked beans [139–141]. The benefits of charcoal on flatus odor are unproved. The combination of charcoal, *Yucca schidigera*, and zinc acetate reduced malodorous flatulence by 86% in one study, but charcoal had no effect in another investigation [142]. Bismuth inhibits the in vitro fermentation of lactose-enriched feces and impairs hydrogen sulfide release. In flatulent patients, bismuth subsalicylate reduces the fermentation of raffinose, suggesting possible benefits in reducing flatus odor [143].

Treatments to modify gut flora

Antibiotics provide benefit to selected patients with gaseous syndromes (Table 15.2). Proven bacterial overgrowth may impressively respond to a single prescription of oral antibiotics, although some individuals require multiple or rotating courses. Antibiotics in several drug classes have shown efficacy in this condition including inexpensive agents such as tetracycline and metronidazole. In patients with systemic sclerosis, ciprofloxacin produces superior symptom control vs trimethoprim [144]. In a second study, amoxicillin–clavulinic acid and cefoxitin were effective for more than 90% of strains responsible for small intestinal bacterial overgrowth [145]. A third investigation observed 70% reductions in breath hydrogen after norfloxacin [146]. Investigators who postulate a pathogenic role for abnormal gut flora in IBS have reported short-term benefits with antibiotic therapy. In an uncontrolled study using whole-body calorimetry, hydrogen production by patients with IBS was reduced by metronidazole [147]. In 111 patients with IBS, neomycin reduced symptoms of IBS by 35% compared with 11% with placebo [148]. In constipation-predominant IBS patients, neomycin was reported to reduce symptoms to a greater degree than placebo – especially in those individuals who exhibited increased

methane production during lactulose breath testing [149]. The recently approved nonabsorbable antibiotic rifaximin has been reported to reduce gaseous symptoms in patients with functional gastrointestinal disorders both in open label and placebo-controlled trials [150,151]. In a more recent, double-blind placebo-controlled trial in 87 patients with IBS, rifaximin was shown to reduce bloating, bowel disturbances, and abdominal discomfort for at least 10 weeks [152].

Another means of modifying the gut flora is to replace pathogenic colonic organisms with ingested innocuous strains (Table 15.2). Physiological benefits of such probiotics may include enhancing the epithelial barrier, decreasing lumenal pH, blocking bacterial adhesion, and releasing neuroactive mediators such as nitric oxide [153]. Placebo-controlled trials of the probiotic preparation VSL#3 in patients with IBS show reductions in flatulence or bloating without improvement in pain or bowel disturbance [154,155]. VSL#3 therapy increases populations of *Lactobacillus*, *Streptococcus thermophilus*, and *Bifidobactera* and reduces fecal β-galactosidase and urease activities [156]. A recent investigation with *Bifidobacterium infantis* reported decreases in pain, discomfort, bloating, distention, and defecatory difficulty in patients with IBS that were associated with the reversal of ratios of proinflammatory interleukin-10 to interleukin-12, suggesting a modulatory effect on gut immune function (Fig. 15.6) [157]. In a follow-up, large, multicenter trial, reductions in scores for bloating, as well as for other symptoms of IBS, with *Bifidobacterium infantis* treatment exceeded those during placebo treatment by more than 20% [158]. In contrast, no similar benefits were seen with *Lactobacillus salivarius* treatment. Other probiotic preparations have been reported to reduce symptoms in some individuals [159, 160].

Dietary modifications may also influence enteric microbial activities. In one study, consumption of an elemental diet reduced breath hydrogen excretion with associated symptom

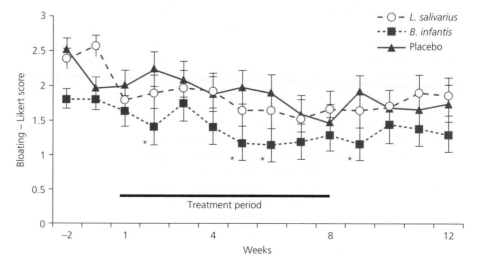

Figure 15.6 The effects of probiotic treatment on Likert scores for bloating are shown as a function of time in patients with irritable bowel syndrome. Probiotics containing *Bifidobacterium infantis* produced significant reductions in bloating at 2, 5, 6, and 9 weeks compared with placebo probiotics. In contrast, preparations containing *Lactobacillus salivarius* produced no benefit. From O'Mahony et al. [157].

improvement [161]. Another potential method to change the gut flora is to administer prebiotic nutrients that promote the growth of beneficial bacteria to the exclusion of pathogenic strains. Inulin, lactulose, oligofructose, and galactooligosaccharides selectively nourish strains of *Lactobacillus* and *Bifidobacterium*, in part as the result of enhanced enzymatic activities in these organisms, including β-fructosidase [162, 163]. In a study of 40 healthy volunteers, short-chain fructooligosaccharide ingestion increased fecal bifidobacteria and total anaerobes but had no effect on *Bacteroides*, *Lactobacillus*, or enterobacterial counts [164]. Bifidobacteria possess significant β-fructosidase levels that hydrolyze β1-2 glycosidic bonds in oligofructose and inulin, which may represent a mechanism for the effect of prebiotic feedings [165]. The utility of therapy with prebiotics alone or in combination with probiotics is being explored [166].

Prokinetic medications

Drugs that stimulate gut propulsion theoretically should benefit patients with pathological gas retention (Table 15.2). The serotonin 5-HT$_4$ agonist tegaserod reduced bloating in controlled trials of constipation-predominant IBS [167]. In patients with IBS who were maintained on tegaserod, withdrawal of medication led to a prompt recurrence of bloating and abdominal discomfort [168]. In healthy volunteers, tegaserod stimulates transit of jejunally perfused gas mixtures, suggesting that its beneficial effects on bloating may relate to its prokinetic capabilities [169]. However, this drug was recently withdrawn from the US market because of observed increases in cardiovascular events. Similarly, the acetylcholinesterase inhibitor neostigmine stimulates the flow of gas perfused into the jejunum in patients with IBS and patients with functional bloating with associated reductions in abdominal distention and symptoms [170]. The clinical utility of this medication to treat gas and bloating has not been confirmed in controlled trials.

Miscellaneous therapies

Other therapies are effective for selected IBS patients with gas and bloating. In placebo-controlled trials, selective serotonin reuptake inhibitors such as citalopram and fluoxetine significantly reduce bloating in patients with IBS independent of effects to reduce anxiety or depression [171,172]. However, in a third study, paroxetine did not produce superior reductions in gastrointestinal symptoms compared with placebo [173]. Herbal extracts containing *Mentha spicata* and *Coriandrum sativum* reduce bloating to greater degrees than placebo in patients with IBS, purportedly because of their antispasmodic effects [174]. Hypnotherapy and acupuncture have been reported to reduce gaseous symptoms in IBS [175,176].

Operative therapies for gas and bloating are usually considered only for the most refractory patients with severe organic disease. Percutaneous endoscopic gastrostomy is effective in selected cases of gas-bloat syndrome after fundo-

plication [177]. Excision of small intestinal diverticula reduced symptoms and vitamin B-12 malabsorption in a patient with small intestinal bacterial overgrowth. Selected patients with localized intestinal pseudoobstruction may benefit from resection of the dysfunctional bowel segment. Patients with more extensive intestinal pseudoobstruction may experience symptom relief with a venting jejunostomy [178]. Similarly, some patients with acute colonic pseudoobstruction may need surgical or radiographic insertion of a decompressing cecostomy to prevent rupture of the organ. Finally, some individuals with advanced pseudoobstruction require surgical or radiographic placement of indwelling central venous catheters for home total parenteral nutrition.

References

1. Tomlin J, Lowis C, Read NW. Investigation of normal flatus production in healthy volunteers. Gut 1991;32:665.
2. Furne JK, Levitt MD. Factors influencing frequency of flatus emission by healthy subjects. Dig Dis Sci 1996;41:1631.
3. Suarez F, Furne J, Springfield J, Levitt M. Insights into human colonic physiology obtained from the study of flatus composition. Am J Physiol 1997;272:G1028.
4. Suarez FL, Springfield J, Levitt MD. Identification of gases responsible for the odour of human flatus and evaluation of a device purported to reduce this odour. Gut 1998;43:100.
5. Bolin TD, Stanton RA. Flatus emission patterns and fibre intake. Eur J Surg Suppl 1998;582:115.
6. Strocchi A, Levitt MD. Factors affecting hydrogen production and consumption by human fecal flora. The critical roles of hydrogen tension and methanogenesis. J Clin Invest 1992;89:1304.
7. Hertzler SR, Savaiano DA, Levitt MD. Fecal hydrogen production and consumption measurements. Response to daily lactose ingestion by lactose maldigesters. Dig Dis Sci 1997;42:348.
8. Serra J, Azpiroz F, Malagelada JR. Intestinal gas dynamics and tolerance in humans. Gastroenterology 1998;115:542.
9. Gonlachanvit S, Coleski R, Owyang C, Hasler WL. Inhibitory actions of a high fibre diet on intestinal gas transit in healthy humans. Gut 2004;53:1577.
10. Gonlachanvit S, Coleski R, Owyang C, Hasler WL. Nutrient modulation of intestinal gas dynamics in healthy humans: dependence on caloric content and meal consistency. Am J Physiol – Gastrointest Liver Physiol 2006;291:G389.
11. Serra J, Azpiroz F, Malagelada JR. Gastric distention and duodenal lipid perfusion modulate intestinal gas transit and tolerance in humans. Am J Gastroenterol 2002;97:2225.
12. Hernando-Harder AC, Serra J, Azpiroz F, Malagelada JR. Sites of symptomatic gas retention during intestinal lipid perfusion in healthy subjects. Gut 2004;53:661.
13. Dianese R, Serra J, Azpiroz F, Malagelada JR. Influence of body posture on intestinal transit of gas. Gut 2003;52:971.
14. Dianese R, Serra J, Azpiroz F, Malagelada JR. Effects of physical activity on intestinal gas transit and evacuation in healthy subjects. Am J Med 2004;116:536.
15. Coleski R, Hasler W. Induction of propagated colonic contractions during jejunal gas perfusion in healthy humans: a possible physiologic enterocolonic reflex for expulsion of excess luminal gas (abstract). Neurogastroenterol Motil 2007;19:423.
16. Tremolaterra F, Villoria A, Serra J, et al. Intestinal tone and gas motion. Neurogastroenterol Motil 2006;18:905.
17. Serra J, Azpiroz F, Malagelada JR. Mechanisms of intestinal gas retention in humans: impaired propulsion versus obstructed evacuation. Am J Physiol – Gastrointest Liver Physiol 2001;281:G138.

18. Harder H, Serra J, Azpiroz F, et al. Intestinal gas distribution determines abdominal symptoms. Gut 2003;52:1708.

19. Harder H, Serra J, Azpiroz F, Malagelada JR. Reflex control of intestinal gas dynamics and tolerance in humans. Am J Physiol – Gastrointest Liver Physiol 2004;286:G89.

20. Kahrilas PJ, Dodds WJ, Dent J, et al. Upper esophageal sphincter function during belching. Gastroenterology 1986;91:133.

21. Bassotti G, Germani U, Morelli A. Flatus-related colorectal and anal motor events. Dig Dis Sci 1996;41:335.

22. Sandler RS, Stewart WF, Liberman JN, et al. Abdominal pain, bloating, and diarrhea in the United States – prevalence and impact. Dig Dis Sci 2000;45:1166.

23. Drossman DA, Li Z, Andruzzi E, at al. US householder survey of functional gastrointestinal disorders. Prevalence, sociodemography, and health impact. Dig Dis Sci 1993;38:1569.

24. Scrimshaw NS, Murray EB. The acceptability of milk and milk products in populations with a high prevalence of lactose intolerance. Am J Clin Nutr 1988;48(4 Suppl.):1079.

25. Suarez FL, Savaiano DA, Levitt MD. A comparison of symptoms after the consumption of milk or lactose-hydrolyzed milk by people with self-reported severe lactose intolerance. N Engl J Med 1995;333:1.

26. Bond JH, Levitt MD, Prentiss R. Investigation of small bowel transit time in man utilizing pulmonary hydrogen (H_2 measurements). J Lab Clin Med 1975;85:546.

27. Ravich WJ, Bayless TM, Thomas M. Fructose: incomplete absorption in humans. Gastroenterology 1983;84:26.

28. Jain NK, Rosenberg DB, Ulahannan MJ, et al. Sorbitol intolerance in adults. Am J Gastroenterol 1985;80:678.

29. Hyams JS. Sorbitol intolerance: an unappreciated cause of functional gastrointestinal complaints. Gastroenterology 1983;84:30.

30. Lee A, Zumbe A, Storey D. Breath hydrogen after ingestion of the bulk sweeteners sorbitol, isomalt and sucrose in chocolate. Br J Nutr 1994;71:731.

31. Bond JH, Currier BE, Buchwald H, Levitt MD. Colonic conservation of malabsorbed carbohydrate. Gastroenterology 1980;78:444.

32. Ouwendijk J, Moolenaar CE, Peters WJ, et al. Congenital sucrase-isomaltase deficiency: identification of a glutamine to praline substitution that leads to a transport block of sucrase-isomaltase in a pre-Golgi compartment. J Clin Invest 1996;97:633.

33. Levitt MD, Hirsh P, Fetzer CA, et al. H_2 excretion after ingestion of complex carbohydrates. Gastroenterology 1987;92:383.

34. Suarez FL, Springfield J, Furne JK, et al. Gas production in human ingesting a soybean flour derived from beans naturally low in oligosaccharides. Am J Clin Nutr 1999;69:135.

35. Kajs TM, Fitzgerald JA, Buckner RY, et al. Influence of methanogenic flora on the breath H_2 and symptom response to ingestion of sorbitol or oat fiber. Am J Gastroenterol 1997;92:89.

36. Levitt MD, Furne J, Olsson S. The relation of passage of gas and abdominal bloating to colonic gas production. Ann Intern Med 1996;124:422.

37. Suau A. Molecular tools to investigate intestinal bacterial communities. J Pediatr Gastroenterol Nutr 2003;3:222.

38. Gorbach SL, Barza M, Giuliano M, Jacobus NV. Colonization resistance of the human intestinal microflora: testing the hypothesis in normal volunteers. Eur J Clin Microbiol Infect Dis 1988;7:98.

39. Gibson GR, Wang X. Regulatory effects of bifidobacteria on the growth of other colonic bacteria. J Appl Bacteriol 1994;77:412.

40. Houghton LA, Green TJ, Donovan UM, et al. Association between dietary fiber intake and the folate status of a group of female adolescents. Am J Clin Nutr 1997;66:1414.

41. Langlands SJ, Hopkins MJ, Coleman N, Cummings JH. Prebiotic carbohydrates modify the mucosa associated microflora of the human large bowel. Gut 2004; 53: 1610–1616.

42. Bauer TM, Steinbruckner B, Brinkmann FE, et al. Small intestinal bacterial overgrowth in patients with cirrhosis: prevalence and relation with spontaneous bacterial peritonitis. Am J Gastroenterol 2001;96:2962.

43. Fried M, Siegrist H, Frei R, et al. Duodenal bacterial overgrowth during treatment in outpatients with omeprazole. Gut 1994;35:23.

44. Virally-Monod M, Tielmans D, Kevorkian JP, et al. Chronic diarrhea and diabetes mellitus: prevalence of small intestinal bacterial overgrowth. Diabetes Metab 1998;24:530.

45. Reddymasu S, Sarosiek I, Sostarich S, McCallum R. Incidence and predictors of small intestinal bacterial overgrowth in gastroparesis (abstract). Gastroenterology 2007;132:686.

46. Lin HC, Van Citters GW, Zhao XT, Waxman A. Fat intolerance depends on rapid gastric emptying. Dig Dis Sci 1999;44:330.

47. Anvari M, Allen C. Postprandial bloating after laparoscopic Nissen fundoplication. Can J Surg 2001;44:440.

48. Lembo T, Naliboff B, Munakata J, et al. Symptoms and visceral perception in patients with pain-predominant irritable bowel syndrome. Am J Gastroenterol 1999;94:1320.

49. Hahn B, Watson M, Yan S, et al. Irritable bowel syndrome patterns: frequency, duration, and severity. Dig Dis Sci 1998;43:2715.

50. Lee OY, Mayer EA, Schmulson M, et al. Gender-related differences in IBS symptoms. Am J Gastroenterol 2001;96:2184.

51. Heitkemper MM, Cain KC, Jarrett ME, et al. Relationship of bloating to other GI and menstrual symptoms in women with irritable bowel syndrome. Dig Dis Sci 2004;49:88.

52. Chang L, Lee OY, Naliboff B, et al. Sensation of bloating and visible abdominal distension in patients with irritable bowel syndrome. Am J Gastroenterol 2001;96:3341.

53. Maxton DG, Whorwell PJ. Abdominal distension in irritable bowel syndrome: the patient's perception. Eur J Gastroenterol Hepatol 1992;4:241.

54. Schmulson M, Lee OY, Chang L, et al. Symptom differences in moderate to severe IBS patients based on predominant bowel habit. Am J Gastroenterol 1999;94:2929.

55. Talley NJ, Dennis EH, Schettler-Duncan VA, et al. Overlapping upper and lower gastrointestinal symptoms in irritable bowel syndrome patients with constipation or diarrhea. Am J Gastroenterol 2003;98.2454.

56. Ragnarsson G, Bodemar G. Division of the irritable bowel syndrome into subgroups on the basis of daily recorded symptoms in two outpatients samples. Scand J Gastroenterol 1999;34:993.

57. Lea R, Reilly B, Whorwell PJ, Houghton LA. The effect of bowel habit and time of day on the relationship between bloating and visible distension in patients with irritable bowel syndrome (abstract). Gastroenterology 2004;126:1634.

58. Azpiroz F, Malagelada JR. Abdominal bloating. Gastroenterology 2005;129:1060.

59. Koide A, Yamaguchi T, Odaka T, et al. Quantitative analysis of bowel gas using plain abdominal radiograph in patients with irritable bowel syndrome. Am J Gastroenterol 2000;95:1735.

60. Chami TN, Schuster MM, Bohlman ME, et al. A simple radiologic method to estimate the quantity of bowel gas. Am J Gastroenterol 1991;86:599.

61. Tolliver BA, Herrera JL, DiPalma JA. Evaluation of patients who meet clinical criteria for irritable bowel syndrome. Am J Gastroenterol 1994;89:176.

62. Tolliver BA, Jackson MS, Jackson KL, et al. Does lactose maldigestion really play a role in the irritable bowel? J Clin Gastroenterol 1996;23:15.

63. Lisker R, Solomons NW, Perez BR, Ramirez MM. Lactase and placebo in the management of the irritable bowel syndrome: a double-blind, cross-over study. Am J Gastroenterol 1989;84:756.

64. Fernandez-Banares F, Esteve-Pardo M, de Lean R, et al. Sugar malabsorption in functional bowel disease: clinical implications. Am J Gastroenterol 1993;88:2044.

65. Goldstein R, Braverman D, Stankiewicz H. Carbohydrate malabsorption and the effect of dietary restriction on symptoms in irritable bowel syndrome and functional bowel complaints. Isr Med Assoc J 2000;2:583.

66. Hotz J, Plein K. Effectiveness of plantago seed husks in comparison with wheat bran on stool frequency and manifestations of irritable colon syndrome with constipation. Med Klin 1994;89:645.

67. Wollner JT, Kirby GA. Clinical audit of the effects of low-fibre diet on irritable bowel syndrome. J Human Nutr Diet 2000;13:249.

68. King TS, Elia M, Hunter DO. Abnormal colonic fermentation in irritable bowel syndrome. Lancet 1998;352:1187.

69. Haderstorfer B, Whitehead WE, Schuster MM. Intestinal gas production from bacterial fermentation of undigested carbohydrate in irritable bowel syndrome. Am J Gastroenterol 1989;84:375.

70. Balsari A, Ceccarelli A, Dubini F, et al. The fecal microbial population in the irritable bowel syndrome. Microbiologica 1982;5:185.

71. Khalif IL, Quigley EM, Konovitch EA, Maximova ID. Alterations in the colonic flora and intestinal permeability and evidence of immune activation in chronic constipation. Dig Liver Dis 2005;37:838.

72. Malinen E, Rinttila T, Kajander K, et al. Analysis of the fecal microbiota of irritable bowel syndrome patients and healthy controls with real-time PCR. Am J Gastroenterol 2005;100:373.

73. Pimentel M, Chow EJ, Lin HC. Eradication of small intestinal bacterial overgrowth reduces symptoms of irritable bowel syndrome. Am J Gastroenterol 2000;95:3503.

74. Pimentel M, Soffer EE, Chow EJ, et al. Lower frequency of MMC is found in IBS subjects with abnormal lactulose breath test, suggesting bacterial overgrowth. Dig Dis Sci 2002;47:2639.

75. Pimentel M, Mayer AG, Park S, et al. Methane production during lactulose breath test is associated with gastrointestinal disease presentation. Dig Dis Sci 2003;48:86.

76. Pimentel M, Lin HC, Enayati P, et al. Methane, a gas produced by enteric bacteria, slows intestinal transit and augments small intestinal contractile activity. Am J Physiol – Gastrointest Liver Physiol 2006;290:G1089.

77. Coleski R, Hasler W. Hydrogen and methane breath testing for small intestinal bacterial overgrowth in patients with unexplained gas and bloating: factors relating to test positivity and response to antibiotics (abstract). Neurogastroenterol Motil 2007;19:433.

78. Pimentel M, Kong Y, Park S. IBS subjects with methane on lactulose breath test have lower postprandial serotonin levels than subjects with hydrogen. Dig Dis Sci 2004;49:84.

79. Walters B, Vanner SJ. Detection of bacterial overgrowth in IBS using the lactulose H2 breath test: comparison with 14C-D-xylose and healthy controls. Am J Gastroenterol 2005;100:1566.

80. Lupascu A, Gabrielli M, Lauritano EC, et al. Hydrogen glucose breath test to detect small intestinal bacterial overgrowth: a prevalence case-control study in irritable bowel syndrome. Aliment Pharmacol Ther 2005;22:1157.

81. Trotman IF, Price CC. Bloated irritable bowel syndrome defined by dynamic ^{99m}Tc bran scan. Lancet 1986; 2:364.

82. Lasser RB, Bond JH, Levitt MD. The role of intestinal gas in functional abdominal pain. N Engl J Med 1975;293:524.

83. Serra J, Azpiroz F, Malagelada JR. Impaired transit and tolerance of intestinal gas in the irritable bowel syndrome. Gut 2001;48:14.

84. Salvioli B, Serra J, Azpiroz F, et al. Origin of gas retention and symptoms in patients with bloating. Gastroenterology 2005;128:574.

85. Serra J, Salvioli B, Azpiroz F, Malagelada JR. Lipid-induced intestinal gas retention in irritable bowel syndrome. Gastroenterology 2002;123:700.

86. Salvioli B, Serra J, Azpiroz F, Malagelada JR. Impaired small bowel gas propulsion in patients with bloating during intestinal lipid perfusion. Am J Gastroenterol 2006;101:1853.

87. Passos M, Serra J, Azpiroz F, et al. Impaired reflex control of intestinal gas transit in patients with abdominal bloating. Gut 2005;54:344.

88. Galati JS, McKee DP, Quigley EM. Response to intraluminal gas in irritable bowel syndrome. Motility versus perception. Dig Dis Sci 1995;40:1381.

89. Lea R, Reilly B, Whorwell PJ, Houghton LA. Abdominal bloating in the absence of physical distension is related to increased visceral sensitivity (abstract). Gastroenterology 2004;126:432.

90. Maxton DG, Martin DF, Whorwell PJ, Godfrey M. Abdominal distension in female patients with irritable bowel syndrome: exploration of possible mechanisms. Gut 1991;32:662.

91. Perez F, Accarino AM, Azpiroz F, et al. Measurement of intestinal gas volume using a new CT-based analysis program (abstract). Gastroenterology 2005;128:A675.

92. Lewis MJ, Reilly B, Houghton LA, Whorwell PJ. Ambulatory abdominal inductance plethysmography: towards objective assessment of abdominal distension in irritable bowel syndrome. Gut 2001;48:216.

93. Reilly BP, Bolton MP, Lewis MJ, et al. A device for 24 hour ambulatory monitoring of abdominal girth using inductive plethysmography. Physiol Meas 2002;23:661.

94. Houghton LA, Lea R, Agrawal A, et al. Relationship of abdominal bloating to distension in irritable bowel syndrome and effect of bowel habit. Gastroenterology 2006;131:1003.

95. McManis PG, Newall D, Talley NJ. Abdominal wall muscle activity in irritable bowel syndrome. Am J Gastroenterol 2001;96:1139.

96. Tremolaterra F, Villoria A, Azpiroz F, et al. Impaired viscerosomatic reflexes and abdominal-wall dystony associated with bloating. Gastroenterology 2006;130:1062.

97. Sanders DS, Carter MJ, Hurlstone DP, et al. Association of adult coeliac disease with irritable bowel syndrome: a case–control study in patients fulfilling ROME II criteria referred to secondary care. Lancet 2001;358:1504.

98. Zar S, Benson MJ, Kumar D. Serum IgG4 antibodies to common food antigens are elevated in irritable bowel syndrome (abstract). Gut 2002;50(Suppl. 11):A25.

99. El Rafei A, Peters SM, Harris N, Bellanti JA. Diagnostic value of IgG4 measurements in patients with food allergy. Ann Allergy 1989;62:94.

100. Sullivan SN. A prospective study of unexplained visible abdominal bloating. NZ Med J 1994;107:428.

101. Levitt MD, Olsson S. Pneumatosis cystoids intestinalis and high breath H_2 excretion: insights into the role of H_2 in this condition. Gastroenterology 1995;108:1560.

102. Tolliver BA, Berry MA, DiPalma JA. Eructation flambe. J Clin Gastroenterol 1994;18:267.

103. Bond JH, Levitt MD. Factors affecting the concentration of combustible gases in the colon during colonoscopy. Gastroenterology 1976;68:1445.

104. Cash BD, Schoenfeld P, Chey WD. The utility of diagnostic tests in irritable bowel syndrome patients: a systematic review. Am J Gastroenterol 2002;97:2812.

105. Spiegel BM, DeRosa VP, Gralnek IM, et al. Testing for celiac sprue in irritable bowel syndrome with predominant diarrhea: a cost-effectiveness analysis. Gastroenterology 2004;126:1721.

106. Mein SM, Ladabaum U. Serological testing for coeliac disease in patients with symptoms of irritable bowel syndrome: a cost-effectiveness analysis. Aliment Pharmacol Ther 2004;19:1199.

107. Lucchinetti CF, Kimmel DW, Lennon VA. Paraneoplastic and oncologic profiles of patients seropositive for type 1 antineuronal nuclear autoantibodies. Neurology 1998;50:652.

108. Maglinte DD, Peterson LA, Vahey TN, et al. Enteroclysis in partial small bowel obstruction. Am J Surg 1984;147:325.

109. Strocchi A, Ellis C, Levitt MD. Reproducibility of measurements of trace gas concentrations in expired air. Gastroenterology 1991;101:175.

110. Barr RG, Watkins JB, Perman JA. Mucosal function and breath hydrogen excretion: comparative studies in the clinical evaluation of children with nonspecific abdominal complaints. Pediatrics 1981; 68:526.

111. Hermans MM, Brummer RJ, Ruijgers AM, Stockbrugger RW. The relationship between lactose intolerance test results and symptoms of lactose intolerance. Am J Gastroenterol 1997;92:981.

112. Choi YK, Johlin FC, Summers RW, et al. Fructose intolerance: an under-recognized problem. Am J Gastroenterol 2003;98:1348.

113. Strocchi A, Corazza G, Ellis CJ, et al. Detection of malabsorption of low doses of carbohydrate: accuracy of various breath H_2 criteria. Gastroenterology 1993;105:1404.

114. Corazza GR, Menozzi MG, Strocchi A, et al. The diagnosis of small bowel bacterial overgrowth. Reliability of jejunal culture and inadequacy of breath hydrogen testing. Gastroenterology 1990;98:302.

115. Riordan SM, McIver CJ, Duncombe VM, et al. Evaluation of the rice hydrogen breath test for small intestinal bacterial overgrowth. Am J Gastroenterol 2000;95:2858.

116. Miller MA, Parkman HP, Urbain JL, et al. Comparison of scintigraphy and lactulose breath hydrogen test for assessment of orocecal transit. Lactulose accelerates small bowel transit. Dig Dis Sci 1997;42:10.

117. Charles F, Camilleri M, Phillips SF, et al. Scintigraphy of the whole gut: clinical evaluation of transit disorders. Mayo Clin Proc 1995;70:113.

118. Metcalf AM, Phillips SF, Zinsmeister AR, et al. Simplified assessment of segmental colonic transit. Gastroenterology 1987;92:40.

119. Levitt MD, Furne J, Aeolus MR, Suarez FL. Evaluation of an extremely flatulent patient: case report and proposed diagnostic and therapeutic approach. Am J Gastroenterol 1998;93:2276.

120. Vesa TH, Korpela RA, Sahi T. Tolerance to small amounts of lactose in lactose maldigesters. Am J Clin Nutr 1996;64:197.

121. Kolars JC, Levitt MD, Aouji M, Savaiano DA. Yogurt – an autodigesting source of lactose. N Engl J Med 1984;310:1.

122. Vesa TH, Marteau P, Zidi S, et al. Digestion and tolerance of lactose from yoghurt and different semi-solid fermented dairy products containing *Lactobacillus acidophilus* and bifidobacteria in lactose maldigesters – is bacterial lactase important? Eur J Clin Nutr 1996;50:730.

123. Nwinuka NM, Abbey BW, Ayalogu EO. Effect of processing on flatus producing oligosaccharides in cowpea (*Vigna unguiculata*) and the troipical African yam bean (*Sphenostylis stenocarpa*). Plant Foods Hum Nutr 1997;51:209.

124. Machaiah JP, Pednekar MD, Thomas P. Reduction in flatulence factors in mung beans (*Vigna raidata*) using low-dose gamma-irradiation. J Sci Food Agricult 1999;79:648.

125. Fernandez-Banares F, Rosinach M, Esteve M, et al. Sugar malabsorption in functional abdominal bloating: a pilot study on the long-term effect of dietary treatment. Clin Nutr 2006;25:824.

126. Shepherd SJ, Gibson PR. Fructose malabsorption and symptoms of irritable bowel syndrome: guidelines for effective dietary management. J Am Diet Assoc 2006;106:1631.

127. Levitt MD. Follow-up of a flatulent patient. Dig Dis Sci 1979;24:652.

128. Wahnschaffe U, Ullrich R, Riecken EO, Schulzke JD. Celiac disease-like abnormalities in a subgroup of patients with irritable bowel syndrome. Gastroenterology 2001;121:1329.

129. Zar S, Mincher M, Benson MJ, Kumar D. Food specific IgG4 antibody guided exclusion diet improves symptoms in irritable bowel syndrome (abstract). Colorect Dis 2002;4(Suppl. 1):P100.

130. Villoria A, Serra J, Azpiroz F, Malagelada JR. Physical activity and intestinal gas clearance in patients with bloating. Am J Gastroenterol 2006;101:2552.

131. Lin MY, DiPalma JA, Martini MC, et al. Comparative effects of exogenous lactase (β-galactosidase) preparations on in vivo lactose digestion. Dig Dis Sci 1993;38:2022.

132. Medow MS, Thek KD, Newman LJ, et al. β-galactosidase tablets in the treatment of lactose intolerance in pediatrics. Am J Dis Child 1990;144:1261.

133. Ramirez FC, Lee K, Graham DY. All lactase preparations are not the same: results of a prospective, randomized, placebo-controlled trial. Am J Gastroenterol 1994;89:566.

134. Ganiats TG, Norcross WA, Halverson AL, et al. Does Beano prevent gas? A double-blind crossover study of oral α-galactosidase to treat dietary oligosaccharide intolerance. J Fam Pract 1994;39:441.

135. Suarez F, Levitt MD, Adshead J, Barkin JS. Pancreatic supplements reduce symptomatic response of healthy subjects to a high fat meal. Dig Dis Sci 1999;44:1317.

136. Treem WR, McAdams L, Stanford L, et al. Sacrosidase therapy for congenital sucrase-isomaltase deficiency. J Ped Gastroenterol Nutr 1999;28:137.

137. Holtmann G, Gschossmann J, Karaus M, et al. Randomised double-blind comparison of simethicone with cisapride in functional dyspepsia. Aliment Pharmacol Ther 1999;13:1459.

138. Kaplan MA, Prior MJ, Ash RR, et al. Loperamide–simethicone vs. loperamide alone, simethicone alone, and placebo in the treatment of acute diarrhea with gas-related abdominal discomfort. A randomized controlled trial. Arch Fam Med 1999;8:243.

139. Hall RG, Thompson H, Strother A. Effects of orally administered activated charcoal on intestinal gas. Am J Gastroenterol 1981;75:192.

140. Jain NK, Patel VP, Pitchumoni CS. Efficacy of activated charcoal in reducing intestinal gas: a double-blind clinical trial. Am J Gastroenterol 1986;81:532.

141. Giffard CJ, Collins SB, Stoodley NC, et al. Administration of charcoal, *Yucca schidigera*, and zinc acetate to reduce malodorous flatulence in dogs. J Am Vet Med Assoc 2001;218:892.

142. Suarez FL, Furne J, Springfield J, Levitt MD. Failure of activated charcoal to reduce the release of gases produced by the colonic flora. Am J Gastroenterol 1999;94:208.

143. Suarez FL, Furne JK, Springfield J, Levitt MD. Bismuth subsalicylate markedly decreases hydrogen sulfide release in the human colon. Gastroenterology 1998;114:923.

144. Kaye SA, Lim SG, Taylor M, et al. Small bowel bacterial overgrowth in systemic sclerosis: detection using direct and indirect methods and treatment outcome. Br J Rheumatol 1995;34:265.

145. Bouhnik Y, Alain S, Attar A, et al. Bacterial populations contaminating the upper gut in patients with small intestinal bacterial overgrowth syndrome. Am J Gastroenterol 1999;94:1327.

146. Attar A, Flourie B, Rambaud JC, et al. Antibiotic efficacy in small intestinal bacterial overgrowth-related chronic diarrhea: a crossover, randomized trial. Gastroenterology 1999;117:794.

147. Dear KL, Elia M, Hunter JO. Do interventions which reduce colonic bacterial fermentation improve symptoms of irritable bowel syndrome? Dig Dis Sci 2005;50:758.

148. Pimentel M, Chow EJ, Lin HC. Normalization of lactulose breath testing correlates with symptom improvement in irritable bowel syndrome. a double-blind, randomized, placebo-controlled study. Am J Gastroenterol 2003;98:412.

149. Pimentel M, Chatterjee S, Chow EJ, et al. Neomycin improves constipation-predominant irritable bowel syndrome in a fashion that is dependent on the presence of methane gas: subanalysis of a double-blind randomized controlled study. Dig Dis Sci 2006;51:1297.

150. Di Stefano M, Strocchi A, Malservisi S, et al. Non-absorbable antibiotics for managing intestinal gas production and gas-related symptoms. Aliment Pharmacol Ther 2000;14:1001.

151. Sharara AI, Aoun E, Abdul-Baki H, et al. A randomized double-blind placebo-controlled trial of rifaximin in patients with abdominal bloating and flatulence. Am J Gastroenterol 2006;101:326.

152. Pimentel M, Park S, Mirocha J, et al. The effect of a nonabsorbed oral antibiotic (rifaximin) on the symptoms of the irritable bowel syndrome: a randomized trial. Ann Intern Med 2006;145:557.

153. Penner R, Fedorak RN, Madsen KL. Probiotics and nutraceuticals: non-medicinal treatments of gastrointestinal diseases. Curr Opin Pharmacol 2005;5:596.

154. Kim HJ, Camilleri M, McKinzie S, et al. A randomized controlled trial of a probiotic, VSL#3, on gut transit and symptoms in diarrhoea-predominant irritable bowel syndrome. Aliment Pharmacol Ther 2003;17:895.

155. Kim HJ, Vazquez Roque MI, Camilleri M, et al. A randomized controlled trial of a probiotic combination VSL# 3 and placebo in irritable bowel syndrome with bloating. Neurogastroenterol Motil 2005;17:687.

156. Brigidi P, Vitali B, Swennen E, et al. Effects of probiotic administration upon the composition and enzymatic activity of human fecal microbiota in patients with irritable bowel syndrome or functional diarrhea. Res Microbiol 2001;152:735.

157. O'Mahony L, McCarthy J, Kelly P, et al. Lactobacillus and bifidobacterium in irritable bowel syndrome: symptom responses and relationship to cytokine profiles. Gastroenterology 2005;128:541.

158. Whorwell PJ, Altringer L, Morel J, et al. Efficacy of an encapsulated probiotic *Bifidobacterium infantis* 35624 in women with irritable bowel syndrome. Am J Gastroenterol 2006;101:1581.

159. Nobaek S, Johansson ML, Molin G, et al. Alteration of intestinal microflora is associated with reduction in abdominal bloating and pain in patients with irritable bowel syndrome. Am J Gastroenterol 2000;95:1231.

160. Kajander K, Hatakka K, Poussa T, et al. A probiotic mixture alleviates symptoms in irritable bowel syndrome patients: a controlled 6-month intervention. Aliment Pharmacol Ther 2005;22:387.

161. Pimentel M, Constantino T, Kong Y, et al. A 14-day elemental diet is highly effective in normalizing the lactulose breath test. Dig Dis Sci 2004;49:73.

162. Gibson GR, Beatty ER, Wang X, Cummings JH. Selective stimulation of bifidobacteria in the human colon by oligofructose and inulin. Gastroenterology 1995;108:975.

163. Bouhnik Y, Attar A, Joly FA, et al. Lactulose ingestion increases faecal bifidobacterial counts: a randomized double-blind study in healthy humans. Eur J Clin Nutr 2004; 58: 462–466.

164. Bouhnik Y, Raskine L, Simoneau G, et al. The capacity of short-chain fructo-oligosaccharides to stimulate faecal bifidobacteria: a dose-response relationship study in healthy humans. Nutr J 2006;5:8.

165. Langlands SJ, Hopkins MJ, Coleman N, Cummings JH. Prebiotic carbohydrates modify the mucosa associated microflora of the human large bowel. Gut 2004;53:1610.

166. Bittner AC, Croffut RM, Stranahan MC. Prescript-Assist probiotic-prebiotic treatment for irritable bowel syndrome: a methodologically oriented, 2-week, randomized, placebo-controlled, double-blind clinical study. Clin Ther 2005;27:755.

167. Muller-Lissner SA, Fumagalli I, Bardhan KD, et al. Tegaserod, a 5-HT$_4$ receptor partial agonist, relieves symptoms in irritable bowel syndrome patients with abdominal pain, bloating, and constipation. Aliment Pharmacol Ther 2001;15:1655.

168. Bardhan KD, Forbes A, Marsden CL, et al. The effects of withdrawing tegaserod treatment in comparison with continuous treatment in irritable bowel syndrome patients with abdominal pain/discomfort, bloating and constipation: a clinical study. Aliment Pharmacol Ther 2004;20:213.

169. Coleski R, Owyang C, Hasler WL. Modulation of intestinal gas dynamics in healthy human volunteers by the 5-HT$_4$ receptor agonist tegaserod. Am J Gastroenterol 2006;101:1858.

170. Caldarella MP, Serra J, Azpiroz F, Malagelada JR. Prokinetic effects in patients with intestinal gas retention. Gastroenterology 2002;122:1748.

171. Tack J, Broekaert D, Fischler B, et al. A controlled crossover study of the selective serotonin reuptake inhibitor citalopram in irritable bowel syndrome. Gut 2006;55:1095.

172. Vahedi H, Merat S, Rashidioon A, et al. The effect of fluoxetine in patients with pain and constipation-predominant irritable bowel syndrome: a double-blind randomized-controlled study. Aliment Pharmacol Ther 2005;22:381.

173. Tabas G, Beaves M, Wang J, et al. Paroxetine to treat irritable bowel syndrome no responding to high-fiber diet: a double-blind, placebo-controlled trial. Am J Gastroenterol 2004;99:915.

174. Vejdani R, Shalmani HR, Mir-Fattahi M, et al. The efficacy of an herbal medicine, Carmint, on the relief of abdominal pain and bloating in patients with irritable bowel syndrome: a pilot study. Dig Dis Sci 2006;51:1501.

175. Gonsalkorale WM, Houghton LA, Whorwell PJ. Hypnotherapy in irritable bowel syndrome: a large-scale audit of a clinical service with examination of factors influencing responsiveness. Am J Gastroenterol 2002;97:954.

176. Palsson OS, Turner MJ, Johnson DA, et al. Hypnosis treatment for severe irritable bowel syndrome: investigation of mechanism and effects on symptoms. Dig Dis Sci 2002;47:2605.

177. Moulis H, Vender RJ. Percutaneous endoscopic gastrostomy for treatment of gas-bloat syndrome. Gastrointest Endosc 1993;39:581.

178. Murr MM, Sarr MG, Camilleri M. The surgeon's role in the treatment of chronic intestinal pseudoobstruction. Am J Gastroenterol 1995;90:2147.

Approach to the patient with acute abdomen

Rebecca M. Minter, Michael W. Mulholland

Neuroanatomy of abdominal pain, 271
Associated gastrointestinal symptoms, 273
History, 274
Physical examination, 274
Confounding factors, 275
Deciding whether to operate, 276
Causes of acute abdomen in adults, 277

The term acute abdomen describes a syndrome of sudden abdominal pain with accompanying symptoms and signs that focus attention on the abdominal region. It is clinically useful to limit discussion to cases in which the pain has been present for less than 24 h. Associated symptoms such as nausea, vomiting, constipation, diarrhea, anorexia, abdominal distention, and fever are often present and may be confusing. Although operative therapy is not required for all cases of acute abdomen, for those in which it is indicated unwarranted operative delay can have serious, potentially fatal, consequences. Successful management of affected patients is based on a careful initial assessment, incorporating history taking and physical examination; delineation of clinical priorities; and concurrent resuscitation, diagnosis, and therapy. The most common causes of the acute abdomen are listed in Tables 16.1 and 16.2.

Neuroanatomy of abdominal pain

Nerve fibers that mediate painful visceral stimuli have cell bodies in the dorsal root ganglia. Processes of first-order sensory neurons pass through the spinal nerves to white rami communicantes and then to sympathetic ganglia, which parallel the spinal cord. Nerve processes then travel from sympathetic ganglia through the splanchnic nerves to reach intraabdominal splanchnic ganglia. The splanchnic ganglia are concentrations of nervous tissue surrounding the origins of the celiac, superior mesenteric, and inferior mesenteric arteries. Sensory nerve fibers traverse the splanchnic ganglia without synapse and accompany blood vessels to reach their target organs. Second-order neurons transmit afferent impulses centrally through the lateral spinothalamic tract on the side opposite to the dorsal root containing the nerve cell body. Neurons in the lateral spinothalamic tract project to the thalamus, where they synapse with tertiary neurons mediating sensory and discriminatory aspects of pain. Tertiary neurons project to the somatosensory cortex. Some secondary neurons in the lateral spinothalamic tract synapse in the brainstem with neurons projecting to the limbic system. Almost all nerve fibers that transmit painful sensations travel in association with sympathetic nerves. As a result, although 80%–90% of vagal fibers are afferent, interruption of parasympathetic innervation by vagotomy does not block abdominal pain.

During normal embryological development, abdominal organs receive bilateral sympathetic innervation, with input to each organ originating from several adjacent spinal levels. As a result, visceral pain is sensed as a midline, poorly localized sensation. The location of the pain is determined by the developmental origin of the affected organ (Fig. 16.1). Visceral pain originating from organs derived from the foregut is sensed in the epigastrium. Foregut structures include the stomach, liver, biliary system, pancreas, spleen, and duodenum. Pain from midgut structures is usually experienced in a periumbilical distribution, whereas organs derived from the hindgut project painful sensations to the hypogastrium and lower midline. The embryonic midgut develops into the

Principles of Clinical Gastroenterology. Edited by Tadataka Yamada, David H. Alpers, Anthony N. Kalloo, Neil Kaplowitz, Chung Owyang, and Don W. Powell. © 2008 Blackwell Publishing. ISBN 978-1-4051-69103

Table 16.1 Abdominal causes of acute abdomen

Gastrointestinal
Appendicitis
Perforated peptic ulcer
Intestinal obstruction
Intestinal perforation
Intestinal ischemia
Colonic diverticulitis
Meckel diverticulitis
Inflammatory bowel disease

Pancreatic, biliary, hepatic, and splenic
Acute pancreatitis
Acute cholecystitis
Hepatic abscess
Ruptured or hemorrhagic hepatic tumor
Acute hepatitis
Acute cholangitis
Splenic rupture

Urological
Ureteral stone
Pyelonephritis

Retroperitoneal
Aortic aneurysm
Retroperitoneal hemorrhage

Gynecological
Ruptured ovarian cyst
Ovarian torsion
Ectopic pregnancy
Acute salpingitis
Pyosalpinx
Endometritis
Uterine rupture

Abdominal wall
Rectus muscle hematoma

Adapted from Mulholland & Debas [55].

Table 16.2 Extraabdominal causes of acute abdomen

Thoracic
Myocardial infarction
Acute pericarditis
Lower lobe pneumonia
Pneumothorax
Pulmonary infarction

Hematological
Sickle cell crisis
Acute leukemia

Neurological
Herpes zoster
Tabes dorsalis
Nerve root compression

Metabolic
Diabetic ketoacidosis
Addisonian crisis
Acute porphyria
Hyperlipoproteinemia

Drug-related
Lead toxicity
Narcotic withdrawal

Adapted from Mulholland & Debas [55].

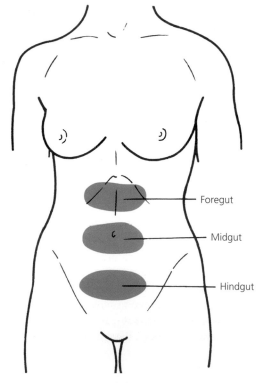

Figure 16.1 Distribution of visceral pain perception based on embryological origin of diseased organ. From Snell RS. Clinical Anatomy for Medical Students, 6th edn. Philadelphia: Lippincott, Williams & Wilkins, 2000.

jejunum, the ileum, the appendix, and the colon to the level of the midtransverse colon. Hindgut structures include the distal transverse, splenic flexure, descending, and sigmoid portions of the colon.

Neuronal pathways that conduct visceral abdominal pain are composed of slowly conducting C-type fibers. Nociceptive fibers may be stimulated by distention, forceful muscular contraction, mesenteric traction or torsion, or by certain noxious chemicals. In hollow organs like the small intestine, sensory fibers are found within the muscular wall. In solid organs, such as the liver, nociceptive fibers are limited to the capsule of the organ. For this reason, mass lesions of the liver parenchyma do not usually cause pain until increasing size causes stretching of the Glisson capsule or traction on the organ.

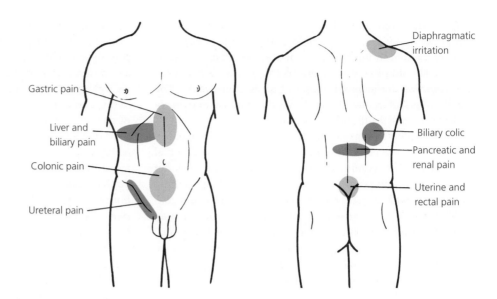

Figure 16.2 Common patterns of referred pain in patients with acute abdominal processes. From Mulholland & Debas [55].

The peritoneum provides a continuous layer over the inner surface of the abdominal wall, reflecting on to the intraperitoneal viscera. Although visceral and parietal peritoneal surfaces have a common mesenchymal derivation, their patterns of innervation are entirely different. The visceral peritoneum is supplied by C-type nociceptive fibers, which transmit painful visceral sensations as outlined above. The parietal peritoneum is supplied by rapidly conducting A-type nerve fibers. The A-type nerve fibers have small receptive fields and produce sharp, well-localized, highly discriminated sensations. The parietal peritoneum is somatically innervated in a unilateral dermatomal distribution. Somatic peritoneal nerves transmit painful impulses in response to changes in temperature or pH and in response to pressure or incision. Somatic pain caused by stimulation of the parietal peritoneum is usually perceived as intense and constant.

Physiological properties of the peritoneum, including particulate and microbial absorption and circulation of intraperitoneal fluid, may affect perception of noxious stimuli. The peritoneal cavity is the largest extravascular space in the body, with an estimated surface area of 1.7 m^2 in adults. Although the entire peritoneal surface can participate in water and low-molecular-weight solute exchange, removal of particulate matter occurs only along the undersurface of the diaphragm. In this area, specialized lymphatic vessels are present beneath the mesothelial layer covering the diaphragmatic surface. Large pores, or lacunae, serve as channels for passage of peritoneal particulate matter up to 10 μm in size into the lymphatic circulation. Negative intrathoracic pressure during inspiration draws fluid into the lymphatic channels; valves in thoracic lymphatic channels prevent reflux during expiration.

The removal of fluid by means of the diaphragmatic lymphatics causes movement of fluid within the peritoneal cavity. Experimentally, injection of contrast material into the right iliac fossa is followed by accumulation of contrast in the right paracolic region, in both subhepatic spaces, and in the pelvis [1]. The patterns of intraperitoneal circulation correspond to the movement of contaminated material after rupture of an abdominal viscus and to subsequent abscess formation. Because the parietal peritoneum is sensitive to chemical irritants, movement of fluid may cause pain to be sensed in an area distinct from the site of pathology. As an example, perforated duodenal ulcer may cause pain in the right lower quadrant as a result of movement of gastric contents along the right paracolic gutter.

A distinctive feature of visceral abdominal discomfort is its association with pain perceived at an extraabdominal site unrelated to the injured organ. This phenomenon is called referred pain. Referred pain associated with intraabdominal or retroperitoneal pathology is usually described as a dull ache near the body surface. In general, referred pain is sensed in a cutaneous area that has its somatic innervation derived from the same spinal segments that supply visceral afferents to the diseased organ. Patterns of referred pain are often stereotypical enough to be diagnostically useful (Fig. 16.2). Gallbladder inflammation is frequently associated with pain referred to the right scapula. Subdiaphragmatic inflammation causes pain referred to the area supplied by cervical dermatomes 3, 4, or 5. Pain from pancreatic disease may be sensed in the posterior midline in the region of the first lumbar vertebra.

Associated gastrointestinal symptoms

Visceral abdominal pain is distressing but is difficult for patients to describe. As a result, patients and physicians may focus on the associated gastrointestinal symptoms that almost invariably accompany acute visceral pain.

Anorexia accompanies almost all acute abdominal processes but is not specific to any pathological process. Anorexia is usually present in most cases of acute appendicitis, and its absence should place that diagnosis in question. Anorexia is also common in the initial phases of acute cholecystitis. The symptom is less frequently found with urological or gynecological causes of acute abdominal pain.

Emesis occurs as a result of reflex stimulation of the medullary vomiting center in the initial phases of acute abdominal processes. Reflex vomiting is not progressive and does not relieve unpleasant symptoms. In contrast, vomiting resulting from mechanical intestinal obstruction is recurrent and progressive. Vomiting caused by intestinal obstruction may cause intravascular volume depletion and prerenal azotemia. Bacterial proliferation proximal to the obstruction causes the vomitus to become feculent in nature.

Abdominal distention associated with acute abdominal pain usually signifies accumulation of swallowed gas in the bowel as a result of mechanical obstruction or ileus. Fluid secreted into the bowel lumen proximal to a mechanical obstruction may also contribute to abdominal distention. Mechanical obstruction may be associated with hyperactive or high-pitched bowel sounds, but the auscultatory finding of diminished bowel sounds is not a reliable sign for the differentiation of ileus from mechanical obstruction. A truly silent abdomen in the presence of distention and tenderness is an ominous sign of bowel necrosis and peritonitis.

Constipation may be a sign of previous health habits (e.g., diet), a disease process (e.g., diverticulitis), or the development of a complication (e.g., perforation). The cessation of intestinal movements or flatus coinciding with the development of acute abdominal pain is more properly referred to as obstipation. Obstipation is associated with both mechanical obstruction and functional ileus.

Watery diarrhea associated with acute abdominal pain suggests acute gastroenteritis or infectious colitis. Bloody diarrhea in the context of the acute abdomen may be associated with exacerbation of chronic inflammatory bowel disease, with mesenteric ischemia, or occasionally with mesenteric venous thrombosis.

History

Treatment for patients with acute abdominal processes differs in a fundamental way from care delivered to patients with long-term complaints. The potential for pathological processes to be rapidly progressive, and for serious adverse consequences to result from therapeutic delay, places a time constraint on diagnosis and treatment. An accurate diagnosis should lead promptly to specific therapy. A complete and accurate history and physical examination is the most important requirement for success.

The treating physician should first focus on the nature and timing of the abdominal pain. The pattern of onset and the progression of pain provide valuable clues to cause. The pain associated with perforation of a duodenal ulcer or rupture of an abdominal aortic aneurysm is incapacitating, begins suddenly, and quickly reaches peak intensity. Because the onset of pain is so dramatic, affected patients may be able to provide detailed information about the time of onset or their activities at that moment. In contrast, pain associated with appendicitis increases over a period of one to several hours. Similarly, pain caused by acute cholecystitis increases over hours before reaching a steady intensity. The duration of painful symptoms is equally important. Biliary colic typically lasts for several hours before rapidly resolving, presumably as a result of the offending stone dislodging from the cystic duct. Pain caused by acute pancreatitis is unrelenting. Initially, patients with mechanical small bowel obstruction may feel remarkably well between episodes of intense and debilitating colic.

Prior symptoms may implicate preexisting pathology. A history of epigastric pain relieved by food may indicate previous duodenal ulceration, whereas previous biliary colic is common in patients presenting acutely with cholecystitis or pancreatitis. Previous abdominal operations influence both the occurrence and manifestations of acute abdominal processes. Adhesions resulting from previous intraperitoneal operation are the most frequent cause of mechanical obstruction of the small intestine. Patients who have undergone hysterectomy, appendectomy, or pelvic colonic resection are at greatest risk for adhesive obstruction.

Physical examination

The physical examination should be conducted in a systematic and unhurried manner. A complete abdominal examination requires unhindered visualization of the area between the nipples and the midthigh, anteriorly and posteriorly. The examination should begin with observation of the patient's expression and behavior. A patient with serious intraperitoneal pathology usually has an anxious, pale face. Sweating, dilated pupils, and shallow breathing are common. In the presence of chemical or bacterial contamination of the peritoneum, the patient tends to lie immobile to minimize movement of inflamed viscera against the parietal peritoneum. Knees may be flexed, the abdomen scaphoid, breathing shallow. Inhaling deeply or coughing aggravates the pain. With ureteral colic or mesenteric ischemia, by contrast, the patient may appear restless, with frequent changes in posture in an attempt to relieve discomfort. During inspection, the location of all surgical scars, masses, external hernias, and stomas should be determined.

Auscultation should precede abdominal palpation. All four quadrants should be auscultated for tone and quantity of bowel sounds and the presence of vascular bruits. Bowel sounds are considered to be absent only if no tones are heard over a 2-min period of auscultation.

Next, the abdomen should be palpated. To determine areas of tenderness and the vigor with which palpation may be pursued, it is useful to first ask the patient to demonstrate the point of maximal discomfort. Palpation should begin in the abdominal quadrant farthest from the area of suspected pathology. Gentle pressure to elicit tenderness and muscular resistance then ensues. Progressively deeper palpation is attempted to delineate masses. Intentional efforts to reproduce abdominal pain by deep palpation and rapid release of pressure, termed rebound tenderness, are not helpful and should not be attempted. Production of rebound tenderness provides no information that is not available through gentle examination, causes the patients to guard voluntarily, and eliminates the possibility of meaningful serial abdominal examinations. The best evidence for a localized inflammatory process is demonstration of point tenderness, caused by the movement of parietal peritoneum against the inflamed surface of a diseased viscus. Point tenderness should be sought by palpation in the area of maximal discomfort but may also be elicited by grasping the patient's hips and gently rocking the pelvis; the movement of inflamed peritoneum is presumed to cause pain. The stethoscope may also be used to palpate the abdominal quadrants with gentle pressure.

Every patient must undergo a digital rectal examination. If an inflamed appendix lies deep within the pelvis, point tenderness may sometimes be elicited only by palpation through the right rectal wall. Stool should be tested for guaiac positivity. In females, manual and speculum vaginal examinations are required; vaginal secretions should be obtained for Gram stain and culture. All external stomas, wounds, and fistulas should be explored digitally.

Confounding factors

Female gender

Almost all series of surgically treated patients with acute abdominal pain report that diagnostic inaccuracy is greatest in young women [2]. Detailed sexual and menstrual histories are crucial; a pregnancy test is mandatory in every female patient of childbearing age who is evaluated with acute abdominal pain. Gynecological causes of acute abdominal pain include ectopic pregnancy, ruptured or twisted ovarian cyst, acute salpingitis, and tuboovarian abscess. On pelvic examination, ectopic pregnancy may present as a tender, unilateral, adnexal mass. Inflammatory disease of the fallopian tubes and uterus produces physical findings of local cervical tenderness, bilateral pelvic pain with displacement of the cervix, adnexal mass, or cervical discharge. All secretions from the cervical os should be submitted for aerobic and anaerobic cultures. Fluid within the pouch of Douglas can be

aspirated and examined for blood or bacteria. For cases in which the distinction between acute appendicitis and salpingitis is difficult, pelvic ultrasound can be diagnostic. If the diagnosis remains in question, further imaging in the form of a computed tomography (CT) scan may be helpful, or alternatively, exploratory laparoscopy can be carried out. Laparoscopy provides a prompt means to evaluate the appendix as well as other pelvic and intraabdominal organs. If appendicitis or tuboovarian pathology is identified, then the majority of these conditions can be easily treated through a laparoscopic approach.

Pregnancy

When evaluating a pregnant woman with abdominal pain, it is most important to remember that the best guarantee for a living, healthy baby is a healthy mother, and clinical decisions should be directed accordingly. The most common cause of the acute abdomen in pregnancy is acute appendicitis, occurring in 1 of 6000 pregnancies. Diagnosis of acute abdominal pain in pregnancy is complicated because uterine enlargement displaces organs from their normal anatomic positions. For example, the appendix is progressively moved from the right lower quadrant superiorly and laterally as it is displaced by the gravid uterus (Fig. 16.3). As a consequence, point tenderness associated with appendicitis may be sensed in a position more cephalad than usual, and in some instances parietal peritoneal irritation may be absent altogether. In addition to altered physical examination findings, there are physiological alterations of laboratory values during pregnancy (mild leukocytosis, anemia, hypoalbuminemia, and

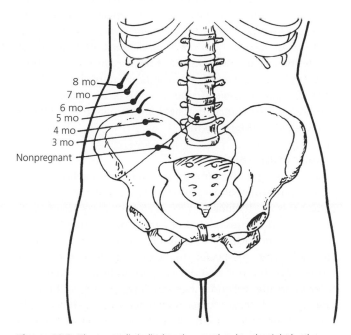

Figure 16.3 The appendix is displaced upward and to the right by the uterus during pregnancy. Movement of the appendix during pregnancy may cause the pain of acute appendicitis to be sensed in an atypical position.

elevated alkaline phosphatase) that add to the confusion [3]. Diagnostic imaging options are also limited during pregnancy. Ultrasound is safe and widely available; however, its sensitivity is often reduced during pregnancy because of the anatomical changes, and CT scans expose the fetus to ionizing radiation. Several recent studies have demonstrated that magnetic resonance imaging is safe during pregnancy and can be useful in identifying both the presence and absence of intraabdominal pathology (i.e., an inflamed or normal appendix) [4–6]. Magnetic resonance imaging is not always readily available, however, and surgery should not be delayed if appendicitis is clinically suspected because perforation significantly increases maternal and infant mortality. In contrast to maternal mortality from appendicitis without perforation, 0.1%, mortality exceeds 4% with perforation. Likewise, fetal mortality is less than 2% without perforation, but exceeds 30% with perforation [3]. Mortality in both instances is typically related to delayed diagnosis.

If operation is indicated, the operative approach will be chosen based on the suspected diagnosis, the surgeon's experience and preference, and the stage of pregnancy. A laparoscopic approach for the treatment of both gallbladder disease and appendicitis during pregnancy has been demonstrated to be safe in the first two trimesters of pregnancy and early in the third with appropriate adjustment of port placement [7,8].

Age

The diagnosis of acute abdominal pain is most difficult at the two extremes of age. Communication is limited in infants, and the temporal progression of symptoms may be impossible to elicit. The abdominal wall in infants is not muscularly well developed, and guarding in response to underlying inflammatory processes is diminished. Because fever and leukocytosis are common accompaniments of many childhood illnesses, their diagnostic utility is reduced. In contrast, fever and elevated leukocyte counts are much less common in elderly patients, even in the presence of advanced disease. Physical signs of intraperitoneal inflammation are likewise diminished in older patients.

Immunosuppression

Patients who are immunosuppressed may not exhibit appropriate clinical responses to acute intraperitoneal inflammatory processes. Included in this category are patients with the acquired immunodeficiency syndrome, patients receiving long-term corticosteroid therapy, and those undergoing chemotherapy. At special risk are recipients of solid organ transplants. The physical signs of peritonitis (e.g., pain, muscular guarding, rebound) may not be apparent, and fever is often absent. Intraperitoneal infection may progress to septic shock as the first manifestation of disease. Leukocytosis is usually present but decreased, and a shift to immature leukocyte forms is apparent. Early use of radiological evaluation, especially CT, is appropriate.

A syndrome of diffuse abdominal pain, fever, and diarrhea has been reported in patients with severe neutropenia (< 500 neutrophils/mL). Patients with acute leukemia or aplastic anemia and those undergoing bone marrow transplantation are at greatest risk. The pathological entity, termed neutropenic colitis, is characterized by diffuse mucosal ulceration, invasive infection with enteric microorganisms, and sepsis [9]. The ascending colon is the intestinal segment most often affected, although the other portions of the colon and the terminal ileum may also demonstrate ulceration. Cecal edema may be demonstrated by CT scan. Operation is indicated if perforation is present or suspected, but recovery correlates more closely with rebound of neutrophil counts than with surgical treatment. If no perforation is suspected then patients are treated with cessation of all chemotherapy, bowel rest, broad-spectrum antibiotics, and granulocyte colony-stimulating factor.

Recent laparotomy

Acute abdominal processes are difficult to evaluate after recent laparotomy. Abdominal pain is universally present, although much decreased if laparoscopic techniques were employed. Leukocytosis is common in the early postoperative period. Numerous sources for fever exist, including pulmonary atelectasis, urinary infection, phlebitis, and infection in the surgical incision. In evaluating abdominal pain in the postoperative period, it is important to consider the signs and symptoms in relation to the time after operation. Uncomplicated recovery should be accompanied by a steady progression: lessening abdominal pain, resolving biochemical abnormalities, mobilization of perioperative fluids, predictable recovery from ileus, and increasing mobility. Failure to achieve this progress warrants investigation. The most common causes of abdominal sepsis after operation relate to inadequacies of surgical technique, such as anastomotic dehiscence. Acute acalculous cholecystitis may also occur in the postoperative setting.

Deciding whether to operate

After the initial history and physical examination, a basic question must be answered: is immediate operation necessary? Immediate operation is indicated if the suspected pathological process is rapidly progressive and potentially fatal. This criterion is met with intraperitoneal hemorrhage – for example, ruptured abdominal aortic aneurysm or ruptured ectopic pregnancy. In these circumstances, laparotomy becomes a method of diagnosis as well as the means of treatment.

If laparotomy is not immediately necessary, the next question becomes will laparotomy ultimately be necessary? If the initial evaluation reveals pneumoperitoneum, radiological evaluations to differentiate perforated ulcer from perforated colonic diverticulum are not required; the processes may easily be distinguished at operation and surgical intervention should not be delayed to perform further diagnostics. Preoperative efforts should be expended to prepare the patient for anesthesia and operation. If the need for operative treatment is uncertain, additional tests to define the diagnosis precisely are justified. As the processes of diagnosis and resuscitation proceed, close observation and a timetable are essential; worsening clinical examination mandates earlier surgical intervention.

Causes of acute abdomen in adults

Appendicitis

Acute appendicitis is the most common cause of the acute abdomen in the United States and should be included in the differential diagnosis for every patient presenting with acute abdominal pain. Approximately 250 000 appendectomies are performed in the United States annually, with 2000 deaths resulting from complications of the disease [10]. The lifetime incidence of developing acute appendicitis is about 7% in the United States [10].

Appendicitis develops as a result of obstruction of the appendiceal lumen by fecalith or appendiceal calculus or by hyperplasia of submucosal lymphatic tissue. In older patients, appendicitis can also develop secondary to obstruction of the appendiceal lumen by a polyp or tumor. In the initial stages, the pathogenesis of appendicitis resembles that of bowel obstruction. Typically, the first symptom is upper midline or periumbilical pain. Discomfort develops over one to several hours and is typically followed by anorexia, nausea, and vomiting. If the appendiceal lumen remains occluded, inflammatory changes, initially confined to the appendiceal mucosa, become transmural. Contact of the inflamed serosal surface of the appendix with the parietal peritoneum is associated with a change in the pain pattern: a shift to the right lower quadrant. When a patient with suspected appendicitis suddenly experiences a sudden relief of their pain, one must worry that the appendix has perforated and pain relief is secondary to decreased appendiceal wall pressure. The usual presentation of midline abdominal pain moving to the right lower quadrant is seen less frequently in older patients, in whom diffuse pain and nonlocalized tenderness are more common.

Approximately 2%–3% of patients with appendicitis have an abdominal mass at the time of initial evaluation [11]. The mass, formed by inflamed omentum and adherent loops of intestine, signifies the development of a phlegmon or an abscess secondary to appendiceal perforation. Perforation should also be suspected if the patient has been symptomatic for more than 24 h, if the temperature exceeds 38°C, or if the leukocyte count is greater than 15 000 cells/mm³. Cross-sectional imaging with CT scan should be obtained in these patients.

Plain films of the abdomen are relatively nonspecific and have a low degree of sensitivity for the diagnosis of appendicitis. Occasionally, a calcified appendicolith may be seen (13%–22% of cases), but more commonly these films will demonstrate the nonspecific findings of an ileus [10]. Pneumoperitoneum is distinctly uncommon, being present in less than 1% of cases.

Appendicitis is a clinical diagnosis, supported by carefully selected laboratory and radiological studies. Patients with compatible historical features and physical examinations do not need additional diagnostic studies, and immediate surgical exploration is appropriate. Ancillary tests are reserved for atypical or equivocal presentations.

Abdominal ultrasonography may be helpful in patients in whom the clinical features of appendicitis are ambiguous. This technique depends on graded compression of the abdomen with the ultrasonographic transducer to displace gas-filled loops of bowel and the appendix is seen in the shape of a round target with the anechoic lumen surrounded by a hypoechoic and thickened (> 2 mm) appendiceal wall. For nonperforated appendicitis, ultrasonography has been reported to have a diagnostic accuracy of 93%, with a negative predictive value of 97%, in selected series, and has proven to be particularly useful in children [12,13]. Ultrasound is attractive as an imaging modality because it does not expose the patient to ionizing radiation, and is inexpensive, rapid, and widely available. However, it is also highly operator-dependent, requires a high level of skill and experience, and may be difficult to perform in patients with significant abdominal pain (when one cannot compress the abdominal wall), with overlying bowel gas, or who are overweight or obese. Additionally, ultrasound does not allow for the differentiation between perforated and nonperforated appendicitis, knowledge of which may alter one's clinical approach.

Helical CT scans are increasingly being used in the diagnosis of acute appendicitis (Fig. 16.4), with reported sensitivities in the range of 91%–98% and diagnostic accuracy ranging from 93%–98% [13–16]. Unlike plain films and ultrasonography, CT scanning increases the clinician's ability to detect other clinical entities that may explain their abdominal pain, as well as to identify those patients with periappendiceal abscess, who may benefit from percutaneous drainage and interval appendectomy in 6–12 weeks. In the absence of a discrete abscess, helical CT has demonstrated a sensitivity of 58.8% and a specificity of 85.7% for the detection of perforation, with extralumenal air and moderate or severe periappendiceal stranding being independent predictors for perforation [17]. Two recent series have demonstrated a significant decrease in the rate of negative appendectomies from a historical rate of 15% to a rate of 2%–4% with the use of CT in the diagnosis of appendicitis [18,19]. Two additional studies have demonstrated net financial savings associated with the use of CT scans for the diagnosis of appendicitis linked to the increased observation time and the prolonged

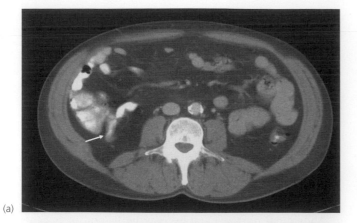

(a)

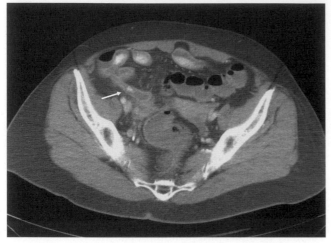

(b)

Figure 16.4 Oral and intravenous contrast-enhanced computed tomography scan shows a normal appendix **(a)** and a thickened, fluid-filled appendix with an appendicolith (arrow) seen within the lumen **(b)**.

hospitalization associated with negative appendectomies [15, 20]. The use of CT scanning in suspected appendicitis is likely to continue to increase given these positive findings; however, its use should still be viewed as complementary to a thorough surgical evaluation, and CT should not be used as a primary diagnostic tool.

Patients presenting with acute appendicitis not complicated by perforation should undergo emergent appendectomy. Either an open or a laparoscopic approach is appropriate, and the approach is chosen based on surgeon's preference and experience as well as on patient characteristics. A laparoscopic approach has distinct benefits in female patients, any patient in whom the diagnosis is in question, and in overweight and obese patients. A recent large review found that laparoscopic appendectomy had significant advantages over open appendectomy with respect to length of hospital stay, rate of routine discharge, and postoperative in-hospital morbidity [21]. Laparoscopy is associated with increased operative costs; however, and may or may not be possible in a patient with a history of previous abdominal surgery.

The overall perioperative mortality rate among patients with appendicitis is approximately 0.5%. Although fewer than 0.2% of nonperforated patients die, the mortality rate rises 10-fold with the occurrence of perforation [22]. Mortality is clearly related to age, with the highest mortality rates occurring in patients older than 50 years. Septic complications occur with increased frequency in the presence of perforation. The wound infection rate is 1.8% when a noninflamed appendix is removed, rising to 8.5% for inflamed appendices and 17% with appendiceal perforation [23]. Pelvic abscess occurs in approximately 15% of patients after resection of a perforated appendix.

An appendiceal mass or abscess may be treated by both operative and nonoperative means [24]. Early operative intervention is not favored by most surgeons treating appendiceal abscesses or phlegmons. Initial treatment should include evaluation using either ultrasound or CT scan, percutaneous drainage of periappendiceal fluid collections, and antibiotic therapy [25,26]. With resolution of periappendiceal inflammation, elective interval appendectomy may be performed in 6–12 weeks. In older patients, a colonoscopy should be performed before interval appendectomy to rule out the presence of an occult cecal malignancy as the cause of the perforation.

Perforated gastric and duodenal ulcer

Although hospitalization rates for peptic ulceration have fallen since 1970, the overall rate of perforation has not decreased in several decades. Furthermore, the introduction of newer antisecretory drugs has not affected rates of perforation. In two-thirds of affected patients, perforation is the first manifestation of duodenal ulcer disease.

Following perforation the patient usually experiences sudden, severe epigastric pain, followed by diffuse abdominal pain. Somatic pain is caused by chemical irritation of the peritoneum by acidic gastric contents. Subphrenic collection of gastric content is associated with right scapular radiation of pain. Respiration worsens symptoms; the patient typically seeks to minimize movement. Physical examination reveals a quiet abdomen with marked muscular rigidity and epigastric tenderness. If perforation has occurred less than 24 h previously, low-grade fever and tachycardia are often present, but hypotension is unusual. Laboratory examinations reveal leukocytosis; mild hyperamylasemia may be present and is attributed to resorption of duodenal contents from the peritoneal cavity. Upright abdominal films demonstrate pneumoperitoneum in 80% of cases (Fig. 16.5). If pneumoperitoneum is absent, water-soluble contrast examination may be used to demonstrate perforation.

The empty, acid-secreting human stomach contains 10^2–10^3 organisms, with lactobacilli and aerobic streptococci predominating. Because the initial bacterial inoculum is low, septic consequences associated with gastric and duodenal perforation are closely related to the length of time that elapses before definitive treatment. Peritoneal fluid samples obtained

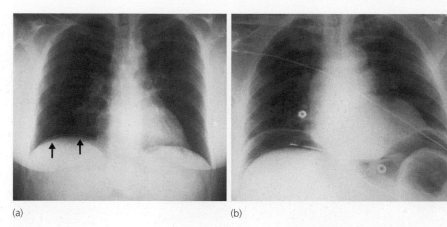

Figure 16.5 Pneumoperitoneum accompanying perforated duodenal ulcer. Upright radiographs from two patients reveal **(a)** minimal pneumoperitoneum (arrows) and **(b)** massive pneumoperitoneum.

(a)   (b)

within 6–12 h of perforation are culturepositive in fewer than 50% of cases; by 24 h more than two-thirds are positive, and after 24 h coliform species predominate. Patients on medications that produce chronic acid suppression, however, will have a gastric flora that is similar to oral flora at baseline [27].

Nonoperative management of documented duodenal ulcer has been described [28], but is only justified in unusual circumstances. Reports of nonoperative management have excluded patients with a history of gastric ulcer, perforations of more than 24 h duration, clinical deterioration, associated shock, diagnostic uncertainty, or serious coexisting medical illnesses. In the remaining patients, initial treatment was intravenous fluids, nasogastric suction, and antibiotics. After 6 h, contrast radiography was used to exclude continued intraperitoneal leakage of gastric contents. Continued extravasation or lack of clinical improvement was considered an indication for immediate operation. In one series, 28% of patients initially managed nonoperatively had clinical deterioration within 24 h and required operation [28]. Perforated neoplasms were discovered in 27% of patients initially presumed to have perforated duodenal ulcer and patients older than 70 years of age were less likely to respond to nonoperative treatment. The length of hospitalization was 35% longer in the group treated nonoperatively; however, complication rates were equivalent in the operative and nonoperative groups. It is unclear, particularly in the era of minimally invasive surgery, which patients would truly benefit from such an approach, and the choice of nonoperative management of perforated ulcer should be used only in select cases where the patient is clinically stable and without signs of peritonitis or clinical deterioration (i.e., evidence of a pneumoperitoneum on radiograph but no clinical signs of perforation).

The surgical approach to perforated peptic ulcer disease has been radically altered in recent years by the knowledge that greater than 90% of patients presenting with peptic ulcer disease are infected with *Helicobacter pylori*, and that with eradication of *H. pylori* the majority of ulcers will heal [29]. This knowledge, combined with the highly effective nature of proton-pump inhibitors for the suppression of gastric acid production, has resulted in a shift in the goals of surgery for perforated ulcers in the stomach and duodenum. Rather than performing a definitive ulcer operation consisting of vagotomy with or without gastric emptying procedure, current surgical goals are primarily directed at closure of the perforation (or resection of the ulcer if it is gastric in location), and peritoneal debridement/drainage of intraabdominal contamination [30]. In the setting of perforated duodenal ulcer, a simple omental patch is performed, increasingly performed laparoscopically [31,32]. Perforated gastric ulcers should be resected to rule out the presence of malignancy. Depending on the location of the ulcer, this may be accomplished with wedge resection, distal gastrectomy, or more complex reconstructions if the ulcer is located more proximally in the stomach. Postoperatively, all patients should be treated for *H. pylori* and placed on proton-pump inhibitors. In addition, all nonsteroidal antiinflammatory medications should be avoided. A definitive antiulcer procedure should be considered for patients with recurrent ulcer disease, particularly those previously treated for *H. pylori*, and for those patients who require chronic nonsteroidal antiinflammatory therapy that cannot be discontinued.

Obstruction of the small intestine

Obstruction of the small intestine accounts for approximately 5% of acute surgical hospitalizations, and despite significant advances in anesthetic and surgical techniques, the mortality rate still ranges from 3% to 7%. In the United States, 70%–80% of cases of small bowel obstruction are a result of postoperative adhesions. In one-fourth of cases, adhesive obstruction is preceded by a gynecological operation, and in one-fourth, the obstruction follows total or segmental colectomy. After adhesions, primary or metastatic carcinoma, external hernias, regional enteritis, and internal hernias occur as causes of small bowel obstruction, in decreasing order of incidence. Less common conditions include previous abdominal or pelvic radiation, intussusception, endometriosis, volvulus, and congenital abnormalities.

Intestinal colic is the cardinal symptom of obstruction of the small intestine. Initially, periods of crampy pain centered

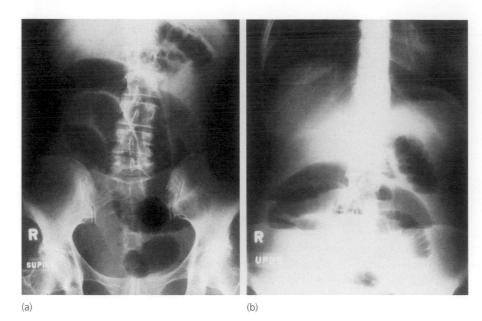

(a)   (b)

Figure 16.6 (a) Supine abdominal radiograph of a patient with small bowel obstruction demonstrates dilated loops of small intestine. **(b)** Upright radiograph of same patient demonstrates air–fluid levels in obstructed small intestinal segments.

in the midabdomen may be interspersed with relatively pain-free intervals. If intestinal distention is unrelieved, pain becomes unrelenting and vomiting is progressive. Bacterial overgrowth in the obstructed segment causes the nature of the vomitus to change with time, becoming feculent. Complete small intestine obstruction is associated with obstipation, although gas and stool distal to the point of obstruction may continue to pass for a short interval after initial symptoms.

The most important diagnostic consideration with these patients is to differentiate partial from complete obstruction. Evaluation begins with plain abdominal radiographs. Complete obstruction is characterized by dilated loops of small intestine with air–fluid levels and no visible gas within the colon (Fig. 16.6). Cases of partial obstruction usually show clear-cut evidence of gas in the colon above the peritoneal reflection in addition to dilated loops of small intestine.

If the diagnosis of complete small intestine obstruction is unequivocal, additional radiological studies to demonstrate the site of obstruction or the nature of the obstructive process are neither appropriate nor necessary in most patients. Barium contrast radiography and CT scanning are useful in clarifying the diagnosis in patients with atypical symptoms, or non-diagnostic plain abdominal films can be used to differentiate paralytic ileus from mechanical obstruction, and to evaluate selected subsets of patients in whom nonoperative management would be desirable. The latter group includes patients with multiple laparotomies for adhesive obstruction, those suffering obstruction in the immediate postoperative period, patients with known intraperitoneal carcinomatosis, patients who have undergone extensive abdominal radiation therapy, and those with Crohn's disease. Imaging by CT scan is typically obtained before barium contrast radiography in these equivocal settings because additional information beyond the point and degree of obstruction can be obtained, and further imaging options are not limited by the retention of barium.

If initial diagnostic studies indicate partial small intestine obstruction, nonoperative management consisting of nasogastric decompression and intravenous hydration is appropriate. Seventy-five per cent of patients treated in this manner have clinical and radiographic improvement within 24 h [33]. An additional 15% respond within 48 h. Failure to achieve clinical improvement by 48 h is an indication for operative treatment. There is no evidence that long intestinal tubes are more effective than standard nasogastric tubes in achieving intestinal decompression. In a series of 91 patients with partial small intestine obstruction treated nonoperatively, none developed strangulation [33].

In contrast to partial obstruction, complete small intestine obstruction is an indication for emergent laparotomy because of the risk associated with the development of intestinal strangulation. The presence of intestinal necrosis doubles operative mortality rates and triples the incidence of serious postoperative complications. In patients with complete obstruction of the small intestine, preoperative diagnosis of strangulation is difficult to exclude by any available radiological test, clinical parameter, or combination of parameters, or by experienced clinical judgment. In one prospective evaluation, preoperative clinical indices and judgments of senior attending surgeons were assessed in 51 consecutive patients about to undergo laparotomy for complete small bowel obstruction [34]. The signs usually considered diagnostic – continuous abdominal pain, fever, peritoneal irritation, leukocytosis, and acidosis – were neither sensitive, specific, nor predictive for strangulation. Senior surgeons, aware of all preoperative data, correctly predicted strangulation in only 10 of 21 affected patients (48% sensitivity). These authors conclude that nonoperative treatment of complete small intestine obstruction entails a calculated risk (30%) of delayed definitive treatment of intestinal ischemia [34]. This represents experience based on a select group of patients all of whom were triaged to operative intervention, however, and may represent a selection bias. Stewardson et al. also report their experience over 10 years in evaluating all patients with a diagnosis of small bowel obstruction. They found that in the absence of the four classic indicators of intestinal strangulation – leukocytosis, localized tenderness, tachycardia, and fever – that it was safe to continue with nonoperative management. However, if any one of these symptoms should develop then immediate operative intervention was recommended [35]. The diagnostic performance of CT in assessing bowel ischemia and complete obstruction was evaluated in a recent review. Fifteen studies and 743 patients were reviewed and the aggregated sensitivity of CT for the detection of small bowel ischemia in the setting of small bowel obstruction was 83%, specificity was 92%, positive predictive value was 79%, and negative predictive value was 93%. For the detection of complete small bowel obstruction, aggregated sensitivity was 92%, specificity was 93%, positive predictive value was 91%, and negative predictive value was 93% [36]. This suggests that CT imaging may be a useful adjunct in the examination of patients with questionable strangulation, but findings must be considered in the context of the clinical examination.

Resuscitation before operative intervention should focus on the correction of hypoxemia caused by respiratory restriction secondary to abdominal distention; replacement of intravascular volume deficits caused by losses through vomiting, bowel wall edema, and extravasation of fluid into the peritoneal cavity; and correction of serum electrolyte abnormalities. Intralumenal bacterial overgrowth and the potential for septic complications associated with intestinal obstruction necessitate the administration of broad-spectrum antibiotics preoperatively. Gastric decompression is necessary to lessen the risk of pulmonary aspiration during anesthetic induction.

Patients who have been treated for cancer and who subsequently develop obstruction of the small intestine present a special challenge. It is important to realize that 25%–40% of such patients do not have recurrent or metastatic cancer as the cause of their obstruction. For these patients, lysis of adhesions or herniorrhaphy provides long-term relief. If localized recurrent or metastatic tumor is the cause of obstruction, significant palliation can be obtained by operative treatment in 63% of patients, with a median survival of 11 months [37]. Advanced metastatic tumor causing small intestine obstruction, exemplified by ovarian carcinomatosis, has a dismal prognosis and may be a contraindication to operative treatment [38].

As with other causes of acute abdomen, elderly patients affected by small bowel obstruction tend to present with more advanced disease and fewer laboratory and physical findings. In one report, 35% of patients older than 70 years of age developing intestinal gangrene had no abnormal physical signs or laboratory parameters [39]. The resultant diagnostic uncertainty in elderly patients is associated with operative delay and a 40% increase in perioperative morbidity.

Colonic diverticulitis

Acute abdominal processes involving the large intestine and emergency surgical procedures used to treat colonic diseases are associated with higher mortality and morbidity rates than are diseases in any other organ system. The treatment of acute diverticulitis illustrates many of these difficulties.

Colonic diverticulae are extremely common and are clearly age-related in the United States. By the seventh decade, more than 50% of the population can be demonstrated to harbor colonic diverticulae. The estimated lifetime risk for the development of diverticulitis in these patients is 10%–25% [40,41]. The sigmoid segment is involved in 90% of cases and is the only site of diverticulosis in half of patients. Isolated right colonic or cecal diverticulae are present much less frequently, being demonstrated in approximately 2% of examinations; they are much more common in Asian populations [42].

The signs and symptoms associated with acute diverticulitis depend on the colonic segment involved, the degree of pericolonic inflammation, and the development of extracolonic complications. Classically, patients present with lower abdominal pain, fever, and obstipation. Nausea and vomiting are usually not prominent. Mild abdominal distention is variably present. Leukocytosis is so common that the diagnosis should be questioned in its absence. Physical examination may reveal a palpable, tender mass in the left lower quadrant, but the absence of a mass does not exclude the diagnosis of diverticulitis.

Acute diverticulitis is a clinical diagnosis. Therapy, consisting of antibiotics and bowel rest, should be initiated if appropriate symptoms exist. In 85% of cases, symptoms abate within 3 days of initiating treatment [40]. After patients have become asymptomatic, radiographic or endoscopic evaluation of the colon should be performed to confirm the diagnosis of diverticulitis and to exclude other diseases, specifically colonic adenocarcinoma. If symptoms do not subside promptly, or if a complication of diverticulitis is suspected, additional radiological evaluation is indicated.

Plain abdominal radiographs, usually obtained in symptomatic patients, do not reveal any abnormality in 70% of cases. Contrast enemas were once the diagnostic standard; however, they are limited by the fact that diverticulitis is largely an extralumenal process. If a contrast enema is to be undertaken then water-soluble contrast should be used and a low-pressure, single-contrast study should be performed. Findings consistent with diverticulitis are localized extravasation of contrast outlining an abscess cavity, intramural sinus tract, or fistula in the setting of other diverticulae.

Contrast enema has been shown in retrospective series to have a sensitivity ranging from 62% to 94%, with false-negative results in 2%–15% of cases [40].

Imaging by CT is increasingly used as the initial test for suspected diverticular complications, and is regarded as the diagnostic imaging modality of choice. It has several advantages in this clinical situation: the study causes much less discomfort than a contrast enema, risk of perforation is negligible, and extracolonic complications of diverticulitis can be evaluated. Pathological changes of diverticulitis detectable by CT include intramural colonic thickening, mesenteric edema, pericolonic and mesenteric abscesses, phlegmon formation, and pneumoperitoneum (Fig. 16.7). If intravenous contrast is not administered, visualization of contrast material

within the bladder is presumptive evidence for colovesical fistula. Sensitivity of CT examination for suspected diverticulitis has been reported to be 93%–98% with specificity ranging from 75% to 100% [40,43].

The ability of CT to accurately define complications of acute diverticulitis in patients, such as pericolonic abscess, allows for CT-guided percutaneous needle aspiration and catheter drainage in properly selected patients. The goal of percutaneous drainage of diverticular abscesses is to minimize the need for colostomy formation and to optimize the conditions for resection with primary anastomosis while not compromising patient safety. Patients successfully treated with percutaneous drainage of an abscess can then safely undergo a bowel preparation, preoperative endoscopic evaluation of their colon, and elective resection of the diseased segment of colon with primary anastomosis 6 to 8 weeks after their initial presentation.

Patients with generalized peritonitis secondary to purulent or fecal contamination, and those presenting with colonic obstruction secondary to diverticulitis, are not candidates for this treatment approach and will require emergent operation. Operative goals include resection of the diseased segment of colon and peritoneal debridement. In the presence of active intraperitoneal infection or a mechanically unprepared bowel, resection of the diseased segment, formation of a proximal colostomy, and closure of the rectum (i.e., Hartmann procedure) is the safest surgical option. In selected obstructed patients, on-table colonic lavage with primary anastomosis may be an option; however, in all other circumstances colostomy will be required with restoration of intestinal continuity in 2–3 months following resolution of the septic process [44].

Acute cholecystitis

Impaction of a gallstone in the cystic duct causes biliary colic, characterized by pain in the epigastrium or right upper quadrant of the abdomen. Biliary colic begins gradually before reaching a plateau of steady pain that typically lasts for several hours. Discomfort relents as the stone dislodges. The pain of biliary colic is severe and is frequently accompanied by nausea and vomiting. Symptoms are classically associated with the ingestion of a fat-containing meal, although they may also begin during fasting.

Continued obstruction of the cystic duct initiates an inflammatory response in the gallbladder wall. The presence of obstruction plus inflammation distinguishes acute cholecystitis from simple colic. Because of continuing ductal obstruction, the pain of acute cholecystitis may persist for many hours to days. If the inflammatory process progresses to involve the serosal surface of the gallbladder then adjacent parietal peritoneum is irritated. In this instance, pain becomes more intense and more clearly localized to the right upper quadrant. Movement of an inflamed gallbladder against the parietal peritoneum during breathing may

(a)

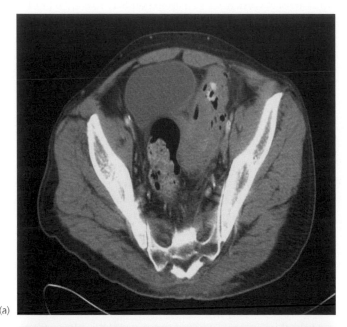

(b)

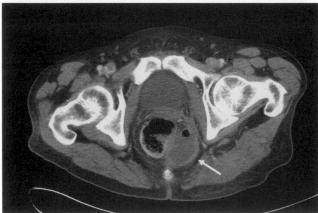

Figure 16.7 Computed tomography scans demonstrating sigmoid diverticulitis **(a)** with adjacent pelvic abscess **(b)**. This was managed with percutaneous drainage.

inhibit deep inspiration, producing a positive Murphy sign. Accompanying fever is usually low-grade. Most patients with uncomplicated cholecystitis have mild leukocytosis, with leukocyte counts ranging from 12 000 to 16 000 cells/mm^3. Levels of serum bilirubin, alkaline phosphatase, and amylase may be nonspecifically elevated, usually not more than twice normal.

Although 95% of patients with acute cholecystitis have calculous biliary disease, the demonstration of cholelithiasis in patients with abdominal pain does not confirm the diagnosis of cholecystitis. Asymptomatic gallstones are present in 30%–40% of persons older than 40 years of age, and only 15%–35% of patients who have symptoms consistent with cholecystitis are proven to have the disease [45]. The high frequency of asymptomatic gallstones make additional tests necessary to support the clinical diagnosis.

Ultrasonography is the preferred initial screening test for acute cholecystitis. Ultrasound has the advantages of low cost, portability, and ease of performance. In addition to detecting gallstones with 95% sensitivity, the procedure also provides information regarding other organs in the upper abdomen. Secondary findings that support the diagnosis of acute cholecystitis include gallbladder wall thickening, distention of the gallbladder, pericholecystic fluid, and sonographic lucency within the gallbladder wall [46]. Thickening of the gallbladder wall greater than 3 mm predicts acute cholecystitis with more than 90% accuracy [47], but this finding must be interpreted within the clinical context because wall thickening has also been reported with portal hypertension, hypoalbuminemia, ascites, and after gallbladder contraction when patients have not fasted.

A sonographic Murphy sign is elicited by placing the ultrasonographic transducer over the gallbladder and applying pressure or asking the patient to inspire deeply. In the presence of gallstones, a positive sonographic Murphy sign predicts acute cholecystitis in 90% of cases [48].

Cholescintigraphy is based on iminodiacetic compounds that are taken up by hepatocytes and secreted into bile. Labeling with technetium 99 permits visualization after intravenous injection. The upper abdomen is imaged for 2–3 h after injection, and delayed images may be obtained for up to 24 h. In normal individuals, the liver is imaged first, followed by the gallbladder, common bile duct, and duodenum. If the common bile duct and duodenum are visible but the gallbladder is not, cystic duct obstruction is presumed to be present. If neither the gallbladder nor the common bile duct can be seen, common duct obstruction may be present. Severe hepatocellular disease and hyperbilirubinemia may also produce this pattern.

The gallbladder cannot be seen by cholescintigraphy in half of patients with chronic cholecystitis, even if the cystic duct is not acutely obstructed. False-positives may also result from failure to fast, alcoholic liver disease, and long-term parenteral nutrition [49]. Because of these limitations, cholescintigraphy is usually reserved for patients with normal ultrasonography but strong clinical suspicion of acute cholecystitis and for those with gallstones who have no ancillary ultrasonographic findings of cholecystitis [50].

Optimal management of patients with acute cholecystitis is cholecystectomy. Most patients may be approached laparoscopically; however, the conversion rate to open cholecystectomy is significantly higher in the setting of acute cholecystitis and approaches 20% [51]. In critically ill or elderly patients with significant comorbidities presenting with acute cholecystitis, percutaneous cholecystostomy is a safe and effective procedure with limited associated morbidity [52]. Whenever possible, these patients should undergo subsequent laparoscopic cholecystectomy if their medical conditions allow for acceptable operative risk.

Mesenteric ischemia

Acute visceral ischemia is a prototypical, common, and frequently misdiagnosed cause of acute abdomen in adults. The four major ischemic syndromes are mesenteric embolism, acute mesenteric thrombosis, nonocclusive mesenteric ischemia, and iatrogenic mesenteric ischemia. Each syndrome is life threatening, with mortality rates exceeding 50%. Early recognition, aggressive resuscitation and monitoring, and directed, specific therapy are essential.

Mesenteric embolism accounts for approximately 50% of cases of acute visceral ischemia. The embolic source is typically cardiac, derived from a mural thrombus associated with atrial fibrillation or myocardial infarction. Embolism to visceral vessels of atheromatous debris from the thoracic aorta is much less common.

Mesenteric embolism is accompanied by sudden severe epigastric and midabdominal pain. Forceful vomiting and evacuation of stool commonly follow the onset of pain. The general physical examination may reveal an irregularly irregular pulse of atrial fibrillation or a cardiac murmur. Early after embolization, physical examination of the abdomen may be entirely unremarkable; a classic presentation is severe abdominal pain out of proportion to physical findings. Abdominal distention, guarding, and absence of bowel sounds are associated with intestinal infarction and imply disease progression.

No laboratory tests are pathognomonic for mesenteric embolism or visceral ischemia. Hemoconcentration, leukocytosis, and acidosis, like definite physical findings, indicate advanced disease. Electrocardiography may demonstrate the cardiac conduction abnormalities that are suspected on physical examination, but does not confirm embolism. Diagnosis is confirmed with either emergent diagnostic angiography or biphasic CT with mesenteric CT angiography [53]. Emboli to the superior mesenteric artery (SMA) typically lodge at branch points of the artery distal to its origin. The inferior pancreaticoduodenal artery and the middle colic artery, the first two branches of the proximal SMA, may be spared with the embolus impacted distally. After diagnosis, systemic heparinization is instituted, vigorous resuscitation with central cardiac monitoring is begun, and the patient is taken emergently for operation. Surgical therapy involves isolation of the proximal SMA and extraction of the embolus through an arteriotomy. Following restoration of flow, an assessment of intestinal viability is performed, and frankly necrotic bowel is resected. Any bowel with questionable viability is left intact and a second-look laparotomy is performed in 24–36 h to reexamine the bowel and determine if additional resection is needed.

Mesenteric thrombosis causes acute visceral ischemia after atherosclerotic narrowing of the SMA exceeds a critical level or becomes complete, typically in the setting of concomitant occlusion of the celiac and inferior mesenteric arteries. Although acute thrombosis can occur without antecedent symptoms, a history of postprandial abdominal pain and weight loss, termed chronic intestinal angina, may exist. Unlike SMA lesions resulting from mesenteric embolism, those associated with thrombosis tend to occur at the origin of the SMA from the aorta (Fig. 16.8). Acute symptoms, abdominal physical findings, and laboratory tests are similar to those listed for mesenteric embolism. Diagnosis again relies on emergent visceral angiography or biphasic CT with mesenteric CT angiography. Biphasic CT with CT angiography provides the ability to evaluate for the presence of acute mesenteric ischemia as well as findings of intestinal ischemia – pneumatosis intestinalis, portal venous gas, and thickened small bowel, as well as to rule out alternative diagnoses [53]. Once the diagnosis of mesenteric thrombosis is confirmed, emergent revascularization procedures are pursued with either construction of an arterial conduit from the aorta to the vessel distal to the point of obstruction (Fig. 16.9) or through endovascular approaches. Exploration with resection of any necrotic bowel is performed after revascularization.

Nonocclusive visceral ischemia occurs in low-flow states that cause intestinal vasoconstriction. Shock, decreased cardiac output, dehydration, hypovolemia, and inappropriate use of vasoconstrictive or inotropic agents can cause nonocclusive mesenteric ischemia. Patients are typically affected by recent myocardial infarction, congestive heart failure, or arrhythmias before the development of intestinal ischemia. Visceral angiography reveals severe vasoconstriction of mesenteric vessels, which typically have a pruned appearance (Fig. 16.10).

Treatment of nonocclusive mesenteric ischemia requires the restoration of intravascular volume and hemodynamic stability, elimination of contributing pharmacological agents, and efforts to relieve mesenteric vasospasm. Operative therapy is not therapeutic in nonocclusive mesenteric ischemia and is reserved for resection of necrotic bowel.

Iatrogenic mesenteric ischemia occurs most commonly after angiographic procedures or operations on the aorta. Angiography may cause intestinal ischemia by dislodging atheroma from a diseased vessel wall or by vessel dissection or intimal flap formation. Aortic aneurysm resection is the operation most often associated with visceral ischemia, because of involvement of the inferior mesenteric artery with the aneurysm. Clinically apparent colonic injury occurs in 1%–2% of cases. Sigmoid colonic ischemia is heralded by bloody diarrhea; the diagnosis may be confirmed by flexible sigmoidoscopy.

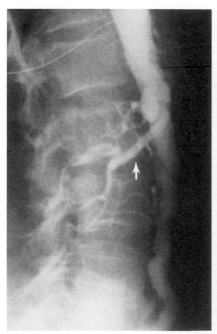
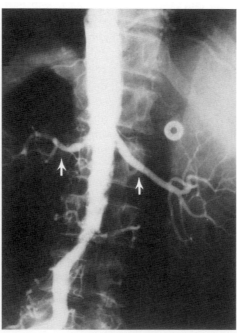

(a)   (b)

Figure 16.8 (a) Lateral and **(b)** anteroposterior emergency visceral angiograms demonstrate the absence of celiac and superior mesenteric artery filling in a patient with acute mesenteric thrombosis. Patent renal arteries are indicated by arrows.

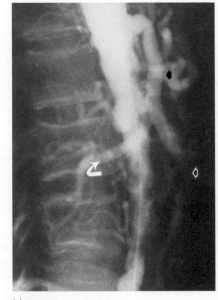

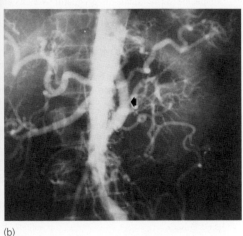

(a)

(b)

Figure 16.9 **(a)** Lateral and **(b)** anteroposterior postoperative angiograms from the patient shown in Fig. 16.8, showing the prosthetic graft (black arrow) supplying the superior mesenteric artery (open arrow). Renal artery (curved arrow) is similar to that shown in Fig. 16.8.

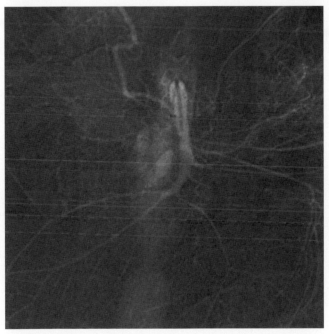

Figure 16.10 Visceral arteriogram demonstrating the classic pruned appearance of mesenteric vessels affected by nonocclusive mesenteric ischemia. Note the vasoconstricted appearance of the mesenteric vessels with loss of visualization of the secondary and tertiary mesenteric radicles.

Abdominal aortic aneurysm

Acute symptoms caused by abdominal aortic aneurysm are usually a result of expansion or rupture or, less commonly, are secondary to dissection, distal embolism, or thrombosis. Through mechanisms that are poorly understood, acute expansion of the aortic wall before rupture is associated with severe pain in the back, flank, or abdomen. Back pain is also typical of small tears, which produce leakage of blood into the retroperitoneum before catastrophic intraperitoneal hemorrhage. Approximately 20% of ruptured abdominal aortic aneurysms present with these prodromal symptoms.

The classic clinical presentation of ruptured abdominal aortic aneurysm is diffuse abdominal pain, hypotension, and pulsatile abdominal mass. Pain may radiate to the back, flank, or groin. Profound shock implies free intraperitoneal leakage of blood. Ultrasound performed in the emergency room can confirm the diagnosis. The most frequent diagnostic errors result from failure to palpate an abdominal mass, and the most frequent misdiagnosis is myocardial infarction.

If ruptured abdominal aortic aneurysm is suspected, an algorithm that includes hypotensive hemostasis, minimizing fluid resuscitation and allowing the systolic blood pressure to fall to 50 mmHg, should be instituted while preparations are made for either endovascular or open operative intervention. The mortality following open repair of a ruptured aortic aneurysm is 50% and acute renal failure, colonic ischemia, and lower extremity ischemia are common postoperative complications. Recent studies utilizing an endovascular, catheter-based approach for the repair of ruptured aortoiliac aneurysms have demonstrated a significant survival advantage over open repair, with a survival rate of 90% and significant reduction in perioperative morbidity reported in the largest endovascular series [54].

References

1. Autio V. The spread of intraperitoneal infection. Studies with Roentgen contrast medium. Acta Chir Scand 1964;36(Suppl. 321):1.
2. Gilmore OJ, Browett JP, Griffin PH, et al. Appendicitis and mimicking conditions. A prospective study. Lancet 1975;2(7932):421.

3. Cappell MS, Friedel D. Abdominal pain during pregnancy. Gastroenterol Clin North Am, 2003;32:1.

4. Birchard KR, Brown MA, Hyslop WB, et al. MRI of acute abdominal and pelvic pain in pregnant patients. Am J Roentgenol 2005;184:452.

5. Oto A, Ernst RD, Shah R, et al. Right-lower-quadrant pain and suspected appendicitis in pregnant women: evaluation with MR imaging – initial experience. Radiology 2005;234:445.

6. Brown MA, Birchard KR, Semelka RC. Magnetic resonance evaluation of pregnant patients with acute abdominal pain. Semin Ultrasound CT MR 2005;26:206.

7. Wu JM, Chen KH, Lin HF, et al. Laparoscopic appendectomy in pregnancy. J Laparoendosc Adv Surg Tech A 2005;15:447.

8. Rollins MD, Chan KJ, Price RR. Laparoscopy for appendicitis and cholelithiasis during pregnancy: a new standard of care. Surg Endosc 2004;18:237.

9. Mulholland MW, Delaney JP. Neutropenic colitis and aplastic anemia: a new association. Ann Surg 1983;197:84.

10. Shelton T, McKinlay R, Schwartz RW. Acute appendicitis: current diagnosis and treatment. Curr Surg 2003;60:502.

11. Skoubo-Kristensen E, Hvid I. The appendiceal mass: results of conservative management. Ann Surg 1982;196:584.

12. Puylaert JB, Rutgers PH, Lalisang RI, et al. A prospective study of ultrasonography in the diagnosis of appendicitis. N Engl J Med 1987;317:666.

13. Kaiser S, Frenckner B, Jorulf HK. Suspected appendicitis in children: US and CT – a prospective randomized study. Radiology 2002;223:633.

14. Hong JJ, Cohn SM, Ekeh AP, et al. A prospective randomized study of clinical assessment versus computed tomography for the diagnosis of acute appendicitis. Surg Infect (Larchmt) 2003;4:231.

15. Rao PM, Rhea JT, Novelline RA, et al. Effect of computed tomography of the appendix on treatment of patients and use of hospital resources. N Engl J Med 1998;338:141.

16. Pinto Leite N, Pereira JM, Cunha R, et al. CT evaluation of appendicitis and its complications: imaging techniques and key diagnostic findings. Am J Roentgenol 2005;185:406.

17. Foley TA, Earnest F 4th, Nathan MA, et al. Differentiation of nonperforated from perforated appendicitis: accuracy of CT diagnosis and relationship of CT findings to length of hospital stay. Radiology 2005;235:89.

18. Kaiser S, Mesas-Burgos C, Söderman E, Frenckner B. Appendicitis in children – impact of US and CT on the negative appendectomy rate. Eur J Pediatr Surg 2004;14:260.

19. Jones K, Peña AA, Dunn EL, et al. Are negative appendectomies still acceptable? Am J Surg 2004;188:748.

20. Flum DR, Koepsell T. The clinical and economic correlates of misdiagnosed appendicitis: nationwide analysis. Arch Surg, 2002;137:799; discussion 804.

21. Guller U, Hervey S, Purves H, et al. Laparoscopic versus open appendectomy: outcomes comparison based on a large administrative database. Ann Surg 2004;239:43.

22. Cooperman M. Complications of appendectomy. Surg Clin North Am 1983;63:1233.

23. Berry J Jr, Malt RA. Appendicitis near its centenary. Ann Surg 1984;200:567.

24. Bagi P, Dueholm S. Nonoperative management of the ultrasonically evaluated appendiceal mass. Surgery 1987;101:602.

25. Barakos JA, Jeffrey RB Jr, Federle MP, et al. CT in the management of periappendiceal abscess. AJR Am J Roentgenol 1986;146:1161.

26. Brown CV, Abrishami M, Muller M, Velmahos GC. Appendiceal abscess: immediate operation or percutaneous drainage? Am Surg 2003;69:829.

27. Karmeli Y, Stalnikowitz R, Eliakim R, Rahav G. Conventional dose of omeprazole alters gastric flora. Dig Dis Sci 1995;40:2070.

28. Crofts TJ, Park KG, Steele RJ, et al. A randomized trial of nonoperative treatment for perforated peptic ulcer. N Engl J Med 1989;320:970.

29. Forbes GM, Glaser ME, Cullen DJ, et al. Duodenal ulcer treated with Helicobacter pylori eradication: seven-year follow-up. Lancet 1994;343(8892):258.

30. Millat B, Fingerhut A, Borie F. Surgical treatment of complicated duodenal ulcers: controlled trials. World J Surg 2000;24:299.

31. Dubois F. New surgical strategy for gastroduodenal ulcer: laparoscopic approach. World J Surg 2000;24:270.

32. Lagoo S, McMahon RI, Kakihara M, et al. The sixth decision regarding perforated duodenal ulcer. JSLS 2002;6:359.

33. Brolin RE. Partial small bowel obstruction. Surgery 1984;95:145.

34. Sarr MG, Bulkley GB, Zuidema GD. Preoperative recognition of intestinal strangulation obstruction. Prospective evaluation of diagnostic capability. Am J Surg 1983;145:176.

35. Stewardson RH, Bombeck CT, Nyhus LM. Critical operative management of small bowel obstruction. Ann Surg 1978;187:189.

36. Mallo RD, Salem L, Lalani T, Flum DR. Computed tomography diagnosis of ischemia and complete obstruction in small bowel obstruction: a systematic review. J Gastrointest Surg 2005;9:690.

37. Osteen RT, Guyton S, Steele G Jr, Wilson RE. Malignant intestinal obstruction. Surgery 1980;87:611.

38. Clarke-Pearson DL, DeLong ER, Chin N, et al. Intestinal obstruction in patients with ovarian cancer. Variables associated with surgical complications and survival. Arch Surg 1988;123:42.

39. Zadeh BJ, Davis JM, Canizaro PC. Small bowel obstruction in the elderly. Am Surg 1985;51:470.

40. Stollman NH, Raskin JB. Diverticular disease of the colon. J Clin Gastroenterol 1999;29:241.

41. Whetsone D, Hazey J, Pofahl WE 2nd, Roth JS. Current management of diverticulitis. Curr Surg 2004;61:361.

42. Law WL, Lo CY, Chu KW. Emergency surgery for colonic diverticulitis: differences between right-sided and left-sided lesions. Int J Colorectal Dis 2001;16:280.

43. Buckley O, Geoghegan T, O'Riordain S, et al. Computed tomography in the imaging of colonic diverticulitis. Clin Radiol 2004;59:977.

44. Practice parameters for sigmoid diverticulitis. The Standards Task Force, American Society of Colon and Rectal Surgeons. Surg Laparosc Endosc Percutan Tech 2000;10:142.

45. Thorpe CD, Olsen WR, Fischer H, et al. Emergency intravenous cholangiography in patients with acute abdominal pain. Am J Surg 1973;125:46.

46. Cohan RH, Mahony BS, Bowie JD, et al. Striated intramural gallbladder lucencies on US studies: predictors of acute cholecystitis. Radiology 1987;164:31.

47. Laing FC, Federle MP, Jeffrey RB, Brown TW. Ultrasonic evaluation of patients with acute right upper quadrant pain. Radiology 1981;140:449.

48. Ralls PW, Colletti PM, Lapin SA, et al. Real-time sonography in suspected acute cholecystitis. Prospective evaluation of primary and secondary signs. Radiology 1985;155:767.

49. Kalff V, Froelich JW, Lloyd R, Thrall JH. Predictive value of an abnormal hepatobiliary scan in patients with severe intercurrent illness. Radiology 1983;146:191.

50. Carroll BA. Preferred imaging techniques for the diagnosis of cholecystitis and cholelithiasis. Ann Surg 1989;210:1.

51. Simopoulos C, Botaitis S, Polychronidis A, et al. Risk factors for conversion of laparoscopic cholecystectomy to open cholecystectomy. Surg Endosc 2005;19:905–9.

52. Pessaux P, Lebigot J, Tuech JJ, et al. [Percutaneous cholecystostomy for acute cholecystitis in high-risk patients]. Ann Chir 2000;125:738.

53. Kirkpatrick ID, Kroeker MA, Greenberg HM. Biphasic CT with mesenteric CT angiography in the evaluation of acute mesenteric ischemia: initial experience. Radiology 2003;229:91.

54. Ohki T, Veith FJ. Endovascular grafts and other image-guided catheter-based adjuncts to improve the treatment of ruptured aortoiliac aneurysms. Ann Surg 2000;232:466.

55. Mulholland MW, Debas HT. Approach to the patient with acute abdomen. In: Kelley WN (ed.). Textbook of Internal Medicine. Philadelphia: Lippincott-Raven, 1997:599.

17 Approach to the patient with ileus and obstruction

Klaus Bielefeldt, Anthony J. Bauer

Epidemiology, 287

Pathophysiology, 288

Changes in motility, 288

Changes in lumenal content, 289

Epithelial changes, 289

Changes in blood flow, 290

Metabolic and systemic consequences, 291

Clinical manifestation, 291

History, 291

Physical findings, 292

Differential diagnosis, 292

Laboratory tests, 293

Radiology, 293

Endoscopy, 297

Motility studies, 298

Therapeutic considerations, 298

Intestinal decompression, 298

Surgical approach, 299

Endoscopic therapy, 299

Pharmacotherapy, 300

Both ileus and obstruction are potentially life-threatening disorders defined by stasis of gastrointestinal contents. The underlying pathophysiology, however, is quite distinct. While ileus is the result of an impaired motility, as highlighted by the more detailed descriptors paralytic or adynamic ileus, intestinal motor function is only secondarily affected in patients with obstruction. Both disorders can occur acutely or develop more slowly in the course of a chronically progressing disease. Independent of the time course of its evolution, a complete mechanical obstruction or ileus is generally fatal unless effective treatment is initiated. With few exceptions, the underlying mechanisms leading to the paralysis of intestinal muscle (adynamic ileus) typically affect multiple regions of the gastrointestinal tract. This differs from cases of mechanical obstruction, where at least during the initial stages of blockage, function and also structure of the gastrointestinal tract distal of the lumenal occlusion remain normal.

Epidemiology

Ileus and intestinal obstruction are among the 10 leading causes of mortality from gastrointestinal diseases [1]. Annually, an estimated 93 000 hospitalizations are primarily the result of ileus or obstruction within the United States [1]. About one-fifth of admissions for acute abdomen are the result of intestinal obstruction with up to 80% located at the level of the small intestine [2]. These numbers likely underestimate the true impact of ileus, as normal motility is at least transiently lost in essentially all patients undergoing intraabdominal

Principles of Clinical Gastroenterology. Edited by Tadataka Yamada, David H. Alpers, Anthony N. Kalloo, Neil Kaplowitz, Chung Owyang, and Don W. Powell. © 2008 Blackwell Publishing. ISBN 978-1-4051-69103

operations. Even with optimal postoperative management strategies, prolonged dysfunction of the gastrointestinal tract occurs in at least 5% of patients after abdominal surgery [3]. Ileus is also among the most common complications requiring prolonged hospitalizations after trauma or surgical interventions not involving the abdominal or pelvic area [4–7]. Severe abdominal diseases, such as pancreatitis, or systemic disorders, such as sepsis, are generally associated with impaired intestinal transit, complicating nutritional support and potentially contributing to additional complications and prolonged hospital stays. Depending on the underlying etiology, the mortality of acute ileus or obstruction ranges between 2% and 20% with even worse outcomes, approaching a 50% mortality rate, in severely ill patients with systemic illnesses and multiple organ dysfunction [8–12].

Pathophysiology

Stasis of lumenal contents and the resulting local and systemic changes define both obstruction and ileus. Obstruction of intestinal transit may be the result of lumenal narrowing, objects occluding the lumen, extralumenal compression, entrapment, or torsion of the intestine (Table 17.1). Torsion around the mesenteric axis with potential proximal and distal occlusion (closed loop obstruction) may compromise the blood supply to the involved area (strangulation) and requires emergent intervention to prevent necrosis and its complications.

Table 17.1 Causes of intestinal obstruction

Lumenal narrowing	Malignancy
	Stricture
	Inflammation
	Intussusception
	Atresia
	Hirschsprung disease
Intralumenal objects	Gallstone ileus
	Meconium ileus
	Foreign body
Extralumenal compression	Peritoneal carcinomatosis
	Pelvic malignancies
	Endometriosis
	Abscess
	Hematoma
	Cysts
Entrapment	Hernia
	Adhesion, congenital bands
Torsion	Strangulated hernia
	Volvulus

Table 17.2 Causes of ileus

Intraabdominal surgery
Trauma (abdominal trauma, retroperitoneal injury, spinal or brain injury)
Sepsis
Severe intestinal or abdominal inflammation or infection (toxic megacolon, pancreatitis)
Intestinal ischemia
Drugs and toxins (opioids, anticholinergics, cytotoxic agents, lead)
Electrolyte abnormalities (hypercalcemia, hypokalemia, hypophosphatemia)
Metabolic disorders (diabetes mellitus, hypothyroidism)
Visceral myopathies
Visceral neuropathies
Connective tissue and infiltrative diseases (scleroderma, amyloidosis)

In the Western world, small bowel diseases account for the majority of patients presenting with obstruction. The leading cause is adhesions, generally a consequence of previous surgeries. Crohn's disease with lumenal narrowing caused by inflammation or stricture formation has surpassed herniations as the second most common cause for intestinal obstruction [13,14]. In contrast to the predominance of benign disorders leading to small bowel obstruction, more than half of the cases of large intestinal obstruction are caused by adenocarcinomas followed by diverticular disease and volvulus. In frail or disabled individuals, impacted fecal material can completely occlude the colonic lumen and present as an obstruction. Drugs, sepsis, abdominal trauma or surgery, ischemia, severe electrolyte or metabolic disorders, primary diseases of intestinal muscle or alterations in the interstitial cells of Cajal or the enteric nervous system can all lead to ileus (Table 17.2).

Changes in motility

Significant alterations in gastrointestinal contractile patterns are caused by intestinal obstruction and develop during ileus. Experimental models of obstruction have demonstrated that contractions increase proximal to the intestinal blockage, whereas distally contractions are inhibited. The resulting proximal accumulation of fluids and gas increases the intralumenal pressure and wall tension, stimulating stretch receptors and enhancing the peristaltic reflex. A major component of this increased proximal motor activity is driven by enteric cholinergic motor neurons. In a prolonged state of obstruction, the enhanced peristaltic motor reflexes, which functionally attempt to overcome the obstruction, are interrupted by periods of clustered contractions, intense aborally migrating contractile pressure waves, or motor quiescence. These alternating contractile patterns produce intermittent colic and borborygmi, particularly in the post-prandial state. The motor patterns are not diagnostic of an obstruction, however, because they also occur in pseudo-obstruction. In chronic obstructive conditions the muscularis externa becomes markedly thickened through both hyper-trophic and hyperplastic mechanisms. Over time, motor activity diminishes, displaying progressively more periods of motor quiescence throughout the gastrointestinal tract, which is most likely caused by inhibitory intestinointest-inal reflexes. In contrast to the enhanced proximal motor activity, distal to the obstruction descending nonadrenergic, noncholinergic (nitric oxide/vasoactive intestinal peptide/adenosine triphosphate) inhibitory motor reflexes maintain this region in a state of hypomotility. Interstitial cells of Cajal within the muscularis externa are known to play a key role in the proper functioning of enteric neuromuscular transmis-sion [15]. It has been shown experimentally that partial bowel obstruction leads to phenotypic changes in the interstitial cells of Cajal, which are slowly reversed after the obstruction is removed [16]. Hence, changes in neuronal activity, inter-stitial cells of Cajal, and the smooth muscle cell itself all appear to contribute to the alterations in motility during chronic intestinal obstruction. The colon has a larger capacity to adapt to obstruction, thus motility abnormalities develop more slowly in the colon. Colonic contractile activity gener-ally follows the pattern discussed for the obstructed small intestine. If the orad right colon is obstructed then the remaining distal regions exhibit hypomotility, whereas if the distal left colon is obstructed then a state of colonic hypermotility consisting of vigorous clustered contractions tends to exist.

Mechanisms causing adynamic ileus may be neurogenic, myogenic, humoral, immunogenic, toxic (bacterial toxins), and pharmacological (narcotics). A common clinical presenta-tion of nonobstructive ileus is exemplified in postoperative ileus, which persists for days after surgery. Although anes-thetics inhibit gastrointestinal motility, experimental models have demonstrated that laparotomy and surgical handling of the bowel trigger the activation of the dense network of macrophages that lie constitutively within the muscularis externa to initiate a complex inflammatory response of transcription factor upregulation, cytokine and chemokine induction, vascular adhesion molecule expression, and leuko-cyte recruitment, which results in a panenteric suppression of neuromuscular function and the activation of inhibitory neural reflexes [17,18]. Uncomplicated clinical postoperative ileus is generally characterized by the return of gastrointest-inal motility first to the small intestine at around 6 h followed by the stomach at 24 h and in the colon after several days. However, bowel dilation from gas and fluid accumulation can additionally activate visceral afferents, which initiates inhibitory reflex responses, further impairing motility. Post-operative ileus persisting for longer than 3 to 4 days indicates that a complication may exist. The intrinsic postoperative

dysmotility response to surgery is often complicated by the use of narcotics for postoperative pain management, as nar-cotics alone are notorious for causing opioid-induced bowel constipation. The mechanism of this appears to be at least in part the result of an abnormal enteric motor suppression of inhibitory nitrergic neuromuscular transmission through activation of μ-opioid and δ-opioid receptors on the postjunc-tional neural membrane [19].

Sepsis-induced ileus represents another major cause of clinical bowel dysfunction. It is appreciated that the dense network of resident muscularis macrophages mediates sepsis-induced ileus [20,21]. Various bacterial toxins that are recog-nized as pathogen-associated molecular patterns (PAMPs) engage and trigger inflammatory responses using the family of Toll-like receptors (TLR) and other PAMP receptors on muscularis macrophages and circulating leukocytes. The classical TLR-4 pathway is the most studied. The resulting generation of cytokines and chemokines, directly through their paracrine interactions within the muscularis and in-directly by recruiting circulating leukocytes to the areas of engagement, causes suppression of gastrointestinal motility.

Infiltrative processes, such as amyloidosis, or progressive replacement of smooth muscle by fibrotic tissues, as may occur in systemic sclerosis, severely alter motility and lead to secondary forms of myogenic pseudoobstruction.

Changes in lumenal content

In cases of intestinal obstruction, ingested materials and swallowed air accumulate proximal to the site of obstruction, resulting in progressive lumenal distention. The normally low number of microorganisms within the proximal gastro-intestinal tract increases with a rise in coliform and anaerobic organisms and contributes to the mucosal damage and inflam-mation [22–24]. In addition, bacteria ferment the intestinal contents, which is associated with generation of hydrogen or methane. The rising lumenal pressure and the developing inflammation trigger secretion, impair the absorptive capac-ity of the intestinal mucosa, and further distend the intestinal lumen (Fig. 17.1).

In patients with chronic intestinal pseudoobstruction or prolonged partial mechanical obstruction, bacterial over-growth may interfere with the absorption of nutrients and micronutrients. The deconjugation of bile acids impairs the absorption of fat and fat-soluble vitamins [25]. In addition, gram-negative bacteria bind intrinsic factor and may cause vitamin B-12 deficiency [26].

Epithelial changes

The intestinal mucosa functions as an active barrier protect-ing the host from microorganisms within the lumen, absorbing

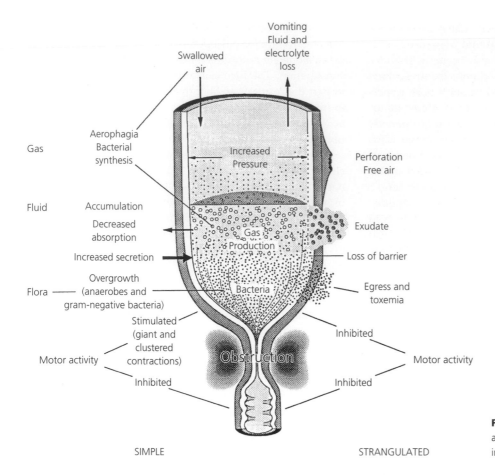

Figure 17.1 Pathophysiology of simple (left) and strangulated (right) obstruction in the small intestine. Courtesy of Dr R.W. Summers.

nutrients, electrolytes and water and producing secretions that are important for the digestive process. Ultrastructural changes in epithelial cells are seen as early as 4 h after experimentally inducing a complete obstruction [27]. Soon afterwards, mucin-producing cells show signs of damage, impairing the production of the protective mucous layer. Consistent with these morphological changes, translocation of bacteria into the gut wall and mesenteric lymph nodes can be seen even in the absence of ischemia and epithelial necrosis [27–30]. The invasion of organisms likely contributes to the inflammation and evidence of focal mucosal damage, as seen under experimental conditions and in patients with chronic intestinal pseudoobstruction [24,27,28]. In parallel with these structural changes, nutrient absorption in the intestine decreases rapidly after the development of obstruction [31]. The initial effect is largely the result of changes in intralumenal pressure, followed by mucosal injury and inflammation as a result of bacterial overgrowth and translocation [32,33]. Inflammatory mediators promote secretion, thereby further exacerbating fluid shifts. In addition, the progressive lumenal distention during ileus or obstruction triggers enteric reflexes, leading to chloride and bicarbonate secretion, thereby worsening the fluid and electrolyte losses [34–38].

Changes in blood flow

The torsion of mesenteric vascular bundles in closed loop obstruction or compression through entrapment or tumors can directly impair venous and arterial blood flow, which may lead to bowel wall gangrene and perforation. In non-strangulated obstruction and ileus, retention of material and increased secretion progressively dilate the intestinal lumen and increase intralumenal pressure. Experimental distention of the intestine to baseline pressures of 20 mmHg significantly increases the vascular resistance, and can impair blood flow in segments with preexisting incomplete obstruction [39,40]. Data obtained in animal experiments and in patients with postoperative ileus demonstrate that baseline pressures remain below 10 mmHg, arguing against a significant effect of intralumenal pressures on blood flow [41,42]. However, hemorrhagic shock represents a quite common cause of motility dysfunction, caused by intestinal ischemia/reperfusion injury [43,44]. Indeed, the intestine has been proposed to be the "motor" of multiple organ failure because of its release of inflammatory factors into the systemic circulation, which results in the dysfunction of distant organs such as the liver, lungs, and kidneys [45].

Metabolic and systemic consequences

Closed loop obstructions with impaired blood flow are true medical emergencies and require rapid correction, generally through surgical intervention. Severe epithelial damage rapidly impairs the barrier function, leading to bacterial translocation and systemic inflammatory response syndrome with cytokine release [46,47]. With persistent ischemia, bowel wall necrosis and perforation ensue, resulting in metabolic acidosis, sepsis, and eventually multiorgan failure.

Even if normal blood flow is preserved, ileus or obstruction can cause significant systemic consequences. While delayed compared to situations with ischemic bowel, bacterial translocation occurs in patients with either ileus or obstruction [28,30]. Stasis of lumenal contents causes a progressive abdominal distention, impeding diaphragmatic excursions and increasing the likelihood of atelectasis or frank respiratory failure. Especially in the case of gastric or small bowel obstruction, patients may regurgitate or vomit retained material, which can further compromise respiratory function. A competent ileocecal valve generally prevents severe vomiting and fluid loss in patients with colonic obstruction. Lumenal distention leads to a shift toward net secretion, exacerbating the fluid and electrolyte losses due to vomiting. If the gastric outlet is occluded, frequent emesis of acidic material results in metabolic alkalosis. In contrast, more distal obstructions are typically associated with acidosis, especially when hypovolemia or systemic inflammatory response syndrome develop. The cardiovascular and other systemic complications largely reflect the consequences of volume loss, systemic inflammatory response, and autonomic reaction caused by significant pain.

Clinical manifestation

When approaching a patient with symptoms of ileus or obstruction, the most important question is whether or not gut perfusion is compromised and may lead to gangrene and perforation. If clinical indicators and test results rule out ischemic bowel, history, physical findings, and diagnostic studies typically allow the differentiation of ileus from mechanical problems, the determination of whether an obstruction is complete or partial, and identification of the location and nature of the underlying anatomical problems.

History

The patient's complaints will depend on the temporal development of ileus or obstruction, the underlying problem, the localization and completeness of a potential mechanical obstruction, complications, and comorbid conditions. Most patients present with abdominal distention and pain or discomfort, often associated with obstipation and nausea or vomiting. While the absence of these symptoms argues against ileus or complete obstruction, the sensitivity of these complaints remains low when used alone or in combination [48]. Patients with proximal obstruction of the gastrointestinal tract may complain about bloating and perhaps distention, although the latter symptom becomes more prominent in individuals with ileus or obstruction of the midgut or distal gut. Patients may mention that they are visibly distended and do not fit into their clothes any longer. Unless complicated by peritonitis, the typical pain of mechanical obstruction is described as a dull pressure or squeezing in nature with cramp- or wave-like exacerbations. The intense pain rarely lasts longer than 1 min before easing up and recurring again within 3–10 min. Food intake generally worsens, while vomiting may alleviate the pain transiently. Intensity and localization of this pain provides additional useful information. Gastric outlet obstruction typically triggers severe nausea and frequent vomiting, which limits distention and typically is associated with mild epigastric pain. The pain of small intestinal obstruction generally projects to the periumbilical area, and is more severe and colicky in character compared to that experienced by patients with gastric obstruction. Patients with colonic obstruction may experience the pain as localized slightly below the umbilicus, and those with distal lesions usually have the pain more localized to the left lower abdomen. Some patients may describe very loud bowel sounds (borborygmi) or movement of dilated intestinal loops visible on the abdominal surface and at times associated with painful exacerbations. If a functioning ileocecal valve does not allow decompression, the pain becomes intense and may eventually be unrelenting. The rapid onset of such a severe and unrelenting pain suggests intestinal ischemia or perforation. Less intense, continuous, and vaguely localized abdominal pain is characteristic of patients with ileus. While nearly all patients experience anorexia and nausea, vomiting is more common in individuals with gastric or small bowel obstruction or ileus. Colonic obstruction typically does not lead to vomiting, as the ileocecal valve only allows limited retrograde escape of colonic contents. Patients with gastric outlet obstruction describe an acidic, non-bilious emesis. In contrast, vomitus of individuals with small bowel obstruction contains bile and is generally perceived as bitter tasting, may become malodorous or feculent. Once a complete obstruction develops, patients become obstipated and eventually do not pass stool or flatus. However, there are exceptions from this general rule, most notably the bloody secretions in infants and children with intestinal intussusception and the often continuous drainage of small amounts of liquid stool in severely ill patients with ileus, acute colonic pseudoobstruction, or fecal impaction. Clearly, information about prior gastrointestinal symptoms, coexisting and prior illnesses, prior surgeries or traumas, medications, and toxin exposure is essential. The combination of abdominal pain and distention with a history of abdominal surgeries significantly increases the likelihood of an acute small bowel obstruction [49]. In an elderly individual, gradual weight loss, change in bowel habits, and hematochezia raise concerns about a malignant obstruction of the distal colon. Finally, the family history may point to hereditary disorders, such as familial polyposis syndromes, mitochondrial myopathies, or visceral neuropathies.

Physical findings

The physical examination provides critical information about the nature and severity of the underlying problem and the presence of potential complications. Significant pain typically leads to distress, which manifests in facial expression and attempts to find a comfortable body position. Behavior and physiognomy may reflect the periodicity of pain exacerbations in patients with mechanical obstruction, which can correlate with audible changes in bowel sounds or even movement of intestinal loops visible on the abdominal surface in thin individuals. There may be signs of chronic, emaciating disease as a result of an advanced malignancy or chronic pseudoobstruction. Some patients may show important signs of volume depletion as a result of impaired intake, repeated vomiting, or fluid shifts, or even indicators of impending circulatory collapse in patients with septic shock. An inspection of the abdomen will reveal distention, potentially visible peristalsis, scars from prior abdominal surgeries or bulges, suggesting herniation of intestinal loops. Gentle percussion may reveal tympanitic sounds, especially in patients with distal colonic obstruction or ileus. A careful palpation of the abdomen may reveal involuntary guarding or rebound tenderness, which indicates the presence of complications that may require emergency surgery. External herniations should be sought in the groin area, umbilicus, and along the borders of the rectus abdominis. In thin individuals, it may be possible to see or feel the above-mentioned intestinal movements through the abdominal wall. During deep palpation, one should try to identify masses due to inflammation or neoplasms. The presence of ascites or an enlarged, nodular liver suggests an advanced malignancy as the potential cause. Especially early in the course of the disease, auscultation is helpful in differentiating ileus from obstruction. The absence of gastrointestinal motility in patients results in few, soft and at times gurgling or tinkling bowel sounds, which can sometimes be triggered by tapping or shaking the abdomen. A characteristic succussion splash, generally attributed to the filled stomach, may also be heard. This is quite distinct from the loud, clustered metallic or tinkling sounds that can be heard every 3 min to 10 min in patients with mechanical obstruction [50]. The intermittent nature of the underlying clustered contractions requires prolonged or repeated listening and may explain the relatively low sensitivity of this characteristic finding in patients with intestinal obstruction [51]. The rectal examination should determine the presence of tenderness or masses in the pelvic area. In some cases of incomplete obstruction associated with fecal soiling, it may identify fecal impaction. The remainder of the physical examination should search for other clues to the underlying problem, such as telangiectasias and skin changes of systemic sclerosis, soft tissue tumors, abnormal pigmentation suggesting malignancies or tumors (Peutz–Jeghers syndrome), or sensory or motor deficits.

Differential diagnosis

The presenting symptoms of patients with ileus and obstruction – abdominal pain and distention – are among the most common gastrointestinal complaints leading to clinic and emergency room visits [1]. With the exception of patients with chronic intestinal pseudoobstruction and individuals with partial intestinal obstruction caused by strictures, ileus and complete intestinal obstruction develop relatively acutely. The main differential diagnoses therefore include other causes of an acute, nontraumatic abdomen, such as perforated viscus, ischemic bowel disease, diverticulitis, aortic dissection, severe inflammatory bowel disease, pancreatitis, renal or biliary colic (see Chapter 16). Some of these diseases may lead to ileus, which potentially confounds the presentation. When symptoms and physical findings are indicative of an obstruction of the gastrointestinal tract, it is important to determine whether the obstruction is complete or associated with ischemia of the affected segment, which generally necessitates immediate intervention. Slowly progressive or intermittent symptoms, continuous passage of flatus or stool, and only minor abnormalities on physical examination argue against the need for emergency surgery. If the clinical presentation suggests a *mechanical obstruction*, then the cause and location needs to be determined (Table 17.1). Most causes of small bowel obstruction are due to *extrinsic lesions*, primarily adhesions, which can entrap loops of intestine and even cause strangulation. Internal and external herniations or congenital bands can similarly lead to closed loop obstruction. Extramural structures, such as abscesses, tumors, hematomas, or vascular abnormalities can obstruct the lumen of large or small intestine. *Intrinsic lesions* with lumenal narrowing, such as strictures, inflammation, or malignancies, are the most common cause of colonic obstruction. Primary malignancies of the small intestine are rare, thus making inflammatory changes due to Crohn's disease the most common cause for mechanical small bowel obstruction, primarily affecting the distal ileum. This differs from the colon, where adenocarcinomas play an important role, with about 15% of the cancers presenting as acute obstruction [11]. In addition to malignancies and the already mentioned Crohn's disease, stricture formation after radiation, ischemia, or diverticulitis can lead to obstruction. Intussusception is rarely seen in adults and is generally caused by an underlying structural abnormality, such as a neoplasm. However, it is more common in children and can be associated with continuing passage of bloody secretions through the anus. *Torsion* or volvulus formation primarily affects the distal gut (sigmoid, less commonly the cecum) and stomach in adults. As a result of the rotation of the mesenteric attachment, the vascular supply can be compromised, potentially resulting in ischemia and perforation. Finally, mobile objects can occlude the lumen. These may include foreign bodies, indigestible materials, or gallstones in patients with cholecystoduodenal fistulae. While strictures, or inflammatory or neoplastic processes can certainly predispose to occlusions, mechanical obstruction may also occur as the result of an intralumenal object.

Should the clinical presentation suggest the presence of an *adynamic ileus*, the underlying problem needs to be identified (Table 17.2). Abdominal surgery clearly remains the most common cause of transient paralysis of the gut. Trauma, radiation, intra-abdominal or severe systemic infections, or ischemia can also severely impair gastrointestinal motility, potentially causing ileus. Toxic megacolon is a feared complication of severe inflammation because of idiopathic inflammatory bowel disease or specific forms of colitis (e.g., pseudomembranous colitis). Retroperitoneal and spinal disorders or surgeries that trigger inhibitory reflexes can complicate and prolong the hospitalization. A variety of drugs, toxins, and metabolic abnormalities affect gastrointestinal motility and can lead to adynamic ileus. Opiates, anticholinergic substances, chemotherapeutic agents, and electrolyte abnormalities are clinically most important in this context. Motility abnormalities, such as chronic intestinal pseudo-obstruction, rarely manifest acutely, thus differentiating them from other disorders causing adynamic ileus. Most patients with chronic intestinal pseudoobstruction present with a long history of gastrointestinal complaints with nausea, vomiting, abdominal distention, and constipation or diarrhea, often complicated by progressive weight loss at later stages.

Laboratory tests

Laboratory testing is of limited value in patients with mechanical obstruction. Hematological parameters, such as the presence of leukocytosis, or other laboratory tests are primarily useful to discern the presence of complications, such as dehydration or electrolyte abnormalities. Several markers of bowel wall ischemia have been proposed, but remain limited in their clinical utility, as significant elevation of specific markers often only occur at later stages in the disease process. However, biochemical tests are important to identify potential underlying problems in patients with ileus, where electrolyte abnormalities, uremia, diabetic ketoacidosis, or other primary disorders may be identified.

Radiology

Radiological imaging is the main diagnostic modality in patients presenting with an acute nontraumatic abdomen. The main goals are to differentiate adynamic ileus from obstruction or other causes of an acute abdomen, to identify the level and cause of a potential obstruction, and to recognize possible complications. Because of the relatively low cost and wide availability of radiography, *plain abdominal radiographs* in the supine and upright positions are most commonly performed as the initial step. The upright image should always include the diaphragm to look for free air as a sign of perforation. For severely ill or frail patients, a radiograph can be taken in the lateral decubitus position. Impaired transit of intestinal contents leads to a progressive distention of small or large bowel loops, which can be recognized if the areas are filled with gas, providing an intrinsic contrast. The intestinal valvulae conniventes can typically be seen as fine and relatively closely spaced structures, differing from colonic haustra, which generally only occupy a portion of the circumference (Fig. 17.2). Diameters of more than 2.5 cm and 8 cm indicate small bowel and colonic distention, respectively [13,52,53].

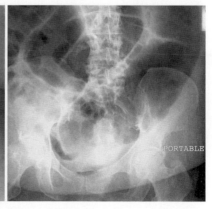

Figure 17.2 Plain abdominal radiographs showing the typical appearance of small bowel loops **(a)** with closely spaced valvulae conniventes, whereas haustra of the distended colon **(b)** are further apart and are often not circumferential.

(a)   (b)

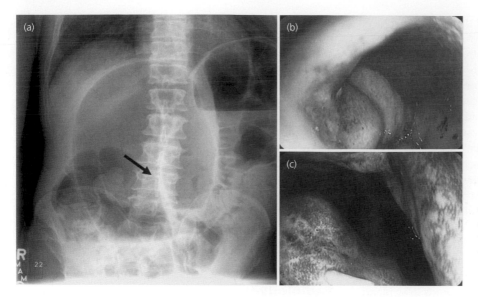

Figure 17.3 The plain abdominal radiograph **(a)** shows a sigmoid volvulus with a very distended loop of colon extending to the right upper quadrant and a distinct midline crease (arrow). The mucosa has a dusky and edematous appearance with spiraling folds as the colonoscope approaches the distal end of the segment **(b)**. Advancement of the scope into the dilated segment reveals a congested, ischemic mucosa **(c)**.

The diameter of the colon is more variable with the sigmoid generally being the narrowest area and the cecum showing the greatest diameter. The position of intestinal loops provides some additional clues about the affected areas with the small intestine primarily occupying the central region and the colon framing the abdomen. With increasing distention, typical features and organ positioning may not be easily identified, thus complicating the interpretation of images. Air–fluid levels, when seen in at least three or more loops of intestine on the upright radiograph or in combination with a dilated segment of small bowel, are suggestive of gastrointestinal obstruction or ileus. However, it is not possible to differentiate obstruction from ileus unless the colon is gasless [13]. The differential height of air–fluid levels in small bowel loops has also been proposed as a sign of mechanical small bowel obstruction, but this feature can also be seen in patients with ileus [52,53]. Sigmoid or the less common cecal volvulus results in a relatively characteristic radiograph with a significantly dilated loop of colon extending from the left lower quadrant toward the diaphragm with the mesenteric root creating a distinct midline crease ("coffee bean" sign) (Fig. 17.3). With a reported sensitivity of about 60%, plain radiographs may be sufficient in many patients presenting with typical symptoms of intestinal obstruction or ileus. However, they are of limited value in determining the location of an obstruction or detecting complications, such as ischemia due to strangulation [13,52,54,55].

Computed tomography (CT) has clearly surpassed the plain X-ray in terms of diagnostic yield [13,55–58]. Especially when ileus or obstruction needs to be differentiated from other potential causes of acute nontraumatic abdominal pain, the detailed image information of abdominal and retroperitoneal organs is invaluable. Unlike plain radiographs, CT imaging can also detect fluid-filled loops of intestine. In addition to dilation, fecal material or small gas bubbles trapped between valvulae conniventes ("string of beads") are abnormal (Fig. 17.4). A distinct transition from dilated to collapsed loops of intestine is diagnostic for an obstruction as the underlying cause (Figs 17.5 and 17.6). Changes in intestinal wall thickness, fat stranding, extralumenal masses, and other findings provide important information about the underlying cause (Fig. 17.7). Closed loop obstruction can be recognized as a C-shaped or U-shaped, fluid-filled segment with tapering ends. The most common cause of small bowel obstruction, adhesions, cannot be directly diagnosed by CT or other imaging techniques. However, a sudden transition point in the absence of identifiable extralumenal structures or abnormalities of the intestinal wall suggests the presence of an adhesive or congenital band. The use of intravenous contrast is especially important if strangulation is suspected. Thickening of the intestinal wall with low contrast compared to the fluid-filled lumen and a lack of enhancement during the contrast phase suggest ischemia [13,52,55,59]. Pneumatosis cystoides intestinalis is a late sign of bowel ischemia and necrosis that can be seen on plain radiographs and CT scans (Fig. 17.8). Pneumatosis can occasionally be seen in patients with chronic intestinal pseudoobstruction. Considering the increasing availability of the CT technology, patients presenting with symptoms of bowel obstruction or ileus should undergo CT, unless the plain radiograph has already established the cause of the problem. Evaluation of early abdominal CT in patients with acute abdomen may actually shorten the time to definitive therapy, thereby reducing morbidity and potentially even mortality in these patients [57]. In cases of incomplete obstruction, *contrast studies* can be helpful in further defining the underlying etiology (Fig. 17.9). To obtain detailed information, barium-containing contrast medium is generally required because water-soluble contrast does not render the lumen sufficiently opaque. Moreover, the high osmolarity of water-soluble contrast may lead to additional

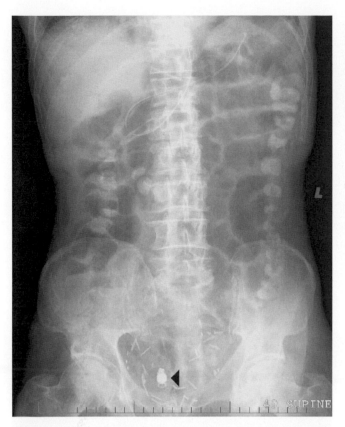

Figure 17.4 The plain abdominal radiograph shows a partial small bowel obstruction in a patient after capsule endoscopy for obscure gastrointestinal bleeding. The dilated loops of small bowel are surrounded by decompressed colon, which is opacified by a residual oral contrast used during a preceding computed tomography scan. The arrowhead points at the retained capsule. Multiple surgical clips and a nasogastric tube can be seen.

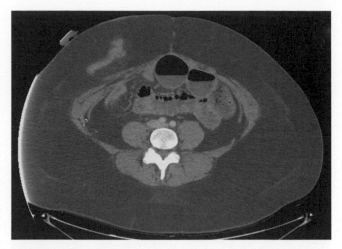

Figure 17.5 The section of an abdominal computed tomography scan shows dilated bowel loops with multiple small air bubbles trapped between valvulae conniventes ("string of beads").

fluid shifts into the lumen. However, if perforation is suspected the use of barium-based contrast material should be avoided because barium causes severe peritonitis. If colonic obstruction is suspected, retained barium may inspissate and lead to impaction. As a result of secretion and the resulting dilution, inspissation of barium is not likely in the small intestine, but even small amounts of retained material may interfere with subsequent imaging using other modalities, primarily CT [13]. If small bowel obstruction is suspected, impaired motility will slow down transit and may not allow appropriate visualization of distal segments. Retained lumenal contents

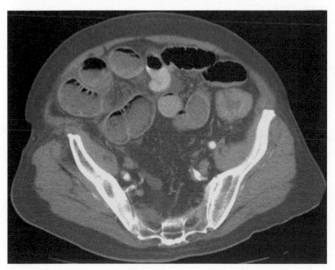

(a)

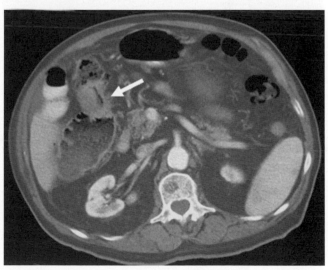

(b)

Figure 17.6 Sections of an abdominopelvic computed tomography scan showing dilated loops of small bowel with the "string of beads" sign **(a)** and wall thickening with lumenal narrowing (arrow) in the ascending colon **(b)**. These findings are consistent with a partial small bowel obstruction due to a proximal colonic malignancy.

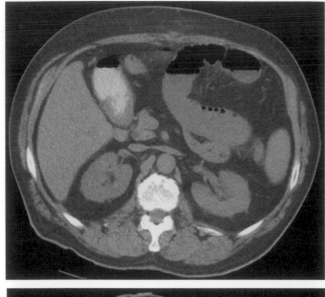

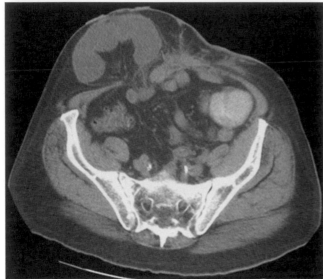

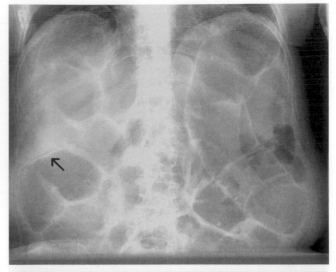

(a)

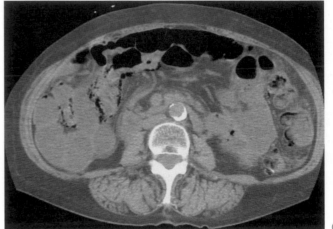

(b)

Figure 17.8 The plain abdominal radiograph **(a)** and section of an abdominal computed tomography (CT) scan **(b)** show dilated loops of large and small bowel consistent with ileus. The arrow points to air trapped within the gut wall (pneumatosis cystoides intestinalis), which is much more prominent on the CT scan.

Figure 17.7 Sections of an abdominopelvic computed tomography scan showing dilated loops of small bowel with the "string of beads" sign **(a)** and a large incisional hernia as the cause of the small bowel obstruction **(b)**.

in the dilated intestine may also dilute the contrast medium, further exacerbating this problem. Therefore, the small bowel contrast study may provide limited information and is inferior to an enteroclysis, perhaps with prior decompression of the distended small bowel [55]. The main niche of small bowel contrast studies is in situations of intermittent or incomplete obstructions with normal findings on CT, where diagnostic gains have been demonstrated with enteroclysis [13,55]. Contrast enemas have a limited role in the evaluation of patients with suspected colonic obstruction. Incomplete filling and retention of fecal material proximal to the obstructing lesion lower detection rates for clinically significant findings. While only a few studies specially examined the use of *virtual colonoscopy* in patients with large bowel obstruc-

tion, this newly evolving technique appears to be superior to conventional contrast examinations of the colon [60,61]. Abdominal ultrasound and magnetic resonance imaging have also been used in patients with ileus or obstruction. The lack of radiation exposure is clearly the main advantage of these modalities. Theoretically, *ultrasound* enables observation of the dynamic intestinal movements, determination of wall thickening and even assessment of blood flow using Doppler probes. However, the often distended and gas-filled loops of intestine interfere with sound penetration, thereby significantly limiting the utility of ultrasound. Initial studies of *magnetic resonance imaging* show performance characteristics comparable with or even superior to those of CT [55,62,63]. However, higher cost and limited availability favor CT scans as the main imaging modality in patients with nontrauma-related abdomen.

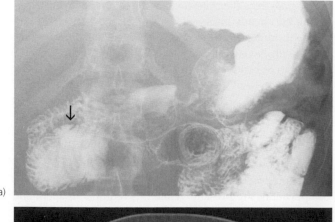

(a)

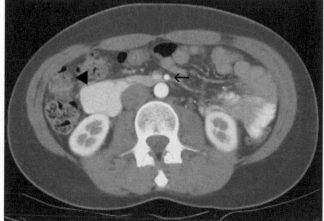

(b)

Figure 17.9 Barium contrast study **(a)** and computed tomography scan **(b)** show a dilated duodenum due to extrinsic compression between the aorta and the superior mesenteric artery (arrow).

Endoscopy

There are no systematic studies on the role of endoscopy in patients with ileus or obstruction. However, in patients with proximal lesions or abnormalities within the reach of the colonoscope, endoscopes may allow inspection, biopsies, and possibly therapeutic interventions (Fig. 17.10). Unless extralumenal processes are suspected, endoscopic examination will certainly be the diagnostic study of choice in such situations. If clinical and radiographic findings are ambiguous or suggest a complete obstruction of the distal colon, colonoscopic examination may still be successful with enemas as preparation. However, it is important to minimize the use of air insufflation, which will further distend the already dilated intestine. While no study has addressed the utility of CO_2 in this clinical setting, randomized trials have demonstrated lower pain ratings and decreased distention in patients after colonoscopy with CO_2 rather than air insufflation [64,65]. Colonoscopy plays an especially important role in patients presenting with sigmoid volvulus. In this situation, the lumen typically tapers in a spiraling way to a

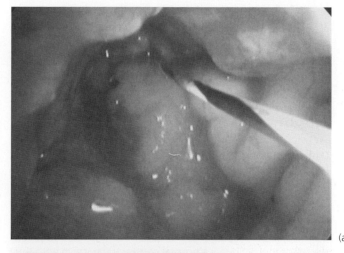

(a)

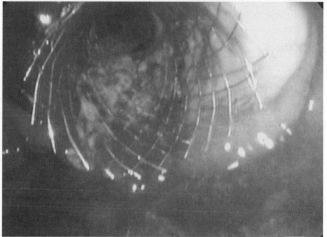

(b)

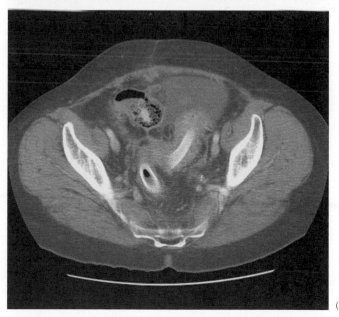

(c)

Figure 17.10 Endoscopic treatment for colonic obstruction caused by a cancer of the distal colon. After insertion of a guidewire **(a)**, the obstruction was successfully treated through stenting **(b,c)**. Images courtesy of Dr A. Slivka.

narrow segment (Fig. 17.3), which can generally be passed by carefully advancing the endoscope, and this may result in reduction of the volvulus. Despite this initial success, the recurrences that occur in more than half of the patients require more definitive therapy [66,67].

Motility studies

If history, physical findings, and radiographic studies suggest a pseudoobstruction, functional studies may be helpful to determine the involvement of different areas of the gastrointestinal tract and differentiate myogenic from neuropathic causes. Small bowel manometry can provide additional information about the underlying motility pattern [68,69]. If the manometry shows a normal contractile pattern with low-amplitude contractions, myogenic problems likely underlie the disease process. In contrast, irregular patterns without the typical migrating motor complex and without conversion from fasting to a fed pattern indicate a neuropathic form of pseudoobstruction. While abnormal motility patterns have also been described in patients with mechanical obstruction [69], functional studies generally provide little useful information in other patients presenting with symptoms suggesting ileus or intestinal obstruction. As the clinical utility of small bowel manometry has not been fully evaluated, the clinical usefulness of small bowel manometry remains to be determined.

Therapeutic considerations

When approaching a patient with ileus or obstruction, the most important therapeutic decision relates to the question whether or not emergent surgical intervention is necessary. Generally, a complete obstruction is a surgical emergency, especially if clinical findings or diagnostic studies indicate strangulation. However, operative interventions in these often severely ill individuals carry a high morbidity and mortality. This has led to the development of alternative approaches [10–12]. In the absence of complications, requiring immediate surgery, symptomatic therapy should be instituted in conjunction with appropriate diagnostic studies. The goal is to improve the overall performance status of the often very ill patient by alleviating pain and discomfort, correcting fluid and electrolyte abnormalities and decreasing the likelihood of complications due to intestinal distention. Intravenous access should be secured to replace fluid and electrolytes and to correct acid–base imbalances. Early decisions should be made about the need for nutritional support, as malnutrition contributes to excess morbidity and mortality in these patients [70,71]. Whenever possible the enteral route should be chosen, as nutrient flowing through the intestine decreases the likelihood of bacterial translocation and sepsis [72–74]. Pain management may be difficult, because centrally

acting analgesics alter intestinal motility, thus potentially worsening the already impaired transit. The most effective management strategy is decompression of the distended intestine, which will alleviate discomfort and associated symptoms.

In cases of complete obstruction, definitive therapy, most often surgery, will be necessary and should be performed after the initial stabilization and decompression. A less aggressive approach is justified in patients with adhesive disease, the most common cause of small bowel obstruction in Western countries [75,76]. As surgery will likely lead to the formation of additional adhesions, conservative management should be tried in patients with adhesive disease unless complications are present. While this requires frequent and careful monitoring to recognize potential signs of worsening or impending complications, repeat operations can be avoided in 60%–90% of the cases [77–80].

Intestinal decompression

Intestinal distention causes significant discomfort with pain, nausea, and vomiting and may impair respiratory function. Therefore, decompression plays an important role in the management of patients with ileus and obstruction. Most commonly, nasogastric suction is employed to relieve gaseous distention. The pylorus may restrict retrograde flow of intestinal contents, thus potentially limiting the effectiveness of nasogastric suction in decompressing the small bowel. Based on these assumptions, long intestinal tubes have been developed, which are placed beyond the ligament of Treitz, but require significant expertise and the use of fluoroscopy or endoscopy [13,79,81]. While the placement distal to the pylorus constitutes a theoretical advantage, the only randomized controlled trial comparing conventional and long tubes for intestinal decompression did not show a difference between the two treatments [80]. Finally, although considered standard of care, no controlled study has directly addressed the importance of nasogastric suction in patients with ileus and obstruction. Especially in patients with significant distention, nausea, and vomiting, decompression clearly alleviates the symptoms and may decrease the potential for complications as a result of regurgitation and aspiration. However, nasogastric tubes themselves are an important cause of patient discomfort. Interestingly, the routine use of nasogastric tube decompression after major abdominal surgery is not associated with an increase in the length of postoperative ileus or an increase in postoperative complications [73,78,82–84]. Only about one-fifth of the patients eventually require brief nasogastric decompression for symptom relief after major abdominal surgery associated with transient postoperative ileus. These results may not be directly applicable to the different clinical scenarios of patients presenting with obstruction. Despite this caveat, it is reasonable to individualize the use of nasogastric tube decompression. Decompression of the proximal gastrointestinal tract is of limited value in patients presenting with colonic distention or obstruction. If the entire colon including the rectum is gas-filled and distended, insertion of a rectal tube can be helpful. However, controlled trials in patients after colonoscopy show conflicting results [85,86]. Several case series report successful decompression of the colon using longer tubes, which can be advanced under fluoroscopic guidance or inserted over a relatively stiff wire placed during colonoscopy [66]. A sufficiently large catheter should be chosen and placed into the proximal colon. When combined with a dilation of strictured areas, the catheter may also be used to lavage the area proximal to the narrowing before possible surgery, thereby decreasing the risk of perforation and septic complications.

Surgical approach

Despite the emergence of other treatment options, complete obstruction remains a surgical emergency, especially when clinical or radiographic findings suggest strangulation. Contrast CT has improved the ability to predict the presence of ischemia with a sensitivity and specificity of about 80%–85% and 90%–95%, respectively [56]. However, surgery is still the gold standard for the diagnosis of ischemia. Considering the significant morbidity and mortality of gangrene formation and perforation, early laparatomy or laparascopic exploration will still be indicated in many patients with findings of complete obstruction, even if CT images do not demonstrate clear evidence of ischemia. The distended and unprepared intestine increases the risk of perforation and often requires a multiple step procedure with initial decompression, temporary diversion of the fecal stream through a stoma and correction or resection of the underlying pathology. Therefore, preoperative decompression should always be attempted. Effective decompression may allow elective single-stage surgery with resection of an obstructing lesion and primary anastomosis. In patients with obstruction due to advanced malignancies, nonoperative management should always be tried first. Surgery carries a high morbidity and mortality in these often severely ill individuals without evidence that it can increase survival or provide better quality of life [87]. With the advent of less invasive systemic or endoscopic treatment options, surgery plays a decreasing role in palliation of patients with malignant obstruction [88–90].

Endoscopic therapy

Several case series have demonstrated that colonoscopic decompression may be useful in patients with acute colonic pseudoobstruction (Ogilvie syndrome) and can resolve sigmoid volvulus [9,66,67,91,92]. However, the objective improvement is often limited and recurrences are common [93]. While not yet shown in appropriately designed trials, long colonic tubes may increase the success rate of colonoscopic decompression [66,94]. Unfortunately, commercially available sets for colonoscopic decompression have a high failure rate because the very flexible wire limits the ability to advance the tube into the proximal colon and fecal material rapidly obstructs the relatively thin tubes. Endoscopic dilation and stent placement increasingly allows nonoperative management of patients with benign or mechanical obstructions. Balloon dilation of anastomotic or inflammatory strictures can be safely performed and is effective in 40%–90% of patients [95–97]. While dilation may allow passage of the endoscope or a decompression tube, malignant obstructions cannot be effectively treated with dilation. Ablative therapy with an argon laser plasma coagulator may transiently restore lumenal patency [98–100]. Expandable metal stents have become the treatment of choice in patients with malignant obstruction of the proximal and distal gastrointestinal tract (Fig. 17.11). Effective palliation can be achieved in 70%–90% of patients. Major complications, such as perforation,

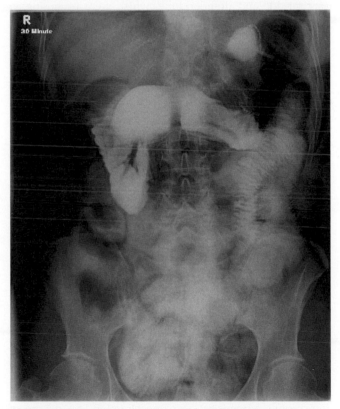

Figure 17.11 Contrast study with water-soluble contrast medium in a patient with partial small bowel obstruction due to adhesive disease. The patient had previously undergone vertical banding gastroplasty. The prolonged retention of contrast in the gastric pouch demonstrates a problem with transit through the narrow pouch outlet. However, the dilated loops of small bowel are only poorly opacified as a result of dilution of the contrast medium.

stent occlusion, or migration, occur in about 20%–25%, but can generally be managed conservatively [88,89,101,102]. Stents can also be used for initial decompression in operative candidates. The decreased distention proximal to the obstruction and the possibility to perform a preoperative antegrade lavage lowers complication rates and often allows single-stage operations.

Pharmacotherapy

Considering the high incidence of postoperative ileus and its associated costs, medical therapy that accelerates the recovery of normal intestinal function has a significant potential in decreasing postoperative morbidity and the length of hospitalizations. Three different strategies have been tried. Initial trials focused on agents stimulating gastrointestinal motility. Only two of the agents tested are approved for clinical use in the United States. *Metoclopramide* and *erythromycin* both affect gastrointestinal transit in healthy volunteers, but do not significantly affect the recovery of normal intestinal motor function after surgery [103–108]. Similarly, other agents such as cisapride and domperidone, which were promising in animal experiments or initial clinical studies, did not yield better results, thus dampening the enthusiasm for the use of prokinetics in the treatment of postoperative ileus [109–111]. Less information is available about the use of these agents in patients with chronic intestinal pseudoobstruction. While some case reports suggest at least transient symptomatic improvement with prokinetics, larger case series generally show limited effectiveness, especially when patients are followed for extended time periods [112–115]. In patients with systemic sclerosis, significant gastrointestinal involvement with progressive weight loss, diarrhea, nausea, and vomiting is seen in up to 8% [116]. In such cases, small bowel manometry typically shows no phase III activity [117]. In a small study, subcutaneous injection of the synthetic somatostatin analogue octreotide triggered phase III-like activity in all patients, improved symptoms, and eliminated the bacterial overgrowth associated with lumenal stasis [118].

The cholinesterase inhibitor *neostigmine* has become the treatment of choice in patients with acute colonic pseudoobstruction (Ogilvie syndrome). In these patients, the initial management should focus on correction of fluid and electrolyte abnormalities, minimize the use of motility suppressant medications, such as opiates or anticholinergic substances, and increase mobilization. If this strategy fails, then a single intravenous administration of neostigmine at a dosage of 2 mg rapidly triggers passage of flatus and stool in 80%–90% of the patients [119]. Considering the potential for adverse effects, patients should always be transferred to a monitored environment with continuous electrocardiogram. Moreover, the antagonist atropine should be readily available, should severe bradycardia develop. Recurrences

are common as immobility or other etiological factors often persist. Current evidence suggests that treatment with polyethyleneglycol may decrease the need for repeat intervention and should be considered [120]. Neostigmine has also been used successfully in patients with postoperative ileus [121,122]. However, the experience remains limited and clinical use cannot be recommended before additional studies confirm the effectiveness and safety of this approach, especially in patients who have undergone gastrointestinal resections. Considering these encouraging results after acute administration, cholinesterase inhibitors have been used in patients with chronic forms of intestinal pseudoobstruction. However, only isolated case reports have been published, which does not allow for appropriate assessment of safety and efficacy using this approach. A few trials report fast recovery of normal gastrointestinal function with the use of osmotic or stimulant *laxatives* [123,124]. However, because of the lack of appropriate control groups or complex interventions with nutritional therapy, aggressive mobilization, and cautious analgesic use, the clinical usefulness of this approach remains to be determined. Postoperative ileus is frequently complicated by the use of opioid analgesics. The use of epidural analgesia and cyclooxygenase inhibitors may achieve good pain control without high dosages of opiates. *Alvimopan*, a peripherally acting μ-opioid receptor antagonist was introduced. This agent can inhibit the inhibitory action of opiates on gastrointestinal motility without affecting their analgesic effects on pain control. In an initial study, performed mainly in patients after abdominal hysterectomy, gastrointestinal function recovered more quickly and likely contributed to a shorter hospital stay in the treatment group [125]. Subsequent studies with larger groups confirmed these results, but showed relatively smaller and less consistent effects with a 15% decrease in the time to the first bowel movement or solid food intake after laparotomy [126,127]. Pharmacotherapy can also serve as an important adjunct in patients with advanced malignancies complicated by bowel obstruction. Several studies support the use of *octreotide*, which inhibits motility and secretion. While more effective than anticholinergic substances, costs and the need for parenteral administration limit its use [128,129]. Based on the assumption that edema may contribute to the obstruction in malignancies, *dexamethasone* has been given, resulting in transient improvement in some patients without affecting the very poor survival in this group of patients with advanced malignancies [90,130].

References

1. Russo MW, Wei JT, Thiny MT, et al. Digestive and liver diseases statistics, 2004. Gastroenterology 2004;126:1448.
2. Welch JP. General consideration and mortality in bowel obstruction. In: Welch JP (ed.). Bowel Obstruction: Differential Diagnosis and Clinical Management. Philadelphia: Saunders, 1990.

3. Kehlet H, Holte K. Review of postoperative ileus. Am J Surg 2001; 182(Suppl. 1):S3.

4. Mythen MG. Postoperative gastrointestinal tract dysfunction. Anesth Analg 2005;100:196.

5. Rajaraman V, Vingan R, Roth P, et al. Visceral and vascular complications resulting from anterior lumbar interbody fusion. J Neurosurg 1999;91:S60.

6. Cetindag IB, Boley TM, Magee MJ, Hazelrigg SR. Postoperative gastrointestinal complications after lung volume reduction operations. Ann Thorac Surg 1999;68:1029.

7. Clarke HD, Berry DJ, Larson DR. Acute pseudo-obstruction of the colon as a postoperative complication of hip arthroplasty. J Bone Joint Surg 1997;79-A:1642.

8. Caprilli R, Latella G, Vernia P, Frieri G. Multiple organ dysfunction in ulcerative colitis. Am J Gastroenterol 2000;95:1258.

9. Tenofsky PL, Beamer L, Smith RS. Ogilvie syndrome as a postoperative complication. Archiv Surg 2000;135:682.

10. Kulah B, Kulacoglu IH, Oruc MT, et al. Presentation and outcome of incarcerated external hernias in adults. Am J Surg 2001;181:101.

11. Tekkis PP, Kinsman R, Thompson MR, Stamatakis JD. The Association of Coloproctology of Great Britain and Ireland study of large bowel obstruction caused by colorectal cancer. Ann Surg 2004;24:76.

12. Biondo S, Pares D, Frago R, et al. Large bowel obstruction: predictive factors for postoperative mortality. Dis Colon Rectum 2004;47:1889.

13. Maglinte DD, Heitkamp DE, Howard TJ, et al. Current concepts in imaging of small bowel obstruction. Radiol Clin North Am 2003;41:263.

14. Miller G, Boman J, Shrier I, Gordon PH. Etiology of small bowel obstruction. Am J Surg 2000;180:33.

15. Ward SM, Sanders KM. Involvement of intramuscular interstitial cells of Cajal in neuroeffector transmission in the gastrointestinal tract. J Physiol 2006;576:675.

16. Chang IY, Glasgow NJ, Takayama I, et al. Loss of interstitial cells of Cajal and development of electrical dysfunction in murine small bowel obstruction. J Physiol 2001;536:555.

17. Kalff JC, Turler A, Schwarz NT, et al. Intra-abdominal activation of a local inflammatory response within the human muscularis externa during laparotomy. Ann Surg 2003;237:301.

18. O'Neill LA. Toll-like receptor signal transduction and the tailoring of innate immunity: a role for Mal? Trends Immunol 2002;23:296.

19. Bauer AJ, Sarr MG, Szurszewski JH. Opioids inhibit neuromuscular transmission in circular muscle of human and baboon jejunum. Gastroenterology 1991;101:970.

20. Overhaus M, Togel S, Pezzone MA, Bauer AJ. Mechanisms of polymicrobial sepsis-induced ileus. Am J Physiol 2004;287:G685.

21. Eskandari MK, Kalff JC, Billiar TR, et al. LPS-induced muscularis macrophage nitric oxide suppresses rat jejunal circular muscle activity. Am J Physiol 1999;277:G478.

22. Gupta S, Reddy KR, Sanyal SC. Bacterial flora in acute small bowel obstruction. Chemotherapy 1980;26:446.

23. Roscher R, Oettinger W, Beger HG. Bacterial microflora, endogenous endotoxin, and prostaglandins in small bowel obstruction. Am J Surg 1988;155:348.

24. Schuffler MD, Kaplan LR, Johnson L. Small-intestinal mucosa in pseudoobstruction syndromes. Am J Dig Dis 1978;23:821.

25. Gregg CR. Enteric bacterial flora and bacterial overgrowth syndrome. Semin Gastrointest Dis 2002;13:200.

26. Festen HP. Intrinsic factor secretion and cobalamin absorption. Physiology and pathophysiology in the gastrointestinal tract. Scand J Gastroenterol 1991;188:S1.

27. Kabaroudis A, Papaziogas B, Koutelidakis I, et al. Disruption of the small-intestine mucosal barrier after intestinal occlusion: a study with light and electron microscopy. J Invest Surg 2003;16:23.

28. Samel S, Keese M, Kleczka M, et al. Microscopy of bacterial translocation during small bowel obstruction and ischemia in vivo – a new animal model. BMC Surg 2002;2:6.

29. O'Boyle CJ, MacFie J, Mitchell CJ, et al. Microbiology of bacterial translocation in humans. Gut 1998;42:29.

30. Deitch EA. Simple intestinal obstruction causes bacterial translocation in man. Arch Surg 1989;124:699.

31. Hajjar JJ, Van Linda B, Fucci J, Tomicic T. Intestinal absorption in the mechanically obstructed rat intestine: protection by prostaglandins. Prostaglandins 1986;31:83.

32. Walshe K, Healy MJ, Speekenbrink AB, et al. Effects of an enteric anaerobic bacterial culture supernatant and deoxycholate on intestinal calcium absorption and disaccharidase activity. Gut 1990;31:770.

33. Enochsson L, Nylander G. Effects of intraluminal hydrostatic pressure on L-methionine absorption in the obstructed small intestine of the rat. Am J Surg 1986;151:391.

34. Nellgard P, Jonsson A, Bojo L, et al. Small-bowel obstruction and the effects of lidocaine, atropine and hexamethonium on inflammation and fluid losses. Acta Anaesthesiol Scand 1996;40:287.

35. Frieling T, Wood JD, Cooke HJ. Submucosal reflexes: distension-evoked ion transport in the guinea pig distal colon. Am J Physiol Gastrointest Liver Physiol 1992;263:G91.

36. Weber E, Neunlist M, Schemann M, Frieling T. Neural components of distension-evoked secretory responses in the guinea-pig distal colon. J Physiol (Lond) 2001;536:741.

37. Schulzke JD, Fromm M, Hegel U, Riecken EO. Ion transport and enteric nervous system (ENS) in rat rectal colon: mechanical stretch causes electrogenic Cl-secretion via plexus Meissner and amiloride-sensitive electrogenic Na-absorption is not affected by intramural neurons. Pflugers Archiv Eur J Physiol 1989;414:216.

38. Harris MS, Ramaswamy K, Kennedy JG. Induction of neurally mediated NaHCO3 secretion by luminal distension in rat ileum. Am J Physiol 1989;257:G191.

39. Enochsson L, Nylander G, Ohman U. Effects of intraluminal pressure on regional blood flow in obstructed and unobstructed small intestines in the rat. Am J Surg 1982;144:558.

40. Ohman U. Studies on small intestinal obstruction. V. Blood circulation in moderately distended small bowel. Acta Chirurg Scand 1975;141:763.

41. Burkitt DS, Donovan IA. Intraluminal pressure adjacent to left colonic anastomoses. Br J Surg 1990;77:1288.

42. Mirkovitch V, Cobo F, Robinson JW, et al. Morphology and function of the dog ileum after mechanical occlusion. Clin Sci Molec Med 1976;50:123.

43. Hierholzer C, Kalff JC, Billiar TR, et al. Induced nitric oxide promotes intestinal inflammation following hemorrhagic shock. Am J Physiol 2004;286:G225.

44. Hassoun HT, Zou L, Moore FA, et al. Alpha-melanocyte-stimulating hormone protects against mesenteric ischemia-reperfusion injury. Am J Physiol 2002;282:G1059.

45. Swank GM, Deitch EA. Role of the gut in multiple organ failure: bacterial translocation and permeability changes. World J Surg 1996;20:411.

46. Heinzelmann M, Simmen HP, Battaglia H, et al. Inflammatory response after abdominal trauma, infection, or intestinal obstruction measured by oxygen radical production in peritoneal fluid. Am J Surg 1997;174:445.

47. Yamamoto T, Umegae S, Kitagawa T, Matsumoto K. The value of plasma cytokine measurement for the detection of strangulation in patients with bowel obstruction: a prospective, pilot study. Dis Colon Rectum 2005;48:1451.

48. Bohner H, Yang Q, Franke C, et al. Simple data from history and physical examination help to exclude bowel obstruction and to avoid radiographic studies in patients with acute abdominal pain. Eur J Surg 1998;164:777.

49. Eskelinen M, Ikonen J, Lipponen P. Contributions of history-taking, physical examination, and computer assistance to diagnosis of acute small-bowel obstruction. A prospective study of 1333 patients with acute abdominal pain. Scand J Gastroenterol 1994;29:715.

50. Arnbjornsson E. Normal and pathological bowel sound patterns. Annal Chirurg Gynaecol 1986;75:314.

51. Gade J, Kruse P, Andersen OT, et al. Physicians' abdominal auscultation. A multi-rater agreement study. Scand J Gastroenterol 1998; 33:773.

52. Taourel P, Kessler N, Lesnik A, et al. Non-traumatic abdominal emergencies: imaging of acute intestinal obstruction. Eur Radiol 2002;12:2161.

53. Lappas JC, Reyes BL, Maglinte DDT. Abdominal Radiography Findings in Small-Bowel Obstruction: Relevance to Triage for Additional Diagnostic Imaging. Am. J. Roentgenol 2001;176:167.

54. Suri S, Gupta S, Sudhakar PJ, et al. Comparative evaluation of plain films, ultrasound and CT in the diagnosis of intestinal obstruction. Acta Radiol 1999;40:422.

55. Burkill G, Bell J, Healy J. Small bowel obstruction: the role of computed tomography in its diagnosis and management with reference to other imaging modalities. Eur Radiol 2001;11:1405.

56. Mallo RD, Salem L, Lalani T, Flum DR. Computed tomography diagnosis of ischemia and complete obstruction in small bowel obstruction: a systematic review. J Gastrointest Surg 2005;9:690.

57. Ng CS, Watson CJE, Palmer CR, et al. Evaluation of early abdominopelvic computed tomography in patients with acute abdominal pain of unknown cause: prospective randomised study. BMJ 2002; 325(7377):1387.

58. Ahn SH, Mayo-Smith WW, Murphy BL, et al. Acute nontraumatic abdominal pain in adult patients: abdominal radiography compared with CT evaluation. Radiology 2002;225:159.

59. Zalcman M, Sy M, Donckier V, et al. Helical CT signs in the diagnosis of intestinal ischemia in small-bowel obstruction. Am J Roentgenol 2000;175:1601.

60. Fenlon HM, McAneny DB, Nunes DP, et al. Occlusive colon carcinoma: virtual colonoscopy in the preoperative evaluation of the proximal colon. Radiology 1999;210:423.

61. Morrin MM, Farrell RJ, Raptopoulos V, et al. Role of virtual computed tomographic colonography in patients with colorectal cancers and obstructing colorectal lesions. Dis Colon Rectum 2000;43:303.

62. Matsuoka H, Takahara T, Masaki T, et al. Preoperative evaluation by magnetic resonance imaging in patients with bowel obstruction. Am J Surg 2002;183:614.

63. Low RN, Chen SC, Barone R. Distinguishing benign from malignant bowel obstruction in patients with malignancy: findings at MR imaging. Radiology 2003;228:157.

64. Bretthauer M, Thiis-Evensen E, Huppertz-Hauss G, et al. NORCCAP (Norwegian colorectal cancer prevention): a randomised trial to assess the safety and efficacy of carbon dioxide versus air insufflation in colonoscopy. Gut 2002;50:604.

65. Sumanac K, Zealley I, Fox BM, et al. Minimizing postcolonoscopy abdominal pain by using CO_2 insufflation: a prospective, randomized, double blind, controlled trial evaluating a new commercially available CO_2 delivery system. Gastrointest Endosc 2002;56:190.

66. Kahi CJ, Rex DK. Bowel obstruction and pseudo-obstruction. Gastroenterol Clin North Am 2003;32:1229.

67. Chung YFA, Eu KW, Nyam DCNK, et al. Minimizing recurrence after sigmoid volvulus. Br J Surg 1999;86:231.

68. Lorenzo CD. Pseudo-obstruction: current approaches. Gastroenterology 1999;116:980.

69. Summers RW, Anuras S, Green J. Jejunal manometry patterns in health, partial intestinal obstruction, and pseudoobstruction. Gastroenterology 1983;85:1290.

70. Howard L, Ashley C. Nutrition in the perioperative patient. Annu Rev Nutr 2003;23:263.

71. Correia MI, da Silva RG. The impact of early nutrition on metabolic response and postoperative ileus. Curr Opin Clin Nutr Metab Care 2004;7:577.

72. Schmidt H, Martindale R. The gastrointestinal tract in critical illness: nutritional implications. Curr Opin Clin Nutr Metab Care 2003;6: 587.

73. Feo CV, Romanini B, Sortini D, et al. Early oral feeding after colorectal resection: a randomized controlled study. ANZ J Surg 2004;74: 298.

74. Lewis SJ, Egger M, Sylvester PA, Thomas S. Early enteral feeding versus "nil by mouth" after gastrointestinal surgery: systematic review and meta-analysis of controlled trials. BMJ 2001;323(7316):773.

75. Lower AM, Hawthorn RJS, Clark D, et al. Adhesion-related readmissions following gynaecological laparoscopy or laparotomy in Scotland: an epidemiological study of 24 046 patients. Hum Reprod 2004; 19:1877.

76. Kossi J, Salminen P, Rantala A, Laato M. Population-based study of the surgical workload and economic impact of bowel obstruction caused by postoperative adhesions. Br J Surg 2003;90:1441.

77. Wolfson PJ, Bauer JJ, Gelernt IM, et al. Use of the long tube in the management of patients with small-intestinal obstruction due to adhesions. Arch Surg 1985;120:1001.

78. Michowitz M, Chen J, Waizbard E, Bawnik JB. Abdominal operations without nasogastric tube decompression of the gastrointestinal tract. Am Surg 1988;54:672.

79. Gowen GF. Long tube decompression is successful in 90% of patients with adhesive small bowel obstruction. Am J Surg 2003;185:512.

80. Fleshner PR, Siegman MG, Slater GI, et al. A prospective, randomized trial of short versus long tubes in adhesive small-bowel obstruction. Am J Surg 1995;170:366.

81. Maglinte DD, Kelvin FM, Micon LT, et al. Nasointestinal tube for decompression or enteroclysis: experience with 150 patients. Abdom Imaging 1994;19:108.

82. Doglietto GB, Papa V, Tortorelli AP, et al. Nasojejunal tube placement after total gastrectomy: a multicenter prospective randomized trial. Arch Surg 2004;139:1309.

83. Wolff BG, Pemberton JH, van Heerden JA, et al. Elective colon and rectal surgery without nasogastric decompression. A prospective, randomized trial. Ann Surg 1989;209:670.

84. Cheatham ML, Chapman WC, Key SP, Sawyers JL. A meta-analysis of selective versus routine nasogastric decompression after elective laparotomy. Ann Surg 1995;221:469.

85. Hilzenrat N, Fich A, Odes HS, et al. Does insertion of a rectal tube after colonoscopy reduce patient discomfort and improve satisfaction? Gastrointest Endosc 2003;57:54.

86. Steinberg EN, Howden CW. Randomized controlled trial of rectal tube placement for the management of abdominal distension following colonoscopy. Gastrointest Endosc 1997;46:444.

87. Feuer DJ, Broadley KE, Shepherd JH, Barton DP. Surgery for the resolution of symptoms in malignant bowel obstruction in advanced gynaecological and gastrointestinal cancer. Cochrane Database Syst Rev 2000;CD002764.

88. Del Piano M, Ballare M, Montino F, et al. Endoscopy or surgery for malignant GI outlet obstruction? Gastrointest Endosc 2005;61:421.

89. Mosler P, Mergener KD, Brandabur JJ, et al. Palliation of gastric outlet obstruction and proximal small bowel obstruction with self-expandable metal stents: a single center series. J Clin Gastroenterol 2005;39:124.

90. Hardy JR. Medical management of bowel obstruction. Br J Surg 2000;87:1281.

91. Rex DK. Colonoscopy and acute colonic pseudo-obstruction. Gastroenterol Clin North Am 1997;7:499.

92. Geller A, Petersen BT, Gostout CJ. Endoscopic decompression for acute colonic pseudo-obstruction. Gastrointest Endosc 1996;44:144.

93. Pham TN, Cosman BC, Chu P, Savides TJ. Radiographic changes after colonoscopic decompression for acute pseudo-obstruction. Dis Colon Rectum 1999;42:1586.

94. Horiuchi A, Maeyama H, Ochi Y, et al. Usefulness of Dennis colorectal tube in endoscopic decompression of acute, malignant colonic obstruction. Gastrointest Endosc 2001;54:229.

95. Di Giorgio P, De Luca L, Rivellini G, et al. Endoscopic dilation of benign colorectal anastomotic stricture after low anterior resection: a prospective comparison study of two balloon types. Gastrointest Endosc 2004;60:347.

96. Thomas-Gibson S, Brooker JC, Hayward CM, et al. Colonoscopic balloon dilation of Crohn's strictures: a review of long-term outcomes. Eur J Gastroenterol Hepatol 2003;15:485.

97. Di ZH, Shin JH, Kim JH, Song HY. Colorectal anastomotic strictures: treatment by fluoroscopic double balloon dilation. J Vasc Intervent Radiol 2005;16:75.

98. Courtney ED, Raja A, Leicester RJ. Eight years experience of high-powered endoscopic diode laser therapy for palliation of colorectal carcinoma. Dis Colon Rectum 2005;48:845.

99. Kimmey MB. Endoscopic methods (other than stents) for palliation of rectal carcinoma. J Gastrointest Surg 2004;8:270.

100. Dohmoto M, Hunerbein M, Schlag PM. Palliative endoscopic therapy of rectal carcinoma. Eur J Cancer 1996;32A:25.

101. Sebastian S, Johnston S, Geoghegan T, et al. Pooled analysis of the efficacy and safety of self-expanding metal stenting in malignant colorectal obstruction. Am J Gastroenterol 2004;99:2051.

102. Khot UP, Lang AW, Murali K, Parker MC. Systematic review of the efficacy and safety of colorectal stents. Br J Surg 2002;89:1096.

103. Davidson ED, Hersh T, Brinner RA, Barnett SM, Boyle LP: The effects of metoclopramide on postoperative ileus. A randomized double-blind study. Ann Surg 1979;190:27.

104. Jepsen S, Klaerke A, Nielsen PH, Simonsen O. Negative effect of Metoclopramide in postoperative adynamic ileus. A prospective, randomized, double blind study. Br J Surg 1986;73:290.

105. Cheape JD, Wexner SD, James K, Jagelman DG: Does metoclopramide reduce the length of ileus after colorectal surgery? A prospective randomized trial. Dis Colon Rectum 1991;34:437.

106. Tollesson PO, Cassuto J, Faxen A, et al. Lack of effect of metoclopramide on colonic motility after cholecystectomy. Eur J Surg 1991;157:355.

107. Bonacini M, Quiason S, Reynolds M, et al. Effect of intravenous erythromycin on postoperative ileus. Am J Gastroenterol 1993;88:208.

108. Smith AJ, Nissan A, Lanouette NM, et al. Prokinetic effect of erythromycin after colorectal surgery: randomized, placebo-controlled, double-blind study. Dis Colon Rectum 2000;43:333.

109. Hallerback B, Bergman B, Bong H, et al. Cisapride in the treatment of post-operative ileus. Aliment Pharmacol Ther 1991;5:503.

110. Roberts JP, Benson MJ, Rogers J, et al. Effect of cisapride on distal colonic motility in the early postoperative period following left colonic anastomosis. Dis Colon Rectum 1995;38:139.

111. Bungard TJ, Kale-Pradhan PB. Prokinetic agents for the treatment of postoperative ileus in adults: a review of the literature. Pharmacotherapy 1999;19:416.

112. Emmanuel AV, Shand AG, Kamm MA. Erythromycin for the treatment of chronic intestinal pseudo-obstruction: description of six cases with a positive response. Aliment Pharmacol Ther 2004;19:687.

113. Mann SD, Debinski HS, Kamm MA. Clinical characteristics of chronic idiopathic intestinal pseudo-obstruction in adults. Gut 1997; 41:675.

114. Heneyke S, Smith VV, Spitz L, Milla PJ. Chronic intestinal pseudo-obstruction: treatment and long term follow up of 44 patients. Arch Dis Child 1999;81:21.

115. Verne GN, Eaker EY, Hardy E, Sninsky CA. Effect of octreotide and erythromycin on idiopathic and scleroderma-associated intestinal pseudoobstruction. Dig Dis Sci 1995;40:1892.

116. Steen VD, Medsger TA. Severe organ involvement in systemic sclerosis with diffuse scleroderma. Arthrit Rheum 2000;43:2437.

117. Greydanus MP, Camilleri M. Abnormal postcibal antral and small bowel motility due to neuropathy or myopathy in systemic sclerosis. Gastroenterology 1989;96:110.

118. Soudah HC, Hasler WL, Owyang C. Effect of octreotide on intestinal motility and bacterial overgrowth in scleroderma. N Engl J Med 1991;325:1461.

119. Ponec RJ, Saunders MD, Kimmey MB. Neostigmine for the treatment of acute colonic pseudo-obstruction. N Engl J Med 1999;341:137.

120. Sgouros SN, Vlachogiannakos J, Vassiliadis K, et al. Effect of polyethylene glycol electrolyte balanced solution on patients with acute colonic pseudo obstruction after resolution of colonic dilation: a prospective, randomised, placebo controlled trial. Gut 2006;55:638.

121. Althausen PL, Gupta MC, Benson DR, Jones DA. The use of neostigmine to treat postoperative ileus in orthopedic spinal patients. J Spinal Disord 2001;14:541.

122. Kreis ME, Kasparek M, Zittel TT, et al. Neostigmine increases postoperative colonic motility in patients undergoing colorectal surgery. Surgery 2001;130:449.

123. Basse L, Madsen J, Kehlet H. Normal gastrointestinal transit after colonic resection using epidural analgesia, enforced oral nutrition and laxative. Br J Surg 2001;88:1498.

124. Fanning J, Yu-Brekke S. Prospective trial of aggressive postoperative bowel stimulation following radical hysterectomy. Gynecol Oncol 1999;73:412.

125. Taguchi A, Sharma N, Saleem RM, et al. Selective postoperative inhibition of gastrointestinal opioid receptors. N Engl J Med 2001;345:935.

126. Wolff BG, Michelassi F, Gerkin TM, et al. Alvimopan, a novel, peripherally acting μ opioid antagonist: results of a multicenter, randomized, double-blind, placebo-controlled, phase III trial of major abdominal surgery and postoperative ileus. Ann Surg 2004;240:728.

127. Delaney CP, Weese JL, Hyman NH, et al. Alvimopan Postoperative Ileus Study Group. Phase III trial of alvimopan, a novel, peripherally acting, mu opioid antagonist, for postoperative ileus after major abdominal surgery. Dis Colon Rectum 2005;48:1114.

128. Ripamonti C, Mercadante S, Groff L, et al. Role of octreotide, scopolamine butylbromide, and hydration in symptom control of patients with inoperable bowel obstruction and nasogastric tubes: a prospective randomized trial. J Pain Symptom Manage 2000;19:23.

129. Mercadante S, Ripamonti C, Casuccio A, et al. Comparison of octreotide and hyoscine butylbromide in controlling gastrointestinal symptoms due to malignant inoperable bowel obstruction. Support Care Cancer 2000;8:188.

130. Feuer DJ, Broadley KE. Corticosteroids for the resolution of malignant bowel obstruction in advanced gynaecological and gastrointestinal cancer. Cochrane Database Syst Rev 2000;CD001219.

Approach to the patient with diarrhea

Don W. Powell

General epidemiology, 304

General definition, 304

Pathophysiology of diarrhea, 305

Acute diarrheas: definition, 311

Acute infectious diarrheas, 311

Prolonged infectious diarrheas, 318

Nosocomial diarrheas, 319

Runner's diarrhea, 321

Chronic diarrheas: definition, classification, and epidemiology, 321

Steatorrhea (malabsorptive diseases), 321

Watery diarrheas, 325

True secretory diarrheas, 327

Inflammatory diarrheas, 329

Clinical evaluation of chronic diarrhea, 331

Antidiarrheal therapy, 345

General epidemiology

Diarrheal diseases affect developed nations differently from developing nations. In developed nations, diarrheal disorders are primarily of economic significance. Over 4 million outpatient visits for diarrhea occurred in the United States in 2000 [1]. Estimated outpatient visits for specific diarrhea-inducing diagnoses in 2000 were 3.4 million for gastroenteritis, 1.6 million for irritable bowel syndrome, 725 000 for Crohn's disease, and 488 000 for ulcerative colitis [1,2]. A similar burden of gastrointestinal disease was reported in Europe in 2003, although celiac disease is a more frequent diagnosis there [3]. The Centers for Disease Control and Prevention (CDC) estimates more than 76 million new cases of food poisoning each year in the United States, accounting for 4000–5000 deaths annually [4]. Although diarrheal diseases are a minor cause of death in industrialized nations, they are among the leading causes of death and morbidity in developing countries. Since the early 1980s, global death rates from diarrheal diseases, mostly affecting infants and small children, have decreased from 5–10 million per year to 3–4 million [5]. Even this reduced rate represents 1 death every 10 seconds.

The approach to suspected acute infectious diarrhea is covered in Chapter 19 of this book.

General definition

Normal stooling frequency ranges from three times a week to three times a day [6,7]. Diarrhea was defined by Roux and Ryle in 1924 as "the too rapid evacuation of too fluid stools," [8]. A decrease in stool consistency or fluidity and stools that cause urgency or abdominal discomfort are more likely to be termed *diarrhea* by patients than increases in frequency alone [6,9]. The physician or clinical investigator often chooses to define diarrhea as a physical sign (24-h excretion weight or volume) rather than a symptom. Healthy children and adults have daily stool weights of less than 200 g [10], and infants have a daily stool weight of less than 10 g/kg [11]. Even though stool consistency probably best defines diarrhea, it cannot be easily measured. Thus, stool weights in

Principles of Clinical Gastroenterology. Edited by Tadataka Yamada, David H. Alpers, Anthony N. Kalloo, Neil Kaplowitz, Chung Owyang, and Don W. Powell. © 2008 Blackwell Publishing. ISBN 978-1-4051-69103

excess of 200 g/24 h may be the most easily obtainable, objective definition of diarrhea. This definition may cause misdiagnosis in 20% of patients with loose stools of less than this weight [9]. Twenty-seven percent of both men and women report having passed one loose stool in the previous month [12]. Stool composition varies from 60%–85% water [9,13,14] so this definition implies that diarrhea is a disease of intestinal water and electrolyte transport.

A stool pattern of increased frequency, with either no change in consistency or a 24-h stool output of less than 200 g, often accompanies motility disorders (irritable bowel syndrome [IBS]) or anorectal disease (proctitis). Some term this *pseudodiarrhea*. *Incontinence* (which is not necessarily diarrhea) is defined as the involuntary release of rectal contents. It is relatively common (2%–10% of the population) and increases with age (15% in the elderly and 1 in 5 women over 50). It is reported to occur in 50% of nursing home patients [14–16]. Incontinence is more common if the stool is liquid, and it is present more often in the setting of abnormal neuromuscular function (abnormalities of afferent sensation or efferent motor function) or pelvic problems (trauma of childbirth or disease of the sphincter or pelvic muscles) [15,16]. It is more common in elderly patients, in persons in poor health, and in women postpartum.

Aside from water content, the factors governing normal stool weight and consistency are not completely understood. *Consistency* is best defined as the ratio of fecal water to the water-holding capacity of insoluble solids [9]. Fiber content and bacterial mass, which make up one-half of the dry weight of stool, are probably the major components of these fecal solids [17]. Increasing fiber (wheat bran) ingestion from 10 to 26 g/24 h increases average stool weight from 100 g/24 h to 149 g/24 h and increases average stool frequency from less than once to twice per day [10]. The weight of women's stool is less than that of men by one half, reflecting differences in dietary fiber intake or hormonal factors [10]. There is some controversy whether the ovarian cycles do [10] or do not [18] influence stool weight and consistency. Both exercise [19] and stress [20] increase stool weight, presumably by decreasing jejunal or colonic fluid and electrolyte absorption. Even personality factors correlate with stool weight [7]. Finally, intralumenal bile acid content may influence stool weight because the ingestion of cholestyramine [21] or aluminum hydroxide [22], both potent bile acid-binding substances, induces constipation. As described later, abnormal stool weight (> 200–300 g/24 h) is almost always the result of a failure of intestinal solute and fluid absorption or actual solute and fluid secretion.

Pathophysiology of diarrhea

Abnormal motor function

In the early 20th century, diarrhea was thought to be caused primarily by increased gastrointestinal motility. Although

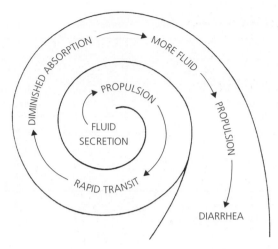

Figure 18.1 The diarrhea spiral. An increase in the amount of intralumenal fluid resulting from abnormalities in intestinal fluid and electrolyte transport initiate propulsive activity both by reflex and as a result of the same pathophysiological processes that disturbed epithelial function. Rapid transit follows with decreased contact time and perhaps also with diminished surface area. This causes diminished absorption, more intralumenal fluid, more propulsion, and finally diarrhea. From Read [609].

gastrointestinal motility plays a role in diarrhea [23,24], most of the diarrheal conditions that have been studied have shown alterations of both intestinal fluid and electrolyte transport and the induction of propagative forms of intestinal motility. What is less clear is whether there is diarrhea caused specifically and only by abnormal motility, a condition termed *diarrhée motrice*. The diarrhea caused by autonomic dysfunction in patients with hexosaminidase B deficiency (Sandhoff disease) may be such a type of diarrhea [25]. Perhaps the "pseudodiarrhea" of anorectal disease and the rapid small intestine transit of IBS are other examples of motility-induced diarrhea. Most clinicians, however, would agree with the concept of the diarrhea spiral shown in Fig. 18.1.

Abnormal fluid and electrolyte transport
Decreased absorption
As shown in Table 18.1, entering the duodenum each 24 h is 8–10 L fluid containing 800 mmol sodium (Na^+), 700 mmol chloride (Cl^-), and 100 mmol potassium (K^+) ions. Two liters of this duodenal load is derived from the diet; the remainder comes from secretions of the salivary glands, stomach, liver, pancreas, and the duodenum itself. The small intestine normally absorbs all but 1.5 L of this fluid, and this is the volume characteristically presented to the colon. The colon, in turn, absorbs all but approximately 100 mL of this fluid, which contains approximately 3, 8, and 2 mmol Na^+, K^+, and Cl^-, respectively. Although the maximum absorptive capacity of the small intestine remains undefined, the capacity of the normal adult human colon is 4–5 L/24 h [26]. Theoretically, diarrhea can result from decreased absorption

Table 18.1 Organ physiology of human intestinal water and solute transport

| Segment | Fluid flow (mL/24 h) | Ionic concentrations (mmol/L) | | | | | |
		Na⁺	K⁺	Ca²⁺ Mg²⁺ NH₄⁺	Cl⁻	HCO₃⁻	OA⁻
Entering duodenum (diet plus endogenous secretions)	8000–10 000	60	15	Variable	60	15	0
Proximal jejunum	3000	130	6	Variable	90	30	0
Entering colon	1500	140	8	10	60	70	~5
Stool	100	40	90	20	15	30	80–180

OA, organic anions.
Adapted from Powell [611].

by either the small intestine or the colon. If either deranged epithelial transport mechanisms or the presence of nonabsorbable solutes in the intestinal lumen reduce the absorptive capacity of the small intestine by 50%, the daily volume of fluid then presented to the normal colon (approximately 5 L) would exceed the colon's absorptive capacity. A stool excretion of up to 1000 mL would result, i.e., diarrhea. Alternatively, if the colon is deranged so that it cannot absorb even the 1.5 L normally presented to it by the small intestine, then diarrhea (stool volume > 200 mL/24 h) would result.

Increased secretion

In the decade after 1965, scientists rediscovered that the intestine could secrete as well as absorb fluid and electrolytes. The result was an entirely new concept: intestinal secretion as a pathophysiological mechanism of diarrhea. The subsequent discoveries that neurotransmitters, hormones, bacterial enterotoxins, inflammatory mediators, and cathartics all stimulated intestinal Cl⁻ and water secretion through changes in intracellular cyclic adenosine monophosphate, cyclic guanosine monophosphate, or ionized calcium (Ca²⁺) further promoted this concept.

Although initially it was thought that bacterial enterotoxins cause secretion only by a direct effect on enterocyte receptors, 50% or more of the intestinal secretion initiated by bacterial enterotoxins in vivo comes about from stimulation of receptors on enterochromaffin cells that release hormones that activate the enteric nervous system, secondarily stimulating the enterocyte [27,28]. Furthermore, inflammatory mediators [proinflammatory cytokines and chemokines, adenosine, histamine, serotonin (5-HT), hydrogen peroxide, leukotrienes, and prostaglandins] released from immune cells (mucosal mast cells and resident phagocytes such as eosinophils, macrophages, and neutrophils) and mesenchymal cells (myofibroblasts, endothelium, and smooth muscle) in the lamina propria and submucosa are also capable of initiating intestinal secretion [29]. These mediators may directly stimulate the enterocyte and may also activate the enteric nervous system.

Studies of intestinal electrolyte and water transport have demonstrated that the intracellular messengers also inhibit electrically neutral NaCl absorption, in addition to stimulating electrogenic Cl⁻ and bicarbonate (HCO₃⁻) secretion by enterocytes of the small intestine and colon [30]. The direction of net fluid movement is in response to the net direction of solute movement [31] so a submaximal secretory stimulus gives the appearance of an inhibition of absorption rather than stimulated secretion.

Normal intestinal physiology

There are three general categories of diarrhea: malabsorption (fatty diarrhea or steatorrhea), watery (secretion and osmotic-induced), and inflammatory diarrhea. To understand the pathophysiology, it is necessary to consider how a normal intestine alters intralumenal ionic concentrations and osmolality and, subsequently, how these parameters are perturbed by secretory agonists or by the presence of nonabsorbable (osmotic) solutes, by failure to digest or absorb nutrients and by inflammation.

Measurements of existing fluid volume in the fasting human gut indicate 45 to 319 mL of free water in the small intestine and 1 to 44 mL in the colon [32]. The fasting intestinal flow rate in healthy humans averages approximately 2.5 mL/min in the upper jejunum and 0.4 to 0.9 mL/min across the ileocecal valve [26]. After meals, flow rates depend on the rate of gastric emptying, the rates of pancreatic and biliary secretion, and the osmolality of the ingested meal. Rates may approximate 20 to 50 mL/min in the upper jejunum and 5 to 10 mL/min across the ileocecal valve. Regardless of whether a subject ingests a hypotonic meal, such as a steak with an osmolality of 230 mOsm/kg H₂O, or a hypertonic meal, such as milk and a doughnut with an osmolality of 630 mOsm/kg H₂O, the very permeable duodenum allows the movement of water and electrolytes into or out of the lumen, rendering the meal approximately isotonic by the time it reaches the proximal jejunum (Fig. 18.2). At this point, the electrolyte content is essentially that of plasma (Fig. 18.3).

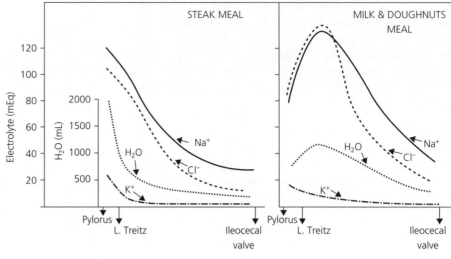

Figure 18.2 Intralumenal volumes and electrolyte content in the human small intestine after a hypotonic (steak) meal and a hypertonic (milk and doughnuts) meal. From Fordtran [13].

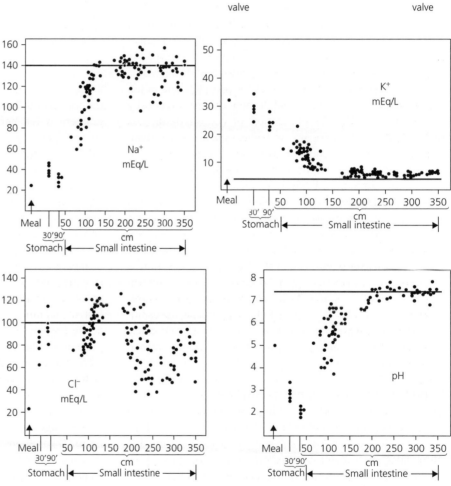

Figure 18.3 Concentrations of Na⁺, K⁺, and Cl⁻ and pH values in human gastric and small intestine fluid after a steak meal. The horizontal line in each figure indicates normal plasma concentrations or pH. From Fordtran [13].

Furthermore, the volume of this meal has been augmented by gastric, pancreatic, biliary, and duodenal secretions such that the 313-mL milk and doughnut meal has expanded to 1200 mL and the 645-mL steak meal approaches 2000 mL by the time it reaches distal duodenum or proximal jejunum. However, the high-carbohydrate hypertonic meal is handled differently from the high-protein hypotonic meal. The rapid digestion of starches and lactose into sugars presents a large osmotic load to the proximal small bowel, and considerable amounts of fluid must passively enter to equilibrate the osmolality. After ingesting this meal, it may be at the midjejunum before efficient absorption of the fluid and electrolytes begins. In contrast, after ingesting the hypotonic steak meal, absorption begins virtually in the duodenum (see Fig. 18.2).

In either case, as the chyme moves toward the colon, the electrolyte concentrations in the lumenal fluid remain approximately those of plasma, except for Cl⁻, which is reduced to concentrations of 60–70 mM, and HCO_3^-, which is increased to a similar concentration, as the result of the Cl⁻ and HCO_3^- transport mechanisms residing in the small intestine (see Fig. 18.3).

In the colon, the amiloride-sensitive Na⁺ transport mechanism of the colonocyte and the low epithelial permeability allow this segment to extract Na⁺ and fluid efficiently from the contents. In fact, the crypts of the distal colon may act like suction devices to extract fluid from the stool efficiently, thus forming solid feces [33]. As a result, the Na⁺ content of stool decreases to approximately 30–40 mM, and poorly absorbed divalent cations such as magnesium (Mg^{2+}) and Ca^{2+} are concentrated to values of 5–100 mM, depending on diet (see Table 18.1). K⁺ values increase from 5–10 mM in the small bowel to 75–90 mM in stool as the result of both the negative electrical potential difference of the lumen, which favors the movement of cations from blood to lumen, and the active K⁺ secretory mechanisms present in the colon [34]. The anion concentrations in the intestinal lumen change drastically in the colon. Bacterial degradation of carbohydrate (i.e., unabsorbed starches, sugars, and fiber) creates short-chain fatty acids that attain concentrations of 80–180 mM [35,36]. At colonic pH, these are present as organic anions, mainly acetate, propionate, and butyrate. Depending on the concentrations and quantities of organic anions created, stool pH may decrease to 4 or lower. Even though colonic bacteria degrade carbohydrates and increase the concentration of organic anions and therefore the number of osmotically active particles, the osmolality of stool, if measured as soon as it is passed, is approximately that of plasma, 280–310 mOsm [35–38]. If stool osmolality is measured hours to days after passage, even if it has been stored in a deep freeze, the osmolality may have increased to greater than 350 mOsm because of continued bacterial degradation of stool carbohydrate in the collecting container.

Pathophysiology of osmotic diarrheas

Contrast the events just described with what transpires after a lactase-deficient subject ingests a lactose test meal [39], or a physiologically normal subject ingests a nonabsorbable solute such as polyethylene glycol (PEG) or Mg^{2+} [37]. Although the same dilution of the meal occurs in the duodenum (Fig. 18.4), the lactase-deficient subject is unable to reabsorb the fluid because the unabsorbable molecule lactose is not metabolized to absorbable glucose and galactose. Similarly, the osmotic activity of ingested PEG, which is nonabsorbable, or of the poorly absorbable Mg^{2+} causes fluid entry into the small bowel, rendering the intralumenal solutions isosmotic with plasma. Intralumenal Na⁺ concentrations drop to less than 80 mM, and the permeable jejunum

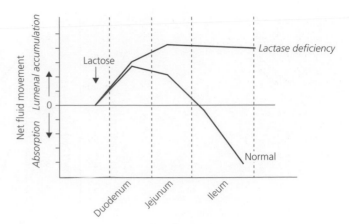

Figure 18.4 Changes in fluid absorption and secretion in the small intestine of normal and lactase-deficient subjects after a lactose meal of 50 g/m² body surface area in 400 mL distilled water. From Binder HJ et al. [610]; data from Christopher & Bayless [39].

cannot absorb Na⁺ against such a steep lumen-to-plasma gradient. What happens to the chyme when it reaches the colon depends on the nature of the unabsorbed solute. If the solute is nonmetabolizable (i.e., PEG or Mg^{2+}), some Na⁺ and water may be absorbed by the colon, which can concentrate Na⁺ from lumenal concentrations of less than 30 mM, but it cannot absorb all the excess stool water. In fact, there is a linear relationship between the ingested osmotic load of PEG and stool water output (stool weight). If the unabsorbed solute is a carbohydrate (i.e., lactulose or lactose) that can be metabolized by colonic bacteria, it affects stool weight differently. The carbohydrate is metabolized to short-chain fatty acids (organic anions) that obligate the retention of inorganic cations, significantly increasing the number of osmotically active particles in the colon. This increases the solute load, promoting the movement of more fluid into the colon. Although some of the organic anions and fluid are absorbed as they traverse the colon, the unabsorbed carbohydrate, the organic anions with their obligate cations, and fluid are excreted in the stool [37].

With ingestion of either unabsorbable solute (i.e., Mg^{2+} or PEG) [37] or unabsorbed carbohydrate (i.e., lactulose [37] or, in some persons, lactose [39]), a considerable amount of the osmolality of stool results from the nonabsorbed solute, so there is a significant difference, or gap, between stool osmolality and the sum of the electrolytes in the stool (see Stool weight, response to fast, and stool osmotic gap).

The osmotic solutes causing osmotic diarrheas can be derived from either exogenous (ingested) or endogenous sources and may result from congenital or acquired malabsorptive disease. The causes are listed in Table 18.2 and are discussed in more detail in later sections.

Table 18.2 Classification of osmotic or malabsorptive diarrhea

Exogenous

Laxatives

Polyethylene glycol/saline (GoLYTELY), Mg(OH)$_2$ (Milk of Magnesia), MgSO$_4$ (Epsom salts), Na$_2$SO$_4$ (Glauber or Carlsbad salt), Na$_2$PO$_4$ (neutral phosphate), lactulose

Antacids

Those containing MgO or Mg(OH)$_2$

Dietetic foods, candy or chewing gum, and elixirs containing sorbitol, mannitol, or xylitol

Acarbose (α-glucosidase inhibitor)

Olestra, orlistat (lipase inhibitor)

Miscellaneous drugs

Long-term ingestion of colchicine, cholestyramine, neomycin, paraaminosalicylic acid, biguanides, methyldopa

Endogenous

Congenital

Specific malabsorptive diseases

Disaccharidase deficiencies (lactase, sucrase–isomaltase, trehalase)

Glucose–galactose or fructose malabsorption

Generalized malabsorptive diseases

Abetalipoproteinemia and hypobetalipoproteinemia

Congenital lymphangiectasia

Enterokinase deficiency

Pancreatic insufficiency (cystic fibrosis or Shwachman syndrome)

Acquired

Specific malabsorptive diseases:

Postenteritis disaccharidase deficiency

Generalized malabsorptive diseases:

Pancreatic insufficiency (alcohol), bacterial overgrowth, celiac Sprue, rotavirus enteritis, parasitic diseases (giardiasis, coccidiosis), Metabolic diseases (thyrotoxicosis, adrenal insufficiency), Inflammatory disease (eosinophilic enteritis, mastocytosis), protein–calorie malnutrition, short bowel syndrome, jejunoileal bypass

Pathophysiology of secretory diarrheas

In secretory diarrheas, particularly in the fasting state, the major solutes in the lumen are Na$^+$, K$^+$, Cl$^-$, and HCO$_3^-$. It is the failure to absorb these electrolytes, their active secretion, or both that determines the amount of fluid entering or leaving the colon. In secretory diarrheas, therefore, the stool osmolality will be close to twice the concentrations of stool Na$^+$ plus K$^+$.

As is the case with osmotic causes of diarrhea, the stimuli causing secretory diarrhea may be of exogenous origin or they may be endogenous (Table 18.3). Endogenous substances such as dihydroxy bile acids [40] and dietary long-chain fatty acids may cause secretory diarrhea [41,42], particularly if they have been hydroxylated by intestinal microflora [43]. The important concept here is that there are "malabsorbed" endogenous detergents that may lend an element of secretory

diarrhea to otherwise malabsorptive diseases. The detergent stool softener dioctyl sodium sulfosuccinate [44] and the cathartic ricinoleic acid (castor oil) [45] are examples of exogenous long-chain fatty acids that stimulate colonic secretion.

Pathophysiology of inflammatory diarrheas

Our understanding of the pathophysiological mechanisms involved in inflammatory diarrhea has increased dramatically with increasing knowledge of mucosal immunology and neuroimmunophysiology. These concepts clarify the mechanisms during gut inflammation that lead to deranged epithelial electrolyte transport, the influx and activation of mucosal inflammatory cells and damage, and ulceration of the intestinal epithelium.

The first concept is that products secreted by activated mast cells, phygocytes, myofibroblasts and T cells in the lamina propria will inhibit NaCl absorption or stimulate Cl$^-$ secretion by the intestinal epithelial cells [28,29,46,47]. These various inflammatory cells secrete meditors such as prostaglandins, leukotrienes, histamine, serotonin, reactive oxygen species (ROS), and other factors that alter the ion exchangers and ion channels, resulting in diarrhea. These cells also secrete factors such as ROS and matrix metalloproteinases that damage enterocytes and proinflammatory cytokines (interleukin-1 [IL-1], tumor necrosis factor-α [TNF-α]) and chemokines (IL-8) that cause chemostaxis and further promote the inflammatory response [28,29,46,49].

Biochemical and structural damage to the enterocyte may be subtle and only interfere with nutrient and electrolyte transport. Alternatively, damage may be severe and result in erosions and frank ulcerations of the epithelium. Cytokines, growth (proliferative) factors, and matrix remodeling factors secreted by mucosal cells result in *villous atrophy* and crypt hyperplasia [48,49].

The second concept is that these lamina propria inflammatory cells and the epithelial cells that first come in contact with lumenal microorganisms are activated initially by a process called innate immunity [50]. In this process, cell surface Toll-like receptors (TLRs), or cytoplasmic receptors such as nucleotide oligomerization domain (NOD) proteins, recognize distinct microbial ligands called pathogen-associated molecular patterns (PAMPs) and transmit activating signals to the epithelial or lamina propria inflammatory or mesenchymal cells [51,52]. These 10 TLRs and NOD proteins are also known as pattern recognition receptors. Subsequent to this inhibition of inflammation by pattern recognition receptors, presentation of specific microorganism antigens by antigen-presenting dentritic cells, macrophages, and B-lymphocytes and by nonprofessional antigen-presenting cells such as enterocytes and myofibroblasts to T lymphocytes augments and sustains the inflammatory response. This process begins to clear the microorganisms through adaptive cellular and humoral immunity.

Table 18.3 Classification of secretory (deranged electrolyte transport) diarrhea

Exogenous

Laxatives

  Phenolphthalein, anthraquinones, bisacodyl, oxyphenisatin, senna, aloe, ricinoleic acid (castor oil), dioctyl sodium sulfosuccinate

Medications

  Diuretics (furosemide, thiazides); asthma medication (theophylline); thyroid preparations; metformin

  Cholinergic drugs: glaucoma eye drops and bladder stimulants (acetylcholine analogues or mimetics); myasthenia gravis medication (cholinesterase
    inhibitors); cardiac drugs (quinidine and quinine); gout medication (colchicine); prokinetic drugs (metoclopramide); antihypertensives
    (ACE inhibitors); H_2 blockers (ranitidine); antidepressants (selective serotonin reuptake inhibitors); antineoplastics; chenodeoxycholic acid

  Prostaglandins (misoprostil); di-5-aminosalicylic acid (azodisal sodium); gold (may also cause colitis), NSAIDs

  Protease inhibitors (HIV medications)

Toxins

  Metals (arsenic); plant (mushroom, e.g., *Amanita phalloides*); organophosphates (insecticides and nerve poisons); seafood toxins (ciguatera, scombroid
    poisoning; paralytic, diarrheal, or neurotoxic shellfish poisoning); coffee, tea, or cola (caffeine and other methylxanthines); ethanol; monosodium
    glutamate

Bacterial toxin (pre-formed)

  Staphylococcus aureus, *Clostridium perfringens*, *Clostridium botulinum*, *Bacillus cereus*

Gut allergy without histological change

Endogenous

Congenital

  Microvillus inclusion disease

  Congenital chloridorrhea (absence of Cl^-/HCO_3^- exchanger)

  Congenital Na diarrhea (absence of Na^+/H^+ exchanger)

  Congenital enterocyte heparan sulfate deficiency

Bacterial enterotoxins (formed after colonization)

  Vibrio cholerae, toxigenic *Escherichia coli* (LT and ST), *Campylobacter jejuni*, *Yersinia enterocolitica*, *Klebsiella pneumoniae*, *Clostridium difficile*,
    S. aureus (toxic shock syndrome)

Endogenous laxatives

Dihydroxy bile acids and long-chain fatty acids, especially hydroxylated ones

Hormone-producing tumors

Pancreatic cholera syndrome and ganglioneuromas (VIP); medullary carcinoma of thyroid (calcitonin and prostaglandins); mastocytosis (histamine); villous
  adenoma (secretagogue unknown, prostaglandins)

ACE, angiotensin-converting enzyme; H_2, histamine; LT, heat-labile toxin; NSAIDs, nonsteroidal antiinflammatory drugs; ST, heat-stable toxin; VIP,
vasoactive intestinal polypeptide.

The third concept is that pathological microorganisms, e.g., *Salmonella*, may invade the cell membrane and cross the epithelial cell [53]. Furthermore, normal flora and noninvasive microorganisms (or antigenic molecules from these organisms) can cross the epithelial barrier between the cells, i.e, across the tight junctions, which join the epithelial cells together into a barrier [54]. These junctions are under pharmacological control: certain cytokines (interferon-γ and TNF-α) [55,56] increase tight junction permeability and other agents (glucocorticoids, prostaglandins, and epidermal growth factor) [57–59] tighten the junctions.

Patients with certain diseases (type 1 diabetes, Crohn's disease, celiac diseases) may have increased junctional permeability, and this may play a fundamental role in the mechanism of the disease by allowing normal dietary or bacterial antigens to join with other genetic or acquired defects to cause clinical disease [54].

The fourth concept is that certain bacteria, e.g., enteropathogenic *Escherichia coli* and others, have molecular protein secretion systems (Types I to VI) that are capable of injecting toxins into epithelial cells [60]. These toxic proteins are capable of altering the electrolyte transport mechanism of the epithelium and futher alter permeability [61–63].

Thus, inflammatory diarrheas may be induced by microorganisms that have the ability to invade and damage the intestinal epithelial cells. Alternatively, bacteria may adhere to epithelial cells and secrete toxin into epithelial cells. Activation of immune cells through both innate and adaptive immunity releases mediators, which damage cells and alter electrolyte transport. Autoimmune inflammatory diarrheas

Table 18.4 Classification of inflammatory diarrheas

With minimal to moderate inflammation

Infections
   Bacteria (enteroadherent or enteropathogenic *Escherichia coli*)
   Viruses (rotavirus and Norwalk agent, human immunodeficiency virus)
   Parasites (*Giardia, Cryptosporidium, Isospora, Cyclospora, Ascaris, Trichinella*)
   Mixed organism (tropical sprue, bacterial overgrowth)
Cytostatic (anticancer) agents
   Chemotherapy (mucositis)
   Radiation therapy (acute or chronic radiation enteritis, radiation sickness)
Hypersensitivity
   Nematode infestation, food allergy
Idiopathic or autoimmune
   Microscopic (lymphocytic) and collagenous colitis, Cronkhite–Canada syndrome, graft-vs-host disease
Medications
   Nonsteroidal antiinflammatory drugs; simvastatin; ticlopidine; cimetidine; lansoprazole; gold (Aurolin); cyclosporine

With moderate to severe inflammation with or without ulceration

Infections
   Destruction of enterocytes (*Shigella*, enteroinvasive *E. coli, Entamoeba histolytica*, hookworm)
   Penetration of mucosa (*Salmonella, Campylobacter jejuni, Yersinia enterocolitica, Mycobacterium avium* complex, Whipple disease)
Hypersensitivity
   Celiac sprue, milk or soybean protein hypersensitivity, eosinophilic gastroenteritis, nematode infestation
   Drug-induced colitis (gold, methyldopa)
Idiopathic or autoimmune disorders
   Ulcerative colitis or proctitis, Crohn's disease, lymphoma

(e.g., Crohn's disease or celiac disease) may have increased epithelial barrier permeability as a primary defect. When coupled to other genetic or acquired defects (NOD proteins or gluten sensitivity), pronounced inflammation with deranged electrolyte transport and mucosal inflammatory cells or epithelial ulceration ensues.

There are four general categories of inflammatory diarrhea: infection, hypersensitivity, cytostatic (anticancer) agents, and idiopathic (possibly autoimmune) diseases (Table 18.4).

Acute diarrheas: definition

Acute diarrheas are defined as those of less than 2–3 weeks' duration and, at most, 6–8 weeks' duration. Whereas no data exist, expert opinion proposes that 80% of acute diarrheas are caused by infectious agents and 20% by drugs or chemicals (toxins). See also Chapter 19 for further details on infectious diarrheas.

Acute infectious diarrheas

Epidemiology
Developing vs developed countries
The most important epidemiological factor for the diagnosis and management of acute infectious diarrhea is whether the diarrhea is occurring in developing countries or in developed countries. Acute infectious diarrheas cause more than 3 million deaths worldwide [5]. This mortality occurs in children younger than 5 years of age in developing nations, where two-thirds of the world's population live in extreme poverty, and in areas of rapid urbanization, crowded substandard housing with inadequate sewage disposal and inadequate water supplies, insufficient food with lack of refrigeration, poor education (particularly with regard to personal hygiene), and a fundamental lack of access to health care. In addition to socioeconomic status and hygienic practices, in developing countries there is a relationship between diarrhea incidence and ambient air temperature [64], which may explain the higher incidence of diarrhea in tropical emerging nations.

Deaths occur in developed nations as well, particularly in infants and the elderly. The incidence of infant diarrheal deaths in the United States decreased by 75% from 1968 to 1991, but diarrhea was still the principal cause of death for more than 500 children each year [65], often secondary to rotavirus infection [66]. It is estimated that acute diarrhea mortality is highest in the elderly and 40% of patient with chronic diarrhea are over 60 years old [67]. The death rate for children and young adults in the United States is 2 to 3 per 100 000 persons and is approximately 15 per 100 000 persons for persons more than 74 years old [67, 68]. Diarrhea also affects United States troops in Iraq and Afghanistan, and was reported in 76% of over 4000 troops [69].

In developing countries, it is estimated that there are 1.8 billion episodes of childhood diarrhea (up to 7 per child per year) each year, accounting for 3 million deaths [5]. In the United States, children have an average of two to three episodes per year. In the total population of the United States, foodborne illness alone accounts for 76 million episodes of diarrhea and 325 000 hospital admissions per year [4]. With improvements in sanitation and education in the United States, rates of parasitic diarrheas have declined, but, in the 1990s, in those diseases with person-to-person transmission (e.g., rotavirus) or foodborne or waterborne transmission (e.g., *Salmonella* or *Campylobacter* organisms), the incidences have doubled [70]. While *Salmonella, Campyolobacter, Shigella, E. coli* O157:H7, and *Cryptosporidium* are the microorganisms most identified by the CDC, it is estimated that viruses account for two-thirds of all foodborne illnesses [71].

Table 18.5 Epidemiological clues to infectious diarrhea

Vehicle	Classic pathogen
Water (including foods washed in such water)	*Vibrio cholerae*, Norwalk agent, *Giardia* organisms, and *Cryptosporidium* organisms
Food	
Poultry	*Salmonella*, *Campylobacter*, and *Shigella* species
Beef, unpasteurized fruit juice	Enterohemorrhagic *Escherichia coli*
Pork	Tapeworm
Seafood and shellfish[a]	*Vibrio cholerae*, *Vibrio parahaemolyticus*, and *Vibrio vulnificus*; *Salmonella* species; hepatitis viruses
(including raw sushi and gefilte fish)	A, B, and C; tapeworm and *Anisakis*
Cheese, milk	*Listeria* species
Eggs	*Salmonella* species
Mayonnaise-containing food and cream pie	Staphylococcal and clostridial food poisonings
Fried rice	*Bacillus cereus*
Fresh berries	*Cyclospora* species
Canned vegetables or fruits	*Clostridium* species
Sprouts, spinach	Enterohemorrhagic *E. coli* and *Salmonella* species
Animal-to-person (pets and livestock)	*Salmonella*, *Campylobacter*, *Cryptosporidium*, and *Giardia* species
Person-to-person (including sexual contact)	All enteric bacteria, viruses, and parasites
Day-care center	*Shigella*, *Campylobacter*, *Cryptosporidium*, and *Giardia* species; viruses; *Clostridium difficile*
Hospital, antibiotics, or chemotherapy	*C. difficile*
Swimming pool	*Giardia* and *Cryptosporidium* species
Foreign travel	*E. coli* of various types; *Salmonella*, *Shigella*, *Campylobacter*, *Giardia*, and *Cryptosporidium* species; *Entamoeba histolytica*, norovirus (cruise ships)

a Also includes fish poisonings such as scombroid, ciguatera, and paralytic, diarrheal, and neurotoxic shellfish poisonings.
Adapted from Parks & Giannella [612].

Sporadic diarrhea

Most infectious diarrheas are acquired by fecal–oral transmission, which can occur by water, food, or person-to-person contact. Although microorganisms can be spread by any of these vehicles, certain classic relations exist between vehicle and disease (Table 18.5). Water systems may be contaminated by human waste as the result of poor sewage systems or by animal feces from farm run-off material. Diarrheal disease results if the water is not properly purified. Beef, pork, or poultry may be the source of infection if it is poorly cooked. More commonly, infection comes from contamination of food-preparing surfaces by organisms present on these meats; the organisms are then spread to uncooked foods, such as salads, that are prepared on these same surfaces. Transmission also comes from minute inoculation of certain foods that is followed by bacterial proliferation because the food is either poorly refrigerated or inadequately heated before serving. This commonly occurs at picnics, banquets, or restaurants. Person-to-person transmission can occur through aerosolization (rotavirus), through contamination of hands (*Clostridium difficile*), or through contamination of fomites [72]. Spread also comes from sexual activity, particularly oral–genital or oral–anal contact.

Patients with infectious diarrhea complain of nausea, vomiting, and abdominal pain and have watery, malabsorptive diarrhea or dysentery (bloody diarrhea and fever). Both large and small bowel infections can present with any combination of these signs and symptoms, but certain patterns tend to occur characteristically (Table 18.6). Patterns of systemic symptoms may be clues to the disease-causing organism. Furthermore, some enteric infections may cause delayed, often severe, complications [73–83] (Table 18.7). Conversely, patients with certain systemic, nonenteric diseases (see Table 18.6) may have diarrhea as a significant component of the illness, either because the gastrointestinal mucosa is the portal of entry, as in hepatitis, listeriosis, and legionellosis, or because of the systemic release of inflammatory mediators, as in several new emerging infectious diseases, causes intestinal secretion.

Foodborne and waterborne diarrheas

Deaths from *E. coli* O157:H7 and *Cyclospora* infections in the United States, United Kingdom, and Japan have produced a

Table 18.6 Correlations between pathophysiology and symptoms of infectious diarrhea

Pathophysiology/microorganisms	Nausea and vomiting	Abdominal pain	Fever	Diarrhea
Toxin producers Preformed toxin *Bacillus cereus, Staphylococcus aureus, Clostridium perfringens*	2–4+ (within 4 h of ingestion)	1–2+	0–1+	3–4+, watery
Enterotoxin *Vibrio cholerae,* enterotoxigenic *Escherichia coli, Klebsiella pneumoniae, Aeromonas* species	(Within 24–72 h of ingestion)			
Enteroadherent Enteropathogenic and enteroadherent *E. coli, Giardia* organisms, *Cryptosporidium* species, helminths	0–1+	1–3+	1–2+	1–2+, watery
Cytotoxin-producing *Clostridium difficile,* hemorrhagic *E. coli* O157:H7	0–1+	3–4+	1–2+	1–3+, usually watery, occasionally or quickly bloody

Invasive organisms
Minimal inflammation
   Rotavirus and Norwalk agent, *Cryptosporidium* and *Cyclospora* species
 	
Variable inflammation
   Salmonella, Campylobacter, and *Aeromonas* species, *Vibrio parahaemolyticus*
 	
Severe inflammation
   Shigella species, enteroinvasive *E. coli, Entamoeba histolytica,* anthrax
	0–3+	2–4+	3–4+	1–4+, watery or bloody

Systemic infection Hepatitis, measles, listeriosis, legionellosis, Rocky Mountain spotted fever, psittacosis, hantavirus, otitis media in infants, toxic shock syndrome, avian influenza (H5N1), severe acute respiratory syndrome (SARS)	Watery diarrhea may accompany these diseases but is often overshadowed by the other disease manifestations			

Note: numbers 0 to 4+ refer to the severity of symptoms.
Adapted from Powell [611].

crisis in public confidence regarding government-regulated food safety [84]. Various factors relating to the industrialization of food consumption and eating habits are responsible for the surge in foodborne illness [84].

Food poisoning occurs not only from invasive organisms but also from toxin producers (see Table 18.5). The infectious food poisonings can occur with ingestion of either fin fish or shellfish [85–90]. Fish can become contaminated in their own environment (especially the filter-feeding bivalve molluscs such as muscles, clams, oysters, and scallops), or fish can be contaminated by food handlers [88]. The infectious organisms contaminating seafood include invasive organisms such as hepatitis virus, Norwalk virus, *Salmonella, Shigella, Campylobacter,* and *Plesiomonas,* and watery diarrhea-producing organisms such as *Aeromonas, Clostridium botulinum,* and *Vibrio cholerae* [88]. Organisms that are specific for seafood are the noncholera vibrios, such as *V. parahemolyticus,* which causes either watery or bloody diarrhea, and *V. vulnificus,* which causes not only watery diarrhea but also fatal septicemia, especially in those with liver disease [90,91].

Food poisoning also occurs with chemicals such as monosodium glutamate, heavy metals or insecticides, and natural toxins found in mushrooms or seafood [85–88]. Ciguatera, diarrhetic, paralytic, neurotoxic, amnestic, and pfiesteria fish

Table 18.7 Systemic symptoms and complications of enteric infections

Organism	Symptoms or complications	References
Vibrio cholerae and *Escherichia coli*	Dehydration, shock, and death	5, 82
Bacillus cereus	Fulminant liver failure	78
Vibrio vulnificus	Shock and death in those with liver disease	89–91
Enteroadherent and enteroaggregative *E. coli*, *Cryptosporidium*, *Cyclospora*, and *Aeromonas* species	Prolonged (> 6 weeks) diarrhea	76, 81, 90, 148, 150–152
Clostridium difficile	Relapse common, protein-losing enteropathy, colonectomy, death	92–100
Enterohemorrhagic *E. coli* (*E. coli* O157:H7)	Hemolytic uremic syndrome or thrombotic thrombocytopenic purpura	139
Salmonella species	Septicemia and invasive (extraintestinal) salmonellosis, e.g., peritonitis, cholecystitis, pancreatitis, intraabdominal abscess, mycotic aneurysm, osteomyelitis	73, 74
Campylobacter species	Guillain–Barré syndrome	77, 79
Shigella species	Seizures and encephalopathy	74, 75, 80
Salmonella, *Shigella*, *Campylobacter*, and *Yersinia* species	Postinfectious reactive arthritis and Reiter syndrome	70, 74, 83
Yersinia species	Thyroiditis, pericarditis, glomerulonephritis, myocarditis, extraintestinal infection, hemolytic uremic syndrome, Guillain–Barré syndrome	152, 153

poisonings are all caused by dinoflagellates ingested by fish or shellfish [85–90]. Puffer fish poisoning is caused by a toxin (tetrodotoxin) contained only in this fish, and scombroid poisoning comes from the breakdown of flesh in certain fish with the release of histamine.

High-risk groups
Antibiotic-associated diarrheas
Diarrhea may occur in up to 20% of patients receiving broad-spectrum antibiotics, but only some (30%–50%) of these diarrheas are the result of *C. difficile* infection (pseudomembranous colitis) (Table 18.8) [92]. *Clostridium difficile*-negative diarrhea has been ascribed to antibiotic-induced abnormalities in colonic carbohydrate fermentation, with resulting decreased short-chain acid production [93], to overgrowth of fungi (*Candida* species) [94], or to overgrowth of other, unidentified microorganisms. Non-*C. difficile* diarrhea is usually mild and self-limited and clears either spontaneously or in response to cholestyramine therapy. *Clostridium difficile* colitis, however, can cause severe diarrhea that has significant morbidity and mortality [95–98] and may present with a relapsing course after seemingly successful therapy with metronidazole or vancomycin [99]. Antibiotic-associated diarrhea can follow treatment with any antibiotic, although broad-spectrum antibiotics such as clindamycin, third-generation cephalosporins, and fluoroquinolones are particularly problematic [95–98]. The disease can be nosocomial and is increasing in frequency, and severity as a result of the

Table 18.8 High-risk groups for infectious diarrhea

Antibiotic use
Outpatient clinics
Hospital

Recent travel
Developing nations
Peace Corps workers
Campers (ground water)
Cruise ships (norovirus)

Homosexuals, sex workers, and intravenous drug users
Gay bowel syndrome
Acquired immunodeficiency syndrome

Day-care facilities
Children
Secondary contacts (family members)

Institutions
Mental institutions
Nursing homes
Hospitals

emergence of a strain that is particularly virulent [95–98]. This new strain causes high morbidity and mortality (over 15%) and must be treated aggressively [95–98]. The incidence of *C. difficile* and other antibiotic-associated diarrheas may be reduced by the concomitant administration of probiotics [99]. Relapses of *C. difficile* colitis not responding to repeated courses and tapering regimens of antibiotics may respond to long-term cholestyramine therapy, intravenous immunoglobulin infusion, or administration of normal, donated stool through the colonoscope [100].

Traveler's diarrhea

Not only are travelers from developed countries at high risk of acute infectious diarrhea, but so are travelers on airplanes and cruise ships, where errors in food preparation or close contact can lead to common-source epidemics. Bacterial agents account for 85% of traveler's diarrhea, with enterotoxigenic *E. coli* (ETEC), *Shigella*, *Campylobacter*, *Aeromonas*, *Plesiomonas*, *Salmonella*, and noncholera vibrios leading the list [101]. Prevention through education or chemoprophylaxis (bismuth subsalicylate, rifaximin, or fluoroquinolones) [101,102], and therapy (fluid and electrolyte replacement and antibiotics) are discussed under Treatment of acute infectious diarrhea (below).

Sexually transmitted diarrheas

Men who have sex with men and sex workers are apt to develop infectious diarrhea through the oral–fecal route.

Day-care diarrhea

Diarrhea is extremely prevalent in the more than 6 million children in the United States attending day care, and it usually involves those organisms that colonize at a low inoculum dose (e.g., *Shigella*, *Giardia*, *Cryptosporidium*) or those that are spread easily (e.g., rotavirus, astrovirus, adenovirus) [72,103]. However, almost any organism can be isolated in outbreaks of day-care diarrhea. The mechanism of transmission in day-care centers is person-to-person contact by way of fecal contamination of hands and fomites (e.g., toys, surfaces in diaper-changing areas, bathroom taps, and flush handles). The secondary attack rate from day-care diarrhea ranges between 10% and 20%, representing an important source of infection for parents and siblings as well [72,104].

Diagnosis of acute infectious diarrheas

Differential diagnosis

An algorithm for the evaluation of acute infectious diarrheas is given in Fig. 18.5. This approach relies heavily on consideration of the epidemiology of acute infectious diarrhea as described earlier and on ruling out other causes of acute watery or bloody diarrhea [105,106].

The differential diagnosis of acute watery diarrhea includes the food toxins, drugs, and medications listed in Tables 18.2 and 18.3. Although these drugs are the most common culprits, any medication can cause diarrhea.

In children, acute appendicitis may be misdiagnosed as "acute gastroenteritis," so delaying surgery [107]. The differ-

ential diagnosis of acute bloody diarrhea in adults includes infectious causes, ischemic colitis, IBD, neoplasms, and drug-induced colitis. Although the patient's age and the presence of manifestations of atherosclerosis may suggest ischemic colitis, older people also may have more severe clinical manifestations with invasive infectious agents. Radiographically, enterohemorrhagic *E. coli* infection can mimic ischemic colitis, with submucosal hemorrhage presenting as thumbprinting on the flat plate of the abdomen. Ulcerative proctitis or colitis and Crohn's disease can present with an acute course that suggests infectious enterocolitis, or vice versa. Although the colonoscopic and radiographic appearance of the various invasive enteritides can mimic IBD with aphthous-like ulcers, segmental colitis, or pancolitis, colonic biopsy will yield histological hallmarks that differentiate IBD from infectious diarrheas. Infection with *C. difficile* may have the classic pseudomembranous enterocolitis appearance by radiography or endoscopy, but on occasion the pseudomembrane is not present, particularly in pancytopenic patients undergoing cancer chemotherapy, and then the disease looks more like IBD. On rare occasions, the opposite mistake is made, and blood-filled macrophages in the stool of a patient with ulcerative colitis are mistaken for blood-filled trophozoites of amebiasis, or chronic ischemic colitis masquerades as pseudomembranous colitis. To complicate matters further, the colonic mucosa inflamed with ulcerative colitis appears to be more susceptible to colonization by pathogenic enteric bacteria. *Salmonella*, *Campylobacter*, or especially *C. difficile* infection may accompany IBD and may confuse the diagnosis and treatment. Drugs that may induce colitis indistinguishable from ulcerative colitis include gold (administered for rheumatoid arthritis) and methyldopa (for hypertension).

Laboratory diagnosis of infectious diarrheas

The cost of making the diagnosis of infectious diarrhea and of delivering specific (antibiotic) therapy is high, especially for a disease that is common and is usually mild and self-limited. Fewer than 10% of stool specimens are positive for pathogens [105,108], so the cost of a single positive stool culture is high (more than $1000) if stools are cultured indiscriminately [108–111]. However, the cost can be reduced to $30 per culture if only *Campylobacter*, *Salmonella*, and *Shigella* are sought and if only liquid stools are cultured. Special rules apply to the culture of stool in hospital-acquired diarrhea [112,113] (see Infectious nosocomial diarrhea). The use of antibiotics in infectious diarrhea is also controversial [90,105, 110]. Therefore, the questions revolve around who should undergo a diagnostic evaluation, who should be treated and when, and whether treatment should consist of only symptomatic therapy or symptomatic therapy plus specific antibiotics.

The algorithm in Fig. 18.5 uses discriminating symptoms to determine whether fecal specimens should be sent for

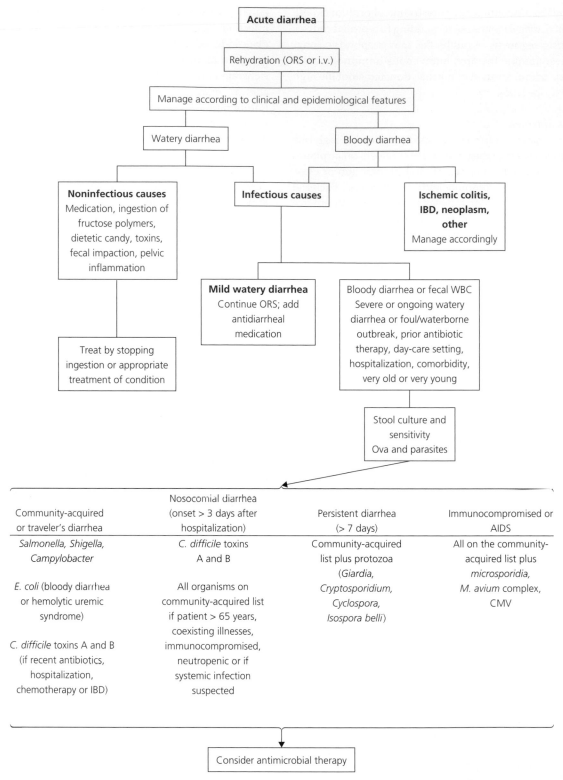

Figure 18.5 Algorithm for the diagnostic approach to acute diarrhea. CMV, Cytomegalovirus; IBD, inflammatory bowel disease; i.v., intravenous; ORS, oral replacement solution; WBC, white blood cell count. Adapted from Thielman & Guerrant [110].

laboratory diagnosis [106,110,111]. Fecal leukocyte stains [114] are not useful for inpatients [115] and have poor sensitivity for ruling out invasive infectious diarrhea [116]. Stool excretion of granulocyte marker proteins is being evaluated as perhaps a better surrogate for fecal leukocytes [110,117–120]. In addition, certain organisms that can cause diarrhea are not generally identified by routine diagnostic methods. For example, certain causes of bloody diarrhea, such as *Yersinia*, *Plesiomonas*, and enterohemorrhagic *E. coli* O157:H7, may require specific special culture techniques or can be identified only with type-specific antisera [121]. Similarly, *Aeromonas*, *Cryptosporidium*, *Cyclospora*, microsporidia, and noncholera *Vibrio* organisms, which cause watery diarrhea, may require special laboratory attention for culture and identification. The enterotoxigenic, enteropathogenic, enteroinvasive, enteroadherent, and enteroaggregative *E. coli* organisms are diagnosed only by methods available in research laboratories. Therefore, the physician may need to communicate the presumptive diagnosis to the laboratory. The enteroadherent bacteria and certain parasites such as *Giardia* and *Strongyloides* may be difficult to detect in stool and may best be diagnosed by intestinal biopsy. *Clostridium difficile* is best diagnosed by toxin assay [92,95,96], although the rapid enzyme-linked immunosorbent assays commonly used in hospitals have a sensitivity of only 70%–90%, so false-negative results can occur [122]. Testing for both *C. difficile* toxins A and B would reduce false negatives. Finally, 20%–40% of all acute infectious diarrheas remain undiagnosed even with the application of all laboratory techniques.

Treatment of acute infectious diarrheas

The treatment of diarrhea can be divided into symptomatic therapy (fluid replacement and antidiarrheal) and specific antimicrobial therapy [90,105,106,110,123]. In most instances where death occurs in acute diarrhea, it is caused by dehydration; for this reason, a cardinal principle in the management of any diarrhea consists of assessment of the degree of dehydration and replacement of fluid and electrolyte deficits [90,105,106,110,123,124]. Severely dehydrated patients, particularly those with altered mental status, should be rehydrated with intravenous Ringer lactate or saline solutions to which additional K^+ and $NaHCO_3$ may be added as necessary. Alert patients should be given oral replacement solution (ORS), which is as effective as intravenous fluid replacement in most instances [125]. Whereas experience in developing countries has demonstrated the efficacy of ORS in treating severe dehydrating diarrhea, ORS use in developed countries has lagged behind. This may account in part for some of the morbidity and mortality still observed in the United States [125–127]. In mild to moderate dehydration, ORS can be given to infants and children in volumes of 50–100 mL/kg over a period of 4–6 h; adults may need to drink up to 1000 mL/h [127]. After the patient is rehydrated, ORS is given at rates equaling stool loss plus insensible losses until the diarrhea ceases. The World Health Organization (WHO) solution is endorsed for use in both rehydration and maintenance therapy worldwide, although some are concerned that the high Na^+ content (90 mM) may lead to hypernatremia and the high osmolarity (311 mOsm/L) may worsen diarrhea. Consequently, many clinicians recommend alternating full-strength WHO ORS with equal volumes of water or giving a mixture of two parts ORS with one part water or formula during the postrehydration, maintenance phase of ORS therapy. There continues to be concern about the proper ORS to use, and the superiority of hypotonic ORS solutions (Na^+ 75 mM, osmolarity 245 mOsm/L) has been questioned [128].

The addition of amino acids to glucose-based ORS or the substitution of rice gruel or cereal for glucose has created "super ORS" solutions that may be even better than the conventional WHO solution [124,128,129]. A newer concept for rehydration is to add amylase-resistant starch (pectin) to the ORS. This starch escapes digestion and absorption in the upper bowel and is then broken down to short-chain fatty acids by bacteria in the colon, where it promotes fluid absorption [130, 131]. Clearly, the WHO solution and the commercial ORS solutions are superior to Gatorade, Coca-Cola, or fruit juices, which were used in the past for rehydration in the United States (Table 18.9). ORS can be used safely with loperamide antidiarrheal medications in traveler's diarrhea [132].

A devastating effect of recurrent diarrheal diseases is malnutrition. At one time, complete or partial bowel rest was recommended during acute diarrhea. It is clear that patients with acute diarrhea should be fed, not starved [133,134]. Continued breast-feeding or half-strength formula for infants is recommended. Ad libitum diets low in fiber, Na^+-rich soups, and foods with high sugar content are preferred for older children and adults.

Bismuth subsalicylate (Pepto-Bismol, Procter & Gamble, Cincinnati, OH) is safe and efficacious in bacterial infectious diarrheas [105,106,110]. It may not have antidiarrheal activity in viral diarrhea, raising the question of whether its main effect in traveler's diarrhea relates to its antibacterial or antiinflammatory action or perhaps to the ability of its clay vehicle to adsorb enterotoxins. Kaolin–pectin preparations, which were previously thought to be minimally effective [135], may be more effective since being reformulated in 2003 to contain bismuth subsalicylate. With the possibility of worsening the colonization or invasion of the organism by paralyzing intestinal motility and with evidence that the use of motility-altering drugs may prolong microorganism excretion time, neither opiates nor anticholinergic drugs are recommended for infectious diarrheas [105,106,110]. However, it has been shown that loperamide can be both useful and safe in traveler's diarrhea, provided it is not given to patients who have high fever or to those with blood or pus in the stool,

Table 18.9 Composition of oral replacement solutions for the treatment of diarrhea

Solution	Na+ (mM)	K+ (mM)	Cl− (mM)	Citrate (mM)	Glucose[a] (mM)
WHO solution	90	20	80	30	111 (20)
Reduced osmolarity ORS	75	20	65	10	75 (13.5)
Glucose plus glycine	120	15	72	48	110 (20) plus 110 glycine
Rehydralyte	75	20	65	30	139 (25)
Pedialyte	45	20	35	30	139 (25)
Resol	50	20	50	34	111 (20)
Ricelyte	50	25	45	34	(30)
Gatorade	23.5	< 1	17		(40)
Coca-Cola	1.6	< 1		13.4[b]	(100)
Apple juice	< 1	25			(120)
Orange juice	< 1	50		50	(120)
Chicken broth	250	8		0	0

a Values in parentheses represent grams of carbohydrate.
b Rice syrup solid rather than glucose.
ORS, oral replacement solution; WHO, World Health Organization.
Adapted from Di John & Levene [613] and Nalin et al. [128].

especially when the drug is administered concomitantly with effective antibiotics [105,106,110,123,124]. The anxiolytics and antiemetics that decrease sensory perception may make symptoms more tolerable and are generally safe. A single oral dose of ondansetron has been recommended for vomiting in pediatric gastroenteritis [136].

Antibiotic therapy in the infectious diarrheas is controversial [105,106,110]. There are certain infectious diarrheas in which treatment is recommended: shigellosis, cholera, traveler's diarrhea, C. difficile colitis, parasitic infections, and sexually transmitted diseases. Patients with mild disease and those who are clearly improving may not need antibiotic treatment. There are other diarrheas in which treatment in the past was not indicated because there was no effective therapy. However, recent reports support the efficacy of treatment with nitazoxanide in both rotavirus diarrhea and cryptosporidiosis [137,138]. Treatment of E. coli O157:H7 infection is not recommended at present because the current antibiotics do not appear to be helpful, and the incidence of hemolytic uremic syndrome may be greater after antibiotic therapy [139]. There are several diseases in which the indications are less clear but in which treatment is usually recommended: infection with the noncholera vibrios, prolonged or protracted infection with Yersinia, early in the course of campylobacteriosis, Aeromonas and Plesiomonas infections, and nursery outbreaks of enteropathogenic E. coli diarrhea. Regardless of the cause of infectious diarrhea, patients should probably be treated if they are debilitated with malignant disease, are immunosuppressed, have an abnormal cardiovascular system or valvular, vascular, or orthopedic prostheses, have hemolytic anemia (especially if salmonellosis is involved), or are extremely young or old. Treatment is

also advised for those with prolonged symptoms and those who relapse. These guidelines were developed for patients with salmonellosis [140], but they are useful guidelines for all infectious diarrheas. The antimicrobial agents of choice are outlined elsewhere [106,107,111]. Aggressive treatment of the new, virulent strain of C. difficile is recommended [95–98]. Although there is evidence that early treatment shortens the course of infectious diarrhea by 2 days [110,140], it usually takes 3 to 5 days after obtaining stools before specific organisms can be grown and identified. If treatment was warranted while awaiting laboratory diagnosis, the quinolones (e.g., ciprofloxacin), which have efficacy against most enteric infections, are the treatments of choice [105,106,110,140]. Trimethoprim-sulfamethoxazole is the second-line therapy in this setting. Resistance to both antibiotics is increasingly recognized. If the symptom complex suggests Campylobacter infection, erythromycin should be added. Prolonged diarrhea suggesting giardiasis or bacterial overgrowth may be treated with a course of metronidazole even if stools are negative for cysts.

Prolonged infectious diarrheas

Severe protracted diarrhea in infants and children
Although classically a severe postinfectious diarrhea syndrome in infants and children of developing countries [141], protracted diarrhea (postenteritis syndrome) can occur in a mild or severe form in developed countries as well [142]. Infection with enteroadherent bacteria, uncleared cryptosporidial, or Cyclospora infection, bacterial overgrowth, or infection with unknown organisms may lead to disaccharidase deficiency

in mild cases and profound generalized malabsorption in severe forms [143]. Severe malnutrition and death (mortality up to 50%) can ensue [141]. Treatment includes dietary lactose exclusion in mild disease [142] and controlled feeding or total parenteral nutrition in those who are severely affected [134]. Metronidazole, tetracycline, trimethoprim-sulfamethoxazole, folic acid, and zinc therapy may also be of help [141,144]. Where this disease ends and tropical sprue begins is uncertain; the difference may be only the age of the patient [143].

Tropical sprue

This disease of unknown origin affects those in certain tropical parts of the world, including the Indian subcontinent and Asia, the West Indies, northern parts of South America, parts of Central America, and central and southern Africa. It can occur in visitors residing in these areas for as short a time as 1–3 months. Its acute onset suggests an infectious origin. Small bowel histology may show minimal villus blunting and inflammatory infiltrate or may reveal severe villus atrophy and crypt hyperplasia. Abnormal pancreatic exocrine function may occur in tropical sprue, as it does in celiac sprue [145]. If the patient is removed from the tropical areas and the mucosal change is mild, the disease may remit spontaneously. A combination of tetracycline and folic acid is effective therapy.

Persistent diarrhea in travelers

Protracted diarrhea lasting more than 3 to 4 weeks has been seen in up to 10% of returned travelers [146,147]. Undiagnosed infection with bacteria or protozoal organisms that typically causes long-lasting diarrhea may be the cause (see Protracted infectious diarrhea in adults), and stool cultures and evaluation for ova and parasites as well as antimicrobial treatment may lead to cure. These patients usually have already received routine traveler's diarrhea antibiotics (e.g., trimethoprim-sulfamethoxazole or quinolones), so tetracycline or metronidazole, which may be effective against enteroadherent E. coli, protozoal organisms, and nonspecific bacterial overgrowth, may be given when the results of stool evaluations for pathogens are negative [146–148]. The pathophysiological mechanisms proposed here are similar to those proposed for severe protracted diarrhea and tropical sprue (see earlier). The point at which protracted traveler's diarrhea ends and tropical sprue begins may be a matter of obtaining a biopsy specimen for small bowel histology.

Protracted infectious diarrhea in adults

In the United States, some organisms typically cause a prolonged course of diarrhea. Organisms that are difficult to diagnose and are known to cause protracted or prolonged diarrheas include enteropathogenic (enteroadherent) E. coli [148], Giardia [149], amoeba [90], Cryptosporidium [150], Aeromonas [81,151], Yersinia enterocolitica [152,153], and Blasto-

cystis hominis [154]. Clostridium difficile infection is often difficult to clear, and five or more relapses have been observed [100]. Patients with chronic diarrhea should have these diagnoses excluded. If none of these organisms are found, a therapeutic trial of metronidazole [146,147] or nitazoxanide [137,138,154] may be indicated.

Infectious diarrhea-induced irritable bowel syndrome and Brainerd or epidemic chronic diarrhea

As many as 25% of patients will experience IBS-like symptoms (pain, bloating, urgency, sense of incomplete evacuation, loose stools) for 6 months or longer after documented infectious diarrhea [155]. The pathophysiology is thought to be unresolved, mild intestinal inflammation [156, 157]. In some patients, the syndrome may be the result of bacterial overgrowth and may be responsive to non-absorbable antibiotics such as Rifaximin [158]. In others, it may be the result of acquired bile acid malabsorption. These latter patients may respond to cholestyramine therapy (see Bile acid diarrhea) [159–161].

Severe and prolonged forms of postinfectious diarrhea after raw milk ingestion were reported in outbreak form in Brainerd, Minnesota in the 1980s [162]. Patients developed prolonged chronic watery diarrhea with weight loss and were often mistakenly diagnosed as having IBS. It also has been reported in other states in association with raw milk ingestion or untreated water ingestion. Many of these patients have microscopic inflammation on colonic biopsy and it is thought that it probably represents a severe form of infectious diarrhea-induced IBS. It may also be the same condition as chronic idiopathic diarrhea discussed in the section on chronic diarrheas.

Nosocomial diarrheas

Diarrhea is either the first or second most common nosocomial illness [163] among hospitalized patients and those residing in chronic-care facilities for the retarded, the mentally disturbed, or the elderly. Often this is a hidden problem, known only by the nurse's aide who changes the bed sheets. In the intensive care setting, it occurs in 30%–50% of patients [164], and in chronic-care facilities more than one-third of patients have a significant diarrheal illness each year [165,166]. This is a multifactorial condition whose recognized causes are discussed in the following subsections.

Fecal impaction

Clinical lore has it that the most common cause of diarrhea in hospitalized or institutionalized patients is fecal impaction. Such paradoxical diarrhea and incontinence appear to be most common in patients with dementia or psychosis [167]. Although the validity of this clinical impression remains uncertain, performing a rectal examination and perhaps a flat and upright abdominal radiograph may be worthwhile in such patients.

Medications and weight-reducing agents

Any of a patient's medications may initiate diarrhea. However, certain medications are more apt to cause diarrhea than others [168] (see Tables 18.2 and 18.3). Antibiotic-associated diarrhea (see "High-risk groups") is certainly the most common manifestation of drug-related diarrhea. Orlistat, a lipase inhibitor used to treat obesity [168], and acarbose, an α-glucosidase inhibitor used to treat diabetes, can both cause diarrhea [169]. Olestra, a nonabsorbable fat substitute used for frying foods, may also cause diarrhea when given at doses greater than 40 g/day [170].

Elixir diarrhea

Drugs such as theophylline or KCl made up in liquid formulations (elixirs) may cause diarrhea because of the high content of sorbitol used to sweeten the elixir [171]. This is the iatrogenic equivalent of "chewing gum diarrhea" (see Sorbitol and fructose diarrhea). Patients receiving medications in the liquid form through feeding tubes may receive more than 20 g of sorbitol daily.

Enteral feeding

An important but poorly understood cause of diarrhea is tube feeding, particularly in the critically ill patient [172–174]. Up to 35% of patients receiving tube feeding develop diarrhea. Various pathophysiological factors are hypothesized: bacterial contamination of the enteral formula; administration of hypertonic solutions that cause diarrhea by inducing a form of "dumping syndrome"; administration of lactose-containing formulas to lactase-deficient subjects; administration of sorbitol-containing elixirs; administration of low-Na^+ formulas that result in considerable blood-to-lumen Na^+ diffusion in addition to fluid movement if the formula is hypertonic as well; and hypoalbuminemia in malnourished patients, a condition that alters the oncotic or Starling forces in the gut capillaries, thus preventing absorption or inducing secretion. Although there are experimental studies that support all these possibilities, there are no clear data supporting any single process or group of pathophysiological processes, and enteral nutrition support should not be discontinued because of watery diarrhea [174]. Furthermore, more mundane causes of diarrhea (e.g., concomitant medication, *C. difficile* infection) can also occur in these patients.

Infectious nosocomial diarrhea

Patients in mental institutions have high incidences of infection by bacterial pathogens, protozoal parasites (*Entamoeba histolytica* and *Giardia*), and helminths [166,175]. Infectious diarrheas also occur in acute-care hospitals; the rates are particularly high in intensive care settings (eight cases per 100 admissions) [176]. In the intensive care setting, a role has been postulated for tube feeding as a source of infection in combination with histamine (H_2) blockers, which eradicate the gastric acid barrier. The most common cause in the past was infection with *Salmonella* species [177]; although it still occurs, since 1980 *C. difficile* has accounted for more than 50% of hospital cases [178]. In addition, shigellosis is a rare nosocomial infection in hospitals [179]. The likelihood of a nosocomial infection caused by *Salmonella* or *Shigella* organisms in the tertiary hospital is so rare that routine cultures for *Salmonella* and *Shigella* and ova or parasite examinations are not cost effective and should not be ordered if diarrhea begins 3 to 4 days after hospital admission, provided the patient is not more than 65 years old and has no preexisting diseases, the patient does not have AIDS or neutropenia, there is no evidence of a nosocomial outbreak, and the patient has no non-diarrheal manifestation of infection (e.g., fever, abdominal pain, erythema nodosum). This dictum is known as the *modified 3-day rule* [111–113].

Immunosuppressed patients are another important group susceptible to nosocomial diarrhea. Viral infections (rotavirus, astrovirus, adenovirus, and coxsackievirus) may be important causes of nosocomial infectious diarrheas in bone marrow transplant units [176,180,181]. In this setting, infectious diarrhea must be differentiated from the diarrhea of graft-vs-host disease.

Outbreaks of hemorrhagic *E. coli* and *C. difficile* infections have been recognized in hospitals and nursing homes [182, 183]. Some of the strokes, injuries from falls, and even myocardial infarctions occurring in nursing home settings could be caused by the hypovolemia and toxic state induced by these nosocomial diarrheas. Infection control measures and restricting use of broad-spectrum antibiotics may reduce the incidence of nosocomial *C. difficile* diarrhea [95,98,184].

Hospital-acquired diarrheas may be a causative factor in other nosocomial hospital infections, such as infection of the urinary tract [185]. The impact of nosocomial diarrhea on the duration and cost of hospitalization and on morbidity is probably substantial.

Cancer treatment

The incidence of acute, mild diarrhea with chemotherapy or radiation therapy is high, approaching 100% with some agents or irradiation regimens [186]. Radiation therapy also causes chronic diarrhea. Nausea, vomiting, and diarrhea are dose- and age-related phenomena. Chemotherapy diarrhea is more likely with specific forms of chemotherapy, such as the following: 5-fluorouracil, irinotecan (CPT-11), interferon-α2A, topotecan, and IL-2 [186–188]. The incidence of diarrhea with some regimens may reach 80%. Neutropenic enterocolitis, which occurs most commonly in association with the chemotherapy of leukemia and lymphoma, is a particularly serious diarrheal disease [189]. The incidence of diarrhea with IL-2 therapy approaches 80% [188]. Radiation may induce diarrhea either through damage to segments of bowel during pelvic irradiation or through damage to the entire bowel if high-dose, total body radiation is received. Total-body radiation at low doses (1.5 Gy) causes only nausea and vomiting; watery or bloody diarrhea ensues at total-body doses greater than 6 Gy. Pelvic irradiation over a period of 4 weeks with doses of 3 to 4 Gy also may cause diarrhea. Current treatment for both chemotherapy- and radiation-induced diarrhea is symptomatic and includes antimotility drugs and cyclooxygenase blockers [186]. Octreotide may be helpful in severe chemotherapy- or radiation-induced diarrhea [186].

Runner's diarrhea

Gastrointestinal disturbances including anorexia, heartburn, nausea, vomiting, cramps, urgency, and diarrhea are common in those who exercise vigorously, particularly marathon runners and triathletes [190]. Watery, self-limiting diarrhea may occur in 10%–25% and is particularly common (40%–70%) in women runners. The mechanisms operative in runner's diarrhea are unclear but may involve the release of gastrointestinal hormones such as gastrin, motilin, or vasoactive intestinal polypeptide (VIP) or release of inflammatory mediators such as prostaglandins [191,192]. A role for ischemia has been postulated because of the occurrence of ischemia colitis in marathon runners [193,194]. Many treatment regimens have been used, but none have been studied thoroughly. Mouth-to-cecum transit time is either normal or delayed with exercise [195] so antimotility drugs may not help, but they may be tried. Nonsteroidal antiinflammatory agents (NSAIDs) are taken by many runners, but it is not clear whether they help in this condition.

Chronic diarrheas: definition, classification, and epidemiology

Definition and classification
Chronic diarrheas are those of at least 4 weeks' duration and, more certainly defined, 6 to 8 weeks' duration. There are three pathophysiological categories of diarrhea: malabsorptive (steatorrheic) diarrhea (see Table 18.2), watery diarrhea, which may be secretory (see Table 18.3) or osmotic, and inflammatory diarrhea (see Table 18.4). It would be convenient clinically if the character of the stool correlated well with the pathophysiology; that is, if an obviously steatorrheic stool occurred with all cases of malabsorptive diarrhea, watery stool only with secretory diarrheas, or bloody stool only with inflammation. Unfortunately, this is not the case. Carbohydrate malabsorption and ingestion of poorly absorbable substances (e.g., $MgSO_4$) causes watery diarrhea, as does inflammation that is not severe enough to cause

intestinal ulceration. Inflammation also may cause malabsorption; for example, celiac sprue, whose hallmark is intestinal malabsorption, is actually caused by inflammation [196]. Furthermore, malabsorptive diseases often have an element of intestinal secretion [197]. For clinical purposes, it is reasonable to classify diarrheas as steatorrhea, watery diarrhea, or inflammatory diarrhea, realizing that these categories are mixed with regard to pathophysiology. Such a categorization directs the physician to certain diagnostic algorithms (see below) [198].

Epidemiology
Although specific prevalence and incidence figures for the major diarrheal diseases are available for certain specific diseases, the precise incidence or prevalence of chronic diarrhea is not known because the appropriate population studies have not been performed. The best estimate is that chronic diarrhea occurs in approximately 5% of the US population [199,200].

Steatorrhea (malabsorptive diseases)

Although all three major nutrients – fat, carbohydrate, and protein – may be malabsorbed, clinical symptoms usually follow from malabsorption of either carbohydrate or fat [198–203]. Protein or amino acid malabsorption (azotorrhea) occurs but is not clinically recognized unless it is severe enough to cause malnutrition or unless specific amino acid transport defects cause congenital systemic disease. Malabsorption of electrolytes and water is also part of the pathophysiology of malabsorptive diarrheas. The gut's limited ability to absorb high concentrations of divalent ions (i.e., magnesium sulfate [$MgSO_4$], and magnesium phosphate [$MgPO_4$]) results in clinically evident diarrhea if these ions are ingested in excess. Nonetheless, the generalized malabsorptive diseases present as steatorrhea. Therefore, an understanding of fat absorption is necessary to understand malabsorptive diseases. Based on the normal physiology of fat absorption, fat malabsorption can be divided into three broad categories: intralumenal maldigestion, mucosal malabsorption, and postmucosal malabsorption related to lymphatic obstruction. The diseases listed in Table 18.2 can be allocated to one or more of these three general categories.

Intralumenal maldigestion
Cirrhosis and bile duct obstruction
Bile duct obstruction from cancer of the pancreas can cause steatorrhea through both pancreatic enzyme and bile salt insufficiency. There is a 25%–100% incidence of mild steatorrhea in patients with cirrhosis as a result of inadequate micelle formation from bile salt insufficiency [204,205]; Secondary factors, including malnutrition, portal hypertension, bacterial overgrowth, and drugs (e.g., neomycin), may also

play a role. In these diseases, the fat malabsorption is usually mild, and diarrhea is not usually a significant clinical problem.

Pancreatic exocrine insufficiency

Chronic pancreatitis may cause weight loss because of anorexia or because of fear that eating will initiate pain by activating pancreatitis. After at least 90% of the exocrine secretory capacity of the pancreas is lost, chronic pancreatic exocrine insufficiency supervenes, and malabsorption may lead to continued weight loss in spite of an excellent appetite. Increased intestinal transit time may add to the poor intralumenal digestion and malabsorption [206]. Up to 70% of patients with pancreatic calcification have chronic pancreatitis severe enough to cause malabsorption. Major degrees of pancreatectomy also cause fat malabsorption that is poorly responsive to pancreatic enzyme replacement [207].

Cystic fibrosis is a childhood equivalent of chronic pancreatic insufficiency, but the weight loss in this disease is probably caused as much by the anorexia of chronic infection [208] as it is by the malabsorption induced by pancreatic enzyme and bile acid deficiencies [209]. Shwachman syndrome is another pediatric cause of pancreatic insufficiency, although some patients improve with age [210].

Somatostatinoma is a rare pancreatic islet tumor with highly variable symptoms that may present with gallstones, diabetes, and diarrhea [211]. It is the one neuroendocrine tumor in which the diarrhea is caused by steatorrhea rather than by intestinal secretion. Presumably, the steatorrhea is secondary to inhibition of pancreatic secretion.

Mucosal malabsorption

Drugs

The chronic ingestion of drugs such as colchicine [212], neomycin [213], paraaminosalicylic acid [214], and the fenamate class of NSAIDs induces steatorrhea by enterocyte damage. Cholestyramine causes mild steatorrhea by binding bile acids [215].

Infectious diseases

Parasites can cause malabsorption through brush border damage, particularly the protozoans *Giardia*, *Cryptosporidium*, and *Isospora* [149,150,216–218] and the helminth *Strongyloides* [219]. These are treatable infections and they must be sought and rigorously excluded by stool examination or small intestine biopsy. Whipple disease and *Mycobacterium avium–intracellulare* complex are infections that cause malabsorption [220,221]. Chronic enteric infections, such as giardiasis associated with the agammaglobulinemias or cryptosporidiosis accompanying AIDS, also cause malabsorption [222].

Autoimmune enteropathies

Autoimmune enteropathy has been described in both newborn infants and children [223] and adults [224]. The histology of the small bowel resembles that in celiac disease, with subtotal or complete villous atrophy and increased lamina propria inflammatory cells, but serological test results for celiac disease are negative, and patients do not respond to a gluten-free diet. Circulating autoantibodies have been found in these patients directed against the enterocytes, goblet cells, smooth muscle, thyroid, islet cells, and parietal cells and against the hemidesmosomes of epithelial cells (the same autoantibodies as in bullous pemphigoid). These patients require glucocorticoids and azathioprine or cyclosporine for control of their disease.

Nongranulomatous chronic idiopathic enterocolitis, also known as *ulcerative jejunitis*, presents with more severe inflammation than autoimmune enteropathy, manifesting superficial ulcerations in addition to the villous atrophy [225]. This disease is prominent in the small intestine but may involve the colon in half of the patients. Patients with nongranulomatous chronic idiopathic enterocolitis may have an abrupt onset of their diarrhea and weight loss in early or middle adult life, and they often develop complications such as obstruction, perforation, and hemorrhage. Mortality is high (approximately 30%), although the patients appear to respond to corticosteroids and immune suppression therapy.

Immunodysregulation, polyendocrinopathy, enteropathy, X-linked (IPEX) syndrome is the result of mutations in the *FOXP3* gene. It presents with diarrhea and malabsorption in childhood, accompanied by type 1 diabetes, thrombocytopenia, hemolytic anemia, arthritis, asthma, and eczema. Those afflicted usually die in infancy or early childhood [226].

Immunoproliferative small intestinal disease is a collective term for immune enteropathies developing in patients in the Middle East or Mediterranean countries who have diseases that are otherwise known as *α-heavy-chain disease* or *Mediterranean lymphoma* [227]. Like patients with the autoimmune enteropathies, these patients present with malabsorption and sprue-like intestinal histology. Though α-heavy-chain disease tends to be benign, it may progress to malignant Mediterranean lymphoma. A common clonal origin of lymphocytes can be detected in both. Current views are that immunoproliferative small intestinal disease is one end of the spectrum of B-cell maltomas.

T-cell lymphomas of the bowel may also be the cause of malabsorption and sprue-like histology, sometimes with intestinal ulcers (see Celiac sprue).

Mastocytosis and eosinophilic gastroenteritis

Infiltrative immune system diseases include systemic mastocytosis [228,229] and eosinophilic gastroenteritis [230], in which gross distortion of the mucosa is associated with fat malabsorption. On occasion, steatorrhea may be profound, and these patients present with a sprue-like syndrome. In other patients, the watery diarrhea, systemic flushing, abdominal pain, tachycardia, and protein-losing enteropathy overshadow the steatorrhea.

Celiac sprue

The term *sprue* comes from the Dutch *spruw*, which means *thrush*, in recognition of the frequently concomitant presence of oral aphthae. The use of highly sensitive and specific antibody tests for celiac disease – immunoglobulin A (IgA) antiendomysial antibodies by immunofluorescent assay and the IgA anti-tissue transglutaminase antibodies test, which both have 90%–99% sensitivity (when coupled with assay of the patient's serum IgA level to rule out IgA deficiency) and specificity – have revolutionized our concept of this disease [231–238]. Instead of being a rare disease (1 in 10 000 population) with a classic "malabsorption/malnutrition" presentation, screening studies suggest that the disease may be as common as 1 in 100–200, with many extraintestinal manifestations (Table 18.10). Five phenotypes of the disease are recognized [237]:

• *Classic* – patients presenting with signs and symptoms of malabsorption or malnutrion
• *Atypical* – patients presenting with the diseases and disorders listed in Table 18.10, or with short stature, infertility, a history of fetal wastage or of low-birth-weight babies
• *Silent* – patients with no gastrointestinal symptoms or diseases associated with celiac disease but some degree of villous atrophy on biopsy
• *Latent* – those who are asymptomatic and have only increased intraepithelial lymphocytes on intestinal biopsy
• *Refractory* – those patients with celiac disease who do not respond to a gluten-free diet and are prone to develop ulcerative jejunoileitis or enteropathy-associated T-cell lymphoma.

Patients with silent and latent disease may present a problem in treatment because of a lack of motivation to adhere to a gluten-free diet.

Currently, physicians do a poor job of diagnosing celiac disease: only 50% of patients consider that they were diagnosed "promptly"; 27% consulted two or more gastroenterologists before the diagnosis; and only 30%–50% consider their physician knowledgeable about diagnosis and treatment [239]. The nonmalabsorptive/nonmalnutrition, extraintestinal manifestations (see Table 18.10) may be an important clue to the disease. The incidence of concomitant celiac disease occurring with most of the conditions listed in Table 18.10 is high enough (> 5%) to warrant screening for celiac disease in these patients. Screening should be considered also for first-degree family members where the prevalence is 5%–23% (and may be as high as 50%, if intraepithelial lymphocytosis on intestinal biopsy lesions is considered diagnostic) [237].

Celiac disease appears to have a significant adverse effect on the onset of menses, fertility, and the outcomes of pregnancy: miscarriage rate, intrauterine growth rate, and eventual birth weight [240]. Low birth rates have also been reported when the father is the one with celiac disease [241].

Patients with a history of active celiac disease have an increased relative risk of small bowel T-cell lymphoma and probably oropharyngeal, esophageal, and small bowel adenocarcinoma [231–238]. However, the incidence is not as high as was once thought, and the higher incidence of these cancers may be related to the severity and duration of untreated disease [242]. Some patients with T-cell lymphomas will present as celiac disease that is unresponsive to gluten-free diet (refractory sprue) [232,237]. Patients labeled as having refractory sprue may be inadvertently or purposely ingesting gluten. A minority of patients may have been misdiagnosed as having celiac disease and really suffer from autoimmune enteropathy [232]. The treatment of true "refractory sprue" is with steroids and immunosuppressive drugs [225,232,237].

Table 18.10 Diseases and conditions associated with celiac disease

Gastrointestinal diseases
Liver diseases
  Primary biliary cirrhosis
  Autoimmune hepatitis
  Autoimmune cholangitis
  Elevated aminotransferases
Others
  Irritable bowel syndrome
  Microscopic colitis
  Lymphocytic gastritis
  Crohn's disease
  Ulcerative colitis

Endocrine disorders
Type 1 diabetes
Autoimmune thyroid disease
Addison disease

Neurological disorders
Neuropathy
Cerebellar ataxia
Epilepsy (with occipital calcifications)

Skin disease
Dermatitis hepatiformis
Alopecia areata

Musculoskeletal disorders
Sjögren syndrome
Arthritis
Osteoporosis/dental enamel hypoplasia
Chronic fatigue syndrome

Cardiac disease
Idiopathic dilated cardiomyopathy
Autoimmune myocarditis

Hematological disorders
Iron deficiency
Hyposplenism

Genetic disorders
Down syndrome
Turner syndrome

Dermatitis herpetiformis

This form of skin disease is associated with sprue-like intestinal morphology in 70%–80% of cases [243]. The specificity and sensitivity of antitissue transglutaminase antibodies in this disease is unclear, with reports ranging from 50% [244] to 90% [245]. This blistering skin disease, which is characterized by IgA deposits in the dermal papilla, usually responds to dapsone, whereas the mucosal lesion responds to a gluten-free diet. The diet also seems to have a beneficial effect on the skin lesion, and about 50% of diet-adherent patients are able to stop dapsone medication [243,244]. Cyclosporine may be useful in patients who are resistant to conventional therapy [246]. These patients may experience many of the same "extraintestinal" complications as patients with celiac disease, including thyroid disease [247] or lymphoma [248]. Most likely, these patients have celiac disease with the skin being the extraintestinal presentation.

Whipple disease

This is a systemic infectious disease caused by an actinomycete, *Tropheryma whippelii*, and classically involving middle-aged men (male-to-female ratio is 5 : 1) [220,221]. The peak incidence occurs at ages 40–50 years, but it has been reported in infants and octogenarians. It presents with all the signs and symptoms of severe mucosal disease (weight loss and diarrhea) but has some additional characteristics: arthralgias in 65% (sacroiliac joints in one-third), chills and fever in up to 40%, hypotension (blood pressure < 110/60 mmHg) in 70%, lymphadenopathy in more than 50%, and, most important, involvement of the central nervous system in a plethora of ways.

Lipoproteinemias

Abetalipoproteinemia and hypobetalipoproteinemia are rare defects in chylomicron formation caused by abnormalities in microsomal transfer proteins or by molecular defects in apolipoprotein B itself [249]. Both conditions present with steatorrhea, acanthocytic red cells, ataxia, and retinitis pigmentosa. Patients with Tangier disease (absence of apolipoprotein A-I and apolipoprotein A-II) have yellow-orange streaks and spots in the tonsils and colonic mucosa. They may have diarrhea but not steatorrhea.

Postmucosal obstruction

Intestinal lymphangiectasia can be either congenital or acquired in association with trauma, lymphoma, carcinoma, or Whipple disease [250]. This condition causes protein-losing enteropathy with significant steatorrhea [250,251]. It is the classic form of postmucosal obstruction malabsorption. The unique clinical presentation – malabsorption of fat with loss of protein and lymphocytes, but normal absorption of carbohydrates – relates to the obstructed lymphatic channels, which are the route of absorption for fat and for the recovery of lymphocyte and protein-laden lymph. The absorption of carbohydrates and amino acids takes place by way of the portal circulation and remains unaffected. Immune deficiency, both humoral and cellular, may result [252]. Octreotide has been used successfully to treat this disease [253]. A primary (non-hereditary) form of lymphangiectasis has been reported [254].

Mixed causes of steatorrhea

Bacterial overgrowth

Stasis syndromes cause steatorrhea as well as an inflammatory and secretory form of diarrhea in patients with surgical gastrojejunal anastomoses, anatomic bowel obstruction (e.g., Crohn's disease), small bowel diverticulosis, and motility disorders, and also in the elderly [255–257]. Steatorrhea results from deconjugation of bile salts, causing poor micelle formation. However, brush border injury, mucosal inflammation, hydroxylation of fat with resulting fatty acid diarrhea, and changes in intestinal motility all play a role in this disease. Surgical correction of obstruction, antibiotics for bacterial overgrowth, and stimulation of motility with octreotide or prokinetic agents may improve symptoms, depending on the cause [256,257]. A role for small intestinal bacterial overgrowth in the pathophysiology and symptoms of irritable bowel syndrome has been proposed [258] and is being tested.

Short bowel syndrome

Extensive intestinal resection that leaves less than 200 cm of jejunum–ileum remaining represents another complicated, multifactorial form of steatorrhea resulting from the lack of sufficient absorptive surface, decreased transit time, and diminished bile salt pool [259–262]. It is part of a larger syndrome called *intestinal failure*, which also includes parenchymal bowel disease (e.g., Crohn's disease) and motility disorders in which nutrition is in peril. The diarrhea is heightened by the osmotic effect of nonabsorbed solutes, by gastric hypersecretion, perhaps by bacterial overgrowth, and conceivably even by intestinal secretion. Nutrition, vitamin, mineral, and electrolyte replacement, antibiotics for bacterial overgrowth, antisecretory and antidiarrheal/antimotility agents are the first-line therapy [262]. Glutamine-rich diets, exogenous growth factors, and long-acting octreotide hormones show promise as new treatments [259–261].

Metabolic diseases

Diseases such as thyrotoxicosis [263], adrenal insufficiency [264], autoimmune polyglandular syndrome [265], protein-calorie malnutrition [266], and prolonged fasting [267] may result in malabsorption through different mechanisms. Thyrotoxicosis may simply shorten transit time and disturb the intralumenal phase of the fat absorption. Adrenal insufficiency appears generally to disturb intralumenal and mucosal absorption, as do protein-calorie malnutrition and prolonged fasting, which also cause villus atrophy. The malabsorption of polyglandular syndrome type I is related to a deficiency of cholecystokinin-producing enteroendocrine cells. As with liver disease, the clinical picture usually overshadows the diarrhea and malabsorption and, certainly, the weight loss in these conditions is only partly related to the malabsorption.

Watery diarrheas

Ingestion of nonabsorbable solutes
Magnesium-induced diarrhea
Persons ingesting significant amounts of magnesium-based antacids or high-potency multimineral–multivitamin supplements may have significant diarrhea with stool weights up to 2000 g/24 h [268,269]. Occasionally, magnesium-containing laxatives are a cause of surreptitious diarrhea [268–270]. Magnesium in tube-feeding preparations may play a role in the diarrhea of patients receiving high-volume liquid feedings [271]. These diarrheas are diagnosed by measurements of stool Mg^{2+} and osmotic gap (see Evaluation of severe or elusive diarrhea).

Sodium anion diarrheas
Nonabsorbable sodium anion laxatives such as Na_2PO_4 (neutral phosphate) or Na_2SO_4 (Glauber or Carlsbad salt) and high concentrations of SO_4^{2-} in naturally occurring drinking water [272] induce osmotic diarrhea. When these substances are ingested factitiously, these diarrheas may be difficult to detect because these substances do not result in a calculated osmotic gap on stool analysis (see Evaluation of severe or elusive diarrhea).

Carbohydrate malabsorption
Sorbitol and fructose diarrhea
Carbohydrate malabsorption may be either specific or generalized (see Table 18.2). Diarrhea can result from the long-term ingestion of dietetic foods, candy, chewing gum, or medication elixirs that are sweetened with unabsorbable carbohydrates such as sorbitol (chewing gum and diarrhea elixir) [273,274]. Sorbitol and fructose are also present in pears, prunes, peaches, and apple juice [275], and excessive ingestion of these foods also results in diarrhea. Long-term ingestion of drugs that cause malabsorption of fat (discussed earlier) also causes carbohydrate malabsorption. Fructose may be malabsorbed if ingested in high concentrations, particularly if it is ingested alone and not as a component of sucrose [276,277]. Primary fructose malabsorption has also been documented secondary to defects in the GLUT 5 transport system [278]. Toddlers' diarrhea in children may be secondary to drinking large amounts of fructose-containing fruit juice [275,279], and colic in infants has been postulated to be caused by carbohydrate malabsorption [280]. Occasional adult diarrhea also appears to be related to ingestion of large volumes of fruit juice or soft drinks that are sweetened with fructose-containing corn polymers ("corn solids").

Glucose–galactose malabsorption and disaccharidase deficiencies
Congenital absence of enterocyte brush border carbohydrate hydrolases and transport proteins may cause diarrheas because of various disaccharidase deficiencies: lactase, sucrase-isomaltase, and trehalase [281]. Lactose intolerance usually presents in childhood or adolescence, but it may not be recognized in adults [282]. The high-risk groups for lactase deficiency include Asians and Native Americans (90% prevalence), African Americans, Jews, Hispanics, and southern Europeans (60%–70% prevalence). However, lactase deficiency should be considered in cases of unexplained watery diarrhea, especially if accompanied by abdominal cramps, bloating, and flatus, even in people not considered to be among the high-risk groups [283,284], because a 10%–15% prevalence of lactase deficiency can be expected in northern or western Europeans and their American descendants. A trial of a lactose-free diet, a breath hydrogen test, or a lactose absorption test may be diagnostic. Disaccharidase deficiency can occur secondary to intestinal insults such as IBD or celiac disease and can last for months [285,286]. Some patients with lactase deficiency are misdiagnosed as having IBS [284,287]. Conversely, many truly lactase-deficient patients attribute intestinal symptoms to lactose intolerance when, in fact, they can tolerate reasonable amounts of lactose and probably do have IBS [287,288]. Patients with low trehalase activity report abdominal symptoms on ingestion of mushrooms, which contain high levels of trehalose [289].

Rapid intestinal transit
As much as 50 g of a normal 200-g carbohydrate diet may be unabsorbed by the normal small intestine and passed into the colon, where it is metabolized by colonic flora [290,291]. Diets high in carbohydrate and low in fat may cause more carbohydrate malabsorption and osmotic diarrhea because the low fat content allows rapid gastric emptying and rapid small intestine motility. A primary intestinal motility abnormality in which the migrating motor complex is not disrupted by eating, resulting in a continuation of the propagative motility pattern, may be the cause of carbohydrate malabsorption and osmotic diarrhea in some children with toddlers' diarrhea [292]. Similar abnormalities of the migrating motor complex have been reported in patients with the painless diarrhea variant of IBS, and a rapid orocecal transit time has been demonstrated [293,294]. Carbohydrate wastage from rapid transit may be part of the pathophysiology of diarrhea in thyrotoxicosis [295] and ulcerative colitis [296]. Carbohydrate is metabolized to H_2 and CO_2 by colonic bacteria, which means that symptoms of excess flatus, abdominal bloating, and cramping abdominal pain may be important clues to the diagnosis of carbohydrate malabsorption.

Prior surgery

Ileostomy diarrhea

Ileostomy patients have high-volume ileostomy output immediately postoperatively, but this usually reverts to between 600 and 700 ml/24 h within 2 weeks [297]. Ileostomy diarrhea is defined as excretion of more than 1 L/24 h in patients who has not undergone extensive (> 50–100 cm) smalll bowel resection. Causes include partial small bowel obstruction, recurrent small bowel disease, bacterial overgrowth, or any routine diarrhea-producing processes (e.g., viral gastroenteritis). Treatment is much the same as conventional diarrhea – with ORS and anti-diarrheal drugs. Oral NaCl supplementation may be required [297].

Bile acid diarrhea

Three types of bile acid-induced diarrhea are proposed: type 1, which results from severe disease, resection, or bypass of the distal ileum; type 2, or primary bile acid malabsorption; and type 3, in which bile acid malabsorption follows upper abdominal surgery, either truncal vagotomy or cholecystectomy [298].

Ileal disease, resection, or bypass (e.g., because of Crohn's disease or postoperative adhesions) allows dihydroxy bile salts to escape absorption. If concentrations higher than 2 mmol are attained in the colon, intestinal secretion and diarrhea ensue [40]. Fasting prevents gallbladder contraction, and large boluses of bile do not, therefore, enter the intestine, so type 1 bile acid diarrhea commonly disappears on fasting. This form of diarrhea can be recognized by the history of previous ileal surgery or the presence of ileal disease. Bile acid diarrhea must be differentiated from fatty acid diarrhea, which occurs if ileal disease or resection involves such a large segment of ileum (> 100 cm) that hepatic synthesis cannot maintain an adequate intralumenal bile salt pool [299,300]. Under these circumstances, steatorrhea ensues, and fatty acid-induced intestinal secretion complicates the picture. It is important to differentiate these two related syndromes because bile acid diarrhea responds to bile salt binders, such as cholestyramine, but the diarrhea of fatty acid malabsorption does not and may worsen with such therapy. Therapy for fatty acid diarrhea is a low-fat diet that is supplemented with medium-chain triglycerides to prevent severe weight loss. Bile acid malabsorption has been associated with active or previous infections of the ileum [159,301], after radiation treatment [302], and with motility disturbance [303,304].

Type 2 bile acid diarrhea, or primary bile acid malabsorption, may be congenital or acquired. The acquired variety is described as a disease of excess bile acid loss that is responsive to cholestyramine, but not associated with other types of ileal dysfunction [305]. It may occur as the result of an absence of bile acid receptors or transport proteins similar to findings in congenital type 2 bile acid diarrhea [306]. Patients have been found with documented bile acid malabsorption who have [307] or do not have [308] histological abnormalities of the terminal ileum, including subtotal villus atrophy and crypt hyperplasia. Some investigators believe that this is a common cause of diarrhea-predominant IBS, and some of these patients clearly have cholestyramine-responsive diarrhea [160,161,309]. There are also well-studied patients with bile acid malabsorption and normal stool fat excretion; however, the diarrhea of these patients did not respond to cholestyramine [302,303]. This appears to be a form of idiopathic diarrhea in which bile acids are malabsorbed, but the diarrhea may not be caused by the bile acids.

Measured increases in fecal bile acids in patients with postcholecystectomy diarrhea suggest that it is one of the type 3 bile acid malabsorption syndromes [310–312]. It is unclear why interruption of gallbladder storage would lead to increased bile acid wastage. Although the diarrhea of many patients responds to cholestyramine, some does not, raising the question whether other pathophysiological mechanisms are involved.

Postvagotomy diarrhea

Truncal vagotomy combined with some type of drainage procedure was previously the most common operation for peptic ulcer disease. It is accompanied by diarrhea in 20%–30% of patients [313,314]. The incidence of diarrhea is much less after selective or superselective vagotomy, so a vagus-mediated discoordination of gastric motility, intestinal secretion, or intestinal absorption may be involved [315,316]. The idea that bile acids play an important role in the diarrhea accounts for its classification as a type of bile acid diarrhea [315]. The treatment for this condition is not always rewarding. Motility-altering drugs (opiates and anticholinergics) or cholestyramine may benefit some patients [315,317]. In addition, celiac sprue may make its first appearance after gastric surgery or vagotomy; it is a diagnosis that is treatable and should not be missed [318].

Functional watery diarrheas (irritable bowel syndrome)

Among patients defined as having IBS, a few (approximately 25%) have a predominant symptom complex of painless diarrhea [319,320]. Over the years, the size of this category of IBS becomes smaller as new conditions are discovered such as occult lactose intolerance, collagenous or microscopic/lymphocytic colitis, primary fructose malabsorption, rapid transit with carbohydrate-wasting diarrhea, primary bile acid malabsorption (type 2), food hypersensitivities, and postinfectious diarrhea-IBS. Adult celiac disease has been added to the list; it has been shown to occur in 10% of patients with IBS who meet the Rome criteria for diagnosis [232–235]. All these examples should give the clinician pause before attributing the painless diarrhea variant of IBS to any psychosocial cause, particularly in men, in whom IBS is rare in the first place. Perhaps such patients are better labeled as having idiopathic chronic diarrhea. Treatment may be symptomatic [321].

Previously, alosetron [322] proved helpful, but this medication has been withdrawn from the market for general use.

True secretory diarrheas

Endocrine tumor diarrheas
Carcinoid syndrome
Patients with metastatic carcinoid tumors of the gastrointestinal tract or, rarely, primary nonmetastatic carcinoid tumors of the bronchial epithelium, may experience a syndrome that includes the following: watery diarrhea; cramping abdominal pain with borborygmus; episodic flushing; skin changes including telangiectasia, cyanosis, and pellagra-like skin lesions; bronchospasm with asthma attacks and dyspnea; and cardiac murmurs, usually related to right-sided valvular lesions [323–325]. The symptoms are caused by secretion of 5-HT, histamine, catecholamines, kinins, prostaglandin, and tachykinins (e.g., substance P) by the tumor mass. All these agents, excluding catecholamines, are potent intestinal secretagogues. Up to one-third of these patients do not report flushing episodes, and the pellagra-like skin changes and heart murmurs may take some time to develop to clinical appearance. Therefore, this disease should be considered in patients with secretory diarrhea, even if the patient does not have the classic history or physical examination findings.

Gastrinoma
Zollinger–Ellison syndrome develops from sporadic, gastric-producing tumors, except in about 20% of cases, when it is part of multiple endocrine neoplasia syndrome 1 (MEN1) [326]. Although 70%–90% of patients with Zollinger–Ellison syndrome present with pain and develop peptic ulcers at some time during the course of their disease, diarrhea also occurs in 25%–75% of patients and may precede the ulcer symptoms [326]. Furthermore, in 10% of patients, diarrhea may be the major pathophysiological manifestation of the disease. The diarrhea is not strictly an intestinal secretory diarrhea [327]. It is caused in part by high volumes of hydrochloric acid (HCl) secretion, and it can be reduced by nasogastric aspiration or effective antisecretory therapy [328]. Maldigestion of fat as a result of inactivation of pancreatic lipase and precipitation of bile acids because of the low pH may also play a role. Zollinger–Ellison syndrome is the most common of the neuroendocrine tumors and it must be definitively ruled out as a cause of secretory diarrhea. Rarely, this syndrome can develop from non-small cell lung cancer [329] or ovarian mucinous cystadenomas [330].

VIPoma or watery diarrhea–hypokalemia–achlorhydria syndrome
Non-β-cell pancreatic adenomas (pancreatic endocrine tumors) secrete a host of peptides, including VIP, pancreatic polypeptide, peptide histidine isoleucine, and occasionally secretin, gastrin inhibitory polypeptide, neurotensin, calcitonin, and prostaglandins [331,332]. Of these, only VIP has been found to be elevated in virtually all patients with watery diarrhea–hypokalemia–achlorhydria (WDHA) syndrome. Infusions of this hormone can produce all the symptoms and it seems likely that VIP is the primary mediator of this syndrome. VIPoma may therefore be a reasonable and perhaps a more descriptive name than pancreatic cholera or WDHA syndrome.

Patients with this tumor have secretory diarrhea, with 70% of patients having more than 3 L of stool per day and virtually all having more than 700 mL/day. Diarrhea with 10–20 L of stool per 24 h has been reported. With high levels of circulating VIP, all segments of the intestine may secrete Na^+, K^+, Cl^-, and HCO_3^-, as well as water, thus accounting for the dehydration, hypokalemia, and acidosis that may accompany this disease [333,334]. Abdominal pain is not an important symptom of this disease. Patients exhibit flushing (20%) and hypercalcemia (without hyperparathyroidism) occurs in more than 70% of patients, probably caused by the release by tumor of neuroendocrine products. Other features of the syndrome include achlorhydria, hypokalemia, hypomagnesemia, enlarged gallbladder, hypokalemic myopathy or nephropathy, hyperglycemia, and lacrimal gland hypersecretion (tearing).

In the pediatric age group, VIPomas may present as neural crest (sympathetic chain) tumors – ganglioneuromas, neuroblastomas, neurofibromas, and pheochromocytomas. Some of these tumors secrete VIP and produce secretory diarrheas that resolve after the tumor is removed [335,336].

A rare patient has pancreatic islet tumors and watery diarrhea with normal VIP levels, suggesting that some other peptide, such as pancreatic polypeptide, neurotensin, calcitonin, or prostaglandins, may cause the intestinal secretion [335].

Medullary carcinoma of the thyroid
This cancer may present in sporadic form or, in 25%–50% of patients, as part of multiple endocrine neoplasia syndrome 2 (MEN2) with pheochromocytomas and hyperparathyroidism [337,338]. MEN2 is caused by activation of the cellular oncogene *RET*, and mutations of this gene are found in a subset of patients with sporadic medullary carcinoma [339]. Watery (secretory) diarrhea is a prominent part of the syndrome. The diarrhea is thought to be caused by the secretion of calcitonin by the tumor; however, these tumors also elaborate other secretagogues, such as prostaglandins, VIP, substance P, and sometimes 5-HT or kallikrein [340]. Although studies in some patients have shown small intestine secretion [340], others have shown severely shortened colonic transit times [341]. Therefore, the pathophysiology in this disease may not always be a straightforward secretory one. Usually, by the time watery diarrhea occurs (30% of cases), it indicates metastasis with poor prognosis.

Glucagonoma

Patients with glucagon-secreting pancreatic islet tumors present with diabetes (90%), a form of eczematous skin rash called migratory necrolytic erythema, and, occasionally, glossitis, cheilitis, mild diarrhea (25%), psychiatric or neurological aberrations, and thromboembolic propensities [342]. The cause of the diarrhea in these patients is unclear.

Nonendocrine malignant diseases
Villous adenomas

Villous adenomas of the rectum or rectosigmoid may cause a secretory form of diarrhea with K^+ loss [343–345]. Diarrhea in the range of 500–3000 mL/24 h has been recorded. Tumors that are capable of causing such secretory diarrhea are usually large – more than 3 to 4 cm in diameter and often as large as 10–12 cm [345]. Although the cause of the secretion may be intrinsic to the nature of this neoplastic epithelium, secretagogues such as prostaglandins have been found in both the tumor and rectal effluent of such patients [346–348], and indomethacin administration reduces the diarrhea in some patients [347–349].

Systemic mastocytosis

If mast cell proliferation is limited to the skin, it is termed *urticaria pigmentosa* [228]. If it involves the bones, liver, spleen, lymph nodes, and gastrointestinal tract, it is known as *systemic mastocytosis*. The diarrhea of systemic mastocytosis may be continuous and accompanied by steatorrhea secondary to infiltration of the mucosa and the resulting villus atrophy [228,229]. However, the diarrhea may be intermittent and may be associated with flushing, tachycardia, hypotension, and, occasionally, headache, cognitive disorders, nausea and vomiting, peptic ulcers, syncope, itching, and urticaria, which may be provoked by alcohol ingestion [228]. In this form of the syndrome, histamine or another mast cell mediators such as prostaglandin D_2 may be the secretagogue responsible, by either stimulating gastric acid secretion (much as occurs in Zollinger–Ellison syndrome) or having a secretory effect on the intestine. Antihistaminics (H_1 blockers), H_2 blockers or proton pump inhibitors, cyclooxygenase inhibitors, and disodium cromoglycate may be helpful in treatment [228,229,350]. Blockade of mast cell mediator receptor or of mast cell degranulation may reduce all these symptoms and the diarrhea, but not the steatorrhea, which may be better treated with corticosteroids [228, 229, 350] .

Factitious diarrhea

Approximately 15% of patients referred to secondary or tertiary centers for diarrhea [351] and 25% of patients with proven secretory diarrheas [352–357] are found to be surreptitiously ingesting either laxatives or diuretics. These patients present with severe chronic watery diarrhea, often with abdominal pain, weight loss, nausea, and vomiting, sometimes with hypokalemic myopathy and acidosis. Occa-

sionally, they have severe protein-losing enteropathy as well. They have 10–20 bowel movements per day, with 24-h stool volumes in the range of 300 to 3000 mL, and may have nocturnal diarrhea as well. The most common drug causing this syndrome in the United States is probably bisacodyl [358]. Anthraquinones, which include senna, cascara, aloe, rhubarb, frangula, and danthron, are other abused laxatives [357–359]. Osmotic laxatives such as Na_2SO_4, Na_2PO_4, $MgSO_4$, and magnesium citrate are occasionally used [356, 357]. There is no readily available assay for dioctyl sodium sulfosuccinate (the docusate salts), one of the more common laxatives, so its frequency of use in this syndrome is uncertain. Some patients ingest large quantities of diuretics.

More than 90% of these patients are women. It is unclear why they ingest these drugs to the point of requiring hospitalization. There appear to be two different clinical syndromes [354,360]:
- women younger than 30 years of age in whom some elements of eating disorders (e.g., anorexia nervosa and bulimia) appear to be part of the psychic abnormality
- middle-aged to elderly women with histories of extensive medical care who seem to gain some kind of secondary benefit from the sick role and the attendant personal attention.

Many of these latter patients are health-care workers, such as nurses' aides, and this is particularly true among the few men who present with this syndrome. On confrontation, patients may either deny the drug ingestion and leave the physician's care or admit the aberrant behavior and submit to psychiatric care. After laxatives are discontinued, these patients develop edema as a result of secondary hyperaldosteronism or pseudo-Bartter syndrome [361], but it subsides spontaneously within 1–2 months if left untreated. Another complication of chronic laxative abuse is the development of ammonium urate renal calculi, presumably secondary also to the dehydration and acidosis of severe diarrhea [362].

This syndrome also exists in pediatrics, where it has been called *Munchausen syndrome by proxy* or *Polle syndrome* [363, 364]. (Polle was Baron von Munchausen's son, who died at an early age of unknown causes.) In these circumstances, it is a form of child abuse in which the guilty parent, usually the mother, again derives some kind of secondary gain from the extensive hospitalizations and evaluations of the child. The frequency of this factitious disorder as a cause of severe diarrhea is high enough to warrant laxative screening to rule out this syndrome before initiating extensive medical evaluation for the other causes of diarrhea.

Chronic idiopathic diarrhea and pseudopancreatic cholera syndrome

Patients in whom extensive evaluation for a cause of secretory diarrhea is negative, including a search for hormone-secreting tumors and laxative and drug ingestion, are said to have either *chronic idiopathic diarrhea* or *pseudopancreatic cholera syndrome*, depending on whether the fasting stool volumes are less than or greater than 700 mL/24 h, respectively [365,366]. Some of the patients with this syndrome are found to have microscopic/lymphocytic colitis, Brainerd diarrhea, or a type 2 bile acid diarrhea variant. Others could be ingesting laxatives or drugs for which assays are not readily available. These cases defy diagnosis, and, importantly, these patients outnumber those with neuroendocrine secretory tumors. If no diagnosis is revealed, symptomatic therapy with bile salt-binding drugs, opiates, or anticholinergic medications may be tried. Follow-up studies suggest that in most of these patients, the diarrhea is self-limiting and disappears spontaneously in 6–24 months [366]. One current hypothesis is that these patients may be suffering from severe, postinfectious IBS, that is, Brainerd diarrhea (see Prolonged infectious diarrheas).

Diabetic diarrhea

The most common gastrointestinal symptom in patients with diabetes of either type is constipation (25% of patients) and not diarrhea (2.5%–3.7%) [367,368]. Nevertheless, up to 20% of young to middle-aged people with type 1 diabetes that has been poorly controlled for more than 5 years (particularly men between 20 and 40 years of age), may have profuse watery, urgent diarrhea, often occurring at night with incontinence [369,370]. These patients usually have severe neuropathy and often have both nephropathy and retinopathy. Some patients have exocrine pancreatic insufficiency or bacterial overgrowth secondary to the motility disturbances of the autonomic neuropathy. Patients with type 1 diabetes may have concomitant celiac disease [235,238], so the single most important test in these patients, at least in terms of diagnosing a potentially treatable disease, is celiac disease serology. The most common cause of "diabetic" diarrhea in those with type 2 diabetes is therapy with metformin [367].

Unfortunately, most diabetic patients with severe diarrhea do not have a treatable cause, and the cause of their diarrheal condition is unknown. Animal studies suggest that diabetes induces specific sympathetic denervation of the bowel [371, 372]. This leaves unopposed cholinergic tone, which impairs fluid and electrolyte absorption or actually stimulates frank intestinal secretion. It is on this basis that clonidine, a specific α_2-adrenergic agent, has been recommended as a treatment for diabetic diarrhea [373]. Diarrhea may improve when patients take this drug, although it is uncertain whether this response is the result of the nonspecific antisecretory effect of α_2-adrenergic agents or whether the response confirms the proposed sympathic denervation. These patients with neuropathy frequently have impaired anal sphincter function, and this contributes to their incontinence [367,374]. Octreotide therapy may be helpful [375].

Alcoholic diarrhea

Binge drinking of alcohol causes a brief episode of diarrhea that usually lasts less than 1 day. This may result from acute damage to both the microvasculature and the epithelium [376–378] and is accompanied by alterations in water, electrolyte, and nutrient absorption [379].

Patients with chronic alcoholism often have severe watery diarrhea that persists for days or even weeks after hospitalization. Physiological abnormalities described in patients with alcoholism include more rapid oral–cecal and colonic transit [380,381], decreased intestinal disaccharidases, decreased bile secretion (particularly in those with cirrhosis), and decreased pancreatic secretion [360]. Folate or vitamin B-12 deficiency or protein malnourishment also may play a role. With abstinence, renourishment, and replenishment of vitamin deficiencies, most patients' diarrhea slowly improves.

Congenital and neonatal diarrheas

Several causes of congenital diarrhea have been documented: a congenital short bowel syndrome [382]; a primary form of ileal dysfunction with bile acid malabsorption, also called *familial microvillus atrophy* [306,307,383]; congenital insulin-dependent diabetes mellitus with secretory diarrhea [384]; congenital chloridorrhea [385–387]; congenital sodium diarrhea [388–390]; microvillus inclusion disease [391, 392]; congenital enterocyte heparan sulfate deficiency [393]; "tufting" enteropathy and epithelial dysplasia [394]; mitochondrial encephalomyelopathies with diarrhea, IPEX syndrome IPEX [226,395]; Satoyoshi syndrome [396], cholecystokinin deficit of type 1 autoimmune polyglandular syndrome [397], and mutant neurogenin-3 congenital malabsorptive diarrhea [398]. A perspective of these diarrheas has been reported by Binder [399].

Inflammatory diarrheas

Inflammatory bowel disease

Patients with either Crohn's disease of the small or large intestine or ulcerative colitis have diarrhea with stool volumes usually less than 1 L/24 h that frequently, but not always, improve with fasting. Decreased Na^+, Cl^-, and water absorption or frank secretion can be demonstrated in both the small intestine and colon of patients with IBD [28,29,46,400]. Patients with severe ulcerative colitis may have water and electrolyte secretion in the unaffected small intestine, suggesting the presence of circulating secretagogues [400]. The abnormalities of transport are caused by inflammatory mediators, such as histamine, prostaglandins, leukotrienes, and cytokines (interleukins) such as TNF-α, IL-1, and interferon-γ, which are released from mast cells, phagocytes, T cells, and mesenchymal cells (see Pathophysiology of inflammatory diarrheas). The abnormalities of electrolyte transport brought about by these secretagogues are further enhanced by a damaged absorptive surface epithelium and even denuded mucosa with leakage of plasma or blood into the lumen. Effective treatment of IBD with salicylates, steroids, antibiotics, antiinflammatory drugs, and immune-mediating drugs such as anti-TNF-α antibodies, is accompanied by reductions in the levels of inflammatory mediators, improved histology, and reduction in diarrhea [401].

Eosinophilic gastroenteritis

Infiltration of the gastrointestinal tract of either adults or children with eosinophils is a recognized clinical entity that is accompanied by diarrhea [402–404]. Diarrhea occurs in 30%–60% of patients with eosinophilic enteritis regardless of whether the eosinophils are infiltrating the mucosa, the muscle, or the serosal layers of the gut [404]. Peripheral eosinophilia is present in 75% of these patients. The disease may involve the entire gastrointestinal tract from esophagus to anus, or it may be isolated to the colon. Abdominal pain, nausea, vomiting, and weight loss are other prominent symptoms of this disease. Steatorrhea and protein-losing enteropathy are present in 10%–30% of these patients. A few patients with peripheral eosinophilia, but no evidence of gastrointestinal infiltration, appear to have symptoms similar to those with gastrointestinal involvement [404]. The cause of this disease is unknown, but approximately 50% of patients have atopic (allergic) histories. Food allergy is suspected in these patients, but elimination diets are only occasionally successful [403]. Parasites, particularly *Strongyloides* [405], and other causes of eosinophilia [406] should be rigorously ruled out before making a diagnosis of eosinophilic gastroenteritis. Steroids remain the mainstay of therapy [402–404]. Sodium cromoglycate may be useful [407].

Milk and soy protein allergy

Intolerance to cows' milk and soy protein is a well-established cause of enterocolitis in infants [408,409]. The disease involves both the small intestine and the colon and may present within the first 6 months of life with either acute or gradual onset of vomiting and diarrhea, occasionally with bloody stools caused by ulcerative proctocolitis. Approximately 50% of the patients who are allergic to one of these proteins are also allergic to the other. In older children, milk allergy can present with constipation [410].

Food allergy

Dietary hypersensitivity is clearly recognized in infants and adults (see earlier), and systemic anaphylaxis has long been recognized in association with peanuts and seafood ingestion [411]. Diarrhea, constipation, and gastroesophageal reflux as a result of food allergy are increasingly recognized [412,413]. Commonly suspected allergens include milk, eggs, seafood, nuts, artificial flavors, and food coloring [412,413].

Microscopic colitides

Collagenous colitis and *lymphocytic colitis* are two reasonably common diarrheal diseases grouped together as atypical or microscopic colitides [414–420]. The diagnosis may be made in 10%–20% of patients studied for non-bloody, chronic watery diarrhea [419]. Microscopic or lymphocytic colitis seems to be equally prevalent in men and women, whereas collagenous colitis occurs 7 to 10 times more often in middle-aged or elderly women. These diseases are categorized as either inflammatory diarrheas, because abdominal pain, weight loss, and intraepithelial lymphocytes and lamina propria lymphocytes are prominent [417–420], or as secretory diarrheas, because intestinal secretion is present in the disease [421]. In many cases, the secretory process is mild, and diarrhea stool volumes may return to normal with fasting, whereas patients with more severe diarrhea continue to have elevated stool volumes on fasting. It is clear that many patients (perhaps 15%) with lymphocytic colitis have celiac sprue [422]. Increased lumenal prostaglandin levels suggest that this inflammatory mediator is being released by the subepithelial immune cells and is causing the diarrhea in this disease [421]. An epidemiological relationship with long-term NSAIDs, lansoprazole, acarbose, sertraline and other drugs has been reported [416–420]. In addition to gluten sensitivity, bile has been proposed as the trigger for such prostaglandin release. Sensitivity to drugs or bile may be the reason that symptoms disappear with fecal stream diversion [423]. Bismuth subsalicylate, cholestyramine, prednisone, 5-aminosalicylates, and immunosuppressants have been successful therapies, but budesonide is the best-documented efficacious therapy [416–420].

Chronic watery diarrhea also occurs in patients whose small intestine and colonic biopsies reveal microscopic eosinophilic infiltration in the crypt region with a normal surface or villous epithelium. Such patients have been labeled as having *pericrypt eosinophilic enterocolitis* [424]. Fifty percent of these patients have a collagen-vascular disease. The diarrhea responds well to corticosteroids.

Protein-losing enteropathy

Severe protein loss through the gastrointestinal tract occurs in a variety of disease states [425–428]:
- Infection – *C. difficile* infection, *Salmonella* infection, enterocolitis, shigellosis, viral gastroenteritis, parasite infestation, bacterial overgrowth, Whipple disease
- Diseases with mucosal erosion or ulcerations – gastritis, gastric cancer, collagenous colitis, IBD
- Diseases marked by lymphatic obstruction – congenital and possibly primary intestinal lymphangiectasia, sarcoidosis, lymphoma, mesenteric tuberculosis, as a sequela of surgical correction of congenital heart disease with Fontan operation, long-term peritoneal dialysis
- Mucosal diseases without ulceration – Ménétrier disease, sprue, eosinophilic gastroenteritis, amyloidosis
- Immune diseases – systemic lupus erythematosus or food allergies, primarily to milk

The condition may respond to octreotide, corticosteroids, or other antiimmune therapy. The epidermal growth factor receptor antibody cetuximab is particularly effective in Ménétrier disease [428].

Chronic radiation enterocolitis

Although acute radiation diarrhea is common (see "Nosocomial diarrheas, Cancer treatment"), patients receiving pelvic radiation for malignant diseases of the female urogenital tract or the male prostate may develop chronic radiation enterocolitis 6 to 12 months after total doses of radiation greater than 4 to 6 Gy. The terminal ileum, cecum, and rectosigmoid are the segments usually involved because they are fixed in the pelvis and therefore may receive the full brunt of the weekly radiation dosages. The histology is one of obliterative arteritis, occasionally with lymphangiectasia, partial villus atrophy, fibrosis, and strictures. With time, severely bleeding rectal telangiectasias develop in many patients. The diarrhea may be caused by bile acid malabsorption if the ileum is involved, by bacterial overgrowth if small intestine strictures occur, or by chronic inflammation of the small intestine and colon [429]. Antiinflammatory drugs such as sulfasalazine and corticosteroids have been tried with little success; occasionally, cholestyramine and NSAIDs may help, as may opiate antidiarrheal medications. The bleeding rectal telangiectasia may respond to electrocoagulation, laser ablation, or intrarectal formalin [430].

Miscellaneous diseases

Although *acute mesenteric arterial* or *venous thrombosis* presents as acute bloody diarrhea, *chronic mesenteric vascular ischemia* may present as watery diarrhea with spotty endoscopic inflammation [431] that can be mistaken for a symptom of IBD. Chronic infections, including gastrointestinal *tuberculosis* [432] and *histoplasmosis* [433], present with diarrhea that may either be bloody or have characteristics of a secretory process. Immunological diseases such as *Behçet disease* [434] may have diarrhea as a symptom. There seems to be geographic heterogeneity among these patients, with those in Japan having more gastrointestinal involvement than those in Turkey or Israel [435]. *Churg–Strauss syndrome* may present with diarrhea [436]. Diarrhea is the hallmark of acute *graft vs host disease* after allogeneic bone marrow transplantation [437]. The triad of dermatitis, hepatic cholestasis, and enteritis with diarrhea define this disease, and the volume of diarrhea has even been proposed as part of clinical staging. *Neutropenic enterocolitis* is ileocolitis occurring in neutropenic patients with leukemia. Some cases of this may be caused by *C. difficile* infection [189,438]. The *Cronkhite–Canada syndrome*, usually listed under the polyposes because of the characteristic retention (inflammatory) polyps, has most of the hallmarks of an immune disorder, and severe gastrointestinal protein loss and diarrhea are present [439,440]. Long-term NSAID use can lead to colonic ulcers (*NSAID colitis*) with diarrhea or right-sided colonic weblike strictures (*diaphragm disease*) [441]. Multiple myeloma can involve the stomach,

small bowel or colon as discrete plasmocytosis or as diffuse myelomatosis with diarrhea [442].

Clinical evaluation of chronic diarrhea

The goal of the gastroenterologist in evaluating a patient with chronic diarrhea is to make a definitive diagnosis as quickly and inexpensively as possible. This section outlines an approach to diagnosis of adult patients; the diagnostic approach in infants and children may be different [222,443]. Experienced clinicians [198–201,444–449] suggest that 75%–80% of cases of chronic diarrheas can be diagnosed by an expert history and physical examination, coupled with certain screening and focused laboratory examinations (Fig. 18.6). This expert opinion is backed by clinical studies [450,451]. The remaining 25% of patients with severe or elusive diarrhea may need hospitalization and extensive testing. Three tests – quantitative stool fat, colonoscopy with biopsy, and the response to fasting with measurement of stool volume and osmotic gap – lead to a definitive diagnosis in most of these remaining patients [445–449].

Malabsorption

History and physical examination

The causes of generalized malabsorption are outlined in Table 18.2, and the signs and symptoms in Tables 18.11 to 18.13 [444,452,453]. The approach to evaluation is shown in Fig. 18.7. Mild degrees of malabsorption may be entirely asymptomatic and may not result in the classic gastrointestinal manifestations of flatulence, bulky or greasy foul-smelling stools, and weight loss. For these reasons, malabsorption sometimes presents as an aberration of one of the other body systems (see Tables 18.11 and 18.12).

Clues that help differentiate clinically severe mucosal disease, such as celiac sprue or Whipple disease, from the malabsorption caused by exocrine pancreatic insufficiency are the presence of cytokine-induced anorexia, lethargy, and malaise as well as extraintestinal signs and symptoms in patients with intestinal mucosal disease. Severe abdominal pain from repeated bouts of pancreatitis and history of chronic alcoholism may be useful clues to pancreatic insufficiency. The character of the stool may be a useful differentiating symptom. The fat content of the stool in pancreatic insufficiency is considerably higher than in mucosal disease (see Table 18.12) [454]. At body temperature, the fat may be present as oil, and the oil may separate from the stool, manifesting as oily seepage from the anus or as oil droplets floating in the toilet bowl after passage of the steatorrheic stool. Patients with pancreatic insufficiency rarely have flatulence and bloating, perhaps because salivary or gastric amylase ameliorates somewhat the carbohydrate malabsorption. Stools tend to float and are difficult to flush in malabsorptive diseases because of the gas content, which is caused by carbohydrate malabsorption and

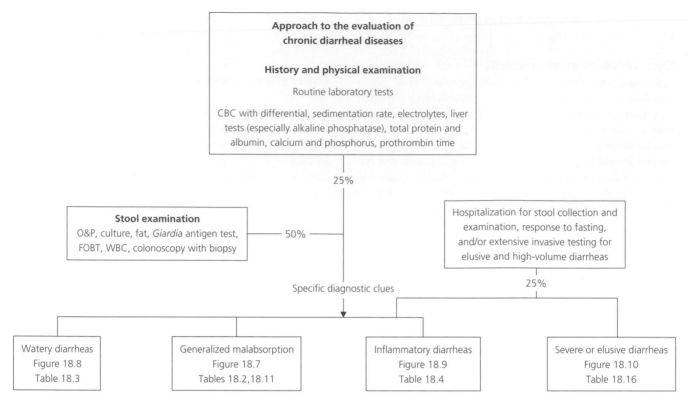

Figure 18.6 Approach to the evaluation of chronic diarrheal disease. CBC, complete blood count; FOBT, fetal occult blood test; O&P, ova and parasite examination; WBC, white blood cell count.

subsequent fermentation and gas formation, and not the fat malabsorption [455]. Total serum protein concentrations are usually lower in intestinal mucosal diseases, most likely because of a chronic disease state and concomitant protein-losing enteropathy, and anemia is more common because of both iron and folate malabsorption.

The association of certain diseases or syndromes with sub-clinical celiac disease (see Table 18.10 and section on celiac sprue) provides a list of conditions for which there should be a low threshold for screening for celiac disease.

Screening tests for malabsorption
Blood tests

Tests that may yield important clues to the presence of significant malabsorption include a complete blood count, prothrombin time, serum protein determination, and alkaline phosphatase (see Table 18.11). These may signal the presence of iron, folate, vitamin B-12, vitamin K, or severe vitamin D malabsorption with osteomalacia. Serum carotene, cholesterol, albumin, serum iron, folate, and vitamin B-12 determinations give additional clues to the presence of malabsorption, and these usually point to intestinal mucosal disease. Serum carotene may be low simply from poor intake, but not usually less than 50 μg/dL, as is commonly seen in severe malabsorption.

Serological tests for celiac disease

Patients suspected of having celiac disease, either because of signs and symptoms of malabsorption or resulting malnutrition, family history, or because of concomitant diseases in which there is a high incidence of celiac disease (see Table 18.10), should be screened with serological tests for celiac disease. IgA tests are highly sensitive (90%) and specific (90%–95%) [231–238]. Enzyme-linked immunosorbent assays for antitissue transglutaminase IgA antibodies using human tissue transglutaminase is considered the best single serological test, with sensitivities and specificities of 95%–100%. It will not diagnose the disease in patients who are IgA-deficient, a not uncommon associated condition in those with celiac disease, so measurements of serum IgA concomitant with serologies is recommended. If IgA levels are low in a given patient, serologies should be repeated testing for IgG antibodies. Screening with anti-endomysial or anti-tissue transglutaminase antibodies alone can underestimate celiac disease, so a panel of anti-IgA and anti-IgG antibodies and even human leukocyte antigen (HLA) typing may be necessary to sort out difficult cases.

Radiography (malabsorption)

Radiology should be viewed as an adjunct to the diagnosis of malabsorption and not as a primary test. A flat plate of the

Table 18.11 Correlation of clinical manifestions, pathophysiology, and laboratory findings in malabsorptive processes

Signs and symptoms	Pathophysiological mechanism	Laboratory abnormalities
Gastrointestinal		
Diarrhea	Malabsorption of fat, carbohydrate, and protein; increased secretion caused by crypt hyperplasia, inflammatory mediators, bile and fatty acids	Stool weight > 200 g; stool weight decreased to normal with fast; stool osmotic gap > 100 mOsm/kg H_2O, [Na] > 60 mmol/L
Weight loss	Nutrient malabsorption, anorexia in mucosal diseases	Increased stool fat, decreased serum proteins
Flatulence, borborygmus, abdominal distention, foul-smelling stools	Bacterial fermentation of malabsorbed carbohydrates and proteins	Increased flatus production
Bulky, greasy stools	Fat malabsorption	Increased stool fat > 7 g/24 h, low serum carotene
Abdominal pain	If severe, from chronic pancreatitis; if mild, distention of bowel and inflammation	
Hematopoietic		
Anemia	Iron, pyridoxine, folate, and vitamin B-12 deficiency	Microcytic, macrocytic, or dimorphic anemia
Hemorrhagic diathesis	Vitamin K deficiency	Prolonged prothrombin time
Musculoskeletal		
Bone pain (osteopenic bone disease)	Calcium, vitamin D, and protein malabsorption	Hypocalcemia, hypophosphatemia, increased serum alkaline phosphatase
Tetany	Calcium, magnesium, vitamin D malabsorption	As for bone pain plus hypomagnesemia
Endocrine		
Amenorrhea, infertility, impotence	Malabsorption with protein-calorie malnutrition	Low serum proteins; may have abnormalities in gonadotropin secretion
Secondary hyperparathyroidism	Probably vitamin D and calcium deficiency	Increased alkaline phosphatase, increased serum parathyroid hormone
Skin and mucous membranes		
Cheilosis, glossitis, stomatitis,	Iron, riboflavin, niacin, folate, and vitamin B-12 deficiency	Low serum iron, folate, vitamin B-12
Purpura	Vitamin K deficiency	Prolonged prothrombin time
Follicular hyperkeratosis	Vitamin A deficiency	Low serum carotene
Scaly dermatitis or acrodermatitis	Zinc and essential fatty acid deficiency	Low serum or urinary zinc
Hyperpigmented dermatitis	Niacin deficiency	
Edema and/or ascites	Protein malabsorption	Low serum albumin
Nervous system		
Xerophthalmia and night blindness	Vitamin A deficiency	Decreased serum carotene
Peripheral neuropathy	Vitamin B, thiamine deficiency	Decreased serum vitamin B-12

Adapted from Trier [452].

abdomen may demonstrate pancreatic calcification. Pancreatic ultrasound, computed tomography, and magnetic resonance cholangiopancreatography can be used if necessary to confirm the presence of pancreatic disease as a cause of malabsorption.

Small intestine disease also can be revealed with lower sensitivity by barium contrast radiographs or by ultrasound [456,457]. Previous gastric surgery, gastrocolic fistulae, blind loops from previous intestinal anastomoses, small intestine

Table 18.12 Comparison of laboratory results in the three types of malabsorption: mucosal disease, impaired intralumenal digestion, and postmucosal or lymphatic obstruction

Test	Mucosal disease	Impaired lumenal digestion		Lymphatic obstruction
		Pancreatic disease	Bacterial overgrowth	
Stool fat	Elevated	Very elevated	Slightly elevated	Elevated
Intestinal biopsy	Abnormal	Normal	Mildly abnormal	Usually abnormal
Screening (blood) tests of malabsorption				
Prothrombin time	May be increased	May be increased	May be increased	May be increased
Serum carotene	Decreased	Decreased	May be decreased	Decreased
Serum cholesterol	Decreased	Decreased	Decreased	Decreased
Serum albumin	Decreased	Normal	May be decreased	Decreased
Serum iron	Decreased	Normal	Normal	Normal
Serum folate	Decreased	Normal	Normal	Normal
Serum vitamin B-12	Normal	Normal	May be decreased	Normal
Specific malabsorption tests				
^{14}C-Triolein breath test	Decreased	Decreased	Decreased	Decreased
D-Xylose absorption	Decreased	Normal	May be decreased	Normal
Schilling test	Normal	Decreased	Decreased	Normal
Breath tests (H$_2$, ^{14}C-xylose, or ^{14}C-cholylglycine)	Normal or abnormal	Normal	Abnormal	Normal
Bentiromide test	Normal or decreased	Normal or decreased		Normal

Adapted from Trier [452].

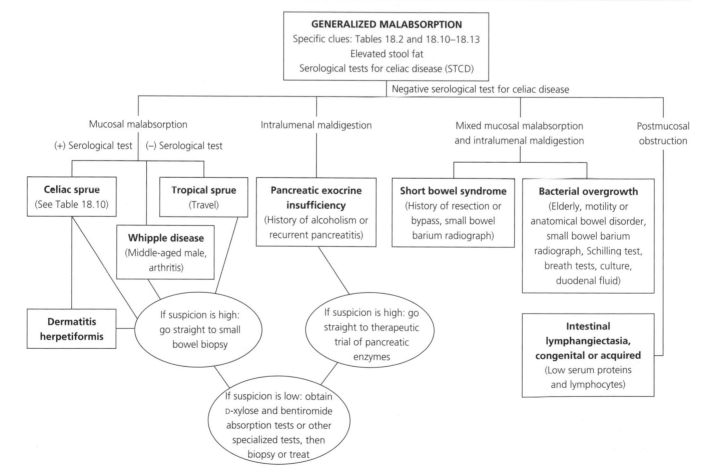

Figure 18.7 Approach to the evaluation of malabsorption.

strictures, multiple jejunal diverticula, and abnormal intestinal motility that could lead to bacterial overgrowth may be demonstrated with higher sensitivity. Certain diseases may present radiographically as uniform thickening of the valvulae conniventes (e.g., amyloidosis, lymphoma, Whipple disease); uniform or patchy diseases such as lymphoma or lymphangiectasia also may be seen. Patients with sprue show fluid-filled loops and dilation of the small intestine with little mucosal abnormality. Segmentation of the barium column also occurs in sprue or in any of the malabsorptive or severe secretory diarrheas if there is sufficient intralumenal fluid to cause precipitation or flocculation of the barium.

Upper gastrointestinal endoscopy and biopsy

Upper gastrointestinal endoscopy with distal duodenal biopsy should be undertaken if diagnostic clues or positive celiac disease serology suggest small bowel mucosal malabsorption, especially in patients with proven steatorrhea (see "Celiac sprue"). Even a negative biopsy result can be helpful if it redirects the clinician to the pancreas. Videocapsule endoscopy has high sensitivity (90%–95%), but low specificity (64%) for small bowel mucosal evaluation [458,459].

Endoscopic appearance

The presence of scalloping or a reduced number of duodenal folds or the presence of a mosaic pattern or nodularity has a positive predictive value in the 95%–100% range for celiac disease in adults [460] and children [461]. However, other diseases may have similar appearances: eosinophilic enteritis, tropical sprue, giardiasis, human immunodeficiency virus-related enteropathy, graft-vs-host disease, and amyloidosis [462–464]. The addition of magnification endoscopy and chromoendoscopy may be useful in the diagnosis of villous atrophy [465,466]. Push enteroscopy may be useful in the evaluation of refractory sprue [465,467], but it does not add much to the evaluation of routine malabsorption [465, 468].

Duodenal histology

When history, physical examination, and screening tests (especially serological tests for celiac disease) strongly suggest malabsorption, and certainly when steatorrhea is documented, small intestine biopsy is probably the most cost-effective way to determine whether the steatorrhea is caused by an intestinal source. Endoscopic grasp biopsies are usually as good as small bowel biopsy instruments, such as the Rubin–Quentin multipurpose tube, the Crosby–Kugler capsule, or the Watson or Carey capsule for distal duodenal biopsy [469]. The capsule technique is still used in infants because of its safety and the ease of passing it orally in the suckling child [470–472].

There are few diseases in which small bowel biopsy is absolutely diagnostic (Table 18.13) [473,474]. Diseases that have a patchy distribution within the gastrointestinal tract may be missed on small bowel biopsies. Our newer

understanding of celiac disease as a mild, occult, or latent disease requires new histological rigor for diagnosis of this disease [474,475]. The presence, location, and number of intraepithelial lymphocytes are becoming important criteria for the diagnosis of subtle celiac disease, although intraepithelial lymphocytes are also seen in other immune-mediated diseases (e.g., tropical sprue, food allergy, autoimmune enteropathy) [473–476]. Miscellaneous lesions not included in Table 18.13 that may be discovered with small bowel biopsy include benign lymphoid hyperplasia, milk or soy protein hypersensitivity, lipid storage diseases such as Fabry or Niemann–Pick disease, histoplasmosis, capillariasis, cytomegalovirus enteritis, schistosomiasis, and Waldenström macroglobulinemia [473–479].

Stool tests for malabsorption
Collection and appearance

Early examination of stools for ova and parasites and a *Giardia* antigen test should be considered before beginning 24-h stool collections or obtaining barium radiographs, although this is not always cost effective. The presence of barium interferes with the ability to find ova or parasites, even 1 to 3 weeks after the procedure.

Outpatient qualitative tests on single stool collections and quantitative tests, usually requiring hospitalization and 48-h to 72-h stool collections, can be useful in defining the cause of diarrhea. Stool can be collected in the outpatient area for analysis. The patient can be given preweighed paint cans and toilet bowl inserts to facilitate separation of stool from urine. The stool is transferred from the insert to the can and kept cold in an inexpensive Styrofoam ice chest containing dry ice or one of the refreezable "blue-ice" packs. Collections are made for 48 h, or better still, for 72 h.

An important adjunct to diagnosing the cause of diarrhea is to look at the stool. The bloody stool of gut inflammation is not easily confused with watery diarrhea. However, the diagnosis of watery diarrhea to the exclusion of steatorrhea can be made with only 80%–95% accuracy [480]. Patients with steatorrhea sometimes have watery diarrhea, so stool appearance and weight can be misleading [480, 481] and it is usually wise to measure stool fat.

Qualitative fecal fat tests

The usual intake of fat in the typical North American diet is 100–150 g/24 h, mostly as triglycerides. Previously, it was thought that 93%–97% of this fat was absorbed and that this percentage capability extended up to an intake of 200 g/24 h [482]. This relationship was recognized not to hold for neonates, whose stool fat may normally exceed 10% of intake [11]. It is clear that the normal coefficient of absorption of dietary triglycerides is 99%, but for phospholipid of endogenous sources (e.g., bile, sloughed enterocytes, bacteria), it is only about 90%. Therefore, 5–6 g of normal fecal fat consists of unabsorbed phospholipid from the 40-g to

Table 18.13 Diagnostic reliability of peroral small intestine biopsy

Diagnostic histology; diffuse lesions; should be present on endoscopic biopsy	
Whipple disease	Periodic acid–Schiff-positive lamina propria macrophages
Mycobacterium avium complex	Acid-fast lamina propria macrophages
Abetalipoproteinemia	Vacuolated, lipid-laden enterocytes with normal architecture
Agammaglobulinemia	Sprue-like histology with *Giardia* organisms
Abnormal but not diagnostic histology; diffuse lesions; should be present on endoscopic biopsy	
Celiac, refractory, and tropical sprue	Varying degrees of villus atrophy and crypt hyperplasia with lamina propria inflammation
Viral enteritis	Same as mild to moderate sprue
Bacterial overgrowth	Same as mild to moderate sprue
Severe, prolonged folate and vitamin B-12 deficiency	Same as sprue, reduced mitoses in crypts
Diagnostic histology; patchy distribution; therefore may be missed on endoscopic biopsy	
Lymphoma	Villi widened and lamina propria filled with malignant lymphoma cells
Lymphangiectasia	Dilated lymphatics in lamina propria and submucosa
Eosinophilic enteritis	Lamina propria infiltrated with eosinophils and neutrophils; mucosa normal to flat
Mastocytosis	Lamina propria infiltrated with mast cells, eosinophils, and neutrophils; mucosa normal to flat
Amyloidosis	Amyloid in lamina propria and submucosa with Congo red stain; normal mucosal architecture
Crohn's disease	Varying inflammation and ulceration with subepithelial granulomas
Giardiasis, coccidiosis, strongyloidiasis	Mucosa normal to flat; *Giardia*, *Cryptosporidium*, or *Strongyloides* organisms on surfaces of villi or crypts; *Eimeria*, *Isospora*, or microsporidia organisms within enterocytes
Abnormal but not diagnostic; patchy distribution; may be missed on endoscopic biopsy	
Acute radiation enteritis, enteropathy of dermatitis herpetiformis	Sprue-like lesion of varying severity

Adapted from Trier [452] and Levitt & Duane [455].

50-g endogenous pool, and 1 g is derived from the diet [483]. When total stool fat exceeds the 7 g/24 h, it is an abnormal finding. Stool fat content exceeding 6–7 g/24 h or triglyceride content exceeding 1 g/24 h can be detected by a simple qualitative fecal fat determination with approximately 90% sensitivity and 90% specificity [484–486]. The test loses some sensitivity with mild steatorrhea (fecal fat in the range of 6–10 g/24 h). There are also false-negative results if fat intake is inadequate; therefore, it is wise to ensure that the patient is ingesting a normal diet (approximately 100 g fat/24 h). False-positive results can occur if mineral oil laxatives, rectal suppositories (cocoa butter), or orlistat are given to the patient before stool collection or if the patient ingests large quantities of olestra [487].

To perform the qualitative stool fat examination, stool is mixed with water and alcohol and is heated; then Sudan stain 3 or 4 is added to stain for neutral fat (triglycerides). Fatty acid soaps can be dissociated by mixing glacial acetic acid and Sudan stain with the stool and heating the mixture to boiling. A positive test is recorded if there are more than 100 orange-red globules of fat at least 6–75 μm in diameter (bigger than red blood cells) per medium-power (40 ×) field. There is a positive correlation between the number of droplets

and the fat content of the stool and a less clear relationship between the size of the droplets and the fat content [486]. The accuracy of the test also depends on the experience of the laboratory personnel, and there seem to be fewer and fewer laboratories that perform this test well.

Complete collection of infants' stools is difficult so various investigators have studied the validity of the steatocrit test, a gravimetric method that is performed on random stool samples [488–490]. The test correlates well with other fecal absorption tests in infants and children and, because of its simplicity, needs to be investigated in adolescents and adults.

Quantitative fecal fat tests
The quantitative fecal fat determination is the standard against which all malabsorption tests are compared. Homogenized stool specimens are analyzed by the techniques of Van de Kamer [491,492]. A patient's bowel movements may vary from day to day so the major problem with the quantitative fecal fat analysis is ensuring that an adequate stool specimen has been collected. This is possible only with a 72-h collection. Even so, fewer than 50% of patients pass more than 90% of ingested stool markers in 3 days [493].

Although stool fat excretion for 24 h may be the same for mucosal and pancreatic disease, mucosal disease usually causes more water malabsorption or outright secretion [454]. The result is stool fat that is increased, but is diluted by the excess fluid. Consequently, the *stool fat concentration* (g fat/100 g wet stool weight) is usually less than 9.5% in mucosal diseases such as celiac sprue and greater than 9.5% in chronic pancreatic insufficiency. Other studies have questioned the value of this refinement of the fecal fat test.

Although it has been repeatedly confirmed that a fecal fat excretion of more than 7 g/24 h exceeds the mean normal fat excretion by more than two standard deviations, it is important to realize that diarrhea of secretory or osmotic origin can wash fat from the bowel lumen and can simulate steatorrhea. Therefore, if diarrhea is severe (> 800 g stool/24 h), stool fat excretion can be as high as 14 g/24 h [494]. Problems arise because patients with mild forms of true steatorrhea have stool fat excretion in the range of 8–14 g/24 h. Obviously, patients with diarrhea whose stool fat excretion falls in this borderline range could have secretory, osmotic, or malabsorptive diarrhea, and these patients need more definitive evaluation.

^{14}C-Triolein breath test for fat maldigestion/malabsorption

Measurements of the respiratory excretion of labeled CO_2 after oral administration and metabolism of radioactive carbon-labeled substrates, or of H_2 after administration of carbohydrates, can be used to assess fat, carbohydrate, and bile salt malabsorption or bacterial overgrowth [495]. All CO_2 breath tests, both those using ^{14}C and those using the stable isotope ^{13}C, are based on the idea that either intralumenal (bacterial) or cellular (intermediary) processes convert the substrate into CO_2, which is excreted in expired air.

After enzymatic hydrolysis by pancreatic proteins and micelle formation with bile salts, triglycerides are absorbed within the first 150 cm of jejunum. In the ^{14}C-triolein breath test, triolein, labeled with ^{14}C at the carboxyl groups, is given with 20–30 g of nonlabeled triolein [496–498]. The triolein is metabolized to CO_2 and water, and the $^{14}CO_2$ appears in the breath. In patients with impaired fat absorption, there is a reduction in the $^{14}CO_2$ excreted, with 85%–95% sensitivity and specificity. The usefulness of the test is limited by the presence of false-positive results in healthy persons (20% in IBS), false-negative results in patients with mild degrees of fat malabsorption and by both false-positive and false-negative tests in diseases that alter gastric emptying, dilute the $^{14}CO_2$ (hypercapnea), or alter fat metabolism [497,498].

D-Xylose absorption tests

D-Xylose is a five-carbon sugar that is incompletely absorbed in the duodenum and jejunum and is metabolized by intralumenal bacteria, so it can be used as a test of both bacterial overgrowth and mucosal disease [499,500]. Xylose is not completely metabolized; therefore, its excretion into urine or its concentration in blood after ingestion of a standardized dose has been used for more than 30 years as a small intestine absorption test [499]. After an overnight fast, either 5 g or 25 g xylose is given orally, and patients with normal renal function excrete more than 4 g after a 25-g dose. The test has poor sensitivity in mild mucosal disease, although sensitivity can be increased by obtaining blood values after the oral dose. A blood level of greater than 25 mg/dL 1 h after the 25-g dose, or greater than 20 mg/dL 1 h after the 5-g dose, can be expected [500]. This test depends on normal renal function so it is less useful in elderly patients, in whom the glomerular filtration rate is reduced, or in patients with known renal disease. Xylose can be distributed into sequestered fluids so this test is also less useful in patients with ascites. Increased portal pressure alone has been shown to decrease xylose absorption and furthermore, NSAIDs impair either absorption or urinary excretion. This test therefore it has false-positive and false-negative rates of 20%–30%. It should be considered in those mucosal diseases in which a patchy distribution of the histological lesion may invalidate the endoscopic biopsy (see Table 18.13).

Pancreatic function tests
Tubeless pancreatic function tests: bentiromide and pancrealauryl tests

Pancreatic chymotrypsin cleaves free paraaminobenzoic acid (PABA) from the synthetic peptide N-benzoyl-L-tyrosyl-paraaminobenzoic acid; this is the principle behind the *Bentiromide test*. If 500 to 1000 mg is administered orally and normal pancreatic chymotrypsin is present, the free PABA should be absorbed, conjugated in the liver, and excreted in the urine. With severe pancreatic insufficiency, less than 57% of the PABA is excreted in 6 h [501–503]. Unfortunately, severe intestinal mucosal disease, renal disease, diabetes, and severe liver disease all diminish PABA absorption or excretion in the absence of pancreatic insufficiency, and the test is not very sensitive in patients with mild pancreatic insufficiency. Furthermore, several ingested substances, including medications (e.g., acetaminophen, benzocaine, lidocaine, procaine, sulfa-containing antibiotics, chloramphenicol, chlorothiazide, furosemide) as well as certain foods (prunes and cranberries), interfere with the laboratory determination [504]. To overcome some of these limitations, the *pancreolauryl test* was developed [501–503]. Fluorescein is conjugated with two molecules of lauric acid. It is given orally and is hydrolyzed by pancreatic cholesterolase. The fluorescein release is absorbed and excreted in the urine. It has many of the same limitations as the bentiromide test.

Blood and stool tests of pancreatic function

The measurement of trypsinogen or pancreatic polypeptide in the blood, or of pancreatic proteases (chymotrypsin) in stool has been used to diagnose chronic pancreatitis. The sensitivity of these tests is poor (< 50%) in mild disease [503–505].

Pancreatic stimulation tests: secretin and Lundh meal tests

After duodenal intubation with a double-lumen tube (one lumen having an aspiration port to remove contaminating gastric juice), the pancreas can be stimulated with intravenous secretin, or cholecystokinin, or by an intragastric liquid meal containing fat, protein, and carbohydrates (Lundh meal) [503,505,506]. Pancreatic juice is aspirated from the duodenal port, and the serially collected samples are analyzed for volume, HCO_3^- concentration, and, in some laboratories, pancreatic enzymes (lipase, colipase, trypsin, or chymotrypsin). An HCO_3^- concentration lower than 90 mM suggests chronic pancreatitis, and in research laboratories there are normal values for specific pancreatic enzyme concentration or output. The secretin test is accurate and sensitive so it has become the "gold standard" for evaluation of exocrine pancreatic function [503]. It requires intestinal intubation and is time consuming; so it is not uniformly available and and may be better suited for research protocols. The test may be accomplished by endoscopic collection of duodenal fluid after intravenous secretin [507].

Tests for bacterial overgrowth

Schilling test

Vitamin B-12 (cobalamin) is not absorbed unless it is bound to intrinsic factor, and intrinsic factor cannot bind if salivary and gastric R proteins are not degraded by the pancreatic proteolytic activity in the upper small intestine. Approximately 50% of patients with severe pancreatic insufficiency are found to have impaired vitamin B-12 absorption, which is measured with the Schilling test. Obviously, this is not specific because vitamin B-12 absorption is diminished in patients with pernicious anemia, bacterial overgrowth, severe mucosal intestinal disease, or extensive ileal disease or resection. The Schilling test may be useful in distinguishing between bacterial overgrowth and mucosal disease in the setting of an abnormal D-xylose test, especially if the test reverts to normal after oral antibiotic treatment [508].

Bacterial growth from duodenal aspirates

The growth of more than 10^6 bacterial colonies per milliliter of duodenal fluid suggests bacterial overgrowth. Care should be taken to collect samples anaerobically, and they should be plated for aerobic and anaerobic cultures immediately [509]. The test has not been standardized, and contamination with oropharyngeal bacteria can be a problem.

H_2 and ^{14}C breath tests for bacterial overgrowth

The H_2 breath test can be used to diagnose bacterial overgrowth and has the advantage of not using radioactive isotopes. However, up to 20% of people are colonized by bacteria that do not produce H_2; thus, the sensitivity and specificity of this test may be poor [510]. The *^{14}C-D-xylose breath test* is said to be more specific for bacterial overgrowth, with 85% of patients having an increase in exhaled $^{14}CO_2$ within 60 min of ingesting 1 g ^{14}C-D-xylose [511]. Most of the ^{14}C-labeled xylose is absorbed in the small intestine so less reaches the colon, where it would be metabolized to CO_2 by bacteria, confounding interpretation of the test results. The test can be complicated by delayed gastric emptying. Champions of the test claim almost 100% specificity and sensitivity and an even greater reproducibility than that found in duodenal intubation with culture [511], but others report little advantage over glucose breath hydrogen tests [512].

The *cholyl-^{14}C-glycine breath test* is based on the rationale that conjugated (glycine or taurine) bile acids are reabsorbed passively throughout the jejunum and are actively absorbed in the terminal ileum [513,514]. Bacterial overgrowth hydrolyzes the peptide bond, releasing the ^{14}C-labeled glycine, which is then absorbed, metabolized to $^{14}CO_2$, and exhaled in expired air. Unfortunately, the test is not specific, and it gives similar results in patients with terminal ileal disease or resection and may be misleading in severe mucosal disease.

Watery diarrheas

History and physical examination

Useful clues to the causes of watery diarrheas include the volume of diarrhea, the number of stools, the presence of nocturnal diarrhea, incontinence, and a history of hypokalemia (Fig. 18.8). A detailed dietary and medication history, history of past surgeries, and positive Rome criteria for IBS may facilitate a diagnosis of diarrheas caused by ingested substances, carbohydrate malabsorption, bile acid diarrhea, postvagotomy status, or IBS. These diarrheas often respond, at least partially, to fasting.

Conversely, a history of 10–20 bowel movements per day, particularly nocturnal bowel movements with incontinence, should suggest the secretory diarrheas, as should documented electrolyte abnormalities (hypokalemia and acidosis) or dehydration, particularly if accompanied by hormone-induced systemic symptoms such as flushing. The presence of long-standing diabetes or alcoholism is necessary for a diagnosis of these forms of diarrhea. Weight loss is not usually a component of most of the watery diarrheas, except for microscopic colitis, advanced neuroendocrine tumors, and mastocytosis. Physical examination is helpful only if the thyromegaly of medullary carcinoma, the cutaneous flushing of the neuroendocrine tumors, and systemic mastocytosis are evident, or if there are the dermatographism of systemic mastocytosis and the migratory necrolytic erythema of glucagonoma [332]. The concomitant presence of peptic ulcer should suggest gastrinoma or systemic mastocytosis. Scars from previous surgery raise the question of postvagotomy diarrhea or terminal ileal resection, causing bile acid diarrhea.

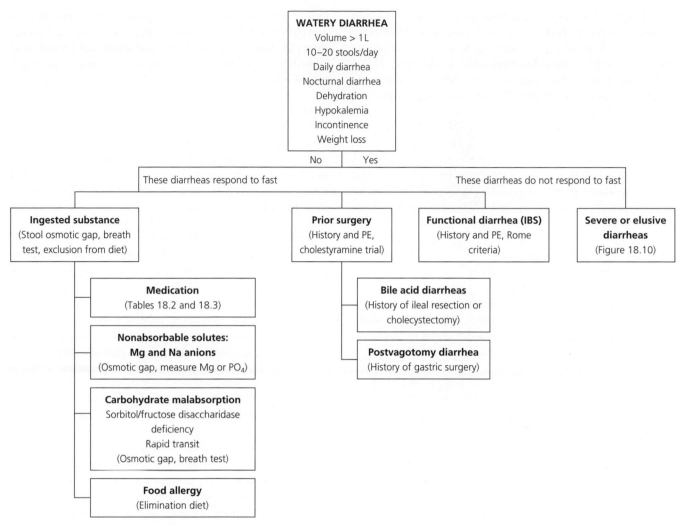

Figure 18.8 Approach to the evaluation of watery diarrheas. PE, physical examination.

Autonomic dysfunction (e.g., postural hypotension, impotence, gustatory sweating) is almost invariably present in diabetic diarrhea.

Screening tests for watery diarrheas

There are no screening tests for these diarrheas. Elimination diets (therapeutic trials) for the carbohydrate diarrheas and food allergy may be used.

Radiography (watery diarrhea)

Contrast radiographs

Routine films of the gastrointestinal tract are not usually helpful in the diagnosis of watery diarrheas unless there is evidence of a previous vagotomy, extensive small bowel resection or cholecystectomy, the presence of a tumor (carcinoid or villous adenoma), or a bowel filled with fluid (endocrine tumor). The radiographic appearance of an ahaustral colon with focal areas of spasm (pseudostrictures) may suggest chronic laxative abuse (the cathartic colon) [515].

Special radiological tests

Suspected pancreatic endocrine tumors and metastatic medullary carcinoma of the thyroid can be accurately localized with a combination of abdominal ultrasound, abdominal computed tomography, magnetic resonance imaging, and selective abdominal angiography, along with radiological somatostatin receptor screening [516,517] and endoscopic ultrasound [518]. Lesions of medullary carcinoma of the thyroid have also been localized with octapeptide (^{111}In-OTPA)-cholecystokinin analogue scanning [519]. Somatostatin receptor scintigraphy has proven to be both sensitive and useful in the diagnosis and evaluation of Zollinger–Ellison syndrome [516].

Flexible sigmoidoscopy or colonoscopy and biopsy

Patients with severe watery or elusive diarrhea should undergo colonoscopy to rule out villous adenomas of the rectosigmoid and biopsy to rule out microscopic or collagenous colitis, mastocytosis, or early Crohn's disease. Colonoscopy and biopsy also may reveal melanosis coli secondary to chronic anthracene laxative use. Melanosis coli can develop as early as 4 months after starting to use such laxatives and may require a year after their discontinuance to resolve [520]. Investigators have suggested that IBD alone can cause melanosis coli [521]. Terminal ileal biopsy may give an indication of type 2 bile acid diarrhea, Crohn's disease, or infectious disease [522]. Colonoscopy and biopsy have proven useful for diagnosis in the tertiary referral setting. However, they have been shown to have poor yield when used as *initial tests* in patients presenting with diarrhea and a normal gross appearance of the colon [523,524]. Biopsy can be useful to distinguish acute self-limited (infectious) colitis from IBD [525,526].

Stool tests for watery diarrhea
Fecal carbohydrate tests and fecal pH
Tests used for the determination of urine sugar can be applied as qualitative tests for stool carbohydrate, although these tests have not been standardized [199]. Urine dipsticks will give a positive reaction to glucose, but not to other sugars. Clinitest tablets (Bayer Corp., Mishawaka, IN) will give a positive reaction to glucose, galactose, fructose, maltose, and lactose, but not to sucrose, lactulose, sorbitol, or mannitol.

Carbohydrate malabsorption can be detected by measuring pH on a homogenized stool sample. The breakdown of unabsorbed carbohydrate by colonic bacteria to short-chain fatty acids reduces stool pH to less than 5.3 in pure carbohydrate malabsorption. However, in generalized malabsorptive disease, stool pH is more than 5.6 and is usually 6.0 or greater [35,36].

Laxative screen
To screen for laxative abuse in factitious diarrhea, it is necessary to send stool or urine to specific reference laboratories for qualitative tests for emetine (a component of ipecac), bisacodyl, castor oil, or anthraquinone [199,356–360]. Screening is not available for the docusate salts (dioctyl sodium sulfosuccinate), which are present in many of the over-the-counter cathartics. Stool SO_4^{2-}, PO_4^{2-}, and Mg^{2+} analysis detects those factitious diarrheas caused by osmotic cathartics. Although there is controversy regarding the ethics and legality of a room search for laxatives and diuretics, most believe that it is warranted because of the expense and risk to the patient of extensive evaluations [199]. Certainly, a room search can be a test with the highest diagnostic yield for surreptitious laxative abuse [351–355].

Tests for carbohydrate malabsorption
Lactose tolerance test
To detect either congenital or acquired lactase deficiency, 50 g lactose is administered, and plasma glucose is measured at 1 h and 2 h. A plasma glucose increase of more than 20 mg/dL is a normal response [282]. Patients who lack lactase and therefore the ability to split lactose into glucose and galactose have little increase in plasma glucose. This test does not have good sensitivity and has largely fallen from favor because of the more sensitive and simple H_2 breath lactose test.

H_2 breath test for carbohydrate malabsorption
Hydrogen breath tests can be used to study carbohydrate malabsorption or bacterial metabolism because the sole source of H_2 in the mammal is bacterial fermentation. In patients in whom a therapeutic trial of carbohydrate-restricted free diet is inconclusive, H_2 breath testing may be indicated [199, 495]. Because H_2 is produced only by bacterial fermentation of carbohydrates, increased H_2 excretion in breath after a carbohydrate challenge can be used to uncover small intestine bacterial overgrowth, disaccharidase deficiency, and even the excess carbohydrate wastage that might occur with motility disorders [527]. Patients with small intestine mucosal disease and pancreatic exocrine insufficiency also may have mild carbohydrate malabsorption. Bacterial overgrowth of the small bowel may cause an early peak of increased H_2 production within 2 h of giving a carbohydrate meal. In disaccharidase deficiency, small intestine mucosal disease, or pancreatic insufficiency, the peak in H_2 may come later, between 3 h and 6 h after ingestion, when the carbohydrate reaches the colonic bacteria [510,528,529]. The increase in H_2 excretion by patients with pancreatic insufficiency can be reduced by concomitant administration of pancreatic enzymes. Therefore, depending on what kind of carbohydrate malabsorption is sought, an oral dose of lactose (0.25–1.0 g/kg body weight), glucose (50 g), lactulose (10 g), fructose (1 g/kg body weight), or rice flour (100 g) may be given after an overnight fast. To test for lactose intolerance, a lactose dose of 25 g is frequently used, although a 50-g test dose may be more sensitive and a 12.5-g dose may be more specific [530]. Hydrogen breath tests must be standardized for each carbohydrate and dose, but generally an increase of more than 20 ppm in exhaled H_2 over baseline values within the first 3–8 h of ingestion is diagnostic. It is important to realize that the H_2 breath test measures only carbohydrate malabsorption, and 10%–20% of people have a gut flora that is incapable of producing H_2 [495].

Tests for bile acid malabsorption
Cholyl-^{14}C-glycine breath test
This test can be used also to identify impaired ileal absorption of bile acids, although it is neither specific nor sensitive [513, 514]. The measurement of cholyl-^{14}C-glycine excreted in the stool may increase the sensitivity but adds to the difficulty of performing the test.

[75]SeHCA test
Selenahomotaurocholic acid (SeHCA) is an analogue of taurocholic acid and has a similar enterohepatic circulation; it

may, therefore, be of value in detecting ileal dysfunction as a cause of bile acid diarrhea. ^{75}Se-labeled HCA is given orally, and the patient is scanned with the γ-camera; those who retain less than 34% of the administered dose after 3 days are considered to have increased bile acid loss [531,532]. This test has not been approved for use in many countries and is not available in the United States.

Serum 7α-hydroxy-4-cholesten-3-one concentration

With impaired bile acid absorption, cholesterol 7α-hydroxylase increases in the liver, and serum levels of 7α-hydroxy-4-cholesten-3-one rise. These levels have been shown to correlate well with the [75]SeHCA test [533].

Blood and urine hormone levels

Endocrine tumors such as carcinoids, gastrinoma, VIPoma, medullary carcinoma of the thyroid, systemic mastocytosis, and glucagonoma can be diagnosed by demonstrating elevated blood levels of 5-HT or urinary 5-hydroxyindoleacetic acid and elevated serum levels of gastrin, VIP, calcitonin, histamine, somatostatin, and glucagon, respectively. These may be obtained through commercial companies (e.g., ARUP Laboratory, Salt Lake City, UT) or research laboratories (the National Institutes of Health, Bethesda, MD). There is little diagnostic usefulness in measuring the other hormones secreted by these tumors [199,534,535]. These tests must be viewed cautiously because no endocrine cause of diarrhea is found in a significant percentage of those with elevated blood hormone levels, while finding an elevated blood hormone level may signify the presence of incurable metastatic disease [534]. Provocative tests such as pentagastrin stimulation for the diagnosis of Zollinger–Ellison syndrome have been developed.

Inflammatory diarrheas

History and physical examination

The important clinical manifestations of inflammatory diarrheas are the signs and symptoms of inflammation and the effects of severe chronic protein loss (Fig. 18.9). Fever with acute or chronic abdominal pain, particularly if it is localized to either the right or the left lower quadrants, may be an important clue to IBD ileitis or colitis. Eosinophilic, allergic, and immunological enteritis usually causes diffuse pain and tenderness. Severe protein-losing enteropathy is manifested either as peripheral edema, ascites, or anasarca in the absence of liver disease or proteinuria. Diarrhea in these inflammatory diseases may be meager (e.g., the pseudodiarrhea of proctitis), or it may be fairly severe. Exsanguinating hemorrhage, as in fulminant colitis, or moderately severe secretory watery-type diarrhea, as in graft-vs-host disease, can occur. Milder watery diarrheas may occur in microscopic or collagenous colitis and eosinophilic gastroenteritis. Crohn's disease,

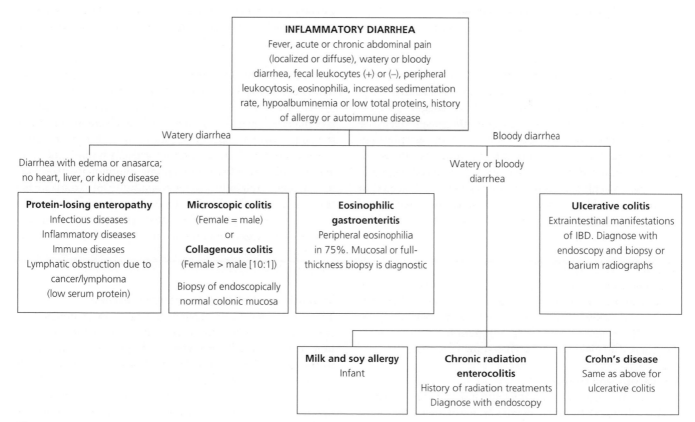

Figure 18.9 Approach to the evaluation of inflammatory diarrheas. IBD, inflammatory bowel disease.

radiation enteritis or colitis, and milk or soy protein allergy may present with either watery or bloody diarrhea.

Systemic, extraintestinal manifestations of inflammatory disease may be prominent in these patients. These include oral aphthous ulcers, polymigratory arthritis, uveitis or scleritis, and various dermatitides, including erythema nodosum, pyoderma gangrenosum, and the palpable purpura of vasculitis. As is the case with the mucosal malabsorptive disease with severe subepithelial inflammation, anorexia can be an important cause of the weight loss.

Screening tests for inflammatory diarrheas

Peripheral blood findings of leukocytosis, eosinophilia, elevated sedimentation rate, C-reactive protein, hypoalbuminemia, or low total serum proteins suggest the presence of inflammation, hypersensitivity, or severe protein-losing enteropathy. Low serum albumin and globulins should always alert one to the possibility of protein-losing enteropathy. The hallmark of the inflammatory diarrheas, however, is the presence of blood, either gross or occult, or leukocytes in the stool. Stool examination for leukocytes should use methylene blue stain and not Gram stain for the best results [114]. Fecal leukocyte tests have poor sensitivity for ruling out inflammatory diarrheas [115,116] and are gradually being supplanted by tests of granulocyte markers such as lactoferrin and calprotectin (see later).

Radiography (inflammatory diarrheas)

Contrast radiographs, computed tomography, and magnetic resonance imaging

Plain films or contrast examinations may show diagnostic evidence of IBD or the inflammation that may be present with eosinophilic gastroenteritis or radiation enterocolitis [536]. Edema of the valvulae conniventes may suggest protein-losing enteropathy. Early or mild gut inflammation may be missed entirely by radiography. Computed tomography may also be used for the detection of inflammatory disease of the colon [537]. Abdominal magnetic resonance imaging is being increasingly evaluated and has proven to be equal to enteroclysis in the accuracy of diagnosis of small bowel Crohn's disease [538] and equal to ileocolonoscopy in evaluating severity [539].

Leukocyte scintigraphy

Indium-labeled or technetium-99m (^{99m}Tc)-labeled leukocyte scans may be useful in detecting bowel inflammation that is not evident by endoscopy or contrast radiography [118, 540–542]. Imaging with ^{99m}Tc antigranulocytic antibodies [543] and ^{123}I-labeled IL-2 [544] has shown promise.

Endoscopy and biopsy

Clues to the diagnosis of any of the inflammatory diseases of the colon and terminal ileum can be made earliest with colonoscopy and biopsy. Thus, colonoscopy and biopsy become useful, if not mandatory, tests. Upper endoscopy and biopsy can be useful to diagnose gastroduodenal inflammatory diseases.

Capsule endoscopy

Wireless (video) capsule endoscopy has been shown to be superior to enteroclysis and push enteroscopy in diagnosing inflammatory disease of the small intestine [545–548]. This technology has demonstrated how common NSAID-induced enteropathy is in patients on these anti-inflammatory drugs [549].

Fecal lactoferrin and calprotectin tests

Excretion of fecal lactoferrin or calprotectin (constituents of leukocytes) in the stools can be used as a quantitative index of fecal leukocyte loss [117,118,550,551]. Fecal calprotectin has reasonable sensitivity (> 60%), specificity (80%–90%), positive predictive value (65%–95%), negative predictive value (70%–95%) and cost effectiveness [551].

Tests for enteric protein loss: ^{51}Cr-albumin clearance, ^{99M}Tc-albumin scintigraphy, and α_1-antitrypsin clearance

Measurements of enteric protein loss are sensitive tests for inflammatory diarrhea. This can be accomplished by measuring 24-h stool excretion or the clearance of ^{51}Cr-labeled albumin [552]. Scintigraphy after labeling albumin with ^{99m}Tc can be useful in determining which gastrointestinal segment (e.g., stomach or small intestine) is weeping protein [553,554]. Unfortunately, these nuclear medicine tests are not available in the United States.

Clearance of the α_1-antitrypsin in native endogenous proteins, particularly, has proven to be as sensitive as ^{51}Cr-labeled protein clearance and avoids the administration of radioactive material [555]. The principle of the clearance studies is the same as with urinary creatinine α_1-clearance and requires the measurement of serum and stool in a 24-h stool collection. When combined with a protein pump inhibitor, it can be used to diagnose protein-losing gastropathy [556]. To avoid the need for 24-h stool collection, the measurement of more than 1.75 mg α_1-antitrypsin per gram of random collected and immediately frozen stool has been proposed as a reasonable substitute for clearance studies [557]. It seems to have good value as a test for protein-losing enteropathy [428].

Evaluation of severe or elusive diarrhea

To evaluate severe or elusive diarrheas, measurements of stool fat, electrolytes, and osmolality on timed stool collections, combined with observing the response of stool volume to fasting, are useful (Fig. 18.10). A 48-h to 72-h stool collection must be obtained while the patient is on a 100-g fat diet and the collection must be repeated while the patient has fasted. The fasting portion of the collection must be performed in the hospital; however, the nonfasting part of

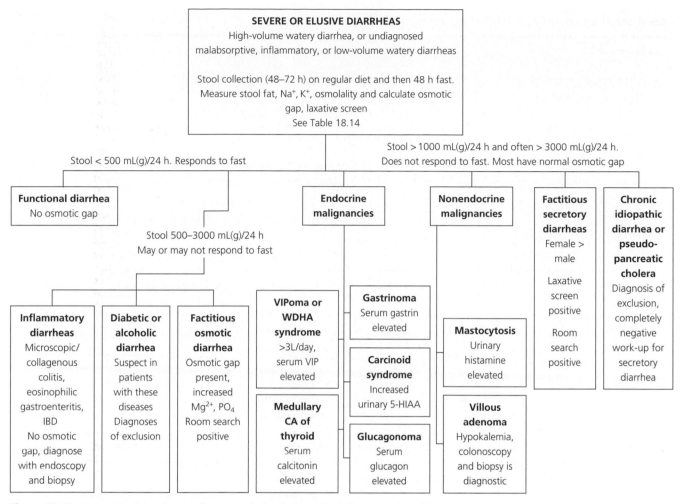

Figure 18.10 Approach to the evaluation of severe or elusive diarrheas. IBD, inflammatory bowel disease.

the collection can be obtained on an outpatient basis. The stool should be analyzed for appearance, weight, quantitative fecal fat, electrolytes (Na^+, K^+, and if thought necessary, Cl^-, PO_4^{2-}, and Mg^{2+}), osmolality, fecal pH, and laxative screen.

Stool weight, response to fast, and stool osmotic gap

There are many theoretical and practical problems encountered in using the response to fasting and feeding and the measurements of stool osmotic gap to diagnose the cause of diarrhea [35–38,199,558–562]. First, in some diseases, the ingestion of a drug or feeding itself initiates the secretory phenomenon. Under these circumstances, the fasting stool may return to normal, and yet the pathophysiology is that of a secretory diarrhea. Examples are the patients who factitiously ingest laxatives and some patients with microscopic or collagenous colitis. Second, the stool specimen may be accidentally contaminated with urine or purposefully diluted with water. Third, there may be malabsorptive diseases that also have a secretory component. For example, in celiac sprue there is secretion by the small intestine, and malabsorbed fat also can initiate active secretion in the colon. Similarly, in

viral diarrhea, there may be simultaneous secretion by the hyperplastic crypts and malabsorption by the damaged villus epithelium.

Nonetheless, there are some general responses of stool volume to fasting in the various diarrheas, especially the watery diarrheas, as shown in Figs 18.8 and 18.10. Steatorrheic stools are usually less than 700 g, and stool weight returns to normal on fasting. Stool osmotic gap measurements are often indeterminate in these patients. Inflammatory diarrheas are variable in weight, but usually less than 1000 g, and have a variable response to fasting. As is the case in steatorrhea, the stool osmotic gap is not usually helpful.

The measurements of stool electrolytes for calculation of osmotic gap are useful only as guidelines for the classification of diarrhea [199,200,270,558–562]. In practice, to calculate the stool osmotic gap, it is not correct to use measured stool osmolality; this may be falsely altered by bacterial degradation of carbohydrate after the stool is passed. Therefore, the use of normal plasma osmolality, 290 mOsm/kg H_2O, is recommended because newly passed stool is essentially isosmotic with plasma. Concentrations of Na^+ and K^+ must be

Table 18.14 Stool osmotic gap as a guide to the pathophysiology and diagnosis of diarrhea

Plasma osmolality or 290 mOsm/kg H$_2$O − 2[Na$^+$ + K$^+$] mM	=	Stool osmotic gap
Stool [Na$^+$] > 90 mM and Osmotic gap < 50 mOsm/kg H$_2$O	=	Secretory diarrhea; or osmotic diarrhea caused by Na$_2$SO$_4$ or Na$_2$PO$_4$ ingestion[a]
Stool [Na$^+$] < 60 mM and Osmotic gap > 125 mOsm/kg H$_2$O	=	Osmotic diarrhea; if stool volume does not return to normal on fast, suspect surreptitious Mg^{2+} ingestion[b]
Stool [Na$^+$] > 150 mM and Stool osmolality > 375–400 mOsm/kg H$_2$O	=	Suspect contamination of specimen with concentrated urine
Stool osmolality < 200–250 mOsm/kg H$_2$O	=	Suspect contamination of specimen with dilute urine or water

a Normal stool SO$_4^{2-}$ and PO$_4^{2-}$ is usually < 10 mmol; exact values not established. In Na$_2$SO$_4$-induced or Na$_2$PO$_4$-induced diarrhea, stool Cl$^-$ concentrations are less than 20 mM.

b Normal stool Mg^{2+} on regular diet is 10–45 mM; during fasting, the concentration should be less than 10 mM. In Mg^{2+}-induced diarrhea, stool Mg^{2+} concentration is always > 45 and usually > 100 mM.

measured in the stool and then multiplied by 2, to account for the obligate (mainly organic) anions in the stool. The osmotic gap, or the difference between 290 mOsm and 2 × [Na$^+$ + K$^+$] concentrations, should normally be less than 125 and is usually less than 50 (Table 18.14). This number takes into account unabsorbed divalent cations (Ca^{2+} and Mg^{2+}) and ammonium and their obligate anions.

In secretory diarrheas, the solute causing the movement of water from blood to bowel lumen is composed of the secreted Na$^+$ and K$^+$ molecules. Thus, in secretory diarrheas, twice the sum of the stool Na$^+$ plus K$^+$ concentrations will approximate stool osmolality. Furthermore, unless the secretory stimulus is being ingested (e.g., laxatives), the diarrhea and stool weight should be only minimally or moderately reduced if the patient fasts; fasting stool weight should remain higher than 200 g/24 h. In general, therefore, if stool Na$^+$ concentrations are greater than 90 mM and the osmotic gap is less than 50, then a secretory diarrhea is present (see Table 18.14). Conversely, if stool Na$^+$ is less than 60 mM and the osmotic gap is greater than 125, then it is likely to be an osmotic form of diarrhea. In osmotic diarrhea, it is the ingestion of nonabsorbable (or nonabsorbed) solutes that displaces Na$^+$ from the stool and causes the osmotic gap and the diarrhea. Osmotic diarrhea should disappear if the patient fasts, and stool weights should return to values of less than 200 g in 24 h. Stools with Na$^+$ concentrations of 60–90 mM and calculated osmotic gaps of 50–100 can result from either secretory or malabsorptive abnormalities or from diseases that have as their pathophysiological basis some element of both secretion and malabsorption [35,38,199,558–562].

Stool osmolality, measured by the freezing-point depression method, may have some utility in diagnosis because a low stool osmolality suggests contamination of the stool, either inadvertently with urine or purposefully with water in the case of factitious diarrhea [35,38,199,558–562] (see Table 18.14).

In patients suspected of having magnesium anion-induced diarrhea, fecal analysis reveals stool Mg^{2+} concentrations greater than 45 mM (usually greater than 100 mM) or Mg^{2+} output greater than 15 mmol/24 h. In patients in whom the magnesium ingestion is innocently motivated, the diarrhea disappears on fasting. In those ingesting magnesium surreptitiously, or in an infant or child being purposefully fed magnesium, stool analysis demonstrates an osmotic gap greater than 100 mOsm/kg H$_2$O, and the excess stool weight and osmotic gap do not disappear on fasting [268–271].

In patients suspected of having sodium anion-induced diarrheas, the stool Na$^+$ concentration is 90 mM or greater, and twice the concentrations of Na$^+$ + K$^+$ is approximately 290 mOsm (see Table 18.14). This type of diarrhea mimics secretory diarrhea, even though it is an osmotic diarrhea, because the stool Na$^+$ content is high (> 90 mM), and there is not an osmotic gap. This type of diarrhea can be diagnosed, in the absence of a history of ingestion of Na$_2$SO$_4$-containing or Na$_2$PO$_4$-containing substances, by determining stool Cl$^-$ concentration. If nonabsorbable anions have been ingested, they displace stool Cl$^-$, and the resulting stool Cl$^-$ value is usually less than 20 mM [35,199].

There are technical and practical problems with using stool analysis as a guide to the diagnosis of diarrhea

[35,38,558–562]. Some hospitals are unable to measure stool electrolytes and osmolality, and therefore an aliquot of the homogenized stool sample must be sent frozen on dry ice to a reference laboratory for analysis. Therefore, the response to fasting may be a more practical way to distinguish secretory from osmotic diarrheas [558].

Antidiarrheal therapy

Mechanisms of action

Antidiarrheal agents can be divided into two categories: agents that are useful for mild to moderate diarrheas (Table 18.15)

Table 18.15 Antidiarrheal agents for mild to moderate diarrheas

Drug	Mechanism of action in humans	Side effects
Proabsorptive agents		
Oral replacement solutions (see Table 18.9)	Stimulate sodium-glucose, galactose, and amino acid absorption and increased water absorption	Though rehydration is improved, may actually increase stool output
Amylase-resistant starch (pectin)	Converted to short-chain fatty acids by colonic bacteria, and these stimulate colon sodium and water absorption	Use has been minimal; therefore, potential side effects are unknown
Bismuth subsalicylate	Antiinflammatory, but not anticyclooxygenase; mechanism not known, has bacteriocidal activity; is suspended in clay that may bind enterotoxins	Salicylate toxicity, encephalopathy in high doses or with impaired renal function, black stools confused with melena
Opiates and opiate-like		
Paregoric	Alters motility, causes dilation and decreased peristalsis of small bowel; ? nonpropulsive contractions of distal colon; increased anal sphincter tone	May enhance bacterial invasion, may precipitate toxic megacolon, may prolong excretion of pathogens, central nervous system (CNS) and respiratory depression, delayed gastric emptying; addiction potential
Deodorized tincture of opium		
Codeine		
Diphenoxylate with atropine[a]		
Loperamide[b]	Experimentally, opiates have proabsorptive and antisecretory effects; loperamide also has calmodulin-binding and calcium channel-blocking activity	
Racecadotril	Inhibits enkephalinase, the enzyme in gut that degrades natural opiates	Does not appear to alter gut motility or have CNS effects (poor ability to cross the blood–brain barrier), so side effects seem minimal; experience is limited, so caution indicated
Bulk-forming agents		
Psyllium	Hydroscopic, partially nonabsorbed bulk added to stool, increasing stool viscosity	Bloating and flatus, intestinal obstruction behind preexisting strictures
Methylcellulose	Alters bacterial cell mass	
Polycarbophil	May bind bacterial enterotoxins	
Silicates		
Kaolin and attapulgite	Hydroscopic, may bind bacterial enterotoxins	None of significance
Anticholinergics	Alters motility, dilation of both small and large intestine	Same as with opiates, plus atropine toxicity, but minus addiction, CNS and respiratory depression
Atropine		
Hyoscyamine		
Synthetic drugs		
Cholestyramine	Binds bile acids	Binds medications and vitamins, steatorrhea with high doses

a Atropine toxicity, especially tachycardia, occurs with overdose.
b Poor passage through blood–brain barrier and good first-pass hepatic metabolism make loperamide the opiate with the fewest side effects.

Table 18.16 Agents helpful in secretory and other severe diarrheas[a]

Drug	Mechanism in humans	Side effects	Diseases used to treat
Octreotide	Suppresses hormone secretion from neuroendocrine cells, mild antisecretory effect, alters motility (dilation and decreased peristalsis)	Suppresses pancreatic secretion (steatorrhea), delays gallbladder emptying (cholelithiasis), suppresses insulin secretion (hyperglycemia)	Carcinoid syndrome, VIPoma and other neuroendocrine tumors, unexplained secretory diarrhea; occasionally helpful in short bowel syndrome
Clonidine	α_2-Adrenergic agonist, mild antisecretory effect, alters motility	Postural hypotension, depression, rebound hypertension when discontinued	Diabetic diarrhea, diarrhea of opiate withdrawal, unexplained secretory diarrheas
Phenothiazines	Calmodulin inhibition, mild antisecretory effect, alters motility	Postural hypotension, depression, tardive dyskinesia	VIPomas and other neuroendocrine tumors, unexplained secretory diarrheas
Calcium-channel blockers	Mild antisecretory effect, alters motility	Postural hypotension, cardiac effects	Neuroendocrine tumors, unexplained secretory diarrheas
H^+, K^+, ATPase inhibitors and H_2 antagonist	Decreases gastric secretion	Encephalopathy, bone marrow toxicity, antiandrogenic effects (cimetidine)	Zollinger–Ellison syndrome, systemic mastocytosis
H_1 antagonist	Decreases intestinal secretion	Somnolence	Systemic mastocytosis
Serotonin antagonist	Decreases intestinal secretion	Bone marrow toxicity	Systemic mastocytosis
Methysergide	Decreases intestinal secretion	Tardive dyskinesia	Carcinoid syndrome
Ketanserin	Alters motility		Carcinoid syndrome
Cyproheptadine	Decreases flushing		Carcinoid syndrome
Indomethacin	Inhibits prostaglandin synthesis and secretion, mild proabsorptive effect	Gastric and intestinal ulceration	Medullary carcinoma of thyroid, villous adenoma, AIDS enteropathy, rare neuroendocrine tumor
Glucocorticoids	Antiinflammatory, proabsorptive	Cushing syndrome	IBD
6-Mercaptopurine	Immunosuppression	Bone marrow depression	IBD
Methotrexate	Immunosuppression	Liver toxicity/cirrhosis	IBD
Infliximab	Antitumor necrosis factor	Infection (tuberculosis); allergic reaction	IBD

a Isolated case reports indicate antisecretory activity of bromocriptine, lithium carbonate, nicotinic acid, and berberine.
AIDS, acquired immunodeficiency syndrome; IBD, inflammatory bowel disease.

and those that are helpful in secretory and other severe diarrheas (Table 18.16). A major drawback of current antidiarrheal drugs is that some have no antisecretory activity; for example, the bulk-forming agents only increase the consistency of stool and do not decrease its elaboration [563]. Other antidiarrheal agents have only mild proabsorptive or antisecretory action [564–566]. Although studies in vitro and in vivo in experimental animals suggest that many of the agents listed in Tables 18.15 and 18.16 have proabsorptive or antisecretory activity, most of them are lacking this effect in human studies, or else it is minimal. The recent development of small-molecule chloride channel (cystic fibrosis transmembrane conductance regulator, CFTR) inhibitors shows great promise of producing effective anti-secretory agents [567–569].

Most of the current antidiarrheal agents act by altering the intestinal motility. Bismuth salicylates, loperamide, clonidine, phenothiazine, and somatostatin have mild antisecretory activity, but they also cause dilation of the small intestine and colon and decrease peristalsis [570–572]. The opiates also cause disordered contractions of the distal large bowel and increased anal sphincter tone [573,574]. The sum of these effects is to trap fluid within the intestine and to put it in contact with the mucosa for a greater period of time, allowing more complete absorption.

It remains to be seen if the recently discovered agents such as enkephalinase inhibitors – like racecadotril (Acetorphan), which inhibits the breakdown of natural endogenous opiates (enkephalins) by intestinal tissue – will be more effective than loperamide. It is effective against experimental secretory diarrheas, and its proabsorptive effect is prevented by naloxone, indicating the role of endogenous opiates in its proabsorptive action [575–579]. Another potential new antisecretory agent is the new 5-HT$_3$ receptor antagonist, alosetron [580–582], which seems to be more effective against the pain and urgency of IBS than against the diarrhea; however, alosetron was recently removed from the market for general use.

Agents for mild diarrhea

Bismuth subsalicylate [105,106,109,123,583] and loperamide [105,106,109,123,584] preparations continue to prove effective and safe in mild to moderate diarrhea of all types (see "Treatment of acute infectious diarrheas"). The antimobility efforts of the opiates listed in Table 18.15 may be symptomatically useful in mild diarrheas, but they may result in inadequate fluid replacement therapy in severe diarrheas if one is relying on stool output as a gauge for replacing fluid losses. The problems may be especially significant in infants and children. Furthermore, the antimotility effects are not desired if the diarrhea is caused by invasive organisms because stasis may enhance their invasion of the intestinal mucosa. These drugs also delay subsequent clearance of the microorganisms from the bowel, thus increasing carriage time. Clinical evidence also suggests that such drugs are dangerous in severe IBD, reportedly precipitating the development of toxic megacolon in severe ulcerative colitis. Therefore, although they appear to be safe, their use must be tempered in severe secretory diarrheas, in invasive infectious diarrheas, and in severe IBD.

The newer antienkephalinase, racecadotril, has been shown to be effective in controlled trials in children [577,578] and adults [585,586]. Similarly, the use of amylase-resistant starch (pectin) has been effective in controlled trials of treatment of protracted infectious diarrheas [130,131]. Experience with these newer agents is limited so potential side effects are unknown.

Agents for secretory diarrhea

The use of drugs with potentially serious side effects (see Table 18.16) can be justified for the treatment of severe secretory diarrheas such as the diarrheas of carcinoid syndrome and neuroendocrine tumors, diabetic diarrhea, graft-vs-host disease, 5-fluorouracil–leucovorin diarrhea, short bowel syndrome, severe dumping syndrome, and AIDS diarrhea [564–566,587–600]. The somatostatin analogue octreotide appears to have its major antisecretory effect in carcinoid syndrome and in some other neuroendocrine tumors because it inhibits hormone secretion by the tumor. It also may prevent some of the other clinical manifestations of hormone release (e.g., flushing, tachycardia, skin rash), and may inhibit tumor growth [600]. Resistance may develop if neuroendocrine tumors are treated for a long period [595]. The newer long-acting preparations, Sandostatin-LAR (Novartis International AG, Basel, Switzerland) and Lanreotide-PR

(Ipsen-Biotech, Milford, MA, USA), have made therapy with this drug more convenient for the patient [592,597].

Although clonidine is useful in the diarrhea of opiate withdrawal and sometimes in patients with diabetic diarrhea, particularly those who already have severe postural hypotension that cannot be made much worse by the agent, such side effects become a limiting factor [373]. Lithium carbonate, bromocriptine, nicotinic acid, and berberine have all been reported to be useful in certain secretory diarrheas [564–566].

Indomethacin, a cyclooxygenase blocker that inhibits prostaglandin production, may occasionally be useful in neuroendocrine tumors and in patients with irritable bowel and possible food allergy (see "Watery diarrheas"), but it may be harmful in IBD. Indomethacin is most useful in patients with acute radiation diarrhea, AIDS diarrhea, and the diarrhea accompanying villous adenomas of the rectum or colon.

Antiinflammatory agents for inflammatory diarrhea

In IBD, glucocorticoids have an effect within 72 h on both prostaglandin and leukotriene production [601], and they can be shown to have a proabsorptive effect on the intestine within 5 h of administration [601–603]. Thus, in IBD, steroids are both antiinflammatory and antidiarrheal.

Treatment options for inflammatory diarrhea include salicylates [604], drugs with immunosuppression and immunomodulation activity such as 6-mecaptopurine, methotrexate, cyclosporine, infliximab, thalidomide, and budesonide [605]. These agents can be considered antidiarrheal medications by virtue of being antiinflammatory agents.

Problotics

Probiotics show promise in inflammatory diarrheas [99, 606–608]. A *probiotic* is defined as a viable microbial dietary supplement that affects the host in a beneficial way through its effects on the intestinal tract. Several different species are available: *Lactobacillus* GG, *Lactobacillus acidophilus*, *Bifidobacterium* species, and *Saccharomyces boulardii* are some of those more widely used. They have been proposed and explored in trials for both prevention and, in some instances, treatment of antibiotic-associated diarrhea, viral diarrhea, bacterial diarrhea, lactose intolerance, IBD, and others [99,606–608]. Level 1 evidence exists for the therapeutic use of probiotics in infectious diarrhea in children, recurrent *C. difficile* diarrhea, and pouchitis [99,606]. Level 2 and 3 evidence only exists for its role in the therapy of inflammatory bowel disease [607].

References

1. Russo MW, Wei JT, Thiny MT, et al. Digestive and liver diseases statistics, 2004. Gastroenterology 2004;126:1448.
2. Sandler RS, Everhart JE, Donowitz M, et al. The burden of selected digestive diseases in the United States. Gastroenterology 2002;122:1500.

3. O'Morain, C. The burden of gastrointestinal disease in Europe. Aliment Pharmacol Therap 2003;18 Suppl. 3.

4. Mead PS, Slutsker L, Dietz V, et al. Food-related illness and death in the United States. Emerg Infect Dis 1999;5:607.

5. Casburn-Jones AC, Farthing MJ. Management of infectious diarrhoea. Gut 2004;53:296.

6. Talley NJ, Weaver AF, Zinsmeister AR, Melton LJ, III. Self-reported diarrhea: what does it mean? Am J Gastroenterol 1994;89:1160.

7. Sandler RS, Drossman DA. Bowel habits in young adults not seeking health care. Dig Dis Sci 1987;32:841.

8. Ryle JA. An address on chronic diarrhea. Lancet 1924;2:101.

9. Wenzl HH, Fine KD, Schiller LR, Fordtran JS. Determinants of decreased fecal consistency in patients with diarrhea. Gastroenterology 1995;108:1729.

10. Davies GJ, Crowder M, Reid B, Dickerson JW. Bowel function measurements of individuals with different eating patterns. Gut 1986;27:164.

11. Rhoads JM, Powell DW. Diarrhea. In: Walker WA, Durie PR, Hamilton JR (eds). Pediatric gastrointestinal disease. Toronto, Ontario: BC Decker, 1991:62.

12. Sandler RS, Stewart WF, Liberman JN, et al. Abdominal pain, bloating, and diarrhea in the United States: prevalence and impact. Dig Dis Sci 2000;45:1166.

13. Fordtran JS. Speculations on the pathogenesis of diarrhea. Fed Proc 1967;26:1405.

14. Phillips SF. Diarrhea: a current view of the pathophysiology. Gastroenterology 1972;63:495.

15. Lunniss PJ, Gladman MA, Hetzer FH, et al. Risk factors in acquired faecal incontinence. J R Soc Med 2004;97:111.

16. Bharucha AE, Zinsmeister AR, Locke GR, et al. Symptoms and quality of life in community women with fecal incontinence. Clin Gastroenterol Hepatol 2006;4:1004.

17. Cummings JH. Short chain fatty acids in the human colon. Gut 1981;22:763.

18. Kamm MA, Farthing MJ, Lennard-Jones JE. Bowel function and transit rate during the menstrual cycle. Gut 1989;30:605.

19. Barclay GR, Turnberg LA. Effect of moderate exercise on salt and water transport in the human jejunum. Gut 1988;29:816.

20. Barclay GR, Turnberg LA. Effect of psychological stress on salt and water transport in the human jejunum. Gastroenterology 1987;93:91.

21. Hofmann AF, Poley JR. Cholestyramine treatment of diarrhea associated with ileal resection. N Engl J Med 1969;281:397.

22. Sali A, Murray WR, MacKay C. Aluminium hydroxide in bile-salt diarrhoea. Lancet 1977;2:1051.

23. Wood JD. Enteric neuroimmunophysiology and pathophysiology. Gastroenterology 2004;127:635.

24. Khan WI, Collins SM. Gut motor function: immunological control in enteric infection and inflammation. Clin Experiment Immun 2006;143:389.

25. Modigliani R, Lemann M, Melancon SB, et al. Diarrhea and autonomic dysfunction in a patient with hexosaminidase B deficiency (Sandhoff disease). Gastroenterology 1994;106:775.

26. Phillips S, Giller J. The contributions of the colon to electrolyte and water conservation in man. J Lab Clin Med 1973;81:733.

27. Turvill JL, Connor P, Farthing MJ. Neurokinin 1 and 2 receptors mediate cholera toxin secretion in rat jejunum. Gastroenterology 2000;119:1037.

28. Crowe SE, Powell DW. Fluid and electrolyte transport during enteric infections. In: Blaser MJ, Smith PD, Ravdin JI et al. (eds). Infections of the gastrointestinal tract. New York: Raven Press, 1994:107.

29. Castro GA, Powell DW. The physiology of the mucosal immune system and immune-mediated responses in the gastrointestinal tract. In: Johnson LR (ed.). Physiology of the gastrointestinal tract. New York: Raven Press, 1994:709.

30. Field M. Intestinal ion transport and the pathophysiology of diarrhea. J Clin Invest 2003;111:931.

31. Masyuk AI, Marinelli RA, LaRusso NF. Water transport by epithelia of the digestive tract. Gastroenterology 2002;122:545.

32. Schiller C, Frohlich CP, Giessmann T, et al. Intestinal fluid volumes and transit of dosage forms as assessed by magnetic resonance imaging. Aliment Pharmacol Ther 2005;22:971.

33. Pedley KC, Naftalin RJ. Evidence from fluorescence microscopy and comparative studies that rat, ovine and bovine colonic crypts are absorptive. J Physiol 1993;460:525.

34. Agarwal R, Afzalpurkar R, Fordtran JS. Pathophysiology of potassium absorption and secretion by the human intestine. Gastroenterology 1994;107:548.

35. Eherer AJ, Fordtran JS. Fecal osmotic gap and pH in experimental diarrhea of various causes. Gastroenterology 1992;103:545.

36. Holtug K, Clausen MR, Hove H, et al. The colon in carbohydrate malabsorption: short-chain fatty acids, pH, and osmotic diarrhoea. Scand J Gastroenterol 1992;27:545.

37. Hammer HF, Santa Ana CA, Schiller LR, Fordtran JS. Studies of osmotic diarrhea induced in normal subjects by ingestion of polyethylene glycol and lactulose. J Clin Invest 1989;84:1056.

38. Shiau YF, Feldman GM, Resnick MA, Coff PM. Stool electrolyte and osmolality measurements in the evaluation of diarrheal disorders. Ann Intern Med 1985;102:773.

39. Christopher NL, Bayless TM. Role of the small bowel and colon in lactose-induced diarrhea. Gastroenterology 1971;60:845.

40. Mekhjian HS, Phillips SF, Hofmann AF. Colonic secretion of water and electrolytes induced by bile acids: perfusion studies in man. J Clin Invest 1971;50:1569.

41. Ammon HV, Phillips SF. Inhibition of colonic water and electrolyte absorption by fatty acids in man. Gastroenterology 1973;65:744.

42. Bright-Asare P, Binder HJ. Stimulation of colonic secretion of water and electrolytes by hydroxy fatty acids. Gastroenterology 1973;64:81.

43. Wiggins HS, Cummings JH, Pearson JR. Hydroxystearic acid and diarrhoea following ileal resection. Gut 1974;15:392.

44. Donowitz M, Binder HJ. Effect of dioctyl sodium sulfosuccinate on colonic fluid and electrolyte movement. Gastroenterology 1975;69:941.

45. Gaginella TS, Chadwick VS, Debongnie JC, et al. Perfusion of rabbit colon with ricinoleic acid: dose-related mucosal injury, fluid secretion, and increased permeability. Gastroenterology 1977;73:95.

46. Sartor RB, Powell DW. Mechanisms of diarrhea in intestinal inflammation and hypersensitivity. In: Field M (ed.). Diarrheal diseases. New York: Elsevier, 1991:75.

47. Powell DW, Mifflin RC, Valentich JD, et al. Myofibroblasts: II. Intestinal subepithelial myofibroblasts. Am J Physiol Cell Physiol 1999;277:C183.

48. Macdonald TT, Bajaj-Elliott M, Pender SL. T cells orchestrate intestinal mucosal shape and integrity. Immunol Today 1999;20:505.

49. Schuppan D, Hahn EG. MMPs in the gut: inflammation hits the matrix. Gut 2000;47:12.

50. Akira S, Uematsu S, Takeuchi O. Pathogen recognition and innate immunity. Cell 2006;124:783.

51. Neish AS. Molecular aspects of intestinal epithelial cell–bacterial interactions that determine the development of intestinal inflammation. Inflamm Bowel Dis 2004;10:159.

52. Cario E. Bacterial interactions with cells of the intestinal mucosa: Toll-like receptors and NOD2. Gut 2005;54:1182.

53. Neish AS. TLRS in the gut. II. Flagellin-induced inflammation and antiapoptosis. Am J Physiol Gastrointest Liver Physiol 2007;292:G462.

54. Arrieta MC, Bistritz L, Meddings JB. Alterations in intestinal permeability. Gut 2006;55:1512.

55. Ye D, Ma I, Ma TY. Molecular mechanism of tumor necrosis factor-alpha modulation of intestinal epithelial tight junction barrier. Am J Physiol Gastrointest Liver Physiol 2006;290:G496.

56. Wang F, Schwarz BT, Graham WV, et al. IFN-gamma-induced TNFR2 expression is required for TNF-dependent intestinal epithelial barrier dysfunction. Gastroenterology 2006;131:1153.

57. Boivin MA, Ye D, Kennedy JC, et al. Mechanism of glucocorticoid regulation of the intestinal tight junction barrier. Am J Physiol Gastrointest Liver Physiol 2007;292:G590.

58. Moeser AJ, Nighot PK, Ryan KA, et al. Prostaglandin-mediated inhibition of Na⁺/H⁺ exchanger isoform 2 stimulates recovery of barrier function in ischemia-injured intestine. Am J Physiol Gastrointest Liver Physiol 2006;291:G885.

59. Clark JA, Doelle SM, Halpern MD, et al. Intestinal barrier failure during experimental necrotizing enterocolitis: protective effect of EGF treatment. Am J Physiol Gastrointest Liver Physiol 2006;291: G938.

60. Yahr TL. A critical new pathway for toxin secretion? N Engl J Med 2006;355:1171.

61. Hecht G, Hodges K, Gill RK, et al. Differential regulation of Na⁺/H⁺ exchange isoform activities by enteropathogenic *E. coli* in human intestinal epithelial cells. Am J Physiol Gastrointest Liver Physiol 2004;287:G370.

62. Sharma R, Tesfay S, Tomson FL, et al. Balance of bacterial pro- and anti-inflammatory mediators dictates net effect of enteropathogenic *Escherichia coli* on intestinal epithelial cells. Am J Physiol Gastrointest Liver Physiol 2006;290:G685.

63. Gill RK, Borthakur A, Hodges K, et al. Mechanism underlying inhibition of intestinal apical Cl/OH exchange following infection with enteropathogenic *E. coli*. J Clin Invest 2007;117:428.

64. Salazar-Lindo E, Pinell-Salles P, Maruy A, Chea-Woo E. El Niño and diarrhoea and dehydration in Lima, Peru. Lancet 1997;350:1597.

65. Kilgore PE, Holman RC, Clarke MJ, Glass RI. Trends of diarrheal disease – associated mortality in US children, 1968 through 1991. JAMA 1995;274:1143.

66. Ciarlet M, Estes MK. Interactions between rotavirus and gastrointestinal cells. Curr Opin Microbiol 2001;4:435.

67. Gangarosa RE, Glass RI, Lew JF, Boring JR. Hospitalizations involving gastroenteritis in the United States, 1985: the special burden of the disease among the elderly. Am J Epidemiol 1992;135:281.

68. Hall KE, Proctor DD, Fisher L, Rose S. American gastroenterological association future trends committee report: effects of aging of the population on gastroenterology practice, education, and research. Gastroenterology 2005;129:1305.

69. Sanders JW, Putnam SD, Riddle MS, Tribble DR. Military importance of diarrhea: lessons from the Middle East. Curr Opin Gastroenterol 2005;21:9.

70. Goldberg MB, Rubin RH. The spectrum of Salmonella infection. Infect Dis Clin North Am 1988;2:571.

71. Gill CJ, Hamer DH. Foodborne illnesses. Curr Treat Options Gastroenterol 2001;4:23.

72. Ekanem EE, DuPont HL, Pickering LK, et al. Transmission dynamics of enteric bacteria in day-care centers. Am J Epidemiol 1983;118:562.

73. Bruce-Jones PN, Allen SC. Variations of invasive Salmonella infection in elderly people. Br J Clin Pract 1996;50:470.

74. Edwards BH. *Salmonella* and *Shigella* species. Clin Lab Med 1999; 19:469.

75. Ferrera PC, Jeanjaquet MS, Mayer DM. *Shigella*-induced encephalopathy in an adult. Am J Emerg Med 1996;14:173.

76. Goodgame RW. Understanding intestinal spore-forming protozoa: cryptosporidia, microsporidia, isospora, and cyclospora. Ann Intern Med 1996;124:429.

77. Hughes RA, Hadden RD, Gregson NA, Smith KJ. Pathogenesis of Guillain–Barré syndrome. J Neuroimmunol 1999;100:74.

78. Mahler H, Pasi A, Kramer JM, et al. Fulminant liver failure in association with the emetic toxin of *Bacillus cereus*. N Engl J Med 1997;336:1142.

79. McCarthy N, Giesecke J. Incidence of Guillain–Barré syndrome following infection with *Campylobacter jejuni*. Am J Epidemiol 2001; 153:610.

80. Perles Z, Bar-Ziv J, Granot E. Brain edema: an underdiagnosed complication of *Shigella* infection. Pediatr Infect Dis J 1995;14:1114.

81. Rautelin H, Hanninen ML, Sivonen A, et al. Chronic diarrhea due to a single strain of *Aeromonas caviae*. Eur J Clin Microbiol Infect Dis 1995;14:51.

82. Sack DA, Sack RB, Chaignat CL. Getting serious about cholera. N Engl J Med 2006;355:649.

83. Thomson GT, DeRubeis DA, Hodge MA, et al. Post-*Salmonella* reactive arthritis: late clinical sequelae in a point source cohort. Am J Med 1995;98:13.

84. Consensus conference statement: *Escherichia coli* O157:H7 infections – an emerging national health crisis, July 11–13, 1994. Gastroenterology 1995;108:1923.

85. Scoging A, Bahl M. Diarrhetic shellfish poisoning in the UK. Lancet 1998;352:117.

86. Becker K, Southwick K, Reardon J, et al. Histamine poisoning associated with eating tuna burgers. JAMA 2001;285:1327.

87. Grattan LM, Oldach DF, Perl TM, et al. Learning and memory difficulties after environmental exposure to waterways containing toxin-producing *Pfiesteria* or *Pfiesteria*-like dinoflagellates. Lancet 1998;352:532.

88. Ahmed FE. Seafood safety. Washington, D.C.: National Academy Press, 1991.

89. Morris JG, Jr. Natural toxins associated with fish and shellfish. In: Blaser MJ, Smith PD, Ravdin JI et al. (eds). Infections of the gastrointestinal tract. New York: Raven Press, 1995:251.

90. American Medical Association. Diagnosis and management of foodborne ilnesses: a primer for physicians. American Medical Association, Centers for Diseases Control and Prevention, Center for Food Safety and Applied Nutrition, Food and Drug Administration, Food Safety and Inspection Service, US Department of Agriculture (eds). Chicago, Illinois, American Medical Association, MMWR.

91. Morris JG, Jr. "Noncholera" *Vibrio* species. In: Blaser MJ, Smith PD, Ravdin JI et al. (eds). Infections of the gastrointestinal tract. New York: Raven Press, 1995:671.

92. Bartlett JG. Clinical practice. Antibiotic-associated diarrhea. N Engl J Med 2002;346:334.

93. Hove H, Tvede M, Mortensen PB. Antibiotic-associated diarrhoea, *Clostridium difficile*, and short-chain fatty acids. Scand J Gastroenterol 1996;31:688.

94. Ponnuvel KM, Rajkumar R, Menon T, Sankaranarayanan VS. Role of *Candida* in indirect pathogenesis of antibiotic associated diarrhoea in infants. Mycopathologia 1996;135:145.

95. Thorpe CM, Gorbach SL. Update on *Clostridium difficile*. Curr Treat Options Gastroenterol 2006;9:265.

96. Mylonakis E, Ryan ET, Calderwood SB. *Clostridium difficile*-associated diarrhea: a review. Arch Intern Med 2001;161:525.

97. Loo VG, Poirier L, Miller MA, et al. A predominantly clonal multi-institutional outbreak of *Clostridium difficile*-associated diarrhea with high morbidity and mortality. N Engl J Med 2005;353:2442.

98. Bartlett JG. Narrative review: the new epidemic of *Clostridium difficile*-associated enteric disease. Ann Intern Med 2006;145:758.

99. Szajewska H, Mrukowicz J. Meta-analysis: non-pathogenic yeast *Saccharomyces boulardii* in the prevention of antibiotic-associated diarrhoea. Aliment Pharmacol Ther 2005;22:365.

100. Maroo S, LaMont JT. Recurrent *Clostridium difficile*. Gastroenterology 2006;130:1311.

101. DuPont AW, DuPont HL. Travelers' diarrhea: modern concepts and new developments. Curr Treat Options Gastroenterol 2006;9:13.

102. DuPont HL, Jiang ZD, Okhuysen PC, et al. A randomized, double-blind, placebo-controlled trial of rifaximin to prevent travelers' diarrhea. Ann Intern Med 2005;142:805.

103. Pickering LK, Woodward WE. Diarrhea in day care centers. Pediatr Infect Dis 1982;1:47.

104. Reves RR, Morrow AL, Bartlett AV, III, et al. Child day care increases the risk of clinic visits for acute diarrhea and diarrhea due to rotavirus. Am J Epidemiol 1993;137:97.

105. Aranda-Michel J, Giannella RA. Acute diarrhea: a practical review. Am J Med 1999;106:670.

106. Scheidler MD, Giannella RA. Practical management of acute diarrhea. Hosp Pract (Off Ed) 2001;36:49.

107. Murch SH. Diarrhoea, diagnostic delay, and appendicitis. Lancet 2000;356:787.

108. Hoshiko M. Laboratory diagnosis of infectious diarrhea. Pediatr Ann 1994;23:570.

109. Guerrant RL, Shields DS, Thorson SM, et al. Evaluation and diagnosis of acute infectious diarrhea. Am J Med 1985;78:91.

110. Thielman NM, Guerrant RL. Clinical practice. Acute infectious diarrhea. N Engl J Med 2004;350:38.

111. Bowman RA, Bowman JM, Arrow SA, Riley TV. Selective criteria for the microbiological examination of faecal specimens. J Clin Pathol 1992;45:838.

112. Bauer TM, Lalvani A, Fehrenbach J, et al. Derivation and validation of guidelines for stool cultures for enteropathogenic bacteria other than Clostridium difficile in hospitalized adults. JAMA 2001;285:313.

113. Wood M. When stool cultures from adult inpatients are appropriate. Lancet 2001;357:901.

114. Harris JC, DuPont HL, Hornick RB. Fecal leukocytes in diarrheal illness. Ann Intern Med 1972;76:697.

115. Savola KL, Baron EJ, Tompkins LS, Passaro DJ. Fecal leukocyte stain has diagnostic value for outpatients but not inpatients. J Clin Microbiol 2001;39:266.

116. Herbert ME. Medical myth: measuring white blood cells in the stools is useful in the management of acute diarrhea. West J Med 2000;172:414.

117. Guerrant RL, Araujo V, Soares E, et al. Measurement of fecal lactoferrin as a marker of fecal leukocytes. J Clin Microbiol 1992;30:1238.

118. Roseth AG, Schmidt PN, Fagerhol MK. Correlation between faecal excretion of indium-111-labelled granulocytes and calprotectin, a granulocyte marker protein, in patients with inflammatory bowel disease. Scand J Gastroenterol 1999;34:50.

119. Ruiz-Pelaez JG, Mattar S. Accuracy of fecal lactoferrin and other stool tests for diagnosis of invasive diarrhea at a Colombian pediatric hospital. Pediatr Infect Dis J 1999;18:342.

120. Vaishnavi C, Bhasin DK, Singh K. Fecal lactoferrin assay as a cost-effective tool for intestinal inflammation. Am J Gastroenterol 2000;95:3002.

121. Mickelsen PA, Tompkins LS. Use of the bacteriology and mycology laboratories to diagnose gastrointestinal infection. In: Blaser MJ, Smith PD, Ravdin JI et al. (eds). Infections of the gastrointestinal tract. New York: Raven Press, 1995:1223.

122. Fedorko DP, Engler HD, O'Shaughnessy EM, et al. Evaluation of two rapid assays for detection of Clostridium difficile toxin A in stool specimens. J Clin Microbiol 1999;37:3044.

123. Rhoads M. Management of acute diarrhea in infants. J Parenter Enteral Nutr 1999;23:S18.

124. Wingate D, Phillips SF, Lewis SJ, et al. Guidelines for adults on self-medication for the treatment of acute diarrhoea. Aliment Pharmacol Ther 2001;15:773.

125. Bellemare S, Hartling L, Wiebe N, et al. Oral rehydration versus intravenous therapy for treating dehydration due to gastroenteritis in children: a meta-analysis of randomised controlled trials. BMC Med 2004;2:11.

126. Endsley S, Galbraith A. Are you overlooking oral rehydration therapy in childhood diarrhea? It's not just for use in developing countries. Postgrad Med 1998;104:159.

127. Snyder JD. Oral therapy for diarrhea. In: Blaser MJ, Smith PD, Ravdin JI et al. (eds). Infections of the gastrointestinal tract. New York: Raven Press, 1995:1417.

128. Nalin DR, Hirschhorn N, Greenough W, III, et al. Clinical concerns about reduced-osmolarity oral rehydration solution. JAMA 2004;291:2632.

129. Fontaine O, Gore SM, Pierce NF. Rice-based oral rehydration solution for treating diarrhoea. The Cochrane Library 2001;CD001264.

130. Ramakrishna BS, Venkataraman S, Srinivasan P, et al. Amylase-resistant starch plus oral rehydration solution for cholera. N Engl J Med 2000;342:308.

131. Rabbani GH, Teka T, Zaman B, et al. Clinical studies in persistent diarrhea: dietary management with green banana or pectin in Bangladeshi children. Gastroenterology 2001;121:554.

132. Caeiro JP, DuPont HL, Albrecht H, Ericsson CD. Oral rehydration therapy plus loperamide versus loperamide alone in the treatment of traveler's diarrhea. Clin Infect Dis 1999;28:1286.

133. Guandalini S. Treatment of acute diarrhea in the new millennium. J Pediatr Gastroenterol Nutr 2000;30:486.

134. Wan C, Phillips MR, Dibley MJ, Liu Z. Randomised trial of different rates of feeding in acute diarrhoea. Arch Dis Child 1999;81:487.

135. Costello AM, Bhutta TI. Antidiarrhoeal drugs for acute diarrhoea in children. BMJ 1992;304:1.

136. Freedman SB, Adler M, Seshadri R, Powell EC. Oral ondansetron for gastroenteritis in a pediatric emergency department. N Engl J Med 2006;354:1698.

137. Rossignol JF, Abu-Zekry M, Hussein A, Santoro MG. Effect of nitazoxanide for treatment of severe rotavirus diarrhoea: randomised double-blind placebo-controlled trial. Lancet 2006;368:124.

138. Rossignol JF, Kabil SM, el Gohary Y, Younis AM. Effect of nitazoxanide in diarrhea and enteritis caused by Cryptosporidium species. Clin Gastroenterol Hepatol 2006;4:320.

139. Wong CS, Jelacic S, Habeeb RL, et al. The risk of the hemolytic–uremic syndrome after antibiotic treatment of Escherichia coli O157:H7 infections. N Engl J Med 2000;342:1930.

140. DuPont HL. Review article: infectious diarrhoea. Aliment Pharmacol Ther 1994;8:3.

141. Ahmed T, Begum B, Badiuzzaman, et al. Management of severe malnutrition and diarrhea. Indian J Pediatr 2001;68:45.

142. Duggan C, Walker WA. Postenteritis syndrome. Gastroenterol Dis Today 1995;4:7.

143. Rastogi A, Malhotra V, Uppal B, et al. Aetiology of chronic diarrhoea in tropical children. Trop Gastroenterol 1999;20:45.

144. Bhutta ZA, Bird SM, Black RE, et al. Therapeutic effects of oral zinc in acute and persistent diarrhea in children in developing countries: pooled analysis of randomized controlled trials. Am J Clin Nutr 2000;72:1516.

145. Morales M, Galvan E, Mery CM, et al. Exocrine pancreatic insufficiency in tropical sprue. Digestion 2001;63:30.

146. Looke DF, Robson JM. 9: Infections in the returned traveller. Med J Aust 2002;177:212.

147. Lima AA. Tropical diarrhoea: new developments in traveller's diarrhoea. Curr Opin Infect Dis 2001;14:547.

148. Bhatnagar S, Bhan MK, Sommerfelt H, et al. Enteroaggregative Escherichia coli may be a new pathogen causing acute and persistent diarrhea. Scand J Infect Dis 1993;25:579.

149. Lebwohl B, Deckelbaum RJ, Green PH. Giardiasis. Gastrointest Endosc 2003;57:906.

150. Chen XM, Keithly JS, Paya CV, LaRusso NF. Cryptosporidiosis. N Engl J Med 2002;346:1723.

151. Wilcox MH, Cook AM, Eley A, Spencer RC. Aeromonas spp as a potential cause of diarrhoea in children. J Clin Pathol 1992;45:959.

152. Baert F, Peetermans W, Knockaert D. Yersiniosis: the clinical spectrum. Acta Clin Belg 1994;49:76.

153. Stolk-Engelaar VM, Hoogkamp-Korstanje JA. Clinical presentation and diagnosis of gastrointestinal infections by Yersinia enterocolitica in 261 Dutch patients. Scand J Infect Dis 1996;28:571.

154. Rossignol JF, Kabil SM, Said M, et al. Effect of nitazoxanide in persistent diarrhea and enteritis associated with Blastocystis hominis. Clin Gastroenterol Hepatol 2005;3:987.

155. Gwee KA. Postinfectious irritable bowel syndrome. Curr Treat Options Gastroenterol 2001;4:287.

156. Spiller RC. Infection, immune function, and functional gut disorders. Clin Gastroenterol Hepatol 2004;2:445.

157. Spiller R, Campbell E. Post-infectious irritable bowel syndrome. Curr Opin Gastroenterol 2006;22:13.

158. Pimentel M, Park S, Mirocha J, et al. The effect of a nonabsorbed oral antibiotic (rifaximin) on the symptoms of the irritable bowel syndrome: a randomized trial. Ann Intern Med 2006;145:557.

159. Niaz SK, Sandrasegaran K, Renny FH, Jones BJ. Postinfective diarrhoea and bile acid malabsorption. J R Coll Physicians Lond 1997;31:53.

160. Sinha L, Liston R, Testa HJ, Moriarty KJ. Idiopathic bile acid malabsorption: qualitative and quantitative clinical features and response to cholestyramine. Aliment Pharmacol Ther 1998;12:839.

161. Ung KA, Kilander AF, Lindgren A, Abrahamsson H. Impact of bile acid malabsorption on steatorrhoea and symptoms in patients with chronic diarrhoea. Eur J Gastroenterol Hepatol 2000;12:541.

162. Osterholm MT, MacDonald KL, White KE, et al. An outbreak of a newly recognized chronic diarrhea syndrome associated with raw milk consumption. JAMA 1986;256:484.

163. DuPont HL, Ribner BS. Infectious gastroenteritis. In: Bennett JV, Brachman PS (eds). Hospital Infections. Boston: Little, Brown, 1992: 641.

164. Kelly TW, Patrick MR, Hillman KM. Study of diarrhea in critically ill patients. Crit Care Med 1983;11:7.

165. McFarland LV. Epidemiology of infectious and iatrogenic nosocomial diarrhea in a cohort of general medicine patients. Am J Infect Control 1995;23:295.

166. Ryan MJ, Wall PG, Adak GK, et al. Outbreaks of infectious intestinal disease in residential institutions in England and Wales 1992–1994. J Infect 1997;34:49.

167. Wrenn K. Fecal impaction. N Engl J Med 1989;321:658.

168. Chassany O, Michaux A, Bergmann JF. Drug-induced diarrhoea. Drug Saf 2000;22:53.

169. Kast RE. Acarbose related diarrhea: increased butyrate upregulates prostaglandin E. Inflamm Res 2002;51:117.

170. McRorie J, Zorich N, Riccardi K, et al. Effects of olestra and sorbitol consumption on objective measures of diarrhea: impact of stool viscosity on common gastrointestinal symptoms. Regul Toxicol Pharmacol 2000;31:59.

171. Edes TE, Walk BE. Nosocomial diarrhea: beware the medicinal elixir. South Med J 1989;82:1497.

172. Montejo JC. Enteral nutrition-related gastrointestinal complications in critically ill patients: a multicenter study. Crit Care Med 1999;27:1447.

173. Gottschlich MM, Warden GD, Michel M, et al. Diarrhea in tube-fed burn patients: incidence, etiology, nutritional impact, and prevention. J Parenter Enteral Nutr 1988;12:338.

174. Thakkar K, Kien CL, Rosenblatt JI, Herndon DN. Diarrhea in severely burned children. J Parenter Enteral Nutr 2005;29:8.

175. Braun TI, Fekete T, Lynch A. Strongyloidiasis in an institution for mentally retarded adults. Arch Intern Med 1988;148:634.

176. Yolken RH, Bishop CA, Townsend TR, et al. Infectious gastroenteritis in bone-marrow-transplant recipients. N Engl J Med 1982;306:1010.

177. Olsen SJ, DeBess EE, McGivern TE, et al. A nosocomial outbreak of fluoroquinolone-resistant salmonella infection. N Engl J Med 2001;344:1572.

178. Samore MH. Epidemiology of nosocomial Clostridium difficile diarrhoea. J Hosp Infect 1999;43 Suppl:S183.

179. Mahoney FJ, Farley TA, Burbank DF, et al. Evaluation of an intervention program for the control of an outbreak of shigellosis among institutionalized persons. J Infect Dis 1993;168:1177.

180. Thom K, Forrest G. Gastrointestinal infections in immunocompromised hosts. Curr Opin Gastroenterol 2006;22:18.

181. Widdowson MA, van Doornum GJ, van der Poel WH, et al. Emerging group-A rotavirus and a nosocomial outbreak of diarrhoea. Lancet 2000;356:1161.

182. Brandt LJ, Kosche KA, Greenwald DA, Berkman D. Clostridium difficile-associated diarrhea in the elderly. Am J Gastroenterol 1999;94:3263.

183. Kohli HS, Chaudhuri AK, Todd WT, et al. A severe outbreak of E. coli O157 in two psychogeriatric wards. J Public Health Med 1994;16:11.

184. Pear SM, Williamson TH, Bettin KM, et al. Decrease in nosocomial Clostridium difficile-associated diarrhea by restricting clindamycin use. Ann Intern Med 1994;120:272.

185. Lima NL, Guerrant RL, Kaiser DL, et al. A retrospective cohort study of nosocomial diarrhea as a risk factor for nosocomial infection. J Infect Dis 1990;161:948.

186. Kornblau S, Benson AB, Catalano R, et al. Management of cancer treatment-related diarrhea. Issues and therapeutic strategies. J Pain Symptom Manage 2000;19:118.

187. Grem JL, Shoemaker DD, Petrelli NJ, Douglass HO, Jr. Severe and fatal toxic effects observed in treatment with high- and low-dose leucovorin plus 5-fluorouracil for colorectal carcinoma. Cancer Treat Rep 1987;71:1122.

188. Rosenberg SA, Lotze MT, Mule JJ. NIH conference. New approaches to the immunotherapy of cancer using interleukin-2. Ann Intern Med 1988;108:853.

189. Davila ML. Neutropenic enterocolitis. Curr Treat Options Gastroenterol 2006;9:249.

190. Riddoch C, Trinick T. Gastrointestinal disturbances in marathon runners. Br J Sports Med 1988;22:71.

191. Sullivan SN, Champion MC, Christofides ND, et al. Gastrointestinal regulatory peptide responses in long-distance runners. Physician Sports Med 1984;12:77.

192. Demers LM, Harrison TS, Halbert DR, Santen RJ. Effect of prolonged exercise on plasma prostaglandin levels. Prostaglandins Med 1981;6:413.

193. Heer M, Repond F, Hany A, et al. Acute ischaemic colitis in a female long distance runner. Gut 1987;28:896.

194. Baska RS, Moses FM, Graeber G, Kearney G. Gastrointestinal bleeding during an ultramarathon. Dig Dis Sci 1990;35:276.

195. van Nieuwenhoven MA, Brouns F, Brummer RJ. The effect of physical exercise on parameters of gastrointestinal function. Neurogastroenterol Motil 1999;11:431.

196. Marsh MN, Hinde J. Inflammatory component of celiac sprue mucosa. I. Mast cells, basophils, and eosinophils. Gastroenterology 1985;89:92.

197. Fordtran JS, Rector FC, Locklear TW, Ewton MF. Water and solute movement in the small intestine of patients with sprue. J Clin Invest 1967;46:287.

198. Camilleri M. Chronic diarrhea: a review on pathophysiology and management for the clinical gastroenterologist. Clin Gastroenterol Hepatol 2004;2:198.

199. Fine KD, Schiller LR. AGA technical review on the evaluation and management of chronic diarrhea. Gastroenterology 1999;116:1464.

200. Schiller LR. Diarrhea. Med Clin North Am 2000;84:1259.

201. Schiller LR. Chronic diarrhea. Gastroenterology 2004;127:287.

202. Harewood GC, Murray JA. Approaching the patient with chronic malabsorption syndrome. Semin Gastrointest Dis 1999;10:138.

203. Ebert EC. Maldigestion and malabsorption. Dis Mon 2001;47:49.

204. Losowsky MS, Walker BE. Liver disease and malabsorption. Gastroenterology 1969;56:589.

205. Salvioli G, Carati L, Lugli R. Steatorrhea in cirrhosis: effect of ursodeoxycholic acid administration. J Int Med Res 1990;18:289.

206. Layer P, der Ohe MR, Holst JJ, et al. Altered postprandial motility in chronic pancreatitis: role of malabsorption. Gastroenterology 1997;112:1624.

207. Ghaneh P, Neoptolemos JP. Exocrine pancreatic function following pancreatectomy. Ann N Y Acad Sci 1999;880:308.

208. Littlewood JM, Wolfe SP. Control of malabsorption in cystic fibrosis. Paediatr Drugs 2000;2:205.

209. Weizman Z, Durie PR, Kopelman HR, et al. Bile acid secretion in cystic fibrosis: evidence for a defect unrelated to fat malabsorption. Gut 1986;27:1043.

210. Cipolli M, D'Orazio C, Delmarco A, et al. Shwachman's syndrome: pathomorphosis and long-term outcome. J Pediatr Gastroenterol Nutr 1999;29:265.

211. Krejs GJ, Orci L, Conlon JM, et al. Somatostatinoma syndrome. Biochemical, morphologic and clinical features. N Engl J Med 1979;301:285.

212. Race TF, Paes IC, Faloon WW. Intestinal malabsorption induced by oral colchicine. Comparison with neomycin and cathartic agents. Am J Med Sci 1970;259:32.

213. Rogers AI, Vloedman DA, Bloom EC, Kalser MH. Neomycin-induced steatorrhea. JAMA 1966;197:935.

214. Halsted CH, McIntyre PA. Intestinal malabsorption caused by aminosalicylic acid therapy. Arch Intern Med 1972;130:935.

215. West RJ, Lloyd JK. The effect of cholestyramine on intestinal absorption. Gut 1975;16:93.

216. Hoskins LC, Winawer SJ, Broitman SA, et al. Clinical giardiasis and intestinal malabsorption. Gastroenterology 1967;53:265.

217. Brandborg LL, Goldberg SB, Breidenbach WC. Human coccidiosis – a possible cause of malabsorption. N Engl J Med 1970;283:1306.

218. Kotcher E, Miranda M, Esquivel R, et al. Intestinal malabsorption and helminthic and protozoan infections of the small intestine. Gastroenterology 1966;50:366.

219. Milner PF, Irvine RA, Barton CJ, et al. Intestinal malabsorption in *Strongyloides stercoralis* infestation. Gut 1965;6:574.

220. Bai JC, Mazure RM, Vazquez H, et al. Whipple's disease. Clin Gastroenterol Hepatol 2004;2:849.

221. Fenollar F, Puechal X, Raoult D. Whipple's disease. N Engl J Med 2007;356:55.

222. Branski D, Lerner A, Lebenthal E. Chronic diarrhea and malabsorption. Pediatr Clin North Am 1996;43:307.

223. Lachaux A, Bouvier R, Cozzani E, et al. Familial autoimmune enteropathy with circulating anti-bullous pemphigoid antibodies and chronic autoimmune hepatitis. J Pediatr 1994;125:858.

224. Corazza GR, Biagi F, Volta U, et al. Autoimmune enteropathy and villous atrophy in adults. Lancet 1997;350:106.

225. Ruan EA, Komorowski RA, Hogan WJ, Soergel KH. Non-granulomatous chronic idiopathic enterocolitis: clinicopathologic profile and response to corticosteroids. Gastroenterology 1996;111:629.

226. De Benedetti F, Insalaco A, Diamanti A, et al. Mechanistic associations of a mild phenotype of immunodysregulation, polyendocrinopathy, enteropathy, X-linked syndrome. Clin Gastroenterol Hepatol 2006;4:653.

227. Fine KD, Stone MJ. Alpha-heavy chain disease, Mediterranean lymphoma, and immunoproliferative small intestinal disease: a review of clinicopathological features, pathogenesis, and differential diagnosis. Am J Gastroenterol 1999;94:1139.

228. Jensen RT. Gastrointestinal abnormalities and involvement in systemic mastocytosis. Hematol Oncol Clin North Am 2000;14:579.

229. Woodward T. Systemic mastocytosis. Curr Treat Options Gastroenterol 2003;6:35.

230. Beishuizen A, van Bodegraven AA, Bronsveld W, Sindram JW. Eosinophilic gastroenteritis – a disease with a wide clinical spectrum. Neth J Med 1993;42:212.

231. Farrell RJ, Kelly CP. Celiac sprue. N Engl J Med 2002;346:180.

232. Green PH, Jabri B. Coeliac disease. Lancet 2003;362:383.

233. Fasano A, Berti I, Gerarduzzi T, et al. Prevalence of celiac disease in at-risk and not-at-risk groups in the United States: a large multicenter study. Arch Intern Med 2003;163:286.

234. Alaedini A, Green PH. Narrative review: celiac disease: understanding a complex autoimmune disorder. Ann Intern Med 2005;142:289.

235. Green PH, Jabri B. Celiac disease. Annu Rev Med 2006;57:207.

236. AGA Institute Medical Position Statement on the Diagnosis and Management of Celiac Disease. Gastroenterology 2006;131:1977.

237. Rostom A, Murray JA, Kagnoff MF. American Gastroenterological Association (AGA) Institute technical review on the diagnosis and management of celiac disease. Gastroenterology 2006;131:1981.

238. Kagnoff MF. Celiac disease: pathogenesis of a model immunogenetic disease. J Clin Invest 2007;117:41.

239. Green PHR, Stavropoulos SN, Panagi SG, et al. Characteristics of adult celiac disease in the USA: results of a national survey. Am J Gastroenterol 2001;96:126.

240. Eliakim R, Sherer DM. Celiac disease: fertility and pregnancy. Gynecol Obstet Invest 2001;51:3.

241. Ludvigsson JF, Ludvigsson J. Coeliac disease in the father affects the newborn. Gut 2001;49:169.

242. Loftus CG, Loftus EV, Jr. Cancer risk in celiac disease. Gastroenterology 2002;123:1726.

243. Hall RP, III. Dermatitis herpetiformis. J Invest Dermatol 1992;99:873.

244. Koop I, Ilchmann R, Izzi L, et al. Detection of autoantibodies against tissue transglutaminase in patients with celiac disease and dermatitis herpetiformis. Am J Gastroenterol 2000;95:2009.

245. Dieterich W, Laag E, Bruckner-Tuderman L, et al. Antibodies to tissue transglutaminase as serologic markers in patients with dermatitis herpetiformis. J Invest Dermatol 1999;113:133.

246. Stenveld HJ, Starink TM, van Joost T, Stoof TJ. Efficacy of cyclosporine in two patients with dermatitis herpetiformis resistant to conventional therapy. J Am Acad Dermatol 1993;28:1014.

247. Zettinig G, Weissel M, Flores J, et al. Dermatitis herpetiformis is associated with atrophic but not with goitrous variant of Hashimoto's thyroiditis. Eur J Clin Invest 2000;30:53.

248. Askling J, Linet M, Gridley G, et al. Cancer incidence in a population-based cohort of individuals hospitalized with celiac disease or dermatitis herpetiformis. Gastroenterology 2002;123:1428.

249. Ohashi KF, Ishibashi SF, Osuga JF, et al. Novel mutations in the microsomal triglyceride transfer protein gene causing abetalipoproteinemia. J Lipid Res 2000;41:1199.

250. Mistilis SP, Skyring AP. Intestinal lymphangiectasia. Am J Med 1966;40:634.

251. Asakura H, Tsuchiya M, Katoh S, et al. Pathological findings of lymphangiectasia of the large intestine in a patient with protein-losing enteropathy. Gastroenterology 1986;91:719.

252. Heresbach D, Raoul JL, Genetet N, et al. Immunological study in primary intestinal lymphangiectasia. Digestion 1994;55:59.

253. Kuroiwa G, Takayama T, Sato Y, et al. Primary intestinal lymphangiectasia successfully treated with octreotide. J Gastroenterol 2001;36:129.

254. Alfano V, Tritto G, Alfonsi L, et al. Stable reversal of pathologic signs of primitive intestinal lymphangiectasia with a hypolipidic, MCT-enriched diet. Nutrition 2000;16:303.

255. Dukowicz AC, Lacy BE, Levine GM. Small intestinal bacterial overgrowth: a comprehensive review. Gastroenterol Hepatol 2007;3:112.

256. Castiglione F, Rispo A, Di Girolamo E, et al. Antibiotic treatment of small bowel bacterial overgrowth in patients with Crohn's disease. Aliment Pharmacol Ther 2003;18:1107.

257. Singh VV, Toskes PP. Small bowel bacterial overgrowth: presentation, diagnosis, and treatment. Curr Treat Options Gastroenterol 2004;7:19.

258. Lin HC. Small intestinal bacterial overgrowth: a framework for understanding irritable bowel syndrome. JAMA 2004;292:852.

259. Buchman AL, Scolapio J, Fryer J. AGA technical review on short bowel syndrome and intestinal transplantation. Gastroenterology 2003;124:1111.

260. Cisler JJ, Buchman AL. Intestinal adaptation in short bowel syndrome. J Investig Med 2005;53:402.

261. O'Keefe SJ, Buchman AL, Fishbein TM, et al. Short bowel syndrome and intestinal failure: consensus definitions and overview. Clin Gastroenterol Hepatol 2006;4:6.

262. Parekh NR, Steiger E. Short bowel syndrome. Curr Treat Options Gastroenterol 2007;10:10.

263. Goswami R, Tandon RK, Dudha A, Kochupillai N. Prevalence and significance of steatorrhea in patients with active Graves' disease. Am J Gastroenterol 1998;93:1122.

264. Oelkers W. Adrenal insufficiency. N Engl J Med 1996;335:1206.

265. Hogenauer C, Meyer RL, Netto GJ, et al. Malabsorption due to cholecystokinin deficiency in a patient with autoimmune polyglandular syndrome type I. N Engl J Med 2001;344:270.

266. James WP. Intestinal absorption in protein-calorie malnutrition. Lancet 1968;1:333.

267. Hernandez G, Velasco N, Wainstein C, et al. Gut mucosal atrophy after a short enteral fasting period in critically ill patients. J Crit Care 1999;14:73.

268. Fine KD, Santa Ana CA, Fordtran JS. Diagnosis of magnesium-induced diarrhea. N Engl J Med 1991;324:1012.

269. Ho J, Moyer TP, Phillips SF. Chronic diarrhea: the role of magnesium. Mayo Clin Proc 1995;70:1091.

270. Crowley VE, Higham AD, Thompson DG, et al. Biochemical investigation of unexplained diarrhoea. J R Soc Med 1996;89:214P.

271. Kandil HE, Opper FH, Switzer BR, Heizer WD. Marked resistance of normal subjects to tube-feeding-induced diarrhea: the role of magnesium. Am J Clin Nutr 1993;57:73.

272. Backer LC. Assessing the acute gastrointestinal effects of ingesting naturally occurring, high levels of sulfate in drinking water. Crit Rev Clin Lab Sci 2000;37:389.

273. Gryboski JD. Diarrhea from dietetic candies. N Engl J Med 1966; 275:718.

274. Badiga MS, Jain NK, Casanova C, Pitchumoni CS. Diarrhea in diabetics: the role of sorbitol. J Am Coll Nutr 1990;9:578.

275. Hoekstra JH, van den Aker JH, Hartemink R, Kneepkens CM. Fruit juice malabsorption: not only fructose. Acta Paediatr 1995;84:1241.

276. Rumessen JJ, Gudmand-Hoyer E. Absorption capacity of fructose in healthy adults. Comparison with sucrose and its constituent monosaccharides. Gut 1986;27:1161.

277. Rumessen JJ, Gudmand-Hoyer E. Functional bowel disease: malabsorption and abdominal distress after ingestion of fructose, sorbitol, and fructose–sorbitol mixtures. Gastroenterology 1988;95:694.

278. Ledochowski M, Widner B, Bair H, et al. Fructose- and sorbitol-reduced diet improves mood and gastrointestinal disturbances in fructose malabsorbers. Scand J Gastroenterol 2000;35:1048.

279. Ament ME. Malabsorption of apple juice and pear nectar in infants and children: clinical implications. J Am Coll Nutr 1996;15:26S.

280. Woolridge MW, Fisher C. Colic, "overfeeding", and symptoms of lactose malabsorption in the breast-fed baby: a possible artifact of feed management? Lancet 1988;2:382.

281. Robayo-Torres CC, Quezada-Calvillo R, Nichols BL. Disaccharide digestion: clinical and molecular aspects. Clin Gastroenterol Hepatol 2006;4:276.

282. Bayless TM, Rothfeld B, Massa C, et al. Lactose and milk intolerance: clinical implications. N Engl J Med 1975;292:1156.

283. Vesa TH, Marteau P, Korpela R. Lactose intolerance. J Am Coll Nutr 2000;19:165S.

284. Shaw AD, Davies GJ. Lactose intolerance: problems in diagnosis and treatment. J Clin Gastroenterol 1999;28:208.

285. Park RH, Duncan A, Russell RI. Hypolactasia and Crohn's disease: a myth. Am J Gastroenterol 1990;85:708.

286. Kochhar R, Mehta SK, Goenka MK, et al. Lactose intolerance in idiopathic ulcerative colitis in north Indians. Indian J Med Res 1993;98:79.

287. Parker TJ, Woolner JT, Prevost AT, et al. Irritable bowel syndrome: is the search for lactose intolerance justified? Eur J Gastroenterol Hepatol 2001;13:219.

288. Suarez FL, Savaiano DA, Levitt MD. A comparison of symptoms after the consumption of milk or lactose-hydrolyzed milk by people with self-reported severe lactose intolerance. N Engl J Med 1995;333:1.

289. Arola H, Koivula T, Karvonen AL, et al. Low trehalase activity is associated with abdominal symptoms caused by edible mushrooms. Scand J Gastroenterol 1999;34:898.

290. Bond JH, Currier BE, Buchwald H, Levitt MD. Colonic conservation of malabsorbed carbohydrate. Gastroenterology 1980;78:444.

291. Stephen AM, Haddad AC, Phillips SF. Passage of carbohydrate into the colon. Direct measurements in humans. Gastroenterology 1983;85:589.

292. Fenton TR, Harries JT, Milla PJ. Disordered small intestinal motility: a rational basis for toddlers' diarrhoea. Gut 1983;24:897.

293. Kellow JE, Phillips SF. Altered small bowel motility in irritable bowel syndrome is correlated with symptoms. Gastroenterology 1987;92:1885.

294. Sellin JH, Hart R. Glucose malabsorption associated with rapid intestinal transit. Am J Gastroenterol 1992;87:584.

295. Tobin MV, Fisken RA, Diggory RT, et al. Orocaecal transit time in health and in thyroid disease. Gut 1989;30:26.

296. Rao SS, Read NW, Holdsworth CD. Is the diarrhoea in ulcerative colitis related to impaired colonic salvage of carbohydrate? Gut 1987;28:1090.

297. DuPont AW, Sellin JH. Ileostomy diarrhea. Curr Treat Options Gastroenterol 2006;9:39.

298. Editorial: Bile acids, diarrhoea, and SeHCAT. Lancet 1991;338:1563.

299. Hofmann AF, Poley JR. Role of bile acid malabsorption in pathogenesis of diarrhea and steatorrhea in patients with ileal resection. I. Response to cholestyramine or replacement of dietary long chain triglyceride by medium chain triglyceride. Gastroenterology 1972;62:918.

300. Hardison WG, Rosenberg IH. Bile-salt deficiency in the steatorrhea following resection of the ileum and proximal colon. N Engl J Med 1967;277:337.

301. Sciarretta G, Bonazzi L, Monti M, et al. Bile acid malabsorption in AIDS-associated chronic diarrhea: a prospective 1-year study. Am J Gastroenterol 1994;89:379.

302. Schiller LR, Hogan RB, Morawski SG, et al. Studies of the prevalence and significance of radiolabeled bile acid malabsorption in a group of patients with idiopathic chronic diarrhea. Gastroenterology 1987;92:151.

303. Schiller LR, Bilhartz LE, Santa Ana CA, Fordtran JS. Comparison of endogenous and radiolabeled bile acid excretion in patients with idiopathic chronic diarrhea. Gastroenterology 1990;98:1036.

304. Suhr O, Danielsson A, Steen L. Bile acid malabsorption caused by gastrointestinal motility dysfunction? An investigation of gastrointestinal disturbances in familial amyloidosis with polyneuropathy. Scand J Gastroenterol 1992;27:201.

305. Westergaard H. Bile Acid malabsorption. Curr Treat Options Gastroenterol 2007;10:28.

306. Heubi JE, Balistreri WF, Fondacaro JD, et al. Primary bile acid malabsorption: defective in vitro ileal active bile acid transport. Gastroenterology 1982;83:804.

307. Williams AJ, Merrick MV, Eastwood MA. Idiopathic bile acid malabsorption – a review of clinical presentation, diagnosis, and response to treatment. Gut 1991;32:1004.

308. Sciarretta G, Furno A, Morrone B, Malaguti P. Absence of histopathological changes of ileum and colon in functional chronic diarrhea associated with bile acid malabsorption, assessed by SeHCAT test: a prospective study. Am J Gastroenterol 1994;89:1058.

309. Smith MJ, Cherian P, Raju GS, et al. Bile acid malabsorption in persistent diarrhea. J R Coll Physicians Lond 2000;34:448.

310. Hearing SD, Thomas LA, Heaton KW, Hunt L. Effect of cholecystectomy on bowel function: a prospective, controlled study. Gut 1999; 45:889.

311. Suhr O, Danielsson A, Nyhlin H, Truedsson H. Bile acid malabsorption demonstrated by SeHCAT in chronic diarrhoea, with special reference to the impact of cholecystectomy. Scand J Gastroenterol 1988;23:1187.

312. Sciarretta G, Furno A, Mazzoni M, Malaguti P. Post-cholecystectomy diarrhea: evidence of bile acid malabsorption assessed by SeHCAT test. Am J Gastroenterol 1992;87:1852.

313. Cuschieri A. Postvagotomy diarrhoea: is there a place for surgical management? Gut 1990;31:245.

314. Raimes SA, Smirniotis V, Wheldon EJ, et al. Postvagotomy diarrhoea put into perspective. Lancet 1986;2:851.

315. al Hadrani A, Lavelle-Jones M, Kennedy N, et al. Bile acid malabsorption in patients with post-vagotomy diarrhoea. Ann Chir Gynaecol 1992;81:351.

316. Schein M. Highly selective vagotomy combined with cholecystectomy: is there an increased risk of diarrhea? World J Surg 1989; 13:782.

317. O'Brien JD, Thompson DG, McIntyre A, et al. Effect of codeine and loperamide on upper intestinal transit and absorption in normal subjects and patients with postvagotomy diarrhoea. Gut 1988;29: 312.

318. Bai J, Moran C, Martinez C, et al. Celiac sprue after surgery of the upper gastrointestinal tract. Report of 10 patients with special attention to diagnosis, clinical behavior, and follow-up. J Clin Gastroenterol 1991;13:521.

319. Camilleri M, Heading RC, Thompson WG. Clinical perspectives, mechanisms, diagnosis and management of irritable bowel syndrome. Aliment Pharmacol Ther 2002;16:1407.

320. Talley NJ, Spiller R. Irritable bowel syndrome: a little understood organic bowel disease? Lancet 2002;360:555.

321. Dellon ES, Ringel Y. Treatment of functional diarrhea. Curr Treat Options Gastroenterol 2006;9:331.

322. Lembo AJ, Olden KW, Ameen VZ, et al. Effect of alosetron on bowel urgency and global symptoms in women with severe, diarrhea-predominant irritable bowel syndrome: analysis of two controlled trials. Clin Gastroenterol Hepatol 2004;2:675.

323. Kulke MH, Mayer RJ. Carcinoid tumors. N Engl J Med 1999;340:858.

324. O'Neil BH, Venook AP. Management of carcinoid tumors and the carcinoid syndrome. Clin Perspect Gastrol 2001;279.

325. Modlin IM, Latich I, Kidd M, et al. Therapeutic options for gastrointestinal carcinoids. Clin Gastroenterol Hepatol 2006;4:526.

326. Roy PK, Venzon DJ, Shojamanesh H, et al. Zollinger–Ellison syndrome. Clinical presentation in 261 patients. Medicine (Baltimore) 2000;79:379.

327. Rambaud JC, Modigliani R, Emonts P, et al. Fluid secretion in the duodenum and intestinal handling of water and electrolytes in Zollinger–Ellison syndrome. Am J Dig Dis 1978;23:1089.

328. Hirschowitz BI, Simmons J, Mohnen J. Clinical outcome using lansoprazole in acid hypersecretors with and without Zollinger–Ellison syndrome: a 13-year prospective study. Clin Gastroenterol Hepatol 2005;3:39.

329. Abou-Saif A, Lei J, McDonald TJ, et al. A new cause of Zollinger–Ellison syndrome: non-small cell lung cancer. Gastroenterology 2001;120:1271.

330. Hirasawa K, Yamada M, Kitagawa M, et al. Ovarian mucinous cystadenocarcinoma as a cause of Zollinger–Ellison syndrome: report of a case and review of the literature. Am J Gastroenterol 2000;95:1348.

331. Gibril F, Jensen RT. Pancreatic endocrine tumors: recent insights. Clin Perspect Gastroenterol 2001;19.

332. Jensen RT. Overview of chronic diarrhea caused by functional neuroendocrine neoplasms. Semin Gastrointest Dis 1999;10:156.

333. Rood RP, DeLellis RA, Dayal Y, Donowitz M. Pancreatic cholera syndrome due to a vasoactive intestinal polypeptide-producing tumor: further insights into the pathophysiology. Gastroenterology 1988;94:813.

334. Eriksson B, Oberg K, Skogseid B. Neuroendocrine pancreatic tumors. Clinical findings in a prospective study of 84 patients. Acta Oncol 1989;28:373.

335. Kimura N, Yamamoto H, Okamoto H, et al. Multiple-hormone gene expression in ganglioneuroblastoma with watery diarrhea, hypokalemia, and achlorhydria syndrome. Cancer 1993;71:2841.

336. Murphy MS, Sibal A, Mann JR. Persistent diarrhoea and occult vipomas in children. BMJ 2000;320:1524.

337. Modigliani E, Franc B, Niccoli-Sire P. Diagnosis and treatment of medullary thyroid cancer. Baillières Best Pract Res Clin Endocrinol Metab 2000;14:631.

338. Gimm O, Sutter T, Dralle H. Diagnosis and therapy of sporadic and familial medullary thyroid carcinoma. J Cancer Res Clin Oncol 2001;127:156.

339. Hansford JR, Mulligan LM. Multiple endocrine neoplasia type 2 and RET: from neoplasia to neurogenesis. J Med Genet 2000;37:817.

340. Isaacs P, Whittaker SM, Turnberg LA. Diarrhea associated with medullary carcinoma of the thyroid. Studies of intestinal function in a patient. Gastroenterology 1974;67:521.

341. Rambaud JC, Jian R, Flourie B, et al. Pathophysiological study of diarrhoea in a patient with medullary thyroid carcinoma. Evidence against a secretory mechanism and for the role of shortened colonic transit time. Gut 1988;29:537.

342. Chastain MA. The glucagonoma syndrome: a review of its features and discussion of new perspectives. Am J Med Sci 2001;321:306.

343. Older J, Older P, Colker J, Brown R. Secretory villous adenomas that cause depletion syndrome. Arch Intern Med 1999;159:879.

344. Duthie HL, Atwell JD. The absorption of water, sodium, and potassium in the large intestine with particular reference to the effects of villous papillomas. Gut 1963;4:373.

345. Stulc JP, Petrelli NJ, Herrera L, Mittelman A. Colorectal villous and tubulovillous adenomas equal to or greater than four centimeters. Ann Surg 1988;207:65.

346. DaCruz GM, Gardner FJ, Peskin GW. Mechanism of diarrhea of villous adenomas. Am J Surg 1968;115:203.

347. Steven K, Lange P, Bukhave K, Rask-Madsen J. Prostaglandin E2-mediated secretory diarrhea in villous adenoma of rectum: effect of treatment with indomethacin. Gastroenterology 1981;80:1562.

348. Pugh S, Thomas GA. Patients with adenomatous polyps and carcinomas have increased colonic mucosal prostaglandin F2. Gut 1994;35:675.

349. Smelt AH, Meinders AE, Hoekman K, et al. Secretory diarrhea in villous adenoma of rectum: effect of treatment with somatostatin and indomethacin. Prostaglandins 1992;43:567.

350. Worobec AS. Treatment of systemic mast cell disorders. Hematol Oncol Clin North Am 2000;14:659.

351. Bytzer P, Stokholm M, Andersen I, et al. Prevalence of surreptitious laxative abuse in patients with diarrhoea of uncertain origin: a cost benefit analysis of a screening procedure. Gut 1989;30:1379.

352. Pollok RC, Banks MR, Fairclough PD, Farthing MJ. Dilutional diarrhoea: under-diagnosed and over-investigated. Eur J Gastroenterol Hepatol 2000;12:609.

353. Phillips SF. Surreptitious laxative abuse: keep it in mind. Semin Gastrointest Dis 1999;10:132.

354. Ewe K, Karbach U. Factitious diarrhoea. Clin Gastroenterol 1986;15:723.

355. Read NW, Krejs GJ, Read MG, et al. Chronic diarrhea of unknown origin. Gastroenterology 1980;78:264.

356. Duncan A, Cameron A, Stewart MJ, Russell RI. Diagnosis of the abuse of magnesium and stimulant laxatives. Ann Clin Biochem 1991;28:568.

357. Duncan A. Screening for surreptitious laxative abuse. Ann Clin Biochem 2000;37:1.

358. Kacere RD, Srivatsa SS, Tremaine WJ, et al. Chronic diarrhea due to surreptitious use of bisacodyl: case reports and methods for detection. Mayo Clin Proc 1993;68:355.

359. Binder HJ. Pharmacology of laxatives. Annu Rev Pharmacol Toxicol 1977;17:355.

360. Fine KD. Diarrhea. In: Felmann M, Scharschmidt BF, Sleisenger MH (eds). Gastrointestinal and liver disease: pathophysiology, diagnosis, management. Philadelphia: W. B. Saunders, 1998:128.

361. Meyers AM, Feldman C, Sonnekus MI, et al. Chronic laxative abusers with pseudo-idiopathic oedema and autonomous pseudo-Bartter's syndrome. A spectrum of metabolic madness, or new lights on an old disease? S Afr Med J 1990;78:631.

362. Dick WH, Lingeman JE, Preminger GM, et al. Laxative abuse as a cause for ammonium urate renal calculi. J Urol 1990;143:244.

363. Chan AA, Salcedo JR, Atkins DM, Ruley EJ. Munchausen syndrome by proxy: a review and case study. J Pediatr Psychol 1986;11:1.

364. Rosenberg DA. Web of deceit: a literature review of Munchausen syndrome by proxy. Child Abuse Negl 1987;11:547.

365. Fordtran JS, Santa Ana CA, Morawski SG, et al. Pathophysiology of chronic diarrhoea: insights derived from intestinal perfusion studies in 31 patients. Clin Gastroenterol 1986;15:477.

366. Afzalpurkar RG, Schiller LR, Little KH, et al. The self-limited nature of chronic idiopathic diarrhea. N Engl J Med 1992;327:1849.

367. Lysy J, Israeli E, Goldin E. The prevalence of chronic diarrhea among diabetic patients. Am J Gastroenterol 1999;94:2165.

368. Talley NJ, Young L, Bytzer P, et al. Impact of chronic gastrointestinal symptoms in diabetes mellitus on health-related quality of life. Am J Gastroenterol 2001;96:71.

369. Ogbonnaya KI, Arem R. Diabetic diarrhea. Pathophysiology, diagnosis, and management. Arch Intern Med 1990;150:262.

370. Valdovinos MA, Camilleri M, Zimmerman BR. Chronic diarrhea in diabetes mellitus: mechanisms and an approach to diagnosis and treatment. Mayo Clin Proc 1993;68:691.

371. Chang EB, Fedorak RN, Field M. Experimental diabetic diarrhea in rats. Intestinal mucosal denervation hypersensitivity and treatment with clonidine. Gastroenterology 1986;91:564.

372. Chang EB, Bergenstal RM, Field M. Diarrhea in streptozocin-treated rats. Loss of adrenergic regulation of intestinal fluid and electrolyte transport. J Clin Invest 1985;75:1666.

373. Fedorak RN, Field M, Chang EB. Treatment of diabetic diarrhea with clonidine. Ann Intern Med 1985;102:197.

374. Schiller LR, Santa Ana CA, Schmulen AC, et al. Pathogenesis of fecal incontinence in diabetes mellitus: evidence for internal-anal-sphincter dysfunction. N Engl J Med 1982;307:1666.

375. Walker JJ, Kaplan DS. Efficacy of the somatostatin analog octreotide in the treatment of two patients with refractory diabetic diarrhea. Am J Gastroenterol 1993;88:765.

376. Rubin E, Rybak BJ, Lindenbaum J, et al. Ultrastructural changes in the small intestine induced by ethanol. Gastroenterology 1972;63:801.

377. Ray M, Dinda PK, Beck IT. Mechanism of ethanol-induced jejunal microvascular and morphologic changes in the dog. Gastroenterology 1989;96:345.

378. Colombel JF, Hallgren R, Venge P, et al. Neutrophil and eosinophil involvement of the small bowel affected by chronic alcoholism. Gut 1988;29:1656.

379. Leddin DJ, Ray M, Dinda PK, et al. 16,16-Dimethyl prostaglandin E2 alleviates jejunal microvascular effects of ethanol but not the ethanol-induced inhibition of water, sodium, and glucose absorption. Gastroenterology 1988;94:726.

380. Wegener M, Schaffstein J, Dilger U, et al. Gastrointestinal transit of solid–liquid meal in chronic alcoholics. Dig Dis Sci 1991;36:917.

381. Bouchoucha M, Nalpas B, Berger M, et al. Recovery from disturbed colonic transit time after alcohol withdrawal. Dis Colon Rectum 1991;34:111.

382. Hamilton JR, Reilly BJ, Morecki R. Short small intestine associated with malrotation: a newly described congenital cause of intestinal malabsorption. Gastroenterology 1969;56:124.

383. Phillips AD, Schmitz J. Familial microvillous atrophy: a clinico-pathological survey of 23 cases. J Pediatr Gastroenterol Nutr 1992;14:380.

384. Jonas MM, Bell MD, Eidson MS, et al. Congenital diabetes mellitus and fatal secretory diarrhea in two infants. J Pediatr Gastroenterol Nutr 1991;13:415.

385. Aichbichler BW, Zerr CH, Santa Ana CA, et al. Proton-pump inhibition of gastric chloride secretion in congenital chloridorrhea. N Engl J Med 1997;336:106.

386. Holmberg C. Congenital chloride diarrhoea. Clin Gastroenterol 1986;15:583.

387. Kere J, Lohi H, Hoglund P. Genetic disorders of membrane transport III. Congenital chloride diarrhea. Am J Physiol 1999;276:G7.

388. Muller T, Wijmenga C, Phillips AD, et al. Congenital sodium diarrhea is an autosomal recessive disorder of sodium/proton exchange but unrelated to known candidate genes. Gastroenterology 2000;119:1506.

389. Holmberg C, Perheentupa J. Congenital Na+ diarrhea: a new type of secretory diarrhea. J Pediatr 1985;106:56.

390. Booth IW, Stange G, Murer H, et al. Defective jejunal brush-border Na+/H+ exchange: a cause of congenital secretory diarrhoea. Lancet 1985;1:1066.

391. Cutz E, Rhoads JM, Drumm B, et al. Microvillus inclusion disease: an inherited defect of brush-border assembly and differentiation. N Engl J Med 1989;320:646.

392. Rhoads JM, Vogler RC, Lacey SR, et al. Microvillus inclusion disease. In vitro jejunal electrolyte transport. Gastroenterology 1991;100:811.

393. Murch SH, Winyard PJ, Koletzko S, et al. Congenital enterocyte heparan sulphate deficiency with massive albumin loss, secretory diarrhoea, and malnutrition. Lancet 1996;347:1299.

394. Sawczenko A, Sandhu BK. Newer diarrheal syndromes. Indian J Pediatr 1999;66:S46.

395. Baud O, Goulet O, Canioni D, et al. Treatment of the immune dysregulation, polyendocrinopathy, enteropathy, X-linked syndrome (IPEX) by allogeneic bone marrow transplantation. N Engl J Med 2001;344:1758.

396. Wisuthsarewong W, Likitmaskul S, Manonukul J. Satoyoshi syndrome. Pediatr Dermatol 2001;18:406.

397. Hogenauer C, Meyer RL, Netto GJ, et al. Malabsorption due to cholecystokinin deficiency in a patient with autoimmune polyglandular syndrome type I. N Engl J Med 2001;344:270.

398. Wang J, Cortina G, Wu SV, et al. Mutant neurogenin-3 in congenital malabsorptive diarrhea. N Engl J Med 2006;355:270.

399. Binder HJ. Causes of chronic diarrhea. N Engl J Med 2006;355:236.

400. Binder HJ, Ptak T. Jejunal absorption of water and electrolytes in inflammatory bowel disease. J Lab Clin Med 1970;76:915.

401. Parkes M, Jewell DP. Review article: the management of severe Crohn's disease. Aliment Pharmacol Ther 2001;15:563.

402. Kelly KJ. Eosinophilic gastroenteritis. J Pediatr Gastroenterol Nutr 2000;30 Suppl:S28.

403. Lake AM. Food-induced eosinophilic proctocolitis. J Pediatr Gastroenterol Nutr 2000;30 Suppl:S58.

404. Talley NJ, Shorter RG, Phillips SF, Zinsmeister AR. Eosinophilic gastroenteritis: a clinicopathological study of patients with disease of the mucosa, muscle layer, and subserosal tissues. Gut 1990;31:54.

405. Corsetti M, Basilisco G, Pometta R, et al. Mistaken diagnosis of eosinophilic colitis. Ital J Gastroenterol Hepatol 1999;31:607.

406. Copeland BH, Aramide OO, Wehbe SA, et al. Eosinophilia in a patient with cyclical vomiting: a case report. Clin Mol Allergy 2004;2:7.

407. Perez-Millan A, Martin-Lorente JL, Lopez-Morante A, et al. Subserosal eosinophilic gastroenteritis treated efficaciously with sodium cromoglycate. Dig Dis Sci 1997;42:342.

408. Sicherer SH. Food protein-induced enterocolitis syndrome: clinical perspectives. J Pediatr Gastroenterol Nutr 2000;30 Suppl:S45.

409. Odze RD, Bines J, Leichtner AM, et al. Allergic proctocolitis in infants: a prospective clinicopathologic biopsy study. Hum Pathol 1993;24:668.

410. Iacono G, Cavataio F, Montalto G, et al. Intolerance of cow's milk and chronic constipation in children. N Engl J Med 1998;339:1100.

411. Sampson HA. Food anaphylaxis. Br Med Bull 2000;56:925.

412. Sicherer SH. Food allergy. Lancet 2002;360:701.

413. Bischoff SC. Food allergies. Curr Treat Options Gastroenterol 2007;10:34.

414. Schiller LR. Microscopic colitis syndrome: lymphocytic colitis and collagenous colitis. Semin Gastrointest Dis 1999;10:145.

415. Nielsen OH, Vainer B, Schaffalitzky de Muckadell OB. Microscopic colitis: a missed diagnosis? Lancet 2004;364:2055.

416. Pardi DS. Microscopic colitis: an update. Inflamm Bowel Dis 2004;10:860.

417. Olesen M, Eriksson S, Bohr J, et al. Lymphocytic colitis: a retrospective clinical study of 199 Swedish patients. Gut 2004;53:536.

418. Stroehlein JR. Microscopic colitis. Curr Opin Gastroenterol 2004;20:27.

419. Freeman HJ. Collagenous mucosal inflammatory diseases of the gastrointestinal tract. Gastroenterology 2005;129:338.

420. Nyhlin N, Bohr J, Eriksson S, Tysk C. Systematic review: microscopic colitis. Aliment Pharmacol Ther 2006;23:1525.

421. Rask-Madsen J, Grove O, Hansen MG, et al. Colonic transport of water and electrolytes in a patient with secretory diarrhea due to collagenous colitis. Dig Dis Sci 1983;28:1141.

422. Matteoni CA, Goldblum JR, Wang N, et al. Celiac disease is highly prevalent in lymphocytic colitis. J Clin Gastroenterol 2001;32:225.

423. Jarnerot G, Tysk C, Bohr J, Eriksson S. Collagenous colitis and fecal stream diversion. Gastroenterology 1995;109:449.

424. Clouse RE, Alpers DH, Hockenbery DM, DeSchryver-Kecskemeti K. Pericrypt eosinophilic enterocolitis and chronic diarrhea. Gastroenterology 1992;103:168.

425. Jeong YS, Jun JB, Kim TH, et al. Successful treatment of protein-losing enteropathy due to AA amyloidosis with somatostatin analogue and high dose steroid in ankylosing spondylitis. Clin Exp Rheumatol 2000;18:619.

426. Greenberger NJ, Tennenbaum JI, Ruppert RD. Protein-losing entero-pathy associated with gastrointestinal allergy. Am J Med 1967;43: 777.

427. Tsutsumi A, Sugiyama T, Matsumura R, et al. Protein losing enteropathy associated with collagen diseases. Ann Rheum Dis 1991;50:178.

428. Settle SH, Washington K, Lind C, et al. Chronic treatment of Ménétrier's disease with Erbitux: clinical efficacy and insight into pathophysiology. Clin Gastroenterol Hepatol 2005;3:654.

429. Andreyev J. Gastrointestinal complications of pelvic radiotherapy: are they of any importance? Gut 2005;54:1051.

430. Hong JJ, Park W, Ehrenpreis ED. Review article: current therapeutic options for radiation proctopathy. Aliment Pharmacol Ther 2001; 15:1253.

431. Brandt LJ. Bloody diarrhea in an elderly patient. Gastroenterology 2005;128:157.

432. Davis GR, Corbett DB, Krejs GJ. Ileal chloride secretion as a cause of secretory diarrhea in a patient with primary intestinal tuberculosis. Gastroenterology 1979;76:829.

433. Cappell MS, Mandell W, Grimes MM, Neu HC. Gastrointestinal histoplasmosis. Dig Dis Sci 1988;33:353.

434. Naganuma M, Iwao Y, Inoue N, et al. Analysis of clinical course and long-term prognosis of surgical and nonsurgical patients with intestinal Behçet's disease. Am J Gastroenterol 2000;95:2848.

435. Bayraktar Y, Ozaslan E, Van Thiel DH. Gastrointestinal manifesta-tions of Behçet's disease. J Clin Gastroenterol 2000;30:144.

436. Memain N, De BM, Guillevin L, et al. Delayed relapse of Churg–Strauss syndrome manifesting as colon ulcers with mucosal granulomas: 3 cases. J Rheumatol 2002;29:388.

437. Ross WA, Couriel D. Colonic graft-versus-host disease. Curr Opin Gastroenterol 2005;21:64.

438. Abbasoglu O, Cakmakci M. Neutropenic enterocolitis in patients without leukemia. Surgery 1993;113:113.

439. Daniel ES, Ludwig SL, Lewin KJ, et al. The Cronkhite–Canada syn-drome. An analysis of clinical and pathologic features and therapy in 55 patients. Medicine (Baltimore) 1982;61:293.

440. Ward EM, Wolfsen HC. The non-inherited gastrointestinal poly-posis syndromes. Aliment Pharmacol Ther 2002;16:333.

441. Puspok A, Kiener HP, Oberhuber G. Clinical, endoscopic, and his-tologic spectrum of nonsteroidal anti-inflammatory drug-induced lesions in the colon. Dis Colon Rectum 2000;43:685.

442. Weintraub R, Pramanik S, Levitt L. Diffuse small-bowel myeloma-tosis. N Engl J Med 2004;350:842.

443. Kneepkens CM, Hoekstra JH. Chronic nonspecific diarrhea of child-hood: pathophysiology and management. Pediatr Clin North Am 1996;43:375.

444. Harewood GC, Murray JA. Approaching the patient with chronic malabsorption syndrome. Semin Gastrointest Dis 1999;10:138.

445. Donowitz M, Kokke FT, Saidi R. Evaluation of patients with chronic diarrhea. N Engl J Med 1995;332:725.

446. Greenberger NJ. Diagnostic approach to the patient with a chronic diarrheal disorder. Dis Mon 1990;36:131.

447. Soergel KH. Evaluation of chronic diarrhea, Part 2. Pract Gastro-enterol 1992;16:25.

448. Headstrom PD, Surawicz CM. Chronic diarrhea. Clin Gastroenterol Hepatol 2005;3:734.

449. Watanabe, JM and Surawicz, CM. Diarrhea in the older patient. Geriatrics & Aging 2004;7:20.

450. Geraedts AA, Esseveld MR, Tytgot GN. The value of noninvasive examination of patients with chronic diarrhea. Scand J Gastroenterol 1988;23:46.

451. Bertomeu A, Ros E, Barragan V, et al. Chronic diarrhea with normal stool and colonic examinations: organic or functional? J Clin Gastroenterol 1991;13:531.

452. Trier JS. Intestinal malabsorption: differentiation of cause. Hosp Pract (Off Ed) 1988;23:195.

453. Caspary WF, Stein J. Diseases of the small intestine. Eur J Gastroenterol Hepatol 1999;11:21.

454. Bo-Linn GW, Fordtran JS. Fecal fat concentration in patients with steatorrhea. Gastroenterology 1984;87:319.

455. Levitt MD, Duane WC. Floating stools – flatus versus fat. N Engl J Med 1972;286:973.

456. Lomoschitz F, Schima W, Schober E, et al. Enteroclysis in adult celiac disease: diagnostic value of specific radiographic features. Eur Radiol 2003;13:890.

457. Rettenbacher T, Hollerweger A, Macheiner P, et al. Adult celiac dis-ease: US signs. Radiology 1999;211:389.

458. Sturniolo GC, Di L, V, Vettorato MG, et al. Small bowel exploration by wireless capsule endoscopy: results from 314 procedures. Am J Med 2006;119:341.

459. Biagi F, Rondonotti E, Campanella J, et al. Video capsule endoscopy and histology for small-bowel mucosa evaluation: a comparison performed by blinded observers. Clin Gastroenterol Hepatol 2006; 4:998.

460. Dickey W, Hughes D. Prevalence of celiac disease and its endoscopic markers among patients having routine upper gastrointestinal endo-scopy. Am J Gastroenterol 1999;94:2182.

461. Ravelli AM, Tobanelli P, Minelli L, et al. Endoscopic features of celiac disease in children. Gastrointest Endosc 2001;54:736.

462. Shah VH, Rotterdam H, Kotler DP, et al. All that scallops is not celiac disease. Gastrointest Endosc 2000;51:717.

463. Ponec RJ, Hackman RC, McDonald GB. Endoscopic and histologic diagnosis of intestinal graft-versus-host disease after marrow trans-plantation. Gastrointest Endosc 1999;49:612.

464. Michael H, Brandt LJ, Tanaka KE, et al. Congo-red negative colonic amyloid with scalloping of the valvulae conniventes. Gastrointest Endosc 2001;53:653.

465. Lee SK, Green PH. Endoscopy in celiac disease. Curr Opin Gastroenterol 2005;21:589.

466. Niveloni S, Fiorini A, Dezi R, et al. Usefulness of videoduo-denoscopy and vital dye staining as indicators of mucosal atrophy of celiac disease: assessment of interobserver agreement. Gastrointest Endosc 1998;47:223.

467. Cellier C, Cuillerier E, Patey-Mariaud DS, et al. Push enteroscopy in celiac sprue and refractory sprue. Gastrointest Endosc 1999;50:613.

468. Cuillerier E, Landi B, Cellier C. Is push enteroscopy useful in patients with malabsorption of unclear origin? Am J Gastroenterol 2001;96:2103.

469. Thomson M, Kitching P, Jones A, et al. Are endoscopic biopsies of small bowel as good as suction biopsies for diagnosis of entero-pathy? J Pediatr Gastroenterol Nutr 1999;29:438.

470. Greene HL, Rosensweig NS, Lufkin EG, et al. Biopsy of the small intestine with the Crosby–Kugler capsule. Experience in 3866 per-oral biopsies in children and adults. Am J Dig Dis 1974;19:189.

471. Gottrand F, Turck D, Mitchell V, Farriaux JP. Comparison of fiberen-doscopy and Watson capsule for small intestinal biopsy in infants and children. Acta Paediatr 1992;81:399.

472. Granot E, Goodman-Weill M, Pizov G, Sherman Y. Histological comparison of suction capsule and endoscopic small intestinal mucosal biopsies in children. J Pediatr Gastroenterol Nutr 1993; 16:397.

473. Babbin BA, Crawford K, Sitaraman SV. Malabsorption work-up: utility of small bowel biopsy. Clin Gastroenterol Hepatol 2006;4: 1193.

474. Owens SR, Greenson JK. The pathology of malabsorption: current concepts. Histopathology 2007;50:64.

475. Oberhuber G, Granditsch G, Vogelsang H. The histopathology of coeliac disease: time for a standardized report scheme for patholo-gists. Eur J Gastroenterol Hepatol 1999;11:1185.

476. Oberhuber G. Histopathology of celiac disease. Biomed Phar-macother 2000;54:368.

477. Freeman HJ. Small intestinal mucosal biopsy for investigation of diarrhea and malabsorption in adults. Gastrointest Endosc Clin N Am 2000;10:739.

478. Trier JS. Diagnostic value of peroral biopsy of the proximal small intestine. N Engl J Med 1971;285:1470.

479. Thomas AG, Phillips AD, Walker-Smith JA. The value of proximal small intestinal biopsy in the differential diagnosis of chronic diarrhoea. Arch Dis Child 1992;67:741.

480. Lankisch PG, Droge M, Hofses S, et al. Steatorrhoea: you cannot trust your eyes when it comes to diagnosis. Lancet 1996;347:1620.

481. Lankisch PG, Droge M, Konig H, et al. Fecal weight determination can unfortunately not replace unpopular and costly fecal fat estimation in the diagnosis of steatorrhea. Int J Pancreatol 1999;25:71.

482. Wiggins HS, Howell KE, Kellock TD, Stalder J. The origin of faecal fat. Gut 1969;10:400.

483. Khouri MR, Huang G, Shiau YF. Sudan stain of fecal fat: new insight into an old test. Gastroenterology 1989;96:421.

484. Drummey GD, Benson JA, Jr., Jones CM. Microscopical examination of the stool for steatorrhea. N Engl J Med 1961;264:85.

485. Ghosh SK, Littlewood JM, Goddard D, Steel AE. Stool microscopy in screening for steatorrhoea. J Clin Pathol 1977;30:749.

486. Rosenberg IH, Sitrin MD. Screening for fat malabsorption. Ann Intern Med 1981;95:776.

487. Balasekaran R, Porter JL, Santa Ana CA, Fordtran JS. Positive results on tests for steatorrhea in persons consuming olestra potato chips. Ann Intern Med 2000;132:279.

488. Phuapradit P, Narang A, Mendonca P, et al. The steatocrit: a simple method for estimating stool fat content in newborn infants. Arch Dis Child 1981;56:725.

489. Guarino A, Tarallo L, Greco L, et al. Reference values of the steatocrit and its modifications in diarrheal diseases. J Pediatr Gastroenterol Nutr 1992;14:268.

490. Lloyd DR, Rawashdeh MO, Booth IW, Brown GA. The steatocrit: an improved procedure. Ann Clin Biochem 1992;29:535.

491. Van de Kamer JH, Ten Bokkel Huinink H, Weyers HA. Rapid method for the determination of fat in feces. J Biol Chem 1949;177:347.

492. Jakobs BS, Volmer M, Swinkels DW, et al. New method for faecal fat determination by mid-infrared spectroscopy, using a transmission cell: an improvement in standardization. Ann Clin Biochem 2000;37:343.

493. Ditchburn RK, Smith AH, Hayter CJ. Use of unabsorbed radioactive marker substances in a re-assessment of the radioactive triolein test of fat absorption. J Clin Pathol 1971;24:506.

494. Fine KD, Fordtran JS. The effect of diarrhea on fecal fat excretion. Gastroenterology 1992;102:1936.

495. Vantrappen G, Ghoos Y, Andriulli A. CO_2- and H_2 breath tests in the diagnosis of intestinal malabsorption. Ital J Gastroenterol 1992;24:212.

496. Newcomer AD, Hofmann AF, DiMagno EP, et al. Triolein breath test: a sensitive and specific test for fat malabsorption. Gastroenterology 1979;76:6.

497. Pedersen NT, Jorgensen BB, Rannem T. The ^{14}C-triolein breath test is not valid as a test of fat absorption. Scand J Clin Lab Invest 1991;51:699.

498. Duncan A, Cameron A, Stewart MJ, Russell RI. Limitations of the triolein breath test. Clin Chim Acta 1992;205:51.

499. Craig RM, Atkinson AJ, Jr. D-xylose testing: a review. Gastroenterology 1988;95:223.

500. Craig RM, Ehrenpreis ED. D-xylose testing. J Clin Gastroenterol 1999;29:143.

501. Manes G, Kahl S, Glasbrenner B, Malfertheiner P. Chronic pancreatitis: diagnosis and staging. Ann Ital Chir 2000;71:23.

502. DiMagno EP. A perspective on the use of tubeless pancreatic function tests in diagnosis. Gut 1998;43:2.

503. Chowdhury RS, Forsmark CE. Review article: pancreatic function testing. Aliment Pharmacol Ther 2003;17:733.

504. Heyman MB. The bentiromide test: how good is it? Gastroenterology 1985;89:685.

505. Toskes PP. Update on diagnosis and management of chronic pancreatitis. Curr Gastroenterol Rep 1999;1:145.

506. Augarten A, Dubenbaum L, Yahav Y, et al. Lundh meal: a single non-invasive challenge test for evaluation of exocrine and endocrine pancreatic function in cystic fibrosis patients. Int J Clin Lab Res 1999;29:114.

507. Stevens T, Conwell DL, Zuccaro G, et al. Electrolyte composition of endoscopically collected duodenal drainage fluid after synthetic porcine secretin stimulation in healthy subjects. Gastrointest Endosc 2004;60:351.

508. Meyers JS, Ehrenpreis ED, Craig RM. Small intestinal bacterial overgrowth syndrome. Curr Treat Options Gastroenterol 2001;4:7.

509. Isaacs PE, Kim YS. The contaminated small bowel syndrome. Am J Med 1979;67:1049.

510. Riordan SM, McIver CJ, Duncombe VM, et al. Evaluation of the rice breath hydrogen test for small intestinal bacterial overgrowth. Am J Gastroenterol 2000;95:2858.

511. Toskes PP. Small intestine bacterial overgrowth, including blind loop syndrome. In: Blaser MJ, Smith PD, Ravdin JI et al. (eds). Infections of the gastrointestinal tract. New York: Raven Press, 1995:343.

512. Fine KD, Seidel RH, Do K. The prevalence, anatomic distribution, and diagnosis of colonic causes of chronic diarrhea. Gastrointest Endosc 2000;51:318.

513. Farivar S, Fromm H, Schindler D, Schmidt FW. Sensitivity of bile acid breath test in the diagnosis of bacterial overgrowth in the small intestine with and without the stagnant (blind) loop syndrome. Dig Dis Sci 1979;24:33.

514. Suhr O, Danielsson A, Horstedt P, Stenling R. Bacterial contamination of the small bowel evaluated by breath tests, ^{75}Se-labelled homocholic-tauro acid, and scanning electron microscopy. Scand J Gastroenterol 1990;25:841.

515. Joo JS, Ehrenpreis ED, Gonzalez L, et al. Alterations in colonic anatomy induced by chronic stimulant laxatives: the cathartic colon revisited. J Clin Gastroenterol 1998;26:283.

516. Jensen RT, Gibril F. Somatostatin receptor scintigraphy in gastrinomas. Ital J Gastroenterol Hepatol 1999;31 Suppl 2:S179.

517. Krausz Y, Rosler A, Guttmann H, et al. Somatostatin receptor scintigraphy for early detection of regional and distant metastases of medullary carcinoma of the thyroid. Clin Nucl Med 1999;24:256.

518. Zimmer T, Scherubl H, Faiss S, et al. Endoscopic ultrasonography of neuroendocrine tumours. Digestion 2000;62 Suppl 1:45.

519. Kwekkeboom DJ, Bakker WH, Kooij PP, et al. Cholecystokinin receptor imaging using an octapeptide DTPA-CCK analogue in patients with medullary thyroid carcinoma. Eur J Nucl Med 2000;27:1312.

520. Wittoesch JH, Jackman RJ, McDonald JR. Melanosis coli: general review and a study of 887 cases. Dis Colon Rectum 1958;1:172.

521. Pardi DS, Tremaine WJ, Rothenberg HJ, Batts KP. Melanosis coli in inflammatory bowel disease. J Clin Gastroenterol 1998;26:167.

522. Cuvelier C, Demetter P, Mielants H, et al. Interpretation of ileal biopsies: morphological features in normal and diseased mucosa. Histopathology 2001;38:1.

523. Marshall JB, Singh R, Diaz-Arias AA. Chronic, unexplained diarrhea: are biopsies necessary if colonoscopy is normal? Am J Gastroenterol 1995;90:372.

524. Patel Y, Pettigrew NM, Grahame GR, Bernstein CN. The diagnostic yield of lower endoscopy plus biopsy in nonbloody diarrhea. Gastrointest Endosc 1997;46:338.

525. Surawicz CM, Haggitt RC, Husseman M, McFarland LV. Mucosal biopsy diagnosis of colitis: acute self-limited colitis and idiopathic inflammatory bowel disease. Gastroenterology 1994;107:755.

526. Lamps LW. Infective disorders of the gastrointestinal tract. Histopathology 2007;50:55.

527. Hoekstra JH. Fructose breath hydrogen tests in infants with chronic non-specific diarrhoea. Eur J Pediatr 1995;154:362.

528. Perman JA. Clinical application of breath hydrogen measurements. Can J Physiol Pharmacol 1991;69:111.

529. Strocchi A, Corazza G, Ellis CJ, et al. Detection of malabsorption of low doses of carbohydrate: accuracy of various breath H_2 criteria. Gastroenterology 1993;105:1404.

530. Newcomer AD, McGill DB, Thomas PJ, Hofman AF. Prospective comparison of indirect methods for detecting lactase deficiency. N Engl J Med 1975;293:1232.

531. Ford GA, Preece JD, Davies IH, Wilkinson SP. Use of the SeHCAT test in the investigation of diarrhoea. Postgrad Med J 1992;68:272.

532. Rudberg U, Nylander B. Radiological bile acid absorption test ^{75}SeHCAT in patients with diarrhoea of unknown cause. Acta Radiol 1996;37:672.

533. Sauter GH, Munzing W, von Ritter C, Paumgartner G. Bile acid malabsorption as a cause of chronic diarrhea: diagnostic value of 7-alpha-hydroxy-4-cholesten-3-one in serum. Dig Dis Sci 1999;44:14.

534. Koch TR, Michener SR, Go VL. Plasma vasoactive intestinal polypeptide concentration determination in patients with diarrhea. Gastroenterology 1991;100:99.

535. Schiller LR, Rivera LM, Santangelo WC, et al. Diagnostic value of fasting plasma peptide concentrations in patients with chronic diarrhea. Dig Dis Sci 1994;39:2216.

536. Almer S, Bodemar G, Franzen L, et al. Use of air enema radiography to assess depth of ulceration during acute attacks of ulcerative colitis. Lancet 1996;347:1731.

537. Horton KM, Corl FM, Fishman EK. CT evaluation of the colon: inflammatory disease. Radiographics 2000;20:399.

538. Schreyer AG, Geissler A, Albrich H, et al. Abdominal MRI after enteroclysis or with oral contrast in patients with suspected or proven Crohn's disease. Clin Gastroenterol Hepatol 2004;2:491.

539. Florie J, Horsthuis K, Hommes DW, et al. Magnetic resonance imaging compared with ileocolonoscopy in evaluating disease severity in Crohn's disease. Clin Gastroenterol Hepatol 2005;3:1221.

540. Weldon MJ, Lowe C, Joseph AE, Maxwell JD. Review article: quantitative leucocyte scanning in the assessment of inflammatory bowel disease activity and its response to therapy. Aliment Pharmacol Ther 1996;10:123.

541. Almer S, Granerus G, Strom M, et al. Leukocyte scintigraphy compared to interaoperative small bowel enteroscopy and laparotomy findings in Crohn's disease. Inflamm Bowel Dis 2007;13:164.

542. Dhekne RD, Chatziioannou SN, Moore WH, et al. Indium-111 leukocyte scintigraphy in suspected bowel ischemia. Am J Gastroenterol 2000;95:1983.

543. Gyorke T, Duffek L, Bartfai K, et al. The role of nuclear medicine in inflammatory bowel disease. A review with experiences of aspecific bowel activity using immunoscintigraphy with ^{99m}Tc anti-granulocyte antibodies. Eur J Radiol 2000;35:183.

544. Signore A, Chianelli M, Annovazzi A, et al. Imaging active lymphocytic infiltration in coeliac disease with iodine-123-interleukin-2 and the response to diet. Eur J Nucl Med 2000;27:18.

545. Melmed GY, Lo SK. Capsule endoscopy: practical applications. Clin Gastroenterol Hepatol 2005;3:411.

546. Marmo R, Rotondano G, Piscopo R, et al. Capsule endoscopy versus enteroclysis in the detection of small-bowel involvement in Crohn's disease: a prospective trial. Clin Gastroenterol Hepatol 2005;3:772.

547. Chong AK, Taylor A, Miller A, et al. Capsule endoscopy vs. push enteroscopy and enteroclysis in suspected small-bowel Crohn's disease. Gastrointest Endosc 2005;61:255.

548. Maunoury V, Savoye G, Bourreille A, et al. Value of wireless capsule endoscopy in patients with indeterminate colitis (inflammatory bowel disease type unclassified). Inflamm Bowel Dis 2007;13:152.

549. Maiden L, Thjodleifsson B, Theodors A, et al. A quantitative analysis of NSAID-induced small bowel pathology by capsule enteroscopy. Gastroenterology 2005;128:1172.

550. Buderus S, Boone J, Lyerly D, Lentze MJ. Fecal lactoferrin: a new parameter to monitor infliximab therapy. Dig Dis Sci 2004;49:1036.

551. Konikoff MR, Denson LA. Role of fecal calprotectin as a biomarker of intestinal inflammation in inflammatory bowel disease. Inflamm Bowel Dis 2006;12:524.

552. Crossley JR, Elliott RB. Simple method for diagnosing protein-losing enteropathies. Br Med J 1977;1:428.

553. Chiu NT, Lee BF, Hwang SJ, et al. Protein-losing enteropathy: diagnosis with (99m)Tc-labeled human serum albumin scintigraphy. Radiology 2001;219:86.

554. Wang SJ, Tsai SC, Lan JL. Tc-99m albumin scintigraphy to monitor the effect of treatment in protein-losing gastroenteropathy. Clin Nucl Med 2000;25:197.

555. Florent C, L'Hirondel C, Desmazures C, et al. Intestinal clearance of alpha 1-antitrypsin. A sensitive method for the detection of protein-losing enteropathy. Gastroenterology 1981;81:777.

556. Takeda H, Nishise S, Furukawa M, et al. Fecal clearance of alpha1-antitrypsin with lansoprazole can detect protein-losing gastropathy. Dig Dis Sci 1999;44:2313.

557. Quigley EM, Ross IN, Haeney MR, et al. Reassessment of faecal alpha-1-antitrypsin excretion for use as screening test for intestinal protein loss. J Clin Pathol 1987;40:61.

558. Binder HJ. The gastroenterologist's osmotic gap: fact or fiction? Gastroenterology 1992;103:702.

559. Duncan A, Robertson C, Russell RI. The fecal osmotic gap: technical aspects regarding its calculation. J Lab Clin Med 1992;119:359.

560. Ladefoged K, Schaffalitzky de Muckadell OB, Jarnum S. Faecal osmolality and electrolyte concentrations in chronic diarrhoea: do they provide diagnostic clues? Scand J Gastroenterol 1987;22:813.

561. Molla AM, Rahman M, Sarker SA, et al. Stool electrolyte content and purging rates in diarrhea caused by rotavirus, enterotoxigenic E. coli, and V. cholerae in children. J Pediatr 1981;98:835.

562. Phillips S, Donaldson L, Geisler K, et al. Stool composition in factitial diarrhea: a 6-year experience with stool analysis. Ann Intern Med 1995;123:97.

563. Eherer AJ, Santa Ana CA, Porter J, Fordtran JS. Effect of psyllium, calcium polycarbophil, and wheat bran on secretory diarrhea induced by phenolphthalein. Gastroenterology 1993;104:1007.

564. Powell DW, Field M. Pharmacological approaches to treatment of secretory diarrhea. In: Field M, Fordtran JS, Schultz S (eds) Secretory diarrhea. Bethesda, MD: American Physiological Society, 1980:187.

565. Schiller LR. Review article: anti-diarrhoeal pharmacology and therapeutics. Aliment Pharmacol Ther 1995;9:87.

566. Powell DW, Szauter KE. Nonantibiotic therapy and pharmacotherapy of acute infectious diarrhea. Gastroenterol Clin North Am 1993;22:683.

567. Thiagarajah JR, Broadbent T, Hsieh E, Verkman AS. Prevention of toxin-induced intestinal ion and fluid secretion by a small-molecule CFTR inhibitor. Gastroenterology 2004;126:511.

568. Sonawane ND, Hu J, Muanprasat C, Verkman AS. Luminally active, nonabsorbable CFTR inhibitors as potential therapy to reduce intestinal fluid loss in cholera. FASEB J 2006;20:130.

569. Thiagarajah JR, Verkman AS. New drug targets for cholera therapy. Trends Pharmacol Sci 2005;26:172.

570. Frantzides CT, Condon RE, Schulte WJ, Cowles V. Effects of morphine on colonic myoelectric and motor activity in subhuman primates. Am J Physiol 1990;258:G247.

571. Sarna SK, Otterson MF. Small intestinal amyogenesia and dysmyogencsia induced by morphine and loperamide. Am J Physiol 1990;258:G282.

572. Szilagyi A, Salomon R, Seidman E. Influence of loperamide on lactose handling and oral-caecal transit time. Aliment Pharmacol Ther 1996;10:765.

573. Goke M, Ewe K, Donner K, Meyer zum Buschenfelde KH. Influence of loperamide and loperamide oxide on the anal sphincter. A manometric study. Dis Colon Rectum 1992;35:857.

574. Musial F, Enck P, Kalveram KT, Erckenbrecht JF. The effect of loperamide on anorectal function in normal healthy men. J Clin Gastroenterol 1992;15:321.

575. Primi MP, Bueno L, Baumer P, et al. Racecadotril demonstrates intestinal antisecretory activity in vivo. Aliment Pharmacol Ther 1999;13 Suppl 6:3.

576. Prado D. A multinational comparison of racecadotril and loperamide in the treatment of acute watery diarrhoea in adults. Scand J Gastroenterol 2002;37:656.

577. Cezard JP, Duhamel JF, Meyer M, et al. Efficacy and tolerability of racecadotril in acute diarrhea in children. Gastroenterology 2001;120:799.

578. Salazar-Lindo E, Santisteban-Ponce J, Chea-Woo E, Gutierrez M. Racecadotril in the treatment of acute watery diarrhea in children. N Engl J Med 2000;343:463.

579. Turck D, Berard H, Fretault N, Lecomte JM. Comparison of racecadotril and loperamide in children with acute diarrhoea. Aliment Pharmacol Ther 1999;13 Suppl 6:27.

580. Watson ME, Lacey L, Kong S, et al. Alosetron improves quality of life in women with diarrhea-predominant irritable bowel syndrome. Am J Gastroenterol 2001;96:455.

581. Chey WD, Chey WY, Heath AT, et al. Long-term safety and efficacy of alosetron in women with severe diarrhea-predominant irritable bowel syndrome. Am J Gastroenterol 2004;99:2195.

582. Chang HY, Kelly EC, Lembo AJ. Current gut-directed therapies for irritable bowel syndrome. Curr Treat Options Gastroenterol 2006;9:314.

583. Tillman LA, Drake FM, Dixon JS, Wood JR. Review article: safety of bismuth in the treatment of gastrointestinal diseases. Aliment Pharmacol Ther 1996;10:459.

584. Dreverman JW, Van der Poel AJ. Loperamide oxide in acute diarrhoea: a double-blind, placebo-controlled trial. The Dutch Diarrhoea Trialists Group. Aliment Pharmacol Ther 1995;9:441.

585. Hamza H, Ben Khalifa H, Baumer P, et al. Racecadotril versus placebo in the treatment of acute diarrhoea in adults. Aliment Pharmacol Ther 1999;13 Suppl 6:15.

586. Vetel JM, Berard H, Fretault N, Lecomte JM. Comparison of racecadotril and loperamide in adults with acute diarrhoea. Aliment Pharmacol Ther 1999;13 Suppl 6:21.

587. Buchanan KD. Effects of sandostatin on neuroendocrine tumours of the gastrointestinal system. Recent Results Cancer Res 1993;129: 45.

588. Davis GR, Camp RC, Raskin P, Krejs GJ. Effect of somatostatin infusion on jejunal water and electrolyte transport in a patient with secretory diarrhea due to malignant carcinoid syndrome. Gastroenterology 1980;78:346.

589. Dharmsathaphorn K, Gorelick FS, Sherwin RS, et al. Somatostatin decreases diarrhea in patients with the short-bowel syndrome. J Clin Gastroenterol 1982;4:521.

590. Ducreux M, Ruszniewski P, Chayvialle JA, et al. The antitumoral effect of the long-acting somatostatin analog lanreotide in neuroendocrine tumors. Am J Gastroenterol 2000;95:3276.

591. Frank-Raue K, Ziegler R, Raue F. The use of octreotide in the treatment of medullary thyroid carcinoma. Horm Metab Res Suppl 1993;27:44.

592. Fried M. Octreotide in the treatment of refractory diarrhea. Digestion 1999;60 Suppl 2:42.

593. Kotler DP. Octreotide therapy for human immunodeficiency virus-associated diarrhea: pitfalls in drug development. Gastroenterology 1995;108:1939.

594. Lamberts SW, Pieters GF, Metselaar HJ, et al. Development of resistance to a long-acting somatostatin analogue during treatment of two patients with metastatic endocrine pancreatic tumours. Acta Endocrinol (Copenh) 1988;119:561.

595. Lamberts SW, van der Lely AJ, de Herder WW, Hofland LJ. Octreotide. N Engl J Med 1996;334:246.

596. Mourad FH, Gorard D, Thillainayagam AV, et al. Effective treatment of diabetic diarrhoea with somatostatin analogue, octreotide. Gut 1992;33:1578.

597. Rubin J, Ajani J, Schirmer W, et al. Octreotide acetate long-acting formulation versus open-label subcutaneous octreotide acetate in malignant carcinoid syndrome. J Clin Oncol 1999;17:600.

598. Simon DM, Cello JP, Valenzuela J, et al. Multicenter trial of octreotide in patients with refractory acquired immunodeficiency syndrome-associated diarrhea. Gastroenterology 1995;108:1753.

599. Penning C, Vecht J, Masclee AA. Efficacy of depot long-acting release octreotide therapy in severe dumping syndrome. Aliment Pharmacol Ther 2005;22:963.

600. Delaunoit T, Rubin J, Neczyporenko F, et al. Somatostatin analogues in the treatment of gastroenteropancreatic neuroendocrine tumors. Mayo Clin Proc 2005;80:502.

601. Lauritsen K, Laursen LS, Bukhave K, Rask-Madsen J. In vivo effects of orally administered prednisolone on prostaglandin and leucotriene production in ulcerative colitis. Gut 1987;28:1095.

602. Sandle GI, Hayslett JP, Binder HJ. Effect of glucocorticoids on rectal transport in normal subjects and patients with ulcerative colitis. Gut 1986;27:309.

603. Sandle GI, McGlone F. Acute effects of dexamethasone on cation transport in colonic epithelium. Gut 1987;28:701.

604. Bergman R, Parkes M. Systematic review: the use of mesalazine in inflammatory bowel disease. Aliment Pharmacol Ther 2006;23:841.

605. Lichtenstein GR, Sbreu MT, Cohen R, Tremaine W. American Gastroenterological Association Institute technical review on corticosteroids, immunomodulators, and infliximab in inflammatory bowel disease. Rev Gastroenterol Mex 2006;71:351.

606. Fedorak RN, Madsen KL. Probiotics and prebiotics in gastrointestinal disorders. Curr Opin Gastroenterol 2004;20:146.

607. Fedorak RN, Madsen KL. Probiotics and the management of inflammatory bowel disease. Inflamm Bowel Dis 2004;10:286.

608. Sartor RB. Probiotic therapy of intestinal inflammation and infections. Curr Opin Gastroenterol 2005;21:44.

609. Read NW. Diarrhée motrice. Clin Gastroenterol 1986;15:657.

610. Binder HJ, Bayless TM, Whiting DS. Pathophysiology of diarrhea. Unit VIIB. In: The undergraduate teaching project in gastroenterology liver disease. Timonium, MD: American Gastroenterological Association, 1979: Unit VIIB.

611. Powell DW. Approach to the patient with diarrhea. In: Kelley WN (ed.). Textbook of internal medicine. Philadelphia: Lippincott–Raven, 1997:617.

612. Parks SI, Giannella R. Approach to the adult patient with acute diarrhea. Gastroenterol Clin North Am 1993;22:483.

613. Di John D, Levene MM. Treatment of diarrhea. Infect Dis Clin North Am 1988;2:719.

19 Approach to the patient with suspected acute infectious diarrhea

John D. Long, Ralph A. Giannella

Definitions, 360
Epidemiology, 360
Etiology and microbiology, 360
Clinical features, 361
Diagnostic evaluation, 364
Treatment, 367

Definitions

Diarrhea is defined as the production of stools of abnormally loose consistency, usually associated with excessive frequency of defecation (three or more times per day) and with excessive stool output [1]. Normal stool output is considered to be less than 200 g/day. Although diarrhea is a common symptom, most cases are self-limiting and if not, they can be successfully treated by patients using over-the-counter medications. Acute diarrhea is defined as an illness lasting up to 14 days. Persistent diarrhea is defined as an illness lasting more than 14 days but less than 30 days, while chronic diarrhea is any illness that lasts more than 30 days [1].

Epidemiology

An estimated 2 million deaths occur annually worldwide from diarrhea, making it the second leading cause of morbidity and mortality. Mortality from diarrhea is declining worldwide. In the United States, an estimated 211 million to 375 million episodes of acute diarrhea occur each year. This works out to be 1.4 episodes per person per year [2]. Such episodes are responsible for 900 000 hospitalizations and 6000 deaths each year [2]. The majority of deaths occur in elderly patients (age over 74 years). Foodborne illnesses alone account for 76 million episodes, 325 000 hospitaliza-

tions, and 5000 deaths each year [3]. The economic costs of infectious diarrheal illnesses are significant. In the United States, an estimated $6 billion is spent each year on medical care and lost productivity as the result of foodborne illnesses, most of which are associated with diarrhea [1].

Etiology and microbiology

The major causes of acute infectious diarrhea include viruses, bacteria, and, less often, protozoa (Table 19.1). The proportion of infections in which the infectious agent is identified is low, however, because most patients with acute diarrhea do not seek medical attention because of the self-limiting nature of most episodes. In addition, in those patients who do seek medical care, diagnostic testing is often not performed. Bacterial stool cultures for unselected patients with acute infectious diarrhea are positive in only 1.5%–5.6% of cases [4]. This suggests that most cases of acute gastroenteritis are probably caused by viruses. Support for a predominance of viral agents as a cause for most cases comes from a study in which stool collection kits were delivered to and from the patients' homes during 54 foodborne outbreaks. In this study, polymerase chain reaction techniques were used to identify noroviruses and, as a result, a pathogen was identified in 71% of outbreaks with norovirus causing three-quarters of cases [5].

In a review of more than 30 000 stool cultures performed at 10 US hospitals from 1990 to 1992, a bacterial pathogen was identified in 5.6% of samples [6]. The frequencies of the common bacterial pathogens were 2.33% for *Campylobacter*, 1.82% for *Salmonella*, 1.06% for *Shigella*, and 0.39% for *Escherichia coli* O157:H7. A similar relative distribution of bacterial causes of acute diarrhea was noted in FoodNet surveys

Principles of Clinical Gastroenterology. Edited by Tadataka Yamada, David H. Alpers, Anthony N. Kalloo, Neil Kaplowitz, Chung Owyang, and Don W. Powell. © 2008 Blackwell Publishing. ISBN 978-1-4051-69103

Table 19.1 Causes of acute infectious diarrhea

Bacteria	Viruses	Protozoa
Campylobacter	Rotavirus	*Giardia lamblia*
Salmonella	Norovirus (Norwalk)	*Cryptosporidum*
Shigella	Adenovirus (enteric)	*Cyclospora*
Enterohemorrhagic *Escherichia coli* (EHEC)	Calicivirus	*Entamoeba histolytica*
Enteroinvasive *E. coli* (EIEC)	Astrovirus	
Enterotoxigenic *E. coli* (ETEC)	Coronavirus	
Enteropathogenic *E. coli* (EPEC)	Herpes simplex virus	
Enteroadherent *E. coli* (EAEC)	Cytomegalovirus	
Clostridium difficile		
Yersinia enterocolitica		
Clostridium perfringens		
Staphylococcus aureus		
Bacillus cereus		
Vibrio parahaemolyticus		
Vibrio cholerae		
Aeromonas		
Plesiomonas shigelloides		

of laboratory-diagnosed cases of foodborne illnesses. The FoodNet group collects data on the incidence of diarrhea attributed to nine pathogens in 13% of the US population (37 million people) living in nine states. Data from 2002 and 2003, respectively, revealed the incidence of the most common pathogens per 100 000 population to be as follows: 16.1 and 14.5 for *Salmonella*; 13.4 and 12.6 for *Campylobacter*; 10.3 and 7.3 for *Shigella*; 1.7 and 1.1 for *E. coli* O157:H7; and 1.4 and 1.9 for *Cryptosporidium* [7, 8]

Patients with a history of bloody diarrhea or a visibly bloody stool specimen have a higher likelihood of a bacterial pathogen being isolated from their stool (20% vs 5.6% in the entire cohort) [6]. In particular, *E. coli* O157:H7 was a common isolate in this subgroup of patients. In patients with visibly bloody specimens, *E. coli* O157:H7 accounted for 63% of all isolates compared with 15% for *Shigella*, 8% for *Campylobacter*, and 5% for *Salmonella* [6]. A more recent study evaluated 877 episodes of reported bloody diarrhea seen in 11 US emergency departments. Cultures were obtained in 63% of episodes, and 31% of these specimens revealed a bacterial pathogen with the following frequency: *Shigella*, 15.3%; *Campylobacter*, 6.2%; *Salmonella*, 5.8%; *E. coli* O157:H7, 2.6%; other, 1.6% [9]. In patients with a history of bloody diarrhea or with a grossly bloody stool specimen, the overall rate of a positive culture increases four- to sixfold.

Clinical features (Tables 19.2 and 19.3)

Person-to-person transmission

Acute infectious diarrhea is acquired mostly through the fecal–oral route and infection occurs through direct contact.

In developed countries acute infectious diarrhea is common in areas where people are housed together, such as day-care centers and nursing homes. Diarrhea is particularly common in the 6 million children who attend day care in the United States, and the mechanism of spread involves person-to-person transmission by fecal contamination of hands and fomites [10]. In developing nations, acute diarrhea is endemic. Transmission occurs primarily in family groups as a result of contamination of food and water with feces. This is especially frequent during natural disasters such as floods and cyclones.

Foodborne and waterborne transmission

The ingestion of food and water contaminated with pathogenic microorganisms is a major source of disease transmission. Several large outbreaks of disease have been reported in the last two decades. Common sources of foodborne illness include contaminated meats (beef, pork, poultry), eggs, shellfish, and raw milk or juice.

The clinical manifestations of an episode of foodborne illness depend on the causative organism.

Traveler's diarrhea

Between 40% and 60% of travelers to any part of the developing world will develop diarrhea. The areas where the risk for developing traveler's diarrhea is highest include Mexico, South and Central America, Asia (with the exception of Singapore), and Africa (with the exception of South Africa). In one series of 30 369 travelers returning from a visit to Jamaica, the attack rate for traveler's diarrhea was 24% [11]. In contrast, the attack rate for approximately 30 000 travelers returning from India and Kenya was much higher (~ 54%)

Table 19.2 Epidemiological features of common community-acquired infectious pathogens

Pathogen	Typical epidemiological settings and risk factors	Usual modes of and sources of transmission
Campylobacter	Picnics Travel	Mode – foodborne Sources – poultry, milk, cheese
Salmonella	Picnics, pets Travel	Mode – foodborne, waterborne Sources – poultry, meats, eggs, alfalfa sprouts, raw milk, unpasteurized juice
Shigella	Day care Travel	Mode – person-to-person, foodborne Sources – salads, green onions
Enterohemorrhagic *Escherichia coli* (EHEC)	Age extremes	Mode – foodborne Sources – hamburger, raw seed sprouts, apple cider
Enterotoxigenic *E. coli* (ETEC)	Travel – Mexico, Central & South America, Africa	Mode – foodborne, waterborne Sources – meats, vegetables
Clostridium difficile	Antibiotic exposure Chemotherapy	Mode – nosocomial, person-to-person
Yersinia enterocolitica	Travel – Scandinavia Hemochromatosis	Mode – foodborne Sources – pork, beef, milk, cheese
Vibrio parahemolyticus	Travel – SE Asia, Japan, Alaska Cirrhosis	Mode – foodborne Sources – undercooked seafood, oysters
Vibrio cholerae	Travel – Tropical regions	Mode – waterborne, foodborne Sources – undercooked seafood
Giardia	Day care Travel – Nepal, Russia, and mountainous areas of US IgA deficiency	Mode – waterborne, person-to-person Sources – surface freshwater, swimming pools
Cryptosporidium	Day care Travel Immunocompromised host	Mode – waterborne, person-to-person Sources – swimming pools
Cyclospora	Travel – Nepal Immunocompromised host	Mode – foodborne Sources – raspberries
Entamoeba histolytica	Travel – tropical regions Emigration from tropical regions	Mode – waterborne Sources – contaminated water
Rotavirus	Day care Nurseries	Mode – person-to-person Sources – fomites
Norovirus	Nursing homes, schools Military barracks, camps Cruise ships	Mode – person-to-person, foodborne Sources – undercooked shellfish

[12]. More than 90% of these types of illnesses in most geographic areas are caused by bacteria, with the most common organism being enterotoxigenic *E. coli* (ETEC) [11,12]. In a study of 636 travelers to Mexico, Jamaica, and India, ETEC was responsible for 30% of cases of diarrhea, while enteroaggregative *E. coli* (EAEC) caused 26% of cases [13]. Parasitic infections rarely cause traveler's diarrhea, with the exception of *Giardia lamblia*, which is more likely to be acquired after travel to Nepal, St Petersburg (Russia), as well as the mountainous regions of the northeast and west United States [14].

The majority of episodes of traveler's diarrhea are self-limiting and last no longer than 5 days, but some episodes may result in significant discomfort and even dehydration. Traveler's diarrhea is usually categorized into three forms:
• *Classic* – passage of three or more unformed stools in a 24-h period plus at least one of the following symptoms or signs: nausea, vomiting, abdominal pain or cramps, fever, bloody stools.
• *Moderate* – passage of one or two unformed stools in a 24-h period plus at least one of the above symptoms or signs,

Table 19.3 Clinical features of common community-acquired infectious pathogens

Pathogen	Incubation period	Fever	Abdominal pain	Nausea and vomiting	Bloody stool	FOBT	WBC	Diagnostic test
Campylobacter jejuni	3 days (1–7 days)	Common	Common	Variable	Variable	Var	Pos	Stool culture
Salmonella	24 h (8–24 h)	Common	Common	Variable	Variable	Var	Pos	Stool culture
Shigella	3 days (1–7 days)	Common	Common	Common	Variable	Var	Pos	Stool culture
EHEC	4 days (1–5 days)	Uncommon	Common	Variable	Common	Pos	Neg	Cytotoxin assay
ETEC	2 days (1–3 days)	Uncommon	Variable	Variable	Uncommon	Neg	Neg	Research lab. only
Clostridium difficile	Unknown	Variable	Variable	Uncommon	Variable	Var	Pos	Enzyme immunoassay
Yersinia enterocolitica	3 days (1–6 days)	Common	Common	Variable	Variable	Var	Var	Stool culture
Vibrio parahemolytica	12 h (2–48 h)	Variable	Variable	Variable	Variable	Var	Var	Stool culture (TCBS)
Vibrio cholerae	2 days (1–3 days)	Variable	Variable	Variable	Uncommon	Neg	Neg	Stool culture (TCBS)
Giardia	9 days (7–14 days)	Uncommon	Common	Variable	Uncommon	Neg	Neg	O&P examination Stool antigen
Cryptosporidium	7 days (1–14 days)	Variable	Variable	Variable	Uncommon	Neg	Neg	Modified acid-fast Stool antigen
Cyclospora	7 days (1–11 days)	Variable	Variable	Variable	Uncommon	Neg	Neg	Modified acid-fast
Entamoeba histolytica	14 days (7–21 days)	Variable	Variable	Variable	Variable	Pos	Var	O&P examination Stool antigen

EHEC, enterohemorrhagic *Escherichia coli*; ETEC, enterotoxigenic *E. coli*; FOBT, fecal occult blood test; neg, negative; O&P, oocyte and parasite; pos, positive; TCBS, thiosulfate/citrate/bile salts/sucrose; var, variable; WBC, white blood cell count.

or three or more unformed stools without any of the above symptoms or signs.

• *Mild* – passage of one or two unformed stools in a 24-h period without any of the above symptoms [12].

Most episodes occur between 4 days and 14 days after arrival but they can occur sooner if a high concentration of bacteria is ingested. Approaches to therapy and prevention are discussed in a recent review by DuPont [15].

Persistent diarrhea

Persistent diarrhea is defined as an episode of acute diarrhea that lasts longer than 14 days. Most forms of bacterial and viral acute diarrhea will resolve before 14 days. Exceptions include diarrhea caused by *Aeromonas*, *Yersinia enterocolitica*, and *Clostridium difficile*. However, the most common pathogens associated with persistent diarrhea in the United States and worldwide are the protozoans *Giardia* and *Cryptosporidium* [1,2].

Nosocomial diarrhea

Nosocomial diarrhea is defined as an episode of acute diarrhea that begins 3 days or more after the onset of hospitalization. The most common cause of nosocomial diarrhea is antibiotic-associated diarrhea resulting from *C. difficile* infection [16]. The major risk factors for *C. difficile* infection include advanced age, hospitalization, and exposure to antibiotics [17]. The antibiotics most frequently implicated in diarrhea associated with *C. difficile* infection include expanded-spectrum penicillins, cephalosporins, and clindamycin. However, ther-

apy with virtually any enteral or parenteral antibiotic can give rise to *C. difficile* infection.

Diarrhea can range from mild symptoms to the life-threatening disease commonly associated with pseudomembranous colitis. Patients may also have fever, abdominal cramping, and peripheral leukocytosis [18]. In severe cases, colitis may be evident on computed tomography or lower endoscopy. Complications include protein-losing enteropathy resulting in hypoalbuminemia and anasarca as well as toxic megacolon [17].

There have been dramatic changes in the epidemiology and clinical aspects of *C. difficile* colitis. The number of cases of *C. difficile* infections has increased markedly in the past several years, associated with a decreased responsiveness of *C. difficile* to metronidazole. The rates of severe complications, intensive-care admissions, toxic megacolon or perforation, and death have also markedly increased. The increase in mortality may be linked to the appearance of a new, hypervirulent strain [19]. This strain has caused widespread epidemic outbreaks and makes between 15 and 20 times the amount of toxins A and B, as well as a binary toxin. There are no clinically available tests to document this strain but suspicious strains can be sent to the Centers for Disease Control (CDC) for documentation. If suspected, vancomycin is the therapy of choice [19,20].

Complications

Several complications may occur as a result of acute bacterial infections. Complications may be either local (i.e., affecting the small or large intestine) or systemic. By far the most serious local complication is toxic megacolon. The syndrome of toxic megacolon is characterized by the presence of fever, with temperature over 38.6°C (> 101.5°F), and tachycardia (heart rate > 120 beats/min) in the setting of abdominal distention and total or segmental nonobstructive dilation of the colon on imaging [21]. Toxic megacolon usually occurs in the setting of idiopathic inflammatory bowel disease and, less commonly, with infectious colitis. Pathogens that have been known to cause toxic megacolon include *Campylobacter*, *Salmonella*, *Shigella*, *Yersinia*, *C. difficile*, and *Entamoeba histolytica* [21]. The major concern in patients with toxic megacolon is the high risk of perforation; up to 50% of patients require subtotal colectomy for definitive treatment. Mortality rates in patients with toxic megacolon caused by *C. difficile* approach 35%. A less serious local complication of acute infectious gastroenteritis is irritable bowel syndrome (IBS). Symptoms compatible with IBS, such as abdominal pain or discomfort associated with altered bowel habits (usually diarrhea), can occur in up to 30% of patients after an episode of acute gastroenteritis [22]. Pathogens that have been associated with postinfectious IBS include *Campylobacter*, *Salmonella*, and *Shigella*.

The most feared systemic complication of acute bacterial colitis is hemolytic uremic syndrome (HUS), which is characterized by hemolytic anemia, thrombocytopenia, and acute renal failure [23]. Twenty-five percent of patients with HUS may also have neurological symptoms. HUS is particularly common in children. The pathogen that causes the majority of cases of postdiarrheal HUS is enterohemorrhagic *E. coli* (EHEC). Of the patients affected by this potentially serious complication 50% require dialysis, 5% develop end-stage renal disease, and 5% die of the condition [23]. A second, less common but still significant complication of acute bacterial colitis is Guillain–Barré syndrome (GBS). This is an acute idiopathic inflammatory demyelinating polyneuropathy that results in progressive muscle weakness and areflexia [24]. *Campylobacter jejuni* is the most common precipitant of GBS and accounts for up to 25% of cases [24].

Finally, an additional pathogen, *Vibrio vulnificus*, occurs in the coastal United States particularly along the Gulf of Mexico. This organism causes a spectrum of illnesses including gastroenteritis, wound infections, necrotizing fasciitis, compartment syndrome, septicemia, and death. Liver disease and alcohol use seem to predispose to infection. Doxycycline and cefotaxime should be used in serious infections [25].

Diagnostic evaluation

History and physical examination

Most cases of acute infectious diarrhea in the United States are caused by viruses. As such, most episodes are self-limited and last less than 48 h. In such cases, diagnostic testing should be kept to a minimum and microbiological investigation is rarely necessary. In patients who ultimately require investigation the choice of diagnostic testing should be directed by the specific epidemiological and clinical clues presented by the patient and testing should be focused toward the most likely pathogens. Important clinical information that should be obtained from the history includes:
• an accurate description of the diarrhea such as the onset, duration, frequency, and appearance (watery, bloody, purulent)
• an assessment of the frequency and severity of associated symptoms including fever, nausea, vomiting, abdominal pain, and tenesmus
• an assessment for symptoms indicative of volume depletion such as thirst, lethargy, orthostasis, and decreased urination [1].
Important epidemiological information that should be obtained from the history includes:
• exposures, occupations, or other activities associated with increased risk for diarrheal illness such as attendance or employment in day-care centers or mental institutions, employment as a food handler, swimming in community pools or freshwater lakes or streams, exposure to animals at farms or petting zoos, and anal intercourse
• recent consumption of high-risk foods such as undercooked meats (beef, poultry, pork), raw shellfish, eggs, and raw milk or juice
• recent travel to regions associated with increased risk for diarrheal illness such as Mexico, Central and South America, Africa, and Southeast Asia
• recent antibiotic use or chemotherapy [1].
The physical examination should focus on detecting fever and abdominal tenderness and on determining whether signs of volume depletion are present (orthostatic pulse or blood pressure changes, dry mucous membranes, decreased skin turgor, and absent jugular venous distention). In patients without a clear history of dysentery or bloody diarrhea, testing the stool obtained by digital rectal examination for the presence of occult blood may be helpful, i.e., it may indicate an inflammatory diarrhea (see Screening for inflammatory diarrhea).

Based on the clinical and epidemiological information gathered from the history and physical examination, an assessment should be made regarding the severity of the episode and the need for medical evaluation. Patients with medically important diarrhea should have either further investigation (stool analysis) or empiric antibiotic treatment. This includes patients with bloody diarrhea, dysentery, duration > 48 h or ≥ six unformed stools per 24 h, severe abdominal pain, fever (T > 101.3° F). In addition, patients who are hospitalized, immunocompromised, or elderly (> 70 years) are included in this group. Furthermore, patients should be categorized into four clinical groups based on the initial evaluation: 1) community-acquired diarrhea; 2) traveler's diarrhea; 3) persistent diarrhea; and 4) nosocomial diarrhea.

Screening for inflammatory diarrhea

The utility of testing stool samples for markers of inflammation in the evaluation of patients with acute diarrhea remains controversial. Proponents of the use of these tests argue that invasive forms of bacterial gastroenteritis often cause colonic inflammation, whereas viral, parasitic, and toxin-mediated etiologies do not [26]. Proposed advantages of a positive assay include the ability to increase the yield of a subsequent stool culture and to select patients who may benefit from empiric antibiotic therapy. Unfortunately, none of the commercially available techniques are sufficiently sensitive, although the fecal lactoferrin assay holds some promise. Fecal testing for the detection of inflammation can be performed using light microscopy for methylene blue-stained polymorphonuclear leukocytes or using an immunoassay for the glycoprotein lactoferrin [26]. Alternatively, stool can be tested for occult blood as a surrogate marker for inflammation. A summary of several studies that reported the prevalence of leukocytes in stool samples from patients with a culture-proven bacterial pathogen found that leukocytes were detected in 73% of samples with *Shigella*, 58% with *Campylobacter*, 52% with *Salmonella*, 54% with *E. coli* O157:H7, and 42% with *C. difficile* [26]. The fecal lactoferrin assay appears to be a more sensitive test to use when screening stool specimens for bacterial pathogens. Lactoferrin is a glycoprotein found in leukocytes and can be detected with a commercially available immunoassay. Two studies showed that the sensitivity of a positive lactoferrin assay in detecting *Salmonella*, *Shigella*, and *Campylobacter* ranged from 83% to 93% [27,28]. Furthermore, a recent study has shown that the sensitivity and specificity for detecting bacterial pathogens by these tests are much higher when employed in developed countries compared with developing countries. For example, the sensitivities of the fecal lactoferrin assay, fecal leukocyte by microscopy, and fecal occult blood test were 92%, 73%, and 71%, respectively, in developed countries. Corresponding sensitivities for each technique in developing countries were 95%, 50%, and 44% [29].

Stool culture

Most cases of acute diarrhea in immunocompetent adults are self-limited and thus do not require investigation. Despite this knowledge, stool cultures are obtained frequently even though their yield is notoriously low. For example, combining data from 10 studies with over 90 000 stool samples revealed that only 5.7% of specimens were positive [30–39]. Attempts have been made to identify clinical factors that increase the yield of stool cultures [14]. Factors such as abrupt onset of diarrhea, more than four stools per day, absence of vomiting before the onset of diarrhea, or the presence of fever, bloody diarrhea, tenesmus, abdominal pain, or raw seafood ingestion all increase the likelihood of recovering a bacterial pathogen from a stool culture. Guidelines from the American College of Gastroenterology for the evaluation and treatment of acute infectious diarrhea suggest that a stool culture positive for bacteria will be obtained only from patients with severe diarrhea (more than six stools in 24 h, or more than 48 h duration, or the presence of clinical volume depletion); bloody diarrhea or dysentery; a temperature over 38.5°C; stools positive for occult blood, leukocytes, or lactoferrin; and immunosuppression [e.g., acquired immunodeficiency syndrome (AIDS), transplant, cancer chemotherapy] [14]. A more recent guideline from the Infectious Diseases Society of America proposed additional indications for stool culture including suspected outbreaks and attendance in day-care centers [1]. Finally, in those patients with known underlying inflammatory bowel disease who are having an acute flare of diarrhea, obtaining a stool culture may help to differentiate between a flare and a superimposed infectious colitis [40,41].

In certain clinical situations, specific stool cultures may need to be requested. These tests are generally not performed in most laboratories unless specifically requested. For example, patients with a clear history of bloody diarrhea or with developing HUS, stool should be tested for Shiga toxin and cultured for *E. coli* O157:H7 [2]. Patients with recent ingestion of raw shellfish should be tested for *Vibrio* using thiosulfate/citrate/bile salts/sucrose (TCBS) agar, while patients with a pseudoappendicitis syndrome should be tested for *Yersinia* using cold enrichment. Finally, patients who develop nosocomial diarrhea should be tested for *C. difficile* toxins [17].

Ova and parasite tests

Sending stool samples for ova and parasite (O&P) examination is not cost-effective for most patients with acute diarrhea. The overall yield is 2%–3%. The yield in patients with persistent diarrhea (14 days or more) may be higher [2]. Practice guidelines from the American College of Gastroenterology suggest that testing for ova and parasites only be employed in patients with the following: recent travel to Russia, Nepal, or mountainous regions of the United States; infants attending day-care centers; men who have sex with men and patients with AIDS; exposure to a possible community waterborne outbreak; bloody diarrhea but few or no fecal leukocytes [14]. In addition, any patient with persistent diarrhea, even without the above specific indications, should be tested for ova and parasites [1].

A complete evaluation of stool for ova and parasites should include an examination of both fresh and fixed specimens. Cysts may be detected in solid stools; however, watery or semisolid stools are usually necessary to detect trophozoites. *Giardia lamblia* is most commonly diagnosed by the identification of cysts or, less frequently, trophozoites in fecal specimens that are stained with trichrome or iron hematoxylin [42]. The cysts are oval and usually between

11 μm and 15 μm in size. These methods depend largely on observer experience and at best are only 60%–70% sensitive in confirming a diagnosis of giardiasis. Analyzing three specimens on consecutive days may increase the yield. Antigen detection tests are commercially available that can diagnose *Giardia* [42]. There are several commercially available enzyme immunoassays (EIA) that are useful; these are directed at detecting the presence of a *Giardia*-specific antigen (GSA) that is present on both cysts and trophozoites [42]. These assays have more than 90% sensitivity and more than 96% specificity in identifying *G. lamblia*.

Direct examination of unstained stool is not useful for the identification of some protozoa such as *Cryptosporidium* and *Cyclospora* because these organisms are too small to be noted. The gastroenterologist should be aware of microbiology laboratory normal practice when ordering a routine O&P examination; many laboratories do not routinely perform the special staining techniques required to detect these pathogens. *Cryptosporidium* and *Cyclospora* can be readily identified by a modified acid-fast stain [43,44]. The oocysts of *Cryptosporidium* are 2–6 μm in size, whereas the oocysts of *Cyclospora* are 8–10 μm in size. In addition, antigen detection tests are available that can diagnose *Cryptosporidium* [43]. There are several useful, commercially available EIAs directed at detecting the presence of a *Cryptosporidium*-specific antigen (CSA), which is present on oocysts [43]. These assays have more than 83% sensitivity and more than 96% specificity in identifying *Cryptosporidium parvum*.

Entamoeba histolytica can be diagnosed in fecal specimens by the identification of trophozoites using wet mounts or the trichrome stain. However, traditional wet mounts or stains are, at best, only 60% sensitive for identifying *E. histolytica*, mainly because this organism is identical in appearance to *Entamoeba dispar*, a nonpathogenic commensal protozoan [45]. One rapid EIA is commercially available that can distinguish *E. histolytica* from *E. dispar* with a 95% sensitivity and 93% specificity. However, polymerase chain reaction techniques are the most sensitive tests for distinguishing these two amebae [45].

Clostridium difficile tests

Clostridium difficile is the most common nosocomial infection of the gastrointestinal tract and tests to detect this pathogen should be used in the evaluation of nosocomial diarrhea. Other frequent causes of diarrhea in hospitalized patients include medications, particularly elixirs that contain sorbitol, and tube feedings. In addition, antibiotics may cause diarrhea in the absence of *C. difficile*. Clinical factors that increase the likelihood of detecting *C. difficile* include recent hospitalization (especially if within the last 2 weeks), antibiotic use within 30 days (particularly cephalosporins), the presence of abdominal pain or severe diarrhea, a white blood cell count greater than 10 000 cells/mm^3, and the presence of fecal leukocytes or lactoferrin [46–48].

The gold standard in the United States for diagnosing *C. difficile* is the tissue culture cytotoxicity assay, which identifies toxin B and carries a sensitivity between 67% and 99% [49]. The cytotoxicity assay detects as little as 10 pg toxin B. However, the test requires 24–48 h to complete. Commercially available EIAs to detect toxins A and B are available and require only 2–3 h to complete. These assays, however, require 100–1000 pg of either toxin A or toxin B and carry sensitivities of 64%–99% and specificities of 93%–100%. Unfortunately, the low sensitivities of some of these assays compromise the ability to detect *C. difficile* if only a single stool specimen is tested. In addition, 1%–2% of cases involve strains of *C. difficile* that produce only toxin B [17]. Therefore, a negative EIA should not deter the clinician from making a diagnosis of *C. difficile* colitis and treating the patient in whom the clinical suspicion is very high.

Lower endoscopy

Lower endoscopy is usually not indicated in the evaluation of most immunocompetent patients with acute diarrhea. There are a few situations, however, in which lower endoscopy may be helpful in subsequent patient management. In patients with severe nosocomial diarrhea and suspected *C. difficile* colitis, flexible sigmoidoscopy may identify pseudomembranous colitis while results of toxin assays are pending or if toxin assays are negative but *C. difficile* infection is highly suspected. In patients with persistent bloody or inflammatory diarrhea of unknown origin (culture-negative), flexible sigmoidoscopy (with or without biopsies) may help to distinguish infectious colitis from ischemic colitis or idiopathic inflammatory bowel disease [50].

Cost issues

Nosocomial diarrhea is rarely caused by community-acquired bacterial or parasitic pathogens. For example, six studies have compared the yield of bacterial stool culture obtained during the first 3 days of hospitalization (2%–12.6%) with the yield after 3 days (0%–1.5%) [30,33–35,37,39]. The yield in the first 3 days is thus two to nine times higher. Similar results are observed with the use of routine O&P examinations in patients with nosocomial diarrhea [51]. Despite this low yield, it has been shown that up to 50% of all bacterial stool cultures submitted to microbiology laboratories have been obtained from patients who have been hospitalized for more than 3 days, which results in substantial costs per positive diagnosis. These issues have helped formulate the "3-day rule," which states that stool samples submitted for routine bacterial culture should be rejected if obtained from a patient who has been hospitalized for more than 3 days [26]. Strict application of this criterion would result in significant reductions in costs by limiting the use of supplies and reagents and decreasing laboratory staff time. Unfortunately, a few cases of clinically important nosocomial diarrhea resulting from bacterial pathogens could be missed.

As a result, a modified 3-day rule has been advocated that allows bacterial cultures to be processed 72 h after admission in certain high-risk patients (age over 65 years with significant comorbid illnesses, human immunodeficiency virus infection, or neutropenia) or in cases in which a nosocomial outbreak of salmonellosis is suspected [52]. It is estimated that widespread application of the modified 3-day rule would save the average hospital per year $10 000 of reagent costs, over $70 000 of patient charges, and 730 h of technologist time [53]. Extrapolation of these figures to the 6000 hospitals in the United States suggests that savings of $27 million to $73 million a year could be achieved by implementation of this policy.

Treatment

General measures

Patients with acute infectious diarrhea of mild-to-moderate severity and without dehydration can usually be managed with simple supportive measures. These include dietary alterations and fluid replacement to prevent dehydration. Oral intake should be encouraged and the misconceptions that oral intake will worsen the diarrhea and that the bowel needs to be at rest should be abandoned [16]. Avoidance of milk and other lactose-containing products is commonly recommended because a transient lactase deficiency may occur in response to infections involving the small bowel. However, supportive evidence for this recommendation is lacking. Caffeine-containing products should also be avoided because caffeine increases cyclic adenosine monophosphate levels, so promoting secretion of intestinal fluid. Initial oral intake should consist of boiled starches/cereals such as noodles, rice, potatoes, and wheat as well as soup, crackers, and toast. The addition of salt is helpful. Fluid replacement may be accomplished with soft drinks, fruit juices, and Gatorade [16]. As stools become less frequent and more formed, the diet can be advanced as tolerated.

Oral rehydration therapy

Patients with severe acute infectious diarrhea, including those with symptoms or signs of dehydration, require more aggressive fluid replacement therapy. Patients with mental status alterations or severe dehydration (at least 10% volume loss) may need intravenous hydration. However, most patients can be treated with oral rehydration with a glucose-based electrolyte solution [1,2]. In particular, infants, the elderly, and immunosuppressed patients are prime candidates for oral rehydration therapy. Glucose in the intestinal lumen facilitates the absorption of sodium and, thereby, water. This cotransport mechanism is usually not damaged by infectious pathogens or their toxins [16]. There are several commercially available oral rehydration solutions that take advantage of the glucose–sodium-coupled transport mechanism. The composition of the oral rehydration solution per liter of water recommended by the World Health Organization (WHO) consists of 3.5 g sodium chloride, 2.5 g sodium bicarbonate, 1.5 g potassium chloride, and 20 g sucrose [1,2]. This makes a solution with 90 mmol/L sodium, 20 mmol/L potassium, 80 mmol/L chloride, 30 mmol/L bicarbonate, and 111 mmol/L glucose. A newer formula with reduced osmolarity may be more appropriate in resource-poor countries for children with acute diarrhea [54,55]. Oral rehydration solutions have been shown to prevent dehydration and reduce mortality from diarrheal disease worldwide. In addition to the WHO oral rehydration solution, other formulations available in the Unites States include Pedialyte (Mead Johnson, Princeton, NJ), Rehydralyte (Ross Labs, Columbus, OH), and Ceralyte (Cera, Columbia, MD).

Antidiarrheal therapy

Antimotility agents such as loperamide (Imodium) and diphenoxylate atropine (Lomotil) may be used for the symptomatic treatment of patients with acute diarrhea in whom fever is absent or low-grade and stools are nonbloody. In general, these agents should be withheld in any patient with symptoms or signs of inflammatory diarrhea because they have been associated with prolonged fever in shigellosis [56], HUS in children infected with enterohemorrhagic E. coli, [57] and toxic megacolon in patients with C. difficile infection [58]. Loperamide works by inhibiting intestinal peristalsis and reducing secretion in the gut, and can reduce stool frequency by as much as 80%. Loperamide does not cross the blood–brain barrier into the central nervous system and has no known potential for addiction. When used in conjunction with antibiotics for the treatment of traveler's diarrhea [59] or bacterial dysentery [60], loperamide may reduce the duration of diarrhea by approximately 1 day. Diphenoxylate atropine is an effective antidiarrheal agent but does have central opiate effects, raising the risk for addiction, and may also cause bothersome anticholinergic side effects.

Bismuth subsalicylate is another option for the symptomatic treatment of acute community-acquired or traveler's diarrhea. This agent works to reduce diarrhea through the antisecretory properties of the salicylate component as well as antibacterial properties [14]. Bismuth subsalicylate may reduce stool frequency by as much as 50% and is particularly useful in patients with significant vomiting along with their diarrhea. In direct comparisons, bismuth subsalicylate is less effective than loperamide as an antidiarrheal agent [61]. Finally, adsorbents such as kaolin–pectin and attapulgite have been used to treat diarrhea, but there are insufficient data from clinical trials to support their use.

Empiric antibiotic therapy

A decision of whether or not to begin empiric antibiotic therapy in a patient presenting with acute infectious diarrhea often emerges as a result of the lack of rapid diagnostic

Table 19.4 Indications for empiric antibiotic therapy for acute infectious diarrhea

Clinical scenario	Antibiotic options and doses	Duration	Comments

Community-acquired, especially if:
– Severe (see text)
– Fever > 38.5°C (> 101.3°F)
– Dysentery
– Stool positive for leukocytes,
  lactoferrin, or occult blood
	Quinolones:
	Ciprofloxacin 500 mg b.i.d.
	Norfloxacin 400 mg b.i.d.
	Levofloxacin 500 mg q.d.
		1–5 days	Antibiotics and should be avoided if infection with
			  Shiga toxin-producing *Escherichia coli* is suspected
			Can use trimethoprim–sulfamethoxazole in children

Moderate-to-severe traveler's diarrhea	Quinolones: Ciprofloxacin 500 mg b.i.d. Norfloxacin 400 mg b.i.d. Levofloxacin 500 mg q.d. Rifaximin 200 mg t.i.d.	1–5 days 3 days	Early treatment with a fluoroquinolone can reduce duration of diarrhea from 3–4 days to 1–2 days Can use trimethoprim–sulfamethoxazole in children
Persistent diarrhea (> 14 days)	Metronidazole: 250–750 mg t.i.d.	7–10 days	Particularly if giardiasis is suspected

Moderate-to-severe nosocomial diarrhea	Metronidazole:
	250 mg q.i.d. or
	  500 mg t.i.d.
		10 days	Causative antibiotics should be discontinued if
			  possible

b.i.d., twice a day; q.d., every day; q.i.d., four times a day; t.i.d., three times a day.

methods to identify potential bacterial pathogens. Furthermore, the potential drawbacks of antibiotic therapy need to be considered before proceeding with such therapy. These include antimicrobial resistance, superinfections, side effects, and the potential for unintended but harmful consequences, such as the induction of Shiga-toxin by certain *E. coli* or the prolongation of shedding of organisms such as *Salmonella* and *C. difficile*. Several specific acute diarrheal syndromes may indicate the need for empiric antibiotic therapy (see Table 19.4). For patients with community-acquired diarrhea, the presence of severe diarrhea, fever (T > 38.5°C), dysentery, or positive fecal markers of inflammation are indications for empiric antibiotic therapy. It is preferable to obtain a stool sample if possible before starting therapy. Antibiotic treatment in this situation may reduce the duration of diarrhea by 1–2 days [62, 63]. For adults, one of the fluoroquinolones is generally used, while trimethoprim/sulfamethoxazole (TMP/SMX) is the first-line therapy in children. Empiric therapy should be withheld in patients who are suspected of having Shiga toxin-producing *E. coli*, mild-to-moderate salmonellosis, and fluoroquinolone-resistant *Campylobacter*. For the latter condition, erythromycin or azithromycin might be used in place of a fluoroquinolone.

Other indications for empiric antibiotic therapy include moderate-to-severe traveler's diarrhea, severe nosocomial diarrhea, and persistent diarrhea in patients with suspected giardiasis [1,2]. For traveler's diarrhea, antibiotics may reduce the duration of diarrhea from 3–4 days to 1–2 days and may require only a single dose [64]. Although a fluoro-

quinolone is usually first-line therapy, for patients who have traveled to areas with high rates of enterotoxigenic *E. coli*, azithromycin [65] and rifaximin (a nonabsorbed antibiotic) [66, 67] have comparable efficacy. Rifaximin is not active against infections associated with dysentery such as *Shigella* and *Campylobacter*. For patients with either severe nosocomial diarrhea or persistent diarrhea, metronidazole is first-line therapy.

Specific antibiotic therapy

Specific antibiotic therapy is given when a treatable pathogen is identified in stool samples submitted to the microbiology laboratory. Antibiotic therapies for specific pathogens are summarized in Table 19.5.

Bacterial pathogens

All patients with confirmed shigellosis should be treated with antibiotic therapy. The initial choice of antibiotic depends on where the infection was acquired. If acquired in the United States, the treatment of choice is TMP/SMX, and if acquired abroad during travel, a fluoroquinolone is the first option [14]. Randomized, controlled trials of antimicrobial treatment of patients with shigellosis have shown that therapy shortens the duration of diarrhea by at least 2.5 days and decreases the duration of fever and tenesmus [2]. In addition, the excretion of infectious organisms is reduced, which decreases the risk of person-to-person transmission. Resistance to TMP/SMX is common outside the United States and limits its efficacy.

Table 19.5 Antibiotic recommendations for specific pathogens

Pathogen	Antibiotic options and dose ranges	Duration	Comments/Alternatives
Campylobacter	Erythromycin 500 mg b.i.d.	5 days	Oral quinolone[a] q.d./b.i.d. × 5 days Quinolone resistance (20%) rising
Salmonella (nontyphoidal)	Not indicated in most cases See below for indications[b]	5–7 days	If indicated, use TMP/SMX 160 mg/800 mg b.i.d. or quinolone q.d./b.i.d. × 5–7 days
Shigella	Quinolone[a] q.d./b.i.d.	3 days	If acquired in the United States, can use TMP/SMX 160 mg/800 mg b.i.d. × 3 days
Enterohemorrhagic *Escherichia coli* (EHEC)	Not indicated in most cases		Antibiotic therapy may increase the risk of hemolytic uremic syndrome
Enterotoxigenic *E. coli* (ETEC)	Quinolone[a] q.d./b.i.d.	3 days	Can use TMP/SMX 160 mg/800 mg b.i.d. × 3 days
Yersinia enterocolitica	Not indicated in most cases See below for indications[c]		If indicated, use doxycycline + aminoglycoside, TMP/SMX, or quinolone
Vibrio parahaemolyticus	Not indicated in most cases Doxycycline 300 mg q.d.	1 day	Can use ciprofloxacin 500 mg b.i.d. × 3 days
Vibrio cholerae 01 or 0139	Doxycycline 300 mg q.d. or quinolone q.d.	1 day	Can use tetracycline 500 mg q.i.d. × 3 days or TMP/SMX 160 mg/800 mg b.i.d. × 3 days
Aeromonas	Quinolone[a] q.d./b.i.d.	3 days	Can use TMP/SMX 160 mg/800 mg b.i.d. × 3 days
Plesiomonas	Quinolone[a] q.d./b.i.d.	3 days	Can use TMP/SMX 160 mg/800 mg b.i.d. × 3 days
Clostridium difficile	Metronidazole 250 mg q.i.d. or 500 mg t.i.d.	10 days	Can use vancomycin 125 mg q.i.d. × 10 days In severe cases or if unable to tolerate oral therapy, can use intravenous metronidazole
Giardia	Metronidazole 250–750 mg t.i.d.	7–10 days	Can use tinidazole 2 g × 1 dose Can use nitazoxanide 500 mg b.i.d. × 3 days
Cryptosporidium	Nitazoxanide 500 mg b.i.d.	3 days	In severe cases, can use combination of paromomycin + azithromycin × 5 days
Cyclospora	TMP/SMX 160/800 mg b.i.d.	7–10 days	
Entamoeba histolytica	Metronidazole 750 mg t.i.d.	5–10 days	Must use along with drug to treat cysts: Iodoquinol 650 mg t.i.d. × 20 days, or Paromomycin 500 mg t.i.d. × 10 days

a Oral quinolone antibiotics include ciprofloxacin 500 mg b.i.d., norfloxacin 400 mg b.i.d., or levofloxacin 500 mg q.d.
b Indications for treatment of nontyphoidal *Salmonella* gastroenteritis include: age under 12 months or over 50 years; predisposing medical conditions such as prostheses, valvular heart disease, severe atherosclerosis, cancer, uremia, immunocompromised, or pregnancy; any patient with severe diarrhea.
c Indications for treatment of *Yersinia* gastroenteritis include: severe diarrhea; bacteremia; immunocompromised.
b.i.d., twice a day; q.d., every day; q.i.d., four times a day; t.i.d., three times a day; TMP/SMX, trimethoprim/sulfamethoxazole.

Patients with confirmed campylobacteriosis should be treated with antibiotic therapy. However, starting therapy 4 days or later after the onset of symptoms has not been shown to reduce the duration of diarrhea [2]. Exceptions include patients who have severe or relapsing diarrhea, are immunocompromised, or are pregnant. Erythromycin remains first-line treatment given its low cost, safety, and minimal rate of *Campylobacter* resistance [24]. The rate of fluoroquinolone-resistant *Campylobacter* continues to rise and approaches 20% [68–70]. The rate of fluoroquinolone resistance appears to be directly related to the increasing use of fluoroquinolones in poultry feeds [24].

Selected patients with nontyphoidal salmonellosis should be treated with antibiotic therapy. The decision to treat these patients should take into account the severity of the episode, the age and health status of the patient, and the presence of risk factors for systemic complications of bacteremia [14]. Patients who are otherwise healthy with mild-to-moderate diarrhea and no signs of dysentery should not be treated because antibiotic therapy is associated with prolonged carriage and relapse [71]. Approximately 5% of patients with acute diarrhea caused by nontyphoidal *Salmonella* will develop bacteremia, a potentially serious complication with mortality rates of 16%–18% [72]. Bacteremia may lead to focal infections such as meningitis, osteomyelitis, septic arthritis, and infectious endarteritis of heart valves or the abdominal aorta. Risk factors for extraintestinal spread in the setting of salmonellosis include age < 12 months or > 50 years, immunosuppression (AIDS, transplant recipients, corticosteroid use), cancer and lymphoproliferative disorders, sickle cell anemia, uremia, atherosclerosis, valvular heart disease, vascular grafts, abdominal aneurysms, and artificial joints [2]. In patients with these risk factors, antibiotic therapy with a fluoroquinolone or TMP/SMX is indicated.

Patients with suspected or confirmed Shiga toxin-producing *E. coli* infection should receive supportive care only and should not receive antibiotic therapy. Shiga toxin-producing *E. coli* infection should be suspected in patients with bloody diarrhea, abdominal pain, little or no fever, and a history of consumption of undercooked hamburger or seed sprouts. A controversial but significant concern exists that antibiotics such as quinolones and TMP/SMX induce the production of Shiga toxin and may increase the risk of HUS [23]. In addition, there is no evidence that patients with Shiga toxin-producing *E. coli* infection benefit from antibiotics.

The initial management step in patients with confirmed *C. difficile*-associated diarrhea should be to discontinue the precipitating broad-spectrum antibiotic if possible. If this is not possible, if symptoms worsen or persist despite discontinuation of antibiotics, or if colitis is present, antibiotics should be initiated with metronidazole or vancomycin as the treatments of choice [17]. Response rates are more than 90% with both agents, although metronidazole is generally the initial choice because of its low cost and low potential for promoting vancomycin-resistant enterococci. The main problem with antibiotic treatment of *C. difficile* is relapse, which occurs in 20%–25% of cases [17].

All patients with documented *Vibrio cholerae* infection should be treated with antibiotics. First-line therapy is a single dose of either doxycycline or a fluoroquinolone [1]. Likewise most patients with *Vibrio parahaemolyticus* infection should be treated with antibiotics, especially patients with severe diarrhea or dysentery, the last of which occurs in 30% of patients [73]. In contrast, most patients with documented *Y. enterocolitica* infection do not require antibiotic therapy. Exceptions include patients with severe diarrhea or dysentery, bacteremia, or who are immunocompromised. Treatments for *Y. enterocolitica* include doxycycline, fluoroquinolones, TMP/SMX, and amino-glycosides [74]. For patients with documented septicemia from *Y. enterocolitica*, combination therapy should be used with a fluoroquinolone and an aminoglycoside.

Protozoal pathogens

Patients with documented giardiasis should be treated with antiparasitic therapy as long as symptoms are present. First-line treatment is metronidazole usually given for 7 to 10 days. Efficacy is greater than 80%–95%. Alternatives with shorter courses of therapy include tinidazole (2-g single dose) and nitazoxanide (500 mg twice a day), the latter agent requires only 3 days of therapy [75]. Patients with documented cryptosporidiosis are much more difficult to treat. Nitazoxanide has been approved by the Food and Drug Administration for the treatment of cryptosporidiosis in children and may decrease diarrhea (80%) and reduce oocyst shedding (67%) [76]. Finally, patients with documented cyclosporiasis should be treated with TMP/SMX with high response rates [44].

Patients with documented intestinal amebiasis should be treated with high-dose metronidazole (750 mg three times a day) for 7–10 days. Patients with mild-to-moderate amebic dysentery will respond to a course of metronidazole in 90% of cases. In the rare case of fulminant amebic colitis, broad-spectrum antibiotics and in some cases surgical intervention may be required [45]. Unfortunately oocysts will persist in the intestine in 50% of cases after a symptomatic response to metronidazole. Therefore, metronidazole therapy should be followed by a course of either paromomycin or iodoquinol to eradicate the residual oocysts [45].

References

1. Guerrant RL, Van Gilder T, Steiner TS, et al. Practice guidelines for the management of infectious diarrhea. Clin Infect Dis 2001;32:331.
2. Thielman NM, Guerrant RL. Acute infectious diarrhea. N Engl J Med 2004;350:38.
3. Mead PS, Slutsker L, Dietz V, et al. Food-related illness and death in the United States. Emerg Infect Dis 1999;5:607.
4. Long JD, Giannella RA. Diagnostic tests in gastrointestinal infections. In: Yamada T (ed.). Textbook of gastroenterology, 4th edn. Philadelphia: Lippincott Williams & Wilkins, 2003;2975.
5. Jones TF, Bulens SN, Gettner S, et al. Use of stool collection kits delivered to patients can improve confirmation of etiology of foodborne disease outbreaks. Clin Infect Dis 2004;39:1454.
6. Slutsker L, Ries AA, Greene KD, et al. *Escherichia coli* O157:H7 diarrhea in the United States: clinical and epidemiologic features. Ann Intern Med 1997;126:505.
7. Preliminary FoodNet data on the incidence of foodborne illnesses – selected sites, United States, 2002. MMWR Morb Mortal Wkly Rep 2003;52:340.
8. Preliminary FoodNet data on the incidence of infection with pathogens transmitted commonly through food – selected sites, United States, 2003. MMWR Morb Mortal Wkly Rep 2004;53:338.
9. Talan DA, Moran GJ, Newdow M, et al. Etiology of bloody diarrhea among patients presenting to United States emergency departments: prevalence of *Escherichia coli* O157:H7 and other enteropathogens. Clin Infect Dis 2001;32:573.
10. Powell DW. Approach to the patient with diarrhea. In: Yamada T

(ed.). Textbook of gastroenterology, 4th edn. Philadelphia: Lippincott Williams & Wilkins, 2003;

11. Steffen R, Collard F, Tornieporth N, et al. Epidemiology, etiology, and impact of traveler's diarrhea in Jamaica. JAMA 1999;281:811.

12. Von Sonnenburg F, Tornieporth N, Waiyaki P, et al. Risk and aetiology of diarrhea at various tourist destinations. Lancet 2000;356:133.

13. Adachi JA, Jiang Z-D, Mathewson JJ, et al. Enteroaggregative *Escherichia coli* as a major etiologic agent in traveler's diarrhea in 3 regions of the world. Clin Infect Dis 2001;32:1706.

14. Dupont HL. Guidelines on acute infectious diarrhea in adults. The Practice Parameters Committee of the American College of Gastroenterology. Am J Gastroenterol 1997;92:1962.

15. DuPont HL. Travellers' diarrhea: contemporary approaches to therapy and prevention. Drugs 2006;66:303.

16. Aranda-Michel J, Giannella RA. Acute diarrhea: a practical review. Am J Med 1999;106:670.

17. Bartlett JG. Antibiotic-associated diarrhea. N Engl J Med 2002;346: 334.

18. Bulusu M, Narayan S, Shetler K, et al. Leukocytosis as a harbinger and surrogate marker of *Clostridium difficile* infection in hospitalized patients with diarrhea. Am J Gastroenterol 2000;95:3137.

19. McDonald LC, Killgore GE, Thompson A, et al. An epidemic, toxin-gene-variant strain of *Clostridium difficile*. N Engl J Med 2005;353:2433.

20. Bartlett JC. Narrative review: the new epidemic of *Clostridium difficile*-associated enteric disease. Ann Intern Med 2006;145:758.

21. Sheth SG, Lamont JT. Toxic megacolon. Lancet 1998;351:509.

22. Marshall JK, Thabane M, Garg AX, et al. Incidence and epidemiology of irritable bowel syndrome after a large waterborne outbreak of bacillary dysentery. Gastroenterology 2006;131:445.

23. Safdar N, Said A, Gangnon RE, et al. Risk of hemolytic uremic syndrome after antibiotic treatment of *Escherichia coli* O157:H7 enteritis. A meta-analysis. JAMA 2002;288:996.

24. Allos BM. *Campylobacter jejuni* infections: update on emerging issues and trends. Clin Infect Dis 2001;32:1201.

25. Klontz KC, Lieb S, Schreiber M, et al. Syndromes of *Vibrio vulnificus* infections: clinical and epidemiologic features in Florida cases, 1981–1987. Ann Intern Med 1988;109:318.

26. Hines J, Nachamkin I. Effective use of the clinical microbiology laboratory for diagnosing diarrheal diseases. Clin Infect Dis 1996;23: 1292.

27. Silletti RP, Lee G, Ailey E. Role of stool screening tests in diagnosis of inflammatory bacterial enteritis and in selection of specimens likely to yield invasive enteric pathogens. J Clin Microbiol 1996;34:1161.

28. Choi SW, Park CH, Silva TMJ, et al. To culture or not to culture: fecal lactoferrin screening for inflammatory bacterial diarrhea. J Clin Microbiol 1996;34:928.

29. Gill CJ, Lau J, Gorbach SL, et al. Diagnostic accuracy of stool assays for inflammatory bacterial gastroenteritis in developed and resource-poor countries. Clin Infect Dis 2003;37:365.

30. Siegel DL, Edelstein PH, Nachamkin I. Inappropriate testing for diarrheal diseases in the hospital. JAMA 1990;263:979.

31. Bowman RA, Bowman JM, Arrow SA, et al. Selective criteria for the microbiologic examination of faecal specimens. J Clin Pathol 1992;45:838.

32. Asnis DS, Bresciani A, Ryan M, et al. Cost-effective approach to evaluation of diarrheal illness in hospitals. J Clin Microbiol 1993;31:1675.

33. Fan K, Morris AJ, Reller LB. Application of rejection criteria for stool cultures for bacterial enteric pathogens. J Clin Microbiol 1993;31:2233.

34. Barbut F, Leluan P, Antoniotti G, et al. Value of routine stool cultures in hospitalized patients with diarrhea. Eur J Clin Microbiol Infect Dis 1995;14:346.

35. Chitkara YK, McCasland KA, Kenefic L. Development and implementation of cost-effective guidelines in the laboratory investigation of diarrhea in a community hospital. Arch Intern Med 1996;156:1445.

36. Valenstein P, Pfaller M, Yungbluth M. The use and abuse of routine stool microbiology. A College of American Pathologists Q-probes study of 601 institutions. Arch Pathol Lab Med 1996;120:206.

37. Rohner P, Pittet D, Pepey B, et al. Etiological agents of infectious diarrhea: implications for requests for microbial culture. J Clin Microbiol 1997;35:1427.

38. Ozerek AE, Rao GG. Is routine screening for conventional enteric pathogens necessary in sporadic hospital-acquired diarrhea? J Hosp Infect 1999;41:159.

39. Bauer TM, Lalvani A, Fehrenbach J, et al. Derivation and validation of guidelines for stool cultures for enteropathogenic bacteria other than *Clostridium difficile* in hospitalized patients. JAMA 2001;285:313.

40. Schumacher G, Kollberg B, Sandstedt B, et al. A prospective study of first attacks of inflammatory bowel disease and non-relapsing colitis. Scand J Gastroenterol 1993;28:1077.

41. Weber P, Koch M, Heizmann WR, et al. Microbic superinfection in relapses of inflammatory bowel disease. J Clin Gastroenterol 1992; 14:302.

42. Ortega YR, Adam RD. *Giardia*: overview and update. Clin Infect Dis 1997;25:545.

43. Chen X-M, Keithly JS, Paya CV, et al. Cryptosporidiosis. N Engl J Med 2002;346:1723.

44. Herwaldt BL. *Cyclospora cayetanensis*: a review, focusing on the outbreaks of cyclosporiasis in the 1990s. Clin Infect Dis 2000;31:1040.

45. Haque R, Huston CD, Hughes M, et al. Amebiasis. N Engl J Med 2003;348:1565.

46. Manabe YC, Vinetz JM, Moore RD, et al. *Clostridium difficile* colitis: an efficient clinical approach to diagnosis. Ann Intern Med 1995;123:835.

47. Cooper GS, Lederman MM, Salata RA. A predictive model to identify *Clostridium difficile* toxin in hospitalized patients with diarrhea. Am J Gastroenterol 1995;91:80.

48. Katz DA, Lynch ME, Littenberg B. Clinical prediction rules to optimize cytotoxin testing for *Clostridium difficile* in hospitalized patients with diarrhea. Am J Med 1996;100:487.

49. Mylonakis E, Ryan ET, Calderwood SB. *Clostridium difficile*-associated diarrhea: a review. Arch Intern Med 2001;161:525.

50. Lamps LW. Infective disorders of the gastrointestinal tract. Histopathology 2007;50:55.

51. Morris AJ, Wilson ML, Reller LB. Application of rejection criteria for stool ovum and parasite examinations. J Clin Microbiol 1992;30:3213.

52. Wood M. When stool cultures from adult inpatients are appropriate. Lancet 2001;357:901.

53. Morris AJ, Murray PR, Reller LB. Contemporary testing for enteric pathogens: the potential for cost, time, and health care savings. J Clin Microbiol 1996;34:1776.

54. Thillainayagam AV, Hunt JB, Farthing MJE. Enhancing clinical efficacy of oral therapy: is low osmolality the key? Gastroenterology 1998;114:197.

55. Hahn S, Kim Y, Garner P. Reduced osmolarity oral rehydration solution for treating dehydration due to diarrhea in children: systematic review. BMJ 2001;323:81.

56. Dupont HL, Hornick RB. Adverse effect of lomotil therapy in shigellosis. JAMA 1973;226:1525.

57. Cimolai N, Basalyga S, Mah DG, et al. A continuing assessment of risk factors for the development of *Escherichia coli* O157:H7-associated hemolytic uremic syndrome. Clin Nephrol 1994;42:85.

58. Trudel JL, Deschenes M, Mayrand S, et al. Toxic megacolon complicating pseudomembranous enterocolitis. Dis Colon Rectum 1995; 38:1033.

59. Petruccelli BP, Murphy GS, Sanchez JL, et al. Treatment of traveler's diarrhea with ciprofloxacin and loperamide. J Infect Dis 1992;165:557.

60. Murphy GS, Bodhidatta L, Echeverria P, et al. Ciprofloxacin and loperamide in the treatment of bacillary dysentery. Ann Intern Med 1993;118:582.

61. Dupont H, Sanchez J, Ericsson C, et al. Comparative efficacy of loperamide hydrochloride and bismuth subsalicylate in the management of acute diarrhea. Am J Med 1990;88:15S.

62. Goodman LJ, Trenholme GM, Kaplan RL, et al. Empiric antimicrobial therapy of domestically acquired acute diarrhea in urban adults. Arch Intern Med 1990;150:541.

63. Wistrom J, Jertborn M, Ekwall E, et al. Empiric treatment of acute diarrheal disease with norfloxacin. A randomized, placebo-controlled study. Swedish Study Group. Ann Intern Med 1992;202:202.

64. Adachi JA, Ostrosky-Zeichner L, DuPont HL, et al. Empirical antimicrobial therapy for traveler's diarrhea. Clin Infect Dis 2000;31:1079.

65. Adachi JA, Ericsson CD, Jiang ZD, et al. Azithromycin found to be comparable to levofloxacin for the treatment of US travelers with acute diarrhea acquired in Mexico. Clin Infect Dis 2003;37:1165.

66. DuPont HL, Jiang ZD, Ericsson CD, et al. Rifaximin versus ciprofloxacin for the treatment of traveler's diarrhea: a randomized, double-blind clinical trial. Clin Infect Dis 2001;33:1807.

67. Steffen R, Sack DA, Riopel L, et al. Therapy of traveler's diarrhea with rifaximin on various continents. Am J Gastroenterol 2003;98:1073.

68. Smith KE, Besser JM, Hedberg CW, et al. Quinolone-resistant Campylobacter jejuni infections in Minnesota, 1992–1998. N Engl J Med 1999;340:1525.

69. Nachamkin I, Ung H, Li M. Increasing fluoroquinolone resistance in Campylobacter jejuni, Pennsylvania, USA, 1982–2001. Emerg Infect Dis 2002;8:1501.

70. Nelson JM, Smith KE, Vugia DJ, et al. Prolonged diarrhea due to ciprofloxacin-resistant Campylobacter infection. J Infect Dis 2004;190:1150.

71. Neill MA, Opal SM, Heelan J, et al. Failure of ciprofloxacin to eradicate convalescent fecal excretion after acute salmonellosis: experience during an outbreak in health care workers. Ann Intern Med 1991;114:195.

72. Hohmann EL. Nontyphoidal salmonellosis. Clin Infect Dis 2001;32:263.

73. Daniels NA, MacKinnon L, Bishop R, et al. Vibrio parahaemolyticus infections in the United States, 1973–1998. J Infect Dis 2000;181:1661.

74. Oldfield EC, Wallace MR. The role of antibiotics in the treatment of infectious diarrhea. Gastroenterol Clin North Am 2001;30:817.

75. Ortiz JJ, Ayoub A, Gargala G, et al. Randomized clinical study of nitazoxanide compared to metronidazole in the treatment of symptomatic giardiasis in children from Northern Peru. Aliment Pharmacol Ther 2001;15:1409.

76. Rossignol J, Ayoub A, Ayers MS. Treatment of diarrhea caused by Cryptosporidium parvum: a prospective randomized, double-blind, placebo-controlled study of nitazoxanide. J Infect Dis 2001;184:103.

20

Approach to the patient with constipation

Satish S.C. Rao

Epidemiology, 373
Psychological distress, abuse, and impact on quality of life, 375
Definition, 375
Etiology, subtypes, and pathophysiology of chronic constipation, 375
Clinical evaluation of chronic constipation, 379
Treatment of chronic constipation, 386
Complications of constipation, 392

Constipation is common and affects 15% of the population [1–4]. It can be mild and transitory, or chronic and unresponsive to treatment and is more prevalent and more severe in women [5]. It places a substantial burden on health-care resources, including physician visits, over-the-counter and prescription medications, and affects quality of life. Over the past decade, significant new knowledge has emerged on several aspects of constipation including its epidemiology, pathophysiology, and treatment.

Epidemiology

The prevalence of chronic constipation varies from 2% to 28% [1–4,6]. It is commonly encountered in primary care (see Fig. 20.1). Telephone interviews with 10 018 individuals, aged at least 18 years, produced an estimated prevalence of 14.7% [2], and if this statistic is applied to the US population, constipation may affect over 33 million adults. Most patients do not seek health care so the prevalence of constipation has been underestimated [7]. Its natural history is not known, and it may not resolve quickly. In one study, 89% had similar symptoms 1 year apart [8]; in another, 45% of subjects interviewed reported having the condition for at least 5 years [2].

Principles of Clinical Gastroenterology. Edited by Tadataka Yamada, David H. Alpers, Anthony N. Kalloo, Neil Kaplowitz, Chung Owyang, and Don W. Powell. © 2008 Blackwell Publishing. ISBN 978-1-4051-69103

Populations at higher risk of constipation

Constipation is more common in women with an estimated female : male ratio of 2.2 : 1 [9–12]. Its occurrence increases with advancing age, particularly after age 65 years, with the elderly reporting more problems with straining and hard stools than with infrequency [10–12]. Its prevalence is twofold higher in African Americans [4,10], in those of lower socioeconomic status (annual income ≤ $20 000) [1,4,10], and in nursing home residents [10,13,14]. Pregnancy is also associated with higher prevalence of constipation, but no differences were found between the first and the last trimester [15].

Familial tendency and other comorbid features

A recent survey showed familial susceptibility, with a higher prevalence in sisters, daughters, and mothers of constipated women with an odds ratio of 3.8 [16]. Chronic constipation is also frequently associated with other functional gastrointestinal disorders including chest pain [17], gastroesophageal reflux disease [18–20], irritable bowel syndrome, and functional dyspepsia [18–20].

Economic and social impact

Chronic constipation has a significant impact on the use of health-care resources, including the cost of inpatient and outpatient care, laboratory tests, and diagnostic procedures [21] (Table 20.1). In the United States, $821 million was spent on laxatives alone in 2002 [22]. Constipation was a reason for seeking care in 5.7 million ambulatory physician visits per year [23] and almost 85% of physician visits resulted in a prescription for laxatives [21]. Also, laxatives are the most

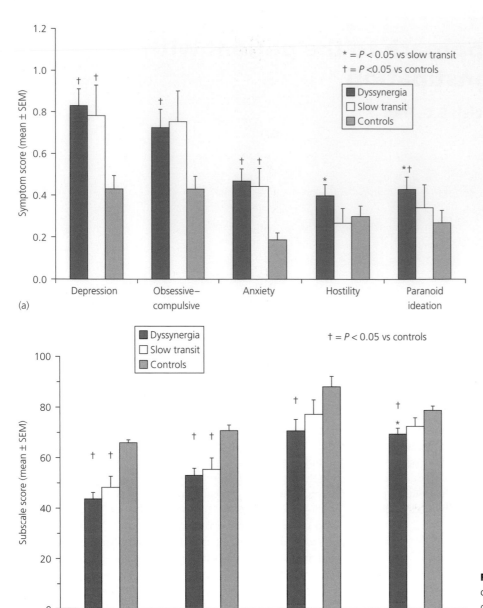

Figure 20.1 **(a)** Effect of chronic constipation on psychological symptoms and **(b)** impact of chronic constipation on quality of life. From Rao et al. [28].

Table 20.1 Socioeconomic and medical consequences of chronic constipation in the United States

Mortality/year	121 deaths (2002)
Hospitalizations/year	398 000 (2002)
Ambulatory care visits/year	1.4 million (1999–2000)
Disability	30 000 (1990–1992)
Physician cost	$3 016 017
Health-care cost	$18 891 008

From Martin et al. [23] and Singh et al. [24].

commonly prescribed medication in long-term care facilities [12]; about 58% of all patients in US nursing homes receive at least one laxative [12].

In a study of 76 854 patients enrolled in Medi-cal program, the total health-care expenditure for patients with constipation over a 15-month period was $18 891 008, with an average cost of $246 per patient [24]. Approximately 0.6% of patients were hospitalized with an average cost of $2993 per admission [24]. In another study, expenditure for constipation was estimated at $235 million/year with 55% incurred from inpatient, 23% from emergency department, and 22% from outpatient care [23]. In a tertiary-care center, average expenditure for diagnostic evaluation was \$2752 [25]. Constipation also resulted in 13.7 million days of restricted activity, missing work or school in 12%, and impaired ability to work in 60% of patients [21].

Psychological distress, abuse, and impact on quality of life

Constipation is associated with increased psychological distress. Several studies have shown higher prevalence for anxiety, depression, obsessive–compulsiveness, psychoticism, and somatization [26–28]. Furthermore, paranoid ideation and hostility subscores were higher (Fig. 20.1a) in patients with dyssynergia than patients with slow transit or healthy controls, providing evidence for significant psychological distress, more so in subjects with dyssynergia than patients with slow-transit constipation.

Sexual abuse was reported by 22%–48% of subjects, mostly women, whereas physical abuse was reported by 31%–74% of constipated subjects [14,29]. Another study found greater incidence of sexual abuse in women with pelvic floor dyssynergia [30]. Also, patients with abuse were more likely to seek health care [7,31] and to report feelings of incomplete evacuation or urge to defecate, but did not demonstrate rectal hypersensitivity [32].

Patients with chronic constipation also showed significant impairment of health-related quality of life (Fig. 20.1b) [13,28,33,34]. Some domains were more affected in subjects with dyssynergia than in those with slow transit [28], suggesting that dyssynergia is associated with greater impact on quality of life. Also, psychological distress and lower quality of life were strongly correlated, suggesting that these dysfunctions have synergistic effects [28].

Definition

Chronic constipation is a heterogeneous disorder that encompasses many symptoms. It has several definitions [5,22], and up to 50% of patients define constipation differently from their physicians [35]. Patients often define constipation as excessive straining, a sense of incomplete bowel evacuation, failed or lengthy attempts to defecate, or hard stools and rarely by stool frequency [10,14,35,36]. Also, patients' perception of constipation may be inaccurate. In one study, 51% of patients considered themselves constipated and reported three or fewer bowel movements per week for at least 6 months, but on prospective stool diaries, they averaged six bowel movements per week [37]. Consequently, stool diaries and physiological measurements may provide a more reliable assessment of bowel function than history by recall.

To improve the diagnosis of constipation, and to facilitate clinical research, consensus criteria have been proposed by

Table 20.2 Diagnostic criteria for functional constipation and dyssynergic defecation

Criteria[a] for functional constipation (Rome III)

1 Must include *two or more* of the following:
  a straining during at least 25% of defecations
  b lumpy or hard stools in at least 25% of defecations
  c sensation of incomplete evacuation in at least 25% of defecations
  d sensation of anorectal obstruction/blockage in at least 25% of defecations
  e manual maneuvers to facilitate at least 25% of defecations (e.g., digital evacuation, support of the pelvic floor)
  f fewer than three defecations per week
2 Loose stools are rarely present without the use of laxatives
3 There are insufficient criteria for irritable bowel syndrome

Criteria for dyssynergic defecation

Patients must fulfill all three criteria:

1 The diagnostic criteria for functional chronic constipation (Rome III)
2 Demonstrate dyssynergia during repeated attempts to defecate (see Fig. 20.4), and a dyssynergic or obstructive pattern of defecation (Types 1–3), which is defined as a paradoxical increase in anal sphincter pressure (anal contraction) or less than 20% relaxation of the resting anal sphincter pressure or inadequate propulsive forces based on manometry, imaging, or electromyography
3 One or more of the following criteria during repeated attempts to defecate:
  a inability to expel an artificial stool (50-mL water-filled balloon) within 1 min
  b a prolonged colonic transit time; i.e., more than five markers (≥ 20% marker retention) on a plain abdominal radiograph taken 120 h after ingestion of one Sitzmarks capsule containing 24 radiopaque markers
  c inability to evacuate or ≥ 50% retention of barium during defecography

a Criteria fulfilled for the last 3 months with symptom onset at least 6 months before diagnosis.
From Bharucha et al. [41], Longstreth et al. [42], and Rao et al. [226].

experts [38–42]. Rome III criteria for functional constipation and diagnostic criteria for dyssynergic defecation are shown in Table 20.2 [41,42]. Observational studies find that many patients do not meet the Rome criteria so the American College of Gastroenterology Chronic Constipation Task Force recommends a broader definition: "unsatisfactory defecation characterized by infrequent stools, difficult stool passage, or both" [43].

Etiology, subtypes, and pathophysiology of chronic constipation

Broadly, constipation can be divided into two groups (Fig. 20.2). Primary constipation results from disordered regulation of

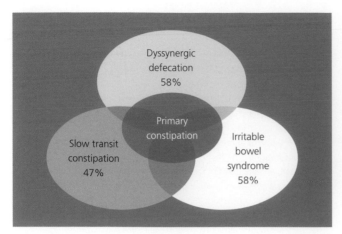

Figure 20.2 Pathophysiological subtypes of primary chronic constipation. From Mertz et al. [266].

Table 20.3 Common causes of secondary constipation

Anorectal and colonic disorders
Anal fissure
Hemorrhoids
Ulcerative (proctitis)
Diverticulitis
Colorectal carcinoma
Inflammatory, postoperative, and radiation strictures

Drugs
Opioids and related agents
Anticholinergic drugs and antispasmodics
Antidepressants
Antihypertensive drugs, particularly calcium channel antagonists, methyldopa
Antiparkinsonian drugs
Anticonvulsants
Antihistamines
Diuretics
Metal ions such as antacids (aluminum or calcium), iron supplements, and calcium supplements
Serotonin 5-HT$_3$ antagonists – alosetron

Endocrine and metabolic disorders
Diabetes mellitus
Hypothyroidism
Hypokalemia
Hypercalcemia
Porphyria

Neuromuscular disorders
Spinal cord lesions
Parkinson disease
Multiple sclerosis
Stroke/cerebrovascular disease
Chagas disease
Hirschsprung disease

From Rao [263].

colonic and anorectal neuromuscular function as well as brain–gut neuroenteric function. Secondary constipation results from a plethora of factors that include diet, drugs, behavioral, endocrine, metabolic, neurological, and other disorders (Table 20.3). Functionally, the right colon serves as a reservoir for mixing, fermentation, salvage, and transport of digestive residues, whereas the left colon serves as a conduit for desiccation and more rapid transport of stool; the rectosigmoid region acts as a sensorimotor organ that stores stool and facilitates defecation. These functions are regulated by neurotransmitters and intrinsic colonic reflexes. Constipation may therefore result from structural, mechanical, metabolic, or functional disorders that affect the colon or anorectum. Healthy subjects can postpone defecation for several days [44] and patients with dyssynergia have impaired gut–brain evoked responses [45], so a dysfunction of the brain–gut axis may play an important role.

At least three subtypes of primary constipation have been recognized, although overlap exists [5,22]. *Slow-transit constipation* (STC) is characterized by prolonged delay in the transit of stool through the colon. This delay may be the result of a primary dysfunction of the colonic smooth muscle (myopathy) or its innervation (neuropathy), or both and can be secondary to dyssynergic defecation. *Evacuation disorders* are characterized by either difficulty or inability with expulsion of stool from the anorectum. They include anorectal functional disorders such as dyssynergic defecation [38], as well as structural disorders such as rectocele, descending perineum syndrome, and rectal prolapse [38]. About 60% of patients with dyssynergic defecation have secondary STC [14,46]. *Constipation-predominant irritable bowel syndrome* (IBS-C), is seen in patients in whom abdominal discomfort or pain is a prominent symptom together with symptoms of constipation [42]. These patients may or may not have coexisting STC or evacuation disorder. It accounts for 24%–58% of chronic constipation cases [47]. Here, patients perceive a difficulty with evacuation or pass hard stools [5] despite normal stool frequency. Approximately 20% of patients with IBS have concurrent constipation [48], making it difficult to distinguish this from chronic constipation [33].

Pathophysiology of slow-transit constipation

In this disorder, the transport of stool across the colon is significantly slower than in normal individuals. Consequently, there is prolonged retention of stool matter. This may occur because of either primary or secondary dysfunction of colonic smooth muscle activity, neurological innervation, colocolonic reflexes, pacemaker cell activity, or neurotransmitters that regulate colonic neuromuscular function. Altered absorption or secretion and alterations in the colonic flora, particularly the presence of methanogenic flora, may also play a role [49–51].

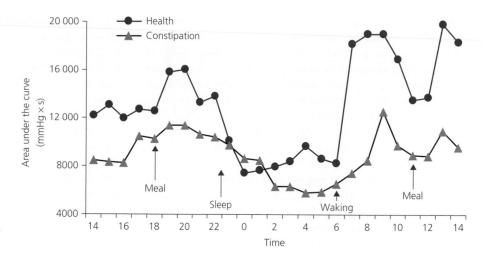

Figure 20.3 Ambulatory 24-h colonic manometry profile in healthy subjects and in patients with chronic slow-transit constipation. From Rao et al. [59].

Colonic dysmotility

Colonic motor activity exhibits temporal and spatial variation [52] and can be influenced by sleep, waking, meals [53–55], physical [56] and emotional stressors [55,57,58], gender, aging, and regional variation [55,59]. Patients with STC exhibit significant reduction in overall colonic motor activity [53,55]. Furthermore, the increased motor activity after meals (gastrocolonic response), and after waking from sleep are significantly diminished or absent, but the diurnal variation of colonic motor activity is preserved (Fig. 20.3) [59]. The colonic motor patterns such as high-amplitude propagated contractions, propagated and simultaneous contractions are all decreased [59,60]. Furthermore, the velocity of propagation of high-amplitude propagated contractions is slower, their amplitude is lower, and they abort prematurely in patients with STC [61]. In contrast, the incidence of periodic rectal motor activity, a 3 cycles per min activity of the rectosigmoid region [62–65] that is often seen at nighttime [63,66], is significantly increased and may serve as a nocturnal brake that retards colonic propulsion of stool [63].

Colonic neuropathy

Recent studies of combined manometry with barostat have shown that the meal-induced colonic tonic and phasic responses are diminished [67–69], and the colocolonic reflexes are impaired [68–72]. There was a greater tendency for retrograde propulsion of colonic contents [70]. Colonic responses to stimulations from a balloon [71] or bisacodyl were diminished [72]. STC may also be the result of dysregulation of the autonomic control of colonic neuromuscular activity [73–75]. The best evidence for this stems from studies that have consistently shown a paucity of interstitial cells of Cajal (ICC), the intestinal pacemaker cells [76,77]. The ICC forms extensive networks of electrically coupled cells that are widely distributed in the submucosal, intramuscular and intermuscular regions of the colonic wall and lie in close proximity to the enteric nerves [78,79]. The ICC regulate the

oscillatory electrical contractile activity of colonic smooth muscle cells [80]. Patients with STC not only exhibit a pancolonic decrease in the ICC volume across the circular and longitudinal muscle layers and submucosa, but also in the number of myenteric ganglion cells [81]. These observations were made on colectomy specimens obtained from patients with chronic constipation so it is unclear whether they represent a primary neuropathy or whether they are secondary to the use of drugs, cathartics or behavioral changes over many years. Rarely, STC is associated with a more generalized dysmotility and forms part of a pseudoobstruction syndrome [82,83].

Neurotransmitter and hormonal disturbances

Constipation is associated with hard stools, so one possible hypothesis is that excessive absorption of water from stool may desiccate the colonic contents. However, the colonic absorptive function is relatively well preserved in patients with constipation [84]. In one study, abnormally impaired hormonal responses to ingested water load were reported, but its significance is unclear [85]. In younger adults, more women than men seek medical help for constipation, suggesting a possible role for endocrine or hormonal imbalance [85]. A decreased level of ovarian and adrenal steroid hormones has been suggested [86], but not confirmed. In fact, routine estrogen and progesterone levels are not altered. Also, the relationship between menstrual cycle and gut transit remains controversial [87]. Both slower transit during the luteal phase [88] and normal transit have been reported [89]. Studies of neurotransmitters have also provided conflicting data [90]. A decrease in vasoactive intestinal polypeptide levels [91], an increase in serotonin levels in the circular muscle [92], and alterations in enteroglucagon, pancreatic polypeptide [93,94] and in other hormones have been reported but whether they are primary or secondary remains unknown [94]. An intriguing study examined G protein-mediated smooth muscle contractility, from colectomy specimens in women with

STC. This study showed down-regulation of progesterone-dependent contractile G proteins and up-regulation of inhibitory G proteins, probably caused by an overexpression of progesterone receptors in constipated patients when compared to nonconstipated controls [95,96]. This study offers some mechanistic insights as to why women are more prone to constipation. Most recently, it has been observed that there is a higher prevalence of methanogenic flora in constipated patients [49–51] and that infusion of methane gas impairs muscle contractions [97]. Whether the presence of methanogenic flora predisposes an individual to develop constipation or whether it is a consequence of altered colonic physiology merits further study. Neuronal and neurotransmitter-mediated excitation and inhibition of colonic smooth muscle activity is largely governed by the ICC and the enteric nervous system. A number of studies suggest that alterations in serotonin (5-hydroxytryptamine [5-HT]) signaling may lead to constipation, but again inconsistencies exist [98]. Serotonin is synthesized and stored in the enterochromaffin cells that are located within the mucosal crypts, and accounts for up to 95% of the total body serotonin [98]. When the mucosa is stimulated, either mechanically, by stroking, or chemically, the enterochromaffin cells release 5-HT and other peptides including calcitonin gene-related peptide [99]. These paracrine neuromediators act on the intrinsic primary afferent neurons that synapse in the myenteric plexus with ascending excitatory and descending inhibitory interneurons. The activation of the ascending cholinergic interneurons releases acetylcholine and substance P, which produces smooth muscle contraction and initiates the peristaltic reflex [98,99]. Simultaneously, the activation of the descending cholinergic interneurons releases nitric oxide, vasoactive intestinal polypeptide, and adenosine triphosphate, which relax the circular muscle. Tegaserod, a 5-HT_4 agonist, stimulates ascending contraction and descending relaxation [100] and accelerates small bowel and colonic transit [101]. In contrast, the gastrocolonic response and ascending contractions of the peristaltic reflex were impaired in patients with STC, and these effects were partially mediated by granisetron, a 5-HT_3 antagonist [102]. These observations support a role for serotonin and its receptors in the pathogenesis of constipation, but it is unclear whether there is decreased availability of serotonin or whether there is decreased receptor density or whether there is altered function of the serotonin reuptake transporter [103]. Clearly, further research is required to better understand the interplay between hormones, neurotransmitters, colonic flora, muscle function, and signaling from the enteric nervous system.

Pathophysiology of evacuation disorders

This group of disorders includes a functional disorder of defecation – dyssynergic defecation – as well as structural disorders such as Hirschsprung disease, rectocele, descending perineum syndrome, and rectal prolapse.

Dyssynergic defecation

Dyssynergia appears to be an acquired behavioral disorder of defecation. In two-thirds of adult patients, it stems from faulty toilet habit, painful defecation, obstetric or back injury, and brain–gut dysfunction [14,45]. In the rest, the process of defecation may not have been learnt since childhood (due to behavioral problems, or parent–child conflicts) [14]. In a prospective study, most patients with dyssynergic defecation showed an inability to coordinate the abdominal, rectoanal, and pelvic floor muscles during attempted defecation [14,104]. This failure of rectoanal coordination consisted of either paradoxical anal contraction, inadequate anal relaxation or impaired rectal/abdominal propulsive forces [14]. Additionally, two-thirds of these patients exhibit rectal hyposensitivity [104,105].

Earlier studies suggested that the paradoxical anal contraction was an involuntary anal spasm (animus) during defecation [106–108]. Of healthy subjects, 20%–30% may also exhibit paradoxical anal contraction [109,110]. In a recent study [111], in the lying position, one-third of healthy subjects showed dyssynergia and one-half could not expel artificial stool, whereas in the sitting position and with a sensation of stooling, most subjects showed a normal pattern of defecation and an ability to expel stool [111]. Thus, body position, sensation of stooling, and stool characteristics can influence defecation.

Based on the notion that dyssynergia is a spasmodic dysfunction of the anal sphincter, myectomy has been performed [107], but it only helped 10%–30% of patients [112]. Similarly, botulinum toxin injection has been ineffective [113,114]. Hence, spasm or inability to relax the anal sphincter is unlikely to be the sole mechanism for dyssynergic defecation.

Manometrically, at least three reproducible types of dyssynergia [38,115] have been recognized (Fig. 20.4). The recognition of these patterns allows the biofeedback therapist to expound patient-specific treatment programs, such as emphasis on pushing effort (Type 2) or improved relaxation (Type 3). In a prospective study of biofeedback therapy, there was no difference in the clinical outcome between the three groups of dyssynergia [116]. Additionally, thresholds for first sensation or desire to defecate or both may be higher in 60% of dyssynergic patients [104].

Hirschsprung disease

This classic neuroenteric disorder often presents by 6 months of age and rarely in adults [117]. It is characterized by absence of intramural ganglion cells in the myenteric plexus of the rectum and stems from developmental arrest of the caudal migration of neural crest cells during embryonic development. Consequently, there is increased acetylcholinesterase activity and depletion of inhibitory neurotransmitter release such as nitric oxide and vasoactive intestinal polypeptide [118]. Manometrically, it is characterized by an absent rectoanal inhibitory reflex [119]. Recent studies have identified mutations in the *RET*, *GDNF*, *EDN3*, and *EDNRB* genes [120].

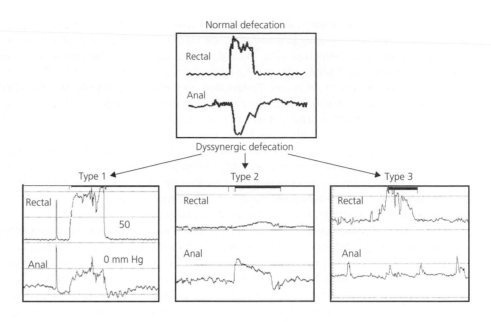

Figure 20.4 Manometric patterns and the intralumenal pressure changes in the rectum and anal canal during attempted defecation in a healthy subject and in patients with dyssynergic defecation. Type 1 – subject can generate an adequate propulsive force (rise in intraabdominal/rectal pressure, ≥ 40 mmHg) along with a paradoxical increase in anal sphincter pressure; Type 2 – subject is unable to generate an adequate propulsive force (inadequate increase in intrarectal pressure) together with either a paradoxical anal contraction or impaired anal relaxation; and Type 3 – subject can generate an adequate propulsive force but either has absent or incomplete (< 20%) anal sphincter relaxation. From Rao et al. [226].

Pathophysiology of IBS-C

Multiple pathophysiological mechanisms have been proposed that include genetic, environmental, social, biological, and psychological factors [121,122]. Altered autonomic regulation and release of neurotransmitters such as serotonin have been proposed, but these lack specificity [121]. Familial aggregation and twin studies have reported the existence of genetic susceptibility for IBS [123]. Although, several candidate genetic markers are associated with IBS, the occurrence of significant genetic polymorphism makes an etiological or pathogenetic relevance less likely [124]. Dietary factors such as fructose intolerance may also lead to IBS symptoms, particularly in those with gas and bloating [125,126]. Small intestinal bacterial overgrowth has been implicated, and its eradication with rifaximin improves symptoms in some patients [50,51]. Also, IBS has been reported in a subset of patients following gastroenteritis, and this postinfectious IBS may be related to up-regulation of intestinal cytokines or antecedent psychiatric problems [127,128]. Recent studies reveal that abnormal cortical perception, hypervigilance and either impaired inhibition of descending efferent signals or dysregulation in the brainstem may play a role [129]. Mucosal serotonin transporter immunoreactivity and messenger systems were all significantly reduced in IBS-C, suggesting altered regulation of enteric serotonin release and reuptake [130].

Clinical evaluation of chronic constipation

Medical history

A detailed medical, surgical, and drug history can help to identify most organic and secondary causes of constipation [5,22]. Constipated patients present with a constellation of symptoms such as excessive straining, passage of hard, pellet-like stool, or decreased stool frequency, or they may misrepresent their symptoms or may feel embarrassed to describe the use of digital disimpaction or vaginal splinting [5,14,33]. However, by establishing a trustworthy relationship and through the use of symptom questionnaires or stool diaries [14,37], it is possible to define the nature of bowel dysfunction. A sensitive and compassionate approach is often the key for unraveling the mind–body interactions and the psychosocial issues of a constipated patient.

Patients should be encouraged to describe their bowel habit – how often they feel the urge to defecate, and if they complete defecation in response to the urge, their definition of constipation – frequency, need for straining, stool consistency, stool size, history of ignoring a call to stool, precipitating events, and how their cultural beliefs and expectations affect their bowel patterns, what they believe is normal bowel habit [131], and whether the problem began in childhood. The history should ascertain how the onset, severity, and duration of each symptom relate to the patient's normal bowel habit. A long history of recurring problems, which is refractory to dietary measures or laxatives, often suggests a functional colorectal disorder, whereas a history of recent onset (rectal bleeding, anemia, guaiac-positive stool, or mass in the abdomen) should alert the physician to seek and exclude an organic illness, including neoplastic disease.

A dietary history should include an assessment of the fiber and fluid intake, the number of meals and when they are consumed, and their caloric and nutrient content. A prospectively maintained food diary for a week and its appraisal by a dietician can be useful. Many patients tend to skip breakfast or do not allow time for defecation because of the "early morning rush" to get to work or school. This may prove to be a handicap. A failure to capitalize on these physiological stimulants such as after waking [55] and after a meal [53,54] may predispose to constipation. The history should also include the number and type of laxatives and frequency of their use. A family history of bowel dysfunction may also be important [16]. Obstetrical, surgical, and back trauma, neurological problems, and drug history may provide clues regarding the etiology of constipation. In the elderly, fecal incontinence may be a presenting feature of stool impaction.

Symptoms alone do not appear to reliably differentiate among the three common pathophysiological subgroups of constipation [132]. In a prospective survey of 120 patients with dyssynergic defecation, the prevalence of constipation symptoms was similar between patients with or without dyssynergia [14]. In another study, two or fewer stools per week, laxative dependency, and constipation since childhood were associated with STC, whereas backache, heartburn, and anorectal surgery and lower prevalence of normal stool frequency were associated with pelvic floor dysfunction [33]. Thus, symptoms were good predictors of transit time, but poor predictors of pelvic floor dysfunction. Also, stool frequency alone was of little value whereas a sense of obstruction or digital assistance for evacuation was specific but not sensitive for difficult defecation [132]. Thus, symptom assessment should be combined with objective testing for optimal assessment of these patients.

Objective measures can facilitate the diagnosis of constipation by providing a common framework for physicians' and patients' understanding of symptoms. Several instruments are available. The Bristol Stool Form scale (Fig. 20.5) allows patients to identify one of seven stool forms for any given bowel movement [133,134]. Other commonly used scales include the Constipation Assessment Scale and the Elderly Bowel Symptom Questionnaire [135]. Assessment of stool form can aid in the assessment of colonic transit time because very loose or hard stools correlate with rapid or slow colonic

transit, respectively [136]. Likewise, assessments of psychological dysfunction or assessments of quality of life and a 1-week prospective stool diary can be useful.

Physical examination

A thorough general physical examination that includes a detailed neurological examination should screen for most organic conditions that cause constipation. The abdomen must be carefully examined for the presence of stool, particularly in the left lower quadrant. A normal physical examination is not uncommon but it is important to exclude a gastrointestinal mass.

Digital rectal examination

A careful perianal and digital rectal examination is not only important but is often the most revealing part of clinical evaluation [5,38]. Anorectal inspection can detect skin excoriation, skin tags, anal fissures, or hemorrhoids. Assessment of perineal sensation and anocutaneous reflex by gently stroking the perianal skin with a cotton bud (Q-tip) or blunt needle in all four quadrants will elicit reflex contraction of the external anal sphincter. If this is absent, a neuropathy should be suspected. Digital rectal examination may reveal a stricture, spasm, tenderness, mass, blood or stool. If stool is present, its consistency should be noted and the patient should be asked if they were aware of its presence. A lack of awareness of stool in the rectum may suggest rectal hyposensitivity. It is useful to assess the resting and squeeze tone of the anal sphincter and puborectalis muscle by asking the subject to squeeze. More importantly, the subject should be asked to push and bear down as if to defecate. During this maneuver, the examiner should perceive relaxation of the external anal sphincter or the puborectalis muscle, together with perineal descent. A hand placed on the abdomen can gauge the abdominal push effort. An absence of these normal findings should raise the index of suspicion for an evacuation disorder

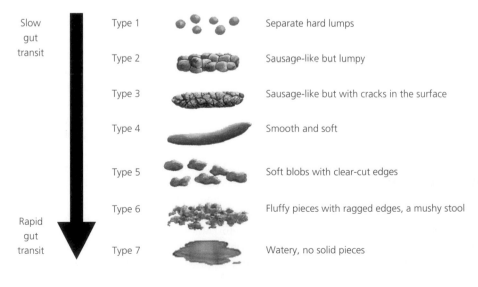

Slow gut transit	Type 1	Separate hard lumps
	Type 2	Sausage-like but lumpy
	Type 3	Sausage-like but with cracks in the surface
	Type 4	Smooth and soft
	Type 5	Soft blobs with clear-cut edges
	Type 6	Fluffy pieces with ragged edges, a mushy stool
Rapid gut transit	Type 7	Watery, no solid pieces

Figure 20.5 Bristol Stool Form Scale – a useful clinical scale for assessing and documenting stool consistency. From Heaton et al. [136].

such as dyssynergic defecation [38]. Digital rectal examination has a high sensitivity for identifying dyssynergia [137]. Even though digital rectal examination is useful clinical tool, there is a lack of knowledge on how to perform a comprehensive evaluation. A survey of 256 final-year medical students revealed that 17% had never performed a digital rectal examination and 48% were unsure of giving an opinion based on their findings [138]. Thus, a concerted effort is needed to improve the training for digital rectal examination.

Diagnostic tests

The first step in making a diagnosis of constipation is to exclude an underlying metabolic or pathological disorder, because constipation may be a symptom of many organic conditions and, rarely, colon cancer. A complete blood count, biochemical profile, serum calcium, glucose levels, and thyroid function tests are usually sufficient for screening purposes. If there is a high index of suspicion, serum protein electrophoresis, urine porphyrins, serum parathyroid hormone, and serum cortisol levels may be requested. However, no studies have assessed the clinical value of the routine use of blood tests [139]. Hence, the American College of Gastroenterology Task Force does not routinely recommend these tests in patients younger than 50 years of age and in whom there are no alarm symptoms or signs of organic disease [140]. Alarm features may include new onset or progressively worsening constipation, onset after age 50 years, bloody stools, weight loss, fever, anorexia, nausea, vomiting, or a family history of inflammatory bowel disease or colon cancer [5,43]. For young patients without alarm features, empiric treatment without diagnostic testing is appropriate [43]. Once an organic disorder has been excluded, most patients have a functional neuromuscular disorder of the colorectum.

Radiographic studies

Plain abdominal radiograph

A plain radiograph of the abdomen is an inexpensive, frequently used test to complement clinical history and physical examination, both in children and adults with a suspicion of constipation [141]. However, systematic reviews have concluded that the evidence is conflicting in constipated children [142], and there is a lack of evidence in adults to support or reject its use [43,139].

Barium enema

This test may be useful for the identification of redundant sigmoid colon, megacolon, megarectum, stenosis, extrinsic compression, and intralumenal masses. However, only two studies have evaluated its clinical utility [43,139]. In one retrospective study of 62 subjects, an organic lesion was not detected with barium enema [143]. In another retrospective study of 791 patients, constipation was reported in 22%, and was equally present in those with an abnormal study as in those with a normal study [144]. Both studies concluded that

barium enema could not exclude organic disease. Hirschsprung disease can be detected by barium enema, although manometry and histology are required to confirm its diagnosis.

Endoscopy

Flexible sigmoidoscopy or colonoscopy

Direct visualization of the colon is indicated in selected patients to exclude mucosal lesions such as solitary rectal ulcer syndrome, inflammation, or malignancy. According to the American Society of Gastrointestinal Endoscopy, a colonoscopy is recommended in constipated patients if they have rectal bleeding, hemepositive stool, iron deficiency anemia, weight loss, obstructive symptoms, recent onset of symptoms, rectal prolapse, or change in stool caliber, and in subjects older than 50 years who have not previously had colon cancer screening [145]. In younger patients, a flexible sigmoidoscopy may be sufficient to exclude distal colonic disease.

Despite its popularity, the diagnostic yield of lower endoscopy in patients with constipation has not been prospectively assessed. In a large retrospective study, in 146 of 563 patients with constipation who underwent endoscopic evaluations (358 colonoscopy and 205 flexible sigmoidoscopy), the range of neoplasia found and the polyp detection rate were comparable to those expected in asymptomatic historical controls [146]. There is therefore little evidence to support the routine use of colonoscopy in patients without alarm features.

Specific diagnostic tests for functional constipation

Detailed physiological testing should be performed in patients whose constipation is refractory to laxatives and dietary changes, and in those with a suspected evacuation disorder. The following tests are routinely performed: colonic transit study, anorectal manometry, balloon expulsion test, and defecography. An evidence-based summary of the various diagnostic approaches for chronic constipation is provided (Table 20.4). Unfortunately, no single test is adequate to define the pathophysiology of constipation, and often more than one test is required [40,139].

Colonic transit study

An assessment of the rate of stool movement through the colon provides an objective measurement of infrequent defecation, because the patient's recall of stool habit is often inaccurate [37,40]. Colonic transit time can be measured using three general methods:

- ingestion of radiopaque markers followed by abdominal radiographs [147]
- radioisotopes and scintigraphy [148,149]
- ingestion of pressure, pH capsule (SmartPill) and tracking its movement [150].

The radiopaque marker test is typically performed by administering a single capsule containing 24 plastic markers (Sitzmarks, Konsyl Pharmaceuticals, Easton, MD, USA) on day 1 and, by obtaining plain abdominal radiographs on

Table 20.4 Evidence-based summary of the utility of the diagnostic tests for chronic constipation

Test	Clinical utility Strength	Weakness	Evidence	Recommendation (Grade)	Comment
Blood tests (thyroid function tests, serum calcium, glucose, electrolytes)	Rule out systemic or metabolic disorder	Is not a cost-effective strategy	No evidence	C	Not recommended for routine evaluation particularly in the absence of alarm features
Imaging tests					
Plain abdominal radiograph	Identify excessive amount of stool in the colon, simple, inexpensive, widely available	Lack of standardization on how to review the image. Lack of controlled studies	Poor	C	Not recommended for routine evaluation particularly in the absence of alarm features
Barium enema	Identify megacolon, megarectum, stenosis, diverticulosis, extrinsic compression, and intralumenal masses	Lack of standardization, embarrassing for patients. Radiation exposure Lack of controlled studies	Poor	C	Not recommended for routine evaluation particularly in the absence of alarm features
Defecography	Identify dyssynergia, rectocele, prolapse, excessive descent, megarectum, Hirschsprung disease	Radiation exposure, embarrassment, availability, interobserver bias, inconsistent methodology	Fair	B3	Used as an adjunct to anorectal manometry
Anorectal ultrasound	Visualization of the internal anal sphincter and puborectalis muscles	Interobserver bias, availability	Poor	C	Experimental
Magnetic resonance imaging	Simultaneously evaluate global pelvic floor anatomy, sphincter morphology, and dynamic motion	Expensive, lack of standardization, availability	Fair	B3	Used as an adjunct to anorectal manometry
Flexible sigmoidoscopy and colonoscopy	Direct visualization of the colon to exclude mucosal lesions such as solitary rectal ulcer syndrome, inflammation, or malignancy	Invasive, risks related to the procedure (perforation, bleeding) and sedation	Poor	C	Indicated in patients younger than 50 years who have alarm symptoms Indicated in all subjects older than 50 years for colorectal cancer screening
Physiological testing					
Colonic transit study with radiopaque markers	Evaluate presence of slow, normal, or rapid colonic transit. Inexpensive and widely available	Inconsistent methodology, validity has been questioned	Good	B2	Useful to classify patients according to the pathophysiological subtypes
Colonic transit study with scintigraphy	Evaluate presence of slow, normal, or rapid colonic transit. Provide evaluation of whole gut transit	Expensive, time consuming, availability, lack of standardization	Good	B2	Useful to classify patients according to the pathophysiological subtypes
Anorectal manometry	Identify dyssynergic defecation, rectal hyposensitivity, rectal hypersensitivity, impaired compliance, Hirschsprung disease	Lack of standardization	Good	B2	Useful to establish the diagnoses of Hirschsprung disease and dyssynergic defecation
Balloon expulsion test (BET)	Simple, nonexpensive, bedside assessment of the ability to expel a simulated stool. Identify dyssynergic defecation	Lack of standardization	Good	B2	Normal BET does not exclude dyssynergia Should be interpreted alongside the results of the other anorectal tests
Colonic manometry	Identify colonic myopathy, neuropathy, or normal function facilitating selection of patients for surgery	Invasive, not widely available, lack of standardization	Fair	B3	Adjunct to colorectal function tests

From Remes-Troche & Rao [264].

Grade A1: Excellent evidence in favor of the test based on high specificity, sensitivity, accuracy, and positive predictive values

Grade B2: Good evidence in favor of the test with some evidence on specificity, sensitivity, accuracy, and predictive values

Grade B3: Fair evidence in favor of the test with some evidence on specificity, sensitivity, accuracy, and predictive values

Grade C: Poor evidence in favor of the test with some evidence on specificity, sensitivity, accuracy, and predictive values

day 6 (120 h later) [40,151,152]. Retention of at least 20% of markers (more than six markers) on day 6 (120 h) is considered abnormal [147,152] and is indicative of STC. Because, 60% of patients with dyssynergic defecation demonstrate excessive retention of markers [104], a diagnosis of STC should only be made after excluding dyssynergia [38,139]. A multiple capsule technique has also been used, but its interpretation is variable and its validity has been questioned [153]. Several studies have assessed the utility of colonic transit in the evaluation of constipation [139,151]. A systematic review of 10 studies concluded that the prevalence of STC varied from 38% to 80% [139]. Also, there were significant differences in study population, methodology, and interpretation, and a gold standard was lacking [139].

Colonic transit scintigraphy is a noninvasive and quantitative method of evaluation of total and regional colonic transit [148,149]. Here, an isotope (^{111}In or ^{99}Tc) is administered either in a coated capsule that dissolves in the colon or terminal ileum or encapsulated in a nondigestive capsule with a test meal. Subsequently, gamma-camera images are obtained at specified time points [148,149]. Assessment and interpretation of the colonic transit time varies among centers. The primary variable of interest is the geometric center at 24 h (normal range 1.7–4.0). A high geometric center represents greater than normal retention of isotope and a slower colonic

transit time. In a recent study, 23 patients diagnosed with STC based on radiopaque marker studies and 13 healthy individuals underwent oral ^{111}indium-diethylenetriaminepentaacetic acid scintigraphy [151]. In this study, there was no difference in transit time in the right colon between the groups of patients and controls whereas patients had significant delay in the left colon. The authors concluded that colonic scintigraphy may help to select patients with STC for hemicolectomy [151]. However, the results of segmental colectomy are less satisfactory [154]. Although scintigraphic studies have been validated, and are reliable and reproducible, they are expensive, time consuming and available in limited centers [139].

Assessment of colonic transit using a novel, ambulatory, capsule technique, SmartPill, provides a noninvasive method of measuring not only colonic transit but also gastric emptying and small bowel transit time (Fig. 20.6) [150]. It also provides information regarding colonic contractile activity and the whole gut pH profile. Studies in healthy controls show good correlation of the colonic transit time between the SmartPill and Sitzmarker techniques [155], and it appears to distinguish controls from patients with STC [155].

Anorectal manometry
Anorectal manometry provides an assessment of pressure activity in the anorectum together with an assessment of

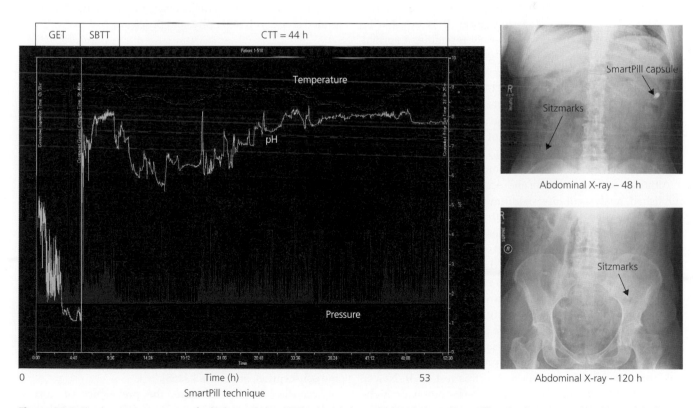

Figure 20.6 Simultaneous assessment of colonic transit time (CTT) using wireless capsule techniques (SmartPill) and radiopaque markers (Sitzmarks). The SmartPill capsule also provides assessment of gastric emptying time (GET), small bowel transit time (SBTT), and CTT. The 48-h plain abdominal radiograph shows both a Sitzmarks marker and the SmartPill capsule, whereas the 120-h radiograph shows only a Sitzmarks marker.

rectal sensation, rectoanal reflexes, and rectal compliance [40,110,156,157]. Manometry can detect dyssynergic defecation and Hirschsprung disease [119]. Normally, when a balloon is distended in the rectum, there is reflex relaxation of the internal anal sphincter. This rectoanal inhibitory reflex is mediated by the myenteric reflex [118] and is absent in Hirschsprung disease [158]. A prospective study of 111 children showed that manometry had a sensitivity of 83% and specificity of 93% when compared to rectal suction biopsy (sensitivity 93% and specificity 100%) [159].

Normally, when healthy subjects attempt to defecate they generate an adequate propulsive force that is reflected by a rise in intrarectal pressure. This movement is synchronized with relaxation of the puborectalis and the external anal sphincter, which is reflected by a decrease in anal sphincter pressure [38,104]. The inability to perform this coordinated maneuver represents the chief pathophysiological abnormality (Fig. 20.4) in patients with dyssynergic defecation [38,104]. However, healthy subjects can also not produce a normal relaxation during attempted defecation [109,110]. The body position, whether sitting or lying down, the presence of stool-like sensation, and the consistency of stool may each influence the occurrence of dyssynergia and the ability to expel artificial stools [111]. Hence, the finding of a dyssynergic pattern alone should not be considered as diagnostic of dyssynergic defecation. Additional features are usually recommended (see Table 20.2). By observing the manometric recordings during attempted defecation, it is possible to identify the sequence that most closely resembles a normal pattern of defecation. This recording can be used to measure the intrarectal pressure, the anal residual pressure, and the percentage of anal relaxation [110,114,115]. From these measurements, it is possible to calculate an index of the forces required to perform defecation – the defecation index [110]; a simple and quantifiable measure of rectoanal coordination (normal index is at least 1.5) [38,110]. Furthermore, rectal sensory testing may reveal rectal hyposensitivity [104,160–162].

Although several studies of anorectal manometry have been published, analysis of nine medium- to high-quality studies [139] has revealed differences in both methodology and interpretation, with dyssynergia prevalence ranging from 20% to 75% [139]. Manometry only detects a dyssynergic pattern, and the diagnosis of dyssynergic defecation requires more [38,41,115], so one should interpret manometric results with caution. Anorectal manometry provides confirmatory evidence for the diagnosis of dyssynergic defecation and paves the way for identifying appropriate subjects for biofeedback therapy. An international consensus panel proposed uniform standards for performing and interpreting anorectal manometry that should help to standardize this test [164]. Newer manometric techniques, such as high-resolution or high-definition manometry with multiple closely spaced solid state sensors, may provide better delineation of the sphincter contours and pressure plots [165].

Balloon expulsion test

The balloon expulsion test provides a simple, bedside assessment of the subject's ability to expel an artificial stool. However, the methodology for this test has not been standardized. Several techniques have been used, including 25-mL or 50-mL balloons filled with warm water or air, 18-mm spheres, silicone-filled artificial stool, or weights attached to a pulley to assess the extra force required to expel a metal sphere in the lying position [111]. The upper limit for normal balloon expulsion time has been variable. Some recommend 1 min or longer, and others at least 5 min. In our laboratory, either a 4-cm long balloon filled with 50 mL warm water or a silicone-filled stool-like device (Fecom) is placed in the rectum, and then, the patient is asked to expel the device in the sitting position in privacy [110]. Most normal subjects will expel the water filled-balloon within 1 min [110].

The prevalence of a positive test in favor of constipation varied between 23% and 67% [139]. A recent study suggested a specificity of 89%, negative predictive value of 97%, sensitivity of 88%, and positive predictive value of 67% [166]. However, this observation is confounded by other studies that have reported that many dyssynergics can expel the balloon and that the test is insufficient to make a diagnosis [38]. Thus, although the failure to expel a balloon strongly suggests dyssynergia, a normal test does not exclude this possibility. Nine studies of balloon expulsion showed impaired expulsion in 23%–67% [139]. Hence, this test should be interpreted along with other physiological tests.

Rectal barostat test

An assessment of rectal sensation, tone, and compliance using a highly compliant balloon that is placed in the rectum and connected to a computerized pressure-distending device (barostat) can be useful. Several studies have revealed rectal hyposensitivity in patients with constipation [160–162]. The test can also be useful for identifying patients with a normal, impaired, or hypercompliant rectum and can facilitate the detection of megarectum. Likewise, rectal barostat studies can reveal rectal hypersensitivity in up to 50% of patients with IBS-C [167].

Defecography

Defecography provides information regarding the anatomical and functional changes of the anorectum. It is performed by infusing 150 mL barium paste into the patient's rectum, and having the subject squeeze, cough, and expel the barium. The most common findings are; poor activation of levator muscles, prolonged retention of or inability to expel the barium, absence of a stripping wave in the rectum, mucosal intussusception, or rectocele [168].

According to the literature, the prevalence of normal defecography varies between 10% and 75% [139]. Although defecography revealed abnormalities in 77% of subjects, there was no relationship between symptoms and abnormalities [169]. Another prospective study found that, the yield of defecography in the diagnosis of constipation was minimal [38]. Among 10 defecography studies, abnormalities were reported in 25%–90% and dyssynergia in 13%–37% [139].

Disadvantages of defecography include radiation exposure, embarrassment, availability, interobserver bias and inconsistent methodology among centers [139]. As a result of these inherent deficiencies, it has been recommended that the test should be considered as an adjunct to clinical and manometric assessment of constipated patients whose symptoms have not responded to conventional therapy or in those with a history of excessive straining, prolapse, or use of digital maneuvers to facilitate defecation.

Colonic manometry

Colonic manometry provides a comprehensive assessment of overall motor activity at rest, during sleep, after waking, after meals, and after provocative stimulation such as drugs, meal, or balloon distentions [55,59]. It is performed by using solid-state probes and portable recorders or water-perfused stationary systems [53,55,59]. It provides reproducible and reliable information regarding the pathophysiology of constipation [55,59,60], and can be used to explore the mechanisms and motor effects of pharmacological agents on the colon. The probes are often placed under endoscopic or fluoroscopic guidance, although other techniques have been described [70]. Prolonged recordings over 24 h are preferred to optimally understand the overall colonic motor profile. Recent studies have confirmed that patients with STC exhibit a significant reduction of phasic colonic motor activity, the gastrocolonic and morning waking responses, and the number of high-amplitude propagated contractions (Figs 20.3 and 20.7) [59,60]. Thus, colonic manometry may reveal an underlying myopathy or neuropathy [59]. In some cases, despite slower colonic transit time, the colonic neuromuscular function is normal [59].

Similar to its utility in children [170], a recent study of adults has shown that the test can facilitate the selection of patients for surgery [59]. In a case-controlled study, most patients with manometric features of colonic neuropathy (i.e., absence of any two of the three normal colonic motor responses: presence of high-amplitude propagated contractions, gastrocolonic response, and morning waking response) failed to respond to aggressive medical treatment and had a better clinical outcome after colectomy [59].

Magnetic resonance imaging

In the last few years several uncontrolled studies have shown that endoanal magnetic resonance imaging (MRI) and dynamic pelvic MRI – "MR defecography" – can be useful [171–173]. In fact, this is the only imaging modality that can simultaneously evaluate global pelvic floor anatomy and dynamic motion. Endoanal MRI may reveal changes in the external anal sphincter that are not identifiable by endoanal ultrasound, whereas MRI fluoroscopy directly shows the pelvic floor and viscera during rectal evacuation and squeeze maneuvers [174]. The free selection of imaging planes, no radiation exposure, a good temporal resolution, and the excellent soft tissue contrast are some of the advantages. Dynamic pelvic MRI in the sitting position provides a more physiological approach than in the supine position [175].

Dynamic MRI is useful for the diagnosis of rectal mucosal intussusception because it can differentiate between a mucosal and a full-thickness rectal prolapse [171]. In dyssynergic patients, dynamic MRI reveals that, the anorectal angle becomes more acute, confirming paradoxical contraction of the puborectalis [172]. In a controlled study, during rectal evacuation, the degree of perineal descent was decreased in 35%, normal in 44%, and increased in 21% of constipated patients [176]. Increased perineal descent was associated with a hypertensive anal sphincter, a normal rectal balloon expulsion test, and a rectocele. Limitations of MRI defecography include its high cost, lack of standardization, and availability.

Conclusions on diagnostic testing

Although several tests are performed to rule out structural and biochemical disorders that cause constipation, there is little evidence to support the use of hematological and biochemical tests, radiographs, or endoscopy in the routine management of constipated patients without alarm features [139]. Hence, the American College of Gastroenterology Task Force concluded that the routine use of a battery of diagnostic tests should be avoided in patients with chronic constipation and that the initial approach should be empiric treatment [140]. Diagnostic tests are indicated for identifying structural or functional causes of constipation in a subgroup of patients with alarm symptoms or signs or in those who do not respond to empirical therapy or a suspicion of dyssynergia. There is good evidence to support the use of physiological tests, such as anorectal manometry or colonic transit, in particular to define the pathophysiological subtypes and to guide the selection of treatment options. However, no single test will provide a pathophysiological basis for constipation, because it is a heterogeneous condition that requires several tests to identify the underlying mechanism(s).

Treatment of chronic constipation

The treatment should be customized for each individual, taking into consideration the etiology of constipation, patient's age, comorbid conditions, underlying pathophysiology, and the patient's concerns and expectations. A survey of 331 primary-care physicians reported that 60% felt that there were inadequate treatments for constipation [177]. In another survey of 4680 patients with self-reported constipation and on medication, 47% reported dissatisfaction with their current treatment [178]. Hence, there is a large unmet need for the treatment of constipation, and the real challenge is to relieve the multiple symptoms and meet the patients' expectations. An algorithmic approach for the diagnosis and management of constipation is shown in Fig. 20.7.

Lifestyle changes, fluid intake, and exercise

Lifestyle changes such as adequate fluid intake, regular nonstrenuous exercise, and dedicated time for passing bowel movements can be useful, but there is limited evidence to

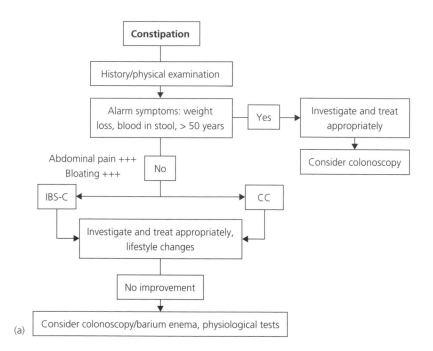

(a)

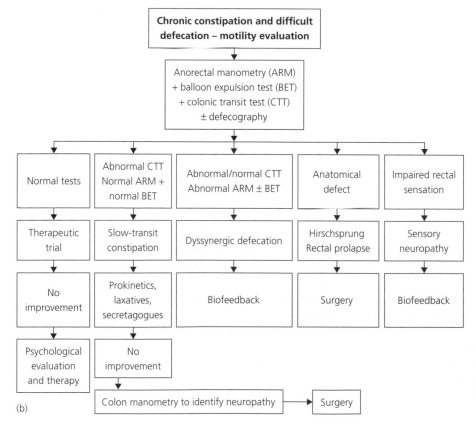

(b)

Figure 20.7 (a) Algorithmic approach to the management of chronic constipation and (b) algorithmic approach to the gastrointestinal motility evaluation and treatment of chronic constipation. CC, chronic constipation; IBS-C, irritable bowel syndrome with concurrent constipation. Modified from Rao [22].

support these measures [94]. Patients should be encouraged to avoid postponing defecation [22], as the urge subsides after a few minutes and may not return for hours. Most patients who have a normal bowel pattern usually empty stool at approximately the same time every day [136]. This observation suggests that the act of defecation is in part a conditioned reflex. Hence, ritualizing the bowel habit is worthwhile and could establish a regular pattern of bowel movement. Colonic motor activity is more active after waking and after a meal [55,59]. Hence, the optimal time for stool evacuation is within the first 2 h after waking and after breakfast. Timed toilet training consists of educating the patient to attempt defecation for approximately 5 min, at least twice a day, usually 30 to 60 min after a meal, irrespective of whether they have an urge or not, and to push at a level of 5 to 7, assuming a maximum straining effort of 10.

Some research suggests that modest exercise can relieve constipation, especially if patients are generally inactive [179]. This recommendation is based on observations that bedridden patients are more prone to constipation and on the premise that exercise shortens gastrointestinal transit time [179]. Exercise changes the colonic motor pattern by increasing the number of propagated contractions in the postexercise period [56]. In a longitudinal study of Australian women, the odds ratio for constipation was lower (0.76) in women who performed low to moderate exercise than in sedentary women [180]. In another study of geriatric patients the relative risks of constipation for those who walked 0.5 km/day, those who walked with help or who were chair-bound or bed-bound were 1.7, 3.4, 6.9, and 15.9 respectively [181]. Thus, bowel function may correlate with exercise activity, particularly in the elderly, but other factors such as diet, cognition, medications, and personality may each play a role [94].

Constipation can be relieved in some patients by increasing daily fluid intake. In a study of 117 adults, intake of 2 L mineral water daily increased stool frequency when compared to controls [182], although baseline stool habit was based on recall and the mineral water contained magnesium and other ions, compromising the validity of this study [94].

Treatment of drug-induced constipation

Many patients with constipation are unaware that they are taking drugs that cause constipation. In a study of 329 individuals with self-reported constipation, 195 (59.3%) were using constipating medications [183]. A common list of drugs is shown in Table 20.3. The physician should seek out medications that cause constipation and, wherever possible, substitute agents that do not. In a study of 46 cancer patients, the percentage of patients taking daily laxatives decreased significantly after patients were switched to a less constipating analgesic [184]. Opioid-induced bowel dysfunction is common and agents such as methyl naltrexone may be useful [185].

Diet and fiber

Organic polymers such as bran or psyllium have the ability to hold extra water and often resist digestion and absorption in the upper gut. Their effectiveness as bulking agents depends on the dosage taken, their water-holding capacity, the extent of breakdown by bacterial fermentation and whether the fermentation products have any supplemental laxation [186]. A high-fiber diet increases stool weight and accelerates colonic transit time [187]. In contrast, a diet that is deficient in fiber may lead to constipation [187,188]. However, there is no evidence that constipated patients in general consume less fiber than nonconstipated patients, and in fact studies show similar levels of fiber intake [94]. Furthermore, constipated patients with slow transit or pelvic floor dysfunction respond poorly to dietary supplementation with 30 g fiber per day, whereas those without an underlying motility disorder improved [189]. A fiber intake of 20–30 g per day is optimal, but it may not be a panacea. Six trials that evaluated bulk laxatives or dietary fiber showed an average weighted increase of 1.4 (95% confidence interval, 0.6–2.2) bowel movements per week, whereas seven trials that evaluated laxative agents other than bulk, showed an increase of 1.5 (95% confidence interval, 1.1–1.8) bowel movements per week [190]. Both the American College of Gastroenterology Task Force [140] and a systematic review [190] concluded that psyllium, a natural fiber supplement, increases stool frequency and they gave this compound a grade B recommendation, but there were insufficient data to make a recommendation for the synthetic polysaccharide methylcellulose, or for calcium polycarbophil or bran in patients with constipation (Table 20.5).

The benefits of added fiber are not evident for days to weeks and its fermentation can produce excessive gas, bloating, and flatulence [186]. It is important to recommend generous fluid intake along with fiber supplementation, failing which, stools could become hard and bulky and difficult to expel. Patients with an obstruction, gastroparesis, fecal impaction, or those confined to bed or requiring fluid restriction should not be given fiber supplements. Inadequate calorie intake can cause constipation [191], and, it is a common problem in patients with anorexia nervosa. Refeeding and restoration of normal weight normalize colonic transit [192].

Pharmacological treatments

These include laxatives, prokinetic agents, serotonergic compounds, chloride channel activators, and others. In one report, $821 million was spent on over-the-counter laxatives in the United States [193]. A summary of these compounds, their mode of action, recommended dosage, and evidence-based recommendations is shown in Table 20.5.

Stool softeners

Sodium and calcium docusate compounds (Colace, SURFAK) are anionic surfactants that lower the surface tension of stool and facilitate the mixing of aqueous and fatty substances and

Table 20.5 Evidence-based summary for the treatment of chronic constipation

Treatment modalities that are commonly used for constipation	Level of evidence	Recommendation
Bulking agents		
Psyllium	II	B
Calcium polycarbophil	III	C
Bran	III	C
Methylcellulose	III	C
Osmotic laxatives		
Lactulose	II	B
Polyethylene glycol	I	A
Wetting agents		
Dioctyl sulfosuccinate	III	C
Stimulant laxatives		
Senna	III	C
Bisacodyl	III	C
Others		
Tegaserod	I	A
Lubiprostone	I	A
Biofeedback therapy for dyssynergic defecation	I	A
Surgery for the treatment of severe colonic inertia	II	B

Modified from Brandt et al. [43], Ramkumar and Rao [190] and Remes-Troche and Rao [265].

also stimulate intestinal fluid secretion [194]. There are four randomized control trials that have compared stool softeners with either placebo or other laxatives. The sample sizes were small and the data were conflicting [190]. Consequently, these compounds were afforded a Grade B recommendation and they were felt to be inferior to psyllium with regards to improvement of stool frequency [43]. Mineral oil is a lubricant used for the treatment of constipation [43]. It provides lubrication by emulsifying the stool mass [195]. There is no published study of the use of mineral oil in adults with constipation, although in children it appears to be more effective than senna-based compounds and less effective than osmotic laxatives [43]. Side effects include lipid pneumonia from aspiration, particularly in elderly subjects, malabsorption of fat-soluble vitamins, foreign-body reactions, and fecal incontinence [195].

Stimulant laxatives

This group consists of anthraquinones (senna, cascara sagrada, danthron, and casanthranol), diphenylmethane derivatives (bisacodyl, sodium picosulphate), and ricinoleic acid (castor oil). Stimulant laxatives affect electrolyte transport across the intestinal mucosa and enhance colonic transport and motility; and usually work within several hours of administration.

The anthraquinones increase fluid and electrolyte secretion

in the small intestine [194] and are absorbed and metabolized by the liver. They cause melanosis coli, a brownish black pigmentation of the colonic mucosa as a result of cell debris inside submucosal macrophages. This is formed during apoptosis of colonic epithelial cells stained by the anthraquinones. Bisacodyl (Dulcolax; Correctol; Carter's Little Pills) is structurally similar to phenolphthalein, increases small intestinal fluid secretion and colonic motor activity, and is approved for the treatment of occasional constipation. It is a gastric irritant so the tablets are enteric coated. It is also available as a suppository. Common side effects include abdominal discomfort or cramps and fecal incontinence [196]. Stimulant laxatives are best reserved for occasional or short-term use [135], are effective, and have been used as rescue agents in many clinical trials. Their long-term safety has not been established. Four randomized control trials were identified but none of them were placebo-controlled, the study design was of low quality and hence, a grade B recommendation was given [190].

Osmotic laxatives

Osmotic laxatives include saline laxatives (salts of magnesium, phosphate, and sulfate), poorly absorbed synthetic disaccharides such as lactulose, sugar alcohols such as sorbitol or mannitol, and an inert polymer, polyethylene glycol (PEG-3350). This group includes ions or molecules that are not well absorbed by the intestine and require retention of water by the intestinal lumen to maintain osmotic balance with plasma. Overuse of osmotic laxatives may induce abdominal cramps, diarrhea, and dehydration [43,190].

Magnesium compounds are commonly used. The typical adult dose of one to two tablespoons of magnesium hydroxide contains 20–40 mmol magnesium ions and can produce an evacuation within 6–12 h. A single, low-quality, 8-week, crossover trial compared magnesium hydroxide with laxamucil and reported 2.8 more bowel movements with magnesium [43,190,197]. Citrate of Magnesia is available as a carbonated drink in 300-mL (10-fluid ounce) bottles and contains 116 mmol magnesium ion, but there are no trials with this compound. Hypermagnesemia can occur in patients with renal failure. Likewise sulfate compounds and phosphate salts (Fleet Phospho-soda, Maryfaxtone) serve as hyperosmolar agents causing laxation. The colon is less permeable to phosphate than is the small intestine so phosphate salts can be used in an enema form to clean the lower colon. A standard phosphate enema (Fleet) contains 120 mL of fluid and 1780 mmol/L of phosphate ion.

Lactulose is a synthetic disaccharide that cannot be hydrolyzed in the small intestine and thereby serves as an osmotic agent and is fermented in the colon by anaerobic flora. Significant diarrhea does not occur until more than 100 g/24 h is consumed [198], and hence standard doses produce mild laxation [186]. Likewise, sorbitol and mannitol are sugar alcohols that are poorly absorbed. In one study of elderly constipated subjects, 70% sorbitol syrup was as effective as lactulose but was approximately one-tenth the cost [199]. Glycerin is another small molecule that can exert osmotic activity in the colon. It is not absorbed by the colon and is often used as a suppository to draw water into the rectum.

Polyethylene glycol, PEG 3350 (MiraLAX; Braintree Labs, Braintree, MA, USA; glycoLax) is a large polymer that is poorly absorbed, metabolically inert, and not degraded by bacteria. It has been widely used as a lavage solution in preparation for colonoscopy. There are at least eight placebo-controlled randomized control trials of PEG compounds and two randomized control trials comparing PEG with lactulose [190]. PEG was superior to placebo in increasing stool frequency and stool consistency [200]. Its efficacy is often greatest in the second week of treatment and a dose–response study showed that a 68-g dose produced reliable laxation within 24 h [201]. Although generally safe it can cause bloating or nausea but no electrolyte changes have been reported. In a 6-month multicenter study, stool frequency increased to 7.7 per week with PEG and 5.4 per week with placebo [202]. A recent study reported relief of constipation in 52% of patients on PEG-3350 vs 11% of patients on placebo [203].

Serotonergic agents
Serotonin is a neurotransmitter that is widely distributed in the body, with more than 90% in the gastrointestinal tract

[98]. Fourteen serotonin receptor subtypes have been identified, including type-4 receptors (5-HT$_4$), which when stimulated, promote peristalsis, induce chloride secretion, and possibly reduce visceral hypersensitivity [204]. In two randomized, placebo-controlled studies of over 1200 patients with chronic constipation, tegaserod 2 mg and 6 mg twice daily, produced a dose-dependent increase in the number of complete spontaneous bowel movements per week in 36%–40% of patients (vs 27% of patients taking placebo; $P < 0.0001$) [205,206]. It also improved stool form, nuisance level of constipation, and satisfaction with bowel habits [206]. Similar improvement was seen in an open-label, 13-month extension study [207]. Diarrhea and headache were the most common adverse effects. There have been post-marketing reports of ischemic colitis [204]. Sales of tegaserod have been suspended because of concerns with coronary and cerebrovascular events.

Chloride channel activators
Chloride channels are located in the apical and serosal membranes of the enterocyte and they facilitate chloride transport [208]. There are four subtypes [209]. Lubiprostone is a gastrointestine-targeted bicyclic fatty acid that selectively activates type 2 chloride channels, resulting in increased secretion of chloride by the intestinal cells lining the small bowel. As the negatively charged chloride ion leaves the cell, sodium and water are also simultaneously excreted into the lumen paracellularly, to maintain enterocyte electrical gradient [208]. Thus, lubiprostone increases fluid secretion, and secondarily increase intestinal motility and enhances stool transport, alleviating symptoms of chronic constipation [208,210,211]. In a randomized controlled trial involving 237 patients, lubiprostone 24 µg twice daily for 28 days was more effective than placebo in increasing the number of spontaneous bowel movements, decreasing straining, improving stool consistency, and relieving symptoms of chronic constipation [212]. Long-term studies show that the compound is efficacious and safe [213]. The most common adverse effects are nausea (31.1%), diarrhea (13.2%), and headache (13.2%) [213]. In guinea pigs, lubiprostone can cause fetal loss so adequate contraceptive measures are recommended for young women taking lubiprostone, and it has been designated a Pregnancy category C drug [214].

Miscellaneous and emerging therapies
Colchicine, a plant alkaloid used to treat gout [186,195], and misoprostol, a prostaglandin analogue used to treat peptic disorders, induce diarrhea as a side effect [186,195]. Consequently, they have been tried in patients with chronic constipation [215,216]. A limited number of studies involving a small number of patients found that colchicine increased stool frequency and accelerated colonic transit, lessening the need for rescue laxatives [190]. Similarly, misoprostol increased intestinal motility, particularly of the left colon, and the rate of intestinal transit [190,216]. Misoprostol can trigger uterine

contractions so it should be avoided by women who are or who could become pregnant [186]. Severe abdominal cramping has also been reported [186].

A novel approach has been the use of neurotropins, which promote maturation of sensory neurons and modulate synaptic transmission at the neuromuscular junction [217]. A 4-week, randomized control trial showed that the neurotropin NT-3 at a dosage of 9 mg three times a week, subcutaneously, increased the number of complete spontaneous bowel movements, improved stool consistency and straining effort, and accelerated colonic transit time in 107 patients with moderately severe, laxative- or enema-dependent STC [218].

Opiates act on postsynaptic receptors to slow peristalsis [219] or increase nonpropagated activity. They also inhibit fluid and electrolyte secretion from the enterocytes through opiate receptors [219]. Hence, peripherally acting, selective opioid antagonists, especially those that do not cross the blood–brain barrier, such as methylnaltrexone may be useful [185]. Another compound, linaclotide, a guanylate cyclase agonist has been shown to accelerate gut transit in healthy subjects [220] and in female patients with IBS-C [221].

Treatment of evacuation disorders

Behavioral approaches using neuromuscular conditioning can be effective in the management of dyssynergic defecation [38].

Treatment of dyssynergic defecation

Treatment of dyssynergic defecation consists of diet, laxatives, timed-toilet training, and other measures outlined above, together with neuromuscular conditioning using biofeedback techniques [38,104]. Biofeedback has been shown to be efficacious [222–224]. Other approaches that have limited efficacy include botulinum toxin injection [113,114], anal myectomy, and surgery [107,225].

Biofeedback therapy is an instrument-based behavioral program that is based on "operant conditioning" techniques. The governing principle is that when any behavior is reinforced, its likelihood of being repeated and perfected increases several fold. In patients with dyssynergic defecation, the goal of neuromuscular conditioning is twofold:
- to correct the incoordination or dyssynergic behavior during defecation, and restore normal coordination of the abdominal, rectal, puborectalis, and anal sphincter
- to improve rectal sensory perception.

Rectoanal coordination training

Three techniques have been used:
- diaphragmatic muscle training with simulated defecation
- manometry-guided pelvic floor retraining
- simulated defecation training.

The biofeedback system consists of placing a manometry or electromyography probe into the anorectum [38]. These sensors pick up pressure or electromyographic signals from the anal sphincter, which are then displayed on a monitor. This provides visual feedback [226]. The simulated defecation technique consists of placing either a water-filled balloon or a silicone-filled balloon, called a Fecom [227], into the rectum, and to train the subject to expel the device by coordinating the abdominal and pelvic floor muscles.

Typically, patients are instructed on diaphragmatic breathing techniques to improve their abdominal pushing effort. Thereafter, visual or auditory feedback techniques are used to provide input to the patient regarding their attempted defecation maneuvers. The patient's posture and breathing techniques are corrected. The number of training sessions is usually customized to the patient's need but an average of six sessions are required. If a patient can demonstrate consistently, i.e., during two consecutive training sessions, a normal pattern of defecation with at least 50% of attempts, together with an improvement in symptoms of difficult defecation, the training sessions may be discontinued [38,224]. Old habits die hard, however, and many patients tend to revert back to their previous pattern of defecation so periodic reinforcement may be required. In a recent long-term assessment of biofeedback therapy, it was shown that compliance with reinforcement sessions decreases with time [163]. Using any one or a combination of these methods, symptomatic improvement has been reported in about 80% of patients [38,222,232].

Sensory training

Sixty percent of patients with dyssynergic defecation have impaired rectal sensation [104,228,229] so rectal sensory conditioning may provide additional therapeutic benefit [163,228]. The goal is to enhance rectal sensory perception by training the patient to perceive a lower volume of rectal balloon distention, but with the same intensity as previously experienced with a larger balloon volume [228,229].

Simulated defecation is a maneuver performed by placing an artificial stool or water-filled balloon into the rectum [38,228]. The patient is asked to sit on a commode and to expel the device. Their posture and breathing techniques are continuously monitored and corrected, and a therapist assists the patient's efforts, if required, by applying gentle traction to the stool-like device while reinforcing their technique of defecation.

Three randomized controlled trials of biofeedback therapy have been reported. Rao and colleagues [224] showed that biofeedback therapy was superior to sham biofeedback and to the standard medical treatment of diet, exercise, and laxatives. Global bowel satisfaction was significantly higher with biofeedback compared to sham treatment (78% vs 48%, $P < 0.05$). Also the number of complete spontaneous bowel movements per week was significantly higher (Fig. 20.8) in the biofeedback group. In another study, Heymen and colleagues [230] showed that biofeedback was more effective than either 5 mg diazepam or a placebo. Response rates, defined by patients' self report of "adequate relief" after 3 months of training, were

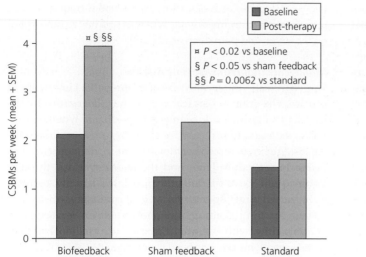
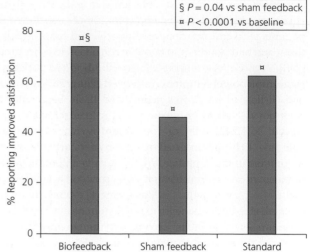

Figure 20.8 Effects of biofeedback therapy on the number of complete spontaneous bowel movements (CSBM) and the proportion of subjects who reported improved bowel satisfaction in a randomized controlled trial that compared biofeedback therapy with sham feedback (relaxation) and standard treatment of diet and laxatives. From Rao et al. [224].

71% for biofeedback, 33% for placebo, and 20% for diazepam. Finally, Chiarioni and colleagues showed that five biofeedback sessions were more effective than continuous PEG (14 g/day) for treating dyssynergia, and benefits lasted for at least 2 years [223]. Two randomized control trials have also reported sustained (1 year) improvement of symptoms [163,223] and colorectal function [163], confirming the long-term efficacy of biofeedback therapy. These studies indicate that biofeedback should be the preferred treatment for dyssynergic defecation.

Biofeedback is a labor-intensive program that is not widely available. To treat the vast number of constipated patients, a home-based, self-training program may be required. Limited studies have demonstrated the feasibility of home training [231,232], but its efficacy has not been assessed.

Treatment of stool impaction

Patients with stool impaction or those with hard stools that are difficult to expel require digital disimpaction. This can be painful and may require sedation or anesthesia. Once the colon has been cleaned, these patients require rigorous bowel conditioning and a regimen of laxatives and suppositories or enemas to prevent stool impaction. Glycerin or bisacodyl suppositories together with enemas (tap water or Fleet) are usually successful, but their efficacy has not been prospectively assessed. Additional measures include saline or osmotic laxatives or PEG solutions. After establishing a bowel regimen, it is important to assess these patients for secondary causes or an underlying colonic or generalized motility disorder.

Surgical treatment

Surgery should be reserved for patients who fail aggressive medical and behavioral treatments under expert supervision, have demonstrable colonic neuropathy [59], and have motility dysfunction that is confined to the colon [233]. The latter two are best assessed by performing a gastric-emptying test, antroduodenojejunal manometry, and colonic manometry. Patients with a generalized motility disorder are more likely to have an unsatisfactory outcome [234,235]. Broadly, the surgical procedures may be considered under three categories; cecostomy, colectomy with anastomosis or construction of a stoma, and surgery for evacuation disorders.

Cecostomy

This procedure is analogous to a gastrostomy. Both surgical [236] and endoscopic [237] techniques have been described and the results appear favorable. The procedure is generally preferred in children, institutionalized patients, and in those with neurological lesions. The Malone or antegrade continent enema procedure consists of fashioning a cecostomy button or appendicostomy [236–238]. The principle is to perform periodic antegrade irrigation of the colon (once every 3 days) so that the colon is adequately cleansed and in a predictable manner. Solutions commonly used include a glycerin : saline solution in a ratio of 1 : 3; a volume of 500–1500 mL as tolerated is infused into the cecostomy. Alternatively, PEG solutions may be used. Satisfactory results range from 40% to 78% [237]. An ileal stoma is felt to cause fewer complications over time [237], but there are no controlled trials.

Colectomy

Several techniques have been advocated that include segmental colectomy, ileorectal anastomosis, ileosigmoid anastomosis, cecorectal anastomosis, ileoanal anastomosis with proctocolectomy, and pouch formation or ileostomy [239].

Subtotal colectomy with ileorectal anastomosis is the most commonly performed technique. A long-term study that compared the outcome of colectomy in patients with constipation, ulcerative colitis, and colon cancer concluded that patients with constipation fared poorly, had more complications, and had poorer quality of life compared to other groups [240]. A more recent series of carefully selected patients reported that bowel symptoms improved in over 80% of patients, and quality of life scores normalized [235]. Segmental colectomy was felt to be unsuccessful in several case–control studies [241,242], although one recent report is more favorable [154]. The rationale for resection of a particular colonic segment is unclear, particularly because segmental retention of markers on a colonic transit study may not accurately predict colonic dysfunction in that segment. An ileostomy may be considered in patients who fail ileorectal anastomosis, but in one series a favorable outcome was seen in only 50% [243]. Many of these patients may have underlying psychological dysfunction [233] or a generalized gut motility disorder [233].

Surgery for evacuation disorders

In patients with structural abnormalities such as rectocele, descending perineum syndrome and mucosal intussusception, several surgical techniques have been tried [244]. Repair of a rectocele using a transrectal approach seems to have fewer side effects [245], although most patients do not require surgery. For patients with mucosal intussusception or rectal prolapse, abdominal rectopexy with sigmoid resection has been recommended [244]. Local excision is not recommended because this procedure does not address the underlying pathophysiology and the lesions tend to recur. Keighley and Shouler [246] described 14 patients who underwent posterior Marlex rectopexy for solitary rectal ulcer syndrome. The ulcer healed in five of six patients (83%) with full-thickness rectal prolapse. A similar result was noted in only two of eight patients (25%) with rectoanal intussusception. The authors concluded that only symptomatic ulcers should be treated by surgery and only after medical treatment has failed. Many of these patients have coexistent dyssynergia for which biofeedback can be effective [247]. A stapling procedure, stapled transanal rectal resection, has been advocated [248]. Initial enthusiasm remains high [249], although in one multicenter series, several complications, including bleeding, incontinence, anal stenosis, and pain, have been reported. Controlled trials are awaited.

Sacral nerve stimulation

Initially used for the treatment of fecal and urinary incontinence, several studies have reported that sacral nerve stimulation may benefit patients with constipation [250–253]. The mechanism by which sacral nerve stimulation improves bowel function is unclear; a recent study of six patients reported that S3 but not S2 nerve stimulation produced more high-amplitude propagated contractions, suggesting that sacral nerve stimulation may alter colonic physiology through neuroenteric pathways [250]. A prospective study of 65 patients who failed

laxatives and biofeedback showed that stool frequency and bowel satisfaction improved, whereas straining, time spent on the toilet, and pain decreased [253].

Management of Hirschsprung disease

Surgery remains the cornerstone of treatment for Hirschsprung disease. The optimal surgical approach is determined by the length of an aganglionic segment, in particular whether it involves the anorectum, rectum, or colon. In patients with significant hindgut involvement, removal of the entire segment, as in Swenson procedure [254] and the endorectal pull-through techniques of Soave and Boley [255], or bypassing the segment, as in the Duhamel operation, have all produced satisfactory results [256]. In patients with a short or ultra-short segment, anal myotomy with or without incision of a variable length of rectal smooth muscle has been reported to be useful [257].

Management of fecal impaction

Fecal impaction can be seen in a variety of clinical settings, including children with prolonged difficulty with defecation, adults with dyssynergia or STC, institutionalized patients, postoperative patients on opioids, patients with psychological and psychiatric comorbidities, and most importantly elderly individuals, many of whom may present with fecal soiling [258]. The first step is to confirm the diagnosis by digital rectal examination. A plain radiograph of the abdomen can reveal stool impaction. Initially, glycerin and bisacodyl suppositories together with phosphosoda or milk of molasses enema should be tried together with gentle disimpaction with fingers. If unsuccessful, manual disimpaction and evacuation should be performed, under sedation sometimes requiring anesthesia (particularly children). Once disimpaction has been achieved, the patient should be placed on an aggressive regimen of oral laxative, prokinetics, and suppositories to ensure frequent soft stools daily. Bulk laxatives and fiber supplements should be avoided [259,260]. Stimulant or osmotic laxatives such as PEG or magnesium compounds are preferred, although newer agents such as tegaserod or lubiprostone may also be effective. After 1 or 2 months, efforts should be made to identify an underlying problem such as dyssynergia, encopresis, mobility, or drugs and appropriate steps should be taken to prevent a recurrence.

Complications of constipation

Several common anorectal conditions such as anal fissure, hemorrhoids, megarectum, megacolon, fecal impaction particularly in the elderly, fecal seepage, stercoral ulcer, solitary rectal ulcer syndrome, and rectoceles may be a consequence of long-standing constipation [261]. Although a causal relationship may sometimes be difficult to establish, based on expert consensus, historical association of these problems and recent evidence of altered anorectal physiology in many of these conditions, it is likely that long-standing constipation or difficulty with defecation or both may predispose to these common problems. Patients may not always describe or be aware of symptoms of coexisting constipation. Consequently, prevention and aggressive treatment of underlying constipation with diet, laxatives, behavioral and other approaches, and sometimes surgery, may lead to longer lasting relief or cure. Colorectal cancer has also been claimed as a potential side effect, either because of long-standing constipation or as the result of unforeseen effects of the medications used to treat constipation [186,262] but there is no concrete evidence. With the recent advances in the pathophysiology of chronic constipation, these complications should be preventable.

References

1. Pare P, Ferrazzi S, Thompson D, et al. An epidemiological survey of constipation in Canada: definitions, rates, demographics, and predictors of health care seeking. Am J Gastroenterol 2001;96:3130.
2. Stewart WF, Liberman G, Sandler RS, et al. A large US national epidemiological study of constipation. Gastroenterology 1998;114:A44.
3. Pare P, Ferrazzi S, Thompson WG. A longitudinal survey of self-reported bowel habits in the United States. Dig Dis Sci 1989;34:1153.
4. Talley NJ, Fleming KC, Evans JM, et al. Constipation in an elderly community: a study of prevalence and potential risk factors. Am J Gastroenterol 1996;91:19.
5. Lembo A, Camilleri M. Chronic constipation. N Engl J Med 2003;349:1360.
6. Sonnenberg A, Koch TR. Physician visits in the United States for constipation: 1958 to 1986. Dig Dis Sci 1989;34:606.
7. Talley NJ. Chronic constipation and irritable bowel syndrome: epidemiology, presentation and diagnosis. Johns Hopkins Adv Stud Med 2006;6:S225.
8. Talley NJ, O'Keefe EA, Zinsmeister AR, Melton LJ. Prevalence of gastrointestinal symptoms in the elderly: a population based study. Gastroenterology 1992;102:895.
9. Drossman DA, Li Z, Andruzzi E, et al. US Householder Survey of Functional Gastrointestinal Disorders. Prevalence, sociodemography and health impact. Dig Dis Sci 1993;38:1569.
10. Higgins PD, Johanson JF. Epidemiology of constipation in North America: a systematic review. Am J Gastroenterol 2004;99:750.
11. Harari D, Gurwitz JH, Avorn J, et al. Bowel habit in relation to age and gender. Findings from the National Health Interview Survey and clinical implications. Arch Intern Med 1996;156:315.
12. Pekmezaris R, Aversa L, Wolf-Klein G, et al. The cost of chronic constipation. J Am Med Dir Assoc 2002;3:224.
13. Chang L, Toner BB, Fukudo S, et al. Gender, age, society, culture, and the patient's perspective in the functional gastrointestinal disorders. Gastroenterology 2006;130:1435.
14. Rao SS, Tuteja AK, Vellema T, et al. Dyssynergic defecation: demographics, symptoms, stool patterns, and quality of life. J Clin Gastroenterol 2004;38:680.
15. Derbyshire E, Davies J, Costarelli V, Dettmar P. Diet, physical inactivity and the prevalence of constipation throughout and after pregnancy. Matern Child Nutr 2006;2:127.
16. Coremans EA. Is there a genetic component in chronic functional constipation? Gastroenterology 2005;128 Supp.2:S1867.
17. Mudipalli RS, Remes-Troche J, Andersen L, Rao SSC. Functional chest pain: esophageal or overlapping functional disorders. J Clin Gastroenterol 2007;41:264.
18. Talley NJ, Waever AL, Zinsmeister AR, Melton LJ. Onset and disappearance of gastrointestinal symptoms and functional gastrointestinal disorders. Am J Epidemiol 1992;136:165.
19. Talley NJ, Dennis EH, Schettler-Duncan VA, et al. Overlapping upper and lower gastrointestinal symptoms in irritable bowel syndrome patients with constipation or diarrhea. Am J Gastroenterol 2003;98:2454.
20. Locke GR, 3rd, Zinsmeister AR, Fett SL, et al. Overlap of gastrointestinal symptom complexes in a US community. Neurogastroenterol Motil 2005;17:29.
21. Dennison C, Prasad M, Lloyd A, et al. The health-related quality of life and economic burden of constipation. Pharmacoeconomics 2005;23:461.
22. Rao SS. Constipation: evaluation and treatment. Gastroenterol Clin North Am 2003;32:659.
23. Martin BC, Barghout V, Cerulli A. Direct medical costs of constipation in the United States. Manag Care Interface 2006;19:43.
24. Singh G, Lingala V, Wang H, et al. Adults with constipation account for significant use of healthcare resources and costs of care. Clin Gastroenterol Hepatol 2007;5:1053.
25. Rantis PC Jr, Vernava AM 3rd, Daniel GL, Longo WE. Chronic constipation – is the work up worth the cost? Dis Colon Rectum 1997;40:280.
26. Mason HJ, Serrano-Ikkos E, Kamm MA. Psychological state and quality of life in patients having behavioral treatment (biofeedback) for intractable constipation. Am J Gastroenterol 2002;97:3154.
27. Nehra V, Bruce BK, Rath-Harvey DM, et al. Psychological disorders in patients with evacuation disorders and constipation in a tertiary practice. Am J Gastroenterol 2000;95:1755.
28. Rao SS, Kinkade K, Schulze K, et al. Psychological profiles and quality of life differ in patients with dyssynergia and those with slow transit constipation. J Psychosom Res 2007;63:441.
29. Drossman DA, Talley NJ, Gelfand MD. Sexual and physical abuse and gastrointestinal illness. Review and recommendations. Ann Intern Med 1995;123:782.
30. Leroi AM, Berkelmans I, Denis P, et al. Anismus as a marker of sexual abuse. Consequences of abuse on anorectal motility. Dig Dis Sci 1995;40:1411.
31. Koloski NA, Talley NJ, Boyce PM. Predictors of health care seeking for irritable bowel syndrome and nonulcer dyspepsia: a critical review of the literature on symptom and psychosocial factors. Am J Gastroenterol 2001;96:1340.
32. Ringel Y, Whitehead WE, Toner BB. Sexual and physical abuse are not associated with rectal hypersensitivity in patients with irritable bowel syndrome. Gut 2004;53:838.
33. Glia A, Lindberg F, Nilsson LH, et al. Clinical value of symptom assessment in patients with constipation. Dis Colon Rectum 1999;42:1401.
34. Irvine EJ, Ferrazzi S, Pare P, et al. Health-related quality of life in functional GI disorders: focus on constipation and resource utilization. Am J Gastroenterol 2002;97:1986.
35. Herz MJ, Kahan E, Zalevski S, et al. Constipation: a different entity for patients and doctors. Fam Pract 1996;13:156.
36. Sandler RS, Drossman DA. Bowel habits in young adults not seeking healthcare. Dig Dis Sci 1987;32:841.
37. Ashraf W, Park F, Quigley EMM, Lof J. An examination of the reliability of reported stool frequency in the diagnosis of idiopathic constipation. Am J Gastroenterol 1996;91:26.
38. Rao SS. Dyssynergic defecation. Gastroenterol Clin North Am 2001;30:97.
39. Thompson WG, Longstreth GF, Drossman DA, et al. Functional bowel disorders and functional abdominal pain. Gut 1999;45:1143.
40. Diamant ND, Kamm MA, Wald A, Whitehead WE. AGA Technical Review on Anorectal Testing Techniques. Gastroenterology 1999;116:735.
41. Bharucha AE, Wald A, Enck P, Rao S. Functional anorectal disorders. Gastroenterology 2006;130:1510.
42. Longstreth GF, Thompson WG, Chey WD, et al. Functional bowel disorders. Gastroenterology 2006;130:1480.
43. Brandt LJ, Prather CM, Quigley EM, et al. Systematic review on the management of chronic constipation in North America. Am J Gastroenterol 2005;100(Suppl. 1):S5.

44. Klauser AG, Voderholzer WA, Heinrich CA, et al. Behavioural modification of colonic function: can constipation be learned? Dig Dis Sci 1990;35:1271.

45. Remes-Troche JM, Paulson J, Yamada T, et al. Anorectal cortical function is impaired in patients with dyssynergic defecation. Gastroenterology 2007;108:A20.

46. Karasick S, Ehrlich SM. Is constipation a disorder of defecation or impaired motility? Distinction based on defecography and colonic transit studies. Am J Roentgenol 1996;166:63.

47. Cash BD, Chey WD. Diagnosis of irritable bowel syndrome. Gastroenterol Clin North Am 2005;34:205,vi.

48. Tillisch K, Chang L. Diagnosis and treatment of irritable bowel syndrome: state of the art. Curr Gastroenterol Rep 2005;7:249.

49. Attaluri A. Is methanogenic flora associated with chronic constipation and altered colonic transit and stool characteristics? Gastroenterology 2007;132(Suppl. 2):T1945.

50. Pimentel M, Chow EJ, Lin HC. Eradication of small intestinal bacterial overgrowth reduces symptoms of irritable bowel syndrome. Am J Gastroenterol 2000;95:3503.

51. Pimentel M, Park S, Mirocha J, et al. The effect of a nonabsorbed oral antibiotic (rifaximin) on the symptoms of the irritable bowel syndrome: a randomized trial. Ann Intern Med 2006;145:557.

52. Sarna SK. Physiology and pathophysiology of colonic motor activity. Part 2. Dig Dis Sci 1991;36:998.

53. Bassotti G, Betti C, Imbimbo BP, et al. Colonic motor response to eating: a manometric investigation in proximal and distal portion of the viscus in man. Am J Gastroenterol 1989;84:118.

54. Rao SS, Kavelock R, Beaty J, et al. Effects of fat and carbohydrate meals on colonic motor response. Gut 2000;46:205.

55. Rao SS, Sadeghi P, Beaty J, et al. Ambulatory 24-h colonic manometry in healthy humans. Am J Physiol Gastrointest Liver Physiol 2001;280:G629.

56. Rao SS, Beaty J, Chamberlain M, et al. Effects of acute graded exercise on human colonic motility. Am J Physiol 1999;276:G1221.

57. Chaudhary NA, Truelone SC. Human colonic motility: a comparative study of normal subjects, patients with ulcerative colitis and patients with irritable bowel syndrome. a resting pattern of motility. Gastroenterology 1961;40:11.

58. Narducci F, Snape WJ, Battle WM, et al. Increased colonic motility during exposure to a stressful situation. Dig Dis Sci 1985;30:40.

59. Rao SS, Sadeghi P, Beaty J, Kavlock R. Ambulatory 24-h colonic manometry in slow-transit constipation. Am J Gastroenterol 2004; 99:2405.

60. Bassotti G, de Roberto G, Castellani D, et al. Normal aspects of colorectal motility and abnormalities in slow transit constipation. World J Gastroenterol 2005;11:2691.

61. Rao SS, Sadeghi P, Kavlock R, Leistikow J. Specialized propagating contractions (SPC) in health and constipation. Gastroenterology 1999;116:G4635.

62. Bassotti G, Chirarioni G, Vantini I, et al. Anorectal manometric abnormalities and colonic propulsive impairment in patients with severe chronic idiopathic constipation. Dig Dis Sci 1994;39:1558.

63. Rao SS, Welcher K. Periodic rectal motor activity: the intrinsic colonic gatekeeper? Am J Gastroenterol 1996;91:890.

64. Rao SS, Sadeghi P, Batterson K, Beaty J. Altered periodic rectal motor activity: a mechanism for slow transit constipation. Neurogastroenterol Motil 2001;13:591.

65. Orkin BA, Hanson RB, Kelly KA. The rectal motor complex. Gastrointest Motil 1989;1:5.

66. Read NW, Sun WM. Coloproctology and pelvic floor. In: Henry M, Swash M, (eds). Anorectal manometry, 2nd edn. London: Buuterworths, 1992:119.

67. Bharucha AE, Phillips SF. Slow transit constipation. Gastroenterol Clin North Am 2001;30:77.

68. Law NM, Bharucha AE, Zinsmeister AR. Rectal and colonic distension elicit viscerovisceral reflexes in humans. Am J Physiol Gastrointest Liver Physiol 2002;283:G384.

69. O'Brien MD, Camilleri M, von der Ohe MR, et al. Motility and tone of the left colon in constipation: a role in clinical practice? Am J Gastroenterol 1996;91:2532.

70. Bampton PA, Dinning PG, Kennedy ML, et al. Spatial and temporal organization of pressure patterns throughout the unprepared colon during spontaneous defecation. Am J Gastroenterol 2000;95:1027.

71. Bassotti G, Iantorno G, Fiorella S, et al. Colonic motility in man: features in normal subjects and in patients with chronic idiopathic constipation. Am J Gastroenterol 1999;94:1760.

72. De Schryver AM, Samsom M, Smout AI. Effects of a meal and bisacodyl on colonic motility in healthy volunteers and patients with slow-transit constipation. Dig Dis Sci 2003;48:1206.

73. Knowles CH, Scott SM, Wellmer A, et al. Sensory and autonomic neuropathy in patients with idiopathic slow-transit constipation. Br J Surg 1999;86:54.

74. Emmanuel AV, Kamm MA. Laser Doppler flowmetry as a measure of extrinsic colonic innervation in functional bowel disease. Gut 2000;46:212.

75. Surrenti E, Rath DM, Pemberton JH, Camilleri M. Audit of constipation in a tertiary referral gastroenterology practice. Am J Gastroenterol 1995;90:1471.

76. He CL, Burgart L, Wang L, et al. Decreased interstitial cell of cajal volume in patients with slow-transit constipation. Gastroenterology 2000;118:14.

77. Lyford GL, He CL, Soffer E, et al. Pan-colonic decrease in interstitial cells of Cajal in patients with slow transit constipation. Gut 2002; 51:496.

78. Sanders KM. A case for interstitial cells of Cajal as pacemakers and mediators of neurotransmission in the gastrointestinal tract. Gastroenterology 1996;111:492.

79. Takaki M. Gut pacemaker cells: the interstitial cells of Cajal (ICC). J Smooth Muscle Res 2003;39:137.

80. Hanani M, Freund HR. Interstitial cells of Cajal – their role in pacing and signal transmission in the digestive system. Acta Physiol Scand 2000;170:177.

81. Yu CS, Kim HC, Hong HK, et al. Evaluation of myenteric ganglion cells and interstitial cells of Cajal in patients with chronic idiopathic constipation. Int J Colorectal Dis 2002;17:253.

82. Mollen RM, Hopman WP, Kuijpers HH, Jansen JB. Abnormalities of upper gut motility in patients with slow-transit constipation. Eur J Gastroenterol Hepatol 1999;11:701.

83. Spiller RC. Upper gut dysmotility in slow-transit constipation: is it evidence for a pan-enteric neurological deficit in severe slow transit constipation? Eur J Gastroenterol Hepatol 1999;11:693.

84. Devroede G, Soffie M. Colonic absorption in idiopathic constipation. Gastroenterology 1973;64:552.

85. Preston DM, Lennard-Jones J. Severe chronic constipation of young women: idiopathic slow transit constipation? Gut 1986;27:41.

86. Kamm MA, Farthing MJ, Lennard-Jones JE, et al. Steroid hormone abnormalities in women with severe idiopathic constipation. Gut 1991;32:80.

87. Kamm MA, Farthing MJ, Lennard-Jones JE. Bowel function and transit rate during the menstrual cycle. Gut 1989;30:605.

88. Wald A, Van Thiel DH, Hoechstetter L, et al. Gastrointestinal transit: the effect of the menstrual cycle. Gastroenterology 1981;80:1497.

89. Turnbull GK, Thompson DG, Day S, et al. Relationships between symptoms, menstrual cycle and orocaecal transit in normal and constipated women. Gut 1989;30:30.

90. Kamm MA. Pathophysiology of constipation. In: Phillips SF, Pemberton JH, Shorter RG (eds). The large intestine. physiology, pathophysiology and disease. New York: Raven Press, 1991:709.

91. Koch TR, Carney JA, Go L, Go VL. Idiopathic chronic constipation is associated with decreased colonic vasoactive intestinal peptide. Gastroenterology 1988;94:300.

92. Lincoln J, Crowe R, Kamm MA, et al. Serotonin and 5-hydroxyindoleacetic acid are increased in the sigmoid colon in severe idiopathic constipation. Gastroenterology 1990;98:1219.

93. Preston DM, Adrian TE, Christofides ND, et al. Positive correlation between symptoms and circulating motilin, pancreatic polypeptide

and gastrin concentrations in functional bowel disorders. Gut 1985; 26:1059.

94. Muller-Lissner SA, Kamm MA, Scarpignato C, Wald A. Myths and misconceptions about chronic constipation. Am J Gastroenterol 2005;100:232.

95. Xiao ZL, Cao W, Biancani P, Behar J. Nongenomic effects of progesterone on the contraction of muscle cells from the guinea pig colon. Am J Physiol Gastrointest Liver Physiol 2006;290:G1008.

96. Xiao ZL, Pricolo V, Biancani P, Behar J. Role of progesterone signaling in the regulation of G-protein levels in female chronic constipation. Gastroenterology 2005;128:667.

97. Pimentel M, Lin HC, Enayati P, et al. Methane, a gas produced by enteric bacteria, slows intestinal transit and augments small intestinal contractile activity. Am J Physiol Gastrointest Liver Physiol 2006;290:G1089.

98. Gershon MD. Review article: serotonin receptors and transporters – roles in normal and abnormal gastrointestinal motility. Aliment Pharmacol Ther 2004;20 Suppl 7:3.

99. Grider JR, Kuemmerle JF, Jin JG. 5-HT released by mucosal stimuli initiates peristalsis by activating 5-HT4/5-HT1p receptors on sensory CGRP neurons. Am J Physiol 1996;270:G778.

100. Grider JR, Foxx-Orenstein AE, Ji-Guang J. 5-Hydroxytryptamine4 receptor agonist initiate the peristaltic reflex in human, rat, and guinea pig intestine. Gastroenterology 1998;115:370.

101. Prather CM, Camilleri M, Zinsmeister AR, et al. Tegaserod accelerates orocecal transit in patients with constipation-predominant irritable bowel syndrome. Gastroenterology 2000;118:463.

102. Bjornsson ES, Chey WD, Hooper F, et al. Impaired gastrocolonic response and peristaltic reflex in slow-transit constipation: role of 5-HT(3) pathways. Am J Physiol Gastrointest Liver Physiol 2002;283:G400.

103. Costedio MM, Hyman N, Mawe GM. Serotonin and its role in colonic function and in gastrointestinal disorders. Dis Colon Rectum 2007;50:376.

104. Rao SS, Welcher KD, Leistikow JS. Obstructive defecation: a failure of rectoanal coordination. Am J Gastroenterol 1998;93:1042.

105. Gladman MA, Scott SM, Williams NS, Lunniss PJ. Clinical and physiological findings and possible aetiological factors of rectal hyposensitivity. Br J Surg 2003;90:860.

106. Preston DM, Lennard-Jones JE. Anismus in chronic constipation. Dig Dis Sci 1985;30:413.

107. Martelli H, Devroede G, Arhan P, Duguay C. Mechanisms of idiopathic constipation: outlet obstruction. Gastroenterology 1978;75:623.

108. Bleijenberg G, Kuijpers HC. Treatment of spastic pelvic floor syndrome with biofeedback. Dis Colon Rectum 1987;30:101.

109. Duthie GS, Bartolo DCC. Anismus: The cause of constipation? Results of investigation and treatment. World J Surg 1992;16:831.

110. Rao SS, Hatfield R, Soffer E, et al. Manometric tests of anorectal function in healthy adults. Am J Gastroenterol 1999;94:773.

111. Rao SS, Kavlock R, Rao S. Influence of body position and stool characteristics on defecation in humans. Am J Gastroenterol 2006;101:2790.

112. Pinho M, Yoshioka K, Keighley MRB. Long term results of anorectal myectomy for chronic constipation. Br J Surg 1989;76:1163.

113. Hallan RI, Williams NS, Melling J, et al. Treatment of animus in intractable constipation with botulinum A toxin. Lancet 1988;ii:714.

114. Ron Y, Avni Y, Lukovetski A, et al. Botulinum toxin type-A in therapy of patients with anismus. Dis Colon Rectum 2001;44:1821.

115. Rao SS, Mudipalli RS, Stessman M, Zimmerman B. Investigation of the utility of colorectal function tests and Rome II criteria in dyssynergic defecation (anismus). Neurogastroenterol Motil 2004;16:589.

116. Paulson J, Miller MJ, Stessman M, Rao SS. Influence of dyssynergia type on the outcome of biofeedback therapy (BT). Neurogastroenterol Motil 2005;17:605.

117. Brocklehurst JC. Colonic disease in the elderly. Clin Gastroenterol 1985;14:725.

118. Rattan S, Regan RF, Patel CA, De Godoy MA. Nitric oxide not carbon monoxide mediates nonadrenergic noncholinergic relaxation in the murine internal anal sphincter. Gastroenterology 2005;129:1954.

119. Tobon F, Reid NC, Talbert JL, Schuster MM. Nonsurgical test for the diagnosis of Hirschsprung's disease. N Engl J Med 1968;278:188.

120. Gath R, Goessling A, Keller KM, et al. Analysis of the RET, GDNF, EDN3, and EDNRB genes in patients with intestinal neuronal dysplasia and Hirschsprung disease. Gut 2001;48:671.

121. Crowell MD, Harris L, Jones MP, Chang L. New insights into the pathophysiology of irritable bowel syndrome: implications for future treatments. Curr Gastroenterol Rep 2005;7:272.

122. American Gastroenterological Association medical position statement: irritable bowel syndrome. Gastroenterology 2002;123:2105.

123. Levy RL, Jones KR, Whitehead WE, et al. Irritable bowel syndrome in twins: heredity and social learning both contribute to etiology. Gastroenterology 2001;121:799.

124. Park MI, Camilleri M. Genetics and genotypes in irritable bowel syndrome: implications for diagnosis and treatment. Gastroenterol Clin North Am 2005;34:305.

125. Choi YK, Johlin FC Jr, Summers RW, et al. Fructose intolerance: an under-recognized problem. Am J Gastroenterol 2003;98:1348.

126. Choi Y, Jackson M, Summers RW, Rao SSC. Fructose intolerance and irritable bowel syndrome (IBS). J Clin Gastroenterol 2008; Jan 24 [epub ahead of print].

127. Gwee KA. Postinfectious irritable bowel syndrome. Curr Treat Options Gastroenterol 2001;4:287.

128. Spiller RC, Jenkins D, Thornley JP, et al. Increased rectal mucosal enteroendocrine cells, T lymphocytes, and increased gut permeability following acute Campylobacter enteritis and in post-dysenteric irritable bowel syndrome. Gut 2000;47:804.

129. Wilder-Smith CH, Schindler D, Lovblad K, et al. Brain functional magnetic resonance imaging of rectal pain and activation of endogenous inhibitory mechanisms in irritable bowel syndrome patient subgroups and healthy controls. Gut 2004;53:1595.

130. Coates MD, Mahoney CR, Linden DR, et al. Molecular defects in mucosal serotonin content and decreased serotonin reuptake transporter in ulcerative colitis and irritable bowel syndrome. Gastroenterology 2004;126:1657.

131. Locke GR III, Weaver AL, Melton LJ III, Talley NJ. Psychosocial factors are linked to functional gastrointestinal disorders: a population based nested case-control study. Am J Gastroenterol 2004;99:350.

132. Koch A, Voderholzer WA, Klauser AG, Muller-Lissner SA. Symptoms in chronic constipation. Dis Colon Rectum 1997;40:902.

133. Heaton KW, Radvan J, Cripps H, et al. Defecation frequency and timing, and stool form in the general population: a prospective study. Gut 1992;33:818.

134. O'Donnell LJ, Virjee J, Heaton KW. Detection of pseudodiarrhoea by simple clinical assessment of intestinal transit rate. BMJ 1990;300:439.

135. Folden SL. Practice guidelines for the management of constipation in adults. Rehabil Nurs 2002;27:169.

136. Heaton KW, Wood N, Cripps HA, Philipp R. The call to stool and its relationship to constipation: a community study. Eur J Gast Hepaol 1994;6:145.

137. Rao P, Tantiphlachiva K, Attaluri A, Rao SS. How useful is digital rectal examination in the diagnosis of dyssynergia? Am J Gastroenterol 2007;102:51.

138. Lawrentschuk N, Bolton DM. Experience and attitudes of final-year medical students to digital rectal examination. Med J Aust 2004;181:323.

139. Rao SS, Ozturk R, Laine L. Clinical utility of diagnostic tests for constipation in adults: a systematic review. Am J Gastroenterol 2005;100:1605.

140. Brandt LJ, Schoenfeld P, Prather CM, et al. Evidence-based position statement on the management of chronic constipation in North America. Am J Gastroenterol 2005;100:S1.

141. van den Bosch M, Graafmans D, Nievelstein R, Beek E. Systematic assessment of constipation on plain abdominal radiographs in children. Pediatr Radiol 2006;36:224.

142. Reuchlin-Vroklage LM, Bierma-Zeinstra S, Benninga MA, Berger MY. Diagnostic value of abdominal radiography in constipated children: a systematic review. Arch Pediatr Adolesc Med 2005;159:671.

143. Patriquin H, Martelli H, Devroede G. Barium enema in chronic constipation: is it meaningful? Gastroenterology 1978;75:619.

144. Gerson DE, Lewicki AM, McNeil BJ, et al. The barium enema; evidence for proper utilization. Radiology 1979;130:297.

145. Qureshi W, Adler DG, Davila RE, et al. ASGE guideline: guideline on the use of endoscopy in the management of constipation. Gastrointest Endosc 2005;62:199.

146. Pepin C, Ladabaum U. The yield of lower endoscopy in patients with constipation: survey of a university hospital, a public county hospital, and a Veterans Administration medical center. Gastrointest Endosc 2002;56:325.

147. Evans RC, Kamm MA, Hinton JM, Lennard-Jones JE. The normal range and simple diagram of recording whole gut transit time. Int J Colorectal Dis 1992;1:15.

148. Stivland T, Camilleri M, Vassallo M, et al. Scintigraphic measurement of regional gut transit in idiopathic constipation. Gastroenterology 1991;101:107.

149. van der Sijp JR, Kamm MA, Nightingale JM, et al. Radioisotope determination of regional colonic transit in severe constipation: comparison with radio opaque markers. Gut 1993;34:402.

150. Rao SS, Kuo B, Chey W, et al. A comparative study of SmartPill® and radioopaque markers for the assessment of colonic transit time in humans. Gastroenterology 2007;DDW 2007.

151. Nam YS, Pikarsky AJ, Wexner SD, et al. Reproducibility of colonic transit study in patients with chronic constipation. Dis Colon Rectum 2001;44:86.

152. Hinton JM, Lennard-Jones JE, Young AC. A new method for studying gut transit times using radio-opaque markers. Gut 1969;24:123–126.

153. Ehrenpreis ED, Jorge JMN, Schiano TD, et al. Why colonic marker studies don't measure transit time. Gastroenterology 1997;110A:728.

154. Lundin E, Karlbom U, Pahlman L, Graf W. Outcome of segmental colonic resection for slow-transit constipation. Br J Surg 2002;89:1270.

155. Rao S, Kuo B, Chey W, et al. Investigation of wireless capsule (Smart Pill) for colonic transit: a comparative study with radiopaque markers in health and constipation. Gastroenterology 2007;1075:S512.

156. Rao SS, Patel RS. How useful are manometric tests of anorectal function in the management of defecation disorders? Am J Gastroenterol 1997;92:469.

157. Karlbom U, Lundin E, Graf W, Pahlman L. Anorectal physiology in relation to clinical subgroups of patients with severe constipation. Colorectal Dis 2004;6:343.

158. Reid JR, Buonomo C, Moreira C, et al. The barium enema in constipation: comparison with rectal manometry and biopsy to exclude Hirschsprung's disease after the neonatal period. Pediatr Radiol 2000;30:681.

159. De Lorijn F, Reitsma JB, Voskuijl WP, et al. Diagnosis of Hirschsprung's disease: a prospective, comparative accuracy study of common tests. J Pediatr 2005;146:787.

160. Gladman MA, Dvorkin LS, Lunniss OJ, et al. Rectal hyposensitivity: a disorder of the rectal wall or the afferent pathway? An assessment using the barostat. Am J Gastroenterol 2005;100:106.

161. Gladman MA, Lunniss PJ, Scott SM, Swash M. Rectal hyposensitivity. Am J Gastroenterol 2006;101:1140.

162. Gladman MA, Scott SM, Williams NS, Lunniss PJ. Clinical and physiological findings, and possible aetiological factors of rectal hyposensitivity. Br J Surg 2003;90:860.

163. Rao SS, Kinkade K, Miller MJ, et al. Randomized controlled trial of long term outcome of biofeedback therapy (BT) for dyssynergic defecation. Am J Gastroenterol 2005;100:386.

164. Rao SS, Azpiroz F, Diamant N, et al. Minimum standards of anorectal manometry. Neurogastroenterol Motil 2002;14:553.

165. Jones MP, Post J, Crowell MD. High-resolution manometry in the evaluation of anorectal disorders: a simultaneous comparison with water-perfused manometry. Am J Gastroenterol 2007;102:850.

166. Minguez M, Herreros B, Sanchiz V, et al. Predictive value of the balloon expulsion test for excluding the diagnosis of pelvic floor dyssynergia in constipation. Gastroenterology 2004;126:57.

167. Delvaux MM. Visceral sensitivity in explaining functional bowel disorders: from concepts to clinical practice. Acta Gastroenterol Belg 2001;64:272.

168. Rao SS. Constipation: evaluation and treatment. Gastroenterol Clin North Am. 2003;32:659.

169. Savoye-Collet C, Savoye G, Koning E, et al. Defecography in symptomatic older women living at home. Age Ageing 2003;32:347.

170. Gertken JT, Cocjin J, Pehlivanov N, et al. Comorbidities associated with constipation in children referred for colon manometry may mask functional diagnoses. J Pediatr Gastroenterol Nutr 2005;41:328.

171. Dvorkin LS, Hetzer F, Scott SM, et al. Open-magnet MR defaecography compared with evacuation proctography in the diagnosis and management of patients with rectal intussusception. Colorectal Dis 2004;6:45.

172. Fletcher JG, Busse RF, Riederer SJ, et al. Magnetic resonance imaging of anatomic and dynamic defects of the pelvic floor in defecatory disorders. Am J Gastroenterol 2003;98:399.

173. Roos JE, Weishaupt D, Wildermuth S, et al. Experience of 4 years with open MR defecography: pictorial review of anorectal anatomy and disease. Radiographics 2002;22:817.

174. Bolog N, Weishaupt D. Dynamic MR imaging of outlet obstruction. Rom J Gastroenterol 2005;14:293.

175. Bertschinger KM, Hetzer FH, Roos JE, et al. Dynamic MR imaging of the pelvic floor performed with patient sitting in an open-magnet unit versus with patient supine in a closed-magnet unit. Radiology 2002;223:501.

176. Bharucha AE, Fletcher JG, Seide B, et al. Phenotypic variation in functional disorders of defecation. Gastroenterology 2005;128:1199.

177. Schiller LR, Dennis E, Toth G. Primary care physicians consider constipation as a severe and bothersome medical condition that negatively impacts patients' lives. Am J Gastroenterol 2004;99:S234.

178. Johanson JF, Kralstein J. Chronic constipation: a survey of the patient perspective. Aliment Pharmacol Ther 2007;25:599.

179. Bi L, Triadafilopoulos G. Exercise and gastrointestinal function and disease: an evidence-based review of risks and benefits. Clin Gastroenterol Hepatol 2003;1:345.

180. Brown WJ, Mishra G, Lee C, Bauman A. Leisure time physical activity in Australian women: relationship with well being and symptoms. Res Q Exerc Sport 2000;71:206.

181. Kinnunen O. Study of constipation in a geriatric hospital, day hospital, old people's home and at home. Aging (Milano) 1991;3:161.

182. Anti M, Pignataro G, Armuzzi A, et al. Water supplementation enhances the effect of high-fiber diet on stool frequency and laxative consumption in adult patients with functional constipation. Hepatogastroenterology 1998;45:727.

183. Rutland T, Di Palma J. Prevalence of medication-associated constipation. Am J Gastroenterol 2004;99(Suppl.):S103.

184. Radbruch L, Sabatowski R, Loick G, et al. Constipation and the use of laxatives: a comparison between transdermal fentanyl and oral morphine. Palliat Med 2000;14:111.

185. Yuan CS, Foss JF. Oral methylnaltrexone for opioid-induced constipation. JAMA 2000;284:1383.

186. Schiller LR. Review article: the therapy of constipation. Aliment Pharmacol Ther 2001;15:749.

187. Burkitt DP, Walker ARP, Painter NS. Effect of dietary fiber on stool and transit times and its role in the causation of disease. Lancet 1972;ii:1408.

188. Tucker DM, Sandstead HH, Logan GM. Dietary fiber and personality factors as determinants of stool output. Gastroenterology 1981; 81:879.

189. Voderholzer WA, Schatke W, Muhldorfer BE, et al. Clinical response to dietary fiber treatment of chronic constipation. Am J Gastroenterol 1997;92:95.

190. Ramkumar D, Rao SSC. Efficacy and safety of traditional medical therapies for chronic constipation: systematic review. Am J Gastroenterol 2005;100:936.

191. Chun AB, Sokol MS, Kaye WH, et al. Colonic and anorectal function in constipated patients with anorexia nervosa. Am J Gastroenterol 1997;92:1879.

192. Chiarioni G, Bassotti G, Monsignori A, et al. Anorectal dysfunction in constipated women with anorexia nervosa. Mayo Clin Proc 2000; 75:1015.

193. Kline C. Non prescription drugs USA. 2000, Little Falls, NJ: Kline

194. Wald A. Approach to the patient with constipation. In: Yamada T, Alpers DH, Owyang C, et al. (eds). Textbook of gastroenterology. Philadelphia: J.B. Lippincott Co, 1991:779.

195. DiPalma JA. Current treatment options for chronic constipation. Rev Gastroenterol Disord 2004;4 Suppl. 2:S34.

196. Siegel J, Di Palma J. Medical treatment of constipation. Clin Colon Rectal Surg. 2005;18:76.

197. Kinnunen O, Salokannel J. Constipation in elderly long-stay patients: its treatment by magnesium hydroxide and bulk-laxative. Ann Clin Res 1987;19:321.

198. Hammer HF, Santa Ana CA, Schiller LR, Fordtran JS. Studies of osmotic diarrhea induced in normal subjects by ingestion of polyethylene glycol and lactulose. J Clin Invest 1989;84:1056.

199. Lederle FA. Epidemiology of constipation in elderly patients. Drug utilization and cost containment strategies. Drugs Aging 1995;6:465.

200. DiPalma JA, DeRidder PH, Orlando RC, et al. A randomized, placebo-controlled, multicenter study of the safety and efficacy of a new polyethylene glycol laxative. Am J Gastroenterol 2000;95:341.

201. Toledo TK, DiPalma JA. Review article: colon cleansing preparation for gastrointestinal procedures. Aliment Pharmacol Ther 2001;15: 605.

202. Corazziari E, Badiali D, Bazzocchi G, et al. Long term efficacy, safety, and tolerability of low daily doses of isosmotic polyethylene glycol electrolyte balanced solution (PMF-100) in the treatment of functional chronic constipation. Gut 2000;46:522.

203. Di Palma J. A randomized, multi-center, placebo controlled trial of polyethylene glycol laxative for chronic treatment of chronic constipation. Am J Gastroenterol 2007;102:1436.

204. Cash BD, Chey WD. Review article: the role of serotonergic agents in the treatment of patients with primary chronic constipation. Aliment Pharmacol Ther 2005;22:1047.

205. Johanson JF, Wald A, Tougas G, et al. Effect of tegaserod in chronic constipation: a randomized, double-blind, controlled trial. Clin Gastroenterol Hepatol 2004;2:796.

206. Kamm MA, Muller-Lissner S, Talley NJ, et al. Tegaserod for the treatment of chronic constipation: a randomized, double-blind, placebo-controlled multinational study. Am J Gastroenterol 2005;100:362.

207. Muller-Lissner S, Kamm MA, Musoglu A, et al. Safety, tolerability, and efficacy of tegaserod over 13 months in patients with chronic constipation. Am J Gastroenterol 2006;101:2558.

208. Cuppoletti J, Malinowska DH, Tewari KP, et al. SPI-0211 activates T84 cell chloride transport and recombinant human ClC-2 chloride currents. Am J Physiol Cell Physiol 2004;287:C1173.

209. Lipecka J, Bali M, Thomas A, et al. Distribution of ClC-2 chloride channel in rat and human epithelial tissues. Am J Physiol Cell Physiol 2002;282:C805.

210. Camilleri M, Bharucha AE, Ueno R, et al. Effect of a selective chloride channel activator, lubiprostone, on gastrointestinal transit, gastric sensory, and motor functions in healthy volunteers. Am J Physiol Gastrointest Liver Physiol 2006;290:G942.

211. Johanson JF, Morton D, Geenen J, Ueno R. Multicenter, 4-week, double-blind, randomized, placebo-controlled trial of lubiprostone, a locally-acting type-2 chloride channel activator, in patients with chronic constipation. Am J Gastroenterol 2008;103:170.

212. Johanson JF. Ueno R. Lubiprostone, a locally acting chloride channel activator, in adult patients with chronic constipation: a double-blind, placebo-controlled, dose-ranging study to evaluate efficacy and safety. Aliment Pharmacol Ther 2007;25:1351.

213. Johanson JF, Holland PC, Ueno R. Long-term efficacy of lubiprostone for the treatment of chronic constipation. Gastroenterology 2006;130:M1171.

214. Lubiprostone: RU 0211, SPI 0211. Drugs 2005;6:245.

215. Verne GN, Eaker EY, David RD. Colchicine is an effective treatment for patients with severe idiopathic constipation. Gastroenterology 1995;108:A705.

216. Roarty TP, Weber F, Soykan I, McCallum RW. Misoprostol in the treatment of chronic refractory constipation: results of a long-term open label trial. Aliment Pharmacol Ther 1997;11:1059.

217. Chalazonitis A. Neurotrophin-3 in the development of the enteric nervous system. Prog Brain Res 2004;146:243.

218. Parkman HP, Rao SS, Reynolds JC, et al. Neurotrophin-3 improves functional constipation. Am J Gastroenterol 2003;98:1338.

219. Staats PS, Markowitz J, Schein J. Incidence of constipation associated with long-acting opioid therapy: a comparative study. South Med J 2004;97:129.

220. Currie M, Kurtz CB, Mahajan-Miklos S. Effects of a single dose administration of MD-1100 on safety, tolerability, exposure, and stool consistency in healthy subjects. Am J Gastroenterol 2005;100: S328.

221. Andresen V, Camilleri M, Busciglio IA, et al. Effect of 5 days on transit and bowel function in females with constipation-predominant irritable bowel syndrome. Gastroenterology 2007;133:761.

222. Chiarioni G, Salandini L, Whitehead WE. Biofeedback benefits only patients with outlet dysfunction, not patients with isolated slow transit constipation. Gastroenterology 2005;129:86.

223. Chiarioni G, Whitehead WE, Pezza V, et al. Biofeedback is superior to laxatives for normal transit constipation due to pelvic floor dyssynergia. Gastroenterology 2006;130:657.

224. Rao SS, Seaton K, Miller M, et al. Randomized controlled trial of biofeedback, sham feedback, and standard therapy for dyssynergic defecation. Clin Gastroenterol Hepatol 2007;5:331.

225. Pinho M, Yoshioka K, Keighley MR. Long term results of anorectal myectomy for chronic constipation. Br J Surg 1989;76:1163.

226. Rao SS. The technical aspects of biofeedback therapy for defecation disorders. The Gastroenterologist 1998;6:96.

227. Pelsang RE, Rao SS, Welcher K. FECOM: a new artificial stool for evaluating defecation. Am J Gastroenterol 1999;94:183.

228. Rao SS, Enck P, Loening-Baucke V. Biofeedback therapy for defecation disorders. Dig Dis 1997;15 Suppl 1:78.

229. Papachrysostomou M, Smith AN. Effects of biofeedback on obstructive defecation – reconditioning of the defecation reflex? Gut 1994; 35:242.

230. Heymen S, Wexner SD, Vickers D, et al. Prospective, randomized trial comparing for biofeedback techniques for patients with constipation. Dis Colon Rectum 1999;42:1388.

231. Patankar SK, Ferrara A, Levy JR, et al. Biofeedback in colorectal practice: a multicenter, statewide, three-year experience. Dis Colon Rectum 1997;40:827.

232. Kawimbe BM, Papachrysostomou M, Binnie NR, et al. Outlet obstruction constipation (anismus) managed by biofeedback. Gut 1991;32:1175.

233. Nyam DC, Pemberton JH, Ilstrup DM, Rath DM. Long-term results of surgery for chronic constipation. Dis Colon Rectum 1997;40:273.

234. Redmond JM, Smith GW, Barofsky I, et al. Physiological tests to predict long-term outcome of total abdominal colectomy for intractable constipation. Am J Gastroenterol 1995;90:748.

235. Hassan I, Pemberton JH, Young-Fadok TM, et al. Ileorectal anastomosis for slow transit constipation: long-term functional and quality of life results. J Gastrointest Surg 2006;10:1330; discussion 1336.

236. Tackett LD, Minevich E, Benedict JF, et al. Appendiceal versus ileal segment for antegrade continence enema. J Urol 2002;167:683.

237. Rivera MT, Kugathasan S, Berger W, Werlin SL. Percutaneous colonoscopic cecostomy for management of chronic constipation in children. Gastrointest Endosc 2001;53:225.

238. Lees NP, Hodson P, Hill J, et al. Long-term results of the antegrade continent enema procedure for constipation in adults. Colorectal Dis 2004;6:362.

239. Pemberton JH, Rath DM, Ilstrup DM. Evaluation and surgical treatment of severe chronic constipation. Ann Surg 1991;214:403.

240. Ghosh S, Papachrysostomou M, Batool M, Eastwood MA. Long-term results of subtotal colectomy and evidence of noncolonic involvement in patients with idiopathic slow-transit constipation. Scand J Gastroenterol 1996;31:1083.

241. Ho YH, Tan M, Seow-Choen F. Prospective randomized controlled study of clinical function and anorectal physiology after low anterior resection: comparison of straight and colonic J pouch anastomoses. Br J Surg 1996;83:978.

242. Preston DM, Hawley PR, Lennard-Jones JE, Todd IP. Results of colectomy for severe idiopathic constipation in women (Arbuthnot Lane's disease). Br J Surg 1984;71:547.

243. van der Sijp JR, Kamm MA, Bartram CI, Lennard-Jones JE. The value of age of onset and rectal emptying in predicting the outcome of colectomy for severe idiopathic constipation. Int J Colorectal Dis 1992;7:35.

244. Rotholtz NA, Wexner SD. Surgical treatment of constipation and fecal incontinence. Gastroenterol Clin North Am 2001;30:131.

245. Altomare DF, Rinalki M, Veglia A, et al. Combined perineal and endorectal repair of rectocele by circular stapler: a novel surgical technique. Dis Colon Rectum 2002;45:1549.

246. Keighley MR, Shouler P. Clinical and manometric features of the solitary rectal ulcer syndrome. Dis Colon Rectum 1984;27:507.

247. Rao SS, Stessman M, De Ocampo S, Ozturk R. Pathophysiology and role of biofeedback therapy in solitary rectal ulcer syndrome. Am J Gastroenterol 2006;101:613.

248. Arroyo A, Perez-Vicente F, Serrano P, et al. Evaluation of the stapled transanal rectal resection technique with two staplers in the treatment of obstructive defecation syndrome. J Am Coll Surg 2007; 204:56.

249. Boccasanta P, Venturi M, Salamina G, et al. New trends in the surgical treatment of outlet obstruction: clinical and functional results of two novel transanal stapled techniques from a randomised controlled trial. Int J Colorectal Dis 2004;19:359.

250. Dinning PG, Fuentealba SE, Kennedy ML, et al. Sacral nerve stimulation induces pan-colonic propagating pressure waves and increases defecation frequency in patients with slow-transit constipation. Colorectal Dis 2007;9:123.

251. Holzer B, Rosen HR, Novi G, et al. Sacral nerve stimulation for neurogenic faecal incontinence. Br J Surg 2007;94:749.

252. Malouf AJ, Wiesel PH, Nicholls T, et al. Short-term effects of sacral nerve stimulation for idiopathic slow transit constipation. World J Surg 2002;26:166.

253. Kamm MA, Dudding TC. Sacral nerve stimulation for constipation: an international multi-center study. Gastroenterology 2007;132 (Suppl. 2):198.

254. Swenson O. A new surgical treatment for Hirschsprung's disease. Surgery 1950;28:371.

255. Boley SJ. An endorectal pull-through operation with primary anastomosis for Hirchsprung's disease. Surg Gynecol Obstet 1968;127:353.

256. Nixon HH. Hirschsprung's disease: progress in management and diagnostics. World J Surg 1985;9:189.

257. Poisson J, Devroede G. Severe chronic constipation as a surgical problem. Surg Clin North Am 1983;63:193.

258. Read NW, Abouzekry L, Read MG, et al. Anorectal function in elderly patients with fecal impaction. Gastroenterology 1985;89:959.

259. Ingebo KB, Heyman MB. Polyethylene glycol-electrolyte solution for intestinal clearance in children with refractory encopresis. A safe and effective therapeutic program. Am J Dis Child 1988;142:340.

260. Puxty JA, Fox RA. Golytely: a new approach to faecal impaction in old age. Age Ageing 1986;15:182.

261. Singh G. Complications and comorbidities of constipation in adults. Gastroenterology 2007;132(Suppl. 2):M2135.

262. Xing JH, Soffer EE. Adverse effects of laxatives. Dis Colon Rectum 2001;44:1201.

263. Rao SS. Constipation – Method of investigation. In: Rakel RE, (ed.). Conn's Current Therapy. Philadelphia: W.B. Saunders Company, 1999:20.

264. Remes-Troche JM, Rao SS. Diagnostic testing in patients with chronic constipation. Curr Gastroenterol Rep 2006;8:416.

265. Remes-Troche JM, Rao SS. Defecation disorders: neuromuscular aspects and treatment. Curr Gastroenterol Rep 2006;8:291.

266. Mertz H, Naliboff B, Mayer E. Physiology of refractory chronic constipation. Am J Gastroenterol 1999;94:609.

267. Lethbridge CM, Schiller JS, Bernadel L. Vital Health Stat 2005;10:1.

21 Approach to the patient with abnormal liver chemistries

Richard H. Moseley

Clinical evaluation, 399
Hepatic function tests, 402
Serum markers of hepatobiliary dysfunction, 405
Disease-specific markers, 407
A general approach to suspected liver disease, 411

The approach to the patient with abnormal liver chemistries is not governed by any well-defined diagnostic algorithms. Instead, a systematic approach to patients with suspected underlying liver disease involves a thorough understanding of the diverse panel of available measurements of liver function and serum markers of hepatobiliary disease. From this panel, a group of indices most appropriate to the particular clinical problem is selected. A single test is rarely sufficient in the approach to most clinical problems. The selection process is, however, facilitated by several distinct patterns of hepatocellular injury. Because diagnostic tests are imperfect, they are usually discussed in terms that allow assessment of their diagnostic value. The *sensitivity* of a test is defined as the likelihood of an abnormal test result in patients known to have a disease, and *specificity* is defined as the likelihood of a normal test result in patients known to be free of the disease. The *false-positive rate* is the likelihood of an abnormal test result in patients without the disease (1 – specificity) and the *false-negative rate* is the likelihood of a normal test result in patients known to have the disease (1 – sensitivity). Thus, sensitivity and the false-negative rate evaluate a diagnostic test in patients with disease, and specificity and the false-positive rate evaluate a test in patients without disease [1]. This chapter discusses representative and commonly used tests and offers guidelines in the interpretation of results.

Clinical evaluation

As in most disease states, an accurate history is critical in the approach to the patient with laboratory evidence of liver disease. Although systemic symptoms of liver disease, such as anorexia, weight loss, chills and fever, nausea, and vomiting, are nonspecific and are typically of little help in the differential diagnosis, valuable information can be elicited by questions regarding family history, use of prescription drugs and over-the-counter medications, alcohol consumption, use or abuse of illicit substances, exposure history, sexual and menstrual history, occupational or environmental history, travel history, past surgery (including anesthesia records, if available), and transfusion history.

A family history of jaundice may be present in Gilbert syndrome, Dubin–Johnson syndrome, Rotor syndrome, benign recurrent intrahepatic cholestasis, and hereditary hemolytic states such as hereditary spherocytosis. Familial forms of chronic intrahepatic cholestasis, such as arteriohepatic dysplasia (Alagille syndrome), and of cirrhosis have been well described. Hemochromatosis, Wilson disease (hepatolenticular degeneration), and α_1-antitrypsin deficiency are examples of liver diseases transmitted by an autosomal recessive mode of inheritance; genetic factors may also play a role in other hepatobiliary disorders, including primary sclerosing cholangitis, primary biliary cirrhosis (PBC), and autoimmune hepatitis.

Given the relatively nonspecific presentation of drug-induced liver disease, drug-related hepatic injury may not be immediately suspected in a patient with impaired liver function. Difficulties in diagnosis are compounded by the unknown hepatotoxicity of newly introduced agents. Nevertheless, the possibility of drug-induced liver injury should be considered in all patients with a seemingly nonspecific

Principles of Clinical Gastroenterology. Edited by Tadataka Yamada, David H. Alpers, Anthony N. Kalloo, Neil Kaplowitz, Chung Owyang, and Don W. Powell. © 2008 Blackwell Publishing. ISBN 978-1-4051-69103

change or worsening in liver chemistries, and such considerations are aided by a complete drug history. Alcohol and nonprescription medication use is an important part of this inquiry. Alcohol intake should be quantified and expressed, if possible, in terms of grams per day of alcohol (daily consumption in milliliters × 0.79 × percentage of alcohol in the form ingested). A threshold for the development of cirrhosis of 80 g/day for 15 years has been described in male patients with alcoholism [2], and it is likely that a lower threshold exists in women [3]. Acetaminophen (paracetamol) hepatotoxicity, secondary to induction of the cytochrome P450-dependent pathway of acetaminophen metabolism by ethanol or to low hepatic glutathione stores in the malnourished patient with alcoholism, is being increasingly recognized [4]. Patients with alcoholism who present with jaundice and profoundly abnormal serum aminotransferase levels should always be questioned regarding the use of acetaminophen. A high incidence of aspirin-induced hepatotoxicity, which appears to correlate with serum salicylate levels, has been observed in patients with rheumatic diseases, including juvenile rheumatoid arthritis and systemic lupus erythematosus [5]. Hypervitaminosis A is a well-recognized clinical syndrome associated with hepatic injury, intracranial hypertension, and desquamative dermatitis [6]. Although most cases of hepatic injury from vitamin A have occurred with massive long-term intakes, hepatotoxicity may be potentiated by ethanol, severe hypertriglyceridemia, and renal failure, and it may occur at vitamin doses as low as 4000 IU/day [6]. Cases of hepatitis following administration of complementary and alternative medications, such as germander (*Teucrium chamaedrys*), Jin Bu Huan Anodyne Tablets (*Lycopodium serratum*), kava, and chaparral, document the need for specific queries about ingestion of herbal products and the use of other unconventional forms of therapy, particularly in the setting of hepatic injury of unknown origin [7].

A history of recent ingestion of raw oysters or steamed clams should suggest infection with the hepatitis A virus (HAV), although specific risk factors that have been associated with HAV infection within the United States also include homosexual contact [8] and contact with children attending day-care centers [9]. In contrast to the well-recognized problem of nosocomial hepatitis B virus (HBV) infection, nosocomial outbreaks of hepatitis A have received little attention [10]. Questions directed at determining the source of water for patients are occasionally relevant, because private water supplies contaminated with sewage have often been implicated in outbreaks of hepatitis A. HBV infection should be suspected in patients with abnormal liver chemistries and a history of exposure to or contact with jaundiced individuals, syringes or needles (including tattoo paraphernalia), or blood or blood products. Intravenous drug users and male homosexuals seem to be particularly susceptible to chronic HBV infection. The development of abnormal liver chemistries in the apparently healthy HBV carrier warrants strong consid-

eration of superinfection with the delta agent (hepatitis D virus, or HDV). In countries with low endemism for HBV, such as the United States, HDV infection is found chiefly among parenteral drug users [11]. Hepatitis C virus (HCV) is parenterally transmitted, and a higher prevalence occurs in individuals with frequent exposure to blood, including patients who received multiple transfusions prior to 1992, patients with hemophilia, and current and former intravenous drug users [12]. Occupational exposure to HCV from needlestick accidents [12] and nosocomial spread of HCV [13] should also be considered. In contrast to HBV, HCV transmission by sexual or close physical contact appears to be inefficient and uncommon [12]. Recent travel to areas endemic for viral hepatitis should be noted; waterborne outbreaks of hepatitis E have been clearly documented in Southeast Asia and the Indian subcontinent. Abnormalities in smell (dysosmia) and taste (dysgeusia) may be noticed by patients afflicted with viral hepatitis. Arthritis, abrupt in onset and with a strong predilection for proximal interphalangeal joints, has been observed during the prodromal phase in approximately 20% of patients with HBV infection [14]. Abnormal liver chemistries may also be a direct manifestation of illicit drug use. The use of the stimulant 5-methoxy-3,4-methylene-dioxymethamphetamine (MDMA), or Ecstasy, has been associated with acute hepatitis and fulminant hepatic failure [15].

Sexually transmitted diseases (STDs) are an important cause of abnormal liver chemistries, and a sexual history should be included in the evaluation of such patients. Efforts to obtain accurate historical information are usually compromised by apprehension felt on the part of the interviewer rather than the patient. Relevant historical elements include information regarding whether the patient is currently sexually active, the number of sexual partners the patient has had in the preceding 6 months, whether the patient's sexual partners are of the same or different sex, whether the patient has recently had a new sexual partner, and the sites of sexual exposure. A sexual history in the female patient should always include information on contraceptive use, which has been associated with intrahepatic cholestasis, hepatic adenoma, and hepatic vein thrombosis (Budd–Chiari syndrome). A menstrual history may reveal the presence of secondary amenorrhea, a frequent complication of chronic liver disease. Infertility may be a presenting symptom in women with autoimmune hepatitis [16].

Although the use of hepatotoxins such as carbon tetrachloride, chloroform, and trinitrotoluene has diminished, liver injury associated with accidental and occupational exposure to workplace chemicals remains a significant problem. Although an itemized list of such chemicals is beyond the scope of this text, a patient's exposure to industrial and environmental hepatotoxins may be elicited by a thorough occupational history. Examples include:
• trichlorethylene – a commonly used solvent in dry cleaning that can cause an acute centrilobular hepatitis

• vinyl chloride – used in the plastics industry and associated with the occurrence of hepatic angiosarcomas

• arsenic – used in insecticide sprays by vineyard workers and implicated in chronic liver diseases, including noncirrhotic portal hypertension and hepatic angiosarcoma

• 2-nitropropane – used in industrial construction, highway maintenance, ship building, and plastic production and implicated in instances of acute liver failure [17].

The liver may be a target organ in a vast array of systemic disorders. In particular, but by no means exclusively, the presence of coexistent cardiac, pancreatic, or inflammatory bowel disease should be considered in the evaluation of any patient with abnormal liver chemistries. Right-sided congestive heart failure, hypotension, and shock are well-recognized causes of abnormal liver chemistries. Prolongation of the prothrombin time, often disproportionately to other signs of liver dysfunction, is the most common abnormality in patients with congestive heart failure, although elevations in serum bilirubin (primarily of the unconjugated form and rarely more than 3 mg/dL) and in serum aminotransferases can also occur [18]. Clinically inapparent left-sided heart failure or cardiac tamponade may present with a picture like that of acute or chronic hepatitis [19]. Hemochromatosis, in turn, may present as a congestive cardiomyopathy [20], or as hypogonadism, arthropathy, diabetes, or hyperpigmentation. Distal common bile duct stenosis is a well-described complication of chronic alcoholic pancreatitis to be considered in the setting of anicteric alkaline phosphatase elevations of a persistent nature [21]. The biliary tree may be similarly affected in cystic fibrosis [22]. Hepatobiliary manifestations of inflammatory bowel disease of clinical import occur in up to 10% of patients [23]. Hematological disorders, such as polycythemia rubra vera, myeloproliferative disorders, and paroxysmal nocturnal hemoglobinuria, may predispose to hepatic vein thrombosis. Hemoglobinopathies, such as sickle cell anemia and thalassemia, have been implicated as risk factors for pigment stone formation. Bacteremia, particularly with gram-negative organisms or *Staphylococcus aureus*, should be considered in any ill individual with direct and total serum bilirubin values that are disproportionately elevated compared with levels of alkaline phophatase and aspartate aminotransferase [24]. Bilirubin elevations may become manifest before the clinical recognition of infection, and persistent or progressive hyperbilirubinemia despite antiinfective therapy portends a poor prognosis and may warrant institution of additional therapeutic agents [25]. Leptospirosis should be regarded with a high index of suspicion in the febrile patient with both hepatic and renal abnormalities and a history of potential contact with animal urine or water. Renal cell carcinoma may present with abnormalities in liver chemistries, primarily elevated alkaline phosphatase levels, in the absence of hepatic metastases (nephrogenic hepatic dysfunction syndrome) [26]. Liver diseases peculiar to gravid women include intrahepatic cholestasis of pregnancy, toxemia, and acute fatty liver of pregnancy, although viral hepatitis is the most common cause of jaundice during pregnancy [27]. Membranoproliferative glomerulonephritis, chronic lymphocytic sialoadenitis, lichen planus, porphyria cutanea tarda, and essential mixed cryoglobulinemia have been associated with chronic HCV infection [28]. A high prevalence of elevated serum aminotransferases has been reported in patients with gluten-sensitive enteropathy; in most cases, these abnormalities resolve on a gluten-free diet [29]. Rarely, abnormal serum aminotransferases may be the sole feature that leads to the diagnosis [29]. Endocrine disorders are rare but recognized causes of abnormal liver function tests. Hyperthyroidism, independent of congestive heart failure or concomitant unrelated liver disease, can result in jaundice and a prolonged prothrombin time [30]; levels of serum aminotransferases and alkaline phosphatase are typically less than 250 IU/L and less than threefold elevated, respectively, although exceptions have been reported [30]. Elevated serum aspartate aminotransferase levels reported in hypothyroidism are secondary to enzyme release from muscle [31]. Moderate elevations in serum aminotransferases and vague constitutional symptoms may suggest the diagnosis of Addison disease [32].

The nature of, and indications for, previous abdominal surgical procedures should be fully ascertained. If it is available, information concerning the gross appearance of the liver at the time of operation may prove valuable. In the postoperative patient, surgical and anesthesia records should be carefully reviewed for the inhalational agent administered, the presence and duration of intraoperative hypotension, and the amount of blood product support required. Hepatic injury has been observed with most of the halogen-substituted inhalation anesthetics (e.g., halothane, methoxyflurane, enflurane); it presents initially with fever and is followed by the appearance of jaundice, with or without eosinophilia, after a latent period of several days [33]. Transfusions, particularly of stored blood, can be a factor in the development of postoperative jaundice. Progressive liver disease, including cirrhosis, has been described as a late complication of jejunoileal bypass surgery [34]. Biliary strictures, retained and recurrent stones, or papillary stenosis should be considered in the diagnosis of abnormal liver chemistries in the patient who has undergone cholecystectomy.

Generalized pruritus may be a presenting symptom in patients with liver disease, particularly cholestatic syndromes. The exact mechanism responsible for this often disabling symptom is unclear. Despite the often favorable response to oral cholestyramine, a bile acid-binding agent, there is no apparent correlation between either serum or tissue levels of bile acids and the degree of pruritus [35]. Clinical experience suggests that pruritus in the jaundiced patient is often nocturnal and is most pronounced on the palms and soles. Muscle cramps, also occurring frequently at night, and affecting largely the gastrocnemius muscle and small muscles of the foot, are common in patients with cirrhosis [36].

The presence, or absence, and character of abdominal pain may provide some clues in the approach to establishing a cause for abnormal liver chemistries. In contrast to the intense and rapidly developing right upper quadrant abdominal pain of acute extrahepatic obstruction, such as occurs in choledocholithiasis, the pain associated with acute viral hepatitis can be best described as a heavy or dragging sensation. Pain from primary and metastatic tumors of the liver may be distinguished by its dull or boring character, although hemorrhage into the tumor may result in the sudden onset of severe pain.

Physical findings of some discriminative value in the patient with abnormal liver chemistries include stigmata of chronic liver disease (e.g., spider angiomas, palmar erythema, parotid gland enlargement, gynecomastia, Dupuytren contracture, and testicular atrophy), hepatomegaly and liver consistency, splenomegaly, gallbladder distention, and abdominal tenderness. However, poor interobserver agreement for several of these clinical signs has been reported [37]; for other signs, such as Dupuytren contracture, the correlation with chronic liver disease is poor [38]. Although the degree of hepatomegaly can vary widely in all forms of hepatobiliary disease, a liver span greater than 15 cm is more often associated with passive congestion from right-sided heart failure or neoplastic and infiltrative processes (e.g., amyloidosis, myeloproliferative disorders, hepatic steatosis, and glycogen and lipid-storage disorders) [39]. A pulsatile liver may be encountered in tricuspid insufficiency. A hepatic bruit or friction rub should alert the examiner to the possibility of an underlying hepatocellular carcinoma; alternatively, a friction rub can occur with a hepatic abscess or in acute cholecystitis [40]. The presence of sunflower cataracts and of Kayser–Fleischer rings (golden-brown or greenish discoloration of the Descemet membrane in the limbic region of the cornea, initially appearing at the superior corneal quadrant) should be sought either with the unaided eye or with slit-lamp ophthalmoscopy, even if Kayser–Fleischer rings are no longer considered pathognomonic for Wilson disease [41]. Conjunctival suffusion, with or without hemorrhage, should suggest leptospirosis. A Murphy sign, or inspiratory arrest during deep palpation of the right upper quadrant, is highly suggestive of acute cholecystitis. Punch or fist percussion tenderness can also be elicited in acute cholecystitis (and in acute hepatocellular injury) and may help to differentiate hepatobiliary from pleural-based pain. A distended gallbladder, detected by either inspection or palpation, may be a presentation of malignant obstruction of the common bile duct (the Courvoisier sign).

Jaundice, manifested by yellow pigmentation of the skin, mucous membranes, and sclerae, typically requires a serum bilirubin concentration of greater than 3 mg/dL for detection. Artificial light makes detection at low levels more difficult.

Similar skin discoloration can be caused by ingestion of foods rich in carotene (e.g., carrots) and lycopene (e.g., tomato juice), by drugs such as Atabrine, quinacrine, or busulfan, or by toxins such as picric acid. This may be readily differentiated from jaundice by the absence of scleral icterus.

In addition to jaundice and excoriations resulting from pruritus, skin manifestations of potential help in the differential diagnosis of patients with abnormal liver chemistries include the hyperpigmentation associated with primary biliary cirrhosis (PBC) and hemochromatosis, the xanthomas and xanthelasmas present in chronic cholestasis, and the hypertrichosis of periorbital and malar regions and eczematoid dermatitis of sun-exposed areas in porphyria cutanea tarda.

Hepatic function tests

Laboratory determinations that reflect hepatic disease are collectively called *liver function tests*. However, only some are true measurements of hepatic function, and the use of this descriptive term should be discouraged. Tests that examine the ability of the liver to excrete substances into bile, particularly organic anions, fall within this strict definition, as do laboratory assessments of the synthetic and metabolic capacity of the liver.

Bilirubin

Because bilirubin is an endogenous organic anion, derived primarily from the degradation of hemoglobin from senescent erythroid cells, tests of bilirubin metabolism are important in the assessment of hepatic function [42]. Photometric determination of the azo derivatives obtained by reaction of plasma with the diazonium ion of sulfanilic acid (the diazo, or van der Bergh, reaction) separates bilirubin into two fractions, a water-soluble direct-reacting conjugated form and a lipid-soluble indirect-reacting form representing unconjugated bilirubin. Normal plasma total bilirubin concentrations in boys and men are significantly higher than in girls and women, and virtually all the bilirubin normally present in serum is in the unconjugated fraction. Hyperbilirubinemia, clinically manifested as jaundice, can accordingly be classified as either predominantly unconjugated or predominantly conjugated, simply by subtracting direct from total serum bilirubin to estimate indirect, or unconjugated, bilirubin. Increased production of bilirubin, impaired transport into hepatocytes, and defective bilirubin conjugation within the hepatocyte characterize disorders associated with unconjugated hyperbilirubinemia. Up to 85% of total serum bilirubin is in the unconjugated form in these disease states [39]. Along with the rate of hemolysis, the ability of the liver to conjugate bilirubin determines the degree of unconjugated hyperbilirubinemia observed. Even in severe hemolytic disorders, total serum bilirubin rarely exceeds 5 mg/dL in the presence of normal hepatic function [39]. Unconjugated hyperbilirubinemia may also be observed in disease states that interfere with the delivery of bilirubin to the liver, such as congestive heart failure, or in the presence of portosystemic shunts. In contrast, in disorders with impaired intrahepatic excretion of bilirubin (the rate-limiting step in overall bilirubin metabolism) and in extrahepatic obstruction, a conjugated hyperbilirubinemia is observed. Typically, in these settings, more than 50% of the serum bilirubin is in the direct-reacting form [39].

A direct-reacting fraction of bilirubin that is apparently covalently bound to albumin has also been identified; it is termed *albumin-bound bilirubin* or *delta bilirubin* [43]. This complex represents a significant fraction of total bilirubin in patients with either hepatocellular or cholestatic forms of jaundice if hepatic excretion of conjugated bilirubin is impaired, but it is not present in disorders associated with a predominant unconjugated hyperbilirubinemia. During recovery from jaundice, albumin-bound bilirubin tends to persist in plasma because the complex is minimally filtered by the kidney [43]. This explains the slow resolution of jaundice in convalescent patients with otherwise apparently normal liver function.

Urine bilirubin is invariably conjugated bilirubin and is encountered only in conditions in which serum levels of direct or conjugated bilirubin are elevated. The tea-colored appearance of urine caused by the presence of bilirubin must be differentiated from similar discoloration caused by hemoglobinuria and myoglobinuria. Prolonged storage before testing may produce false-negative results; phenothiazine administration can cause false-positive findings [39]. Bilirubinuria may precede the clinical appearance of jaundice, largely because of the low (< 1.0 mg/dL) renal threshold for conjugated bilirubin.

Serum bile acids

Two primary bile acids, cholic acid and chenodeoxycholic acid, are synthesized in the liver from cholesterol and converted by intestinal bacteria to the secondary bile acids, deoxycholic acid and lithocholic acid. Chenodeoxycholate can also be transformed into the tertiary bile acid, ursodeoxycholate. Serum bile acid determination in the assessment of patients with liver disease has been advocated. Although serum bile acid levels are almost always elevated in moderate to severe liver disease, poor diagnostic sensitivity in patients with mild liver disease has prevented widespread application of this test [44]. The finding of normal fasting levels of cholic acid conjugates may, however, be helpful in supporting a diagnosis of Gilbert syndrome in patients with unconjugated hyperbilirubinemia [45]. Greater sensitivity of serum bile acid levels, compared with conventional tests, has also been demonstrated in the detection of patients with cirrhosis [46], reflecting decreased first-pass elimination resulting from portosystemic shunting [47]. Elevated serum levels of bile acids in these patients may also have prognostic implications

[48]. The increase in serum bile acids that uniformly occurs as a result of diminished hepatic uptake or biliary excretion may be absent in patients with coexisting ileal disease that interferes with the intestinal phase of the enterohepatic circulation of bile acids. Conversely, small intestinal bacterial overgrowth may elevate serum bile acid levels [49]. Furthermore, serum bile acid determination appears to be of no value in assessing the patency of surgical portosystemic shunts [50].

Dye tests

Sulfobromophthalein (BSP) is a cholephilic organic anion previously used to assess hepatic function. The only current clinical application of the BSP plasma disappearance test is in the diagnosis of the inherited conjugated hyperbilirubinemic states, Dubin–Johnson syndrome and Rotor syndrome [51]. Anaphylactic reactions have been reported after BSP injection, largely limiting studies of BSP uptake and biliary excretion to research settings.

Indocyanine green (ICG) is a less toxic dye with hepatic uptake and excretion characteristics similar to those of BSP. However, because of greater hepatic clearance, ICG appears to be a less sensitive indicator of mild hepatic dysfunction than BSP [52]. Negligible removal by extrahepatic tissues makes ICG an ideal indicator of hepatic blood flow [53].

Clotting factors

Liver disease is a common cause of impaired coagulation. Normal serum activities of the vitamin K-dependent coagulation-factor proenzymes (factors II, VII, IX, and X), as assessed by the one-stage prothrombin time, depend on both intact hepatic synthesis and adequate intestinal absorption of lipid-soluble vitamin K. Vitamin K is required for the post-translational formation of γ-carboxyglutamyl residues that are essential for physiological activation of the factors [54]. Prolonged prothrombin times can be observed in both hepatocellular disorders that impair hepatic synthetic function, such as hepatitis and cirrhosis, and in cholestatic syndromes that interfere with lipid absorption. Hepatocellular injury can be differentiated from cholestatic causes of prothrombin time prolongation by the parenteral administration of vitamin K [55]; intact hepatic function is established by an improvement in prothrombin time greater than 30% within 24 h of administration. A prolonged prothrombin time may occur in the absence of liver disease, for example in: consumption coagulopathies; anticoagulant, antibiotic, or cholestyramine use; steatorrhea; and, rarely, dietary deficiency of vitamin K. Correction of the abnormal prothrombin time by parenteral vitamin K is observed in these conditions. Prolongation of prothrombin time in acute hepatocellular injury signifies severe hepatocellular necrosis, may antedate other manifestations of hepatic failure, and is associated with a poor prognosis [56]. Similarly, in chronic liver disease, a prolonged prothrombin time carries a poor long-term prognosis [57]. Plasma concentrations of individual proteins may be useful clinical guides; because of its short half-life, factor VII is considered the best index of severity of liver disease and of prognosis [58]. A characteristic pattern of hemostatic abnormalities occurs in patients with severe liver dysfunction; it consists of a low plasma fibrinogen level, a prolonged prothrombin time, and a normal or prolonged partial thromboplastin time. A hepatoma-associated dysfibrinogen, similar to fetal fibrinogen, has been described that produces prolonged prothrombin, thrombin, and reptilase times and inhibition of normal plasma coagulation [59].

Albumin

Albumin is quantitatively the most important of several plasma proteins formed in the liver. Accordingly, measurement of total concentration of serum albumin is a useful test of hepatic synthetic function. The relatively long half-life of serum albumin (20 days) makes the serum albumin level a better index of severity and prognosis in patients with chronic liver disease than in patients with acute hepatic injury, in whom levels are usually normal or only minimally depressed [52]. Nutritional factors, namely, the availability of amino acids, are crucial determinants of the rate of albumin synthesis [60]. Moreover, alterations in serum albumin levels may reflect not only disturbances in synthesis but also changes in the rate of catabolism, dilution by expanded plasma volume (e.g., in cirrhosis), or enhanced loss from the gastrointestinal tract or kidneys. Serum albumin levels are also decreased during normal pregnancy [61]. The shorter half-life (1.9 days) of prealbumin, a glycoprotein synthesized by the liver with a faster electrophoretic migration than albumin, was exploited to demonstrate that serum prealbumin levels may be a sensitive index of liver function after acetaminophen overdose [62].

Immunoglobulins

Although measurement of serum globulins does not fulfill the operational definition of a liver function test, the hypergammaglobulinemia that is commonly observed in patients with liver disease indirectly represents functional impairment of the reticuloendothelial cells of the hepatic sinusoids [52]. Nondiagnostic immunoglobulin abnormalities can be detected in most acute and chronic forms of liver disease, with drug-induced and extrahepatic cholestasis being notable exceptions. Although there is considerable overlap, hypergammaglobulinemia greater than 3.0 g/dL in a patient with chronic hepatitis is more consistent with autoimmune liver disease than with viral hepatitis. Rarely, the hypergammaglobulinemia in autoimmune hepatitis may be so pronounced that it causes the hyperviscosity syndrome [63]. A predominant rise in the IgA fraction is observed in hypergammaglobulinemia associated with alcoholic cirrhosis, whereas a disproportionate elevation of IgM is a feature that differentiates PBC from other liver diseases, specifically chronic active hepatitis, that are associated with prominent hypergammaglobulinemia [64]. However, a specific diagnosis is rarely established by quantitative determinations of immunoglobulins. The demonstration of hyperglobulinemia on serum protein electrophoresis is only a clue to the presence of chronic liver disease [52]. Conversely, hypoglobulinemia should suggest a protein-losing enteropathy.

Lipoproteins

The pivotal role of the liver in normal lipoprotein and cholesterol metabolism is reflected in the characteristic finding of abnormal lipoproteins and mild hypertriglyceridemia in acute forms of hepatocellular injury. Decreases in hepatic lecithin–cholesterol acyltransferase activity appear to account for the absence of α and pre-β bands on lipoprotein electrophoresis commonly associated with acute viral hepatitis and alcoholic hepatitis [65]. Alterations in hepatic triglyceride lipase activity may result in the characteristic elevation in low-density lipoprotein triglyceride, which, in turn, gives rise to the broad β electrophoretic band observed in these disorders [66]. Abnormalities in serum lipoproteins in chronic forms of liver disease reflect the degree of ongoing liver injury [52]. Hypocholesterolemia is observed in acute and chronic forms of hepatic insufficiency and is associated with a poor prognosis [67]. In contrast, cholestasis is associated with hypercholesterolemia, as a result of increases in unesterified cholesterol, and the appearance of an abnormal lipoprotein, lipoprotein X [68]. The origin of lipoprotein X appears to be biliary vesicles destined for canalicular secretion that in the setting of cholestasis are instead transcytosed to the sinusoidal membrane and released into the blood [69].

Tests of hepatic metabolism

Drug metabolism is another critical hepatic function, and liver disease is frequently associated with impaired drug metabolism. The most widely performed tests of hepatic metabolic capacity are the antipyrine clearance determination and the aminopyrine demethylation breath test. Antipyrine is a minor analgesic that, on the basis of rapid and complete absorption from the gastrointestinal tract, distribution in total body water, and minimal nonhepatic elimination, would seem to qualify as an ideal probe for studies of hepatic drug metabolism. Impaired antipyrine metabolism by the cytochrome P450 oxidase system, however, appears to be more a reflection of chronic active liver disease; the extent of impairment correlates well with serum albumin and prothrombin time determinations and with the degree of necrosis and inflammation on liver biopsy [70]. Little or no impairment in antipyrine metabolism is observed in patients with acute hepatitis or well-compensated cirrhosis [70]. The aminopyrine breath test avoids the need for multiple blood determinations. [^{14}C]aminopyrine is demethylated, through a [^{14}C]formaldehyde intermediate, to $^{14}CO_2$, which is measured in expired air. Single-sample, 2-h breath $^{14}CO_2$ determinations (expressed as a percentage of the administered dose) are significantly decreased in patients with both acute and chronic hepatocellular injury but are normal to minimally decreased in patients with intrahepatic and extrahepatic cholestasis without hepatocellular injury [71]. The aminopyrine breath test has also been used as a prognostic test in patients with alcoholic hepatitis, a value exceeding 1% of the administered dose correlating with improved 3-week survival [72]. Additional measurements of functional hepatic mass include the galactose elimination capacity, which demonstrates significant correlation with albumin synthesis in patients with cirrhosis [73], the caffeine and phenacetin breath tests, and measurement of the hepatic conversion of lidocaine to its primary metabolite, monoethylglycinexylodide. Although these quantitative tests may be noninvasive predictors of hepatic histology, interindividual differences in the metabolism of a single drug and intraindividual differences in the metabolism of different drugs make interpretation difficult, and it is unlikely that these tests will supplant percutaneous liver biopsy, for example, in the diagnostic approach to the patient with liver disease.

There is increasing evidence to suggest that susceptibility of individuals to hepatotoxic drug reactions or disease states is related to a genetically determined capacity for oxidative metabolism [74]. Noninvasive tests have been developed that identify significant interpatient differences in hepatic concentrations and activities of certain forms of cytochrome P450 underlying this polymorphism in oxidative drug metabolism [75]. The high incidence of impaired sulfoxidation in patients with PBC [76] may be a pathophysiological manifestation of this polymorphism.

Serum markers of hepatobiliary dysfunction

As has been discussed, routine biochemical laboratory tests are not true indices of hepatic function. Instead, they serve as markers of hepatobiliary dysfunction resulting from hepatocellular necrosis, cholestasis, or infiltrative processes.

Aminotransferases (transaminases)

Aspartate aminotransferase (AST) and alanine aminotransferase (ALT), measured by the serum glutamic–oxaloacetic transaminase (SGOT) and serum glutamic–pyruvic transaminase (SGPT) tests, respectively, are important markers of hepatocellular injury. Whereas AST can be found in various tissues, notably cardiac and skeletal muscle, kidney, and brain, ALT is limited primarily to the liver. Within the liver cell, AST is present in two isozymic forms, one in mitochondria and one in the cytosol [77], but ALT is localized to the cytosol. In normal serum, most of the AST activity is accounted for by the cystolic isoenzyme [78]. Serum ALT levels vary according to gender and body mass index, with higher values found in male patients and in persons whose body mass index is greater than 23 [79]. Serum ALT activity also decreases with age [80], and consumption of coffee and caffeine has been associated with a lower risk of elevated ALT activity [81]. A revised upper limit of normal serum ALT activity (30 U/L [500 nkat/L] for men; 19 U/L [317 nkat/L] for women) lower than current limits (40 U/L [667 nkat/L] for men; 30 U/L [500 nkat/L] for women) has been proposed to account for the presence of subclinical liver disease from nonalcoholic fatty liver disease and chronic hepatitis C in populations [82]. Furthermore, a graded increase in the risk of mortality from liver disease for both sexes has been reported in a large prospective cohort study from Korea even with serum AST and ALT levels within the normal range of 20–40 IU/L [83].

Given the tissue distribution of these two enzymes, elevations of serum ALT are a more specific reflection of hepatocellular disease than elevated serum AST level. The latter is more often elevated after acute myocardial infarction, and elevations in serum ALT levels in this setting are commonly the result of hepatic ischemia brought on by extensive myocardial injury, congestive heart failure, or cardiogenic shock [84]. Patients with idiopathic inflammatory myopathies, such as polymyositis and dermatomyositis, may, however, present with elevated serum ALT levels in association with elevated serum creatine phosphokinase as a reflection of muscle, and not hepatic, injury [85]. Elevated serum ALT levels have also been reported in patients with acute rhabdomyolysis [86]. The greatest serum elevations of both enzymes are seen in patients with viral, toxin-induced, and ischemic hepatitis, whereas smaller (< 300 U/L) elevations relative to the degree of histological necrosis are usually encountered in alcoholic hepatitis [84]. The AST/ALT ratio in serum is also regarded as a useful indicator, with a ratio greater than 2 being highly suggestive of alcohol-induced hepatic injury [87]. In contrast, in patients with acute or chronic viral hepatitis or extrahepatic biliary obstruction, an AST/ALT ratio of less than 1 is typically observed, although a correlation between an AST/ALT ratio greater than 1 and the presence of underlying cirrhosis has been described in patients with chronic hepatitis B infection [88]. An AST/ALT ratio of greater than 1 in the setting of nonalcoholic chronic liver disease should raise suspicion regarding underlying cirrhosis, but in the presence of cirrhosis the AST/ALT ratio may be less useful in differentiating alcoholic from nonalcoholic forms of liver disease.

Several mechanisms have been proposed for the disproportionate elevation of serum AST levels in alcoholic liver disease. Hepatic ALT activity in this setting is diminished to a greater extent than hepatic AST activity [89]. Pyridoxal 5′-phosphate is necessary for the activity of both aminotransferases, and there may be enhanced sensitivity of hepatic ALT to alcohol-induced pyridoxine deficiency [90]. Preferential alcohol-induced injury to mitochondria enriched in AST is an alternative hypothesis. Impaired plasma clearance of AST by sinusoidal cells [91] may play a role in the relative increase in serum AST levels observed in cirrhosis [88].

Although these indices of hepatocellular injury are not predictive of histological findings, serial determinations of serum AST and ALT levels may reflect the extent of hepatocellular injury and are useful in following the progression of liver disease. However, decreases in AST and ALT levels in serum may be either a sign of recovery from an acute injury or, particularly in the case of fulminant hepatic failure, an indication of limited hepatic reserve after overwhelming hepatocyte necrosis. In addition, hypoaminotransferasemia in patients with chronic renal failure who are undergoing hemodialysis has been found to obscure the diagnosis of HCV infection [92]. False elevations of AST have been observed in patients receiving *para*-aminosalicylic acid and erythromycin, and AST may, rarely, exist as a macroenzyme by forming a complex with immunoglobulin, leading to an otherwise unexplained elevation in serum AST activity [93].

Serum levels of the mitochondrial isoenzyme of aspartate aminotransferase (mAST) and the ratio of mAST to total AST have been reported to be specific and sensitive markers of chronic alcoholism [94]. Until these and other new markers of alcohol abuse, such as desialyated transferrin, are better evaluated, the γ-glutamyltransferase determination, in combination with mean corpuscular volume and serum AST levels, remains the recommended biochemical indicator of recent alcohol abuse [95].

Other enzyme markers of hepatocellular injury

Within the liver, the mitochondrial enzyme, glutamate dehydrogenase (GDH), is preferentially localized in centrizonal hepatocytes. The observation that alcohol exerts a toxic effect predominantly on mitochondria in centrizonal hepatocytes may account for the finding, in a large series of patients with alcoholism, that serum GDH determination was more useful than serum AST levels in diagnosing patients with histologically documented alcoholic hepatitis [96]. Serum GDH levels have also been reported to be increased in the congestive hepatopathy observed in acute right-sided heart failure [96]. However, the specificity of GDH as a marker of pericentral hepatocellular necrosis in alcoholic liver disease is open to question [97], and serum GDH determinations have not gained widespread application.

Alkaline phosphatase

In the liver, alkaline phosphatase appears to be an integral enzyme of the exterior surface of the bile canalicular membrane [98]. Although hepatocellular injury invariably results in increases in serum aminotransferase activity, significant (fourfold or greater) elevations of serum alkaline phosphatase activity are typically observed in patients with cholestatic syndromes. Lesser increases in serum alkaline phosphatase levels lack specificity and may be present in all forms of liver disease. The major mechanism underlying these

elevations is increased synthesis, through enhanced mRNA translation [99], of hepatic alkaline phosphatase rather than impaired biliary secretion of the enzyme. The mechanisms by which increased hepatic alkaline phosphatase activity leads to elevations in serum activity are less clear. Alkaline phosphatase contained within the bile canalicular membrane may be solubilized by bile acids that accumulate during cholestasis; these, in turn, alter the permeability characteristics of the intercellular tight junctions [100]. Alternatively, the distribution of hepatic alkaline phosphatase activity may be altered, again by the high intrahepatic concentrations of bile acids in patients with cholestasis, so that the enzyme is found in all domains of the hepatocyte plasma membrane and enters serum directly from the plasma membrane [100].

Alkaline phosphatase activity can also be demonstrated in bone, placenta, intestine, kidney, and leukocytes. Liver and bone are the predominant sources of serum alkaline phosphatase activity in normal subjects, with less than 20% derived from the intestine. Elevations of the intestinal isoenzyme occur in several disorders, including chronic renal failure, and in individuals secreting the ABH red blood cell antigen and in those of B and O blood groups [101]. In pregnancy, a substantial fraction may be derived from the placenta. Low levels of serum alkaline phosphatase have received comparatively less attention but may be encountered in hypothyroidism, pernicious anemia, zinc deficiency, and congenital hypophosphatasia. Decreased serum alkaline phosphatase levels have also been observed in acute hemolytic anemia complicating Wilson disease [102]. Benign familial elevation of serum alkaline phosphatase in a pattern suggesting autosomal dominant inheritance has been reported [103]. Ectopic production of an alkaline phosphatase isoenzyme (Regan isoenzyme) occurs in patients with cancer, and elevations in serum alkaline phosphatase levels may, therefore, be observed in the absence of bony or hepatic metastases [104]. Similarly, patients with stage I and II Hodgkin disease, osteomyelitis, and congestive heart failure have been found to have marked elevations in serum alkaline phosphatase levels in the absence of hepatic involvement [105].

Other enzyme markers of cholestasis

Although the alkaline phosphatase isoenzymes exhibit varied susceptibility to heat inactivation, and separation is possible with polyacrylamide gel electrophoresis [106], alternative approaches are commonly used to determine the source of an elevated serum alkaline phosphatase level. Serum γ-glutamyltransferase determination establishes the hepatic origin of an elevated alkaline phosphatase by virtue of its localization within the hepatobiliary tree, as well as kidney, pancreas, and intestine. Alcohol ingestion produces elevated serum levels of γ-glutamyltransferase, presumably by enzyme induction, and this finding has been invoked as a sensitive marker of chronic alcohol consumption that occurs independently of any liver damage [107]. However, sensitivity varies from 30% to 80%, depending on the population studied, and elevated serum γ-glutamyltransferase levels are also encountered in pancreatic disorders, myocardial infarction, uremia, chronic obstructive pulmonary disease, rheumatoid arthritis, and diabetes mellitus, as well as in patients using microsomal enzyme-inducing drugs such as barbiturates, phenytoin, and warfarin.

Determination of serum 5′-nucleotidase or leucine aminopeptidase levels fulfills a role similar to that of serum γ-glutamyltransferase determination. Despite the presence of these enzymes in a wide variety of other body tissues, elevated enzyme levels in the nonpregnant patient are specific for hepatobiliary disease and correlate well with elevated alkaline phosphatase levels of hepatic origin. Serum leucine aminopeptidase levels are elevated in pregnancy [108], and conflicting data exist concerning 5′-nucleotidase levels in pregnancy. In patients with cancer, elevated 5′-nucleotidase levels are a sensitive marker in the diagnosis of metastatic disease to the liver [109]. A normal 5′-nucleotidase level does not exclude liver disease in the setting of an elevated alkaline phosphatase, because these enzyme markers may not increase in parallel in early or mild hepatic injury [110].

Lactate dehydrogenase

Although commonly available, measurement of total serum lactate dehydrogenase (LDH) has limited diagnostic specificity for hepatocellular disease, and fractionation of LDH to determine levels of the isoenzyme of hepatic origin (LDH$_5$) is rarely indicated. Moderate elevations of LDH are frequently encountered in hepatocellular disorders such as viral hepatitis and cirrhosis and are less common in cholestatic disorders. However, marked elevations of serum LDH are observed in ischemic hepatitis, and an ALT/LDH ratio of less than 1.5 may differentiate ischemic hepatitis from acute viral hepatitis [111].

Disease-specific markers

The laboratory tests outlined earlier alert the physician to the presence of hepatobiliary disease. In the sections that follow, additional markers of specific disorders are discussed.

Viral serology

Diagnosis of acute hepatitis A is based on serological detection of HAV-specific IgM antibody (anti-HAV IgM). Seropositivity first becomes detectable at the onset of clinical illness and is invariably present at the onset of jaundice. This serological marker typically persists for 120 days, far exceeding both clinical and biochemical resolution of illness, and prolonged periods of seropositivity (> 200 days) have been observed [112]. Nevertheless, it is best regarded as a marker of acute or recent HAV infection. In contrast, anti-HAV IgG is present primarily in convalescent sera and persists for long periods after infection, perhaps for life.

Certain serological tests are available to establish a diagnosis of HBV infection. Hepatitis B surface antigen (HBsAg) is the first marker detectable in serum, preceding elevations in serum aminotransferases and the onset of symptoms. This antigenemia typically lasts for 1–2 months in self-limited infections. The titer of HBsAg, although not routinely reported, appears to be inversely related to the degree of hepatic inflammation. Persistence of HBsAg beyond 24 weeks is associated with a chronic carrier state, although persistence of HBV may also occur in the absence of any conventional serological marker [113].

Antibody to hepatitis B core antigen (anti-HBc) is detected in serum approximately 2 weeks after the appearance of HBsAg; typically, a window or lag period then occurs before the appearance of specific antibody to HBsAg (anti-HBs). During this period, and in the 10% of patients who do not manifest detectable levels of HBsAg, anti-HBc may be the only detectable serological marker of recent infection with HBV. The highest titers of anti-HBc occur in patients with the longest periods of HBsAg positivity. Antibody to the HBV core antigen of the IgM class (anti-HBc IgM) is the most sensitive marker of acute hepatitis B [114]. The specificity of anti-HBc IgM as a test, however, is lessened by its persistence, at low levels, in some patients with chronic active hepatitis B [115]. In acute hepatitis B, the hepatitis B e antigen (HBeAg) and the other direct marker of viral replication, HBV DNA, are detectable in serum shortly after HBsAg can be detected. However, tests of these markers of active viral replication should be reserved for patients with chronic hepatitis B, in whom they are used for determining and monitoring treatment. Testing for HBV DNA is also useful in the identification of HBV as the cause of liver disease in HBsAg-negative patients, including: patients with fulminant hepatitis B, who have early clearance of HBsAg; patients with cryptogenic cirrhosis [113] and hepatocellular carcinoma [116]; and patients infected with HBV mutants [117]. "Occult" hepatitis B infection has also been documented in several other patient populations, including those with HCV and human immunodeficiency virus (HIV) infection [118], and HBV DNA testing should be considered for all HIV-infected patients who have isolated positivity for anti-HBc [119]. The HBV genotype has been associated with both clinical outcome and response to antiviral therapy, but HBV genotyping is not routinely performed or recommended [120].

Diagnosis of bloodborne non-A, non-B hepatitis previously relied on the serological exclusion of HAV, HBV, and other hepatotropic viruses such as cytomegalovirus, herpes simplex virus (HSV), and Epstein–Barr virus (EBV). With the identification of HCV, initial screening relies on detection of circulating antibody to HCV using enzyme-linked immunosorbent assays (ELISAs). Hypergammaglobulinemia and connective tissue disorders are associated with false-positive results, and a recombinant immunoblot assay (RIBA) can be used to confirm ELISA results [121]. False-negative ELISA results may occur in immunocompromised patients and patients on chronic hemodialysis [122]. Qualitative HCV RNA by polymerase chain reaction (PCR) confirms the diagnosis and is particularly useful in patients with acute hepatitis C, before an antibody response is detectable, and in monitoring during and after treatment. Genotyping and quantitative HCV RNA tests are performed only before treatment.

Hepatitis D should be considered in any HBsAg-positive patient with acute or chronic hepatitis, especially if the disease is severe or the patient is in a high-risk group. Serological confirmation of hepatitis D coinfection or superinfection is accomplished by testing for HDV antigen (HDV RNA) and anti-HDV antibodies. A minimum of one acute and one convalescent serum sample should be assayed, because anti-HDV antibodies can be transient, present at low titer, and appear late in infection. Total (predominantly IgG) antibodies to HDV are usually detectable at high titer in superinfections. Persistence of anti-HDV IgM typically predicts progression to chronic HDV infection. Detection of HDV RNA by reverse transcriptase-PCR (RT-PCR) is the method of choice for the diagnosis of ongoing HDV infection [11].

Acute hepatitis E infections typically occur in the United States and Western Europe in persons returning from endemic areas in Asia and Africa, although serological studies suggest that hepatitis E virus (HEV) may also be endemic in more industrialized countries [123]. Diagnosis rests on detection of antibodies to hepatitis E viral antigens (anti-HEV).

Similar to other forms of acute viral hepatitis, EBV hepatitis typically manifests as a hepatocellular form of injury. However, cholestatic hepatitis induced by EBV has been described; diagnosis is confirmed with EBV-specific antibodies, such as serum IgM EBV-viral capsid antigen (VCA) [124].

The diagnosis of HSV hepatitis requires a high index of suspicion and may be distinguished from other forms of acute viral hepatitis by disproportionately low serum bilirubin levels in the face of marked serum AST>ALT levels [125]. Although the diagnosis of HSV hepatitis can be based on liver biopsy, which shows parenchymal necrosis, characteristic viral inclusions, and nuclear changes, HSV may also be identified by a PCR assay and culture of blood and mucocutaneous lesions, although such lesions are not always present. Tests for IgM antibody against HSV may be negative in patients with reactivated infection and early primary infection; therefore, serological findings may be used to support the diagnosis but cannot be used to exclude it [126].

Immunological tests

Immunological abnormalities occur in a wide spectrum of liver diseases. The antinuclear antibody (ANA) reaction in type 1 autoimmune hepatitis is of the homogeneous pattern by immunofluorescence, and a titer of 1:80 or higher is usually required for diagnosis. However, ANAs are observed in various liver diseases and their presence is not diagnostic of type 1 autoimmune hepatitis. Antimitochondrial antibodies (AMA) are present in more than 90% of patients with PBC and in about 25% of patients with type 1 autoimmune hepatitis and drug-induced liver injury [127]. An AMA titer higher than 1:40, even in the absence of serum alkaline phosphatase elevation or symptoms, is strongly suggestive of PBC [128]. Four major mitochondrial antigens related to PBC have been described: M2 antigen on the inner mitochondrial membrane, identified as the dihydrolipoamide acyltransferase of the branched-chain α-keto acid dehydrogenase complex [129]; and M4, M8, and M9 antigens on the outer mitochondrial membrane. The specific profile of antibodies to these antigens in patients may have clinical and prognostic importance [130]. Antibodies to the soluble Ro antigen [131] (often present in patients with Sjögren syndrome and systemic lupus erythematosus) and anticentromere antibodies [132] have also been identified in patients with PBC, particularly those with extrahepatic autoimmune disorders such as sicca syndrome and limited scleroderma, respectively.

Anti-smooth muscle antibodies (SMA), reactive to S actin, may be detected in up to 70% of patients with type 1 autoimmune hepatitis, in approximately 50% of patients with PBC, and occasionally in patients with acute viral hepatitis [133]. They may be the only immunological marker present in 33% of patients with autoimmune hepatitis [134]. The presence of anti-liver/kidney microsomal antibodies (anti-LKM1), along with absent or low-titer antiactin or antinuclear antibodies, serves to identify a subset of patients with idiopathic autoimmune hepatitis characterized by a more aggressive course and a predominance in young women [135]. The antigen to which anti-LKM1 is directed has been identified as the polymorphic cytochrome P450 isozyme, CYP2D6 [135]. This form of autoimmune hepatitis, termed type 2, is most prevalent in Western Europe and is rare in the United States [135]. Similarly, anti-LKM2 antibodies directed against cytochrome CYP2C9 were described in patients with hepatitis who were treated with the diuretic tienilic acid (Ticrynafen) [135].

Unlike the case of PBC, a specific autoantibody useful in the diagnosis of primary sclerosing cholangitis has not been identified. Although more than 80% of patients with primary sclerosing cholangitis have detectable perinuclear antineutrophil cytoplasmic antibodies, considerable overlap with autoimmune hepatitis limits determination of these antibodies as a diagnostic tool [136].

Human leukocyte antigens (HLA) have been associated with a wide spectrum of liver diseases. Specifically, HLA-DR3 and HLA-DR4 have been associated with autoimmune hepatitis, and HLA-DR4 may be associated with milder disease, a better response to corticosteroid therapy but an increased incidence of extrahepatic manifestations [137]. However, the increased frequencies of these HLA haplotypes are neither absolute nor diagnostic. Although HLA typing provides information on gene frequencies, it is neither routinely performed nor recommended.

Copper storage parameters

Determination of the serum concentration of ceruloplasmin, a copper transport protein in plasma, is particularly useful in the diagnosis of Wilson disease. Although not directly involved in the pathogenesis of this autosomal recessively inherited copper storage disorder, low levels of ceruloplasmin (< 20 mg/dL) are found in approximately 90% of homozygotes and in about 10% of heterozygotes. By contrast, serum ceruloplasmin is typically elevated in PBC, another disorder associated with increased hepatic copper concentrations [138]. Increased serum levels in this disorder and other forms of liver disease reflect the role of ceruloplasmin as a nonspecific acute-phase reactant. Accordingly, normal values may occasionally be observed during the chronic active hepatitis phase of Wilson disease [139]. Pregnancy and exogenous estrogen administration may also lead to elevated values for this protein [140]. Likewise, hypoceruloplasminemia may result from the diminution in hepatic synthetic function observed in non-Wilsonian fulminant hepatic injury [141], in chronic hepatitis [142], and, less commonly, in severe malnutrition, other protein-losing states, and Menkes syndrome [140]. A high incidence of low ceruloplasmin levels has been described in otherwise healthy members of a single family; this benign disorder has been termed *hereditary hypoceruloplasminemia* to differentiate it from Wilson disease [143]. By contrast, an autosomal recessive disorder of iron metabolism has been described in which serum ceruloplasmin is absent [144]. Excessive iron deposition, predominantly in the brain, liver, and pancreas in patients with aceruloplasminemia, leads to movement disorders and diabetes and may be mistaken for nonclassical forms of Wilson disease [144].

Alternative diagnostic tests in Wilson disease include determinations of urinary copper excretion, serum copper levels, and quantitative hepatic copper content in a liver biopsy specimen. In almost all patients with symptomatic Wilson disease, urinary copper excretion exceeds 100 μg/24 h. Total serum copper comprises a predominant (~ 90%) fraction that is irreversibly bound to ceruloplasmin and a small fraction that is loosely bound to albumin and to amino acids. The latter, termed the *free* or *nonceruloplasmin copper*, is calculated by subtracting the amount of copper associated with ceruloplasmin (0.047 mmol/mg) from the total amount of serum copper. Normally this value is less than 10 μg/dL; it is markedly elevated in Wilson disease, although total serum copper concentrations may be normal given the profound decrease in ceruloplasmin-bound copper [145,146]. The concentration of ceruloplasmin-bound serum copper can also be calculated by multiplying the ceruloplasmin concentration (in mg/dL), determined by an oxidase assay, by three [146]. Because copper is preferentially excreted in bile, caution is advisable in the interpretation of the results of these two tests in patients with chronic cholestasis or cirrhosis. Liver biopsy with quantitative copper determination is used to confirm the diagnosis; patients with untreated Wilson disease have hepatic copper levels greater than 250 μg/g dry weight.

Despite the discovery of the gene for Wilson disease, designated *ATP7B*, molecular diagnosis by direct mutation analysis has been complicated by the lack of a single dominant mutation among the more than 60 disease-specific mutations identified [147]. However, analysis of inheritance of highly polymorphic satellite markers surrounding the *ATP7B* gene has been useful in confirming or refuting Wilson disease in family members of affected patients [148,149].

Iron storage parameters

Measurements of serum iron level and total iron-binding capacity (or transferrin) are useful in the diagnosis of hereditary hemochromatosis (HHC). Transferrin is normally 20%–45% saturated, and both the serum iron level and percentage of saturation of transferrin are elevated early in the course of this disorder. A transferrin saturation of 45% or greater is a useful screening threshold because it identifies 98% of affected persons while producing few false-positive results [150]. However, these tests have a relatively low degree of specificity in patients with liver disease; increased serum iron levels, with normal transferrin saturation, are commonly observed in patients with alcohol-induced liver injury [151]. Acute elevations in serum iron levels have also been observed in acute viral hepatitis [152]. Transferrin synthesis is inversely correlated with total body iron stores; hence transferrin levels decrease in iron overload and increase in iron deficiency [153]. Factors other than iron balance, however, affect transferrin levels. Transferrin levels are decreased in inflammation and chronic disease and are increased during pregnancy and with estrogen therapy [153]. False-positive elevations in transferrin saturation are frequently observed if a nonfasting specimen is obtained [153]. Assays of serum ferritin may more closely estimate hepatic and total body iron stores [154], and elevated serum ferritin levels are commonly observed early in the course of HHC, even before there is any histological evidence of liver injury [155]. Ascorbic acid deficiency in patients with iron overload may lead to inappropriately low serum ferritin levels [156], and several families have been described in which asymptomatic relatives of patients with HHC had normal serum ferritin levels despite evidence of moderate hepatic iron overload [157]. Because serum ferritin is an acute-phase reactant, other forms of hepatocellular necrosis and systemic infection can be associated with elevated serum ferritin levels disproportionate to body iron stores [158]. Furthermore, in chronic hepatitis, elevated serum iron and ferritin levels in the absence of increased hepatic iron stores most likely represent increased release of iron from damaged hepatocytes [159]. Increases in serum vitamin B-12 levels reflect release from necrotic hepatocytes and may be used to interpret elevated serum ferritin levels [160]. As a general guideline, in the presence of inflammation, ferritin levels of less than 50 µg/L usually reflect iron deficiency and levels above 500 µg/L, in association with a transferrin saturation of more than 50%, usually represent HHC. A fasting transferrin saturation level threshold associated with the homozygous genotype of more than 62% in men and more than 50% in women was exceeded in 4% of men and in 8% of women heterozygous for HHC on the basis of HLA typing [161]. For these reasons, quantitative determination of tissue iron concentration on liver biopsy had been previously required; a hepatic iron index was calculated by dividing the hepatic iron concentration (in mmol/g dry weight) by the patient's age (in years); an index value greater than 1.9 was considered diagnostic of HHC [162]. However, with the identification of the hemochromatosis gene, HFE, and a mutation that leads to the substitution of tyrosine for cysteine at position 282 (C282Y) associated with HHC (in addition, a small percentage of individuals with compound heterozygosity for C282Y and a mutation in which aspartic acid replaces histidine at position 63 (H63D) seem predisposed to HHC) [163], liver biopsy is rarely required for the diagnosis and instead is used to assess the degree of liver injury. In certain C282Y homozygous patients, liver biopsy may be avoided completely, because age under 40 years, absence of hepatomegaly, normal serum AST and ALT levels, and, in particular, serum ferritin levels less than 1000 µg/L, reliably predicts the absence of severe fibrosis [164]. In addition, magnetic resonance imaging has been validated to determine liver iron concentration noninvasively [165].

Since the discovery of the HFE gene it has become clear that mutations in other genes that control iron metabolism can cause similar forms of iron overload. Besides classical hereditary hemochromatosis (type 1) associated, in most cases, with a C282Y mutation in HFE, other types of hereditary hemochromatosis, each caused by mutations involving a different gene, are recognized. These include: type 2a, associated with mutations in the hemojuvelin gene (HJV); type 2b, associated with mutations in the hepcidin gene (HAMP); and type 3, associated with mutations in the transferrin receptor 2 gene (TfR2), all of which are autosomal recessive disorders. Additionally there is the autosomal dominant type 4, associated with mutations in the ferroportin gene (SLC40A1) [166]. As a result, second-line genetic testing, not widely available, should be considered for patients with HFE genotypes other than C282Y/C282Y or C282Y/H63D and persistently elevated serum ferritin levels.

α-Fetoprotein

A sensitive radioimmunoassay for α-fetoprotein (AFP), a major serum protein during fetal life, is employed in the screening for primary hepatocellular carcinoma. About 70%–90% of patients with hepatocellular carcinoma have elevations in serum AFP, and significant elevations are also observed in patients with germ-cell tumors, other gastrointestinal malignancies, and nonneoplastic hepatic disorders such as autoimmune, viral, and alcoholic hepatitis, and PBC [167]. In particular, serum AFP values are frequently elevated in patients with advanced chronic hepatitis C, even in the absence of hepatocellular carcinoma [168]. To enhance the specificity of this test in the diagnosis of hepatocellular carcinoma, a minimum concentration for positivity of 400 ng/mL has usually been assumed [169], although this arbitrary cutoff may exclude up to one-third of patients with biopsy-proven hepatocellular carcinoma. A monoclonal radioimmunoassay may improve the specificity of AFP screening [170]. Although not widely available, assays for des-γ-carboxyprothrombin, an abnormal prothrombin, may also be useful in the detection of primary hepatocellular carcinoma [171].

α₁-Antitrypsin

α₁-Antitrypsin is a 52-kDa glycoprotein that is synthesized in the liver and, to a lesser extent, in monocytes and macrophages [172], and migrates in the α₁-globulin fraction on serum protein electrophoresis. Normal serum levels (150–350 mg/dL) may increase postoperatively and in association with inflammation, malignant disease, pregnancy, or estrogen therapy. The principal function of this protein is the inhibition of leukocyte elastase. The single gene encoding the synthesis of α₁-antitrypsin is contained within a 10-kb segment of five exons on chromosome 14 [173]. More than 25 codominantly expressed alleles have been described at this locus, and the normal phenotype for the protease inhibitor (Pi) system has been designated Pi MM by electrophoretic mobility. Individuals homozygous for the electrophoretically slowest of the genetic variants of this protein, designated Pi ZZ, exhibit markedly decreased serum α₁-antitrypsin levels and are predisposed to the early onset of chronic active hepatitis and cryptogenic cirrhosis [174]. Heterozygotes (Pi MZ) demonstrate serum levels that are 50%–60% of normal values [175]. The inability of the hepatocyte to process and secrete the Z protein, which differs from the normal M protein by a single amino acid substitution [176], results in the characteristic presence of periodic acid–Schiff (PAS)-positive diastase-resistant globules in periportal hepatocytes on percutaneous liver biopsy. The diagnosis of α₁-antitrypsin deficiency should be entertained in a patient with a pattern of liver chemistry abnormalities consistent with hepatocellular injury if there is an absent α₁-globulin peak on serum electrophoresis; the diagnosis is confirmed by serum α₁-antitrypsin activity determination and genetic Pi typing.

Serum ammonia

Urea formation in the liver, through the Krebs–Henseleit cycle, is required for the disposal of ammonia, the toxic product of nitrogen metabolism. Elevated serum ammonia levels are often observed in both acute and chronic forms of liver disease. The striking elevations seen in fulminant hepatic failure are the result of impaired conversion of ammonia to urea in the setting of severe hepatocellular necrosis, whereas the hyperammonemia present in patients with cirrhosis and portal hypertension primarily reflects portosystemic shunting of ammonia derived from colonic bacteria [177]. Additional factors that influence the level of serum ammonia in patients with cirrhosis include:

- intestinal production of ammonia by bacterial deamination of blood or dietary protein
- renal production of ammonia by glutaminase in response to metabolic alkalosis or hypokalemia
- intestinal production of ammonia from urea by urease-forming bacteria in the setting of diminished renal function
- hepatic production of ammonia from amino acids in response to increased glucagon secretion [178].

Although routinely determined in patients with suspected hepatic encephalopathy and used as an index of the success of therapy, serum ammonia levels only roughly correlate with the degree of encephalopathy [178]. Hyperammonemia and encephalopathy in the absence of liver disease have been reported in patients with urea cycle enzyme deficiencies, after ureterosigmoidostomy, and in a patient with a neurogenic bladder infected with urease-producing bacteria [179]. Serum ammonia determination is best regarded merely as an aid in the differential diagnosis of encephalopathy, and serial determinations have little role in clinical practice. One exception may be patients with acute liver failure, in whom high arterial ammonia levels can be correlated with cerebral herniation [180].

Additional abnormalities that can be observed in hepatic encephalopathy include decreased serum levels of branched-chain amino acids and elevated serum levels of aromatic amino acids, methanethiol, and short-chain fatty acids [181]. This serum amino acid profile contrasts with that observed in severe autoimmune hepatitis, in which both aromatic and branched-chain amino acid levels are increased, but it does not distinguish between patients with and without clinical manifestations of hepatic encephalopathy [181].

Liver biopsy

Unlike most of the laboratory tests discussed above, a predictive value cannot be assigned to a specific morphological feature observed with a liver biopsy. Yet liver biopsy can be extremely useful in the diagnostic approach to the patient with abnormal liver chemistries. Proper biopsy interpretation is assisted by the availability of all clinical, biochemical, immunological, and radiographic data to correlate histological features with an etiological diagnosis. As a general rule, direct forms of liver injury tend to cause predominant centrizonal necrosis; immunologically mediated forms of hepatocyte injury are localized to the periportal regions; and cholestatic liver injury can be recognized by the accumulation of canalicular bile and feathery degeneration of hepatocytes in the absence of a significant inflammatory infiltrate. Major applications of liver biopsy, other than in the evaluation of a patient with persistently abnormal liver chemistries, include the following:

- establishing the diagnosis in patients with unexplained hepatomegaly
- assisting diagnosis in patients with suspected systemic disease, such as tuberculosis, sarcoidosis, or fever of unknown origin [182]
- establishing a diagnosis in patients with suspected primary or metastatic carcinoma.

Contraindications to percutaneous liver biopsy include an uncooperative or unstable patient, ascites, right-sided empyema, and suspected hemangioma or echinococcal cyst. Transjugular liver biopsy is an alternative to the percutaneous approach in patients with severe coagulopathy and massive ascites [183].

A general approach to suspected liver disease

Numerous tests have been described above and in other chapters. Initially, nonhepatic causes of any observed abnormalities must be considered (Table 21.1). The dilemma then faced is in selecting a proper diagnostic approach to the patient with suspected liver disease. Liver disease can be classified into four major types: cholestatic, hepatocellular, and immunological injuries and infiltrative processes. Depending on the target of the immune response, immunological injury results in either a cholestatic picture (if the bile ducts are preferentially involved, as in PBC) or a hepatocellular form of injury (if the primary insult is to the hepatocyte membrane, as in viral and autoimmune hepatitis). Cholestasis can be further categorized as either a functional defect in bile formation at the level of the hepatocyte (intrahepatic cholestasis) or a structural impairment in bile secretion and flow (extrahepatic cholestasis). Evaluation is aided by the presence of these relatively discrete patterns of liver injury and tests of discriminative value in the detection of these patterns. Routinely, the results of the following tests should be determined in all patients with suspected liver disease before disease-specific markers are sought:

- serum aminotransferase (AST and ALT) activity
- serum alkaline phosphatase
- serum total and direct bilirubin
- serum total protein, with albumin and globulin fractionation
- prothrombin time.

Patterns of abnormalities typical of the various forms of hepatobiliary injury emerge from this battery of tests, as outlined in Table 21.2. Cholestatic liver injury is typically characterized by a ratio of serum ALT to alkaline phosphatase of 2 or less, whereas a ratio of 5 or greater suggests the presence of hepatocellular injury. Mixed cholestatic–hepatocellular injury is characterized by ratios of between 2 and 5. Testing for disease-specific markers, as listed in

Table 21.1 Nonhepatic causes of abnormal liver chemistries

Test	Nonhepatic causes	Discriminating tests
Albumin	Protein-losing enteropathy	Serum globulins, α_1-antitrypsin clearance
	Nephrotic syndrome	Urinalysis, 24-h urinary protein
	Malnutrition	Clinical setting
	Congestive heart failure	Clinical setting
Alkaline phosphatase	Bone disease	GGT, SLAP, 5'-NT
	Pregnancy	GGT, 5'-NT
	Malignant disease	Alkaline phosphatase electrophoresis
Serum aspartate aminotransferase	Myocardial infarction	MB-CPK
	Muscle disorders	Creatine kinase, aldolase
Bilirubin	Hemolysis	Reticulocyte count, peripheral smear, urine bilirubin
	Sepsis	Clinical setting, cultures
	Ineffective erythropoiesis	Peripheral smear, urine bilirubin, hemoglobin electrophoresis, bone marrow examination
	"Shunt" hyperbilirubinemia	Clinical setting
GGT	Alcohol, drugs	History
Ferritin	Systemic disease, chronic inflammation	Clinical setting
Prothrombin time	Antibiotic and anticoagulant use, steatorrhea, dietary deficiency of vitamin K (rare)	Response to vitamin K, clinical setting

GGT, γ-glutamyltransferase; MB-CPK, MB isoenzyme of creatine phosphokinase; 5'-NT, 5'-nucleotidase; SLAP, serum leucine aminopeptidase.

Table 21.2 Routine biochemical tests in the patient with idealized hepatobiliary disease

Test	Hepatocellular necrosis	Cholestasis	Infiltrative process
Aminotransferase	++ to +++	0 to +	0 to +
Alkaline phosphatase	0 to +	++ to +++	++ to +++
Total/direct bilirubin	0 to +++	0 to +++	0 to +
Prothrombin time	Prolonged	Prolonged; responsive to vitamin K	Normal
Albumin	Decreased in chronic disorders	Normal	Normal

0, normal; + to +++, increasing degrees of abnormality.

Table 21.3, may provide additional diagnostic information. Further laboratory evaluation of any patient with evidence of chronic (> 6 months) elevation in serum aminotransferases should, at the minimum, include the following tests:
• serum protein electrophoresis
• serum ferritin
• ANA and anti-smooth muscle antibodies
• serum ceruloplasmin
• hepatitis B viral serology
• antibody to HCV and, if positive, HCV RNA by PCR
• endomysial and tissue transglutaminase antibodies.
The cause of the chronic elevation in serum aminotransferases is suggested by these and other tests, as outlined in Fig. 21.1. The management of minor elevations in serum ALT

levels, for example, of less than 6 months' duration is less defined, although in asymptomatic individuals this may represent clinically insignificant fluctuation and may resolve over time [184].

The differential diagnosis of a patient with abnormal liver chemistries consistent with cholestatic injury (i.e., elevations of serum alkaline phosphatase and bilirubin levels, with or without moderate elevations of ALT or AST) represents a formidable clinical challenge. Hyperbilirubinemia resulting from extrahepatic biliary obstruction, in contrast to that observed in acute and chronic forms of hepatocellular injury, tends to level off over time and the bilirubin concentration rarely exceeds 35 mg/dL in the absence of oliguria or hemolysis. The mechanism for this plateau effect appears to be

Table 21.3 Diagnosis of selected hepatobiliary disorders

Form of liver injury	Supporting laboratory data	Role of liver biopsy
Hepatocellular		
Viral hepatitis	Viral serology	Usually required in hepatitis B and C
Drug-induced hepatitis	Eosinophil count	Rarely diagnostic
Autoimmune hepatitis	Immunoelectrophoresis Antinuclear antibody Anti-smooth muscle antibody	Usually required
Wilson disease	Serum ceruloplasmin	Usually required
Hemochromatosis	Serum iron/total iron-binding capacity Serum ferritin	Usually required
α_1-Antitrypsin (AAT) deficiency	Protein electrophoresis Serum AAT level Protease inhibitor typing	Usually required
Cholestatic		
Primary biliary cirrhosis	Antimitochondrial antibody Immunoelectrophoresis	Essential
Infiltrative		
Hepatocellular carcinoma	α-Fetoprotein	Essential

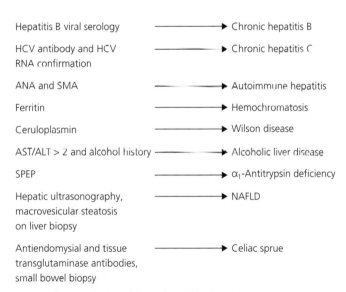

Figure 21.1 Evaluation of the patient with elevated serum aminotransferase levels. Liver biopsy should be considered in most cases to confirm suspected disorders. ALT, alanine aminotransferase; ANA, antinuclear antibody; AST, aspartate aminotransferase; HCV, hepatitis C virus; NAFLD, nonalcoholic fatty liver disease; SMA, smooth muscle antibody; SPEP, serum protein electrophoresis.

related to altered bilirubin metabolism, including enhanced renal excretion of conjugated bilirubin. In addition, a daily increase of 1.5 mg/dL in total serum bilirubin is characteristic of extrahepatic biliary obstruction [185]. Nevertheless, none of the routine biochemical laboratory tests can reliably differentiate intrahepatic cholestasis from extrahepatic biliary obstruction. Furthermore, within 24–48 h of acute extrahepatic obstruction, profound elevations in serum ALT and AST levels may be observed, followed by a rapid decline [186]. An elevated serum bilirubin level in the absence of elevations of AST or alkaline phosphatase levels is an unusual finding and more commonly is a marker of underlying cardiac disease than any liver or biliary tract disease [187].

Although no symptoms or signs are pathognomonic for intrahepatic or extrahepatic forms of cholestasis, a history of previous biliary tract surgery, the presence of abdominal pain or significant weight loss, palpable gallbladder or abdominal mass, fever or other signs of cholangitis, and an elevated serum amylase should point to an extrahepatic cause such as choledocholithiasis, pancreatitis, cholangiocarcinoma, or carcinoma of the pancreas. Partial obstruction or obstruction involving only a portion of the intrahepatic biliary tree may result in an elevated serum alkaline phosphatase level in the absence of hyperbilirubinemia. Conversely, a normal alkaline phosphatase level in a jaundiced patient strongly rules against the presence of extrahepatic biliary obstruction [39]. Fever and right upper quadrant abdominal pain may occur in drug-induced cholestasis and lead to confusion if a detailed drug history is not available. A cholestatic biochemical profile with fluctuating levels of serum alkaline phosphatase in a patient with inflammatory bowel disease should suggest primary sclerosing cholangitis. Marked cholangiographic changes in the presence of advanced histological stage may, however, occur without a concomitant increase in serum alkaline phosphatase activity [188]. In the setting of acute pancreatitis, marked elevations in ALT and γ-glutamyltransferase levels point to a biliary origin [189].

Additional laboratory tests, even liver biopsy, may not further differentiate between intrahepatic and extrahepatic cholestasis. Moreover, in drug-induced cholestasis, one of the more common causes of intrahepatic cholestasis, discontinuation of the offending drug may not be immediately followed by resolution of the cholestatic picture. As discussed in greater detail in other chapters, the most direct approach to the differential diagnosis of cholestatic injury is the use of abdominal ultrasonography to assess bile duct size, followed, if biliary dilation is present, by endoscopic retrograde cholangiopancreatography (ERCP) or percutaneous transhepatic cholangiography (PTC). Biliary tract obstruction of short duration may not be accompanied by detectable dilation of the bile ducts, and, when there is a strong clinical suspicion of an extrahepatic cause of cholestasis, ERCP or PTC may be indicated even in the presence of a normal ultrasonographic examination [190].

Isolated elevation of serum alkaline phosphatase, confirmed by either serum leucine aminopeptidase, 5'-nucleotidase, or γ-glutamyltransferase to be of hepatic origin, is strongly suggestive of an infiltrative process, whether a localized (i.e., PBC) or systemic granulomatous disease, such as sarcoidosis, miliary tuberculosis, coccidiomycosis, histoplasmosis, brucellosis, Q fever, or a drug reaction (e.g., allopurinol, quinidine); alternatively, it may be the first indication of metastatic carcinoma of the liver. A greater than threefold elevation in serum alkaline phosphatase levels in patients with cirrhosis should raise concern for the development of hepatocellular carcinoma. The triad of an elevated serum alkaline phosphatase level, detectable titers of AMA, and an elevated serum IgM level in a middle-aged woman is of considerable discriminative value in the diagnosis of PBC. In a patient with a history of malignant disease, particularly breast or colon cancer, the presence of an elevated serum alkaline phosphatase warrants an evaluation for metastases. The absence, in this setting, of diagnostic findings on abdominal ultrasound, computed tomography of the abdomen, technetium sulfur colloid nuclear imaging, and invasive tests such as ERCP, is one of the major indications for percutaneous or laparoscopic liver biopsy. A decision tree that can be used in the approach to the patient with an elevated alkaline phosphatase is provided in Fig. 21.2.

Although other features, such as serum bilirubin levels and prolongation of the prothrombin time, may vary and correlate with the severity of the injury, elevated serum

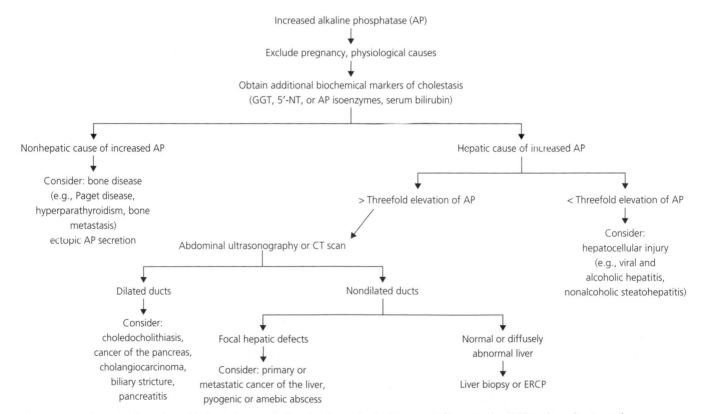

Figure 21.2 Diagnosing the patient with elevated serum alkaline phosphatase levels. CT, computed tomography; ERCP, endoscopic retrograde cholangiopancreatography; GGT, serum γ-glutamyltransferase; 5'-NT, 5'-nucleotidase.

aminotransferases are characteristically associated with hepatocellular forms of injury and reflect release of intracellular enzymes from hepatocytes undergoing necrosis. As a general rule, aminotransferase levels greater than 400 U/L are indicative of hepatocellular injury. In contrast, milder degrees of serum aminotransferase elevation (< 300 U/L) are of little diagnostic benefit because they are seen in cholestatic disorders as often as in acute and chronic hepatocellular disease. Establishing the cause of hepatocellular necrosis usually requires more information than routine laboratory results can provide.

As discussed previously, the nature and degree of aminotransferase elevation may be helpful in differentiating alcoholic hepatitis from ischemic, viral-induced, or drug-induced hepatitis. Leukocytosis can be a prominent feature associated with alcoholic hepatitis. Ischemic liver injury is, at times, indistinguishable from acute viral hepatitis. A disproportionate and marked elevation in serum aminotransferases in the setting of generalized malaise, anorexia, jaundice, and tender hepatomegaly characterize both disorders. However, measures to improve hepatic blood flow (e.g., correction of hypotension or congestive heart failure) are accompanied by a faster fall in serum aminotransferase levels than is observed in the course of acute viral hepatitis [191]. Normal values are occasionally found within 48–72 h in cases of ischemic hepatitis. Associated mild to moderate renal impairment also suggests ischemic hepatitis [191]. Features suggestive of drug-related hepatotoxicity include a history of recent institution of therapy and indirect evidence of a hypersensitivity reaction, such as rash, arthralgia, or eosinophilia. Profoundly abnormal aminotransferase activities, with preservation of an elevated AST/ALT ratio, are observed in patients with alcoholism and acetaminophen hepatoxicity [192], and a positive response to questions regarding the use of acetaminophen mandates measurement of the blood level of this drug. The liver is commonly involved in patients with typhoid fever. Lower peak serum ALT and AST, higher peak serum alkaline phosphatase, an ALT/LDH ratio of less than 4, fever, and relative bradycardia may help to distinguish *Salmonella* hepatitis from acute viral hepatitis [193]. A high index of suspicion is required in the diagnosis of Wilson disease, and ceruloplasmin levels should be routinely determined in patients under 40 years of age with hepatic (variable elevations in serum.aminotransferases in the presence of mild hyperbilirubinemia and hypoalbuminemia suggesting HBsAg-negative chronic active hepatitis, autoimmune hepatitis, or cryptogenic cirrhosis) and neurological abnormalities. Reports of patients diagnosed with Wilson disease in their seventh or eighth decade of life point out that screening for this disorder with serum ceruloplasmin determination should be performed, if appropriate symptoms or signs are present, regardless of age [194]. Although a reduced serum ceruloplasmin level may be observed in other disorders, as has been discussed, its presence in an asymptomatic individual with elevated serum aminotransferase levels is highly suggestive of Wilson disease. Hemolytic anemia, with or without low alkaline phosphatase activity [102], and hypo-uricosemia are additional clues to the diagnosis of this disorder. However, establishing such a diagnosis in the setting of fulminant hepatic failure is difficult. The specificity of an alkaline phosphatase/total bilirubin ratio of less than 2 in distinguishing fulminant hepatic failure secondary to Wilson disease from that resulting from other causes is open to question [195].

With the development of serological tests for HCV, up to 17% of volunteer blood donors with asymptomatic elevations in serum ALT were found to have evidence of HCV infection [196]. Determination of antibody to HCV is routinely performed as part of the evaluation of patients with elevated serum ALT and AST levels. Asymptomatic patients who test positive for anti-HCV antibodies often demonstrate chronic liver disease on liver biopsy even in the absence of serum ALT elevations. However, liver biopsy need not be performed in antibody-positive patients with normal ALT levels whose serum HCV RNA evaluation is negative [197].

Criteria and a scoring system have been proposed to standardize the diagnosis of autoimmune hepatitis that includes historical, biochemical, serological, and histopathological parameters [198]. Considerable weight is given to seropositivity for ANA, SMA, or LKM-1; seronegativity for markers of viral hepatitis; hypergammaglobulinemia with selective elevation of serum IgG; and interface (periportal or periseptal) hepatitis with a predominantly lymphoplasmacytic necroinflammatory infiltrate on liver biopsy [198].

Unexplained elevation of serum aminotransferases is an indication for serological testing for celiac disease. Tests for IgA endomysial and tissue transglutaminase (tTG) antibodies are favored over tests for antigliadin antibodies because of their higher specificity and sensitivity. Because selective IgA deficiency occurs more commonly in patients with celiac disease, a total IgA level and a test based on IgG antibody, preferably IgG-tTG, is recommended [199]. The prevalence of celiac disease in patients with chronic asymptomatic elevations in serum aminotransferases has been estimated to be of the order of 4% [200]. False positive anti-tissue transglutaminase antibodies have, however, been reported in chronic liver disease [201], and celiac disease has been clearly linked to PBC and autoimmune hepatitis [202,203].

Several studies performed prior to the identification of HCV addressed the issue of evaluating asymptomatic patients with moderate elevations in serum aminotransferase levels [204,205]. Apart from determinations of ferritin, ceruloplasmin, α_1-antitrypsin, and markers for HBV, blood tests had little discriminative value. A high incidence of obesity and regular alcohol use was demonstrated in these patients. Fatty infiltration, consequently, was the most common finding on liver biopsy; however, histological findings of chronic persistent or active hepatitis in 20% of patients in one study [204] lent support for the use of percutaneous liver biopsy in the diagnostic approach to patients with persistently elevated levels of serum aminotransferases. Furthermore, examination of a select population of individuals with unexplained chronic serum ALT elevations, in whom viral, alcohol-related, or drug-related disease was excluded, demonstrated histological features of chronic active hepatitis, including cirrhosis, in more than two-thirds of patients [206]. Steatohepatitis was the most frequent alternative diagnosis, with clinical and laboratory findings, including seropositivity for ANAs, indistinguishable from those of patients with chronic active hepatitis [206].

Nonalcoholic steatohepatitis (NASH), as described in these studies, is part of the spectrum of nonalcoholic fatty liver disease (NAFLD), which ranges from asymptomatic steatosis to cryptogenic cirrhosis. It is well established that NAFLD is the most common cause of abnormal serum aminotransferases; estimated prevalence rates up to 33% and 5% have been reported for NAFLD and NASH, respectively [207–209]. NAFLD is frequently associated with the metabolic syndrome consisting of obesity, diabetes, hypertension, and hyperlipidemia. The diagnosis of NAFLD is made in the appropriate clinical context after other forms of liver disease have been excluded. Confirmation of NASH relies on the presence of macrovesicular steatosis and parenchymal inflammation with or without Mallory bodies, fibrosis, and cirrhosis in liver biopsy specimens in the absence of a history of excessive alcohol consumption [210,211]. However, the role of liver biopsy in patients with suspected NAFLD is controversial, and may be best reserved for those patients with clinical features (BMI > 30, type 2 diabetes mellitus, age > 45, and an AST/ALT ratio > 1) suggestive of a higher risk for NASH [211]. Serum aminotransferases are the most common biochemical abnormalities in this disorder, although there is a lack of association between biochemical abnormalities and the degree of steatosis. In general, serum aminotransferase levels are only mildly to moderately increased; fewer than one-third of patients have serum AST or ALT levels greater than threefold elevated [210]. In contrast to patients with alcoholic liver disease, patients with NASH usually have an AST/ALT ratio less than 1 [212], and an AST/ALT ratio greater than 1 is a significant predictor of severe liver fibrosis or cirrhosis [212,213]. Serum albumin levels are normal; hyperbilirubinemia is unusual and, when present, levels of bilirubin are less than 2 mg/dL [210]. Increased transferrin saturation and serum ferritin levels have been described but most likely result from underlying necroinflammatory activity [210]. Although the determination method is not widely available, the ratio of desialylated transferrin to total transferrin, if normal, helps distinguish patients with NASH from patients with excessive alcohol ingestion [214]. A model using mean corpuscular volume, AST/ALT ratio, BMI, and gender also accurately differentiates alcoholic liver disease

from NAFLD [215]. Weight reduction and regular exercise in patients with NAFLD may lead to improvement in serum aminotransferase abnormalities [216].

The role of liver biopsy is not well established in asymptomatic patients with chronic liver chemistry abnormalities in whom specific liver disorders have been excluded by serological evaluation. Although a liver biopsy may establish a diagnosis, frequently NASH, the results of the liver biopsy are infrequently different from the presumptive pre-biopsy diagnosis, and no proven therapy is available for the majority of these patients [217,218]. Therefore, the decision to perform a liver biopsy under these circumstances needs to be individualized, taking into account the risks and benefits of this procedure. Effective therapy may soon become available for NASH [211], but until that time, liver biopsy is unlikely to have a significant impact on patient management.

Patients who have undergone liver transplantation are frequently evaluated for abnormal liver chemistries. The differential diagnosis is extensive and includes acute cellular rejection, hepatic artery thrombosis, infectious complications such as cytomegalovirus and opportunistic infections, drug-induced hepatotoxicity (e.g., cyclosporine [ciclosporin]-induced cholestasis), and biliary complications. Abnormal liver chemistries in the posttransplant patient may also herald recurrence of their primary liver disease. For example, autoimmune hepatitis may recur in up to 33% of patients who undergo liver transplantation for chronic disease [219]. Liver biopsy and Doppler ultrasonography are frequently required because a specific pattern of biochemical changes corresponding to a particular diagnosis cannot usually be identified [220].

The extent of hepatic dysfunction in any form of injury is routinely assessed by the prothrombin time and serum albumin concentration. Prolongation of the prothrombin time without improvement after parenteral vitamin K administration and a serum albumin concentration lower than 3 g/dL both reflect a worse prognosis and greater severity of underlying liver disease. The prothrombin time is a component of both the Model for End-stage Liver Disease (MELD) score ($9.57 \times \log_e$ [creatinine mg/dL] + $3.78 \times \log_e$ [bilirubin mg/dL] + $11.20 \times \log_e$ [INR] + 6.43) and the Maddrey discriminant function [$4.6 \times$ (prothrombin time [PT] in seconds − control PT) + serum bilirubin in mg/dL], used to predict prognosis, particularly in alcoholic hepatitis [221].

In conclusion, the diagnostic tests discussed in this chapter suggest but rarely provide a specific diagnosis in a patient with suspected liver disease. Nevertheless, information obtained from these tests should facilitate the efficient and proper use of other noninvasive and invasive tests such as ultrasonography, computed tomography, radionuclide hepatobiliary scanning, PTC, ERCP, liver biopsy, and laparoscopy.

References

1. Pauker SG, Eckman MH. Principles of diagnostic testing. In: Kelley WN (ed.). Textbook of internal medicine. Philadelphia: J.B. Lippincott, 1989:16.
2. Lelbach WK. Cirrhosis in the alcoholic and its relation to the volume of alcohol abuse. Ann NY Acad Sci 1975;252:85.
3. Saunders JB, Davis M, Williams R. Do women develop alcoholic liver disease more readily than men? Br Med J 1981;282:1140.
4. Zimmerman HJ, Maddrey WC. Acetaminophen (paracetamol) hepatotoxicity with regular intake of alcohol: analysis of instances of therapeutic misadventure. Hepatology 1995;22:767.
5. Zimmerman HJ. Effects of aspirin and acetaminophen on the liver. Arch Intern Med 1981;141:333.
6. Leo MA, Lieber CS. Hypervitaminosis A: a liver lover's lament. Hepatology 1988;8:412.
7. Stickel F, Patsenker E, Schuppan D. Herbal hepatotoxicity. J Hepatol 2005;43:901.
8. Corey L, Holmes KK. Sexual transmission of hepatitis A in homosexual men: incidence and mechanism. N Engl J Med 1980;302:435.
9. Hadler SC, Webster HM, Erben JJ, et al. Hepatitis A in day-care centers: a community-wide assessment. N Engl J Med 1980;302:1222.
10. Goodman RA. Nosocomial hepatitis A. Ann Intern Med 1985;103:452.
11. Farci P. Delta hepatitis: an update. J Hepatol 2003;39:S212.
12. Wong W, Terrault N. Update on chronic hepatitis C. Clin Gastroenterol Hepatol 2005;3:507.
13. Allander T, Gruber A, Naghavi M, et al. Frequent patient-to-patient transmission of hepatits C virus in a haematology ward. Lancet 1995;345:603.
14. Inman RD. Rheumatic manifestations of hepatitis B virus infection. Semin Arthritis Rheum 1982;11:406.
15. Dykhuizen RS, Brunt PW, Atkinson P, et al. Ecstasy-induced hepatitis mimicking viral hepatitis. Gut 1995;36.939.
16. Steven MM, Buckley JD, MacKay IR. Pregnancy in chronic active hepatitis. Q J Med 1979;48:519.
17. Zimmerman HJ, Lewis JH. Chemical- and toxin-induced hepatotoxicity. Gastroenterol Clin North Am. 1995;24:1027.
18. Ware AJ. The liver when the heart fails. Gastroenterology 1978;74:627.
19. Rex DK, Rogers DW, Mohammed Y, Williams ES. Post-cardiac surgery tamponade mimicking acute hepatitis. J Clin Gastroenterol 1992;14:136.
20. Skinner C, Denmure ACF. Hemochromatosis presenting as congestive cardiomyopathy associated with hemochromatosis. N Engl J Med 1972;287:866.
21. Petrozza JA, Dutta SK, Latham PS, et al. Prevalence and natural history of distal common bile duct stenosis in alcoholic pancreatitis. Dig Dis Sci 1984;29:890.
22. Gaskin KJ, Waters DLM, Howman-Giles R, et al. Liver disease and common-bile-duct stenosis in cystic fibrosis. N Engl J Med 1988;318:340.
23. Danzi JT. Extraintestinal manifestations of idiopathic inflammatory bowel disease. Arch Intern Med 1988;148:297.
24. Franson TR, Hierholzer WJ, LaBrecque DR. Frequency and characteristics of hyperbilirubinemia associated with bacteremia. Rev Infect Dis 1985;7:1.
25. Franson TR, LaBrecque DR, Buggy BP, et al. Serial bilirubin determinations as a prognostic marker in clinical infections. Am J Med Sci 1989;297:149.
26. Strickland RC, Schenker S. The nephrogenic hepatic dysfunction syndrome: a review. Dig Dis 1977;22:49.
27. Steven MM. Pregnancy and liver disease. Gut 1981;22:592.
28. Agnello V, De Rosa FG. Extrahepatic disease manifestations of HCV infection: some current issues. J Hepatol 2004;40:341.
29. Bardella MT, Vecchi M, Conte D, et al. Chronic unexplained hypertransaminasemia may be caused by occult celiac disease. Hepatology 1999;29:654.
30. Fong T-L, McHutchison JG, Reynolds TB. Hyperthyroidism and hepatic dysfunction. J Clin Gastroenterology 1992;14:240.
31. Babb RR. Associations between diseases of the thyroid and the liver. Am J Gastroenterol 1984;79:421.
32. Boulton R, Hamilton MI, Dhillon AP, et al. Subclinical Addison's disease: a cause of persistent abnormalities in transaminase values. Gastroenterology 1995;109:1324.
33. Lewis JH, Zimmerman HJ, Ishak KG, et al. Enflurane hepatotoxicity: a clinicopathologic study of 24 cases. Ann Intern Med 1983;98:984.
34. Hocking MP, Duerson MC, O'Leary JP, et al. Jejunoileal bypass for morbid obesity: late follow-up in 100 cases. N Engl J Med 1983;308:995.
35. Freedman MR, Holzbach RT, Ferguson DR. Pruritus in cholestasis: no direct causative role for bile acid retention. Am J Med 1981;70:1011.
36. Angeli P, Albino G, Carraro P, et al. Cirrhosis and muscle cramps: evidence of a causal relationship. Hepatology 1996;23:264.
37. Espinoza P, Ducot B, Pelletier G, et al. Interobserver agreement in the physical diagnosis of alcoholic liver disease. Dig Dis Sci 1987;32:244.
38. Attali P, Ink O, Pelletier G, et al. Dupuytren's contracture, alcohol consumption, and chronic liver disease. Arch Intern Med 1987;147:1065.
39. Lumeng L, O'Connor KW. Differential diagnosis of jaundice. In: Ostrow JD (ed.). Bilirubin, bile pigments and jaundice. New York: Marcel Dekker, 1986:475.
40. Nicholas GG, Williams E. Friction rub in acute cholecystitis: an unusual finding. JAMA 1971;218:1945.
41. Frommer D, Morris J, Sherlock S, et al. Kayser-Fleischer-like rings in patients without Wilson's disease. Gastroenterology 1977;72:1331.
42. Tiribelli C, Ostrow JD. New concepts in bilirubin chemistry, transport and metabolism. Hepatology 1993;17:715.
43. Weiss JS, Gautam A, Lauff JJ, et al. The clinical importance of a protein-bound fraction of serum bilirubin in patients with hyperbilirubinemia. N Engl J Med 1983;309:147.
44. Ferraris R, Colombatti G, Fiorentini MT, et al. Diagnostic value of serum bile acids and routine liver function tests in hepatobiliary diseases: sensitivity, specificity, and predictive value. Dig Dis Sci 1983;28:129.
45. Vierling JM, Berk PD, Hofmann A, et al. Normal fasting-state levels of serum cholyl-conjugated bile acids in Gilbert's syndrome: an aid to the diagnosis. Hepatology 1982;2:340.
46. Festi D, Labate AMM, Roda A, et al. Diagnostic effectiveness of serum bile acids in liver diseases as evaluated by multivariate statistical methods. Hepatology 1983;3:707.
47. Ohkubo H, Okuda K, Iida S, et al. Role of portal and splenic vein shunts and impaired hepatic extraction in the elevated serum bile acids in liver cirrhosis. Gastroenterology 1984;86:514.
48. Mannes GA, Thieme C, Stellaard F, et al. Prognostic significance of serum bile acids in cirrhosis. Hepatology 1986;6:50.
49. Setchell KDR, Harrison DL, Gilbert JM, et al. Serum unconjugated bile acids: qualitative and quantitative profiles in ileal resection and bacterial overgrowth. Clin Chim Acta 1985;152:297.
50. Tabibian N, Reynolds TB. Serum bile acid determination for assessing patency portosystemic shunts: lack of value. Arch Intern Med 1987;147:911.
51. Wolpert E, Pascasio FM, Wolkoff AW, et al. Abnormal sulfobromophthalein metabolism in Rotor's syndrome and obligate heterozygotes. N Engl J Med 1977;296:1099.
52. Stolz A, Kaplowitz N. Biochemical tests for liver disease. In: Zakim D, Boyer TD (eds). Hepatology: a textbook of liver disease. Philadelphia: W.B. Saunders, 1990:637.
53. Groszmann RJ. The measurement of liver blood flow using clearance techniques. Hepatology 1983;3:1039.

54. Friedman PA. Vitamin K-dependent proteins. N Engl J Med 1984; 310:1458.

55. Lord JW, Andrus WW. Differentiation of intrahepatic and extrahepatic jaundice: response of the plasma prothrombin to intramuscular injection of menadione (2-methyl-1,4-naphthaquinone) as a diagnostic aid. Arch Intern Med 1941;68:199.

56. Clark R, Rake MO, Flute PT, et al. Coagulation abnormalities in acute liver failure: pathogenetic and therapeutic implications. Scand J Gastroenterol 1973;8:63.

57. Christensen E, Schlichting P, Andersen PK, et al. Updating prognosis and therapeutic effect evaluation in cirrhosis with Cox's multiple regression model for time-dependent variables. Scand J Gastroenterol 1986;21:163.

58. Kelly DA, Summerfield JA. Hemostasis in liver disease. Semin Liver Dis 1987;7:182.

59. Gralnick HR, Givelber H, Abrams E. Dysfibrinogenemia associated with hepatoma: increased carbohydrate content of the fibrinogen molecule. N Engl J Med 1978;299:221.

60. Rothschild MA, Oratz M, Schreiber SS. Alcohol, amino acids, and albumin synthesis. Gastroenterology 1974;67:1200.

61. Bacq Y, Zarka O, Brechot J-F, et al. Liver function tests in normal pregnancy: a prospective study of 103 pregnant women and 103 matched controls. Hepatology 1996;23:1030.

62. Hutchinson DR, Smith MG, Parke DV. Prealbumin as an index of liver function after acute paracetamol poisoning. Lancet 1980;2:121.

63. Lee WM, Lebwohl O, Chien S. Hyperviscosity syndrome attributable to hyperglobulinemia in chronic active hepatitis. Gastroenterology 1978;74:918.

64. Feizi T. Immunoglobulins in chronic liver disease. Gut 1968;9:193.

65. Harry DS, Day RC, Owen JS, et al. Plasma lecithin: cholesterol acyltransferase activity and the lipoprotein abnormalities of liver disease. Scand J Clin Lab Invest Suppl 1978;150:223.

66. Muller PR, Fellin R, Lambrecht J, et al. Hypertriglyceridemia secondary to liver disease. Eur J Clin Invest 1974;4:419.

67. D'Arienzo A, Manguso F, Scaglione G, et al. Prognostic value of progressive decrease in serum cholesterol in predicting survival in Child-Pugh C viral cirrhosis. Scand J Gastroenterol 1998;33:1213.

68. Seidel D, Alaupovic P, Furman RH. A lipoprotein characterizing obstructive jaundice. I. Method for quantitative separation and identification of lipoproteins in jaundiced subjects. J Clin Invest 1969;48:1211.

69. Elferink RP, Ottenhoff R, van Marle J, et al. Class III P-glycoproteins mediate the formation of lipoprotein X in the mouse. J Clin Invest 1998;102:1749.

70. Branch RA, Herbert CM, Read AE. Determinants of serum antipyrine half-lives in patients with liver disease. Gut 1973;14:569.

71. Hepner GW, Vesell EJ. Quantitative assessment of hepatic function by breath analysis after oral administration of [^{14}C]aminopyrine. Ann Intern Med 1975;83:632.

72. Schneider JF, Baker AL, Haines NW, et al. Aminopyrine N-demethylation: a prognostic test of liver function in patients with alcoholic liver disease. Gastroenterology 1980;79:1145.

73. Ballmer PE, Reichen J, McNurlan MA, et al. Albumin but not fibrinogen synthesis correlates with galactose elimination capacity in patients with cirrhosis of the liver. Hepatology 1996;24:53.

74. Jacqz E, Hall SD, Branch RA. Genetically determined polymorphisms in drug oxidation. Hepatology 1986;6:1020.

75. Watkins PB, Murray SA, Winkelman LG, et al. Erythromycin breath test as an assay of glucocorticoid-inducible liver cytochromes P-450: studies in rats and patients. J Clin Invest 1989;83:688.

76. Olomu AB, Vickers CR, Waring RH, et al. High incidence of poor sulfoxidation in patients with primary biliary cirrhosis. N Engl J Med 1988;318:1089.

77. Morino Y, Kagamiyama H, Wada H. Immunochemical distinction between glutamic-oxaloacetic transaminase from the soluble and mitochondrial fractions of mammalian tissues. J Biol Chem 1964; 239:943.

78. Boyde TRC, Latner AL. Starch gel electrophoresis of transaminase in human tissue extracts and serum. Biochem J 1961;82:52.

79. Piton A, Poynard T, Imbert-Bismut F, et al. Factors associated with serum alanine transaminase activity in healthy subjects: consequences for the definition of normal values, for selection of blood donors, and for patients with chronic hepatitis C. Hepatology 1998;27:1213.

80. Elinav E, Ben-Dov IZ, Ackerman E, et al. Correlation between serum alanine aminotransferase activity and age: an inverted U curve pattern. Am J Gastroenterol 2005;100:2201.

81. Ruhl CE, Everhart JE. Coffee and caffeine consumption reduce the risk of elevated serum alanine aminotransferase activity in the United States. Gastroenterology 2005;128:24.

82. Prati D, Taioli E, Zanella A, et al. Updated definitions of healthy ranges for serum alanine aminotransferase levels. Ann Intern Med 2002;137:1.

83. Kim HC, Nam CM, Jee SH, et al. Normal serum aminotransferase concentration and risk of mortality from liver diseases: prospective cohort study. BMJ 2004. doi:10.1136/bmj.38050.593634.63.

84. Reichling JJ, Kaplan MM. Clinical use of serum enzymes in liver disease. Dig Dis Sci 1988;33:1601.

85. Morton BD, Statland BE. Serum enzyme alterations in polymyositis: possible pitfalls in diagnosis. Am J Clin Pathol 1980;73:556.

86. Nathwani RA, Pais S, Reynolds TB, Kaplowitz N. Serum alanine aminotransferase in skeletal muscle diseases. Hepatology 2005;41:380.

87. Cohen JA, Kaplan MM. The SGOT/SGPT ratio – an indicator of alcoholic liver disease. Dig Dis Sci 1979;24:835.

88. Williams AL, Hoofnagle JH. Ratio of serum aspartate to alanine aminotransferase in chronic hepatitis: relationship to cirrhosis. Gastroenterology 1988;95:734.

89. Matloff DS, Selinger MJ, Kaplan MM. Hepatic transaminase activity in alcoholic liver disease. Gastroenterology 1980;78:1389.

90. Diehl AM, Potter J, Boitnott J, et al. Relationship between pyridoxal 5' phosphate deficiency and aminotransferase levels in alcoholic hepatitis. Gastroenterology 1984;86:632.

91. Kamimoto Y, Horiuchi S, Tanase S, et al. Plasma clearance of intravenously injected aspartate aminotransferase isozymes: evidence for preferential uptake by sinusoidal liver cells. Hepatology 1985;5:367.

92. Yasuda K, Okuda K, Endo N, et al. Hypoaminotransferasemia in patients undergoing long-term hemodialysis: clinical and biochemical appraisal. Gastroenterology 1995;109:1295.

93. Litin SC, O'Brien JF, Pruett S, et al. Macroenzyme as a cause of unexplained elevation of aspartate aminotransferase. Mayo Clin Proc 1987;62:681.

94. Nalpas B, Vassault A, Charpin S, et al. Serum mitochondrial aspartate aminotransferase as a marker of chronic alcoholism: diagnostic value and interpretation in a liver unit. Hepatology 1986;6:608.

95. Menon KVN, Gores GJ, Shah VH. Pathogenesis, diagnosis, and treatment of alcoholic liver disease. Mayo Clin Proc 2001;76:1021.

96. Van Waes L, Lieber CS. Glutamate dehydrogenase: a reliable marker of liver cell necrosis in the alcoholic. Br Med J 1977;2:1508.

97. Jenkins WJ, Rosalki SB, Foo Y, et al. Serum glutamate dehydrogenase is not a reliable marker of liver cell necrosis in alcoholics. J Clin Pathol 1982;35:207.

98. Blitzer BL, Boyer JL. Cytochemical localization of Na$^+$,K$^+$-ATPase in the rat hepatocyte. J Clin Invest 1978;62:1104.

99. Seetharam S, Sussman NL, Komoda T, et al. The mechanism of elevated alkaline phosphatase activity after bile duct ligation in the rat. Hepatology 1986;6:374.

100. Kaplan MM. Serum alkaline phosphatase – another piece is added to the puzzle. Hepatology 1986;6:526.

101. Robinson JC, Goldsmith LA. Genetically determined variants of serum alkaline phosphatase: a review. Vox Sang 1967;13:289.

102. Shaver WA, Bhatt H, Combes B. Low serum alkaline phosphatase activity in Wilson's disease. Hepatology 1986;6:859.

103. Wilson JW. Inherited elevation of alkaline phosphatase activity in the absence of disease. N Engl J Med 1979;301:983.

104. Stolbach LL, Krant MJ, Fishman WH. Ectopic production of an alkaline phosphatase isoenzyme in patients with cancer. N Engl J Med 1969;281:757.

105. Brensilver HL, Kaplan MM. Significance of elevated liver alkaline phosphatase in serum. Gastroenterology 1975;68:1556.

106. Kaplan MM, Rogers L. Separation of human serum alkaline phosphatase isoenzymes by polyacrylamide gel electrophoresis. Lancet 1969;2:1029.

107. Kristensson H, Trell E, Eriksson S, et al. Serum gamma-glutamyltransferase in alcoholism. Lancet 1977;1:609.

108. Bressler R, Forsyth BR. Serum leucine aminopeptidase activity in normal pregnancy and in patients with hydatidiform mole. N Engl J Med 1959;261:746.

109. Kim NK, Yasmineh WG, Freier EF, et al. Value of alkaline phosphatase, 5'-nucleotidase, γ-glutamyltransferase and glutamate dehydrogenase activity measurements (single and combined) in serum in diagnosis of metastasis to the liver. Clin Chem 1977;23:2034.

110. Connell MD, Dinwoodie AJ. Diagnostic use of serum alkaline phosphatase isoenzymes and 5'-nucleotidase. Clin Chim Acta 1970;30:235.

111. Cassidy WM, Reynolds TB. Serum lactic dehydrogenase in the differential diagnosis of acute hepatocellular injury. J Clin Gastroenterol 1994;19:118.

112. Kao HW, Aschcavai M, Redeker AG. The persistence of hepatitis A IgM antibody after acute clinical hepatitis A. Hepatology 1984;4:933.

113. Brechot C, Degos F, Lugassy C, et al. Hepatitis B virus DNA in patients with chronic liver disease and negative tests for hepatitis B surface antigen. N Engl J Med 1985;312:270.

114. Lemon SM, Gates NL, Simms TE, et al. IgM antibody to hepatitis B core antigen as a diagnostic parameter of acute infection with hepatitis B virus. J Infect Dis 1981;143:803.

115. Banninger P, Altorfer J, Frosner GG, et al. Prevalence and significance of anti-HBc IgM (radioimmunoassay) in acute and chronic hepatitis B and in blood donors. Hepatology 1983;3:337.

116. Paterlini P, Gerken G, Nakajima E, et al. Polymerase chain reaction to detect hepatitis B virus DNA and RNA sequences in primary liver cancers from patients negative for hepatitis B surface antigen. N Engl J Med 1990;323:80.

117. Lee WM. Hepatitis B virus infection. N Engl J Med 1997;337:1733.

118. Torbenson M, Thomas DL. Occult hepatitis B. Lancet Infect Dis 2002;2:479.

119. Alberti A, Clumeck N, Collins S. Short statement of the first European Consensus Conference on the treatment of chronic hepatitis B and C in HIV co-infected patients. J Hepatol 2005;42:615.

120. Keeffe EB, Dieterich DT, Han ST, et al. A treatment algorithm for the management of chronic hepatitis B virus infection in the United States. Clin Gastroenterol Hepatol 2004;2:87.

121. Chapko MK, Sloan KL, Davison JW, et al. Cost effectiveness of testing strategies for chronic hepatitis C. Am J Gastroenterol 2005;100:607.

122. Poynard T, Yuen MF, Ratziu V, Lai CL. Viral hepatitis C. Lancet 2003;362:2095.

123. Emerson SU, Purcell RH. Hepatitis E virus. Rev Med Virol 2003;13:145.

124. Hinedi TB, Koff RS. Cholestatic hepatitis induced by Epstein-Barr virus infection in an adult. Dig Dis Sci 2003;48:539.

125. Peters DJ, Greene WH, Ruggiero F, McGarrity TJ. Herpes simplex-induced fulminant hepatitis in adults: a call for empiric therapy. Dig Dis Sci 2000;45:2399.

126. Bliss SJ, Moseley RH, Del Valle J, Saint S. Clinical problem-solving: a window of opportunity. N Engl J Med 2003;349:1848.

127. Klatskin G, Kantor FS. Mitochondrial antibody in primary biliary cirrhosis and other diseases. Am Intern Med 1972;77:533.

128. Mitchison HC, Bassendine MF, Hendrick A, et al. Positive antimitochondrial antibody but normal alkaline phosphatase: is this primary biliary cirrhosis? Hepatology 1986;6:1279.

129. Surh CD, Danner DJ, Ahmed A, et al. Reactivity of primary biliary cirrhosis sera with a human fetal liver cDNA clone of branched-chain α-keto acid dehydrogenase dihydrolipoamide acyltransferase, the 52 kD mitochondrial autoantigen. Hepatology 1989;9:63.

130. Weber P, Brenner J, Stechemesser E, et al. Characterization and clinical relevance of a new complement-fixing antibody – anti-M8 – in patients with primary biliary cirrhosis. Hepatology 1986;6:553.

131. Penner E. Demonstration of immune complexes containing the ribonucleoprotein antigen Ro in primary biliary cirrhosis. Gastroenterology 1986;90:724.

132. Bernstein RM, Callender ME, Neuberger JM, et al. Anticentromere antibody in primary biliary cirrhosis. Ann Rheum Dis 1982;41:612.

133. Whittingham S, Irwin J, MacKay DR, et al. Smooth muscle autoantibody in "autoimmune" hepatitis. Gastroenterology 1966;51:499.

134. Czaja AJ, Norman GL. Autoantibodies in the diagnosis and management of liver disease. J Clin Gastroenterol 2003;37:315.

135. Manns MP, Strassburg CP. Autoimmune hepatitis: clinical challenges. Gastroenterology 2001;120:1502.

136. Bansi D, Chapman R, Fleming K. Antineutrophil cytoplasmic antibodies in chronic liver diseases: prevalence, titre, specificity and IgG subclass. J Hepatol 1996;24:581.

137. Krawitt EL. Autoimmune hepatitis. N Engl J Med 2006;354:54.

138. Kaplan MM. Primary biliary cirrhosis. N Engl J Med 1987;316:521.

139. Scott J, Gollan JL, Samourian S, et al. Wilson's disease, presenting as chronic active hepatitis. Gastroenterology 1978;74:645.

140. Scheinberg IH, Sternlieb I. Wilson's disease. Philadelphia: W.B. Saunders, 1984.

141. McCullough AJ, Fleming CR, Thistle JL, et al. Diagnosis of Wilson's disease presenting as fulminant hepatic failure. Gastroenterology 1983;84:161.

142. Spechler SJ, Koff RS. Wilson's disease: diagnostic difficulties in the patient with chronic hepatitis and hypoceruloplasminemia. Gastroenterology 1980;78:803.

143. Edwards CQ, Williams DM, Cartwright GE. Hereditary hypoceruloplasminemia. Clin Gen 1979;15:311.

144. Nittis T, Gitlin JD. The copper-iron connection: hereditary aceruloplasminemia. Semin Hematol 2002;39:282.

145. Stremmel W, Meyerrose KW, Niederau C, et al. Wilson disease: clinical presentation, treatment, and survival. Ann Intern Med 1991;115:720.

146. Schilsky ML, Sternlieb I. Overcoming obstacles to the diagnosis of Wilson's disease. Gastroenterology 1997;113:350.

147. Loudianos G, Gitlin JD. Wilson's disease. Sem Liver Dis 2000;20:353.

148. Maier-Dobersberger T, Mannhalter C, Rack S, et al. Diagnosis of Wilson's disease in an asymptomatic sibling by DNA linkage analysis. Gastroenterology 1995;109:2015.

149. Vidaud D, Assouline B, Lecoz P, et al. Misdiagnosis revealed by genetic linkage analysis in a family with Wilson disease. Neurology 1996;46:1485.

150. McLaren CE, McLachlan GJ, Halliday JW, et al. Distribution of transferrin saturation in an Australian population: relevance to the early diagnosis of hemochromatosis. Gastroenterology 1998;114:543.

151. Brissot P, Bourel M, Herry D, et al. Assessment of liver iron content in 271 patients: a reevaluation of direct and indirect methods. Gastroenterology 1981;80:557.

152. Turnberg LA. Iron absorption in acute hepatitis. Am J Dig Dis 1966;11:20.

153. Bacon BR, Brown KE. Iron metabolism and disorders of iron overload. In: Kaplowitz N (ed.). Liver and biliary diseases, 2nd edn. Baltimore: Williams & Wilkins, 1996.

154. Powell LW, Halliday JW, Cowlishaw JL. Relationship between serum ferritin and total body iron stores in idiopathic hemochromatosis. Gut 1978;19:583.

155. Halliday JW, Russo AM, Cowlishaw JL, et al. Serum ferritin in the diagnosis of hemochromatosis. Lancet 1977;2:621.

156. Chapman RW, Hussain MAM, Gorman A, et al. Effect of ascorbic acid deficiency on serum ferritin concentration in patients with β-thalassaemia major and iron overload. J Clin Pathol 1982;35:487.

157. Wands JR, Rowe JA, Mezey SE, et al. Normal serum ferritin concentrations in precirrhotic hemochromatosis. N Engl J Med 1976;294:302.

158. Prieto J, Barry M, Sherlock S. Serum ferritin in patients with iron overload and with acute and chronic liver diseases. Gastroenterology 1975;68:525.

159. Di Bisceglie AM, Axiotis CA, Hoofnagle JH, Bacon BR. Measurements of iron status in patients with chronic hepatitis. Gastroenterology 1992;102:2108.

160. Zimmerman HJ. Function and integrity of the liver. In: Henry JB (ed.). Clinical diagnosis and management by laboratory methods. Philadelphia: W.B. Saunders, 1984.

161. Bulaj ZJ, Griffen LM, Jorde LB, et al. Clinical and biochemical abnormalities in people heterozygous for hemochromatosis. N Engl J Med 1996;335:1799.

162. Summers KM, Halliday JW, Powell LW. Identification of homozygous hemochromatosis subjects by measurement of hepatic iron index. Hepatology 1990;12:20.

163. Feder JN, Gnirke A, Thomas W, et al. A novel MHC class I-like gene is mutated in patients with hereditary haemochromatosis. Nature Genetics 1996;13:399.

164. Morrison ED, Brandhagen DJ, Phatak PD, et al. Serum ferritin level predicts advanced hepatic fibrosis among U.S. patients with phenotypic hemochromatosis. Ann Intern Med 2003;138:627.

165. St Pierre TG, Clark PR, Chua-anusorn W, et al. Noninvasive measurement and imaging of liver iron concentrations using proton magnetic resonance. Blood 2005;105:855.

166. Pietrangelo A. Hereditary hemochromatosis – a new look at an old disease. N Engl J Med 2004;350:2383.

167. Bloomer JR, Waldmann TA, McIntre KR, et al. α-Fetoprotein in nonneoplastic hepatic disorders. JAMA 1975;233:38.

168. Di Bisceglie AM, Sterling RK, Chung RT, et al. Serum alpha-fetoprotein levels in patients with advanced hepatitis C: results from the HALT-C trial. J Hepatology 2005;43:434.

169. Chen D-S, Sung J-L. Serum alphafetoprotein in hepatocellular carcinoma. Cancer 1977;40:779.

170. Bellet DH, Wands JR, Isselbacher KJ, et al. Serum α-fetoprotein levels in human disease: perspective from a highly specific monoclonal radioimmunoassay. Proc Natl Acad Sci U S A 1984;81:3869.

171. Weitz IC, Liebman HA. Des-γ-carboxy (abnormal) prothrombin and hepatocellular carcinoma: a critical review. Hepatology 1993;18:990.

172. Perlmutter DH, Cole FS, Kilbridge P, et al. Expression of the α$_1$-proteinase inhibitor gene in human monocytes and macrophages. Proc Natl Acad Sci USA 1985;82:795.

173. Darlington GJ, Astrin KH, Muirhead SP, et al. Assignment of human α$_1$-antitrypsin to chromosome 14 by somatic cell hybrid analysis. Proc Natl Acad Sci U S A 1982;79:870.

174. Berg NO, Eriksson S. Liver disease in adults with alpha$_1$-antitrypsin deficiency. N Engl J Med 1972;287:1264.

175. Erikkson S, Carlson J, Velez R. Risk of cirrhosis and primary liver cancer in alpha$_1$-antitrypsin deficiency. N Engl J Med 1986;314:736.

176. Brantly M, Nukiwa T, Crystal RG. Molecular basis of alpha$_1$-antitrypsin deficiency. Am J Med 1988;84:13.

177. Black M. Hepatic detoxification of endogenously produced toxins and their importance for the pathogenesis of hepatic encephalopathy. In: Zakim D, Boyer TD (eds). Hepatology: a textbook of liver disease. Philadelphia: W.B. Saunders, 1982:397.

178. Fraser CL, Arieff AI. Hepatic encephalopathy. N Engl J Med 1985;313:865.

179. Drayna CJ, Titcomb CP, Varma RR, et al. Hyperammonemic encephalopathy caused by infection in a neurogenic bladder. N Engl J Med 1981;304:766.

180. Clemmesen JO, Larsen FS, Kondrup J, et al. Cerebral herniation in patients with acute liver failure is correlated with arterial ammonia concentration. Hepatology 1999;29:648.

181. McCullough AJ, Czaja AJ, Jones JD, et al. The nature and prognostic significance of serial amino acid determinations in severe chronic active liver disease. Gastroenterology 1981;81:645.

182. Mitchell DP, Hanes TE, Hoyumpa AM, et al. Fever of unknown origin: assessment of the value of percutaneous liver biopsy. Arch Intern Med 1977;137:1001.

183. Bravo AA, Sheth SG, Chopra S. Liver biopsy. N Engl J Med 2001;344:495.

184. Kundrotas LW, Clement DJ. Serum alanine aminotransferase (ALT) elevation in asymptomatic US Air Force basic trainee blood donors. Dig Dis Sci 1993;38:2145.

185. Schiff L. Jaundice: a clinical approach. In: Schiff L, Schiff ER (eds). Diseases of the liver, 6th edn. Philadelphia: J.B. Lippincott, 1987:209.

186. Nathwani RA, Kumar RA, Reynolds TB, Kaplowitz N. Marked elevation in serum transaminases: an atypical presentation of choledocholithiasis. Am J Gastroenterol 2005;100:295.

187. Brown AN, Sheiner LB, Cohen SN. Evaluation of bilirubin in a liver screening panel. JAMA 1992;268:1542.

188. Balasubramaniam K, Wiesner RH, LaRusso NF. Primary sclerosing cholangitis with normal serum alkaline phosphatase activity. Gastroenterology 1988;95:1395.

189. Ros E, Navarro S, Bru C, et al. Occult microlithiasis in "idiopathic" acute pancreatitis: prevention of relapses by cholecystectomy or ursodeoxycholic acid therapy. Gastroenterology 1991;101:1701.

190. Scharschmidt BF, Goldberg HI, Schmid R. Approach to the patient with cholestatic jaundice. N Engl J Med 1983;308:1515.

191. Gitlin N, Serio KM. Ischemic hepatitis: widening horizons. Am J Gastroenterol 1992;87:831.

192. Himmelstein DU, Woolhandler SJ, Adler RD. Elevated SGOT/SGPT ratio in alcoholic patients with acetaminophen hepatoxicity. Am J Gastroenterol 1984;79:718.

193. El-Newihi HM, Alamy ME, Reynolds TB. Salmonella hepatitis: analysis of 27 cases and comparison with acute viral hepatitis. Hepatology 1996;24:516.

194. Ala A, Borjigin J, Rochwager A, Schilsky M. Wilson disease in septuagenarian siblings: raising the bar for diagnosis. Hepatology 2005;41:668.

195. Sallie R, Katsiyiannakis L, Baldwin D, et al. Failure of simple biochemical indexes to reliably differentiate fulminant Wilson's disease from other causes of fulminant liver failure. Hepatology 1992;16:1206.

196. Katkov WN, Friedman LS, Cody H, et al. Elevated serum alanine aminotransferase levels in blood donors: the contribution of hepatitis C virus. Ann Intern Med 1991;115:882.

197. Alberti A, Morsica G, Chemello L, et al. Hepatitis C viraemia and liver disease in symptom-free individuals with anti-HCV. Lancet 1992;340:697.

198. Alvarez F, Berg PA, Bianchi FB, et al. International Autoimmune Hepatitis Group Report: review of criteria for diagnosis of autoimmune hepatitis. J Hepatol 1999;31:929.

199. Green PH, Jabri B. Celiac disease. Annu Rev Med 2006;57:207.

200. Lo Iacono O, Petta S, Venezia G, et al. Anti-tissue transglutaminase antibodies in patients with abnormal liver tests: is it always coeliac disease? Am J Gastroenterol 2005;100:2472.

201. Vecchi M, Folli C, Donato MF, et al. High rate of positive anti-tissue transglutaminase antibodies in chronic liver disease: role of liver decompensation and of the antigen source. Scand J Gastroenterol 2003;38:50.

202. Villalta D, Girolami D, Bidoli E, et al. High prevalence of celiac disease in autoimmune hepatitis detected by anti-tissue tranglutaminase autoantibodies. J Clin Lab Anal 2005;19:6.

203. Stevens FM, McLoughlin RM. Is coeliac disease a potentially treatable cause of liver failure? Eur J Gastroenterol Hepatol 2005;17:1015.

204. Hultcrantz R, Glaumann H, Lindberg G, et al. Liver investigation in 149 asymptomatic patients with moderately elevated activites of serum aminotransferases. Scand J Gastroenterol 1986;21:109.

205. Friedman LS, Dienstag JL, Watkins E, et al. Evaluation of blood donors with elevated serum alanine aminotransferase levels. Ann Intern Med 1987;107:137.

206. Hay JE, Czaja AJ, Rakela J, et al. The nature of unexplained chronic aminotransferase elevations of a mild to moderate degree in asymptomatic patients. Hepatology 1989;9:193.

207. Clark JM, Brancati FL, Diehl AM. The prevalence and etiology of elevated aminotransferase levels in the United States. Am J Gastroenterol 2003;98:960.

208. Browning JD, Szczepaniak LS, Dobbins R, et al. Prevalence of hepatic steatosis in an urban population in the United States: impact of ethnicity. Hepatology 2004;40:1387.

209. Pendino GM, Mariano A, Surace P, et al. Prevalence and etiology of altered liver tests: a population-based survey in a Mediterranean town. Hepatology 2005;41:1151.

210. Bacon BR, Farahvash MJ, Janney CG, et al. Nonalcoholic steatohepatitis: an expanded clinical entity. Gastroenterology 1994;107:1103.

211. Cortez-Pinto H, de Moura MC, Day CP. Non-alcoholic steatohepatitis: from cell biology to clinical practice. J Hepatol 2006;44:197.

212. Sorbi D, Boynton J, Lindor KD. The ratio of aspartate aminotransferase to alanine aminotransferase: potential value in differentiating nonalcoholic steatohepatitis from alcoholic liver disease. Am J Gastroenterol 1999;94:1018.

213. Angulo P, Keach JC, Batts KP, Lindor KD. Independent predictors of liver fibrosis in patients with nonalcoholic steatohepatitis. Hepatology 1999;30:1356.

214. Fletcher LM, Kwoh-Gain I, Powell EE, et al. Markers of chronic alcohol ingestion in patients with nonalcoholic steatohepatitis: an aid to diagnosis. Hepatology 1991;13:455.

215. Dunn W, Angulo P, Sanderson S, et al. Utility of a new model to diagnose an alcohol basis for steatohepatitis. Gastroenterology 2006;131:1057.

216. Suzuki A, Lindor K, St Saver J, et al. Effect of changes on body weight and lifestyle in nonalcoholic fatty liver disease. J Hepatol 2005;43:1060.

217. Daniel S, Ben-Menachem T, Vasudevan G, et al. Prospective evaluation of unexplained chronic liver transaminase abnormalities in asymptomatic and symptomatic patients. Am J Gastroenterology 1999;94:3010.

218. Sorbi D, McGill DB, Thistle JL, et al. An assessment of the role of liver biopsies in asymptomatic patients with chronic liver test abnormalities. Am J Gastroenterology 2000;95:3206.

219. Reich DJ, Fiel I, Guarrera JV, et al. Liver transplantation for autoimmune hepatitis. Hepatology 2000;32:693.

220. Henley KS, Lucey MR, Appelman HD, et al. Biochemical and histopathological correlation in liver transplant: the first 180 days. Hepatology 1992;16:688.

221. Dunn W, Jamil LH, Brown LS, et al. MELD accurately predicts mortality in patients with alcoholic hepatitis. Hepatology 2005;41:353.

Bilirubin, 423

Hyperbilirubinemia, 426

Approach to the patient with jaundice, 430

Diagnostic approach, 434

Complications of cholestasis, 438

Jaundice (icterus) is the yellow discoloration of skin, sclera, and mucous membranes caused by the excessive accumulation of bilirubin pigments. It is usually apparent when bilirubin levels exceed 3 mg/dL or 50 µmol/L [1]. Hyperbilirubinemia results from one or more derangements in the complex, multistep process that balances bilirubin formation with bilirubin clearance. Consequently, jaundice can indicate a disorder in bilirubin metabolism, hepatic function, or biliary disease or combinations thereof. The optimal approach to the patient with jaundice demands precise determination of the site of disordered bilirubin handling and appropriate diagnostic tests. A review of the causes and management of jaundice logically begins with a precise understanding of the structure, formation, uptake, and conjugation of bilirubin, its clearance through the liver, and its subsequent excretion into the biliary tree and gastrointestinal tract.

Cholestasis is characterized by the constellation of physiological, morphological, and clinical manifestations that result from the impairment of the bile excretory system in the liver and biliary tree [2,3]. Reduced bile flow resulting in the accumulation of conjugated bilirubin, bile salts, and cholesterol in the blood is the hallmark of cholestasis. However, an impairment of organic ion transport, decreased excretion of biliary lipids, a release of liver plasma-membrane enzymes, and a decrease in intestinal bile also occur. In patients with cholestasis, total serum bilirubin may be normal whereas serum alkaline phosphatase and bile acids are elevated [4].

Bile acids, or bile salts, are soluble, amphipathic end products of cholesterol metabolism formed in the pericentral hepatocytes and accounting for approximately 85% of the constituents of bile [5]. The primary bile acids (formed in the hepatocyte), chenodeoxycholic and cholic acids, are the most common. The secondary bile acids are formed by anaerobic bacterial dehydratase conversion of primary bile acids to lithocholic and deoxycholic acids, respectively. Primary and secondary bile acids account for 99% of the bile acids in human bile. Another bile acid, ursodeoxycholic acid, so termed after its initial isolation from bile of the polar bear, is present in trace amounts. The hydroxyl groups of bile acids are water soluble and thus hydrophilic, whereas the opposite pole is relatively hydrophobic, giving bile acids their detergent properties. The hydrophilic activity of bile salts increases as the number of hydroxyl groups increases. Thus, lithocholic acid is more hydrophobic than chenodeoxycholic acid and cholic acid, with ursodeoxycholic acid the most hydrophilic.

Bile acids are absorbed in the distal small intestine and are returned to the liver mostly protein bound and resecreted, constituting the *enterohepatic circulation*. The bile acid pool is 2–3 g in adults and cycles several times with each meal. Although bile acid synthesis averages 0.3 g/day, total bile acid secretion is 12–18 g/day. Bile acids are critical for cholesterol elimination, by conversion of cholesterol to bile acids, by stimulation of biliary cholesterol and phospholipid secretion, and by micellar solubilization of cholesterol and phospholipids within bile, ultimately facilitating fecal elimination. Bile acids also induce bile flow, and through negative feedback, they can inhibit bile and cholesterol biosynthesis. Bile is a major conduit for the elimination of other endogenous and exogenous pigments including porphyrins and urobilins, in addition to the elimination of most rare metals (copper, zinc, manganese, chromium, selenium, molybdenum, and cadmium) and organic anions [6]. In the small intestine, bile acids promote dietary lipid absorption through the formation of mixed micelles.

Principles of Clinical Gastroenterology. Edited by Tadataka Yamada, David H. Alpers, Anthony N. Kalloo, Neil Kaplowitz, Chung Owyang, and Don W. Powell. © 2008 Blackwell Publishing. ISBN 978-1-4051-69103

Bilirubin

Structure and formation

Bilirubin, a yellow tetrapyrrole pigment, is the principal end product of the degradation of the heme moiety of hemoglobin and other hemoproteins. Heme catabolism occurs largely within the reticuloendothelial cells of the liver, spleen, and bone marrow. The heme iron protoporphyrin IX ring is opened by oxidation of the α-bridge carbon by heme oxygenase, present in many cell types, particularly Kupffer cells, macrophages, hepatocytes, and renal epithelial cells. The reaction forms biliverdin, a green tetrapyrrolic pigment, and equimolar quantities of carbon monoxide, which binds to hemoglobin and is excreted through the lungs (Fig. 22.1). Biliverdin is then rapidly reduced to bilirubin by biliverdin reductase. Bilirubin IXα, derived from protoporphyrin isomer IX with cleavage at the α bridge, is the predominant bile pigment in plasma, where its concentration generally does not exceed 1 mg/dL (17 μmol/L) in healthy people [7]. Hydrogen bonds stabilize the molecule in a folded, ridge-tile conformation restricting exposure of the molecule's polar groups to aqueous solvents. These structures form the basis of bilirubin's hydrophobic behavior and slow (indirect) diazo reactivity [8]. Opening of the heme ring at non-α-carbon positions would lead to isomeric pigments that are more water-soluble and do not require conjugation for efficient excretion in bile and urine. However, although heme catabolism generates almost exclusively a single form of bilirubin, other stereoisomers are formed from this by exposure to light as the pigment circulates through peripheral tissues. Being more polar, these photoisomers do not require conjugation for excretion in bile. Their formation is clinically important in phototherapy of neonatal jaundice, in which they accelerate bilirubin elimination, but otherwise they have no known significance [8]. With the exception of bilirubin IXβ found in meconium, significant quantities of these isomers are not detectable.

Most bilirubin (80%) derives from senescent and sequestered erythrocytes [1]. The remainder is largely derived from the degradation of hepatic and renal heme, which constitutes a cytosolic pool of heme destined for incorporation into specific heme proteins including cytochrome P450, peroxidase, and catalase. One-third of the bilirubin derived from

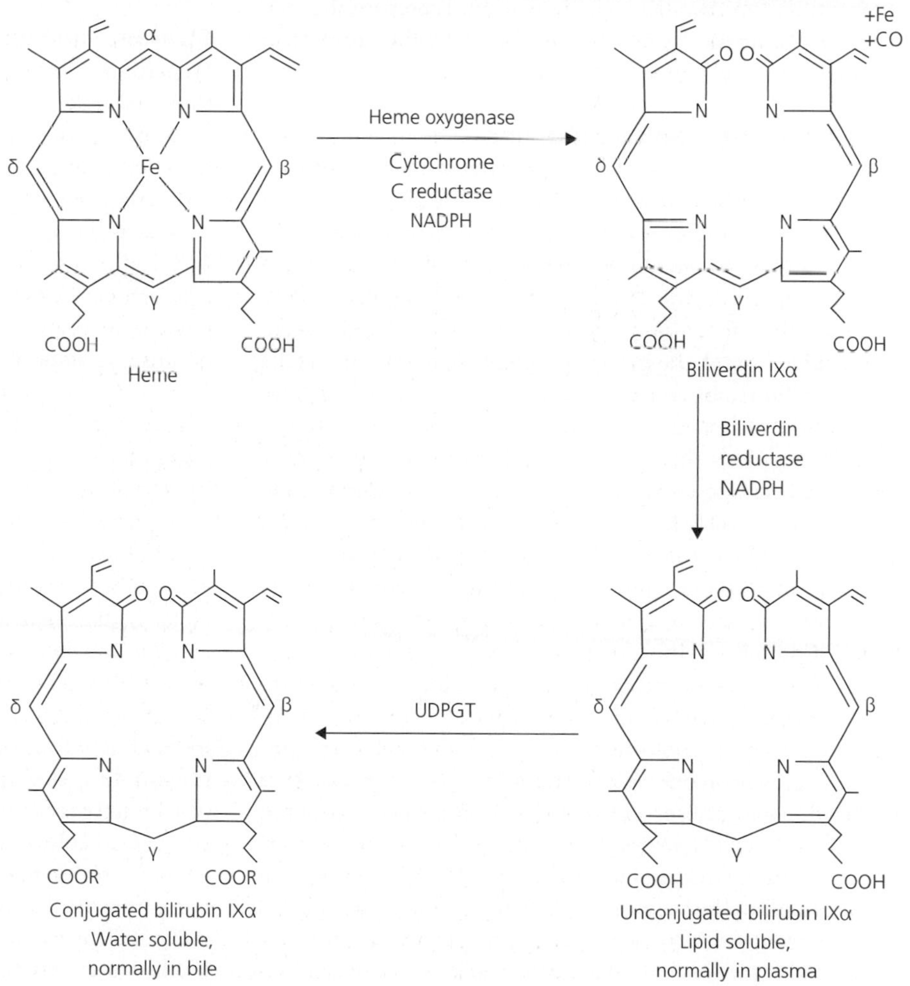

Figure 22.1 Bilirubin metabolism. The first step in the degradation of the heme group to bilirubin is the cleavage of its α-methene bridge to form biliverdin, a reaction catalyzed by heme oxygenase. The enzyme is a monooxygenase, and O$_2$ and NADPH are required for the cleavage reaction. The reaction releases CO, iron, and biliverdin. The CO binds to hemoglobin and is excreted through the lungs, and most of the iron is reincorporated into new heme proteins. The second step in heme catabolism is the reduction of biliverdin IXα to bilirubin IXα by biliverdin reductase and NADPH. The result is unconjugated bilirubin. After bilirubin IXα is formed, it is released into the bloodstream, where it rapidly binds to plasma proteins, especially albumin. These complexes are poorly filtered by the glomerulus. Bilirubin is rendered more soluble in the liver by conjugation: the attachment of sugar residues such as glucuronates to its propionate side chains. This reaction requires the enzyme bilirubin UDP-glucuronosyltransferase (bilirubin UGT).

the hepatic heme proteins passes directly into bile as conjugated bilirubin, and the rest refluxes into plasma [9]. Myoglobin heme, because of its slow turnover, contributes less than 1% to bilirubin formation. Normally, less than 3% of bilirubin is derived from ineffective erythropoiesis in the bone marrow, but this fraction may be considerably increased in hemoglobinopathies, congenital and acquired dyserythropoietic anemias, and megaloblastic anemia. Normal daily human bilirubin production averages 4 mg/kg body weight, equivalent to approximately 250 mg of bile pigment.

Unconjugated bilirubin is normally insoluble in water. In bile, however, it is solubilized by weak interactions with mixed micelles of bile salts and other lipids [6]. When the capacity for bilirubin solubilization is exceeded in bile, the unbound pigment may precipitate as a calcium salt and may form bilirubin pigment stones. Most bilirubin formed peripherally is transported in plasma tightly bound to albumin. The concentration of unbound bilirubin remains small until the bilirubin concentration exceeds 35 mg/dL [10]. Increased unbound bilirubin pigment may cross cell membranes resulting in tissue injury, a key factor in the pathogenesis of bilirubin encephalopathy and kernicterus in the newborn [11]. In its albumin-bound state, bilirubin is poorly filtered at the glomerulus, limiting its renal elimination. Therefore, the conjugation of bilirubin by hepatocytes facilitates the excretion in bile of a potentially toxic substance.

Uptake, binding, and conjugation

The hepatocyte has evolved specialized mechanisms to facilitate the uptake of the nonpolar, tightly albumin-bound molecule across the sinusoidal membrane, to maintain solubility by binding to cytosolic proteins and to convert it to more polar compounds by conjugation, permitting subsequent excretion. Initially, albumin spontaneously dissociates from its bilirubin ligand, the principal determinant of which is the unbound bilirubin concentration [12]. Subsequent hepatocyte uptake of unconjugated bilirubin is often considered a facilitated process involving several transporters, possibly including liver-specific forms of the organic anion-transporting polypeptide (OATP) family, a sodium-independent transport system [13]. Once inside the hepatocyte, hydrophobic bilirubin is maintained in solution by binding nonenzymatically to the cytosolic fatty acid binding proteins and ligandins (isoforms of proteins of the glutathione S-transferase [GST] gene family) [14]. GSTs are important in creating intracellular gradients, in determining bilirubin's movement, in compartmentalization, and in presentation to microsomes for conjugation.

The conjugation of bilirubin in the endoplasmic reticulum is the physiological process whereby bilirubin is rendered soluble and more hydrophilic for ultimate excretion into the bile canaliculus. Conjugation is achieved by the esterification of one or both of the propionic side chains through the addition of polar groups. Glucuronic acid esterification predominates, but xylose or glucose esterification can also occur. Bilirubin is conjugated with uridine 5'-diphospho (UDP)-glucuronic acid by bilirubin UDP-glucuronosyltransferase (bilirubin UGT, also known as UGT1A1). This produces bilirubin monoglucuronides and subsequently the diglucuronide. Normal human bile principally contains bilirubin diglucuronide (70%–90%) and smaller amounts of monoglucuronides (5%–25%). Their proportions change when the ratio of unconjugated bilirubin to available enzyme is increased (with an increased bilirubin load in hemolysis or reduced enzyme activity in Gilbert syndrome), favoring the formation of monoglucuronides [15]. It is becoming apparent that there are many distinct UGT isoforms. However, in humans, conjugation of bilirubin is exclusively carried out by the substrate-specific microsomal enzyme UGT1A1, encoded by the UGT1 gene subfamily, which is located on chromosome 2 [16]. Apart from bilirubin, other substrates for glucuronidation include drugs such as testosterone, estradiol, 1,25-dihydroxyvitamin D-3, digoxin, and propranolol, in addition to thyroid hormones and catecholamines. Determining the sequence of bilirubin UGT and subsequent identification of mutations have facilitated understanding of several disorders characterized by deficient bilirubin conjugation, such as Gilbert syndrome and Crigler–Najjar syndrome, as described later.

Clearance and excretion

Hyperbilirubinemia results from either increased bilirubin turnover or decreased bilirubin clearance or a combination of both. Isotope labeling studies permit an estimation of daily hepatic bilirubin clearance but are available only in a research setting [7]. Hepatic extraction of unconjugated bilirubin from plasma is 4.6 µg/min/kg under normal conditions. Almost 40% refluxes unaltered back into plasma, as does a small proportion of esterified bilirubin. The proportion of unconjugated to conjugated can change from more than 9:1 in nondisease states to 1:1 in cholestatic disease. Bile flow and transporters are described elsewhere in this volume.

The generation of bile flow is highly regulated and involves the coordinated action of several transporter proteins located at canalicular and sinusoidal domains in the hepatocyte. The canalicular ATP-dependent export pumps include the multidrug resistance 1 P-glycoprotein (MDR1/ABCB1), the phospholipid multidrug resistance 3 P-glycoprotein (MDR3/ABCB4), the canalicular bile salt export pump (BSEP/ABCB11), and the canalicular multispecific organic anion transporter (MRP2/cMOAT/ABCC2), all members of the ATP-binding cassette family, in addition to several putative ATP-independent transport systems [13]. The transporters are the rate-limiting step in bile salt export. Conjugated bilirubin is excreted across the canalicular membrane by a saturable process capable of functioning against a concentration gradient of 40- to 100-fold. Bilirubin monoglucuronides and diglucuronides are excreted into bile by the transporter MRP2/ABCC2. This carrier is also responsible for excreting leukotriene 4, some hydrophobic bile acids, oxidized glutathione, indocyanine green, sulfobromophthalein, and cholecystographic contrast. Definitive evidence of a potential sensitive membrane transporter is lacking.

After conjugated bilirubin reaches the bile ducts, it flows into the gallbladder, where sodium, bicarbonate, and water are actively absorbed. Cholecystokinin coordinates gallbladder contraction and sphincter of Oddi relaxation, permitting the controlled flow of bile into the small intestine to participate in the digestive process. Conjugated bilirubin is not absorbed from the gastrointestinal tract. However, it may be deconjugated and degraded by bacterial β-glucuronidases and other enzymes in the terminal ileum and colon to form a large variety of urobilinogens. Some urobilinogen is reabsorbed from the colon resulting in small plasma concentrations. Most of this is reexcreted by the liver, although the kidney filters a small proportion. Increased urine urobilinogen may represent increased bilirubin formation and subsequent enterohepatic circulation of urobilinogen or decreased hepatic clearance of urobilinogen, and therefore does not distinguish between hemolysis and liver disease [17]. In circumstances of complete biliary obstruction, jaundice may be apparent in the absence of urobilinogens because of the lack of delivery of bilirubin to the intestine. Urine urobilinogen levels may rise before jaundice becomes clinically apparent. Because unconjugated bilirubin is tightly bound to albumin, the free fraction is small and consequently never appears in the urine. Bilirubin conjugates are much less tightly bound to albumin. Therefore, in the presence of cholestasis, bilirubin conjugates formed in the hepatocyte are diverted back into the circulation, and the larger unbound fraction is filtered in the kidney. Thus, urine bilirubin is an absolute indication of conjugated hyperbilirubinemia. In the neonate, increased β-glucuronidases and deconjugation may contribute unconjugated bilirubin to the physiological jaundice of the newborn. In the colon, the unstable urobilinogens are oxidized to urobilins, orange pigments that are excreted in the feces. Bilirubin itself is rarely found in human feces unless the intestinal flora is underdeveloped or altered by antibiotics. Although the reticuloendothelial system has the capacity to metabolize heme from hemoglobin to form up to 1500 mg of bilirubin daily, a substantial increase in hemoglobin turnover is necessary before an increase in bilirubin levels becomes apparent. Consequently, jaundice seldom results from hemolysis unless it is severe or accompanied by hepatic dysfunction [18].

Measurement

The upper limit of normal for total plasma bilirubin concentration is 1.0–1.5 mg/dL (17–26 μM), with indirect-reacting bilirubin 0.8–1.2 mg/dL (14–21 μM) and direct-reacting bilirubin usually less than 0.2 mg/dL (largely a technical artifact); the ranges reflect variations in analytical methods [19]. The distribution of plasma bilirubin in the population is not normal, but it is skewed toward the upper end values. Males have slightly higher values than females. Unconjugated bilirubin IXα accounts for 95% of circulating isomers, and bilirubin monoesters and diesters account for about 4% [20].

Diazo method

Accurate measurement of total bilirubin and its fractions in serum is a crucial first step in the approach to a patient with jaundice [21]. The formation of diazo derivatives of bilirubin, as originally described by van den Berg in 1913, provides the basis for most clinical methods of quantifying bilirubin [7]. The addition of the diazo reagent (e.g., diazotized sulfanilic acid) ultimately results in the generation of two azopyrromethane molecules from the tetrapyrrole, the amount of which formed can be determined spectrophotometrically. van den Bergh and Müller first noted in 1916 that conjugated bilirubin reacted rapidly with the diazo reagent. The direct-reacting bilirubin (a proxy for conjugated bilirubin) and total bilirubin were measured, and indirect-reacting bilirubin (a proxy for unconjugated bilirubin) was then calculated by subtraction. However, this methodology was abandoned because of inadequate specificity and sensitivity.

Delta bilirubin

Glucuronides are chemically reactive metabolites. In adults, with prolonged cholestasis, especially if it is accompanied by renal failure, a fraction of the bilirubin conjugates reacts nonenzymatically and irreversibly with serum albumin to give yellow biliproteins in which bilirubin is covalently bound to albumin [22]. This fraction increases with the duration of cholestasis. Designated *delta bilirubin*, it retains its direct-reacting properties. Because delta bilirubin is irreversibly bound to albumin, it is not filtered at the glomerulus, and its half-life reflects that of albumin (14 days). Consequently, it remains in plasma long after other bilirubin esters have been eliminated. Clinically, this is suggested by persistent conjugated hyperbilirubinemia in the absence of bilirubinuria and is particularly evident in the recovery phase of cholestasis [23]. Delta bilirubin can be calculated as follows: delta bilirubin = total bilirubin − (conjugated + unconjugated bilirubin).

Dry film method

The adoption of dry film technology represented a major advance in accuracy and is standard in most clinical laboratories [24]. Using the Ektachem or Fuji dry chemistry slides, diazo coupling proceeds on a buffered porous layer, and the azo derivatives become bound to a cationic polymeric mordant, resulting in a spectral change. Spectrophotometric measurements are usually made at two different wavelengths. Protein-conjugated bilirubin is retained on only one of the slides and therefore can be removed from the sample being measured. One slide is used to measure total bilirubin, and a second slide measures both unconjugated bilirubin and conjugated bilirubin, the difference being delta bilirubin. The methodology is accurate, reproducible, and amenable to automation.

Hyperbilirubinemia

Hyperbilirubinemia results from a disruption at one or more steps in the complex metabolic pathways previously described, extending from excess bilirubin formation, altered uptake, defective conjugation, and diminished excretion into the biliary tree and subsequently into the gastrointestinal tract. Bilirubin levels correlate directly with bilirubin production and inversely with hepatic bilirubin plasma clearance. Practically, hyperbilirubinemia is classified as excess of either conjugated (direct-reacting) or unconjugated (indirect-reacting) bilirubin. This distinction is crucial to guide the evaluation of the patient, the differential diagnoses to be considered, and subsequently the optimal investigative approach. A pure increase in unconjugated bilirubin is usually indicative of defective conjugation. A parallel increase in both fractions in proportion to normal is usually indicative of increased pigment production. A normal or increased unconjugated bilirubin level with a markedly increased conjugated bilirubin level occurs in hepatobiliary disease [21]. Mixed conjugated and unconjugated hyperbilirubinemia may occur in the setting of multiple transfusions postoperatively, in fulminant liver failure with hemolysis resulting from Wilson disease, and in bacteremia. Many patients with chronic hemolytic disorders such as sickle cell anemia or thalassemia have underlying liver disease from transfusion-related iron overload or transfusion-related viral hepatitis, resulting again in a mixed pattern of hyperbilirubinemia.

Unconjugated hyperbilirubinemia

Overproduction of bilirubin may occur with excess destruction of red cells, with ineffective erythropoiesis, or with increased catabolism of heme compounds in the liver. Hemolysis may be intravascular (heme in plasma), extravascular (in cells of the reticuloendothelial system), or a combination of both. The bone marrow is capable of an eightfold increase in erythrocyte production in times of chronic hemolysis, with a maximum achievable steady-state bilirubin turnover of approximately 40 mg/kg/day, resulting in a serum unconjugated bilirubin level of 4 mg/dL [19]. With normal hepatic function, a 50% reduction in erythrocyte survival does not result in jaundice [25]. Even in the context of more severe hemolysis, unconjugated bilirubin levels rarely exceed 4–5 mg/dL unless there is concomitant impairment of hepatic clearance.

Hemolysis and ineffective erythropoiesis

Hemolysis and ineffective erythropoiesis are the only relevant causes of bilirubin overproduction in humans. Hemolysis, even if severe, usually results in mild hyperbilirubinemia (< 5 mg/dL) unless there is coexistent liver disease, which may contribute to concomitant conjugated hyperbilirubinemia. Hemolytic anemia may result from inherited disorders

of the red cell membrane (sickle cell anemia), of hemoglobin (thalassemia), or of red cell enzymes (glucose-6-phosphate dehydrogenase or pyruvate kinase deficiency). Acquired hemolytic conditions may result from ABO blood group incompatibility, iron or vitamin B-12 deficiency, and lead toxicity. Ineffective erythropoiesis shortens red cell life span and can be associated with hyperbilirubinemia. Impaired hepatic blood flow from congestive heart failure, cirrhosis, and portacaval shunting decreases bilirubin delivery to the liver and decreases clearance with resulting increased unconjugated hyperbilirubinemia. Other causes include hypothyroidism and hyperthyroidism, sepsis, and drugs (e.g., isoniazid, α-methyldopa, phenothiazines, nonsteroidal antiinflammatory drugs, rifampicin, sulfonamides, thiazides, and ribavirin).

Bilirubin uridine diphosphate glucuronosyltransferase deficiencies

These disorders are characterized by abnormalities of the bilirubin UGT enzyme UGT1A1 and consequently are manifest by unconjugated hyperbilirubinemia. Whereas Gilbert syndrome is common, the other disorders remain rare, but their study has provided invaluable insights into the complexities of bilirubin metabolism.

Gilbert syndrome

This condition is a characterized by unconjugated hyperbilirubinemia occurring in the absence of overt hemolysis or liver disease [26]. Typically, there are mild, chronic, or intermittent episodes of jaundice that increase with intercurrent illness, fasting, stress, fatigue, menses, and ethanol and nicotinic acid intake. Gilbert syndrome affects 3%–8% of the population, with a male predominance. It is usually inherited in an autosomal recessive pattern and is rarely manifest before puberty. Patients are generally asymptomatic, and nonspecific symptoms of fatigue and abdominal pain do not correlate with bilirubin levels. Mildly lemon-tinged sclerae are usually the only physical findings although splenomegaly is occasionally noted. About 50% of patients may have mild hemolytic anemia of uncertain origin [26].

Serum bilirubin concentrations are usually higher than 3 mg/dL but may increase to 5–8 mg/dL during stress. However, bilirubin levels may fluctuate in anyone, and it may be difficult to differentiate these from the higher end of the normal spectrum. Other hepatic biochemical indices are normal. A presumptive diagnosis can be made in a patient with isolated, asymptomatic, unconjugated hyperbilirubinemia if a careful history and physical examination do not suggest alternative diagnoses. Provocative fasting studies to confirm the diagnosis are seldom indicated or useful. Routine use of liver biopsy is not indicated. The significance of reports of increased lipofuscin pigment within the centrilobular cells is uncertain. Fasting serum bile acid levels are normal, in contrast to the hyperbilirubinemia of liver disease.

Bilirubin UGT activity is reduced to approximately one-fourth of normal [27]. Patients have reduced bilirubin diesters and increased bilirubin monoglucuronides. Molecular studies have indicated that the phenotype results from different mutations. One mutation is an expansion of thymidine-adenosine (TA) repeats in the promoter region of the *UGT1A1* gene (autosomal recessive) for which homozygosity is predicted in 16% of whites. Another mutation is found in exon 1A1 of the same gene, occurring in Japanese and Asian populations (autosomal dominant), and is associated with serum bilirubin levels in the range 3–10 mg/dL [28]. The genetic variation described in Gilbert syndrome may lead to pharmacological variation in drug glucuronidation and may explain the occasional unexpected drug toxicities reported [28–30]. The use of pharmacological agents that induce hepatic microsomal enzymes, such as phenobarbital, which normalizes plasma unconjugated bilirubin levels and corrects ratios of monoesters and diesters but does not increase UGT1A1 activity, leaves questions regarding the true mode of action of phenobarbital. Gilbert syndrome is a benign condition, and no therapy is routinely required.

Crigler–Najjar syndrome
This syndrome is characterized by unconjugated hyperbilirubinemia, which may occur from birth [31]. Crigler–Najjar type I is a rare autosomal recessive disorder and is characterized by a complete deficiency of the enzyme bilirubin UGT. It results from a mutation in one of the five exons of the gene encoding bilirubin UGT. Mutations may occur in exon 1A1 or exons 2 to 5 of the *UGT1* gene locus encoding the enzyme UGT1A1, resulting in complete absence of the enzyme in type I. Crigler–Najjar type I bile contains only traces of bile conjugates. Heterozygotes have normal bilirubin levels. Infants develop severe unconjugated hyperbilirubinemia within 7 days of birth, followed by kernicterus and bilirubin encephalopathy if prompt therapy is not initiated. Death follows within 18 months if the disorder is untreated. Treatment consists of the rapid initiation of phototherapy with exchange transfusions. Type I does not respond to phenobarbital. Orthotopic liver transplantation is curative. Reports have indicated temporary success with isolated hepatocyte transplants [32].

Type II (Arias disease) is an autosomal dominant disorder with variable penetrance that results in various levels of unconjugated hyperbilirubinemia. Type II is caused by a variety of mutations in exons 1A1, 2, and 5 of the *UGT1* gene locus, the functional consequence of which is partial inactivation of bilirubin UGT. Affected persons have about 10% of normal bilirubin UGT activity. Bilirubin monoconjugates and even some diconjugate are present in bile. Jaundice often is not apparent until the second year of life. Bilirubin levels rarely exceed 20 mg/dL. Therapy with phenobarbital results in a decrease in serum bilirubin by 30% but is usually unnecessary unless there is a risk of kernicterus.

Conjugated hyperbilirubinemia
Conjugated hyperbilirubinemia is defined by a conjugated bilirubin level greater than 30% of the total bilirubin level [18,25]. Broadly, causes may be congenital, familial, or acquired (Table 22.1).

Congenital hyperbilirubinemias
Rotor syndrome
First described in 1948, Rotor syndrome is a rare, asymptomatic, benign, congenital disorder that is manifested as conjugated or mixed hyperbilirubinemia [33]. It is an autosomal recessive disorder that becomes apparent in childhood. Total bilirubin levels are usually 2–5 mg/dL, consisting of more than 50% conjugated bilirubin, with bilirubinuria and exacerbation of hyperbilirubinemia during illness. Other liver tests, including bile acids, are normal, as is liver histology. Although the result of an oral cholecystogram is normal, radionuclide scans show absent or markedly delayed excretion. It is unclear whether the primary defect is impaired secretion or impaired storage of bilirubin. Urinary coproporphyrins are markedly increased, especially type I. Therapy is not required for Rotor syndrome.

Dubin–Johnson syndrome
This is an autosomal recessive syndrome resulting in impaired ATP-mediated transport of bilirubin diglucuronide and other organic ions [34]. Bilirubin refluxes back into plasma, and hyperbilirubinemia results. Total bilirubin levels are usually between 2 and 5 mg/dL; other liver tests are normal. Patients usually present after puberty, and exacerbations occur during intercurrent illness and with some drugs. The secretory defect in patients with Dubin–Johnson syndrome results in abnormal radionuclide scans and oral cholecystographic studies. Bile salt secretion is normal. Although total urinary coproporphyrin levels are normal, there is an increase in type I levels in the urine and a decrease in type III levels. Liver histology reveals a darkly pigmented liver that is black on gross inspection. The importance of diagnosing Rotor or Dubin–Johnson syndrome is to reassure the patient that there is not a more serious problem, and to avoid repetitive testing for more serious disorders, including porphyrias.

Familial cholestasis
The disorders collectively termed *progressive familial intrahepatic cholestasis* (PFIC) have disparate pathogeneses but share the following common features: chronic, persistent hepatocellular cholestasis usually leading to cirrhosis; exclusion of other metabolic and anatomical defects; autosomal recessive inheritance patterns; and characteristic combined clinical, biochemical, and histological features. All these disorders share a defect in the generation of bile flow. Identification, cloning, and characterization of numerous bile transport proteins have allowed a more precise definition of the diverse PFIC syndromes [35,36].

Table 22.1 Causes of conjugated hyperbilirubinemia

Congenital conjugated hyperbilirubinemias
Rotor syndrome
Dubin–Johnson syndrome

Intrahepatic cholestasis
Familial and congenital
    Progressive familial intrahepatic cholestasis types 1 to 3
    Benign recurrent intrahepatic cholestasis
    Cholestasis of pregnancy
    Choledochal cysts, Caroli disease
    Congenital biliary atresia

Hepatocellular conditions
    Alcohol-related disorders
    Viral hepatitis
    Autoimmune hepatitis
    Cirrhosis
    Drug-related hepatitis
    Wilson disease
    Hereditary hemochromatosis

Infiltrative conditions
    Granulomatous
    Carcinoma
    Hematological malignant disease
    Amyloidosis

Cholangiopathies
    Primary biliary cirrhosis
    Idiopathic adult ductopenia
    Autoimmune (overlap) cholangiopathies

Infections
    Bacterial
    Fungal
    Parasitic
    HIV-related

Miscellaneous causes
    Postoperative sepsis
    Pregnancy
    Total parenteral nutrition
    Cholestasis after liver transplantation
    Drug hepatotoxicity

Extrahepatic cholestasis
Inside bile ducts
    Calculi
    Parasites

Inside wall
    Stricture
    Cholangiocarcinoma
    Sclerosing cholangitis
    Choledochal cysts

Outside duct wall
    Tumor in porta hepatis
    Tumor in pancreas
    Pancreatitis, acute or chronic

Briefly, PFIC1 describes syndromic forms of defects in the *FIC1/ATP8B1* gene. Byler disease is the best-known form of FIC1 disease and is named after Jacob Byler, of Amish ancestry. Patients typically have persistent cholestasis, evolving to cirrhosis. Clinically, the disease is characterized by jaundice, steatorrhea, growth retardation, hepatosplenomegaly, and watery diarrhea. Biochemically, although bilirubin, alkaline phosphatase, and serum bile acids are elevated, γ-glutamyl-transferase and biliary bile acid concentrations are low. *FIC1* encodes a member of the subfamily of P-type ATPases involved in aminophospholipid transport [37].

Benign recurrent intrahepatic cholestasis

Mutations in *FIC1* have also been identified in some patients with benign recurrent intrahepatic cholestasis (BRIC), which has different phenotypic manifestations. BRIC is a familial disorder characterized by recurrent episodes of painless intrahepatic cholestasis, beginning in early childhood or adulthood [38,39]. Episodes last weeks to months and may be associated with steatorrhea and weight loss, but they resolve spontaneously without permanent liver injury. Biochemical alterations are similar to those of PFIC1. Mutation analyses suggest that phenotypic differences between PFIC1 and BRIC relate to quantitative differences in FIC1 protein function [37,40].

Other types of PFIC

PFIC2 designates a group of patients with phenotypic features similar but not identical to those with PFIC1. In PFIC2, the initial presentation and progression are more severe. Liver biopsy often shows evidence of giant-cell hepatitis. The disorder is caused by mutations in a gene encoding the canalicular bile salt export protein (BSEP/ABCB11), a gene related to the MDR/ABC family of the ATP-binding cassette transporter superfamily [41]. These mutations result in defective canalicular excretion of bile acids with accumulation within hepatocytes and ongoing injury that is unresponsive to treatment with ursodeoxycholic acid.

PFIC3 shares features with PFIC1 and PFIC2, except for elevated serum levels of γ-glutamyltransferase and extensive bile ductular proliferation. Patients have less jaundice, often present later in life, and may respond to ursodeoxycholic acid. Mutations have been described in the MDR3/ABCB4, a canalicular phospholipid transporter [42] whose absence permits toxic bile acid accumulation and exposure to hepatocytes and cholangiocytes. Other rare syndromes that may mimic PFIC are 3-β-OH steroid dehydrogenase deficiency and cholestasis with lymphedema or hypertrichosis [35]. There are also likely to be other as-yet-unidentified PFIC genes.

Choledochal cystic disorders

These disorders, including Caroli disease, are inherited anomalies of the biliary ducts. Caroli disease involves the congenital dilation of the segmental intrahepatic biliary tree, whereas choledochal cysts involve the cystic dilation of the common bile duct. Patients can present at any age with jaundice or with symptoms of cholangitis, such as fever and right upper quadrant pain. Choledochal cysts are three times more frequent in female patients. Jaundice in a patient with Caroli disease or a choledochocele should raise suspicion of cholangiocarcinoma because these patients are at increased risk of developing such tumors.

Hepatocellular diseases

Hyperbilirubinemia may accompany acute or chronic hepatocellular disease and must be considered in the differential diagnosis and distinguished from diseases whose manifestations are predominantly cholestatic. All hepatocellular diseases may present as cholestasis, especially when severe, and they constitute the most common causes of intrahepatic cholestasis. Therefore, cholestatic forms of viral hepatitis and alcoholic liver disease are more common than primary sclerosing cholangitis or primary biliary cirrhosis. These hepatocellular diseases are described individually elsewhere in this book. Viral hepatitis may have a prolonged cholestatic phase after acute infection. Patients may come to medical attention only during this phase of lowered serum aminotransferases and high bilirubin, with or without prolonged prothrombin time. Patients with elevation in prothrombin time resulting from poor absorption will respond to parenteral vitamin K, whereas those with submassive necrosis or fulminant hepatic failure will not. Even patients with hepatitis A, which never becomes chronic, may rarely have a prolonged cholestatic phase up to 18 months after acute infection [43]. Bilirubin may be elevated in 10%–20% of patients with alcoholic hepatitis, and usually right upper quadrant pain, fever, and leukocytosis accompany this condition [44]. Finally, with end-stage liver disease of any cause, bilirubin may become elevated. However, physical signs of cirrhosis should be readily apparent. Patients with cholestatic immune-mediated liver diseases, such as primary biliary cirrhosis, primary sclerosing cholangitis, and autoimmune cholangiopathy, are cholestatic early (elevated serum alkaline phosphatase) but develop jaundice only later in the course of disease [45,46]. Drug hepatotoxicity is an increasingly common cause of liver injury that can include jaundice, cholestasis, or bile duct damage [47].

Infiltrative disorders

These disorders may also result in cholestasis. When jaundice occurs in patients with primary or metastatic tumors, much of the liver is usually replaced, and the prognosis is poor [48]. However, if a tumor obstructs a major bile duct, such as in cholangiocarcinoma, jaundice may occur earlier. Diffuse lymphomatous infiltration occurs with Hodgkin disease and periportal lymphadenopathy with non-Hodgkin lymphoma, and both may cause jaundice. Granulomatous hepatitis has a diverse etiology, and patients may occasionally present with jaundice [49,50]. In systemic amyloidosis, either primary or secondary, histological evidence of hepatic involvement is common but usually clinically quiescent. However, a subgroup may develop marked cholestasis, which often portends a poor prognosis [51].

Renal disease

The association between renal dysfunction and cholestatic jaundice is long established. A postoperative fall in glomerular filtration rate is observed in 60%–75% of patients undergoing surgery for obstructive jaundice [52]. Acute renal failure may occur in 8%–10% of those patients and is a contributing cause of death in 70%–80% of those who develop it [53]. The pathophysiology is complex and multifactorial, and not surprisingly, no clearly effective therapeutic strategy has emerged. Intrahepatic cholestasis, with or without jaundice, can occur as a paraneoplastic manifestation of renal cell carcinoma (Stauffer syndrome) in the absence of liver metastases [54].

Infection

Infections may cause jaundice through extrahepatic obstruction (e.g., ascariasis), granulomatous inflammation (e.g., tuberculosis), or, more commonly, through intrahepatic cholestasis [55]. The predominant mechanism of sepsis-associated cholestasis (especially gram-negative sepsis) is related to endotoxins derived from the bacterial cell wall, which are potent inducers of proinflammatory cytokines, tumor necrosis factor-α and interleukin-1 (IL-1) and IL-6 [56,57]. A disproportionate elevation of bilirubin in relation to alkaline phosphatase and aminotransferases is suggestive of sepsis-related cholestasis [58]. Persistent or increasing hyperbilirubinemia with ongoing infection correlates with the worst outcome. Patients infected with human immunodeficiency virus (HIV) are susceptible to various hepatic processes related to immunosuppression or shared risk factors. These disorders include hepatic granulomas, cytomegalovirus hepatitis, syphilis, multimicrobial HIV cholangiopathy, Kaposi sarcoma, and lymphoma. The differential diagnosis also includes other opportunistic infections and neoplasms, and concomitant chronic viral hepatitis B, C, and D and drug-related (including antiretroviral) hepatotoxicity [59]. Systematic evaluation and treatment are necessary to ensure that morbidity and mortality are minimized and quality of life and medical care costs are optimized [60].

Bone marrow transplantation

Bone marrow transplant recipients may develop jaundice for many reasons. Venoocclusive disease is a common cause of hyperbilirubinemia, especially after autologous bone marrow transplantation [61], and it is associated with increased morbidity and mortality. Other complications include drug- and chemotherapy-induced hepatitis, sepsis-related liver injury, and recurrent disease. Acute or chronic graft-vs-host disease affects up to half of long-term transplant survivors and is associated with elevated alkaline phosphatase levels and a poor prognosis.

Total parenteral nutrition

Total parenteral nutrition (TPN) is associated with a spectrum of hepatobiliary complications that are a major cause of morbidity and mortality and increase with the duration of therapy, although modifications to TPN formulation have reduced the prevalence of these. Cholestasis is the most common hepatic complication in infants receiving TPN. Although cholestasis is less common in adults, steatosis and steatohepatitis in addition to biliary sludge and gallstone formation predominate [62,63]. The cause of TPN-induced cholestasis is uncertain but is probably multifactorial [64,65]. Direct hepatotoxicity may result from individual TPN components including excess lipids and amino acids such as tryptophan and peroxides. Cholestasis may be related to specific nutritional deficiencies in TPN of substances such as taurine and methyl-donor molecules. Defective or altered bile acid secretion may be relevant and may have therapeutic implications. The lack of enteral intake and inadequate stimulation of the enterohepatic circulation and gut function lead to diminished cholecystokinin release and understimulation of the gallbladder. This has numerous potential pathological consequences including gallbladder and bile stasis. Gut hypomotility and small bowel bacterial overgrowth results, with production and absorption of lithocholic acid, a cholestatic bile salt, and enhanced endotoxin absorption, often exacerbated by concomitant sepsis.

Liver biochemical tests are of limited use as sensitive or specific indicators of TPN-related hepatobiliary disease. Liver biopsy is rarely necessary. Jaundice may reflect the development of biliary sludge (50% incidence at 4–6 weeks of TPN and present in 100% of patients after more than 6 weeks) and calculous or acalculous biliary tract disease (the former occurring particularly with preexisting ileal disease). With long-term TPN, a rising alkaline phosphatase level may reflect the development of intrahepatic cholestasis or, alternatively, progression of TPN-associated steatohepatitis to decompensated cirrhosis [66].

Approaches that may ameliorate the hepatobiliary impact include minimizing the duration of TPN, cycling of TPN, optimizing caloric components, and reducing excess lipids and amino acids. Attempted limited enteral intake, selective gut decontamination, and the use of ursodeoxycholic acid and cholecystokinin may further limit the TPN injury.

Approach to the patient with jaundice

The investigation of a patient with jaundice begins with a thorough review of the history of presentation, medication use, past medical history, examination, and evaluation of liver-related laboratory tests. With an understanding of the pathophysiology of cholestasis, a systematic approach to the jaundiced patient can be applied. Identification of the correct diagnosis can lead to an appropriate therapeutic intervention. The implications of jaundice in certain conditions can be life threatening, and thus a timely diagnosis is important. Several questions must be answered initially:

• Is the elevated bilirubin conjugated or unconjugated? In general, most jaundiced patients will not have isolated unconjugated hyperbilirubinemia.
• If the hyperbilirubinemia is unconjugated, is it caused by increased production, decreased uptake, or impaired conjugation?
• If the hyperbilirubinemia is conjugated, is the problem intrahepatic or extrahepatic?
• Is the process acute or chronic?

Patients with conjugated hyperbilirubinemia usually have acquired disease, and the physician must identify an intrahepatic or obstructive cause. Acute disease can usually be differentiated from chronic disease by the patient's history, physical examination, and laboratory tests. For example, clinical evaluation may demonstrate xanthelasmas, spider angiomas, ascites, or hepatosplenomegaly. Laboratory evidence of chronic disease may consist of a hypoalbuminemia, thrombocytopenia, and a prolonged prothrombin time that is not corrected with vitamin K administration.

Chronic cholestasis may arise from such diseases as cirrhosis, primary sclerosing cholangitis, primary biliary cirrhosis, or carcinoma, or it may result from drugs. Patients with chronic cholestasis do not usually have hepatitis or gallstones [67]. The presence of fever, right upper quadrant pain, tenderness, hepatomegaly, and new-onset bilirubinuria usually indicates acute disease. An adult with asymptomatic, isolated unconjugated hyperbilirubinemia who is not taking any drugs and has no evidence of hemolysis probably has Gilbert syndrome and can be monitored with bilirubin determinations for 12 months. If no abnormality develops, no further evaluation is needed.

The patient's history, physical examination, and laboratory tests are crucial to the diagnosis of hyperbilirubinemia [68]. Physicians are 80%–90% accurate in diagnosing extrahepatic disease by these means, but obstruction is often overdiagnosed [69]. When first evaluating a patient with hyperbilirubinemia, the physician must make a quick assessment of the emergency of the situation. Fever, leukocytosis, and hypotension point to ascending cholangitis, which requires immediate therapy. Asterixis, confusion, or stupor may indicate severe hepatocellular dysfunction or fulminant hepatic failure and mandates immediate therapy. After immediate life-threatening causes of hyperbilirubinemia have been excluded, a systematic approach to the patient helps to make the diagnosis.

Diagnosis by age of the patient

The most common causes of jaundice differ according to the age of the patient. In neonates, physiological jaundice is overwhelmingly the most common form, with biliary atresia, infections (toxoplasmosis, other [*Treponema pallidum*, varicella-zoster virus, parvovirus B19], rubella virus, cytomegalovirus, herpes simplex virus, and syphilis [TORCHES]), and metabolic diseases together accounting for less than 25% of cases. In adolescents, Gilbert syndrome and viral hepatitis account for 80% of cases, with the remainder including toxins, drugs, and autoimmune and biliary tract diseases. A careful history will elicit drug use or abuse, risk factors for viral hepatitis, amenorrhea associated with autoimmune hepatitis, or symptoms associated with biliary tract disease.

In young adults, viral hepatitis is the most common cause of jaundice, followed by biliary tract disease, alcoholic liver disease, and autoimmune diseases. Genetic diseases (hemochromatosis and Wilson disease) may present solely as an elevation in aminotransferases but rarely as cholestasis at this age, and evaluation should include ceruloplasmin, urine copper, ferritin, and transferrin saturation in these patients.

By contrast, malignant disease accounts for half of the cases of jaundice seen in elderly patients. Drug toxicity is common with increasing polypharmacy in the elderly and should always be included in the history of these patients with jaundice. Multiple drugs have been associated with hyperbilirubinemia, whether hepatocellular (acetaminophen [paracetamol]), cholestatic (anabolic steroids), or mixed (sulfonamides). Drug toxicity is associated with 10% of abnormal liver tests in hospitalized patients. Autoimmune disease has a second peak in the elderly and should be sought. Antinuclear antibodies may be weakly elevated in healthy elderly patients, and other laboratory evidence of autoimmune disease should be sought (elevated IgG in autoimmune hepatitis, IgM in primary biliary cirrhosis). Biliary tract disease, viral hepatitis, and alcoholic liver disease also occur in elderly patients.

Neonatal and childhood jaundice

The neonate is predisposed to the development of jaundice because of an increased production of bilirubin, reduced bilirubin UGT levels, and impaired excretory ability. Physiological jaundice (with a serum bilirubin of 5–6 mg/dL) occurs in full-term infants in the first few days of life but is more common in premature infants, usually resolving over several weeks. Exaggerated physiological jaundice is characterized by hyperbilirubinemia up to 17 mg/dL, but higher levels in a term infant should prompt a search for a pathological cause [11]. The consequences and optimal treatment of neonatal hyperbilirubinemia are controversial [70]. Neonates should have follow-up examinations 2–5 days after delivery, and jaundiced infants require early measurement of total bilirubin. Phototherapy is the mainstay of therapy. Exchange transfusions are rarely necessary.

Neonatal infection, birth trauma, and hypothyroidism may compound hyperbilirubinemia. Increased bilirubin production occurs in certain racial groups such as Native Americans. Inherited defects in red cell enzymes such as glucose-6-phosphate dehydrogenase deficiency, red cell structural defects such as elliptocytosis, or blood group incompatibility

may result in pathological jaundice. Icterus in neonates may be related to Gilbert syndrome. In Crigler–Najjar syndrome type I, bilirubin encephalopathy may occur in the first few days or months of life, whereas in Crigler–Najjar syndrome type II, bilirubin levels rarely exceed 20 mg/dL. Neonates, particularly if they are not feeding well or are exclusively breast-fed, have lower levels of intestinal bacteria. As a result, bilirubin deconjugated in the gut is not reduced to urobilinogen and excreted but undergoes enhanced enterohepatic circulation. Later-onset breast-milk jaundice is seen in 0.5%–1% of newborns during days 4–10 after birth. Unconjugated bilirubin levels may rise to 10–20 mg/dL. The infant remains well, interruption of breast-feeding will result in a rapid decline in bilirubin levels, and resolution occurs by 4–6 weeks [71]. Transient familial neonatal hyperbilirubinemia (Lucy–Driscoll syndrome) results from a serum inhibitor of bilirubin UGT that disappears by 2 weeks of life.

Severe neonatal hyperbilirubinemia has neurotoxic sequelae in the form of bilirubin encephalopathy. *Kernicterus* describes the pathological findings of yellow staining and necrosis of neuronal cells of the basal ganglia, hippocampal cortex, and subthalamic area, and clinically it may follow an acute or chronic course with potentially debilitating outcomes. Early hospital discharge and a less aggressive approach to treatment may have contributed to a possible reemergence of this disorder [72,73]. The free fraction of unconjugated bilirubin crosses the blood–brain barrier, especially if it is impaired by infection, prematurity acidosis, or hyperoxia. The neurotoxic effects are related to the concentration of bilirubin in the brain and the duration of exposure, although serum bilirubin levels correlate poorly with encephalopathy in nonhemolytic hyperbilirubinemia. Hypoalbuminemia and drugs that displace bilirubin from albumin further exacerbate the toxicity.

In the older neonate and infant, the diagnostic algorithm must reflect knowledge of the age-specific onset of disorders and their predominant presenting features, combined with the use of selected diagnostic tests [74]. Whereas jaundice may be obvious, more subtle manifestations of chronic cholestasis may exist, such as the consequences of fat-soluble vitamin deficiency (neurological and hematological), xanthomas, and growth failure. In the initial evaluation of an infant with cholestasis, if hepatic synthetic function is impaired, causes of liver failure must be considered such as neonatal iron storage disease, tyrosinemia, galactosemia, fructosemia, and mitochondrial cytopathies. In the absence of liver failure, other metabolic causes such as α_1-antitrypsin deficiency and cystic fibrosis, and viral causes, must be sought.

Anatomical causes of cholestasis that may be corrected surgically must be distinguished. Biliary atresia is the single most common cause of neonatal cholestasis and accounts for 50%–60% of pediatric liver transplantations. Two phenotypes are apparent: the less common (congenital) form presents in the first few weeks of life, whereas the more common phenotype (acquired form) presents in the first to second month of life. Numerous theories attempt to provide rational etiological explanations [75]. Jaundice, pale stools, and hepatomegaly are the dominant clinical features. Rapid diagnosis is essential for definitive surgical intervention. Portoenterostomy results in successful biliary drainage in 80% of patients, but it must be performed as early as possible. In infants, idiopathic neonatal hepatitis is the second most common cause of cholestasis and refers to a heterogeneous group of disorders that includes infectious, toxic, metabolic, and genetic defects in bile acid synthesis [35].

Alagille syndrome is a cause of cholestasis in infants before the age of 6 months. The five main features are hepatic, cardiovascular, vertebral, and ocular signs, and a peculiar facies [76]. Expression is variable, and the first two manifestations are most common. Jaundice may be intermittent, but cholestasis is persistent, with its attendant complications. Histologically, paucity of interlobular bile ducts is typical. The mode of transmission is autosomal dominant with reduced penetrance. Mutations in the coding sequence of the *JAG1* gene have been identified in a large proportion of patients with the Alagille syndrome. *JAG1* encodes a ligand for the Notch1 receptor, implicated in a fundamental mechanism controlling cell fate during embryogenesis and leading to overexpression of hepatocyte growth factor [77].

Liver disease in pregnancy

Liver disease in pregnancy includes disorders unique to pregnancy and those coincident with or exacerbated by pregnancy [78–80]. Normal changes during pregnancy include a lower mean serum albumin (3.1 g/dL) resulting from hemodilution, and a higher alkaline phosphatase level (two to four times normal), mainly of placental origin. Fibrinogen, transferrin, and cholesterol levels are also increased. Serum aminotransferases, bilirubin, serum bile acids, and γ-glutamyltransferase levels are unchanged. Spider angiomas and palmar erythema may be seen in more than 60% of pregnant women [81]. The differential diagnosis of hepatic disorders of pregnancy depends on the time of onset in relation to the stage of gestation and the type of symptoms and signs. A careful history of present and past pregnancies, and parity, including a family history of complicated pregnancies, may provide important clues to diagnosis.

Liver disease unique to pregnancy
Hyperemesis gravidarum

Intractable nausea and vomiting in the first trimester are key features of hyperemesis gravidarum, which may result in dehydration, electrolyte disturbances, and malnutrition. More common in young women with a multiple gestation, it may be associated with increased fetal wastage. Mild elevations of alkaline phosphatase and hyperbilirubinemia (< 4 mg/dL) occur, although aminotransferases may rarely increase markedly. Treatment includes hydration and careful management of electrolytes and nutrition.

Intrahepatic cholestasis of pregnancy

Intense, often debilitating pruritus is the hallmark of intrahepatic cholestasis of pregnancy (ICP), which typically begins in the third trimester [82]. Although rare in most countries, the endemic occurrence in Chilean Indians and Scandinavians suggests a strong genetic predisposition in some persons. ICP recurs in 45%–70% of subsequent pregnancies and with the use of birth control pills. It is more common in twin pregnancies. Defects in the MDR3 transporter involved in phospholipid salt secretion may contribute to a subset of women with ICP who also have increased γ-glutamyltransferase levels [83]. Hyperbilirubinemia, up to 5 mg/dL, is detected in 20% of cases, with minimal elevations in hepatic alkaline phosphatase. An increase in total serum bile acids (often up to 100-fold) with pruritus is highly suggestive of ICP [84]. Fetal morbidity is increased because of premature births (19%–60%) and intrapartum fetal distress (22%–33%). The perinatal mortality of 10%–11% is poorly predicted by maternal disease severity or conventional antepartum fetal testing [82]. Limited controlled data suggest that early treatment with ursodeoxycholic acid is safe, improves pruritus, lowers bilirubin and aminotransferases, normalizes some bile acid ratios, and may contribute to improved fetal outcome [85–87]. Early delivery in cases of fetal distress, preferably after establishment of fetal lung maturity, is usually followed by complete resolution.

Other disorders

In the third trimester (and rarely in the postpartum period), three other disorders unique to pregnancy have predominantly hepatocellular patterns of injury with elevated aminotransferases. If severe, they may be associated with cholestasis and significant maternal and perinatal morbidity and mortality [78,79,88].

Acute fatty liver of pregnancy is characterized by a spectrum of disease that may extend from mild disease to fulminant hepatic failure. Histology reveals a microvesicular steatosis. In some cases, inherited disorders of mitochondrial β-oxidation of long-chain fatty acids are evident in the fetus and mother [89]. *Preeclampsia* is a multisystem disorder associated with proteinuria, hypertension, peripheral edema, and hyperreflexia. It is common (5%–7%) among primigravidas, especially those with a multiple gestation. Hepatic involvement indicates severe disease and increased risk of eclampsia. Serum aminotransferases may be massively increased. Acute, severe, right upper quadrant pain may raise the specter of complicating hepatic infarction or rupture. *HELLP syndrome*, characterized by hemolysis, elevated liver enzymes, and low platelet counts, may occur in a subset of patients with preeclampsia/eclampsia or acute fatty liver of pregnancy. Indeed, it may be difficult to distinguish the latter three disorders because they share many overlapping features [79]. However, prompt recognition and expedited delivery remain the cornerstone of management of the more severe cases.

Liver biopsy is reserved for patients in whom the result will affect immediate obstetrical management. Oil red O staining of fresh tissue is required for confirmatory diagnosis of microvesicular steatosis. Complete recovery usually follows delivery.

Diseases coincident with pregnancy

Liver disorders that are exacerbated by pregnancy include acute hepatitis E virus in travelers from endemic areas, where maternal mortality may approach 29% in the third trimester. Herpes simplex hepatitis may be more common in pregnancy; it has a high mortality rate, and prompt antiviral therapy improves survival. Some patients with Dubin–Johnson syndrome may experience asymptomatic, isolated, conjugated hyperbilirubinemia during the third trimester. A hypercoagulable state exists in pregnancy and can be associated with the development of Budd–Chiari syndrome. Pregnancy is associated with increased gallstone formation, and extrahepatic cholestasis from choledocholithiasis or biliary sludge may be encountered, extending into the postpartum period. Surgical management may be appropriate only in the second trimester. For women with known severe chronic liver disease, amenorrhea may be present. However, autoimmune hepatitis and primary biliary cirrhosis are usually better controlled in pregnancy because of increased endogenous glucocorticoid production. Patients with portal hypertension may develop variceal bleeding, and there is a higher degree of fetal wastage [90].

Postoperative jaundice

Jaundice is uncommon after elective abdominal surgery (< %), but it may occur in up to 17% of patients who are in the intensive care unit or after major surgery. The cause is multifactorial, and liver failure is rarely associated with the jaundice. Specific treatment is not usually required. Postoperative jaundice falls into three major categories [91].

1 Bilirubin overproduction may result from hemolysis of transfused blood or absorption of hematomas; hemolysis may be related to administered drugs, prosthetic valves, or underlying hemolytic anemias; or Gilbert syndrome may become manifest. One liter of transfused blood will generate 5 g of bilirubin. Ten percent of red blood cells within a transfused unit are hemolyzed within 24 h of storage.

2 Hepatocellular dysfunction may result from a diverse group of insults [92]: anesthesia, ischemia, drugs, and TPN. Ischemia, related to cardiogenic or noncardiogenic shock, may be apparent only after careful examination of the anesthetic records. Most forms of anesthesia reduce blood flow. Anesthetic drugs, especially the halogenated hydrocarbon anesthetics such as halothane, typically cause acute hepatitis within 21 days of initial exposure. Seventy-five percent of cases have an accompanying fever, and 20%–60% of patients have peripheral eosinophilia [93]. Recurrent exposure may result in icterus within 7 days. Features predictive of

an adverse outcome include age older than 60 years, obesity, multiple exposures, short latent period to the development of jaundice, serum bilirubin more than 10 mg/dL, and prothrombin time longer than 20 s. A careful review of drugs (including TPN) employed in the perioperative period is essential. Posttransfusion hepatitis is rarely encountered because of screening of the donor population. Preexisting liver disease is an important risk factor and may be exacerbated by an operative procedure, potentially leading to decompensation if the patient has cirrhosis. Ascites is frequent in cirrhotic patients who decompensate after surgery as a result of poor volume handling. Jaundice with abnormal biochemical test results is commonly seen in patients who have bacteremia, especially with intraabdominal sources of infection. The mechanisms are uncertain and may relate to direct infection of the liver, endotoxin production, or hemolysis [94].

3 Acalculous cholecystitis is a cause of jaundice in hospitalized patients, especially after vascular surgery, trauma, or burns. The mortality is high, usually related to comorbid conditions. Proposed etiological mechanisms include bile stasis, infection, and gallbladder ischemia. Patients affected are often volume depleted, receiving opiates and hyperalimentation. A high index of suspicion is necessary in a hospitalized patient with right upper quadrant pain, fever, leukocytosis, and cholestatic hepatic biochemical abnormalities. Ultrasound is usually the favored and feasible imaging study, and typical sonographic features include a thickened wall, pericholecystic fluid, intramural gas, and sloughed mucosal membrane [95]. Treatment should consist of antibiotics and possible cholecystostomy.

Any evaluation of postoperative jaundice should include a careful review of the operative notes, blood products requirements, microbiology culture results, and medications. In patients with cholestasis, an ultrasound interrogation of the biliary tree should be performed.

Cholestasis after liver transplantation

Cholestasis occurring after liver transplantation may be categorized as related to conditions occurring early (within 6 months of transplantation) or late (after 6 months from transplantation), although overlap may occur [96,97]. Early cholestasis may be related to the condition of the donor liver, vascular and biliary problems, infections, and acute rejection. Functional cholestasis related to donor liver preservation injury (cold or rewarming ischemia or reperfusion injury) peaks between 10 and 16 days postoperatively and usually resolves with supportive management. Prolonged ischemia, especially cold type, is associated with an increased risk of later biliary strictures. Bacterial infection may result in cholestasis and mandates a systematic evaluation of potential sources, particularly the biliary tree. Cholestasis may result from viral infection, especially by cytomegalovirus, chiefly within 3 months of transplantation. Direct viral culture, the faster shell vial culture technique, or histological documentation of the cytopathic effects and microabscesses may confirm the diagnosis. Most transplant recipients experience at least one episode of acute cellular rejection, although a predominant cholestatic pattern of liver enzyme abnormalities is uncommon. Complex drug regimens used after transplantation predispose to drug-related cholestasis. Cyclosporine (ciclosporin), tacrolimus, and azathioprine (but not mycophenolate mofetil) have been implicated, in addition to sulfonamides. The integrity of the bile ducts depends on the hepatic arterial supply. Subacute or incomplete hepatic arterial thrombosis can result in chronic ductal ischemia, bacteremia from cholangitis, and ultimately nonanastomotic biliary strictures.

Cholestasis after 6 months may result from chronic rejection, recurrent disease, and bile duct damage. Chronic rejection is characterized histologically by bile duct atrophy and loss leading to progressive cholestasis and graft failure that is unresponsive to antirejection therapy. Primary biliary cirrhosis may recur in 17% of patients [98]. Fibrosing cholestatic hepatitis is an early aggressive posttransplantation form of recurrent viral hepatitis, especially hepatitis B and C. It rapidly leads to graft failure and is characterized histologically by intrahepatic cholestasis with perisinusoidal fibrosis and minimal inflammation [99]. Risk factors for severe recurrent hepatitis C include advanced donor age and ischemia time, high pretransplantation viral load, type of immunosuppression, treatment of acute cellular rejection, and cytomegalovirus (CMV) infection [100]. Retransplantation in this setting is controversial.

Diagnostic approach

Figures 22.2 and 22.3 depict algorithms intended to be useful in the differential diagnosis and evaluation of a patient with jaundice, respectively. The initial step is to determine whether the jaundice is conjugated or unconjugated. The causes of conjugated hyperbilirubinemia range anatomically from the ampulla of Vater to the hepatocyte. If the history and physical examination do not provide a clue to the cause, the initial

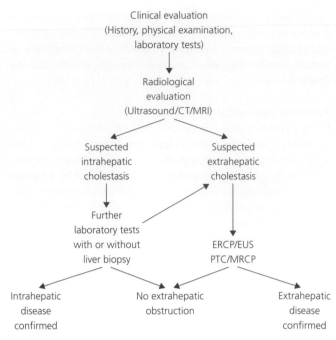

Figure 22.3 The evaluation of the jaundiced patient. CT, computed tomography; EUS, endoscopic ultrasound; ERCP, endoscopic retrograde cholangiopancreatography; MRCP, magnetic resonance cholangiopancreatography; MRI, magnetic resonance imaging; PTC, percutaneous transhepatic cholangiography.

approach should be a right upper quadrant ultrasound scan to evaluate the liver, the biliary system, and the porta hepatis.

History

A family history of liver disease, alcohol and drug history, sexual history, transfusion history, and nutrition history are important clues to the possible cause of hyperbilirubinemia. Exposure to environmental toxins, persons with jaundice, drugs (e.g., prescription, nonprescription, intravenous drugs and nutritional herbal supplements), and outbreaks or epidemics in the community should be sought. Previous liver biochemical tests are valuable, as is a history of biliary or pancreatic disease.

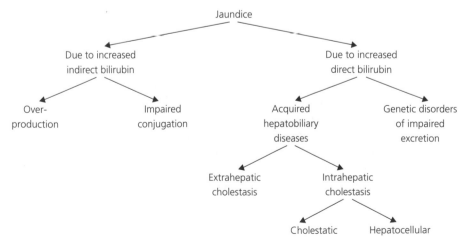

Figure 22.2 Differential diagnosis of the jaundiced patient.

Constitutional symptoms, such as fever, chills, weight loss, and flu-like symptoms, are also important clues. For instance, shaking chills or fevers point toward cholangitis or bacterial infection and should steer the clinician away from viral hepatitis. Abdominal pain may indicate pancreatic disease, especially if it radiates to the back, but it is otherwise not helpful [101]. Viral hepatitis can cause a right upper quadrant ache, but it is not usually described as a pain. Weight loss, anorexia, nausea, and vomiting are not helpful signs because most patients with hepatobiliary disease or obstruction have anorexia and some weight loss [25]. The absence of weight loss does not rule out a diagnosis of malignant disease. Pruritus can be associated with intrahepatic cholestasis and biliary obstruction, especially if the latter lasts longer than 3–4 weeks.

The patient's age may be helpful in constructing a differential diagnosis, as discussed earlier. Patients younger than 30 years are more likely to have acute parenchymal disease. Patients older than 65 years are more likely to have stones or malignant diseases. Patients between 30 and 50 years of age are more likely to have chronic liver disease. In general, children and young adults are more likely to have viral hepatitis. Women older than 30 years and men older than 50 years are likely to have biliary tract disease in the form of stones or carcinoma, respectively. In middle adulthood, cirrhosis and drug effects are common causes. Men are more likely to develop cirrhosis secondary to alcohol use, pancreatic cancer, hepatocellular carcinoma, or hemochromatosis. Women are more likely to have primary biliary cirrhosis, gallstones, and chronic active hepatitis.

Physical examination

Physical examination should include examination of the liver and examination for evidence of chronic liver disease and extrahepatic disease. Jaundice is differentiated from other abnormalities in skin color, such as hypercarotenemia, uremic pigmentation, picric acid ingestion, or quinacrine therapy on the basis that only bilirubin stains the sclera, because of its high affinity for elastin [25]. Later, and especially if the jaundice is severe, the skin color can be greenish. The general appearance of the patient may suggest chronic liver disease, with cachexia, muscle wasting, palmar erythema, Dupuytren contracture, leukonychia, parotid enlargement, skin pigmentation, or xanthelasmas. Chest evaluation may reveal gynecomastia, spider nevi, or dilated veins.

The size and consistency of the liver may be helpful. A shrunken, nodular liver may enable the examiner to identify cirrhosis, and a palpable mass may indicate an abscess or malignant tumor. If the liver span is greater than 15 cm, the physician should consider fatty infiltration, congestion, other infiltrative diseases, or malignant disease. Liver tenderness may denote acute disease but is generally not helpful. The presence of a friction rub or bruit suggests malignant disease. A bruit may be found in alcoholic hepatitis and liver cancer. Spider angiomas, palmar erythema, and distended abdominal veins in a patient with jaundice indicate cirrhosis [101]. Ascites in the presence of jaundice usually indicates cirrhosis, although it can be seen with malignant disease and severe acute disease, such as viral or alcoholic hepatitis. Splenomegaly may be seen in patients with infections, infiltrative diseases, congestive heart failure, viral hepatitis, or cirrhosis. A palpable, distended gallbladder suggests biliary obstruction, often malignant in origin. Asterixis is an unusual finding, except in fulminant hepatic failure and end-stage liver disease.

Laboratory tests

Laboratory tests can confirm suspicions formed during the history and physical examination. The clinician must differentiate conjugated from unconjugated hyperbilirubinemia by using total and direct bilirubin assays. Patients with unconjugated hyperbilirubinemia should be evaluated for evidence of hemolysis, which includes a reticulocyte count, examination of the peripheral smear, serum level of lactic dehydrogenase, and haptoglobin levels. An abnormality in any of these values may lead the clinician to look for evidence of ineffective erythropoiesis, such as vitamin B-12 deficiency, lead toxicity, thalassemia, or sideroblastic anemia. When hemolysis is excluded in patients with unconjugated hyperbilirubinemia, most asymptomatic healthy patients have Gilbert syndrome.

For conjugated hyperbilirubinemia, initial serum tests should include assays of serum aminotransferases and alkaline phosphatase. These test results can differentiate hepatocellular from cholestatic disease. Bilirubin levels consistently less than 5 mg/dL are not seen in obstruction, unless early, but they are common in patients with cirrhosis [101]. Bilirubin levels greater than 20 mg/dL in the presence of normal renal function, especially in elderly patients, should make the clinician suspect malignant biliary obstruction.

Although neither aspartate aminotransferase nor alanine aminotransferase levels are specific for liver disease, they rarely rise to more than 300 IU/mL in any other diseases [25]. An acute myocardial infarction can raise the serum aspartate aminotransferase level because of necrotic cardiac muscle. In a jaundiced patient, serum aminotransferase levels less than 300 IU/mL are seen in alcoholic hepatitis and drug-induced injury, although these levels also are seen in chronic liver disease and obstruction. Levels greater than 400 IU/mL indicate hepatocellular injury, and levels greater than 1000 IU/mL usually indicate acute hepatitis, drug hepatotoxicity, or prolonged hypotension. A level of serum alanine aminotransferase greater than the aspartate aminotransferase level suggests viral hepatitis or nonalcoholic steatohepatitis.

Second-line tests for jaundice help to evaluate the patient for evidence of obstruction and exclusion of bone disease (e.g., γ-glutamyltransferase, 5′-nucleotidase, leucine aminopeptidase), specific liver diseases (e.g., antimitochondrial antibody, hepatitis serologies, α₁-antitrypsin, iron levels, ceruloplasmin), malignant disease (e.g., α-fetoprotein), and autoimmune phenomena (e.g., immunoglobulins, sedimentation rate, antinuclear antibody). Bile acids are increased in virtually all forms of hepatobiliary disease and are not usually useful in determining the cause of jaundice (except in inherited disorders of bilirubin metabolism, when they are normal).

The alkaline phosphatase level can signal the cause of hyperbilirubinemia. If the alkaline phosphatase level is normal, extrahepatic obstruction is unlikely, with the exception of early acute obstruction [101]. If the alkaline phosphatase level is more than three times the upper limit of normal, cholestasis or extrahepatic obstruction probably exists. The level of alkaline phosphatase may be elevated disproportionately compared with bilirubin in partial biliary obstruction or early intrahepatic cholestasis (e.g., primary biliary cirrhosis or primary sclerosing cholangitis) because the large reserve of nonobstructed parenchyma remains intact to excrete bilirubin. The elevation in alkaline phosphatase and bile acids reflects enzyme shedding in the hepatocyte and altered permeability in the biliary tree [2,102]. If the alkaline phosphatase and bilirubin levels are markedly elevated, a common bile duct stone should be excluded. Therefore, the alkaline phosphatase level is a more sensitive test for biliary obstruction than bilirubin.

Bilirubin remains normal until most of the bile ducts are obstructed. γ-Glutamyltransferase is found in the liver, pancreas, heart, and lungs and its plasma concentration is raised in a multitude of disorders. It is elevated in patients with hepatobiliary disease, alcohol intake, pancreatitis, chronic lung disease, renal failure, diabetes, and congestive heart failure and as a result of a variety of drugs.

Albumin levels and prothrombin time should be determined to assess liver function. Protein levels help to differentiate acute from chronic liver disease. Elevated globulin with hypoalbuminemia supports the diagnosis of cirrhosis, as does failure of the prothrombin time to correct after oral or parenteral administration of vitamin K. A trial of vitamin K should be given and administered parenterally to ensure adequate absorption. Hypercholesterolemia is often seen in patients with cholestasis.

Urine tests that signal cholestasis or elevated bilirubin include urinary urobilinogen and urinary conjugated bilirubin. In acute hyperbilirubinemia, jaundice can lag behind bilirubinuria [25]. The renal threshold for conjugated bilirubin is 1 mg/dL, which is less than that needed to produce clinical jaundice. False-positive urine test results occur with salicylates and phenothiazines, and false-negative results occur if the urine is not analyzed promptly. A positive urine test result is a sensitive indicator of conjugated hyperbilirubinemia and should prompt further investigation [103].

Noninvasive tests

After the history has been taken, physical examination performed, and laboratory test results obtained, an informed choice must be made regarding further diagnostic tests. These tests incur substantial cost and therefore should not be ordered indiscriminately for any abnormal biochemistry value. These diagnostic tests can be invasive or noninvasive. Noninvasive tests include ultrasound, computed tomography (CT), magnetic resonance imaging (MRI), and technetium 99 (^{99}Tc) scans.

Ultrasound

Ultrasound is the first test used to detect biliary obstruction. Ultrasound is of low cost, widely available, noninvasive, and easy to perform. The diagnostic accuracy ranges from 77% to 94%, and the result is most accurate when the bilirubin level exceeds 10 mg/dL. In a comparative study of 131 patients, ultrasound had a diagnostic accuracy of 80% with a sensitivity of 71% and specificity of 96% for cholelithiasis [104], with less reported accuracy in the distal common bile duct and in obese patients. In cases of acute obstruction, it may take 4 h to 4 days for ducts to dilate, and the ducts of some patients with partial or intermittent obstruction may not dilate. Not all patients with dilated ducts have obstruction; conversely, between 24% and 40% of patients with common bile duct stones have normal-sized bile ducts. The variability in sensitivity reflects limitations from overlying bowel gas, obesity, site and size of the stones, and presence or absence of duct dilation. Ultrasound is inconsistent in determining the site of obstruction, partly because of its inability to see the distal duct well in 30%–50% of patients [105,106]. Despite these caveats and the fact that ultrasound is operator dependent, it remains the preferred initial screening test for evaluating biliary obstruction.

Computed tomography

CT imaging has a sensitivity of 60%–90% and results rely less on the operator's proficiency. CT is not impeded by fat. However, CT scanning is more expensive than ultrasound and requires intravenous contrast medium in many instances. Unless the patient is obese, ultrasound should be the initial test of choice [104,107].

Magnetic resonance imaging

MRI relies on the physical properties of unpaired protons in tissues to generate images, without use of ionizing radiation [108,109]. MRI is generally insufficiently sensitive or specific in the assessment of diffuse liver disease, except for the assessment of fat and iron. It appears that MRI is more sensitive and specific than CT with contrast for the detection and evaluation of focal and malignant lesions. Using the tissue contrast inherent in the technique, MRI avoids the potentially nephrotoxic contrast agents used with CT imaging. This is particularly relevant in patients with jaundice or cholestasis. The MRI characteristics of stationary and mobile liquids makes MR cholangiopancreatography (MRCP) and MR angiography powerful noninvasive diagnostic tools. Bile duct calculi are seen particularly well with MRCP, and this technique should be used in patients with negative sonography and a high index of suspicion [104]. With MRI, imaging of the biliary tree is feasible both proximal and distal to the site of obstruction. MRCP is more accurate than ultrasound in disease staging and evaluation of distal common bile duct lesions. Use of ultrasound and MRCP has decreased the use of diagnostic ERCP and aided in directing patients to therapeutic ERCP or surgery.

Radiolabeled technetium–sulfur colloid

This sulfur colloid is rapidly taken up by the reticuloendothelial system. Radionuclide imaging with hepatic iminodiacetic acid scan (HIDA) is a good method for detecting cystic duct obstruction and is the test of choice if acute cholecystitis with cystic duct obstruction or biliary leakage is suspected. However, it has little value in differentiating intrahepatic from extrahepatic causes of cholestasis and is rarely used for diagnosis of cholestasis.

Invasive tests

Invasive tests used include ERCP, percutaneous transhepatic cholangiography (PTC), endoscopic ultrasound (EUS), and liver biopsy. ERCP and PTC use cholecystographic dye and radiography to visualize the biliary tree. They are excellent tests to verify ductal dilation and permit concomitant therapeutic intervention.

PTC visualizes the biliary tree in 90%–100% of patients with dilated ducts and localizes the site of obstruction in 90% of cases. To perform the test safely, PTC usually requires a prothrombin time of less than 16 s, a platelet count greater than 50 000, and the absence of ascites. Minor complications occur in 30% of patients. Major complications, including sepsis, bleeding, biliary leak, pneumothorax, arteriovenous fistula, hematoma, abscess, and peritonitis, occur in 1%–10% of patients who undergo PTC.

ERCP can localize the site of obstruction in more than 90% of patients. It is particularly helpful in diagnosing patients with common duct stones. Because it has therapeutic capabilities, it allows some patients to avoid surgery. ERCP is also helpful if a stricture resulting from chronic pancreatitis is suspected. The major reasons for nonvisualization of the biliary tree during ERCP are prior surgery (e.g., Roux-en-Y loop) and an inability to cannulate the sphincter of Oddi. The morbidity rate is 2%–3%, somewhat less than with PTC. The most common complications are pancreatitis, bleeding, and cholangitis. The rate of sepsis is less than 1% if prophylactic antibiotics are given when an obstruction is suspected.

EUS combines endoscopy with real-time, high-resolution ultrasound and provides excellent sonographic visualization of the biliary tree without bowel gas interference. EUS is superior to ultrasound and CT for diagnosing bile duct stones [110]. EUS is comparably accurate but safer and less expensive than ERCP when evaluating patients with suspected choledocholithiasis. If available, EUS should be considered, particularly if there is a contraindication to ERCP or if prior ERCP was unsuccessful [111]. The widespread use of EUS has altered the diagnostic approach and management of extrahepatic biliary obstruction [112], especially obstruction caused by extrabiliary disease, permitting real-time imaging and sonographic-guided sampling. Deciding among ERCP, PTC, or EUS should depend on the presumed site of obstruction, the presence of coagulopathy or ascites, and the local expertise of the radiologists and gastroenterologists [113]. PTC and ERCP rarely are used in combination. Benign strictures should be differentiated from cholangiocarcinoma, which often requires cytological analysis or biopsy of the lesion.

Liver biopsy

If high-grade extrahepatic obstruction has been excluded or hepatocellular disease is strongly suspected, a liver biopsy should be performed [114]. Liver biopsy can correct 20% of errors in clinical diagnosis. Liver biopsy kits usually include the Jamshidi (suction) needle, Klatskin needle, or Tru-Cut needle. Complications after liver biopsy occur with an incidence ranging from 0.1% to 3.0% [115]. The liver biopsy complications warranting hospital admission include pain, hypotension, hemoperitoneum, hemobilia, pneumothorax or hemothorax, and intrahepatic arteriovenous fistula. Overall, this is a safe procedure, but the risk-to-benefit ratio needs to be carefully assessed and explained to the patient. The use of ultrasound before the procedure may reduce the complication rate [116]. Patients with coagulopathy, thrombocytopenia, or ascites may require blood products or an alternative route for biopsy, such as the transjugular approach [117]. For patients with renal insufficiency or patients who were taking warfarin (Coumadin), an ultrasound-guided liver biopsy with desmopressin acetate or a gelatin foam plug may reduce the risk of serious bleeding complications.

In the workup of a patient with hyperbilirubinemia, a liver biopsy can be useful if other diagnostic tests are unrevealing. This diagnostic strategy is essential. If the ERCP result is nondiagnostic, a liver biopsy should be performed. Five percent of the cases of extrahepatic cholestasis are diagnosed by liver biopsy because of inadequate clinical suspicion of obstruction or an inability to visualize the ducts adequately [118]. For 15% of cases, a liver biopsy is not helpful in determining the cause of the hyperbilirubinemia. If the clinician's level of suspicion is high but the ultrasound scan is negative, a cholangiogram should be performed.

The decision tree that the clinician follows depends to a great extent on pretest probability (see Fig. 22.3). If there is a low suspicion of extrahepatic obstruction and the ultrasound scan is negative, further evaluation of possible dilated ducts probably is not warranted and intrahepatic disease would be assessed with liver biopsy. Clinical instinct should not be ignored, however, if the radiographic tests do not confirm the physician's suspicions, and further assessment with MRCP or CT should be performed. Judgment based on the patient's history and physical examination is required in evaluating patients with jaundice. Diagnostic accuracy with subsequent adequate care relies on the judicious use of appropriate confirmatory tests and radiographic studies.

Complications of cholestasis

Pruritus

Pruritus is commonly associated with cholestasis and may limit activity, cause anxiety, disturb sleep patterns, and result in secondary skin infection. The presence and severity of pruritus in cholestasis do not necessarily correlate with the degree of cholestasis and may have genetic influences. The pathogenesis of cholestasis-associated pruritus is uncertain. Formerly it was proposed that accumulated endogenous pruritogens of cholestasis interacting with cutaneous nerve endings were implicated. More recently, the concept that pruritus is of central origin, mediated by endogenous opioid or serotonin ligands, has been largely accepted [119]. Conventional agents have not been adequately or objectively evaluated using reliable and validated outcome measures, but they are generally safe, modestly effective, and usually the agents of first choice. Studies using objective quantitative behavioral methodologies have suggested the efficacy of opioid antagonists [120,121]. Table 22.2 outlines current management options for pruritus.

Hepatic osteodystrophy

Hepatic osteodystrophy is the metabolic bone disease that occurs in patients with chronic liver disease, particularly cholestatic disease, and can lead to pain and immobility as a result of the development of fractures [122,123]. Hepatic osteodystrophy can encompass both osteoporosis and osteomalacia, although the former is dominant. Risk factors for osteoporosis include the following: older age, female gender, Caucasian race, low body mass index, immobility, prolonged corticosteroid use, excessive alcohol intake, and cigarette smoking. Cholestatic liver disease and the presence of cirrhosis are associated with more severe disease. The roles of vitamin D receptor polymorphisms, osteoblast trophic factors such as insulin-like growth factor type I, and osteoprotegerin, an osteoclast regulator, are being actively explored [124]. Whereas calcium and vitamin D metabolism is often altered, especially in cholestatic liver disease, bone mineralization appears unaffected [125]. The management of hepatic osteodystrophy is outlined in Table 22.3. Bone mineral density assessment using dual-energy X-ray absorptiometry (DEXA) is used to screen for fracture risk and should be performed in all patients with cirrhosis and especially with cholestatic

---

Table 22.2 Management of pruritus of cholestasis

Topical therapy
Lower bathing water temperature and use fewer or lighter clothes and bed coverings
Minimize dry skin by using moisturizing soaps (e.g., Dove) and applying topical moisturizers liberally (e.g., Eucerin cream)

Anion-exchange resins
Cholestyramine or colestipol: start with 4 g (one scoop or packet) p.o. twice daily, starting before and after breakfast, and increasing to six packets or scoops daily, separated from other medications by 2 h (esp. ursodeoxycholic acid)

Bile salts
Ursodeoxycholic acid, 15 mg/kg/day p.o.

Doxepin
25–50 mg p.o. daily taken at night

Hepatic microsomal enzyme induction
Rifampin, 150 mg p.o., two to three times daily

Opioid receptor antagonists
Naltrexone, 12.5 mg p.o. daily, increasing slowly to 50 mg p.o. daily
Naloxone and nalmefene are only commonly available for parenteral use

---

Table 22.3 Management of hepatic osteodystrophy

Baseline DEXA scanning

Normal (T score):	< 1 SD below the mean
Osteopenia:	1–2.5 SD below the mean
Osteoporosis:	> 2.5 SD below the mean or one or more fragility fractures (thoracolumbar radiographs should be performed to screen for compression fractures)

Laboratory testing
Baseline: 25-OH vitamin D level (normal range 10–55 mg/mL), calcium, phosphate, thyroid function tests, intact parathyroid hormone (free serum testosterone in men and estradiol and luteinizing hormone in women)

Treatment
(Relative contraindication: patients with history of renal stones)
Adequate calcium (1–1.5 g per day), protein calorie nutrition and regular exercise
Before transplantation: calcidiol (Calderol), 20–50 µg three times weekly
After transplantation: calcidiol (Calderol), 20–50 µg weekly
If coexistent renal disease: calcitriol (Rocaltrol), 0.25–0.5 µg p.o.,
Estrogen replacement (if no contraindications exist) or selective estrogen receptor modulators
If bone density worsens rapidly or if there is evidence of osteoporosis or symptomatic fractures, treat with bisphosphonates or calcitonin

Monitoring
DEXA
For osteoporosis: repeat 6 months after treatment initiated and then yearly
For normal study: repeat every 2 years
Repeat 25-OH vitamin D and 24-h urine calcium yearly and treat accordingly

---

DEXA, dual-energy X-ray absorptiometry; SD, standard deviation.

Table 22.4 Management of fat-soluble vitamin deficiency in prolonged cholestasis

Monitoring fat-soluble vitamins

25-OH vitamin D level (normal range 10–55 mg/mL). If renal disease, check 1,25-(OH)$_2$ vitamin D

Vitamin A level (normal range 360–1200 µg/L)

Vitamin E level, with fasting total lipid profile (normal range 5.5–17.0 mg/L). Total lipids = cholesterol plus triglycerides (in grams). To calculate vitamin E level: serum vitamin E (mg)/ total lipid (g). If ≥ 0.8, normal; if < 0.6, supplement

Vitamin K: measure prothrombin time (normal range 11.4–13.2 s)

Replacement

Vitamin D: calcium, 1–1.5 g p.o. per day

Calcidiol (Calderol) 20–50 µg p.o., three times weekly, before transplantation. If coexistent renal disease, use calcitriol (Rocaltrol) 0.25–0.5 µg p.o. daily

Vitamin A: β-carotene 15 mg (25 000 U vitamin A) p.o., q.i.d., or Aquasol A 50 000 U i.m., daily for 2 weeks

Vitamin E: liquid E (D-α-tocopherol), water-soluble, 100 IU p.o., daily

Vitamin K: 10 mg subcutaneously daily, for 3 days, then monthly if cholestatic

ADEK p.o. 1–2 daily

Evaluation of therapy

After 3 months: 24-h urine calcium (normal range 50–250 mg/day)

Yearly: 25-OH vitamin D (1,25-(OH)$_2$ vitamin D if renal disease), vitamins A and E, and prothrombin time

liver disease [123]. Despite limited data, it would appear that intervention with antiresorptive medications, especially bisphosphonates, is indicated for those with symptomatic fractures or confirmed osteoporosis based on bone density measurement [126]. The rate of bone loss increases rapidly in the first 6 months after liver transplantation – this may be reduced by the use of intravenous bisphosphonates such as zeledronic acid [127].

Fat-soluble vitamin deficiency

This condition is common in patients with prolonged cholestasis, and management is outlined in Table 22.4. Oral or parenteral vitamin replacement will depend on the extent of deficiency and response to therapy. Care should be taken to inform patients of the risks and benefits of therapy, including the need for assessment of hypercalcuria after therapeutic intervention.

References

1. Bissell DM. Heme catabolism and bilirubin formation. In: Ostrow JD (ed.). Bile pigments and jaundice. New York: Marcel Dekker, 1986; 133.
2. Sherlock S. Overview of chronic cholestatic conditions in adults: terminology and definitions. Clin Liver Dis 1998;2:217,vii.
3. Duffy MC, Boyer JL. Pathophysiology of intrahepatic cholestasis and biliary obstruction. In: Ostrow JD (ed.). Bile pigments and jaundice. New York: Marcel Dekker, 1986;333.
4. Wulkan RW, Leijnse B. Alkaline phosphatase and cholestasis. Ann Clin Biochem 1986;23:405.
5. Hofmann AF. The continuing importance of bile acids in liver and intestinal disease. Arch Intern Med 1999;159:2647.
6. Carey MC, Spivak W. Physical chemistry of bile pigments and porphyrins with particular reference to bile. In: Ostrow JD (ed.). Bile pigments and jaundice. New York: Marcel Dekker, 1986;81.
7. Blanckaert N, Heirwegh KPM. Analysis and preparation of bilirubins and biliverdins. In: Ostrow JD (ed.). Bile pigments and jaundice. New York: Marcel Dekker, 1986;31.
8. Berk PD. Structure, formation, and sources of bilirubin and its transport in plasma. Semin Liver Dis 1994;14:325.
9. Berlin NI. Overproduction of bilirubin. In: Ostrow JD (ed.). Bile pigments and jaundice. New York: Marcel Dekker, 1986;271.
10. Brodersen R. Aqueous solubility, albumin binding, and tissue distribution of bilirubin. In: Ostrow JD (ed.). Bile pigments and jaundice. New York: Marcel Dekker, 1986;157.
11. Dennery PA, Seidman DS, Stevenson DK. Neonatal hyperbilirubinemia. N Engl J Med 2001;344:581.
12. Sorrentino D, Zifroni A, van Ness K, Berk PD. Unbound ligand drives hepatocyte taurocholate and BSP uptake at physiological albumin concentration. Am J Physiol 1994;266:G425.
13. Trauner M, Meier PJ, Boyer JL. Molecular pathogenesis of cholestasis. N Engl J Med 1998;339:1217.
14. Berk PD. Hepatic uptake, binding, conjugation, and excretion of bilirubin. Semin Liver Dis 1994;14:331.
15. Fevery J, Blanckaert N, Heirwegh KP, et al. Unconjugated bilirubin and an increased proportion of bilirubin monoconjugates in the bile of patients with Gilbert's syndrome and Crigler-Najjar disease. J Clin Invest 1977;60:970.
16. Iyanagi T, Emi Y, Ikushiro S. Biochemical and molecular aspects of genetic disorders of bilirubin metabolism. Biochim Biophys Acta 1998;1407:173.
17. Berk PD. Bile pigments in the gastrointestinal tract and urine. Semin Liver Dis 1994;14:344.
18. Powell LW. Clinical aspects of unconjugated hyperbilirubinemia. Semin Hematol 1972;9:91.
19. Berk PD. Clinical chemistry and physiology of bilirubin. Semin Liver Dis 1994;14:346.
20. Muraca M, Fevery J, Blanckaert N. Analytic aspects and clinical interpretation of serum bilirubins. Semin Liver Dis 1988;8:137.
21. Westwood A. The analysis of bilirubin in serum. Ann Clin Biochem 1991;28:119.
22. Fukunaga FH. Delta bilirubin. Hawaii Med J 1989;48:302.
23. Weiss JS, Gautam A, Lauff JJ, et al. The clinical importance of a protein-bound fraction of serum bilirubin in patients with hyperbilirubinemia. N Engl J Med 1983;309:147.
24. Wu TW, Dappen GM, Spayd RW, et al. The Ektachem clinical chemistry slide for simultaneous determination of unconjugated and sugar-conjugated bilirubin. Clin Chem 1984;30:1304.
25. Lumeng L, O'Connor KW. Differential diagnosis of jaundice. In: Ostrow JD (ed.). Bile pigments and jaundice. New York: Marcel Dekker, 1986;475.
26. Berk PD. The familial unconjugated hyperbilirubinemias. Semin Liver Dis 1994;14:356.
27. Tukey RH, Strassburg CP. Human UDP-glucuronosyltransferases: metabolism, expression, and disease. Annu Rev Pharmacol Toxicol 2000;40:581.
28. Burchell B, Hume R. Molecular genetic basis of Gilbert's syndrome. J Gastroenterol Hepatol 1999;14:960.
29. Wasserman E, Myara A, Lokiec F, et al. Severe CPT-11 toxicity in patients with Gilbert's syndrome: two case reports. Ann Oncol 1997; 8:1049.
30. Zucker SD, Qin X, Rouster SD, Yu F, et al. Mechanism of indinavir-induced hyperbilirubinemia. Proc Natl Acad Sci USA 2001;98: 12671.

31. Jansen PL. Diagnosis and management of Crigler-Najjar syndrome. Eur J Pediatr 1999;158(Suppl. 2):S89.

32. Fox IJ, Chowdhury JR, Kaufman SS, et al. Treatment of the Crigler-Najjar syndrome type I with hepatocyte transplantation. N Engl J Med 1998;338:1422.

33. Berk PD. The familial conjugated hyperbilirubinemias. Semin Liver Dis 1994;14:386.

34. Toh S, Wada M, Uchiumi T, et al. Genomic structure of the canalicular multispecific organic anion-transporter gene (MRP2/cMOAT) and mutations in the ATP-binding-cassette region in Dubin-Johnson syndrome. Am J Hum Genet 1999;64:739.

35. Bezerra JA, Balistreri WF. Cholestatic syndromes of infancy and childhood. Semin Gastrointest Dis 2001;12:54.

36. Jacquemin E. Progressive familial intrahepatic cholestasis. Genetic basis and treatment. Clin Liver Dis 2000;4:753.

37. Bull LN, van Eijk MJ, Pawlikowska L, et al. A gene encoding a P-type ATPase mutated in two forms of hereditary cholestasis. Nat Genet 1998;18:219.

38. Brenard R, Geubel AP, Benhamou JP. Benign recurrent intrahepatic cholestasis. A report of 26 cases. J Clin Gastroenterol 1989;11:546.

39. van Mil SW, van der Woerd WL, van der BG, et al. Benign recurrent intrahepatic cholestasis type 2 is caused by mutations in ABCB11. Gastroenterology 2004;127:379.

40. Klomp LW, Vargas JC, van Mil SW, et al. Characterization of mutations in ATP8B1 associated with hereditary cholestasis. Hepatology 2004;40:27.

41. Strautnieks SS, Bull LN, Knisely AS, et al. A gene encoding a liver-specific ABC transporter is mutated in progressive familial intrahepatic cholestasis. Nat Genet 1998;20:233.

42. Deleuze JF, Jacquemin E, Dubuisson C, et al. Defect of multidrug-resistance 3 gene expression in a subtype of progressive familial intrahepatic cholestasis. Hepatology 1996;23:904.

43. Gordon SC, Reddy KR, Schiff L, Schiff ER. Prolonged intrahepatic cholestasis secondary to acute hepatitis A. Ann Intern Med 1984;101:635.

44. Tung BY, Carithers RL, Jr. Cholestasis and alcoholic liver disease. Clin Liver Dis 1999;3:585.

45. Angulo P, Lindor KD. Primary biliary cirrhosis and primary sclerosing cholangitis. Clin Liver Dis 1999;3:529.

46. Vierling JM. Autoimmune cholangiopathy. Clin Liver Dis 1999;3:571.

47. Lewis JH, Zimmerman HJ. Drug- and chemical-induced cholestasis. Clin Liver Dis 1999;3:433,vii.

48. Rowbotham D, Wendon J, Williams R. Acute liver failure secondary to hepatic infiltration: a single centre experience of 18 cases. Gut 1998;42:576.

49. Devaney K, Goodman ZD, Epstein MS, et al. Hepatic sarcoidosis. Clinicopathologic features in 100 patients. Am J Surg Pathol 1993;17:1272.

50. Sartin JS, Walker RC. Granulomatous hepatitis: a retrospective review of 88 cases at the Mayo Clinic. Mayo Clin Proc 1991;66:914.

51. Rockey DC. Striking cholestatic liver disease: a distinct manifestation of advanced primary amyloidosis. South Med J 1999;92:236.

52. Fogarty BJ, Parks RW, Rowlands BJ, Diamond T. Renal dysfunction in obstructive jaundice. Br J Surg 1995;82:877.

53. Green J, Better OS. Systemic hypotension and renal failure in obstructive jaundice – mechanistic and therapeutic aspects. J Am Soc Nephrol 1995;5:1853.

54. Dourakis SP, Sinani C, Deutsch M, et al. Cholestatic jaundice as a paraneoplastic manifestation of renal cell carcinoma. Eur J Gastroenterol Hepatol 1997;9:311.

55. Cunha BA. Systemic infections affecting the liver. Some cause jaundice, some do not. Postgrad Med 1988;84:148,166.

56. Moseley RH. Sepsis and cholestasis. Clin Liver Dis 2004;8:83.

57. Moseley RH. Mechanisms of bile formation and cholestasis: clinical significance of recent experimental work. Am J Gastroenterol 1986;81:731.

58. Franson TR, Hierholzer WJ, Jr, LaBrecque DR. Frequency and characteristics of hyperbilirubinemia associated with bacteremia. Rev Infect Dis 1985;7:1.

59. Lefkowitch JH. The liver in AIDS. Semin Liver Dis 1997;17:335.

60. Poles MA. HIV-related hepatic disease: when and why to biopsy. Gastrointest Endosc Clin N Am 1998;8:939.

61. Wasserheit C, Acaba L, Gulati S. Abnormal liver function in patients undergoing autologous bone marrow transplantation for hematological malignancies. Cancer Invest 1995;13:347.

62. Quigley EMM, Marsh MN, Shaffer JL, Markin RS. Hepatobiliary complications of total parenteral nutrition. Gastro 1993;104:286.

63. Kelly DA. Intestinal failure-associated liver disease: what do we know today? Gastroenterology 2006;130:S70.

64. Alpers DH. Liver complications and failure in patients on home parenteral nutrition. Curr Opin Gastroenterol 2001;17:147.

65. Angelico M, Della GP. Review article: hepatobiliary complications associated with total parenteral nutrition. Aliment Pharmacol Ther 2000;14(Suppl. 2):54.

66. Sandhu IS, Jarvis C, Everson GT. Total parenteral nutrition and cholestasis. Clin Liver Dis 1999;3:489,viii.

67. Elias E. Clinical and biochemical diagnosis of jaundice. Baillière Clin Gastr 1989;3:357.

68. Frank BB. Clinical evaluation of jaundice. A guideline of the patient care committee of the American Gastroenterological Association. JAMA 1989;262:3031.

69. Olen R, Pickleman J, Freeark RJ. Less is better. The diagnostic workup of the patient with obstructive jaundice. Arch Surg 1989;124:791.

70. Berk PD. Practice parameter: management of hyperbilirubinemia in the healthy term newborn. American Academy of Pediatrics. Provisional Committee for Quality Improvement and Subcommittee on Hyperbilirubinemia. Pediatrics 1994;94:558.

71. Lee K-S, Gartner LM. Fetal bilirubin metabolism and neonatal jaundice. In: Ostrow JD (ed.). Bile pigments and jaundice. New York: Marcel Dekker, 1986;373.

72. Gourley GR. Bilirubin metabolism and kernicterus. Adv Pediatr 1997;44:173.

73. Newman TB, Maisels MJ. Less aggressive treatment of neonatal jaundice and reports of kernicterus: lessons about practice guidelines. Pediatrics 2000;105:242.

74. el Youssef M, Whitington PF. Diagnostic approach to the child with hepatobiliary disease. Semin Liver Dis 1998;18:195.

75. Ohi R. Surgery for biliary atresia. Liver 2001;21:175.

76. Crosnier C, Lykavieris P, Meunier-Rotival M, Hadchouel M. Alagille syndrome. The widening spectrum of arteriohepatic dysplasia. Clin Liver Dis 2000;4:765.

77. Yuan ZR, Kobayashi N, Kohsaka T. Human Jagged 1 mutants cause liver defect in Alagille syndrome by overexpression of hepatocyte growth factor. J Mol Biol 2006;356:559.

78. Wolf JL. Liver disease in pregnancy. Med Clin North Am 1996;80:1167.

79. Knox TA, Olans LB. Liver disease in pregnancy. N Engl J Med 1996;335:569.

80. Riely CA. Liver disease in the pregnant patient. American College of Gastroenterology. Am J Gastroenterol 1999;94:1728.

81. Knox TA. Evaluation of abnormal liver function in pregnancy. Semin Perinatol 1998;22:98.

82. Davidson KM. Intrahepatic cholestasis of pregnancy. Semin Perinatol 1998;22:104.

83. Lammert F, Marschall HU, Glantz A, Matern S. Intrahepatic cholestasis of pregnancy: molecular pathogenesis, diagnosis and management. J Hepatol 2000;33:1012.

84. Heikkinen J, Maentausta O, Ylostalo P, Janne O. Changes in serum bile acid concentrations during normal pregnancy, in patients with intrahepatic cholestasis of pregnancy and in pregnant women with itching. Br J Obstet Gynaecol 1981;88:240.

85. Palma J, Reyes H, Ribalta J, et al. Ursodeoxycholic acid in the treatment of cholestasis of pregnancy: a randomized, double-blind study controlled with placebo. J Hepatol 1997;27:1022.

86. Meng LJ, Reyes H, Palma J, et al. Effects of ursodeoxycholic acid on conjugated bile acids and progesterone metabolites in serum and urine of patients with intrahepatic cholestasis of pregnancy. J Hepatol 1997;27:1029.

87. Elias E. URSO in obstetric cholestasis: not a bear market. Gut 1999;45:331.

88. Pereira SP, O'Donohue J, Wendon J, Williams R. Maternal and perinatal outcome in severe pregnancy-related liver disease. Hepatology 1997;26:1258.

89. Ibdah JA, Bennett MJ, Rinaldo P, et al. A fetal fatty-acid oxidation disorder as a cause of liver disease in pregnant women. N Engl J Med 1999;340:1723.

90. Steven MM, Buckley JD, Mackay IR. Pregnancy in chronic active hepatitis. Quarterly J Med 1979;48:519.

91. Molina EG, Reddy KR. Postoperative jaundice. Clin Liver Dis 1999;3:477.

92. Becker SC, Lamont JT. Postoperative jaundice. Semin Liver Dis 1988;8:183.

93. Zimmerman HJ, Ishak KG. General aspects of drug-induced liver disease. Gastroenterol Clin North Am 1995;24:739. [Review, with 54 refs.]

94. Jansen PL, Muller M. Early events in sepsis-associated cholestasis. Gastroenterology 1999;116:486.

95. Mirvis SE, Vainright JR, Nelson AW, et al. The diagnosis of acute acalculous cholecystitis: a comparison of sonography, scintigraphy, and CT. AJR Am J Roentgenol 1986;147:1171.

96. Heneghan MA, Sylvestre PB. Cholestatic diseases of liver transplantation. Semin Gastrointest Dis 2001;12:133.

97. Heneghan MA. Long-term outcome of hepatitis C infection after liver transplantation. N Engl J Med 1996;335:522.

98. Liermann Garcia RF, Evangelista GC, McMaster P, Neuberger J. Transplantation for primary biliary cirrhosis: retrospective analysis of 400 patients in a single center. Hepatology 2001;33:22.

99. Zylberberg H, Carnot F, Mamzer MF, et al. Hepatitis C virus-related fibrosing cholestatic hepatitis after renal transplantation. Transplantation 1997;63:158.

100. Charlton M. Approach to recurrent hepatitis C following liver transplantation. Curr Gastroenterol Rep 2007;9:23.

101. Schenker S, Balint J, Schiff L. Differential diagnosis of jaundice: report of a prospective study of 61 proved cases. J Dig Dis 1962;7:449.

102. Pellegrini CA, Thomas MJ, Way LW. Bilirubin and alkaline phosphatase values before and after surgery for biliary obstruction. Am J Surg 1982;143:67.

103. Kupka T, Binder LS, Smith DA, et al. Accuracy of urine urobilinogen and bilirubin assays in predicting liver function test abnormalities. Ann Emerg Med 1987;16:1231.

104. Ferrari FS, Fantozzi F, Tasciotti L, et al. US, MRCP, CCT and ERCP: a comparative study in 131 patients with suspected biliary obstruction. Med Sci Monit 2005;11:MT8.

105. Pedrosa CS, Casanova R, Lezana AH, Fernandez MC. Computed tomography in obstructive jaundice. Radiology 1981;139:635.

106. Scott BB, Evans JA, Unsworth J. The initial investigation of jaundice in a district general hospital: a study of ultrasonography and hepatobiliary scintigraphy. Brit J Radiol 1980;53:557.

107. Wolcott JK, Chen PS. Radiologic evaluation of the jaundiced patient.

Diagnostic and therapeutic role of current procedures. Radiol Eval 1988;84:233.

108. Macdonald GA, Peduto AJ. Magnetic resonance imaging and diseases of the liver and biliary tract. Part 2. Magnetic resonance cholangiography and angiography and conclusions. J Gastroenterol Hepatol 2000;15:992.

109. Macdonald GA, Peduto AJ. Magnetic resonance imaging (MRI) and diseases of the liver and biliary tract. Part 1. Basic principles, MRI in the assessment of diffuse and focal hepatic disease. J Gastroenterol Hepatol 2000;15:980.

110. Amouyal P, Amouyal G, Levy P, et al. Diagnosis of choledocholithiasis by endoscopic ultrasonography. Gastroenterology 1994;106: 1062.

111. Canto MI, Chak A, Stellato T, Sivak MV, Jr. Endoscopic ultrasonography versus cholangiography for the diagnosis of choledocholithiasis. Gastrointest Endosc 1998;47:439.

112. Kahaleh M, Hernandez AJ, Tokar J, et al. Interventional EUS-guided cholangiography: evaluation of a technique in evolution. Gastrointest Endosc 2006;64:52.

113. Rubens DJ. Hepatobiliary imaging and its pitfalls. Radiol Clin North Am 2004;42:257.

114. Tobkes AI, Nord HJ. Liver biopsy: review of methodology and complications. Dig Dis 1995;13:267.

115. Janes CH, Lindor KD. Outcome of patients hospitalized for complications after outpatient liver biopsy. Ann Intern Med 1993;118:96.

116. Lindor KD, Bru C, Jorgensen RA, et al. The role of ultrasonography and automatic-needle biopsy in outpatient percutaneous liver biopsy. Hepatology 1996;23:1079.

117. Brenard R, Horsmans Y, Rahier J, et al. Transjugular liver biopsy. An experience based on 500 procedures. Acta Gastroenterol Belg 1997; 60:138.

118. Lindberg G, Nilsson L, Thulin L. Decision theory as an aid in the diagnosis of cholestatic jaundice. Acta Chir Scand 1983;149:521.

119. Bergasa NV. The pruritus of cholestasis. J Hepatol 2005;43:1078.

120. Bergasa NV, Alling DW, Talbot TL, et al. Effects of naloxone infusions in patients with the pruritus of cholestasis. A double-blind, randomized, controlled trial. Ann Intern Med 1995;123:161.

121. Wolfhagen FH, Sternieri E, Hop WC, et al. Oral naltrexone treatment for cholestatic pruritus: a double-blind, placebo-controlled study. Gastroenterology 1997;113:1264.

122. Hay JE. Bone disease in cholestatic liver disease. Gastro 1995;108: 276.

123. Hay JE, Guichelaar MM. Evaluation and management of osteoporosis in liver disease. Clin Liver Dis 2005;9:747,viii.

124. Rouillard S, Lane NE. Hepatic osteodystrophy. Hepatology 2001;33: 301.

125. Guichelaar MM, Malinchoc M, Sibonga J, et al. Bone metabolism in advanced cholestatic liver disease: analysis by bone histomorphometry. Hepatology 2002;36:895.

126. Guanabens N, Pares A, Ros I, et al. Alendronate is more effective than etidronate for increasing bone mass in osteopenic patients with primary biliary cirrhosis. Am J Gastroenterol 2003;98:2268.

127. Crawford BA, Kam C, Pavlovic J, et al. Zoledronic acid prevents bone loss after liver transplantation: a randomized, double-blind, placebo-controlled trial. Ann Intern Med 2006;144:239.

23

Approach to the patient with ascites and its complications

Guadalupe Garcia-Tsao

The patient with suspected ascites, 442

The patient with new-onset ascites, 444

The patient with cirrhosis and ascites, 448

The patient with cirrhosis and hepatic hydrothorax, 455

The patient with spontaneous bacterial peritonitis, 455

The patient with cirrhosis and acute renal failure, 457

The patient with hepatorenal syndrome, 459

Ascites is the accumulation of fluid in the peritoneal cavity. In the Western world, cirrhosis is the main cause of ascites, accounting for more than 75% of the cases (Table 23.1). Other less common causes of ascites are peritoneal malignancy, which accounts for ~ 12%, cardiac failure in 5%, and peritoneal tuberculosis in only 2% of the cases [1], although the latter is still an important cause of ascites in many developing countries. Approximately 5% of patients will have more than one cause of ascites, such as cirrhosis and heart failure, cirrhosis and tuberculous peritonitis, or cirrhosis and malignancy [2].

In patients with cirrhosis, ascites is one of the complications that mark the transition from a compensated to a decompensated stage [3]. Initially, ascites is "uncomplicated," that is, it responds well to diuretics and is not infected. As cirrhosis progresses and the mechanisms that lead to ascites formation worsen, ascites ceases to respond to diuretics (refractory ascites). Bacteria may infect ascites, an entity known as spontaneous bacterial peritonitis (SBP), which occurs mainly in hospitalized patients with severe liver disease. With further progression of cirrhosis, the patient with ascites may develop hyponatremia and functional renal failure (hepatorenal syndrome). The hemodynamic alterations that lead to ascites and refractory ascites are the same as those that lead to hyponatremia and hepatorenal syndrome, differing only in the degree of abnormality, with the latter complications denoting a more deranged circulatory status.

The approach to a patient with ascites depends on the setting surrounding its presentation. In a patient with new-onset ascites, the priority is to determine the etiology of ascites, because this will determine its management. In a patient with ascites caused by cirrhosis, management depends on the phase that the patient has reached, ranging from uncomplicated ascites to hepatorenal syndrome.

The patient with suspected ascites

History and physical examination are important in determining the presence and etiology of ascites, but they are not definitive.

The most frequent symptoms associated with the development of ascites are increased abdominal girth, described as tightness of the belt or garments around the waist, associated with weight gain. However, sometimes weight gain is masked by concomitant loss of muscle mass as a result of cirrhosis or malignancy. The rapid onset of symptoms in a matter of weeks helps to distinguish ascites from obesity, which develops over a period of months to years.

Physical examination is relatively insensitive for detecting ascitic fluid, particularly when the amount is small or the patient is obese. When present in small to moderate amounts

Principles of Clinical Gastroenterology. Edited by Tadataka Yamada, David H. Alpers, Anthony N. Kalloo, Neil Kaplowitz, Chung Owyang, and Don W. Powell. © 2008 Blackwell Publishing. ISBN 978-1-4051-69103

Table 23.1 Etiology of ascites and classification by serum–ascites albumin gradient (SAAG) and ascites protein level

	SAAG	Ascites protein
Main etiological factors of ascites		
Cirrhosis or alcoholic hepatitis	High	Low
Congestive heart failure	High	High
Peritoneal malignancy	Low	High
Peritoneal tuberculosis	Low	High
Other etiologies of cirrhosis (account for < 2% of all cases)		
Massive hepatic metastases	High	Low
Nodular regenerative hyperplasia	High	Low
Fulminant liver failure	High	Low?
Budd–Chiari syndrome (late)	High	Low
Budd–Chiari syndrome (early)	High	High
Constrictive pericarditis	High	High
Venoocclusive disease	High	High
Myxedema	High	High
Nephrogenous (dialysis) ascites	High	High
Mixed ascites (cirrhosis + peritoneal malignancy)	High	Variable
Pancreatic ascites	Low	High
Serositis (connective tissue disease)	Low	High
Chlamydial/gonococcal	Low	High
Biliary	Low	High?
Ovarian hyperstimulation syndrome	Low?	High
Nephrotic syndrome	Low	Low

Those assessments followed by a question mark are theoretical and have not been confirmed by data in the literature.

(> 1500 mL), ascites can be identified on examination by bulging flanks, flank dullness, and shifting dullness. Shifting dullness is the most sensitive finding in the clinical diagnosis of ascites (compared with abdominal distention, bulging flanks and fluid wave) and its absence can rule out ascites with over 90% accuracy [4]. The presence of an umbilical hernia or diastasis recti suggests that the patient has had tense ascites.

Imaging investigations

The initial, least invasive, and most cost-effective method to confirm the presence of ascites is *abdominal ultrasonography*. It can detect amounts as small as 100 mL and is considered the gold standard for the diagnosis of ascites [5]. Abdominal ultrasound is also useful in locating the optimal site to perform a paracentesis, particularly in patients with a small amount of ascites or in those with loculated ascites. Additionally, ultrasound can be accompanied by Doppler examination of the hepatic venous system – an important initial test to rule out the presence of hepatic vein obstruction, a frequently overlooked cause of ascites [6].

Abdominal *computed tomography (CT) scan* is also highly sensitive and specific in diagnosing the presence of intra-abdominal fluid; however, its cost precludes it as a first-line diagnostic method to confirm the presence of ascites. Abdominal CT scan is more sensitive than ultrasonography in determining the presence of cirrhosis or malignancy. Finding a small nodular liver, splenomegaly, and collaterals on CT scan establishes the diagnosis of cirrhosis.

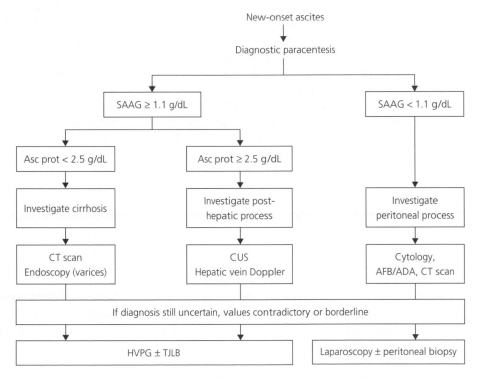

Figure 23.1 Approach to the patient with new-onset ascites. ADA, adenosine deaminase; AFB, acid-fast bacilli; Asc prot, ascites total protein levels; CT, computed tomography; CUS, cardiac echosonography; HVPG, hepatic venous pressure gradient; SAAG, serum–ascites albumin gradient; TJLB, transjugular liver biopsy.

The patient with new-onset ascites

In a patient with new ascites, the priority is to establish the cause of ascites because this will determine its management.

Initial evaluation

The history and physical examination are important in guiding the evaluation of ascites. Several aspects of the physical examination should receive special attention. The presence of spider angiomas, palmar erythema, and muscle wasting in addition to jaundice or signs of portal hypertension, such as splenomegaly and abdominal wall collaterals, suggests cirrhosis. Finding a palpable (or ballotable) left lobe of the liver (in the epigastric area) is almost pathognomonic of cirrhosis. Distended neck veins, gallop rhythm (S3), and uniform hepatomegaly with hepatojugular reflux or peripheral edema suggests congestive heart failure. The presence of a small nodule at the umbilicus (Sister Joseph Mary nodule) or an enlarged supraclavicular lymph node (Virchow node) suggests malignant ascites. Large veins with an upward flow localized in the back suggest obstruction of the inferior vena cava.

Diagnostic paracentesis

The simplest and most inexpensive way to orient the diagnostic workup of a patient with new-onset ascites is through the analysis of ascitic fluid. A diagnostic paracentesis should be the first test performed in a patient with new-onset ascites (see Fig. 23.1). It is a safe procedure with a low incidence of serious complications, the most serious being the development of large hematomas, which occurs in 0.2%–0.9% of cases [7,8]. Coagulopathy is not a contraindication to performing a diagnostic paracentesis particularly if it is performed with a small-gauge needle [7,8]. Care should always be taken to avoid surgical scars, abdominal wall collaterals, and the area of the inferior hypogastric artery, which lies midway between anterior superior iliac spine and pubic tubercle. If there are doubts about the presence of ascites or if no fluid is obtained in the first attempt, paracentesis should be performed under sonographic guidance.

In a diagnostic paracentesis, 20–50 mL of ascitic fluid is obtained. Tests that should be performed on the fluid are shown in Table 23.2, and their use in the differential diagnosis of ascites is detailed below.

Appearance of ascitic fluid

Uncomplicated "normal" ascitic fluid is transparent, straw colored to slightly yellow. In patients with marked jaundice, the fluid may have a deeper yellow color. Fluids with a leukocyte count greater than 5000/mm^3 appear cloudy, and those with a leukocyte count exceeding 50 000/mm^3 appear frankly purulent and indicate the presence of a gross intraabdominal infection (secondary peritonitis) or an abscess [1].

Table 23.2 Tests performed in diagnostic paracentesis
Routine analysis of ascitic fluid
Gross appearance
Total protein
Albumin (with simultaneous estimation of serum albumin) so that the ascites–serum albumin gradient can be calculated by subtracting the ascitic fluid value from the serum value
White blood cell count and differential
Bacteriological cultures
Focused analysis of ascitic fluid
Cytology (to exclude malignant ascites)
Amylase (if pancreatic ascites is suspected)
Acid-fast bacilli smear and culture and adenosine deaminase determination (if peritoneal tuberculosis is suspected)
Glucose and lactic dehydrogenase (if secondary peritonitis is suspected in a patient with ascites PMN > 250/mm^3)
Triglycerides (if the fluid has a milky appearance, i.e., chylous ascites)
Red blood cell count (if the fluid is bloody)
PMN, polymorphonuclear leukocytes.

Purulent ascites may be confused with the milky fluid associated with a high fat content (chylous ascites). Lack of odor and a triglyceride level greater than 200 mg/dL establishes the diagnosis of chylous ascites. An easier way to confirm the presence of chylous ascites is to refrigerate a tube with ascites – in case of chylous ascites, a creamy layer will separate at the top.

Fluids with a red blood cell count exceeding 10 000/mm^3 will appear pink, whereas frank bloody fluid is usually associated with a red blood cell count greater than 20 000/mm^3. In the presence of bloody fluid, the question will be whether it is the result of a traumatic tap or whether it is due to hemoperitoneum. Blood in the fluid resulting from a traumatic tap will clot, whereas fluid from a hemoperitoneum will not clot because blood has already clotted (intraperitoneally) and the clot has lysed. A tap performed immediately in the opposite flank will also clarify the situation. Hemoperitoneum suggests malignant ascites.

A tea-colored fluid can be seen in pancreatic ascites and the result of breakdown of ascitic fluid red cells. This phenomenon is more pronounced in hemorrhagic pancreatitis, resulting in a black fluid. Bile-stained fluid is green and can be seen with gallbladder or intestinal perforation.

Serum–ascites albumin gradient and ascites total protein levels

These two inexpensive tests taken *together* are the most useful in determining the etiology of ascites and thereby in further directing the workup of patients with ascites (see Table 23.1).

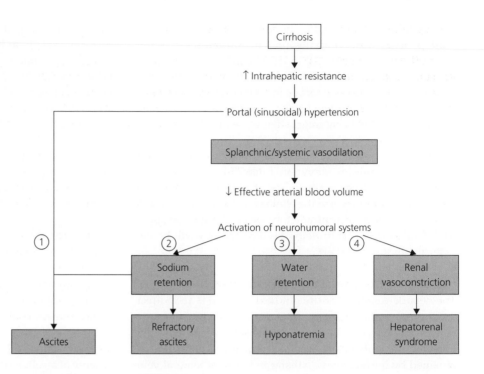

Figure 23.2 Common pathogenesis of ascites, hyponatremia and hepatorenal syndrome. Ascites (1) results from increased sinusoidal pressure and sodium retention. Sinusoidal pressure increases as a result of increased intrahepatic resistance. Sodium retention results from splanchnic and systemic vasodilation that leads to decreased effective arterial blood volume and subsequent upregulation of sodium-retaining hormones. With progression of cirrhosis and portal hypertension, vasodilation is more pronounced, leading to further activation of the renin–angiotensin–aldosterone and sympathetic nervous systems. The resulting increase in sodium and water retention can lead to refractory ascites (2) and hyponatremia (3), respectively, while the resulting increase in vasoconstrictors can lead to renal vasoconstriction and hepatorenal syndrome (4).

The *serum–ascites albumin gradient (SAAG)* is obtained by subtracting the concentration of ascites albumin from that of serum albumin (ideally determined from specimens obtained on the same day) and is a reflection of hepatic sinusoidal pressure [9,10]. The SAAG concept is based on Starling forces. When sinusoidal hypertension (hydrostatic pressure) is the cause of ascites, the colloidosmotic gradient (exerted mainly by serum and ascites albumin) has to increase to counterbalance the high hydrostatic pressure that is driving fluid into the peritoneal cavity. SAAG correlates well with the hepatic venous pressure gradient ($r = 0.72$), a measure of hepatic sinusoidal pressure [9]. The cutoff value that best distinguishes patients in whom ascites is caused by sinusoidal hypertension vs ascites caused by peritoneal malignancy is a SAAG of 1.1 g/dL, with a SAAG greater than 1.1 g/dL indicating ascites resulting from sinusoidal hypertension (e.g., cirrhosis, heart failure) [11]. Interestingly, the SAAG value of 1.1 g/dL roughly corresponds to a hepatic venous pressure gradient (HVPG, a measure of sinusoidal pressure) of 11–12 mmHg [9], which is the threshold pressure necessary for the development of ascites in cirrhosis (see below). The accuracy of SAAG is reduced if samples are not obtained simultaneously, if serum albumin levels are low or if ascites is chylous (falsely high SAAG). Serum hyperglobulinemia (> 5 g/dL) leads to a high ascitic fluid globulin concentration and can narrow the albumin gradient by contributing to the oncotic forces. To correct the SAAG in the setting of a high serum globulin level, the uncorrected SAAG should be multiplied by (0.16) × (serum globulin [in g/dL] + 2.5) [12].

The *ascites total protein content* at different cutoff values (2.5–3.0 g/dL) has been traditionally used to divide ascitic fluid into "exudates" secondary to peritoneal processes (malignancy, tuberculosis) or "transudates" in case of ascites secondary to sinusoidal portal hypertension. It is increased in peritoneal processes because of leakage of high-protein mesenteric lymph from obstructed lymphatics or from an inflamed peritoneal surface [13]. However, exudative ascites is also present in ascites secondary to heart failure [2], in which the mechanism is an increased hepatic sinusoidal pressure. In this situation, the process that leads to sinusoidal hypertension is posthepatic and therefore the hepatic sinusoids are normal. Normal hepatic sinusoids are uniquely permeable ("leaky") and hepatic congestion secondary to hepatic vein or inferior vena cava obstruction or cardiac failure has been shown to lead to profuse outpouring of protein-rich lymph into the peritoneal cavity [14]. In cirrhosis, there is deposition of fibrous tissue in the sinusoids ("capillarization of the sinusoid") that renders the sinusoid less leaky to macromolecules, and this leads to an abnormally low protein content of liver lymph [15,16]. Therefore, in addition to identifying peritoneal causes of ascites (high protein), the ascites total protein enables differentiation of intrahepatic (e.g., cirrhosis) causes of ascites (low protein) from posthepatic causes (e.g., heart failure, Budd–Chiari) of ascites (high protein), in both of which the SAAG is elevated [2]. This differential is extremely important because constrictive pericarditis is one of the few curable causes of ascites. Also, the distinction between cardiac or hepatic origin of ascites is especially important in alcoholic patients, who can have ascites secondary to alcoholic cardiomyopathy or from cirrhosis, with significant management implications.

In addition to being useful in determining the etiology of ascites, total protein levels in ascites are useful to determine susceptibility of developing bacterial infection [17]; cirrhotic patients with an ascites protein concentration below 1.0 g/dL have a higher risk of developing infection (spontaneous bacterial peritonitis). Contrary to what occurs with pleural fluid, ascites does not become an "exudate" with infection [18]; however, protein levels greater than 1.0 g/dL have been described as being suggestive of secondary (surgical) peritonitis.

All causes of ascites and their known/expected SAAG and total protein levels are shown in Table 23.1. The diagnostic workup for the three main causes of ascites is outlined in Fig. 23.1. In cases in which the etiology of ascites is still undetermined because of contradictory or borderline results of SAAG or ascites total protein, the ultimate test will be the determination of the HVPG.

Hepatic venous pressure gradient measurement

The hepatic venous pressure gradient (HVPG) is an indirect measure of portal pressure and a direct measure of hepatic sinusoidal pressure. The concept is the same as the measurement of the pulmonary wedged pressure. The HVPG is obtained by introducing a catheter in the right femoral vein or the internal jugular vein and advancing a balloon catheter into the right main hepatic vein. Pressures are recorded with the balloon inflated (wedged hepatic venous pressure, or WHVP) and deflated (free hepatic venous pressure, or FHVP). The WHVP is the direct measurement of sinusoidal pressure but it is usually corrected by subtracting the FHVP (a measure of systemic pressure that acts as an internal zero) thereby yielding the HVPG. Normal WHVP is 5–7 mmHg, normal FHVP is 1–2 mmHg, and normal HVPG is 3–6 mmHg. Portal hypertension is defined as an HVPG greater than 6 mmHg; however, the development of ascites requires that a threshold portal pressure gradient of 12 mmHg is exceeded [19,20]. Importantly, patients in whom the HVPG is reduced below 12 mmHg, or at least 20% from baseline values, show a decrease in the development of ascites [21].

Therefore, and as shown in Table 23.3, in cirrhotic ascites the HVPG will be elevated at the expense of an elevated WHVP and a normal FHVP, and the levels are usually greater than or equal to 12 mmHg. In cases of cardiac ascites, both the WHVP and the FHVP will be elevated (reflecting elevated systemic pressures) and therefore the HVPG will be normal [22]. In cases of peritoneal ascites (i.e., malignancy or tuberculosis), all hepatic venous pressure measurements (WHVP, FHVP, and HVPG) will be normal, unless the patient has coexisting cirrhosis or heart failure. When performed properly, HVPG measurements are reproducible and safe [23]; in fact, hepatic vein catheterization for measurement of hepatic vein pressures enables the performance, in the same procedure, of a transjugular liver biopsy, which will further define the etiology of ascites [24].

Evaluation of infection

Tests to investigate infection should be performed if the ascites is purulent or in any patient with cirrhotic ascites with symptoms or signs suggestive of spontaneous bacterial peritonitis (SBP) or who is admitted to the hospital [25]. A low ascites protein content (< 1.0 or 1.5 g/dL), present in most patients with cirrhosis, is the most important predictor of ascites infection [17]. SBP is the infection of ascitic fluid in the absence of an obvious local source, and it is the most common bacterial infection in hospitalized patients with cirrhosis. Importantly, the development of SBP is not associated with a significant change in ascites protein levels [18].

Total and differential cell counts

A predominance of neutrophils or polymorphonuclear leukocytes (PMN) in the ascitic fluid indicates the presence of an acute intraabdominal inflammatory process. Processes such as cholecystitis, appendicitis or diverticulitis can lead to ascites with a high neutrophil count, but in the absence of cirrhosis, the amount of fluid is generally minimal.

The diagnosis of SBP, that is, the infection of cirrhotic ascites, is established with an ascites PMN count greater than 250/mm^3 [25]. In patients with bloody ascites (i.e., ascites RBC count > 10 000/mm^3), 1 PMN per 250 RBC should be subtracted to adjust for the presence of blood in ascites.

Ascites PMN cell counts are performed manually and this may take several hours and not be available outside regular work hours. Although the use of reactive strips for leukocyte esterase has been proposed as an alternative to manual counting [26], several studies (mostly including small numbers of patients with SBP) show sensitivities that range widely between 50% and 100% [27]; therefore these strips cannot be recommended until larger studies are performed and the method is standardized.

A predominance of mononuclear cells indicates a chronic process and would suggest the presence of tuberculous peritonitis.

Smears and bacteriological culture

Sample collection at the bedside inoculating blood culture bottles (both aerobic and anaerobic) with 10 mL of ascitic

Table 23.3 Differential of ascites based on hepatic venous pressure gradient (HVPG) measurements

Cause of ascites	WHVP	FHVP	HVPG
Cirrhosis	Increased	Normal	Increased
Cardiac ascites	Increased	Increased	Normal
Peritoneal malignancy or TB	Normal	Normal	Normal

FHVP, free hepatic venous pressure; TB, tuberculosis; WHVP, wedged hepatic venous pressure.

fluid is more likely to yield an infecting organism compared with samples that are centrifuged and plated [28]. Although ascites culture is negative in approximately 40% of patients with clinical manifestations suggestive of SBP and increased ascites PMN [25], it is important to isolate an infecting microorganism, as this will further guide management [29]. Gram stain is positive in less than one-third of cases of SBP.

Ascites glucose and lactate dehydrogenase levels

In contrast to pleural fluid, ascites glucose and lactate dehydrogenase (LDH) levels are of little value in determining the cause of ascites or in determining the presence of infection. The ascites/serum LDH ratio is approximately 0.4–0.5 in uncomplicated cirrhotic ascites and increases in SBP, presumably because of the release of LDH from PMNs [18]; however, its diagnostic accuracy is low. It has been proposed that a ratio greater than 1.0 (i.e., if the ascites LDH is higher than serum LDH) and an ascites glucose below 50 mg/dL would suggest the presence of secondary bacterial peritonitis, although the specificity of these criteria is low [30] and they have not been validated prospectively.

Ascites lactate and pH

These tests were thought to be useful in the rapid diagnosis of SBP. However, several studies have demonstrated that they are no more useful than the ascites PMN determination [31].

Evaluation of malignancy

This should be undertaken in patients with a compatible clinical presentation. It is important to distinguish malignant ascites secondary to an infiltrated peritoneum (peritoneal carcinomatosis) from ascites secondary to massive liver metastases or "pseudocirrhosis" secondary to profound desmoplastic response to infiltrating breast cancer [32] or secondary to nodular regenerative hyperplasia related to chemotherapy [33]. In patients with cancer and ascites, peritoneal carcinomatosis is the cause of ascites in two-thirds of the patients [34].

Cytology

Cytological examination of ascites should be performed in all patients with suspected malignancy, particularly in those with low SAAG and high ascites protein, findings that suggest the presence of peritoneal carcinomatosis (as opposed to hepatic malignancy or pseudocirrhosis). In peritoneal carcinomatosis, SAAG is low, total protein high, and the diagnostic yield of cytology is as high as 97% (but could be as low as 42% [35]), whereas in patients with massive liver metastases, SAAG is high, ascites protein is low, and cytology is often negative [34].

It has been suggested that flow cytometry may be a useful adjunct to cytology in the diagnosis of peritoneal carcinomatosis, particularly when related to lymphoma or pancreatic cancer [35,36]; however, in a patient with suspected malignancy, low SAAG, high ascites protein, and negative results on cytological examination, the test of choice is probably a peritoneoscopy with peritoneal biopsies.

Tumor markers in ascites

Although CA-125 levels may be considered a sensitive tumor marker in patients with ovarian cancer, high serum CA-125 levels are elevated in *any* patient with ascites regardless of etiology. In fact, serum and ascites CA-125 levels were comparable among patients with cirrhotic ascites, patients with malignant ascites, and those with "benign" ascites [37]. Awareness of this association can prevent unnecessary workup and cost.

Other ascites markers such as carcinoembryonic antigen, fibronectin, and cholesterol have been found to be nonspecific and unhelpful in the diagnosis of malignant ascites, mostly because in the studies analyzing such markers patients were not stratified by the type of malignant ascites [38].

Evaluation of peritoneal tuberculosis

Although the incidence of peritoneal tuberculosis (PTB) appears to be rising in the United States, it remains an uncommon cause of ascites although it commonly occurs in patients with cirrhosis [39]. This makes its identification more problematic. In a noncirrhotic patient, ascites secondary to peritoneal tuberculosis is associated with a low SAAG and a high ascites protein. In a cirrhotic patient, findings associated with cirrhosis will predominate, that is, high SAAG and low protein. A diagnostic algorithm of patients with suspected PTB has been proposed [40].

Acid-fast bacilli culture and smear

Although isolating acid-fast bacilli (AFB) in ascites is the gold standard in the diagnosis of PTB, less than 10% of patients with PTB have positive ascitic fluid cultures, and Ziehl–Neelsen staining of the ascitic fluid for mycobacterial detection is positive in only about 3% of cases with proven PTB [40]. Additionally, conventional culture media require 4–8 weeks to detect AFB, which can lead to a delay in the initiation of specific therapy. Newer methods of identifying mycobacterial isolates include liquid chromatography and DNA probes, which reduce the turnaround time, and rapid amplification-based tests like polymerase chain reaction (PCR), which can yield results in days. However, their diagnostic value requires further analysis.

Ultimately, laparoscopy is the best test to diagnose PTB, either by visualization alone (typical findings) or in combination with biopsy, culture, and histological examination. This test should be considered at an early stage whenever PTB is suspected.

Adenosine deaminase ascitic fluid activity

With difficulties in the bacteriological diagnosis of PTB, there has been an ongoing search for alternative rapid and noninvasive tests, with adenosine deaminase (ADA) activity in the ascitic fluid being the most promising.

Adenosine deaminase is an enzyme related to proliferation and differentiation of lymphocytes, and establishing its activity appears to be a fast and discriminating test for diagnosing PTB, as shown by a metaanalysis of 12 studies (some performed in countries with a higher prevalence of PTB) including 264 patients, of which 50 (18.9%) had peritoneal tuberculosis. ADA levels showed high sensitivity (100%) and specificity (97%) using cutoff values from 36 to 40 IU/L, with an optimal cutoff point of 39 IU/L [41]. Although a retrospective study suggested that ADA activity is much less sensitive in detecting PTB in the setting of cirrhosis [39], other systematic reviews have not confirmed this contention [42]. Given its diagnostic accuracy and easy availability, performance of this test is recommended in suspected PTB.

Evaluation of pancreatic ascites

Pancreatic ascites is caused by extravasation of pancreatic fluid from the pancreatic ductal system, either from a leaking pseudocyst or from a ruptured pancreatic duct. Therefore, this fluid has high amylase levels (much higher than serum amylase) and a protein content greater than 2.5 g/dL. Because pancreatic ascites is not secondary to sinusoidal hypertension, the SAAG will be lower than 1.1 g/dL. In a relatively large series, only about two-thirds of the patients experienced abdominal pain [43], and it has been suggested that pancreatic ascites occurs more often than reported and a workup for it should be done even in the face of unconvincing radiographic evidence [44]. Of note, nonpancreatic tumors (e.g., ovarian) may cause an increase in the serum and ascitic fluid amylase, which may be incorrectly diagnosed as pancreatic ascites. However, isoenzyme analysis of this amylase will show that it is salivary isoamylase [45].

Evaluation of chylous ascites

Chylous ascites is an uncommon form of ascites resulting from an accumulation of peritoneal fluid rich in triglycerides, due to the presence of lymph in the abdominal cavity. A triglyceride level greater than 200 mg/dL is diagnostic of chylous ascites.

It occurs because of disruption of the lymphatic system resulting from obstruction (malignant infiltration or inflammatory process) or traumatic injury (surgery, trauma) with leakage of chylomicron-rich fluid into the peritoneum. Altered hemodynamics leading to increased caval (constrictive pericarditis) and hepatic venous pressures (cirrhosis) can also lead to an increased formation of hepatic duct lymph.

The most common cause of nontraumatic chylous ascites in adults is abdominal malignancy, with non-Hodgkin lymphomas accounting for at least one-third to half of these malignancies [46,47]. In addition to lymphomas other tumors that cause chyloperitoneum may arise from the ovary, colon, kidney, prostate, pancreas, and stomach. The most common inflammatory causes of chylous ascites are abdominal or pelvic radiation, pancreatitis, and tuberculosis. Surgical procedures that involve extensive retroperitoneal dissection are most commonly associated with postoperative chylous ascites, including the distal splenorenal shunt. Blunt trauma, stab wounds, and gunshot wounds can also lead to traumatic chylous ascites.

Cirrhotic ascites has chylous characteristics in only 0.5–1.3% of cases. Spontaneous transformation of previously clear ascites appears to be associated with a poor prognosis. In contrast, the appearance of chylous ascites de novo in a cirrhotic patient appears to indicate a more favorable outcome [48].

Given the multiple etiologies of chylous ascites, workup of the patient is directed by clinical and ascitic fluid findings as described for nonchylous ascites. The only caveat is that the SAAG may be falsely elevated in chylous ascites. Additional tests to determine the presence of lymphatic disruption include lymphangiography and lymphoscintigraphy.

The patient with cirrhosis and ascites

To understand the natural history of the patient with cirrhosis and ascites and its management at each stage it is important to understand the pathophysiology of ascites.

Pathogenesis and natural history of cirrhotic ascites

In cirrhosis, ascites results from two main pathogenic mechanisms: sinusoidal hypertension and sodium retention (Fig. 23.2). Ascitic fluid leaks into the peritoneal space as a result of sinusoidal hypertension, which in turn results from hepatic venous outflow block secondary to regenerative nodules, fibrosis, and active vasoconstriction. As mentioned previously, there is a minimal sinusoidal pressure necessary for ascites formation [19,20]. This would be a self-limited process but for the continuous replenishment of the intravascular volume through sodium and water retention. Sodium retention results from splanchnic and peripheral vasodilation resulting in a decrease in effective arterial blood volume, and activation of neurohumoral systems (angiotensin, renin, aldosterone) that leads to renal sodium retention [49]. As liver disease worsens, vasodilation also worsens leading to the nonosmotic release of antidiuretic hormone, which then leads to water retention and hyponatremia [50]. In the final stage of cirrhosis, vasodilation is extreme and in addition to marked sodium and water retention (refractory ascites with or without hyponatremia) there is renal vasoconstriction, which leads to a decrease in glomerular filtration rate and renal failure (hepatorenal syndrome, HRS).

Therefore, a patient with cirrhosis goes through a sequence of diuretic-responsive ascites, followed by refractory ascites, and then hyponatremia and HRS [51], with each stage reflecting a more deranged circulatory state. Overall, most cirrhotic patients with ascites have "uncomplicated" ascites, that is, ascites that is not infected, is not associated with renal dysfunction, and responds to diuretic therapy [52]. However, the

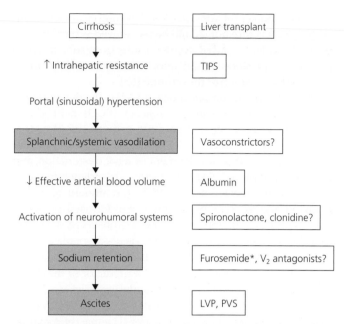

Figure 23.3 Site of action of different therapies for ascites. *Furosemide should only be used in conjunction with spironolactone. LVP, large-volume paracentesis; PVS, peritoneovenous shunt; TIPS, transjugular intrahepatic portosystemic shunt; V_2, arginine vasopressin type 2 receptor.

prevalence of uncomplicated ascites is lower in certain settings (e.g., transplant centers, in hospital).

Therapies for ascites

Different therapies for ascites and their site of action are depicted in Fig. 23.3. Except for transplant, none of the different treatments of ascites has resulted in significant improvements in survival. However, treating ascites is important, not only because it improves the quality of life of the cirrhotic patient but also because SBP, a lethal complication of cirrhosis, does not occur in the absence of ascites.

Liver transplant

The development of ascites in a patient with cirrhosis denotes a poor prognosis, with a median survival of about 1.5 years, compared with a median survival of more than 12 years in patients who remain compensated [3]. In the presence of ascites, mortality in cirrhosis is about 20% per year [53]. Patients with cirrhosis who develop ascites should therefore be evaluated for liver transplantation because this constitutes the ultimate treatment for ascites and its complications.

Sodium restriction and diuretics

Sodium restriction is recommended in all cirrhotic patients with ascites. Restriction to approximately 90 mEq/day (i.e., 2 g sodium/day = 5.2 g of dietary salt/day) is the recommended goal [52]. Further restriction of sodium is unrealistic and difficult to achieve. Nonpalatability of a salt-restricted diet may lead to inadequate food intake. In these cases, liberalizing sodium restriction and adding or increasing diuretics

is preferable to compromising the already compromised nutrition of the cirrhotic patient with ascites.

Although loop diuretics such as furosemide are the most potent natriuretics, randomized controlled trials have demonstrated that spironolactone is significantly more effective than furosemide alone in the treatment of cirrhotic ascites [54,55]. When furosemide is used alone, sodium not reabsorbed in the loop of Henle is taken up at the distal and collecting tubules as a result of the hyperaldosteronism present in most cirrhotic patients with ascites. Therefore, spironolactone, which acts by blocking aldosterone, is the diuretic of choice in the treatment of ascites. Furosemide can be used together with spironolactone but should not be used alone.

There is no evidence that other diuretics such as metolazone, thiazides, or torasemide offer an advantage over spironolactone and furosemide.

In contrast to the treatment of acute heart failure, where the response to therapy needs to be fast and an intravenous (i.v.) route is preferable, elimination of cirrhotic ascites should be slow (only about 500 mL/day can be eliminated) and an oral route is preferred. Nonsteroidal antiinflammatory drugs or aspirin blunt the natriuretic effect of diuretics and should be avoided in cirrhotic patients with ascites [56,57]. Although selective cyclooxygenase-2 (COX-2) inhibitors have not been shown to impair natriuresis or to induce renal dysfunction in cirrhotic rats [58], preliminary data in patients indicate that celecoxib may be related to a decrease in renal function [59] and therefore COX-2 inhibitor use should also be avoided until more clinical data become available.

Complications of diuretic therapy

Common complications are renal impairment caused by intravascular volume depletion (25%), hyponatremia (28%), and hepatic encephalopathy (26%) [60–62]. Spironolactone is often associated with adverse events, mainly painful gynecomastia, related to its antiandrogenic activity. Potassium canrenoate, one of the major metabolites of spironolactone, has a comparable diuretic effect and a lower antiandrogenic activity and could be used in cases in which gynecomastia and mastalgia are side effects of spironolactone therapy. However, this drug is not available in the United States. Amiloride, another potassium-sparing diuretic, does not produce gynecomastia and is recommended in patients with intolerable painful gynecomastia, but it has significantly less natriuretic effect than spironolactone [63]. Amiloride is used at an initial dose of 20 mg/day and can be increased to 60 mg/day. In patients in whom the natriuretic response with amiloride is suboptimal it may be worthwhile to attempt retreatment with spironolactone.

Large-volume paracentesis

Several randomized studies have demonstrated that large-volume paracentesis (LVP) associated with i.v. albumin is as effective as standard therapy with diuretics in patients with

449

uncomplicated ascites but with a significantly faster resolution and the same or a lower rate of complications [60,61]. However, LVP is a local therapy that does not act on the mechanisms of ascites formation (Fig. 23.3) and ascites recurrence is the rule. Additionally, the procedure is more costly and requires more resources than the administration of diuretics.

The standard therapy for refractory ascites is LVP + albumin. Although initially the recommendation was to perform daily 5-L paracenteses until the disappearance of ascites, it was subsequently determined that total paracentesis (i.e., removal of all ascites in a single procedure accompanied by the concomitant infusion of 6–8 g albumin per liter of ascites removed) was as safe as repeated partial paracenteses [64].

The frequency of LVP is determined by the rate of ascites reaccumulation and, ultimately, on the need to relieve the patient's discomfort. The rate of ascites reaccumulation depends largely on the patient's compliance with salt restriction and diuretics and the degree of sodium retention. A randomized controlled study showed that the administration of diuretics after LVP is associated with longer time to recurrence of ascites without any differences in complications [65]. Notably, in this study the urinary sodium of patients in the diuretic group in whom ascites recurred by day 30 was significantly lower at 3 days and 2 weeks (8 and 15 mEq/L, respectively) compared with that of patients in whom ascites had not recurred by day 30 (109 and 67 mEq/L, respectively). This suggests that although sodium restriction and diuretics should be used after LVP, in patients with a urinary sodium less than 30 mEq/L diuretics are not useful and should be discontinued, particularly if associated with complications [52].

Complications of large-volume paracentesis

Procedure-related complications consist mainly of bleeding and ascites leakage. Major *bleeding* occurs rarely but may be lethal [66] and has been related to rupture of mesenteric varices rather than as a result of coagulopathy. In fact, in a series of over 1000 LVPs there was no significant bleeding, not even in patients with marked thrombocytopenia or prolongation in the prothrombin time [67]. Renal dysfunction, more than coagulopathy, appears to be associated with a higher risk of post-LVP hemorrhage [8]. LVP should probably be avoided in patients with renal failure and clinically evident severe coagulopathy. Care should be taken to avoid abdominal wall collaterals and to avoid the area of the inferior hypogastric artery, which lies midway between anterior superior iliac spine and pubic tubercle. Technically, the midline below the umbilicus is often recommended as a site for paracentesis because of its presumed avascularity. However, a laparoscopic study in 20 patients with cirrhosis demonstrated that, in patients with portal hypertension, this area is commonly vascular [68].

Leakage of ascitic fluid is rare and occurs when extraction of ascites is incomplete. Therefore, this complication can be resolved by completing the LVP preferably in a site remote from the leaking puncture site. Another complication of paracentesis that is rare but should be recognized is the development of sudden *scrotal edema* that results from subcutaneous tracking of peritoneal fluid into the scrotum. This can be resolved by elevation of the scrotum [69].

One of the main complications of LVP is the development of *postparacentesis circulatory dysfunction* (PCD), defined as a significant increase in plasma renin activity (PRA) 6 days after LVP. Development of PCD is associated with a faster recurrence of ascites, development of renal dysfunction, and a higher mortality [70,71]. Two factors are independent predictors of the development of PCD: the amount of ascites removed and the type of volume expander used in association with LVP [70]; the lowest rates are observed when less than 5 L is removed or when albumin is used as a plasma volume expander (rate around 16%) [70,72–74]. The presence (or absence) of peripheral edema is not a predictor of the development of PCD. Albumin should be administered at a dose of 6–8 g of albumin i.v. per liter of ascites removed. For LVP less than 5 L, a synthetic plasma expander (Haemaccel, Dextran-70) or even saline solution can be used instead of albumin, and it has been suggested that no plasma expansion may be necessary in this setting [52,70,74]. The pathogenesis of PCD appears to be a worsening of the vasodilatory state of the cirrhotic patient with a consequent further decrease in effective arterial blood volume and marked activation of neurohumoral systems that lead to further sodium retention, renal vasoconstriction, renal dysfunction, and death [71]. Therefore LVP should not be performed in the setting of conditions that have been associated with a worsening in the vasodilatory state of cirrhosis, such as SBP.

Regarding the possibility of infection in outpatients undergoing serial LVP, three studies have shown that SBP is not a significant complication in this setting [75–77].

Transjugular intrahepatic portosystemic shunt

Transjugular intrahepatic portosystemic shunt (TIPS) is a nonsurgical, percutaneous procedure performed by an interventional radiologist by which a portosystemic shunt is established inside the liver parenchyma by connecting, through a metal stent, a main portal branch with a large hepatic vein. By acting as a side-to-side portocaval shunt, it relieves sinusoidal pressure, the main driving force in the formation of ascites. Although TIPS placement is associated early on with a worsening in systemic hemodynamics (increase in cardiac output, further decrease in systemic vascular resistance) and a worsening of liver synthetic function, these changes are no longer present 3 months after TIPS insertion [78]. Additionally, despite deterioration of the hyperdynamic circulatory state and of liver synthetic function, urinary sodium excretion increases significantly as soon as 7 days after TIPS placement and correlates closely with a decrease in plasma renin activity (PRA) and aldosterone levels [78–84]. In addition to sinusoidal decompression, TIPS placement has the advantage of, at least transiently, increasing the effective arterial blood volume by transferring blood volume from the splanchnic to the systemic circulation.

Five prospective randomized trials have compared TIPS (using uncovered stents) with LVP in the treatment of refractory ascites [81,85–88]. Metaanalysis of these trials demonstrates that an uncovered TIPS stent is more effective at preventing ascites from recurring; however, it is associated with an increased occurrence of hepatic encephalopathy without differences in survival [89]. However, when the trial that included Child C patients [81] is excluded, metaanalysis showed a tendency for an improved survival with TIPS [89]. In these trials, the rate of post-TIPS shunt morbidity was an important issue that increased its cost [86]. However, new polytetra-fluoroethylene (PTFE)-covered stents are associated with improved TIPS patency, and a decrease in the number of clinical relapses and reinterventions, without increasing the risk of encephalopathy [90]. In fact, a case–control study suggested that patients undergoing TIPS with covered stents have higher 2-year survival rates when compared with patients with uncovered TIPS [91]. This benefit needs to be prospectively evaluated in patients with refractory ascites. Until then, the consensus recommendation is to consider TIPS placement when the frequency of LVP is greater than two to three times per month [52].

Complications of transjugular intrahepatic portosystemic shunt

The procedure-related complication rate is around 9%, with the most common being intraperitoneal hemorrhage [92]. Other important complications are heart failure and hemolysis, which may develop in 10%–15% of patients. As mentioned above, long-term complications of TIPS are new onset or worsening of hepatic encephalopathy and shunt dysfunction. Each occurs in about one-third of the patients, with a mean follow-up of about 1 year [78]; the incidence for both complications appears to be lower with covered TIPS stents. Resolution of ascites post-TIPS has been associated with the development of abdominal wall hernia incarceration [93].

Contraindications to transjugular intrahepatic portosystemic shunt

TIPS can precipitate death secondary to liver failure. The strongest predictor of survival post-TIPS placement for patients with refractory ascites is the serum bilirubin concentration [78,89], and a cutoff level of 3 mg/dL has been proposed [94]. Consensus recommendations also suggest that an age greater than 70 years, preexisting cardiac dysfunction, and a Child–Turcotte–Pugh (CTP) score greater than 11 should be considered contraindications to TIPS placement in the setting of refractory ascites [52]. Serum bilirubin may be the decisive factor in reaching the CTP cutoff score of 11 because patients with refractory ascites have, by definition, the highest score for ascites (i.e., tense ascites) and most have the highest score

for albumin [78]. TIPS is not recommended in patients with heart failure (ejection fraction < 55%), firstly because with high right-sided pressures there may not be an adequate pressure gradient between the portal and the systemic venous systems for TIPS to function, and secondly because TIPS placement in this setting may precipitate exacerbation of heart failure. Patients with alcoholic cirrhosis who are drinking alcohol may improve with alcohol abstinence and therefore TIPS should be delayed in these patients.

Peritoneovenous shunt

The peritoneovenous (PVS) shunt is a therapy that combines removal of intraperitoneal fluid and replenishment of the intravascular volume. It consists of a silicone tube system and a one-way valve that transfers ascites from the peritoneal cavity to the internal jugular vein (i.e., the systemic circulation). The increase in fluid return to the cardiopulmonary circulation can lead sequentially to decreased activity of sodium-retaining and vasoconstrictive mechanisms (such as the renin–angiotensin–aldosterone system), a marked rise in urinary sodium excretion, and a modest elevation in glomerular filtration rate.

In randomized controlled trials of refractory ascites PVS has been shown to be more effective than diuretics [95] (a predictable result) and as effective as LVP + albumin [96,97]. In these studies, no differences in survival have been observed among therapies. However, as a result of its high obstruction rate, PVS requires frequent admissions for shunt revision or for the management of other more serious complications. The use of PVS has been progressively abandoned over the years because LVP + albumin is a simpler procedure that can be performed in the outpatient setting and because of the advent of TIPS. In a small randomized trial comparing PVS with uncovered TIPS, control of ascites was achieved sooner after PVS, but longer-term (3-year) efficacy favored TIPS, with numerous interventions required to assist patency with both shunts. This study suggests that PVS is a reasonable option for a short (< 1-year) period, particularly because the mean patency of the shunt is around 6 months [95,96]. In fact, a case series of 36 patients listed for liver transplantation who had PVS placed for refractory ascites and who were followed for a mean of 9 months, reported adequate palliation (i.e., no need for further LVP until transplant) in 83% with a lower occurrence of renal failure (compared with historical controls) [98]. Although PVS might complicate liver transplant surgery given its ability to produce peritoneal adhesions, none of the 16 patients who were transplanted in this series had intraoperative complications secondary to PVS [98].

Traditionally, placement of PVS has been performed by surgeons under general anaesthesia and employing venous cutdown. But there is increasing experience of these shunts being placed by radiologists in the interventional suite, with successful revision in case of dysfunction in the majority of patients [99].

Therefore, placement of PVS should clearly be considered in patients who are not TIPS candidates, and it can also be considered (based on local surgeon preference) for patients on the transplant list.

Complications of peritoneovenous shunt
The major problem with PVS is the relatively high rate of complications, although in randomized controlled trials PVS has a similar rate of complications as LVP + albumin [96,97]. The complications related to PVS include disseminated intravascular coagulation (due to introduction of endotoxins and other procoagulants from ascites into the systemic circulation), infection of the shunt (which can can lead to bacteremia and requires shunt removal), variceal bleeding or heart failure resulting from volume expansion and a concurrent rise in systemic and portal venous pressure, and small bowel obstruction from peritoneal adherences [100]. The transoperative drainage of ascites can minimize the complications related to massive ascites infusion, such as disseminated intravascular coagulation and increased systemic and portal pressures [101].

Therapies under investigation for the treatment of ascites
Sympathetic system antagonists
Clonidine is a centrally acting α_2-agonist with antiadrenergic activity in cirrhosis. In a small randomized pilot study, the administration of clonidine, at a dose of 0.075 mg orally (p.o.) twice a day, plus spironolactone to patients with refractory ascites increased natriuresis and significantly decreased plasma norepinephrine (noradrenaline) and aldosterone levels and plasma renin activity. In a mean follow-up of 10.5 months and compared with patients who were treated with LVP + albumin ($n = 10$), patients who received clonidine plus spironolactone ($n = 10$) had fewer readmissions for ascites, a longer time to ascites reaccumulation, and decreased spironolactone requirements [102].

A single-center randomized double-blind placebo-controlled trial from the same group of investigators evaluated the efficacy of clonidine in patients with uncomplicated ascites and an activated sympathetic nervous system (as defined by serum norepinephrine levels > 300 pg/mL). Patients randomized to clonidine ($n = 32$) had a significantly lower number of readmissions for ascites and a longer time to readmission, and lower requirements for LVP, spironolactone, and furosemide compared with patients randomized to placebo ($n = 32$), with a lower rate of hyperkalemia and renal impairment [103]. These promising results require further investigation before clonidine can be widely recommended.

V_2 receptor antagonists
Selective inhibition of arginine vasopressin type 2 receptors (V_2) was considered important only in the treatment of dilutional hyponatremia in cirrhosis. However, data from experimental animals show that V_2 receptor antagonists also have a natriuretic effect [104–106]. In fact, a phase II study of satavaptan, a V_2 receptor antagonist, in 148 patients with cirrhosis and ascites without hyponatremia demonstrated a dose-related increase in urine volume and a dose-related decrease in body weight without changes in serum creatinine [107]. Furthermore, in a randomized double-blind placebo-controlled study in 151 patients treated with LVP plus spironolactone, satavaptan was associated with a longer time to recurrence of ascites requiring LVP and a significantly lower number of paracenteses [108].

Therefore, V_2 receptor antagonists could be useful adjuvants to diuretics in the treatment of ascites (refractory or nonrefractory ascites) by preventing diuretic-induced hyponatremia and by a synergistic natriuresis. However, further analysis is required.

Vasoconstrictors
Because vasodilation is one of the main mechanisms in the formation of cirrhotic ascites, a rational therapeutic approach is the use of vasoconstrictors. There is limited experience with these agents. A pilot study shows that a 7-day course of midodrine (at a dose of 10 mg p.o. three times a day) was associated with significant increases in urinary sodium, mean arterial pressure, and creatinine clearance and with significant decreases in plasma renin activity and plasma aldosterone levels [109]. Its effect as an adjuvant to diuretics in the treatment of ascites remains to be determined.

Two small randomized studies have compared terlipressin with albumin in the prevention of postparacentesis circulatory dysfunction [110,111]. Both studies showed that the postparacentesis circulatory dysfunction (i.e., plasma renin activity before and 4–6 days after LVP) did not differ between the study groups; however, given the small numbers of patients included in these studies, results are not conclusive.

The patient with cirrhosis and uncomplicated ascites
The approach to the patient with cirrhosis and uncomplicated ascites is depicted in Fig. 23.4.

In contrast to the treatment of heart failure, where achieving a negative sodium and water balance demands a certain urgency given the risk/presence of pulmonary edema, therapy of cirrhotic ascites is not an emergency because the risk of death is not implicit unless the fluid is infected. Therefore, most patients with uncomplicated ascites should treated in a stepwise, unhurried fashion, and treatment should only be initiated in a "stable" cirrhotic patient, that is, one in whom complications such as gastrointestinal hemorrhage, bacterial infection, or renal dysfunction are absent or have resolved. One exception is the patient with tense ascites who experiences not only abdominal discomfort but also respiratory distress. In these patients, a single large-volume paracentesis should be performed prior to or concomitant with starting diuretic therapy.

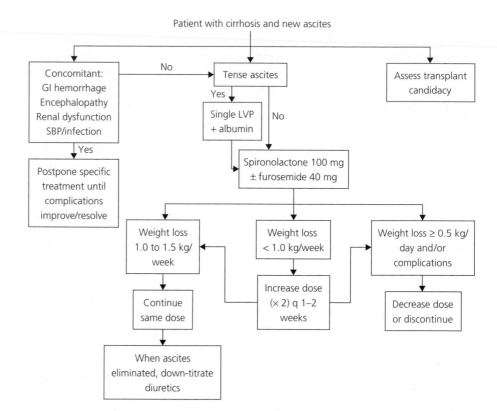

Figure 23.4 Approach to the patient with cirrhosis and uncomplicated ascites. GI, gastrointestinal; LVP, large-volume paracentesis; SBP, spontaneous peritonitis.

Because renal dysfunction secondary to diuretics results from a reduction in effective arterial blood volume, diuretics should not be initiated in patients with concomitant complications of cirrhosis known to be associated with a decreased effective arterial blood volume, such as variceal hemorrhage and SBP.

Treatment aimed at achieving a negative sodium balance (i.e., sodium restriction and diuretics) still constitutes the mainstay of therapy in patients with uncomplicated ascites, given its general applicability, low cost, and ease of administration. However, in hospitalized patients with moderate/tense ascites in whom other complications have been resolved, it is reasonable to initiate therapy with total paracentesis as this will accelerate discharge from the hospital.

Diuretic therapy can be initiated with spironolactone alone (initial dose of 100 mg p.o. daily) or with spironolactone (100 mg p.o. daily) plus furosemide (40 mg p.o. daily). Both schedules are equally effective; however, dose adjustments are needed more frequently in patients in whom treatment is initiated with combination therapy because of a more rapid mobilization of fluid with consequent increases in blood urea nitrogen or decreases in serum sodium [54,112]. In an inpatient setting, where renal function can be monitored more frequently, combination therapy can be used. However, in the outpatient setting it is preferable to initiate therapy with spironolactone alone at a daily dose of 100 mg p.o. Because spironolactone takes several days to act it should be administered in a single daily dose. If weight loss is not optimal (weight loss < 1 kg in the first week and < 2 kg/week in subsequent weeks) the dose should be increased in a stepwise manner with increases of 100 mg every 1–2 weeks to a maximum of 400 mg p.o., q.i.d [52]). If hyperkalemia develops before the maximal dose is reached, furosemide should be added at an initial single daily dose of 40 mg, increased in a stepwise fashion in increments of 40 mg to a maximum of 160 mg/day.

Before considering that ascites is refractory to diuretics, it is necessary to ascertain whether the patient has adhered to the prescribed sodium-restricted diet and has restrained from using nonsteroidal antiinflammatory drugs. Nonadherence to dietary sodium restriction or diuretics should be suspected if patients fail to lose weight despite an adequate 24-h urine sodium excretion (> 50 mEq/L or greater than daily sodium intake). In a patient in whom ascites disappears, one can attempt to downtitrate the dose of diuretics and maintain it at the minimal effective dose so that complications can be minimized.

In patients who develop renal dysfunction (elevation in creatinine > 50% to a creatinine > 1.5 mg/dL) or encephalopathy, diuretics should be temporarily discontinued and restarted at a lower dose when creatinine returns to baseline. Patients who develop hyponatremia (serum sodium < 130 mEq/L) while on diuretics should be managed with fluid restriction and a decrease in the dose of diuretics. The role of V_2 receptor antagonists in this setting is promising [106,113]. To minimize the rate of complications, patients without edema should not lose more than 0.5 kg/day, whereas in patients with edema a weight loss of 1 kg/day is allowable.

There are insufficient data to support the use of long-term antibiotic prophylaxis to prevent SBP and other bacterial infections in patients with uncomplicated ascites who are not hospitalized with gastrointestinal hemorrhage or who have not had a previous episode of SBP, even in those with an ascites protein concentration < 1 g/dL [27]. Limiting the use of prophylactic antibiotics is important given the increased rate of infections with quinolone-resistant and trimethoprim–sulfamethoxazole (cotrimoxazole)-resistant organisms observed in patients on long-term norfloxacin prophylaxis [114,115].

The patient with cirrhosis and refractory ascites

The approach to the patient with cirrhosis and refractory ascites is depicted in Fig. 23.5.

Refractory ascites assumes either diuretic-resistant ascites (ascites that is not eliminated even with maximal diuretic therapy) or diuretic-intractable ascites (ascites that is not eliminated because maximal doses of diuretics cannot be reached given the development of complications) [116]. The majority of patients with refractory ascites have the diuretic-intractable type [51]. Vasodilation is more pronounced in patients with refractory ascites (Fig. 23.2), thereby leading to a further decrease in effective arterial blood volume and further activation of the renin–angiotensin–aldosterone and sympathetic nervous systems. Further alteration in hemodynamics results in a greater susceptibility to develop hyponatremia or renal dysfunction in these patients. In fact, hepatorenal syndrome (HRS) type 2, in which renal dysfunction is characterized by a moderate and steady or slowly progressive renal failure (serum creatinine < 2.5 mg/dL), is almost exclusively seen in patients with refractory ascites [116]. Patients with type 2 HRS are predisposed to develop type 1 HRS following infections or other precipitating events.

The median survival of patients with type 2 HRS (4–6 months) is worse than that of patients with nonazotemic cirrhosis with ascites [117]. Therefore, a patient with refractory ascites who has not yet been evaluated for liver transplant candidacy should be evaluated without delay.

First-line therapy for patients with refractory ascites is serial LVP, adding albumin if more than 5 L is removed at once. In patients in whom 5 L or less is being removed, a plasma volume expander can be used. To increase the time between paracenteses, patients should continue on maximally tolerated diuretic dose provided that the urinary sodium is greater than 30 mEq/L. Otherwise, diuretics can be discontinued [52].

Routine cell count and culture analysis are not warranted in asymptomatic cirrhotic patients undergoing outpatient paracenteses for refractory ascites because studies have shown a low prevalence (0%–3.5%) of SBP in this setting [75–77]. Data from a randomized double-blind placebo-controlled trial suggest, however, that in patients with a low concentration of ascites protein (< 1 g/dL) who also have evidence of deranged circulatory status (creatinine > 1.2 mg/dL or blood urea nitrogen (BUN) > 25 mg/dL or a serum sodium ≤ 130 mEq/L) or severe liver disease (CTP score ≥ 9 and a serum bilirubin concentration ≥ 3 mg/dL) primary prophylaxis with norfloxacin at a daily dose of 400 mg p.o. is associated with a significantly lower incidence of first SBP and a reduced 3-month mortality [118]. These criteria will probably be met by most patients with refractory ascites.

In patients who require LVP more than two to three times per month or in whom ascites is loculated and cannot be entirely removed with a single LVP, evaluation for TIPS placement should be undertaken. In general, TIPS should not be

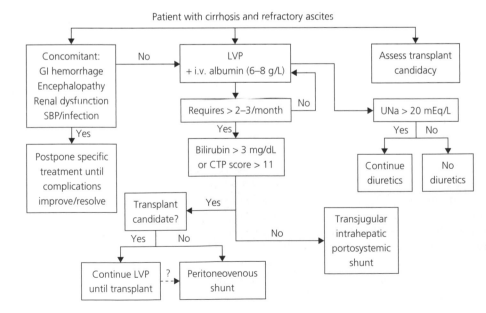

Figure 23.5 Approach to the patient with cirrhosis and refractory ascites. CTP, Child–Turcotte–Pugh; GI, gastrointestinal; i.v., intravenous; LVP, large-volume paracentesis; SBP, spontaneous bacterial peritonitis; UNa, urine sodium concentration.

performed in patients with serum bilirubin greater than 3 mg/dL, a CTP score greater than 11, age over 70 years, or evidence of heart failure [52,78] because these factors are associated with a poorer survival and a poorer shunt function. Although studies of TIPS for refractory ascites were performed using uncovered stents, covered stents should be used because of the lower rate of shunt dysfunction and potential benefits regarding development of encephalopathy and survival [90].

Although the goal of TIPS is to reduce the portosystemic pressure gradient to less than 12 mmHg (the threshold for the formation of ascites), too low a reduction (e.g., to levels < 5 mmHg) carries a higher risk of post-TIPS portosystemic encephalopathy [119] and should therefore be avoided.

Most cases of post-TIPS encephalopathy respond to standard therapy, and only about 3%–10% develop recurrent, severe encephalopathy that can be treated with stent reduction [120], with preliminary evidence suggesting that covered reduction stents are better than uncovered reduction stents [121]. In a randomized controlled trial, prophylactic therapy with lactitol or rifaximin for 1 month after TIPS placement was ineffective in preventing portosystemic encephalopathy [119], and prophylaxis is therefore not recommended.

Because TIPS placement improves but does not normalize sodium excretion [82], peripheral edema may continue to be a problem and the use of diuretics after the procedure is advisable. Diuretic therapy immediately after the procedure also has the theoretical advantage of improving the pressure gradient across the shunt by reducing central pressure more than portal pressure.

Serial assessment of shunt patency is not necessary after TIPS unless there is recurrence of ascites, a clinically obvious event indicative of stent dysfunction.

In patients requiring frequent LVP and who are not TIPS candidates, a peritoneovenous shunt (PVS) should be considered. Placement of a PVS may hinder future placement of TIPS. The intraabdominal limb of the PVS is associated with the formation of peritoneal adhesions and may complicate transplant surgery; therefore it has also been considered a contraindication in patients who are candidates for transplant. However, a case series of pretransplant patients showed that PVS is not associated with surgical complications [98].

The patient with cirrhosis and hepatic hydrothorax

Pleural effusion (hepatic hydrothorax) develops in approximately 5%–10% of patients with cirrhosis, most probably as the result of the transdiaphragmatic movement of fluid from the peritoneum to the pleural space through diaphragmatic defects [122,123]. The negative intrathoracic pressure favors the movement of fluid across these defects, and patients usually have minimal or mild ascites. In fact, hepatic hydrothorax may be present in patients without detectable ascites [124].

Pleural effusion is right-sided in 85%, left-sided in 13%, and bilateral in 2% of the cases [125].

Although large amounts of ascites can accumulate in the peritoneal cavity before resulting in significant patient discomfort, the accumulation of smaller amounts of fluid (1–2 L) in the pleural space results in severe shortness of breath and hypoxemia. A diagnostic radionuclide ascites scan is useful in the diagnosis of hepatic hydrothorax, particularly in cases where ascites is absent [126]. It consists of the injection of technetium-99m-labeled sulfur colloid [127] or macroaggregated serum albumin [126] into the peritoneal cavity followed by chest imaging every 15–30 min. Transdiaphragmatic movement of ascites into the pleural space is demonstrated generally within 2 h of intraperitoneal injection of the radiotracer.

Hepatic hydrothorax should be treated in the same manner as cirrhotic ascites, that is, the mainstay of therapy is sodium restriction and diuretics. Before determining that hydrothorax is refractory, a trial of in-hospital diuretic therapy should be attempted. In patients with refractory hepatic hydrothorax other therapeutic options such as repeated thoracenteses, TIPS, or pleurodesis should be considered. Regarding thoracentesis, and given that no more than 2 L is removed at a time because of the risk of reexpansion pulmonary edema, the procedure may need to be repeated frequently. When thoracentesis is required every 2–3 weeks, alternative strategies such as TIPS should be considered. Uncontrolled studies of TIPS have shown resolution of the pleural effusion or a decrease in the need for thoracentesis in 67% of patients; however, mortality is high, particularly in nonresponders to TIPS [128]. In patients who have not responded to TIPS, an option is video-assisted thoracoscopy to repair diaphragmatic defects and to perform pleurodesis. However, information is available on only a small number of patients, and the procedure is associated with significant morbidity and mortality [123]. Placement of a chest tube should be avoided in patients with hepatic hydrothorax because it has been associated with multiple complications, mainly volume and electrolyte disturbances.

The patient with spontaneous bacterial peritonitis

Spontaneous bacterial peritonitis (SBP) is the most common type of bacterial infection in hospitalized cirrhotic patients, occurring in about 9% of the patients and accounting for about 25% of all infections [115].

SBP is an infection of ascitic fluid that occurs in the absence of perforation of a hollow viscus or of an intraabdominal inflammatory focus, such as an abscess, acute pancreatitis, or cholecystitis.

Bacterial translocation – the migration of bacteria from the intestinal lumen to mesenteric lymph nodes and other extraintestinal sites – is the main mechanism implicated in the pathogenesis of SBP. Impaired local and systemic immune defenses and intestinal bacterial overgrowth promote bacterial translocation and, together with shunting of blood away from the hepatic Kupffer cells through portosystemic collaterals, allow a transient bacteremia to become more prolonged, subsequently colonizing ascitic fluid. Bacterial translocation and the development of SBP in cirrhosis worsen the hyperdynamic circulatory state by a cytokine-mediated aggravation of vasodilation [129–131]. By worsening vasodilation, SBP can lead to renal dysfunction and the hepatorenal syndrome [132].

SBP occurs in patients with reduced ascites defense mechanisms, such as low ascites complement levels. Because ascites complement levels correlate with ascites protein levels, it follows that the most important predictor in the development of SBP is a low concentration of ascites protein (< 1 g/dL) [17,133].

When first described, the mortality of SBP exceeded 90%; however, with early recognition of the disease and prompt and appropriate antibiotic therapy, mortality has been reduced to around 20%–30% [134], a much lower but still significant mortality.

The approach to the patient with cirrhosis and SBP is depicted in Fig. 23.6. Early recognition of SBP involves the performance of a diagnostic paracentesis (for total and differential cell counts and bacteriological culture) in any patient in whom SBP is suspected. Suspicion of SBP should be raised in patients with symptoms or signs directly due to SBP, such as fever, abdominal pain or tenderness, and leukocytosis, but should also be raised in the presence of unexplained encephalopathy, jaundice, or worsening renal failure – complications of sepsis. Simultaneous blood and urine cultures and a chest radiograph should also be obtained because any bacterial infection in cirrhosis can lead to similar manifestations.

In patients with hepatic hydrothorax in whom an infection is suspected and SBP has been ruled out, a diagnostic thoracentesis should be performed to rule out spontaneous bacterial empyema, an entity akin to SBP that may occur in the absence of ascites or SBP and that should be managed as described below for SBP [135].

Isolation of an infecting organism is definitive in establishing the diagnosis of SBP. The most common organisms isolated in SBP are gram-negative bacteria, and the infections are mostly monomicrobial [31,115]. However, despite the use of sensitive culture methods that include inoculation of ascites into blood culture bottles, ascites cultures are negative in up to 60% of patients with clinical manifestations compatible with SBP and increased ascites PMN counts [115].

Therefore, the diagnosis of SBP is established with an ascites PMN count greater than 250/mm^3, and treatment should be initiated before obtaining bacteriological culture results [25]. If the PMN count is below 250/mm^3, culture results must be awaited. If ascites culture is positive (bacterascites), the ascites cell count should be repeated and, if the repeat PMN count is greater than 250/mm^3, SBP has developed and should be treated. However, if the PMN count remains below 250/mm^3, the results of a second bacteriological culture should be awaited. In most cases, the repeat culture will be negative but if it continues to be positive for the same organism it is assumed that bacteria are being seeded into ascites from an extraabdominal source and, although it is not causing peritonitis, bacterascites should then be treated [25].

The most effective (~ 90% resolution rate) and safe antibiotics are intravenous cefotaxime (2 g i.v. every 12 h) or other third-generation cephalosporins, such as ceftriaxone (1–2 g i.v. every 24 h) or ceftazidime (1 g i.v. every 12–24 h)

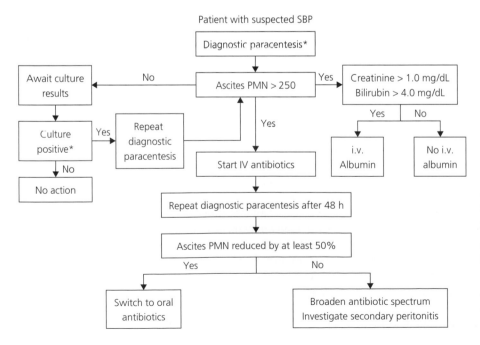

Figure 23.6 Approach to the patient with suspected spontaneous bacterial peritonitis (SBP). *A diagnostic paracentesis should be performed in any patient with symptoms or signs suggestive of SBP, any patient with unexplained renal dysfunction or encephalopathy, and in any hospitalized patient with cirrhosis and ascites. i.v., intravenous; PMN, polymorphonuclear leukocytes.

[136–139]. The combination of amoxicillin/clavulanic acid (1 g/0.2 g i.v. every 8 h) has been shown to be as effective and safe as cefotaxime in the treatment of SBP [140]. Patients who develop SBP on prophylactic quinolones have been shown to respond as well to cefotaxime as patients not on prophylaxis [141]. The antibiotics recommended above have been associated with few side effects and no renal toxicity. By contrast, aminoglycosides should be avoided in patients with cirrhosis because of their increased propensity to develop aminoglycoside-induced nephrotoxicity [142,143].

Renal dysfunction is the main cause of death in SBP and both can be prevented by the use of intravenous albumin [144]. Because renal dysfunction and death in SBP occur almost exclusively in patients with a baseline concentration of serum bilirubin greater than 4 mg/dL and a serum creatinine level exceeding 1 mg/dL [144,145], the prophylactic use of albumin in SBP can probably be restricted to this subgroup of high-risk patients [146]. The dose of albumin used is arbitrary: 1.5 g/kg of body weight during the first 6 h, followed by 1 g/kg on day 3, with a maximum of 100 g/day. There is a subgroup of patients with SBP – those with community-acquired infection, no encephalopathy, and normal renal function – that have a 100% cure rate and 100% survival with antibiotic therapy alone [147]. Albumin would not be indicated in these patients [146].

A control paracentesis performed 48 h after starting therapy is recommended to assess the response to therapy and the need to modify antibiotic therapy (depending on the isolation of a causative organism) or to initiate investigations to rule out secondary peritonitis [25]. If clinical improvement is obvious, this control paracentesis may not be necessary. Failure of initial therapy, defined as a decrease in PMN of less than 25% from baseline, occurs in up to 23% of the cases and is associated with a poor prognosis. In the presence of either clinical or cytological improvement, intravenous antibiotics can be switched to oral antibiotics after 2 days of therapy. This strategy has been shown to be as effective as continuous intravenous antibiotic therapy in two trials that used ciprofloxacin (first intravenous and then oral) [148,149]. Although a growing number of infections involving quinolone-resistant organisms may limit the use of quinolones as first-line antibiotic therapy in SBP [115], switching from intravenous cephalosporins to oral quinolones is a common practice recommended in complicated urinary tract infection in adults [150].

Total duration of antibiotic therapy should be for a minimum of 5 days. However, in prospective trials in which ascites PMN counts were carefully monitored, the median time to SBP resolution (i.e., a decrease in PMN count below 250/mm³) was 8 days and therefore this duration of therapy is probably more recommendable [151].

In patients who survive an episode of SBP, the one-year cumulative SBP recurrence rate is high, at about 70%. Recurrence, particularly secondary to gram-negative organisms, is significantly and markedly lower with the use of norfloxacin at a dose of 400 mg p.o. per day [152,153]. It is therefore essential that patients surviving an episode of SBP are started on antibiotic prophylaxis to prevent recurrence. The use of weekly quinolones is not recommended because it has been shown to be less effective in preventing SBP recurrence and is associated with a higher rate of development of quinolone-resistant organisms [153]. Prophylaxis should be continuous until disappearance of ascites (i.e., patients with alcoholic hepatitis), death, or transplant.

The patient with cirrhosis and acute renal failure

Acute renal failure occurs in 14%–25% of hospitalized patients with cirrhosis [143,154,155]. There are three types of acute renal failure: prerenal failure, which results from renal hypoperfusion without a glomerular or tubular lesion; intrinsic renal failure, which results from tubular necrosis (ischemic or toxic), glomerulonephritis, or interstitial nephritis; and postrenal failure, which results from urinary tract obstruction.

In hospitalized patients with cirrhosis, the most common cause of acute renal failure is prerenal (accounting for 60%–80% of the cases) [154,156,157], followed by acute tubular necrosis (20%–40%) [154,156,157], with postrenal causes accounting for less than 1% of the cases [156,157].

Prerenal failure results from any factor that will further decrease the already decreased effective arterial blood volume of the patient with cirrhosis. Therefore prerenal failure can result from factors that cause hypovolemia, such as gastrointestinal hemorrhage, overdiuresis, or diarrhea; factors that worsen vasodilation, such as sepsis, use of vasodilators, and the postparacentesis circulatory dysfunction; and factors that cause renal vasoconstriction, such as nonsteroidal antiinflammatory drugs or intravenous contrast agents. These factors account for up to 80% of the causes of prerenal failure [154]. The persistence of acute renal failure despite exclusion or reversal of the above-mentioned precipitant factors indicates the presence of type 1 hepatorenal syndrome (HRS), which accounts for only about 20% of cases of acute renal failure in cirrhosis [156]. HRS type 1 is a type of prerenal failure because it results from hemodynamic abnormalities (extreme vasodilation) leading to renal vasoconstriction [49] (Fig. 23.2). The other type of HRS, type 2, although also resulting from vasodilation, is a chronic form of renal failure associated with refractory ascites and is not considered in the differential diagnosis of acute renal failure in cirrhosis.

In patients with cirrhosis, acute tubular necrosis (ATN) is mainly caused by an ischemic insult to the renal tubules, mostly as a result of a hypotensive event, although the use of aminoglycosides (which cause renal failure by direct toxicity to renal tubules) was found to be the most important predictor of renal failure in cirrhosis in a study performed in US

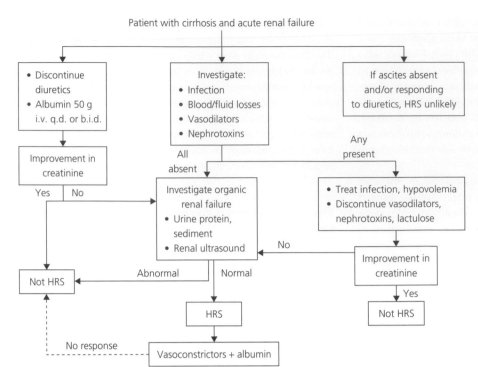

Patient with cirrhosis and acute renal failure

- Discontinue diuretics
- Albumin 50 g i.v. q.d. or b.i.d.

Improvement in creatinine

Yes   No

Investigate:
- Infection
- Blood/fluid losses
- Vasodilators
- Nephrotoxins

All absent

If ascites absent and/or responding to diuretics, HRS unlikely

Any present

Investigate organic renal failure
- Urine protein, sediment
- Renal ultrasound

- Treat infection, hypovolemia
- Discontinue vasodilators, nephrotoxins, lactulose

No

Improvement in creatinine

Yes

Not HRS

Abnormal   Normal

Not HRS

HRS

No response

Vasoconstrictors + albumin

Figure 23.7 Approach to the patient with cirrhosis and acute renal failure. b.i.d., twice a day; HRS, hepatorenal syndrome; i.v., intravenous; q.d., once a day.

veterans [143]. Studies are needed on the natural course, diagnosis, and treatment (e.g., hemodialysis) of acute tubular necrosis in patients with cirrhosis.

The approach to a patient with cirrhosis and acute renal failure is depicted in Fig. 23.7 [132,158].

In a patient with cirrhosis who presents with an acute deterioration in renal function as evidenced by a doubling of serum creatinine to more than 2.5 mg/dL within a 2-week period [116], the main issue is to rule out HRS as this entity involves a totally separate therapeutic approach (see below). Indirect estimates of glomerular filtration rate such as the Modification of Diet in Renal Disease (MDRD) equation have not yet been evaluated in the assessment of renal failure in patients with cirrhosis.

Urine indices (urine osmolality, urinary sodium concentration, and fractional excretion of sodium) may help to distinguish prerenal failure (including HRS) from acute tubular necrosis. The tubular ability to reabsorb sodium and to concentrate urine is preserved in prerenal azotemia and is impaired in acute tubular necrosis. Therefore, patients with prerenal failure have low urinary sodium concentrations (< 20 mEq/L) and elevated urine osmolality (> 500 mOsm/kg) whereas patients with tubular necrosis have high urinary sodium concentrations (> 40 mEq/L) and a urine osmolality below 350 mOsm/kg. However, the urinary sodium concentration may be low early in the course of certain processes that lead to tubular necrosis, such as sepsis, and some cases of HRS with elevated urinary sodium concentrations have been reported [158].

If the patient with acute renal failure does not have ascites, the diagnosis of HRS is highly unlikely, because HRS is the result of maximal derangement in the hemodynamics that lead to ascites formation (Fig. 23.2) [49].

A first step in the diagnostic workup is to discontinue diuretics and to expand the intravascular volume with albumin at a dose of 50 g i.v. This dose can be repeated in 12 h if the creatinine has not normalized. A reduction in creatinine will rule out HRS.

At the same time, investigations to rule out the precipitants of renal dysfunction should be undertaken, specifically diagnostic paracentesis (to rule out SBP), blood and urine bacteriological cultures and chest radiograph to rule out a bacterial infections other than SBP, and stool investigations to rule out gastrointestinal hemorrhage. If any of these precipitants is identified, the patients should be treated accordingly.

Once precipitants of renal dysfunction are excluded or treated and if creatinine does not improve or continues to worsen despite diuretic discontinuation and continued volume expansion the differential diagnosis is between intrinsic renal failure, postrenal failure, or HRS. To rule out intrinsic renal failure, urinary sediment and urine protein should be analyzed. To rule out postrenal failure, a renal ultrasound should be obtained. To ensure that volume has been adequately expanded, it is reasonable to perform central venous pressure measurements at this point.

If ATN or other organic or postobstructive causes of renal failure are ruled out, the patient has HRS type 1. The differentiation between acute tubular necrosis and HRS is the most difficult, and it has been suggested that the response to vasoconstrictors plus albumin (see below) may be used to establish this differential [158].

The patient with hepatorenal syndrome

HRS is a potentially reversible functional renal failure that occurs in patients with cirrhosis, ascites, and liver failure and in patients with acute liver failure and alcoholic hepatitis [132]. HRS is secondary to renal vasoconstriction that results from markedly decreased effective arterial blood volume and the resultant activation of renal vasoconstrictive systems. Decreased effective blood volume is in turn the result of intense vasodilation (Fig. 23.2) and, as postulated, of a relatively low cardiac output [132]. Because HRS represents the extreme of the spectrum of abnormalities that lead to sodium and water retention, ascites unresponsive to diuretics is universal, and dilutional hyponatremia is almost always present (Fig. 23.2).

HRS is divided into two types based on clinical characteristics and prognosis. Type 1 HRS is characterized by rapidly progressive renal failure defined by doubling of the serum creatinine concentrations to a level greater than 2.5 mg/dL in less than 2 weeks. It may appear spontaneously, but often develops after a precipitating event, particularly SBP. Its prognosis is poor, with a median survival of 2–4 weeks [159,160]. Type 2 HRS is a moderate renal failure (serum creatinine 1.5–2.5 mg/dL), with a steady or slowly progressive course, and is associated with refractory ascites. Survival of patients with type 2 HRS is shorter than that of nonazotemic cirrhotic patients with ascites but better than that of patients with type 1 HRS (median survival about 6 months) [132,160]. Type 2 HRS will not be considered in this section.

Patients with ascites have 1- and 5-year probabilities of developing HRS of around 20% and 40% respectively [159]. The likelihood of developing HRS is highest in patients with more marked sodium and water retention and more marked activation of vasoconstrictive systems (renin–angiotensin and sympathetic nervous system) [159], indicative of marked vasodilation (Fig. 23.2). A low cardiac output and high plasma renin activity were found to be independent predictors of HRS in patients with cirrhosis and uncomplicated ascites [161].

As mentioned previously, HRS is diagnosed by exclusion of other known causes of acute renal failure (Fig. 23.8).

Therapies for hepatorenal syndrome

Different therapies for HRS and their site of action are depicted in Fig. 23.8. Except for transplant, none of the different treatments of HRS has resulted in significant improvements in survival. However, treating HRS is important because patients who respond to therapy have a better survival and because the presence of renal disease has an impact on post-liver transplant outcomes [162].

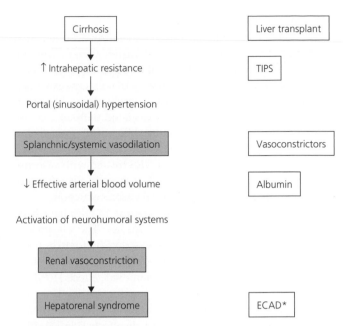

Figure 23.8 Site of action of different therapies for hepatorenal syndrome. *ECAD (extracorporeal albumin dialysis) is an experimental therapy that seems to improve hepatorenal syndrome; it probably acts by decreasing the amount of circulating vasodilators. TIPS, transjugular intrahepatic portosystemic shunt.

Liver transplant

The first and only definitive therapy for HRS is liver transplantation because it is the only therapy that will provide long-term survival. With the implementation of the Model for End-stage Liver Disease (MELD) score in the allocation of organs in the United States, priority for transplant is given to patients with a high creatinine [163]. In a study aimed at assessing prognostic factors in HRS, MELD score and the type of HRS (type 1 or 2) were independent predictors of death. Whereas all patients with type 1 HRS had a high MELD score (> 20) and had a poor outcome (median survival 1 month), survival of patients with type 2 HRS was longer and depended on their MELD score [160]. This suggests that the development of HRS type 1 per se should indicate a high priority for transplant, independent of MELD.

Patients with HRS who are transplanted have more complications and a higher in-hospital mortality rate than those without HRS [164–167]. Therefore, HRS should be treated before transplantation in an attempt to improve renal function. In fact, the outcome of liver transplantation in patients with HRS treated with vasopressin analogues prior to transplant is similar to that of patients transplanted without HRS [168]. HRS alone should not be a reason for combined kidney and liver transplant; however, this is being considered in patients with HRS who become dialysis-dependent and show no recovery after 8 weeks of dialysis (the usual recovery time for acute renal failure) [162]. The need for dialysis should theoretically be prevented by the early treatment of HRS with the "bridging" therapies outlined below.

Vasoconstrictors plus albumin

The rationale behind this approach is to improve the deranged circulatory function by ameliorating vasodilation thereby improving effective arterial blood volume and decreasing renal vasoconstriction. Albumin, an intravascular volume expander, has been used to increase effective blood volume. However, albumin dialysis (see below) is associated with an increase in blood pressure attributable to the ability of albumin to bind vasodilators. It is therefore conceivable that an improvement of renal function in patients with HRS treated with vasoconstrictors and albumin is the result of the additive effects of both agents in producing peripheral vasoconstriction.

Data about the use of vasoconstrictors in HRS have been mostly derived from uncontrolled studies. The vasopressin analogue ornipressin was the first vasoconstrictor to be used, and although it was found to be effective, its use was abandoned because of a high rate of ischemic side effects [169,170]. Terlipressin, another vasopressin analogue, has been the most widely used vasoconstrictor agent in type 1 HRS and is associated with a low incidence of side effects [156,171–175]. The combination of midodrine plus octreotide has been effective in two small uncontrolled studies [176,177]. It is uncertain whether the effectiveness of this therapy is the result of midodrine alone (an α-adrenergic agonist) or the combination, because octreotide alone has been shown to have no effect in HRS when compared with placebo [178] or with a vasopressin infusion [179]. The combination of intravenous noradrenaline (another α-adrenergic agonist) plus albumin was effective and safe in a small uncontrolled study [180]; however, the need for medication infusion in an intensive care setting limits its applicability.

In most of these studies, albumin was associated with the vasoconstrictor, and one of them showed that treatment with terlipressin and albumin was associated with a significant decrease in the serum creatinine level and an increase in arterial pressure, changes that were not observed in a nonconcurrent group of patients treated with terlipressin alone [181].

In total, 11 uncontrolled studies have been published using vasoconstrictors and including 215 patients with HRS type 1. Reversal of HRS (decrease in creatinine below 1.5 mg/dL) was observed in 64% of the cases and, interestingly, HRS recurred in only a minority (23%) of these patients once therapy was discontinued. One-month survival was 39%, with a better survival in patients who responded to vasoconstrictors [156,179]. Terlipressin may induce ischemic side effects and arrhythmias requiring drug discontinuation.

A small, nonblinded, placebo-controlled study suggested that terlipressin (compared with placebo) was associated with an improvement in HRS (5/12 vs 0/12) and in survival (5/12 vs 0/12) [182]. However, a large multicenter, randomized, placebo-controlled double-blind trial of terlipressin vs placebo in the treatment of type 1 HRS showed that, although reversal of HRS was significantly better in patients in the terlipressin group (19/56, or 34%, in the terlipressin group vs 7/56, or 13%, in the placebo group), survival was identical in both treatment groups (27/56, or 48%, survival at 60 days for both groups) and, notably, HRS reversal rate (34%) was much lower than that demonstrated in uncontrolled studies [183]. The study also confirms that survival is significantly better in patients who responded to terlipressin.

Transjugular intrahepatic portosystemic shunt

Only three small prospective but uncontrolled studies have assessed the role of TIPS in HRS type 1, using 6, 14, and 5 patients (who had responded to octreotide/midodrine), respectively [177,184,185]. All studies showed a decrease in serum creatinine in most patients and a decrease in plasma renin activity. The rate of decrease in creatinine in most patients was slower than that obtained using terlipressin plus albumin. Recurrence of HRS was rare as long as the shunt remained patent but portosystemic encephalopathy was a frequent complication. Post-TIPS resolution of HRS type 1 appeared to improve survival. Long-term success was demonstrated in the study that explored sequential treatment with vasoconstrictors and albumin followed by TIPS [177]. Notably, a great majority of patients included in these three studies had alcoholic cirrhosis, many with active alcoholism, and therefore the improvement observed could have resulted from improvement in an acute-on-chronic process. Also, all three studies excluded patients with a CTP score equal to or greater than 12.

Given the paucity of data, TIPS could be used as a treatment of type 1 HRS only in the setting of prospective randomized trials.

Extracorporeal albumin dialysis

In a small, randomized study, the molecular adsorbent recirculating system, a modified dialysis method using an albumin-containing dialysate (eventually combined with intermittent venovenous hemofiltration), was shown to improve 30-day survival in eight patients with HRS type 1 compared with five patients treated with intermittent venovenous hemofiltration alone [186]. Because extracorporeal albumin dialysis (ECAD) incorporates a standard dialysis machine or a continuous venovenous hemofiltration monitor and glomerular filtration rate was not measured, the decrease in serum creatinine observed in most patients could be related to the dialysis process. However, clear beneficial effects on systemic hemodynamics and on hepatic encephalopathy were observed. ECAD is still considered an experimental therapy and its use in patients with type 1 HRS cannot be recommended outside prospective pathophysiological or therapeutic investigations.

The patient with suspected hepatorenal syndrome

Patients with suspected type 1 HRS should be managed as inpatients for diagnostic investigation and treatment. Vital signs, urine output, and blood chemistry should be closely monitored. Diuretics should continue to be withheld in these patients to prevent further decreases in effective arterial blood volume. Saline solution should not be administered as it will lead to significant increases in ascites and edema because sodium retention is severe in these patients. Because most patients have dilutional hyponatraemia, fluids (both oral and intravenous) should be restricted to approximately 1000 mL/day. Early identification of bacterial infections and treatment with broad-spectrum antibiotics is fundamental, because severe infections are common and contribute to death in these patients. The patient should be evaluated for liver transplantation and, if already on a transplant list, his or her status should be updated.

Specific treatment with vasoconstrictors plus albumin should be initiated as soon as the diagnosis is suspected. The best evidence supports the use of terlipressin, which should be started at a dose 0.5–1 mg i.v. every 4–6 h. If there is no early response (> 25% decrease in creatinine levels after 2 days), the dose can be doubled every 2 days up to a maximum of 12 mg/day (i.e., 2 mg i.v. every 4 h). Treatment can be stopped if serum creatinine does not decrease by at least 50% after 7 days at the highest dose, or if there is no reduction in creatinine after the first 3 days. In patients with early response, treatment should be extended until reversal of HRS (decrease in creatinine below 1.5 mg/dL) or for a maximum of 14 days [132].

A more rational method for adjusting the dose of vasoconstrictors is by monitoring mean arterial blood pressure (an indirect indicator of vasodilation). This method has been used for adjusting the dose of midodrine plus octreotide [176], an alternative to terlipressin in places such as the United States where terlipressin is not available. In this study, the doses of octreotide and midodrine were titrated to obtain an increase in mean arterial pressure of at least 15 mmHg; midodrine was administered orally at an initial dose of 7.5 mg t.i.d and, if necessary, increased to 12.5 mg t.i.d; octreotide was administered subcutaneously at an initial dose of 100 µg t.i.d and, if necessary, increased to 200 µg t.i.d [176]. In another study, different doses of midodrine (2.5 mg p.o., t.i.d) and octreotide (i.v. infusion of 25 µg/h after an initial bolus of 25 µg) were used [177].

Other alternatives to terlipressin are vasopressin or noradrenaline. Noradrenaline is used as a continuous intravenous infusion at an initial dose of 0.5 mg/h, adjusted to achieve an increase in mean arterial pressure of at least 10 mmHg or an increase in 4-h urine output to more than 200 mL. If these goals are not reached, the dose is increased every 4 h in steps of 0.5 mg/h, up to the maximum dose of 3 mg/h [180]. Vasopressin is also used as a continuous intravenous infusion, starting at a low dose of 0.01 U/min and titrating up to a dose of 0.5 U/min, depending on changes in mean arterial pressure and urine output and the presence of ischemic side effects. In the study that assessed vasopressin for HRS, the mean vasopressin dose in the group of responders was 0.23 ± 0.19 U/min [179].

Albumin should be administered with the vasoconstrictor. The maintenance dose, once the diagnosis of HRS is established and vasoconstrictors are initiated, is 20–40 g/day. Albumin may be discontinued if the serum albumin concentration exceeds 45 g/L and should be withdrawn in case of pulmonary edema. Because this complication is uncommon, catheterization to monitor central venous pressure is not mandatory, but careful physical and radiological monitoring of cardiopulmonary function is recommended [132].

In early responders, treatment with vasoconstrictors and albumin should be maintained until normalization of serum creatinine (< 1.5 mg/dL). Once reversal of HRS is obtained (creatinine < 1.5 mg/dL), the dose of vasoconstrictors can be titrated down until discontinuation.

Renal replacement therapy should be considered in patients who develop pulmonary edema, severe hyperkalemia, or metabolic acidosis not responding to medical therapy.

Prophylaxis of hepatorenal syndrome

Three randomized controlled studies suggest that HRS can be prevented in three specific clinical settings: SBP, ascites with low protein associated with severe liver and/or renal dysfunction, and alcoholic hepatitis.

In a non-placebo-controlled study in patients with SBP, the intravenous administration of albumin (1.5 g/kg at the diagnosis of the infection and 1 g/kg 48 h later) together with antibiotics decreased the risk of HRS by 66% compared with treatment using antibiotics alone (10% vs 33%) and improved hospital survival [144]. The beneficial effect of albumin is probably related to its capacity to improve effective arterial blood volume, as shown by a decrease in plasma renin activity, and is mainly observed in high-risk patients (i.e., those with a serum creatinine > 1.0 mg/dL or a serum bilirubin > 4 mg/dL) [145].

In a placebo-controlled study, the daily administration of norfloxacin (400 mg p.o.) in patients with low ascites protein (< 1.5 g/dL) and either renal or severe liver dysfunction was associated with a lower probability of developing HRS than placebo-treated patients [118].

In a double-blind, placebo-controlled study in patients with alcoholic hepatitis, the administration of pentoxifylline (400 mg t.i.d) was associated with significantly lower rates of HRS (8% vs 35%) and mortality (24% vs 46%) compared with patients randomized to placebo [187]. The beneficial effect of pentoxifylline could be related to its capacity to inhibit production of tumor necrosis factor and the resultant vasodilation; however, the study failed to show significant changes in plasma levels of tumor necrosis factor and did not report on hemodynamics.

In these three studies, the relation between prevention of HRS and improved survival is further proof that renal failure is an important determinant of death in patients with decompensated cirrhosis [3].

References

1. Runyon BA. Ascites. In: Schiff L, Schiff ER (eds). Diseases of the liver. Philadelphia: Lippincott, 1993:990.
2. Runyon BA, Montano AA, Akriviadis EA, et al. The serum-ascites albumin gradient is superior to the exudate-transudate concept in the differential diagnosis of ascites. Ann Intern Med 1992;117:215.
3. D'Amico G, Garcia-Tsao G, Pagliaro L. Natural history and prognostic indicators of survival in cirrhosis. A systematic review of 118 studies. J Hepatol 2006;44:217.
4. Cummings S, Papadakis M, Melnick J, et al. The predictive value of physical examinations for ascites. West J Med 1985;142:633.
5. Goldberg BB, Goodman GA, Clearfield HR. Evaluation of ascites by ultrasound. Radiology 1970;96:15.
6. Black M, Friedman AC. Ultrasound examination in the patient with ascites. Ann Intern Med 1989;110:253.
7. Runyon BA. Management of adult patients with ascites caused by cirrhosis. Hepatology 1998;27:264.
8. McVay PA, Toy PT. Lack of increased bleeding after paracentesis and thoracentesis in patients with mild coagulation abnormalities. Transfusion 1991;31:164.
9. Hoefs JC. Serum protein concentration and portal pressure determine the ascitic fluid protein concentration in patients with chronic liver disease. J Lab Clin Med 1983;102:260.
10. Henriksen JH. Colloid osmotic pressure in decompensated cirrhosis. A 'mirror image' of portal venous hypertension. Scand J Gastroenterol 1985;20:170.
11. Pare P, Talbot J, Hoefs JC. Serum-ascites albumin concentration gradient: a physiologic approach to the differential diagnosis of ascites. Gastroenterology 1983;85:240.
12. Hoefs JC. Globulin correction of the albumin gradient: correlation with measured serum to ascites colloid osmotic pressure gradients. Hepatology 1992;16:396.
13. Hirabayashi K, Graham J. Genesis of ascites in ovarian cancer. Am J Obstet Gynecol 1970;106:492.
14. Witte CL, Witte MH, Dumont AE, et al. Lymph protein in hepatic cirrhosis and experimental hepatic and portal venous hypertension. Ann Surg 1968;168:567.
15. Dumont AE, Witte CL, Witte MH. Protein content of liver lymph in patients with portal hypertension secondary to hepatic cirrhosis. Lymphology 1975;8:111.
16. Henriksen JH, Horn T, Christoffersen P. The blood-lymph barrier in the liver. A review based on morphological and functional concepts of normal and cirrhotic liver. Liver 1984;4:221.
17. Runyon BA. Low-protein-concentration ascitic fluid is predisposed to spontaneous bacterial peritonitis. Gastroenterology 1986;91:1343.
18. Runyon BA, Hoefs JC. Ascitic fluid chemical analysis before, during and after spontaneous bacterial peritonitis. Hepatology 1985;5:257.
19. Morali GA, Sniderman KW, Deitel KM, et al. Is sinusoidal portal hypertension a necessary factor for the development of hepatic ascites? J Hepatol 1992;16:249.
20. Casado M, Bosch J, Garcia-Pagan JC, et al. Clinical events after transjugular intrahepatic portosystemic shunt: correlation with hemodynamic findings. Gastroenterology 1998;114:1296.
21. Abraldes JG, Tarantino I, Turnes J, et al. Hemodynamic response to pharmacological treatment of portal hypertension and long-term prognosis of cirrhosis. Hepatology 2003;37:902.
22. Myers RP, Cerini R, Sayegh R, et al. Cardiac hepatopathy: clinical, hemodynamic, and histologic characteristics and correlations. Hepatology 2003;37:393.
23. Groszmann RJ, Wongcharatrawee S. The hepatic venous pressure gradient: Anything worth doing should be done right. Hepatology 2004;39:280.
24. Trejo R, Alvarez W, Garcia-Pagan JC, et al. The applicability and diagnostic effectiveness of transjugular liver biopsy. Medicina Clinica 1996;107:521.
25. Rimola A, Garcia-Tsao G, Navasa M, et al. Diagnosis, treatment and prophylaxis of spontaneous bacterial peritonitis: a consensus document. J Hepatol 2000;32:142.
26. Castellote J, Lopez C, Gornals J, et al. Rapid diagnosis of spontaneous bacterial peritonitis by use of reagent strips. Hepatology 2003;37:893.
27. Ghassemi S, Garcia-Tsao G. Prevention and treatment of infections in patients with cirrhosis. Baillière's Best Pract Res Clin Gastroenterol 2007;21:77.
28. Runyon BA, Canawati HN, Akriviadis EA. Optimization of ascitic fluid culture technique. Gastroenterology 1988;95:1351.
29. Bobadilla M, Sifuentes J, Garcia-Tsao G. Improved method for bacteriological diagnosis of spontaneous bacterial peritonitis. J Clin Microbiol 1989;27:2145.
30. Akriviadis EA, Runyon BA. Utility of an algorithm in differentiating spontaneous from secondary bacterial peritonitis. Gastroenterology 1990;98:127.
31. Garcia-Tsao G. Spontaneous bacterial peritonitis. Gastro Clin North Am 1992;21:257.
32. Young ST, Paulson EK, Washington K, et al. CT of the liver in patients with metastatic breast carcinoma treated by chemotherapy: findings simulating cirrhosis. AJR Am J Roentgenol 1994;163:1385.
33. Sass DA, Clark K, Grzybicki D, et al. Diffuse desmoplastic metastatic breast cancer simulating cirrhosis with severe portal hypertension: a case of "pseudocirrhosis." Dig Dis Sci 2007;52:749.
34. Runyon BA, Hoefs JC, Morgan TR. Ascitic fluid analysis in malignancy-related ascites. Hepatology 1988;8:1104.
35. Both CT, de Mattos AA, Neumann J, et al. Flow cytometry in the diagnosis of peritoneal carcinomatosis. Am J Gastroenterol 2001;96:1605.
36. Weissman GS, McKinley MJ, Budman DR, et al. Flow cytometry. A new technique in the diagnosis of malignant ascites. J Clin. Gastroenterol 1987;9:599.
37. Zuckerman E, Lanir A, Sabo E, et al. Cancer antigen 125: a sensitive marker of ascites in patients with liver cirrhosis. Am J Gastroenterol 1999;94:1613.
38. Runyon BA. Malignancy-related ascites and ascitic fluid "humoral tests of malignancy". J Clin Gastroenterol 1994;18:94.
39. Hillebrand DJ, Runyon BA, Yasmineh WG, et al. Ascitic fluid adenosine deaminase insensitivity in detecting tuberculous peritonitis in the United States. Hepatology 1996;24:1408.
40. Sanai FM, Bzeizi KI. Systematic review: tuberculous peritonitis – presenting features, diagnostic strategies and treatment. Aliment Pharmacol Ther 2005;22:685.
41. Riquelme A, Calvo M, Salech F, et al. Value of adenosine deaminase (ADA) in ascitic fluid for the diagnosis of tuberculous peritonitis: a meta-analysis. J Clin Gastroenterol 2006;40:705.
42. Burgess LJ, Swanepoel CG, Taljaard, JJ. The use of adenosine deaminase as a diagnostic tool for peritoneal tuberculosis. Tuberculosis (Edinb.) 2001;81:243.
43. Sankaran S, Walt AJ. Pancreatic ascites: recognition and management. Arch Surg 1976;111:430.
44. Munoz JN, Bose S. Pancreatic ascites. A case report and review of the literature. Am J Dig Dis 1975;20:1178.
45. Joseph J, Viney S, Beck P, et al. A prospective study of amylase-rich pleural effusions with special reference to amylase isoenzyme analysis. Chest 1992;102:1455.
46. Press OW, Press NO, Kaufman SD. Evaluation and management of chylous ascites. Ann Intern Med 1982;96:358.
47. Aalami OO, Allen DB, Organ CH, Jr. Chylous ascites: a collective review. Surgery 2000;128:761.
48. Rector WG, Jr. Spontaneous chylous ascites of cirrhosis. J Clin Gastroenterol 1984;6:369.
49. Schrier RW, Arroyo V, Bernardi M, et al. Peripheral arterial vasodilation hypothesis – A proposal for the initiation of renal sodium and water retention in cirrhosis. Hepatology 1988;8:1151.
50. Gines P, Berl T, Bernardi M, et al. Hyponatremia in cirrhosis: from pathogenesis to treatment. Hepatology 1998;28:851.

51. Planas R, Montoliu S, Balleste B, et al. Natural history of patients hospitalized for management of cirrhotic ascites. Clin Gastroenterol Hepatol 2006;4:1385.

52. Moore KP, Wong F, Gines P, et al. The management of ascites in cirrhosis: report on the consensus conference of the International Ascites Club. Hepatology 2003;38:258.

53. Salerno F, Borroni G, Moser P, et al. Survival and prognostic factors of cirrhotic patients with ascites: a study of 134 outpatients. Am J Gastroenterol 1993;88:514.

54. Fogel MR, Sawhney VK, Neal A, et al. Diuresis in the ascitic patient: a randomized controlled trial of three regimens. J Clin Gastroenterol 1981;3(Suppl. 1):73.

55. Perez-Ayuso RM, Arroyo V, Planas R, et al. Randomized comparative study of efficacy of furosemide versus spironolactone in non-azotemic cirrhosis with ascites. Relationship between the diuretic response and the activity of the renin-aldosterone system. Gastroenterology 1983;84:961.

56. Mirouze D, Zipser RD, Reynolds TB. Effects of inhibitors of prostaglandin synthesis on induced diuresis in cirrhosis. Hepatology 1983;3:50.

57. Planas R, Arroyo V, Rimola A, et al. Acetylsalicylic acid suppresses the renal hemodynamic effect and reduces the diuretic action of furosemide in cirrhosis with ascites. Gastroenterology 1983;84:247.

58. Bosch-Marce M, Claria J, Titos E, et al. Selective inhibition of cyclooxygenase 2 spares renal function and prostaglandin synthesis in cirrhotic rats with ascites. Gastroenterology 1999;116:1167.

59. Guevara M, Abecasis R, Terg R: Effect of celecoxib on renal function in cirrhotic patients with ascites. A pilot study. Scand J Gastroenterol 2004;39:385.

60. Gines P, Arroyo V, Quintero E, et al. Comparison of paracentesis and diuretics in the treatment of cirrhotics with tense ascites: Results of a randomized study. Gastroenterology 1987;93:234.

61. Salerno F, Badalamenti S, Incerti P, et al. Repeated paracentesis and i.v. albumin infusion to treat "tense" ascites in cirrhotic patients: A safe alternative therapy. J Hepatol 1987;5:102.

62. Sola R, Vila MC, Andreu M, et al. Total paracentesis with dextran 40 vs. diuretics in the treatment of ascites in cirrhosis: a randomized controlled study. J Hepatol 1994;20:282.

63. Angeli P, Dalla Pria M, DeBei E, et al. Randomized clinical study of the efficacy of amiloride and potassium canrenoate in nonazotemic cirrhotic patients with ascites. Hepatology 1994;19:72.

64. Tito L, Gines P, Arroyo V, et al. Total paracentesis associated with intravenous albumin management of patients with cirrhosis and ascites. Gastroenterology 1990;98:146.

65. Fernandez-Esparrach G, Guevara M, Sort P, et al. Diuretic requirements after therapeutic paracentesis in non-azotemic patients with cirrhosis. A randomized double-blind trial of spironolactone versus placebo. J Hepatol 1997;26:614.

66. Arnold C, Haag K, Blum HE, et al. Acute hemoperitoneum after large-volume paracentesis. Gastroenterology 1997;113:978.

67. Grabau CM, Crago SF, Hoff LK, et al. Performance standards for therapeutic abdominal paracentesis. Hepatology 2004;40:484.

68. Oelsner DH, Caldwell SH, Coles M, et al. Subumbilical midline vascularity of the abdominal wall in portal hypertension observed at laparoscopy. Gastrointest Endosc 1998;47:388.

69. Conn HO. Sudden scrotal edema in cirrhosis: a postparacentesis syndrome. Ann Intern Med 1971;74:943.

70. Gines A, Fernandez-Esparrach G, Monescillo A, et al. Randomized trial comparing albumin, dextran-70 and polygeline in cirrhotic patients with ascites treated by paracentesis. Gastroenterology 1996;111:1002.

71. Ruiz del Arbol L, Monescillo A, Jimenez W, et al. Paracentesis-induced circulatory dysfunction: mechanism and effect on hepatic hemodynamics in cirrhosis. Gastroenterology 1997;113:579.

72. Gines P, Tito L, Arroyo V, et al. Randomized comparative study of therapeutic paracentesis with and without intravenous albumin in cirrhosis. Gastroenterology 1988;94:1493.

73. Planas R, Gines P, Arroyo V, et al. Dextran-70 versus albumin as plasma expanders in cirrhotic patients with tense ascites treated with total paracentesis. Results of a randomized study. Gastroenterology 1990;99:1738.

74. Sola-Vera J, Minana J, Ricart E, et al. Randomized trial comparing albumin and saline in the prevention of paracentesis-induced circulatory dysfunction in cirrhotic patients with ascites. Hepatology 2003;37:1147.

75. Jeffries MA, Stern MA, Gunaratnam NT, et al. Unsuspected infection is infrequent in asymptomatic outpatients with refractory ascites undergoing therapeutic paracentesis. Am J Gastroenterol 1999;94:2972.

76. Evans LT, Kim WR, Poterucha JJ, et al. Spontaneous bacterial peritonitis in asymptomatic outpatients with cirrhotic ascites. Hepatology 2003;37:897.

77. Romney R, Mathurin P, Ganne-Carrie N, et al. Usefulness of routine analysis of ascitic fluid at the time of therapeutic paracentesis in asymptomatic outpatients. Results of a multicenter prospective study. Gastroenterol Clin Biol 2005;29:275.

78. Garcia-Tsao G. The transjugular intrahepatic portosystemic shunt for the management of refractory ascites. Nat Clin Pract Gastroenterol Hepatol 2006;3:380.

79. Somberg KA, Lake JR, Tomlanovich SJ, et al. Transjugular intrahepatic portosystemic shunts for refractory ascites: assessment of clinical and hormonal response and renal function. Hepatology 1995;21(3):709.

80. Wong F, Sniderman K, Liu P, et al. The mechanism of the initial natriuresis after transjugular intrahepatic portosystemic shunt. Gastroenterology 1997;112:899.

81. Lebrec D, Giuily N, Hadengue A, et al. Transjugular intrahepatic portosystemic shunts: comparison with paracentesis in patients with cirrhosis and refractory ascites: a randomized trial. J Hepatol 1996;25:135.

82. Quiroga J, Sangro B, Nunez M, et al. Transjugular intrahepatic portal-systemic shunt in the treatment of refractory ascites: effect on clinical, renal, humoral, and hemodynamic parameters. Hepatology 1995;21(4):986.

83. Wong F, Sniderman K, Liu P, et al. Transjugular intrahepatic portosystemic stent shunt: effects on hemodynamics and sodium homeostasis in cirrhosis and refractory ascites. Ann Intern Med 1995;122(11): 816.

84. Wong W, Liu P, Blendis L, et al. Long term renal sodium handling in patients with cirrhosis treated with transjugular intrahepatic portosystemic shunts for refractory ascites. Amer J Med 1999;106:315.

85. Rossle M, Deibert P, Haag K, et al. Randomised trial of transjugular-intrahepatic-portosystemic shunt versus endoscopy plus propranolol for prevention of variceal rebleeding. Lancet 1997;349:1043.

86. Gines P, Uriz J, Calahorra B, et al. Transjugular intrahepatic portosystemic shunting versus repeated paracentesis plus intravenous albumin for refractory ascites in cirrhosis: A multicenter randomized comparative study. Gastroenterology 2002;123:1839.

87. Sanyal AJ, Genning C, Reddy KR, et al. The North American Study for the Treatment of Refractory Ascites. Gastroenterology 2003;124:634.

88. Salerno F, Merli M, Riggio O, et al. Randomized controlled study of TIPS versus paracentesis plus albumin in cirrhosis with severe ascites. Hepatology 2004;40:629.

89. D'Amico G, Luca A, Morabito A, et al. Uncovered transjugular intrahepatic portosystemic shunt for refractory ascites: a meta-analysis. Gastroenterology 2005;129:1282.

90. Bureau C, Garcia-Pagan JC, Otal P, et al. Improved clinical outcome using polytetrafluoroethylene-coated stents for TIPS: results of a randomized study. Gastroenterology 2004;126:469.

91. Angermayr B, Cejna M, Koenig F, et al. Survival in patients undergoing transjugular intrahepatic portosystemic shunt: ePTFE-covered stentgrafts versus bare stents. Hepatology 2003;38:1043.

92. Boyer TD: Transjugular intrahepatic portosystemic shunt: current status. Gastroenterology 2003;124:1700.

93. Trotter JF, Suhocki PV. Incarceration of umbilical hernia following transjugular intrahepatic portosystemic shunt for the treatment of ascites. Liver Transpl Surg 1999;5:209.

94. Gerbes AL, Gulberg V. Benefit of TIPS for patients with refractory or recidivant ascites: serum bilirubin may make the difference. Hepatology 2005;41:217.

95. Stanley MM, Ochi S, Lee KK, et al. Peritoneovenous shunting as compared with medical treatment in patients with alcoholic cirrhosis and massive ascites. N Engl J Med 1989;321:1632.

96. Gines P, Arroyo V, Vargas V, et al. Paracentesis with intravenous infusion of albumin as compared with peritoneovenous shunting in cirrhosis with refractory ascites. N Engl J Med 1991;325:829.

97. Gines A, Planas R, Angeli P, et al. Treatment of patients with cirrhosis and refractory ascites by LeVeen shunt with titanium tip. Comparison with therapeutic paracentesis. Hepatology 1995;22:124.

98. Dumortier J, Pianta E, Le Derf Y, et al. Peritoneovenous shunt as a bridge to liver transplantation. Am J Transplant 2005;5:1886.

99. Bratby MJ, Hussain FF, Lopez AJ. Radiological insertion and management of peritoneovenous shunt. Cardiovasc Intervent Radiol 2007;30:415.

100. Bernhoft RA, Pellegrini CA, Way LW: Peritoneovenous shunt for refractory ascites: operative complications and long-term results. Arch Surg 1982;117:631.

101. Zervos EE, McCormick J, Goode SE, et al. Peritoneovenous shunts in patients with intractable ascites: palliation at what price? Am Surg 1997;63:157.

102. Lenaerts A, Codden T, Henry JP, et al. Comparative pilot study of repeated large volume paracentesis vs the combination on clonidine-spironolactone in the treatment of cirrhosis-associated refractory ascites. Gastroenterol Clin Biol 2005;29:1137.

103. Lenaerts A, Codden T, Meunier JC, et al. Effects of clonidine on diuretic response in ascitic patients with cirrhosis and activation of sympathetic nervous system. Hepatology 2006;44:844.

104. Jimenez W, Gal CS, Ros J, et al. Long-term aquaretic efficacy of a selective nonpeptide V(2)-vasopressin receptor antagonist, SR121463, in cirrhotic rats. J Pharmacol Exp Ther 2000;295:83.

105. Ros J, Fernandez-Varo G, Munoz-Luque J, et al. Sustained aquaretic effect of the V2-AVP receptor antagonist, RWJ-351647, in cirrhotic rats with ascites and water retention. Br J Pharmacol 2005;146:654.

106. Gerbes AL, Gulberg V, Gines P, et al. Therapy of hyponatremia in cirrhosis with a vasopressin receptor antagonist: a randomized double-blind multicenter trial. Gastroenterology 2003;124:933.

107. Gines P, Wong F, Watson H, et al. Effects of a selective vasopressin V2 receptor antagonist, satavaptan (SR121463B), in patients with cirrhosis and ascites without hyponatremia. Hepatology 2006;44 (Suppl. 1):445A.

108. Wong F, Gines P, Watson H et al. Effects of a selective vasopressin V2 receptor antagonist, satavaptan (SR121463B) on recurrence of ascites after large volume paracentesis. Hepatology 2006, 44 (Suppl 1): 256A.

109. Kalambokis G, Fotopoulos A, Economou M, et al. Effects of a 7-day treatment with midodrine in non-azotemic cirrhotic patients with and without ascites. J Hepatol 2007;46:213.

110. Moreau R, Asselah T, Condat B, et al. Comparison of the effect of terlipressin and albumin on arterial blood volume in patients with cirrhosis and tense ascites treated by paracentesis: a randomized pilot study. Gut 2002;50:90.

111. Singh V, Kumar R, Nain CK, et al. Terlipressin versus albumin in paracentesis-induced circulatory dysfunction in cirrhosis: a randomized study. J Gastroenterol Hepatol 2006;21:303.

112. Santos J, Planas R, Pardo A, et al. Spironolactone alone or in combination with furosemide in the treatment of moderate ascites in nonazotemic cirrhosis. A randomized comparative study of efficacy and safety. J Hepatol 2003;39:187.

113. Wong F, Blei AT, Blendis LM, et al. A vasopressin receptor antagonist (VPA-985) improves serum sodium concentration in patients with hyponatremia: a multicenter, randomized, placebo-controlled trial. Hepatology 2003;37:182.

114. Novella M, Sola R, Soriano G, et al. Continuous versus inpatient prophylaxis of the first episode of spontaneous bacterial peritonitis with norfloxacin. Hepatology 1997;25:532.

115. Fernandez J, Navasa M, Gomez J, et al. Bacterial infections in cirrhosis: epidemiological changes with invasive procedures and norfloxacin prophylaxis. Hepatology 2002;35:140.

116. Arroyo V, Gines P, Gerbes AL, et al. Definition and diagnostic criteria of refractory ascites and hepatorenal syndrome in cirrhosis. Hepatology 1996;23:164.

117. Arroyo V, Terra C, Gines P. Advances in the pathogenesis and treatment of type-1 and type-2 hepatorenal syndrome. J Hepatol 2007;46: 935.

118. Fernandez J, Navasa M, Planas R, et al. Primary prophylaxis of spontaneous bacterial peritonitis delays hepatorenal syndrome and improves survival in cirrhosis. Gastroenterology 2007;133:818.

119. Riggio O, Masini A, Efrati C, et al. Pharmacological prophylaxis of hepatic encephalopathy after transjugular intrahepatic portosystemic shunt: a randomized controlled study. J Hepatol 2005;42:674.

120. Kochar N, Tripathi D, Ireland H, et al. Transjugular intrahepatic portosystemic stent shunt (TIPSS) modification in the management of post-TIPSS refractory hepatic encephalopathy. Gut 2006;55:1617.

121. Maleux G, Verslype C, Heye S, et al. Endovascular shunt reduction in the management of transjugular portosystemic shunt-induced hepatic encephalopathy: preliminary experience with reduction stents and stent-grafts. AJR Am J Roentgenol 2007;188:659.

122. Lieberman FL, Hidemura R, Peters RL, et al. Pathogenesis and treatment of hydrothorax complicating cirrhosis with ascites. Ann Intern Med 1966;64:341.

123. Cardenas A, Kelleher T, Chopra S. Review article: hepatic hydrothorax. Aliment Pharmacol Ther 2004;20:271.

124. Rubinstein D, McInnes IE, Dudley FJ. Hepatic hydrothorax in the absence of clinical ascites: diagnosis and management. Gastroenterology 1985;88:188.

125. Strauss RM, Boyer TD. Hepatic hydrothorax. Semin Liver Dis 1997;17:227.

126. Schuster DM, Mukundan S, Jr, Small W, et al. The use of the diagnostic radionuclide ascites scan to facilitate treatment decisions for hepatic hydrothorax. Clin Nucl Med 1998;23:16.

127. Bhattacharya A, Mittal BR, Biswas T, et al. Radioisotope scintigraphy in the diagnosis of hepatic hydrothorax. J Gastroenterol Hepatol 2001;16:317.

128. Garcia-Tsao, G. Transjugular intrahepatic portosystemic shunt (TIPS) for the management of refractory ascites in cirrhosis. In: Gines P, Arroyo V, Rodes J, Schrier RW (eds). Ascites and renal dysfunction in liver disease. Pathogenesis, diagnosis and treatment. Oxford: Blackwell Publishing, 2005:251.

129. Wiest R, Das S, Cadelina G, et al. Bacterial translocation to lymph nodes of cirrhotic rats stimulates eNOS-derived NO production and impairs mesenteric vascular contractility. J Clin Invest 1999;104:1223.

130. Navasa M, Follo A, Filella X, et al. Tumor necrosis factor and interleukin-6 in spontaneous bacterial peritonitis in cirrhosis: relationship with the development of renal impairment and mortality. Hepatology 1998;27:1227.

131. Ruiz-del-Arbol L, Urman J, Fernandez J, et al. Systemic, renal, and hepatic hemodynamic derangement in cirrhotic patients with spontaneous bacterial peritonitis. Hepatology 2003;38:1210.

132. Salerno F, Gerbes A, Gines P, et al. Diagnosis, prevention and treatment of the hepatorenal syndrome in cirrhosis. A consensus workshop of the international ascites club. Gut 2007;53:1310.

133. Llach J, Rimola A, Navasa M, et al. Incidence and predictive factors of first episode of spontaneous bacterial peritonitis in cirrhosis with ascites: relevance of ascitic fluid protein concentration. Hepatology 1992;16:724.

134. Garcia-Tsao G. Spontaneous bacterial peritonitis: a historical perspective. J Hepatol 2004;41:522.

135. Xiol X, Castellvi JM, Guardiola J, et al. Spontaneous bacterial empyema in cirrhotic patients: a prospective study. Hepatology 1996;23:719.

136. Felisart J, Rimola A, Arroyo V, et al. Cefotaxime is more effective than is ampicillin-tobramycin in cirrhotics with severe infections. Hepatology 1985;5:457.

137. Runyon BA, McHutchison JG, Antillon MR, et al. Short-course versus long-course antibiotic treatment of spontaneous bacterial peritonitis. Gastroenterology 1991;100:1737.

138. Gomez-Jimenez J, Ribera E, Gasser I, et al. Randomized trial comparing ceftriaxone with cefonicid for treatment of spontaneous bacterial peritonitis in cirrhotic patients. Antimicrob Agents Chemother 1993; 37:1587.

139. Rimola A, Salmeron JM, Clemente G, et al. Two different dosages of cefotaxime in the treatment of spontaneous bacterial peritonitis in cirrhosis: results of a prospective, randomized, multicenter study. Hepatology 1995;21:674.

140. Ricart E, Soriano G, Novella M, et al. Amoxicillin-clavulanic acid versus cefotaxime in the therapy of bacterial infections in cirrhotic patients. J Hepatol 2000;32:596.

141. Llovet JM, Rodriguez-Iglesias P, Moitinho E, et al. Spontaneous bacterial peritonitis in patients with cirrhosis undergoing selective intestinal decontamination. A retrospective study of 229 spontaneous bacterial peritonitis episodes. J Hepatol 1997;26:88.

142. Garcia-Tsao G. Further evidence against the use of aminoglycosides in cirrhotic patients. Gastroenterology 1998;114:612.

143. Hampel H, Bynum GD, Zamora E, et al. Risk factors for the development of renal dysfunction in hospitalized patients with cirrhosis. Am J Gastroenterol 2001;96:2206.

144. Sort P, Navasa M, Arroyo V, et al. Effect of intravenous albumin on renal impairment and mortality in patients with cirrhosis and spontaneous bacterial peritonitis. N Engl J Med 1999;341:403.

145. Terg R, Gadano A, Lucero R, et al. Serum creatinine and bilirubin levels at admission are useful to select patients with SBP who should be treated with plasma expansion with albumin. Hepatology 2006; 44(Suppl. 1):441A.

146. Garcia-Tsao G. Bacterial infections in cirrhosis: treatment and prophylaxis. J Hepatol 2005;42(Suppl.):S85.

147. Navasa M, Follo A, Llovet JM, et al. Randomized, comparative study of oral ofloxacin versus intravenous cefotaxime in spontaneous bacterial peritonitis. Gastroenterology 1996;111:1011.

148. Terg R, Cobas S, Fassio E, et al. Oral ciprofloxacin after a short course of intravenous ciprofloxacin in the treatment of spontaneous bacterial peritonitis: results of a multicenter, randomized study. J Hepatol 2000;33:564.

149. Angeli P, Guarda S, Fasolato S, et al. Switch therapy with ciprofloxacin vs. intravenous ceftazidime in the treatment of spontaneous bacterial peritonitis in patients with cirrhosis: similar efficacy at lower cost. Aliment Pharmacol Ther 2006;23:75.

150. Stamm WE, Hooton TM. Management of urinary tract infections in adults. N Engl J Med 1993;329:1328.

151. Garcia-Tsao, G. Spontaneous bacterial peritonitis. In: Weinstein WM, Hawkey CJ, Bosch J (eds). Clinical gastroenterology and hepatology. Philadelphia: Elsevier, 2005:723.

152. Gines P, Rimola A, Planas R, et al. Norfloxacin prevents spontaneous bacterial peritonitis recurrence in cirrhosis: results of a double-blind, placebo-controlled trial. Hepatology 1990;12:716.

153. Bauer TM, Follo A, Navasa M, et al. Daily norfloxacin is more effective than weekly rufloxacin in prevention of spontaneous bacterial peritonitis recurrence. Dig Dis Sci 2002;47:1356.

154. Peron JM, Bureau C, Gonzalez L, et al. Treatment of hepatorenal syndrome as defined by the international ascites club by albumin and furosemide infusion according to the central venous pressure: a prospective pilot study. Am J Gastroenterol 2005;100:2702.

155. Terra C, Guevara M, Torre A, et al. Renal failure in patients with cirrhosis and sepsis unrelated to spontaneous bacterial peritonitis: value of MELD score. Gastroenterology 2005;129:1944.

156. Moreau R, Durand F, Poynard T, et al. Terlipressin in patients with cirrhosis and type I hepatorenal syndrome: a retrospective multicenter study. Gastroenterology 2002;122:923.

157. Moreau R, Lebrec D. Acute renal failure in patients with cirrhosis: perspectives in the age of MELD. Hepatology 2003;37:233.

158. Moreau R, Lebrec D. Diagnosis and treatment of acute renal failure in patients with cirrhosis. Best Pract Res Clin Gastroenterol 2007;21:111.

159. Gines A, Escorsell A, Gines P, et al. Incidence, predictive factors, and prognosis of the hepatorenal syndrome in cirrhosis with ascites. Gastroenterology 1993;105:229.

160. Alessandria C, Ozdogan O, Guevara M, et al. MELD score and clinical type predict prognosis in hepatorenal syndrome: relevance to liver transplantation. Hepatology 2005;41:1282.

161. Ruiz-del-Arbol L, Monescillo A, Arocena C, et al. Circulatory function and hepatorenal syndrome in cirrhosis. Hepatology 2005;42: 439.

162. Davis CL. Impact of pretransplant renal failure: when is listing for kidney-liver indicated? Liver Transpl 2005;11:S35.

163. Wiesner R, Edwards E, Freeman R, et al. Model for end-stage liver disease (MELD) and allocation of donor livers. Gastroenterology 2003;124:91.

164. Rimola A, Gavaler JS, Schade RR, et al. Effects of renal impairment on liver transplantation. Gastroenterology 1987;93:148.

165. Gonwa TA, Klintmalm GB, Levy M, et al. Impact of pretransplant renal function on survival after liver transplantation. Transplantation 1995;59:361.

166. Nair S, Verma S, Thuluvath PJ. Pretransplant renal function predicts survival in patients undergoing orthotopic liver transplantation. Hepatology 2002;35:1179.

167. Gonwa TA, McBride MA, Anderson K, et al. Continued influence of preoperative renal function on outcome of orthotopic liver transplant (OLTX) in the US: where will MELD lead us? Am J Transplant 2006;6:2651.

168. Restuccia T, Ortega R, Guevara M, et al. Effects of treatment of hepatorenal syndrome before transplantation on posttransplantation outcome. A case-control study. J Hepatol 2004;40:140.

169. Guevara M, Gines P, Fernandez-Esparrach G, et al. Reversibility of hepatorenal syndrome by prolonged administration of ornipressin and plasma volume expansion. Hepatology 1998;27:35.

170. Gulberg V, Bilzer M, Gerbes AL. Long-term therapy and retreatment of hepatorenal syndrome type I with ornipressin and dopamine. Hepatology 1999;30:870.

171. Uriz J, Gines P, Cardenas A, et al. Terlipressin plus albumin infusion: an effective and safe therapy of hepatorenal syndrome. J Hepatol 2001;33:43

172. Mulkay JP, Louis H, Donckier V, et al. Long-term terlipressin administration improves renal function in cirrhotic patients with type I hepatorenal syndrome: a pilot study. Acta Gastroenterol Belg 2001; 64:15.

173. Ortega R, Gines P, Uriz J, et al. Terlipressin therapy with and without albumin for patients with hepatorenal syndrome: results of a prospective, non-randomized study. Hepatology 2002;36:941.

174. Colle I, Durand F, Pessione F, et al. Clinical course, predictive factors and prognosis in patients with cirrhosis and type 1 hepatorenal syndrome treated with Terlipressin: a retrospective analysis. J Gastroenterol Hepatol 2002;17:882.

175. Halimi C, Bonnard P, Bernard B, et al. Effect of terlipressin (Glypressin) on hepatorenal syndrome in cirrhotic patients: results of a multicentre pilot study. Eur J Gastroenterol Hepatol 2002;14: 153.

176. Angeli P, Volpin R, Gerunda G, et al. Reversal of type 1 hepatorenal syndrome with the administration of midodrine and octreotide. Hepatology 1999;29:1690.

177. Wong F, Pantea L, Sniderman K. Midodrine, octreotide, albumin, and TIPS in selected patients with cirrhosis and type 1 hepatorenal syndrome. Hepatology 2004;40:55.

178. Pomier-Layrargues G, Paquin SC, Hassoun Z, et al. Octreotide in hepatorenal syndrome: a randomized, double-blind, placebo-controlled, crossover study. Hepatology 2003;38:238.

179. Kiser TH, Fish DN, Obritsch MD, et al. Vasopressin, not octreotide, may be beneficial in the treatment of hepatorenal syndrome: a retrospective study. Nephrol Dial Transplant 2005;20:1813.

180. Duvoux C, Zanditenas D, Hezode C, et al. Effects of noradrenalin and albumin in patients with type I hepatorenal syndrome: A pilot study. Hepatology 2002;36:374.

181. Ortega R, Gines P, Uriz J, et al. Terlipressin therapy with and without albumin for patients with hepatorenal syndrome: results of a prospective, nonrandomized study. Hepatology 2002;36:941.

182. Solanki P, Chawla A, Garg R, et al. Beneficial effects of terlipressin in hepatorenal syndrome: a prospective, randomized placebo-controlled clinical trial. J Gastroenterol Hepatol 2003;18:152.

183. Sanyal AJ, Boyer TD, Garcia-Tsao G, et al. A prospective, randomized, double-blind, placebo-controlled trial of terlipressin for type 1 hepatorenal syndrome. Hepatology 2006;44(Suppl. 1):694A.

184. Guevara M, Gines P, Bandi JC, et al. Transjugular intrahepatic portosystemic shunt in hepatorenal syndrome: effects on renal function and vasoactive systems. Hepatology 1998;28:416.

185. Brensing KA, Textor J, Perz J, et al. Long-term outcome after transjugular intrahepatic portosystemic stent-shunt in non-transplant cirrhotics with hepatorenal syndrome: a phase II study. Gut 2000;47:288.

186. Mitzner SR, Stange J, Klammt S, et al. Improvement of hepatorenal syndrome with extracorporeal albumin dialysis MARS: results of a prospective randomized, controlled clinical trial. Liver Transpl 2000;6:277.

187. Akriviadis E, Botla R, Briggs W, et al. Pentoxifylline improves short-term survival in severe acute alcoholic hepatitis: a double-blind, placebo-controlled trial. Gastroenterology 2000;119:1637.

24

Approach to the patient with central nervous system and pulmonary complications of end-stage liver disease

Javier Vaquero, Andres T. Blei, Roger F. Butterworth

Hepatic encephalopathy, 467
Hepatopulmonary syndrome, 475
Portopulmonary hypertension, 481

End-stage liver disease and advanced portal hypertension result in blood from the splanchnic circulation accessing the systemic circulation without being adequately detoxified by the liver. In addition, the injured liver may be a source of abnormal mediators or fail to produce essential metabolites. The consequence of these alterations is the exposure of peripheral organs to an altered composition of blood. Hepatic encephalopathy, hepatopulmonary syndrome, and portopulmonary hypertension are the result of the exposure of brain and lungs to this altered milieu. Together with variceal bleeding, ascites, and hepatorenal syndrome they are the major manifestations of advanced liver disease and can cause significant deterioration of quality of life, morbidity, and mortality. Medical therapies often attenuate the symptoms or delay the progression of these complications, but liver transplantation is considered the only definitive cure.

Hepatic encephalopathy

Definition and classification

Hepatic encephalopathy (HE) is a serious neuropsychiatric complication of both acute and chronic liver failure, with a significant impact on quality of life. Results of a working group were published in 2002 and they include a definition of HE and a new system of classification (Table 24.1). HE is defined as a spectrum of neuropsychiatric abnormalities seen in patients with liver dysfunction after exclusion of other known brain diseases [1]. This multiaxial definition of HE

defines both the type of hepatic dysfunction and the characteristics of the neurological manifestations. Three types of hepatic abnormalities are defined, namely:

- Type A: HE associated with **a**cute liver failure
- Type B: HE associated with portosystemic **b**ypass with no intrinsic hepatocellular disease
- Type C: HE associated with **c**irrhosis and portal hypertension or portosystemic shunts.

In the case of chronic liver disease, the terms *episodic HE* and *persistent HE* were coined and the term *minimal HE* was invoked to replace *subclinical encephalopathy*. It is anticipated that this new system of classification of HE will help to dispel the confusion frequently present in classical textbook definitions and to facilitate recruitment of patients into multicenter clinical trials.

Table 24.1 Classification of hepatic encephalopathy (HE)

Type **A**	Encephalopathy associated with **a**cute liver failure
Type **B**	Encephalopathy associated with portosystemic **b**ypass and no intrinsic hepatocellular disease
Type **C**	Encephalopathy associated with **c**irrhosis and portal hypertension or portosystemic shunts **1** Episodic HE 　**a** Precipitated 　**b** Spontaneous 　**c** Recurrent **2** Persistent HE 　**a** Mild 　**b** Severe 　**c** Treatment-dependent **3** Minimal HE

Principles of Clinical Gastroenterology. Edited by Tadataka Yamada, David H. Alpers, Anthony N. Kalloo, Neil Kaplowitz, Chung Owyang, and Don W. Powell. © 2008 Blackwell Publishing. ISBN 978-1-4051-69103

Diagnosis

Neuropsychiatric symptoms characteristic of HE include shortened attention span, sleep abnormalities, and motor incoordination progressing through lethargy to stupor and coma. Psychiatric symptoms, particularly anxiety and depression, are not uncommon. Type B HE is, in practice, uncommon. In type C HE, symptoms take an undulating course progressing relatively slowly. In type A HE associated with acute liver failure, the neurological disorder may progress from altered mental status to coma within days, seizures may occur, and mortality rates are high. In these patients, death is frequently the result of brain herniation caused by brain edema and intracranial hypertension.

In patients with an episode or worsening of HE, it is essential to identify potential precipitating factors and to initiate corresponding treatment immediately. Common precipitating factors are gastrointestinal bleeding, hypovolemia, hyponatremia, hypokalemia, hypoxia, hypoglycaemia, infection, and the use of sedative drugs [2].

Diagnosis of HE in chronic liver failure is generally based on clinical and laboratory criteria following exclusion of other causes of neuropsychiatric dysfunction (Table 24.2). Differential diagnosis may require the use of computed tomography (CT) scans to eliminate other causes of encephalopathy such as traumatic brain injury, tumors, or edema.

Grading of HE in clinical practice is generally performed using the West Haven criteria (Table 24.3), which assess mental status on a scale of I to IV based on levels of consciousness, intellectual function, and personality changes [3]. Asterixis or flapping tremor (common in patients in stage II and III) refers to the presence of rapid involuntary flexion and extension movements of the wrist when the patient is told to maintain them actively in dorsiflexion with the fingers extended. Flapping tremor may also be observed during tongue protrusion or pedal dorsiflexion. Patients in stage IV of the West Haven classification may be better assessed using the Glasgow coma scale (Table 24.4).

Psychometric testing is commonly used to quantify the degree of impairment of neurological function, particularly in mild or minimal HE. Tests most commonly used include the Number Connection Test (NCT) and measurement of reaction times to visual or auditory stimuli. The Psychometric Hepatic Encephalopathy Score (PHES) consists of a series of psychometric tests including NCT-A, NCT-B, line tracing test, digit symbol test, and the serial dotting test. This battery of tests examines such entities as visual perception, construction, and visuospatial orientation in addition to motor speed, accuracy, attention, and memory function [4].

Electroencephalographic (EEG) changes in HE start with a bilateral synchronous decrease in wave frequency, increase in amplitude, and loss of normal α rhythm. Computer-assisted spectral EEG analysis facilitates measurement of mean dominant EEG frequency and decreases interoperator variability. Other more sophisticated tests used for grading of

HE in chronic liver failure include the use of event-related evoked responses (typically the P300 peak following auditory stimuli) [5] and measurement of critical flicker frequency [6].

Table 24.2 Differential diagnosis of hepatic encephalopathy.

Metabolic encephalopathies
  Hypoglycemia
  Electrolyte imbalance
  Hypoxia
  Carbon dioxide narcosis
  Azotemia
  Ketoacidosis

Toxic encephalopathies
  Alcohol
    Acute intoxication
    Withdrawal syndrome
    Wernicke–Korsakoff syndrome
  Psychoactive drugs
  Salicylates
  Heavy metals

Intracranial lesions
  Subarachnoid, subdural, or intracerebral hemorrhage
  Cerebral infarction
  Cerebral tumor
  Cerebral abscess
  Meningitis
  Encephalitis
  Epilepsy or postseizure encephalopathy

Neuropsychiatric disorders

Adapted from Riordan and Williams [238], with permission from the Massachusetts Medical Society.

Table 24.3 West Haven criteria for clinical grading of hepatic encephalopathy

Stage 0	No abnormality detected
Stage I	Trivial lack of awareness, euphoria, or anxiety Shortened attention span Impairment of addition or subtraction
Stage II	Lethargy Disorientation for time Obvious personality change Inappropriate behavior
Stage III	Somnolence to semistupor, but responsive to stimuli Confusion Gross disorientation Bizarre behavior
Stage IV	Coma Tests of mental state not possible

Table 24.4 Glasgow coma scale

Criteria	Points awarded
Eyes open	
Spontaneous (eyes open does not imply awareness)	4
To speech (any speech, not necessarily a command)	3
To pain (should not use supraorbital pressure for pain stimulus)	2
Never	1
Best verbal response	
Oriented (to time, person, place)	5
Confused speech (disoriented)	4
Inappropriate (swearing, yelling)	3
Incomprehensible sounds (moaning, groaning)	2
None	1
Best motor response	
Obeys commands	6
Localizes pain (deliberate or purposeful movement)	5
Withdrawal (moves away from stimulus)	4
Abnormal flexion (decortication)	3
Extension (decerebration)	2
None (flaccidity)	1

Neuropathology and neuroimaging

Neuropathology

The principal neuropathological finding in type C HE is altered astrocyte morphology. The term *Alzheimer type II astrocyte* is used to describe the characteristic morphological features manifested by astrocytes in type C HE, which consist of large, pale (watery-looking) nuclei, margination of the chromatin, and prominent nucleoli. The nuclei take on a variety of shapes from round (in cerebral cortex) to irregular or lobulated forms (in basal ganglia), and in many cases occur in pairs or triplets suggestive of hyperplasia [7]. Intranuclear glycogen inclusions are also evident in these cells. The number of cells that manifest the Alzheimer type II phenotype is significantly correlated with the severity of encephalopathy [8,9].

Mixed glial-neuronal cultures exposed to sera from HE patients develop morphological changes characteristic of Alzheimer type II astrocytes [10]. Although rare, neuronal cell death and severe neuronal dysfunction have been documented in several clinical entities in chronic liver failure, which include acquired (non-Wilsonian) hepatocerebral degeneration, postshunt myelopathy, cerebellar degeneration, and extrapyramidal disorders (parkinsonism) [11].

Neuroimaging

Bilateral signal hyperintensities have been described in globus pallidus on T1-weighted magnetic resonance imaging (MRI) (see Fig. 24.2a; see also "Manganese" below), and T2-weighed Fast-FLAIR MRI reveals white matter lucencies along the cor-

ticospinal tract in cirrhotic patients with overt HE [12]. Both of these MRI alterations resolve following liver transplantation.

Studies using positron emission tomography (PET) and $^{13}NH_3$ have been used to investigate brain ammonia metabolism in cirrhotic patients. In one study, patients with mild HE presented a significant increase in the cerebral metabolic rate for ammonia, accompanied by an increase of the blood–brain barrier permeability to ammonia, which suggested an increased ease of ammonia for entering the brain in patients with HE [13]. This could explain the hypersensitivity of cirrhotic patients to ammoniagenic conditions such as protein loading, gastrointestinal bleeding, and constipation, and the occurrence of HE in patients with near normal arterial ammonia levels. Results of a subsequent $^{13}NH_3$ PET study, however, suggested that increased cerebral trapping of ammonia in cirrhotic patients with HE was primarily the result of increased circulating ammonia rather than altered blood–brain ammonia kinetics [14].

Pathophysiology

Bloodborne toxins

Ammonia

There is evidence for a pathogenetic link between hyperammonemia and the phenomenon of Alzheimer type II astrocytosis, because the latter phenotype has been described in hyperammonemic syndromes associated with congenital urea cycle enzyme defects, in experimental animals with urease-induced hyperammonemia, and in primary cultures of rat cortical astrocytes exposed to ammonia [9].

A network of organs is involved in ammonia homeostasis (Fig. 24.1) and there is a convincing body of evidence to suggest that hyperammonemia in liver failure results from altered interorgan trafficking of ammonia [15]. In chronic liver failure, hyperammonemia results primarily from reduced hepatic urea synthesis rather than increased intestinal ammonia production [16]. Urea is synthesized in the liver from ammonia by the urea cycle in periportal hepatocytes, whereas perivenous hepatocytes also transform ammonia into glutamine by glutamine synthetase. Cirrhotic patients have intra- and extrahepatic portosystemic shunts that account for a large portion of portal blood flow. This, in addition to the loss of hepatocytes and impaired residual hepatocyte function, results in decreased ammonia removal by the liver. Increased renal ammonia synthesis reported in liver failure is offset by increased ammonia excretion into the urine [16].

In contrast to the liver, skeletal muscle and brain are devoid of an effective urea cycle and rely only on glutamine synthesis for ammonia removal. In liver failure, muscle becomes the major route for ammonia detoxification [17], because chronic hyperammonemia results in increased glutamine synthetase (GS) activity because of a posttranslational increase of GS [18]. In contrast to skeletal muscle, brain does not adapt its ammonia removal capacity by induction of GS. On the contrary, GS activities are consistently decreased in brains of

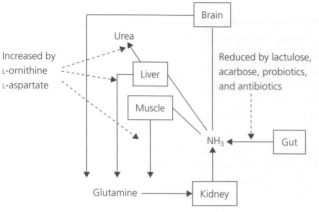

Figure 24.1 Interorgan trafficking of ammonia. Ammonia (NH₃) produced by the gut and kidney is, under normal physiological conditions, removed primarily by the liver (as urea and glutamine) and to a lesser extent by muscle and brain (as glutamine). In liver failure, liver urea and glutamine production is severely impaired, and muscle (not brain) becomes the organ principally responsible for removal of circulating ammonia. Ammonia production in the gut is lowered by treatment with lactulose, acarbose, probiotics, and antibiotics. Hepatic ammonia removal as urea and glutamine together with muscle ammonia removal (as glutamine) are stimulated with L-ornithine L-aspartate.

animals with experimental chronic liver failure [18] and in autopsied brain tissue from cirrhotic patients who died in hepatic coma [19]. This decreased GS activity in brain may be explained by increased GS protein tyrosine nitration, as demonstrated in both in vitro and in vivo models of hyperammonemia and liver failure [20]. Moreover, NMR spectroscopic studies in liver-impaired animals [21] have been unable to demonstrate significant increases of de novo glutamine synthesis in the brain, suggesting that the increased brain glutamine reported in liver failure results primarily from decreased glutamine release from astrocytes or decreased glutamine degradation by glutaminase.

Manganese

Evidence suggests that manganese deposition is the cause of the bilateral T1-weighed hyperintensities of basal ganglia observed in the MRI of cirrhotic patients (Fig. 24.2). Manganese, which is normally eliminated by the hepatobiliary route, is increased in the blood of cirrhotic patients, who manifest pallidal signal hyperintensities on MRI. Similar MRI pallidal signals probably caused by manganese deposition have been reported in other cholestatic conditions such as Alagille syndrome [22], intrahepatic bile duct paucity, and in patients during total parenteral nutrition [23]. Direct measurements using neutron activation analysis reveal up to sevenfold increases in manganese content of dissected pallidus globus obtained postmortem from cirrhotic patients who died in hepatic coma (Fig. 24.2b) [24]. Experimental animals with surgical portacaval shunts also manifest selective accumulation of manganese in pallidus globus and in other basal ganglia structures [25].

Cerebral blood flow and energy metabolism

Alterations of brain glucose utilization, of cerebral blood flow, and of brain glucose metabolic pathways have consistently been reported in HE resulting from chronic liver failure. PET studies using ¹⁸F-deoxyglucose revealed significant decreases in glucose utilization localized to the anterior cingulate cortex in cirrhotic patients with mild HE [26], and the extent of such decreases correlated with the reduced performance in attention-demanding tasks such as NCT and digit symbol psychometric tests. Anterior cingulate cortex is known to be implicated in the control of the anterior attention system responsible for monitoring the selection of responses to visual stimuli.

Measurement of cerebral blood flow using ¹⁵[O]H₂O-PET reveals a redistribution of flow from cortical regions such as the anterior cingulate to subcortical structures such as the thalamus [27].

Precipitation of severe encephalopathy and coma in experimental animals with chronic liver failure following the

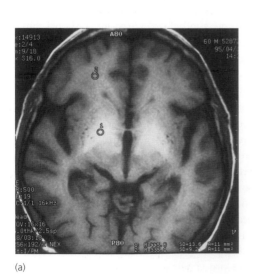

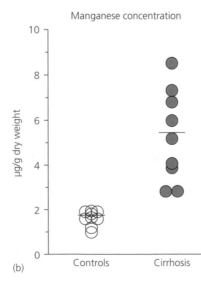

(a)   (b)

Figure 24.2 **(a)** Typical bilateral signal hyperintensities in pallidus globus on T1-weighted magnetic resonance imaging of a 47-year-old cirrhotic patient with minimal hepatic encephalopathy. Signal hyperintensities resolved following liver transplantation. **(b)** Increased pallidal manganese concentrations in autopsied brain tissue from cirrhotic patients who died in hepatic coma. Data from Pomier-Layrargues et al. [24].

administration of ammonium salts results in severe alterations of brain glucose metabolism leading to accumulation of lactate [28]. Increased brain lactate concentrations are consistent with impaired oxidation of pyruvate in brain in liver failure. Increased brain and cerebrospinal fluid lactate concentrations have consistently been reported in HE patients [29,30].

Neurotransmitters

Neurotransmission defects in HE have been ascribed to direct neurotoxic effects of the ammonium ion (NH_4^+) on inhibitory (GABA[γ-aminobutyric acid]ergic) and excitatory (glutamatergic) neurotransmission, to the accumulation of neuroactive metabolites of tryptophan, to altered glutamatergic synaptic regulation, and to activation of "peripheral-type" benzodiazepine receptors resulting in the synthesis of neuroactive steroids with potent GABA agonist properties.

Glutamate

In a report by Schmidt et al. [31], the exposure to blood obtained from cirrhotic patients with varying degrees of HE resulted in a dose-dependent inhibition of the uptake of D-aspartate (a nonmetabolizable glutamate analogue) in rat hippocampal slices, and the relative potency of the inhibition correlated with blood ammonia concentrations. Other studies demonstrate ammonia-induced inhibition of high-affinity glutamate uptake into rat synaptosomal preparations [32] and cultured rat astrocytes [33]. Alterations of several subclasses of glutamate binding sites expressed by both neurons and astrocytes have been reported in experimental models of chronic liver failure [34,35].

Serotonin (5-hydroxytryptamine, 5-HT)

Tryptophan is increased in the cerebrospinal fluid (CSF) of patients with hepatic coma [36], and its blood–brain barrier transport is enhanced in dogs with portacaval anastomosis [37]. Because tryptophan hydroxylation (the rate-limiting step in brain 5-HT synthesis) is not saturated at normal blood and brain tryptophan concentrations, increased availability of tryptophan has the potential to result in increased 5-HT synthesis in brain. Supporting an increased synthesis and turnover of 5-HT in the brain in HE, the concentration of 5-hydroxyindoleacetic acid (a metabolite of 5-HT) is increased in the CSF of cirrhotic patients in hepatic coma [36], and in autopsied brain tissue from both HE patients [38] and portacaval-shunted rats [39]. Measurement using an in vivo decarboxylase inhibition assay also revealed increased 5-HT turnover [40] in the brains of portacaval-shunted animals. Increased brain 5-HT turnover correlates with the degrees of portosystemic shunting and hyperammonemia in rats with variable portal vein stenosis [41], an animal model of minimal HE. Other evidence for altered 5-HT metabolism and function in human HE include the report of increased activity and mRNA of monoamine oxidase A (MAO-A; the enzyme responsible for 5-HT breakdown in human brain) [42] and

of increased concentration of 5-hydroxyindoleacetic acid in brain tissue from patients who died in hepatic coma [38]. Increased densities of postsynaptic $5-HT_2$ receptors were also described in this material [43]. Together, these findings suggest a serotonin synaptic deficit in HE. $5-HT_2$ plays a key role in the regulation of sleep, and altered serotoninergic neurotransmission is present in a range of psychiatric disorders in humans. Changes in cerebral $5-HT_2$ turnover in HE, therefore, could underlie some early signs and symptoms, such as altered sleep patterns and depression.

γ-Aminobutyric acid

Throughout the 1980s a great deal of attention was focused on the theory that HE was the result of alterations of the GABA neurotransmitter system in brain. Abnormalities of the brain GABA system were initially reported in animal models of acute liver failure [44]. In animal models of chronic liver failure, however, no alterations of this system have been reported, whether reflected by GABA content, its related enzymes, or receptor sites [45–48]. Autopsied brain tissue from cirrhotic patients who died in hepatic coma also contains normal activities of GABA-related enzymes and unchanged densities and affinities of GABA binding sites [19,49,50].

In the central nervous system, benzodiazepine binding sites form part of the GABA-A receptor complex. Stimulation of the benzodiazepine binding site "facilitates" the action of GABA on the functionally linked GABA-A site of the complex, and results in increased chloride channel opening leading to hyperpolarization and inhibition. Administration of the benzodiazepine antagonist flumazenil has been noted to ameliorate the neurological status in cirrhotic patients with HE [51,52]. It was suggested that the beneficial action of flumazenil in HE was the result either of inhibition of increased densities of benzodiazepine binding sites or of inhibition of the action of an "endogenous" ligand at these sites. Subsequent investigations revealed no alterations of densities or affinities of binding sites in either experimental or human HE [50], leaving open the possibility that the beneficial effects of flumazenil were the result of the blockage of "endogenous" benzodiazepines [53]. Initial reports demonstrated that CSF and sera from patients with advanced HE contained significant amounts of "benzodiazepine-like" substances, among which were isolated two known benzodiazepines that are positive allosteric modulators of GABA neurotransmission (diazepam and its NN-desmethyl metabolite) [54]. Unfortunately, the interest generated by these reports was tempered by the fact that these benzodiazepines were in most cases pharmaceutical in origin. Moreover, the concentrations of benzodiazepines reported in blood, CSF, and brain extracts of HE patients were well below levels associated with their sedative actions.

An alternative theory to explain increased GABAergic neurotransmission in HE has emerged. Two distinct types of benzodiazepine receptors are expressed in brain. The first type, mentioned in the previous paragraph, forms part of the

GABA–benzodiazepine receptor complex and is situated on the postsynaptic neuronal membrane. The second type is the "peripheral-type" benzodiazepine receptor (PTBR), so-called because of its initial discovery in peripheral tissues but subsequently identified on the outer mitochondrial membrane of astrocytes. Increased densities of PTBRs have been reported in autopsied brain tissue from cirrhotic patients who died in hepatic coma [55], and increased PTBR binding sites and mRNA have been reported in the brain of portacaval-shunted rats [56,57]. Endogenous ligands for the PTBR include the neuropeptide diazepam binding inhibitor and its processing peptide octadecaneuropeptide (ODN) [58]. Portacaval anastomosis in the rat results in increased ODN-immunolabeling of astrocytes and other nonneuronal elements in several brain regions [59]. Exposure to PTBR ligands results in proliferation and swelling of mitochondria in cultured glioma cells [60] and, because mitochondrial proliferation and swelling are observed in astrocytes in liver failure, PTBR activation could play a role in the pathogenesis of this astrocytic response.

Activation of PTBRs in brain in liver failure results in increased synthesis of a novel class of compounds known as neurosteroids, many of which (e.g., allopregnanolone) are potent GABA-A receptor agonists and consequently potent inhibitory agents. Allopregnanolone concentrations are increased up to sevenfold in autopsied brain tissue from cirrhotic patients who died in hepatic coma [61].

Histamine

Histamine is involved in a wide range of physiological functions including sleep, arousal, and circadian rhythmicity. In rats, portosystemic shunting results in increased hypothalamic concentrations of both histamine and its principal metabolite, tele-methylhistamine, and in increased hypothalamic release of histamine [62], suggesting increased histaminergic activity. Increased brain histamine could result from increased brain availability of the precursor amino acid L-histidine. Postsynaptic histamine H_1 receptors are implicated in the entrainment of circadian rhythms to the light–dark cycle in mammals [63], and their activation suppresses deep slow-wave sleep [64]. Upregulation of histamine H_1 receptors has been reported in cerebral cortex of patients with HE and of portacaval-shunted rats. Therefore, it is plausible that increased histaminergic activity through H_1 receptors contributes to the disorganization of the normal sleep cycle and decreased total duration of slow-wave sleep that are characteristically observed in cirrhotic patients with HE [65]. Similar changes in sleep patterns and diurnal rhythms have been reported in portacaval-shunted rats [66]. Histamine H_1 receptor blockade, known to affect sleep quality in humans, significantly improved circadian rhythmicity in these animals [66].

Dopamine

Studies in autopsied brain tissue from cirrhotic patients who died in hepatic coma reveal several-fold increases in the dopamine metabolite homovanillic acid [38]. Similar findings, consistent with increased dopamine metabolism or turnover, were reported in the brains of rats following portacaval anastomosis [67]. A possible explanation for these findings could relate to the increased activities of the monoamine metabolizing enzyme MAO-A [42]. Densities of postsynaptic dopamine (D_2) receptors are significantly reduced in brain tissue obtained at autopsy of cirrhotic patients who died in hepatic coma [68], and in living patients with mild HE studied by PET using [11C]methylspiperone [69].

Opioids

Cirrhotic patients are particularly sensitive to morphine, and portacaval shunting is known to increase pain sensitivity, which involves the endogenous opioid neurotransmitter system. Increased circulating levels of endogenous opioid [Met]enkephalin have been reported in patients with primary biliary cirrhosis [70], and brain levels of β-endorphin are increased in experimental chronic liver failure [71]. Portacaval anastomosis in the rat results in region-selective increases of μ and δ opioid receptor sites in brain [72], a finding that has been linked to increased ethanol consumption in these animals [73].

Oxidative/nitrosative stress

Portacaval anastomosis in the rat results in increased expression of neuronal nitric oxide synthase (nNOS) in brain [74]. NOS activities are also increased by ammonia-induced stimulation of L-arginine uptake into neuronal preparations both in vitro and in vivo. Exposure of cultured astrocytes to millimolar concentrations of ammonia results in oxidative stress and protein tyrosine nitration [20], a process dependent on increases in the inducible isoform of NOS (iNOS). Astrocytic protein tyrosine nitration was also described in the brains of rats following portacaval anastomosis [20], confirming the presence of nitrosative stress under these conditions.

Inflammation

It is becoming increasingly evident that ammonia and manganese neurotoxicity are not the only pathophysiological processes with the potential to affect adversely cerebral function in liver failure. In particular, there is evidence that infection and inflammation also play a significant role.

The severity of HE in acute liver failure is significantly influenced by the so-called systemic inflammatory response syndrome (SIRS) [75], which is a response to the action of proinflammatory cytokines such as tumor necrosis factor-α (TNF-α) or the interleukins IL-1β and IL-6. Infection and inflammation are also common in cirrhotic patients, in whom increased circulating levels of TNF-α and IL-6 have been described [76]. Shawcross et al. studied 10 patients with cirrhosis who had evidence of infection and SIRS but no clinically evident HE [77]. In these patients, exogenously induced hyperammonemia was associated with significant deterioration in neuropsychological testing during the inflammatory state but not after its resolution, indicating that SIRS may modulate the effects of ammonia on brain function.

Therapy

Therapy for HE continues to be a challenge. The reasons for this include a lack of standardization of assessment of mental status, the hesitation by some ethics boards to sanction placebo-controlled trials, confounding issues such as the presence of precipitating factors (infection, hyponatremia, unidentified neuroactive drugs, and others), and difficulties related to the

effective blinding of patients and clinical investigators to the treatment regimen. A schematic approach to the management of HE is shown in Fig. 24.3.

Nutritional support

Severe restriction of dietary protein is no longer recommended as a means of preventing HE in cirrhotic patients [78]. Long-term nitrogen restriction is potentially harmful, and a positive nitrogen balance is essential to promote liver regeneration and to increase the capacity for ammonia removal by skeletal muscle. Protein intake in the 1–2 g/kg/day range is generally

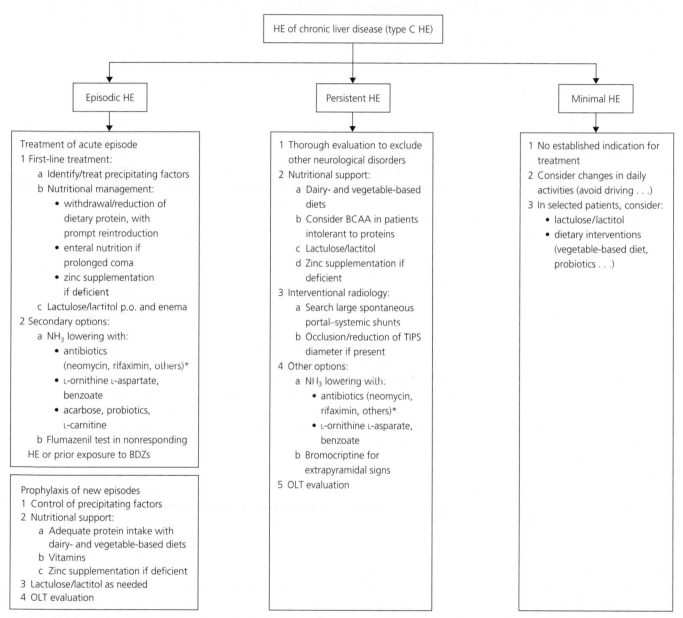

Figure 24.3 General management of hepatic encephalopathy (HE) of chronic liver disease (type C HE). No therapy has conclusively been shown to improve HE compared with placebo in randomized clinical trials. A majority of patients with HE, however, are effectively managed by following the present orientative scheme, based on published guidelines [2,238]. The

management of the recurrent type of episodic HE would be similar to that of persistent HE. *Neomycin for chronic use requires periodic monitoring to avoid toxicity (renal, otological). BCAA, branched-chain amino acids; BDZ, benzodiazepine; OLT, orthotopic liver transplant; p.o., orally; TIPS, transjugular intrahepatic portosystemic shunt.

recommended to maintain an adequate nitrogen balance [2]. Oral supplements of branched-chain amino acids have been suggested to offer significant improvement in severely protein-intolerant patients with chronic HE [79].

Ammonia-lowering strategies (Fig. 24.1)

Nonabsorbable disaccharides, such as lactulose and lactitol, are routinely used to decrease ammonia production in the gut despite a paucity of adequate controlled clinical trials. In the case of lactulose, the ammonia-lowering effect involves increased fecal nitrogen excretion by facilitation of the incorporation of ammonia into bacteria as well as a cathartic effect. In the colon, lactulose and lactitol are catabolized, respectively, to lactic and acetic acids, leading to a lowering of colonic pH to around 5.0. This reduction in pH favors the formation of the less absorbable NH_4^+ from NH_3 thus effectively trapping ammonia in the colon. The dose of lactulose (45–90 g/day) is titrated to achieve 2–3 soft stools per day. Major side effects include abdominal cramps, flatulence, and diarrhea. Antibiotics such as neomycin are also traditionally used to lower blood ammonia by inhibiting bacterial ammonia production. However, neomycin therapy is associated with significant side effects and is increasingly being replaced by alternative antibiotics such as rifaximin.

Significant lowering of blood ammonia and concomitant improvement in neuropsychiatric status in cirrhotic patients with grade I–II HE has been demonstrated following administration of the novel hypoglycemic agent acarbose [80]. One suggested mechanism of action of acarbose involves inhibition of proteolytic flora responsible for gut ammonia production. Along these same lines, there is renewed interest (after a 40-year hiatus) in the area of lowering gut ammonia production by oral supplementation of probiotics [81]. The objective of probiotics is to increase the intestinal proportion of urease-negative bacteria thereby decreasing gut ammonia production. Lactic acid-producing probiotics have the advantage of reducing gut ammonia absorption. Synbiotic preparations consist of both lactic acid-producing probiotics and fermentable fiber. Controlled clinical trials with these agents reveal significant improvement of neurological status and lowering of venous ammonia [81].

An alternative means of lowering blood ammonia in chronic liver failure involves the stimulation of ammonia fixation. Ammonia is normally removed by urea formation (periportal hepatocytes) and by glutamine formation (perivenous hepatocytes, muscle and brain) (Fig. 24.1). Several strategies are aimed at stimulating residual urea or glutamine synthesis. One of the most successful, L-ornithine L-aspartate, has been shown to lower blood ammonia and concomitantly improve neuropsychiatric status in cirrhotic patients in controlled clinical trials in Europe and Asia [82]. Studies in experimental chronic liver failure reveal that this beneficial effect is primarily due to the stimulation of urea and glutamine formation in the liver and in the stimulation of glutamine formation by

skeletal muscle [83]. In experimental acute liver failure, the ammonia-lowering effect of L-ornithine L-aspartate appears to be due predominantly to the stimulation of muscle glutamine synthetase. Successful lowering of blood ammonia concentrations in cirrhotic patients has also been accomplished using sodium benzoate, an agent that combines with glycine to form hippurate. A controlled clinical trial with 5 g sodium benzoate twice daily in patients with acute HE found it to be as effective as lactulose but 25 times less expensive [84].

Studies in both experimental animal models of HE [85] and in cirrhotic patients [86] demonstrate that L-carnitine is effective in lowering blood ammonia and improving neurological status. The mechanism of action probably involves improvements in mitochondrial metabolism.

Neuropharmacology

As the precise pathophysiological mechanisms and alterations in neurotransmitter systems responsible for the pathogenesis of HE become more clearly defined, novel pharmacological approaches are starting to emerge.

Agents acting on the GABA-receptor complex

A number of controlled clinical trials have evaluated the efficacy of the benzodiazepine receptor antagonist flumazenil in HE patients [2]. In a subset of HE patients, improvements following flumazenil are spectacular [51]. However, enthusiasm for this approach has been tempered by the possible confounding effects of prior exposure to pharmaceutical benzodiazepines (used as sedatives or as part of an endoscopic workup) and by the poor correlation between the clinical response and blood levels of benzodiazepines in these patients. Adding to these difficulties is the short half-life and lack of an oral formulation for flumazenil.

Benzodiazepine partial inverse agonists display weak negative intrinsic activity and act as mild GABA-A receptor antagonists [87]. One such agent, Ro15-4513, ameliorates the symptoms of HE in rats with thioacetamide-induced [88] and ischemic [89] acute liver failure (ALF), and similar results were obtained with a second benzodiazepine partial inverse agonist, sarmazenil. A major mechanism responsible for the beneficial effect of these agents appears to involve the attenuation of the effects of neurosteroids such as allopregnanolone at the GABA-A receptor complex [90]. Surprisingly, no studies have so far been undertaken to test the efficacy of benzodiazepine partial inverse agonists in patients with acute or chronic liver failure.

Dopamine receptor agonists

Both L-DOPA (the amino acid precursor of dopamine) and the dopamine receptor agonist bromocriptine have been used in clinical trials in patients with portosystemic encephalopathy [2]. Although results were not encouraging in terms of overall cognitive improvement, it is possible that these agents have a beneficial effect on motor performance.

Histamine H₁ receptor antagonists

Following up on the demonstration of a beneficial effect of histamine H_1 antagonists on neurological function in an experimental animal model of HE [66], results of a controlled clinical trial revealed improvements in sleep quality in cirrhotic patients with minimal HE following administration of the H_1 blocker hydroxyzine [91].

Liver assist devices

In chronic liver disease, the role of liver assist devices to treat HE is likely to be relevant only to a small proportion of patients, because of the complexity, associated adverse effects, and discontinuous use of these devices, in addition to the frequent resolution of HE episodes with standard medical therapy. These devices have been used mainly in patients who had advanced chronic liver disease with superimposed acute injury (so-called acute-on-chronic liver failure) [92]. Dialysis against albumin, which allows the removal of water-soluble and non-water-soluble toxins bound to albumin in the blood, has received most attention. In one study of patients with acute-on-chronic liver failure, treatment with albumin dialysis was associated with an improvement of HE, which was not observed in those treated only with standard medical therapy [93]. In a preliminary report of 70 patients with advanced cirrhosis and severe HE, those randomized to albumin dialysis presented significant improvements of HE compared with those receiving standard medical therapy alone [94]. The use of liver assist devices for treating HE, however, is still experimental.

Liver transplantation

The appearance of HE in a patient with cirrhosis is a poor prognostic factor and should prompt evaluation of the patient for liver transplantation [95]. Elective liver transplantation should not be performed during an acute episode of HE; it is preferable to wait until the episode and its precipitating factors are corrected.

Liver transplantation corrects the majority of alterations related to HE, including neuropsychiatric symptoms and altered neuropsychometric tests [96,97], alterations of electroencephalogram [96], alterations of regional cerebral blood flow [98] and regional brain glucose metabolism [99], cerebral osmolyte disturbances [100], basal ganglia hyperintensities [100], and the decrease of the magnetization transfer ratio in the brain [100]. The posttransplant normalization of the cerebral osmolyte disturbances correlates well with the correction of the neuropsychological alterations [100].

Despite the reversibility of HE, neurological complications are common (~ 30%) following liver transplantation, especially within the first weeks [101,102]. In one study, the presence of HE pretransplant was an independent risk factor for developing these complications [101], which include central pontine myelinolysis, cerebrovascular disease, anoxia, seizures, and infections [101,102]. Neurotoxicity from immunosuppressive medications is also common in the early postoperative period [103], but it usually responds to the reduction or discontinuation of the drug. Liver transplantation candidates may also have neurological impairment related to the etiology of liver disease, such as frontal lobe and cerebellar atrophy in alcohol consumption [104], or cognitive and ^{1}H-NMR spectroscopic alterations associated with hepatitis C virus infection [105]. The posttransplant evolution of these preexisting conditions has not been completely characterized.

Hepatopulmonary syndrome

The association between liver disease and pulmonary dysfunction has been known for more than 100 years, since Fluckiger described in 1884 the case of a woman with chronic liver disease presenting cyanosis and digital clubbing [106]. Subsequently, similar cases were reported, and a wide range of structural alterations in the pulmonary vascular tree of patients with liver disease were described [107]. The term *hepatopulmonary syndrome* (HPS) was coined in 1977 by Kennedy and Knudson as an analogy to the *hepatorenal syndrome*, recognizing the vascular nature of the altered gas exchange in these patients [108].

Today, HPS distinguishes a subgroup of patients with liver disease or portal hypertension who present alterations of arterial oxygenation caused by the development of intrapulmonary vascular dilations (IPVDs). The term IPVD reflects the variety of pulmonary vascular alterations leading to altered gas exchange in HPS, from diffuse peripheral dilations of pulmonary capillaries to true anatomical arteriovenous shunts.

Definition

HPS is defined by the three following criteria, all of which must be present to establish the diagnosis [109,110]:
- presence of chronic liver disease or portal hypertension
- alteration of arterial oxygenation, usually defined as a widened age-corrected alveolar–arterial oxygen gradient on room air with or without arterial hypoxemia
- evidence of IPVDs.

In early definitions, the presence of other cardiopulmonary causes of hypoxemia was incompatible with the diagnosis of HPS. However, it is generally accepted that HPS can be diagnosed in patients with coexisting intrinsic cardiopulmonary disease [110]. Increased experience and the ability to detect specifically the presence and degree of IPVDs has made it possible to distinguish HPS in such a setting.

Epidemiology

Most patients with HPS have underlying liver cirrhosis with variable degrees of portal hypertension. A prevalence of HPS of approximately 10%–20% has been reported in cirrhotic patients evaluated for liver transplantation [111–115] and in less selective populations [116–120]. HPS is not associated with any specific etiology of liver disease, and there is no clear relation between HPS and the degree of hepatic dysfunction [110]. Therefore, HPS should be suspected independently of the stage of liver disease.

HPS has also been diagnosed in noncirrhotic portal hypertension (extrahepatic portal vein thrombosis, Budd–Chiari syndrome, and others) and in liver diseases where portal hypertension is not a significant feature, such as in acute and chronic viral hepatitis without cirrhosis [110]. In a series of critically ill patients with diverse cardiopulmonary diseases, criteria of HPS were fulfilled by almost 50% of those who developed hypoxic hepatitis compared with 0% of patients without liver disease [121]. Structural pulmonary vascular changes characteristic of HPS have also been described in patients with fulminant hepatic failure [122]. These reports underscore that both portal hypertension and liver dysfunction (acute or chronic) are important factors in the pathogenesis of HPS.

Natural history

The natural history of HPS has not been completely elucidated. Approximately 10%–20% of cirrhotic patients present evidence of IPVDs without alterations of arterial oxygenation [112,116–118], not fulfilling the diagnostic criteria of HPS. This situation may represent an initial phase of HPS, but its evolution is unknown.

Once established, the diagnosis of HPS has important implications for the patient with liver disease. Although spontaneous improvement of HPS has been reported [123], progressive deterioration of arterial oxygenation occurs in most cases even in the setting of stable liver disease [124,125]. In patients with HPS awaiting liver transplantation, a mean P_aO_2 decline of 5.2 mmHg per year has been estimated [125]. Diagnosis of HPS is also associated with increased mortality [115,125]. In a prospective study of 111 patients with cirrhosis, the median survival time was 10.6 months in those with HPS compared with 40.8 months in those without HPS ($P < 0.05$), with the survival disadvantage for HPS being independent of the severity of liver disease [115]. In patients who do not undergo liver transplantation, the 5-year survival is significantly diminished in those who have HPS (20% vs 32%–63% in those without HPS) [115,125]. The severity of HPS also influences prognosis, with a $P_aO_2 < 60$ mmHg being correlated with worse survival [115,125]. The causes of mortality, including respiratory failure, are similar in patients with and without HPS and are mainly liver- or portal hypertension-related events [115,125].

Pathophysiology
Pathology

Alterations in the pulmonary vascular tree, generally within a normal lung parenchyma, are the distinctive pathological feature of HPS. In 1956, Hoffbauer and Rydell first described numerous abnormal vascular channels connecting the pulmonary arteries and veins in a patient with cirrhosis and cyanosis [126]. In subsequent years, a range of pulmonary vascular abnormalities were described in necropsy studies of patients with hypoxemia and liver disease. A diffuse dilation of pulmonary vessels mainly at the precapillary and capillary levels was the most conspicuous finding [127–129]. Other common alterations included pleural and subpleural spider nevi [127,129], thickening of walls of pulmonary capillaries and venules by collagen [128], discrete or multiple anatomical pulmonary arteriovenous communications [127,130], and communications between pulmonary veins with portal [131] or systemic veins [132]. All these alterations allow venous or mixed venous blood to pass directly to the pulmonary veins without being fully oxygenated.

Mechanisms of altered arterial oxygenation

Early studies suggested that the cause of hypoxemia in patients with cirrhosis was a decreased affinity of hemoglobin for oxygen, but subsequent research has shown that it was not a sufficient explanation and pointed instead to pulmonary causes of hypoxemia [133]. Among these, hypoventilation can be dismissed because hyperventilation is commonly found in HPS. The other theoretical pulmonary causes of hypoxemia, namely ventilation/perfusion mismatch, diffusion impairment, and vascular shunt, may all play a role in HPS (Fig. 24.4) [133]. Determination of which mechanism is more relevant in individual patients may have therapeutic implications.

Ventilation/perfusion mismatch is the most common cause of hypoxemia in clinical medicine. In normal conditions, the relation between ventilation and perfusion is maintained constant in each lung unit by the modulation of tone in pulmonary arterioles. Thus, arterioles that perfuse poorly ventilated alveoli undergo vasoconstriction and divert blood to better ventilated areas where it can be adequately oxygenated. The presence of abnormally elevated perfusion due to IPVDs results in areas with a low ventilation/perfusion ratio, or "physiological" shunts, which is considered the predominant mechanism of hypoxemia in mild-to-moderate HPS [134]. Characteristically, hypoxemia due to alterations of ventilation/perfusion mismatch has an excellent response ($P_aO_2 > 500$ mmHg) to breathing 100% oxygen (Fig. 24.4). In addition, an impaired pulmonary vasoconstrictive response to hypoxia is present in many patients with cirrhosis [135,136], and it has been associated with more advanced hypoxemia, pulmonary and systemic vasodilation, and ventilation/perfusion mismatch [135]. The extent to which a blunted hypoxic pulmonary vasoconstriction contributes to ventilation/perfusion mismatch in patients with HPS is, however, controversial [136].

Diffusion impairment is common in patients with liver disease, with up to 55% of candidates for liver transplantation [111,118,137–139] and almost 100% of patients with HPS

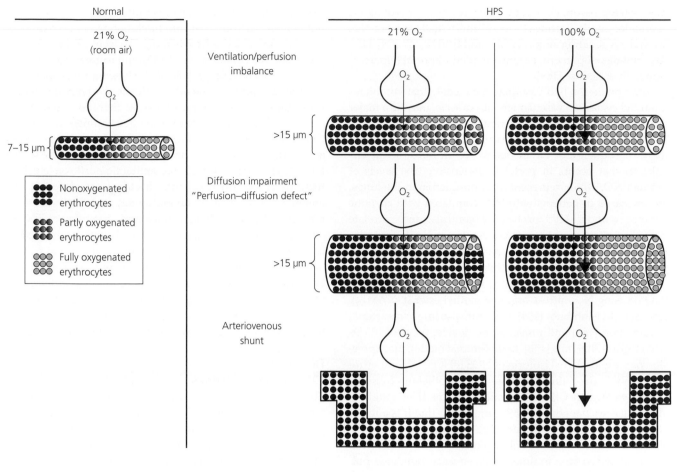

Figure 24.4 Schematic representation of the major mechanisms of hypoxemia in hepatopulmonary syndrome (HPS) and response to breathing 100% oxygen.

[111,124,140] presenting an abnormal diffusing capacity for carbon monoxide. A so-called diffusion-perfusion defect has been suggested in HPS [141], where the oxygen pressure within the alveoli would not be sufficient to oxygenate the erythrocytes that travel in the central portion of pulmonary precapillaries and capillaries, because of their abnormal dilation (Fig. 24.4). Based on this hypothesis, the excellent response to 100% oxygen in HPS could be explained by the increased oxygen pressure enhancing the oxygenation of those central erythrocytes. Interestingly, impaired diffusion persists after liver transplantation in many patients despite the reversibility of the hypoxemia and the IPVDs [142], suggesting that the impairment of diffusion is multifactorial.

True anatomical arteriovenous shunts may be present in patients with HPS. Large arteriovenous fistulae between the pulmonary artery and veins are occasionally detected in pulmonary angiography [143]. These arteriovenous communications separate blood from the respiratory interface and, therefore, breathing 100% oxygen does not improve arterial oxygenation (Fig. 24.4). Vascular plexuses between bronchial arteries and veins are common in the pleural surface of patients with cirrhosis, and may be recognized on visual inspection at autopsy as spider nevi [127]. The contribution of portopulmonary anastomoses to the hypoxemia in HPS is likely to be small, because portal venous blood is relatively rich in oxygen (~ 50 mmHg) and the flow through these vessels is small [133].

Importantly, *extrapulmonary factors* also influence gas exchange in these patients. In particular, increased cardiac output may impair arterial oxygenation by decreasing the transit time of erythrocytes through the dilated alveolar capillaries [144].

Mechanisms of pulmonary vasodilation

Pulmonary vascular alterations similar to those of HPS occur in rare cases of congenital heart malformations with anomalous drainage of hepatic veins [145]. Such alterations are reversible after surgical correction, indicating that factors produced or cleared by the liver strongly influence the pulmonary vascular structure. Mechanisms involved in the development of HPS include altered regulation of pulmonary vascular tone and processes of vascular remodeling and angiogenesis [146]. The cellular and molecular factors implicated have been investigated in humans and in an animal model of HPS, the rat with common bile duct ligation (CBDL) [147,148]. CBDL rats develop severe cholestatic liver disease, hyperdynamic circulation, and, starting 2 weeks after CBDL, progressive arterial oxygenation abnormalities and IPVDs [147,148]. HPS does not develop in other animal models of portal hypertension or liver disease [149].

Nitric oxide (NO), a vasodilator molecule that stimulates guanylyl cyclase in vascular smooth muscle, may be a major mediator of the pulmonary vascular abnormalities of HPS [110,150,151]. The development of HPS, however, is not a mere consequence of the increased NO in the systemic circulation that occurs in portal hypertension. The levels of exhaled NO, which represent local production in the lungs, are increased in patients with HPS compared with cirrhotic patients without HPS or healthy controls, and correlate with the alterations of arterial oxygenation [117]. Transient improvements of arterial oxygenation have been reported in patients with HPS after the inhibition of guanylyl cyclase (using methylene blue) [152,153] or nitric oxide synthases (NOS) (using $N_{(G)}$-nitro-L-arginine methyl ester [L-NAME]), a nonselective inhibitor [154]. L-NAME also improves arterial oxygenation [155] and prevents the development of IPVDs and HPS in CBDL rats [156]. In this animal model, the expression of the endothelial isoform of NOS (eNOS) increases progressively in the pulmonary vascular endothelium from the second week after CBDL in parallel with the IPVDs and the altered gas exchange [157–159], suggesting that it is a major source of increased NO production. An important but transient increase of the inducible isoform of NOS (iNOS) can also be detected later in time, localized in accumulated pulmonary intravascular monocyte/macrophages [158–160]. Alterations of the endothelin-1 system, a major regulator of vascular tone, may determine the altered pulmonary expression of NOS and NO production in CBDL rats [110,150]. In particular, the combination of increased circulating levels of endothelin-1 [149,159] and increased expression of endothelin type B (ETB) receptors in pulmonary vascular endothelium [159] appears to be unique to CBDL rats. Signaling of endothelin-1 through ETB receptors mediates vasodilation by stimulating endothelial NOS activity and NO production. Inhibition of ETB receptors in CBDL rats reduces the expression of both endothelial NOS and ETB receptors, and ameliorates HPS [159]. Rats with prehepatic portal hypertension, which have increased pulmonary expression of the ETB receptor but normal circulating endothelin-1, also develop increased pulmonary expression of endothelial NOS, altered oxygenation and IPVDs when they are infused with low doses of endothelin-1 [149]. Whether these mechanisms are relevant to human HPS, however, is unknown.

Carbon monoxide is another molecule that can induce vasodilation by stimulating guanylyl cyclase. Patients with cirrhosis and HPS present higher arterial levels of carboxyhemoglobin than those without HPS, and the levels moderately correlate with gas exchange abnormalities [114]. In CBDL rats, the expression of heme oxygenase 1, an enzyme that produces carbon monoxide from heme, is induced in liver tissue and pulmonary macrophages, and inhibition of heme oxygenase activity normalizes carboxyhemoglobin levels, attenuates gas-exchange abnormalities and IPVDs, and restores hypoxic pulmonary vasoconstriction [158,161]. These findings, therefore, suggest that carbon monoxide production by heme oxygenase contributes to the pulmonary vascular alterations of HPS.

Other factors may influence the development of HPS. In CBDL rats, the presence of bacterial translocation is associated with higher levels of circulating TNF-α and more severe HPS [162]. Treatment with the antibiotic norfloxacin selectively decreases gram-negative bacterial translocation and attenuates gas-exchange abnormalities and IPVDs in these rats [160]. Pentoxifylline, a nonspecific inhibitor of TNF-α, also prevents the development of HPS in CBDL rats [163]. In rats with prehepatic portal hypertension that receive an intravenous (i.v.) infusion of endothelin-1, the development of HPS is associated with an increase of circulating TNF-α [149]. Overall, these studies suggest that inflammation and bacterial translocation, which are frequent in patients with portal hypertension, may play a role in the development of HPS.

Diagnosis
Clinical manifestations

The diagnosis of HPS requires a high index of suspicion. Symptoms related to HPS may be erroneously attributed to progression of the underlying liver disease, which in most cases had been diagnosed years before, or to other conditions common in these patients, such as anemia, malnutrition, ascites, or intrinsic lung disease. This may delay the diagnosis of HPS, and thus it is common to find significant hypoxemia when the diagnosis is finally established.

There are no symptoms or physical signs pathognomonic of HPS. Many patients with HPS may be asymptomatic. The most common complaint (57%–78% of patients) is the insidious onset of dyspnea on exertion and subsequently at rest, but dyspnea is also frequent in cirrhotic patients without HPS (25%–46%) [111,112,164]. Platypnea (worsening of dyspnea in the standing position) is more specific for HPS, but it is present in only a few patients [111]. Spider angiomas, cyanosis, and finger clubbing are signs associated with HPS. Spider nevi are found in the majority of patients with HPS (> 80%) [111,112,165], and have been associated with more severe liver disease, prominent hyperdynamic circulation, and worse arterial oxygenation [112,135]. However, spider nevi can also be found in 40%–70% of cirrhotic patients without HPS [111,112]. Cyanosis and finger clubbing, by contrast, are highly specific for advanced HPS, reflecting the impact of chronic hypoxemia. Their sensitivity for HPS, however, is low as they are absent in many patients [111,164].

Arterial blood gases

Demonstration of altered arterial oxygenation is required for establishing the diagnosis of HPS. Several thresholds and parameters of arterial oxygenation have been used for defining HPS, partly explaining the variable prevalence reported [112]. In general, HPS can be diagnosed if the age-corrected alveolar–arterial oxygen pressure gradient is higher than normal (age-corrected upper limit of normal = $10 + [0.26 \times age - 0.43]$) with or without hypoxemia ($P_aO_2 < 70$ mmHg) [110]. The use of the alveolar–arterial oxygen gradient increases the sensitivity, as it includes in its calculation a correction for the value of P_aCO_2. This gradient is known to increase with age and, therefore, an age correction is necessary to avoid HPS overdiagnosis. The ERS Task Force on Pulmonary-Hepatic Vascular Disorders has staged the severity of HPS based on the P_aO_2 value on room air into mild (≥ 80 mmHg), moderate (≥ 60 and < 80 mmHg), severe (≥ 50 and < 60 mmHg), and very severe (< 50 mmHg; < 300 mmHg if on 100% oxygen), a classification that has prognostic significance [109].

Orthodeoxia (worsening of arterial oxygenation in the standing position) is relatively common in patients with HPS [124], but it can also be encountered in other medical conditions. In patients with HPS, orthodeoxia has been defined as a fall in $P_aO_2 \geq 5\%$ or ≥ 4 mmHg from supine, and it is caused by a gravity-induced heterogeneous redistribution of blood flow to lung bases that increases intrapulmonary shunt and ventilation/perfusion imbalance [165]. To maximize the chance of revealing HPS, the determination of arterial blood gases should be done in the sitting or standing position.

Analysis of arterial blood gases while breathing 100% oxygen may add valuable information, and also allows the quantification of the "physiological shunt." Many patients with HPS present an excellent response to 100% oxygen ($P_aO_2 > 500$ mmHg), indicating that ventilation/perfusion imbalance or diffusion impairment are the principal mechanisms of hypoxemia. A poor response to 100% oxygen ($P_aO_2 < 300$ mmHg) indicates the presence of perfusion without ventilation, and suggests (especially if $P_aO_2 < 150$ mmHg) the presence of anatomical arteriovenous shunts.

Chest radiography and lung function tests

Chest radiography and lung function tests must be done to detect other cardiopulmonary conditions that may cause hypoxemia (see Table 24.5). These conditions may be related to liver disease, such as a hepatic hydrothorax, or may be secondary to intrinsic cardiopulmonary diseases. Importantly, one-third of patients with HPS have coexisting chronic pulmonary conditions, such as chronic obstructive pulmonary disease or bronchial asthma [166,167]. If liver transplantation is being considered it is crucial to evaluate the extent to which these conditions are responsible for the hypoxemia.

The chest radiograph of patients with HPS may reveal bilateral interstitial and pulmonary vascular markings in lower lobes that correspond to the presence of IPVDs [124], but this finding is not specific.

In lung function tests, the majority of patients with HPS present mild to moderate alterations of the diffusing capacity

of carbon monoxide [111,124,140], but this is also frequent in patients without HPS [111,118,137–139]. A restrictive pattern can be found in patients who have ascites, pleural effusions, or muscular wasting. In patients with coexisting intrinsic pulmonary diseases, lung function tests will present the corresponding patterns.

Assessment of intrapulmonary vascular dilations

The diagnosis of HPS requires the documenting of the presence of intrapulmonary vascular dilations (IPVDs).

Transthoracic contrast-enhanced echocardiography

Transthoracic contrast-enhanced echocardiography (TT-CEE) is the preferred screening method, because it is noninvasive, highly sensitive for IPVDs, and allows the simultaneous detection of cardiac anomalies and the estimation of right ventricular systolic pressure. Approximately 20% of patients with cirrhosis and a positive TT-CEE for IPVDs, however, do not present alterations of arterial oxygenation [112,116–118]. TT-CEE is usually performed by injecting 10 mL of agitated saline i.v., which produces echogenic microbubbles 24–180 μm in diameter [119]. The microbubbles can be detected in right heart chambers within seconds, they are then trapped in lung capillaries (7–15 μm in diameter) and, in normal conditions, no contrast is observed in left heart chambers. If they are detected in left heart chambers after three heartbeats of their detection in the right chambers, it indicates intrapulmonary shunting. If detected before three heartbeats, it is indicative of intracardiac communication, such as a patent foramen ovale. Different contrast agents, such as indocyanine green solution, may have slightly different sensitivity for IPVDs [119]. TT-CEE cannot quantify the degree of shunt or determine the type of intrapulmonary shunt present (microdilation of fine vessels vs arteriovenous fistula). Transesophageal CEE (TE-CEE) may provide more anatomical information by visualizing specific pulmonary veins, and it is also more sensitive for detecting IPVDs, especially when image quality is bad with the transthoracic approach [118]. However, TE-CEE is more invasive and expensive than TT-CEE, and therefore its main use is in patients with a high suspicion of HPS and negative TT-CEE [118].

Radionuclide lung perfusion scanning

Evidence of right-to-left shunting can be obtained by the intravenous injection of technetium-labeled macroaggregated albumin particles (^{99m}Tc-MAA, 20–90 μm in diameter) combined with whole-body scintigraphy. In normal subjects, ^{99m}Tc-MAA particles are trapped in lung capillaries, and less than 6% of the isotopic activity can be detected in brain, kidneys, spleen, or liver. When the ^{99m}Tc-MAA activity in extrapulmonary tissues (usually calculated from the activity in the brain) is higher than 6% of the total, it indicates the presence of a right-to-left shunt. The ^{99m}Tc-MAA technique permits quantification of the shunt fraction, allowing a better evaluation of the contribution of HPS to the hypoxemia in patients with coexisting cardiopulmonary diseases [140,167]. The calculated ^{99m}Tc-MAA shunt fraction is strongly correlated with arterial oxygenation parameters in patients with HPS [140]. Compared with TT-CEE, the main disadvantages of ^{99m}Tc-MAA are that it may be negative in patients with less severe disease ($P_aO_2 > 60$ mmHg) [140], and that it cannot distinguish between intracardiac or intrapulmonary shunt, evaluate cardiac disease, or estimate the pulmonary arterial pressure.

Pulmonary angiography

Pulmonary angiography is an invasive, nonsensitive test for the detection of IPVDs. Low pulmonary arterial pressure and low pulmonary vascular resistance are common findings in HPS. Two different angiographic patterns of IPVDs have been described. Type I (diffuse) is characterized by a diffuse dilation of small peripheral branches of the pulmonary artery, mainly in lower lobes. The less common type II (focal) refers to the presence of discrete pulmonary arteriovenous communications [124]. The main indication for pulmonary angiography is patients with a poor response to 100% oxygen ($P_aO_2 < 150$ mmHg), who may have pulmonary arteriovenous communications amenable to embolization [168]. In patients with a good response to 100% oxygen, the likelihood of finding discrete arteriovenous communications is minimal [167].

High-resolution chest computed tomography (CT)

High-resolution chest CT is useful to diagnose coexisting intrinsic cardiopulmonary disease. When evaluated with this technique, patients with HPS present greater peripheral pulmonary artery diameters and pulmonary artery/bronchus ratios compared with healthy controls and normoxemic patients with cirrhosis [169,170]. The degree of dilation is correlated to some extent with the severity of gas exchange abnormalities [169]. The reliability of this technique for diagnosing IPVDs in HPS, however, requires further study.

Screening

All candidates for liver transplantation should be screened for HPS. Detection of HPS allows a better evaluation of the prognosis and the risk of perioperative complications in individual patients. Guidelines also support the expedited transplantation of patients with severe HPS ($P_aO_2 < 60$ mmHg on room air) by providing additional points for the Model for End-stage Liver Disease (MELD) [171], because of the unacceptable posttransplant mortality if P_aO_2 falls below 50 mmHg [172]. Under these conditions, screening for HPS in liver transplant candidates is cost-effective, especially with pulse oximetry, and may improve survival [173]. In patients who are not candidates for liver transplantation, general screening for HPS is not recommended, but the diagnostic evaluation of those presenting dyspnea, finger clubbing, or cyanosis should include consideration of HPS.

A general diagnostic approach is shown in Fig. 24.5. If pulse oximetry is used, arterial blood gases should be obtained if oxygen saturation is $\leq 97\%$. Lower thresholds could miss the diagnosis in many patients because pulse oximetry overestimates arterial oxygenation [113]. Most diagnostic strategies recommend the use of TT-CEE for the detection of IPVDs, reserving the use of ^{99m}Tc-MAA lung perfusion scanning to evaluate those patients with positive TT-CEE and coexisting cardiopulmonary disease [109,110].

Therapy

Oxygen therapy

Mortality in HPS increases with the severity of hypoxemia and is mainly due to liver-related complications [115,125], suggesting that hypoxemia may accelerate the progression of liver disease. Experimental studies suggest that hepatocellular hypoxia enhances fibrogenesis [174]. For these reasons, oxygen therapy is used in patients with significant hypoxemia. Improvement of liver function after long-term oxygen therapy has been reported in two patients with HPS [175]. Despite the rationality behind its use, no study has assessed the effects of oxygen supplementation on the evolution of HPS or liver disease.

Pharmacological therapy

There are no effective pharmacological agents for treating HPS. Somatostatin analogues, indometacin (indomethacin), almitrine bismesylate (a pulmonary vasoconstrictor), inhaled NO, and norfloxacin, have all been tested in small numbers of patients showing minimal (or no) beneficial effects [110,164]. Inhibitors of the NO–guanylyl cyclase pathway (L-NAME, methylene blue) transiently improved hypoxemia, intrapulmonary shunt fraction, and systemic hemodynamics in some studies [152–154], but no effects or even worsening of hypoxemia have also been reported [176,177]. Of note, improvement of arterial oxygenation has been noted in a total of 16 of 33 patients (49%) with HPS treated with garlic powder [178–182]. Despite some promising observations, no clear conclusions can be made regarding the efficacy or safety of any of these agents, because they were all tested in noncontrolled, small series of patients.

Interventional radiology

Pulmonary angiography with coil embolotherapy may improve oxygenation in selected patients with HPS and discrete pulmonary arteriovenous fistulae [168].

Transjugular intrahepatic portosystemic shunts (TIPS) could theoretically improve HPS by relieving portal hypertension, but reports of both improvement and no improvement of HPS have appeared [110]. Short follow-up times and coexistence of hepatic hydrothorax limit the interpretation of the case reports. In general, significant IPVDs persist in most patients after TIPS, suggesting that oxygenation is improved because of blood flow redistribution to regions with normal

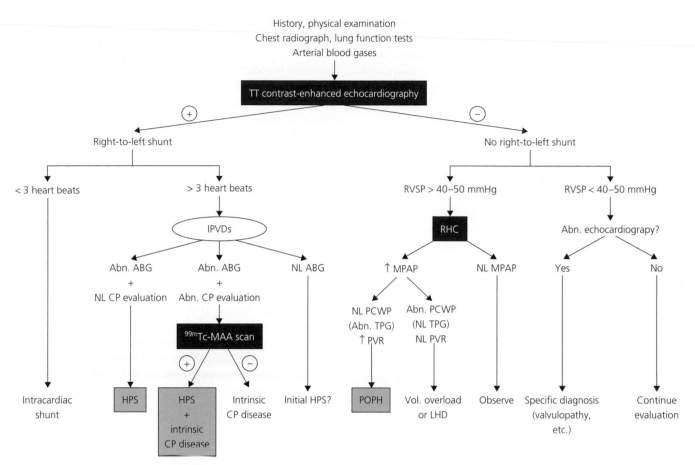

Figure 24.5 General diagnostic approach for hepatopulmonary syndrome (HPS) and portopulmonary hypertension (POPH). Patients with liver disease or portal hypertension presenting with respiratory symptoms or specific signs should be evaluated. All patients being evaluated for major surgical procedures (including liver transplantation) should undergo screening for HPS and POPH, even if asymptomatic. ABG, arterial blood gases; Abn., abnormal; CP, cardiopulmonary; IPVD, intrapulmonary vascular dilation; LHD, left heart dysfunction; MPAP, mean pulmonary arterial pressure; NL, normal; PCWP, pulmonary capillary wedge pressure; PVR, pulmonary vascular resistance; RHC, right heart catheterization; RVSP, right ventricular systolic pressure; 99mTc-MAA, technetium-labeled macroaggregated albumin; TPG, transpulmonary gradient; TT, transthoracic; Vol., volume.

ventilation/perfusion ratios rather than a true reversal of HPS [164]. Consequently, TIPS should not be considered a therapy for HPS until more evidence of its efficacy and safety is provided [109].

Liver transplantation

Liver transplantation is the only effective therapy for HPS, based on the resolution of hypoxemia and intrapulmonary shunt noted in the majority of reported cases [125,133,183]. In some patients with stable liver disease, severe HPS may constitute the indication per se for liver transplantation. The reversibility of HPS after liver transplantation may be slow (> 1 year), probably reflecting the presence of important structural alterations in the pulmonary vasculature [146]. In general, patients with HPS who undergo liver transplantation have better survival than those who do not, but the effect of comorbid conditions in the latter cannot be dismissed [125]. In patients undergoing liver transplantation, mortality tends to be higher in those with HPS compared with those

without HPS [125,172], and it increases with the severity of HPS. A $P_{a}O_2 \leq 50$ mmHg and a 99mTc-MAA shunt fraction $\geq 20\%$ are strong predictors of postoperative mortality [172]. The most common posttransplant complications in patients with HPS include infections and respiratory failure with persistent or worsening hypoxemia [172], but more specific complications of HPS may occur, such as cerebral embolic hemorrhages [184] or the development of portopulmonary hypertension [185]. Despite the beneficial influence of liver transplantation, the criteria used for selecting or prioritizing patients with HPS in the waiting list still require refinement to optimize outcomes and organ allocation [171].

Portopulmonary hypertension

In the early 1950s, Mantz and Craige first described cor pulmonale in a patient with portal vein thrombosis, portal hypertension, and portosystemic shunt [186]. Today, portopulmonary hypertension (POPH) refers to a pathological obstructive process in the pulmonary vasculature of patients who have portal hypertension, resulting in increased resistance to blood flow and pulmonary arterial hypertension. In common with HPS, POPH is also a complication of portal hypertension. In contrast to HPS, however, POPH is characterized by pulmonary vasoconstriction rather than vasodilation.

Definition

POPH is defined as pulmonary arterial hypertension (PAH) associated with portal hypertension, with or without underlying liver disease [109,187]. POPH is not considered a "secondary" form of PAH, but is classified in the same group as idiopathic PAH, familial PAH, and PAH associated with diverse conditions (collagen vascular disease and others) [187].

The following traditional criteria must be fulfilled to diagnose POPH:

- presence of portal hypertension with or without cirrhosis
- mean pulmonary arterial pressure (MPAP) > 25 mmHg (3.33 kPa) at rest
- pulmonary capillary wedge pressure (PCW) < 15 mmHg (2.0 kPa)
- pulmonary vascular resistance (PVR) > 240 dyn·s·cm^5 (3.0 mmHg/L/min).

Performance of right heart catheterization with complete hemodynamic study is, therefore, required to diagnose POPH correctly.

Epidemiology

By definition, the diagnosis of POPH is made in patients with portal hypertension. Most patients have underlying cirrhosis, but POPH can also develop in patients with noncirrhotic portal hypertension, such as nodular regenerative hyperplasia or portal vein obstruction [188]. The diagnosis of portal hypertension usually precedes by more than 4 years that of POPH [189]. POHP may occur at any age, including childhood, but the diagnosis is most common in the fifth decade, compared with the fourth decade in idiopathic PAH [188].

POPH is a rare complication of portal hypertension, but it appears to be more common than reported in early studies. In 1983, a series of 17 901 unselected autopsies noted changes characteristic of idiopathic PAH more commonly in patients with cirrhosis than in the whole series (0.73% vs 0.13%) [190]. In a cohort of 507 patients with portal hypertension (of cirrhotic origin in 85%) undergoing hemodynamic studies, the prevalence of POPH was 2% [189]. In two studies in candidates for liver transplantation, the prevalence of POPH was more than double these rates (5%–6%) [191,192], maybe reflecting a longer duration of portal hypertension. No clear correlations exist, however, between the severity of POPH and the etiology or severity of liver disease, degree of portal hypertension, or hyperdynamic circulation [188,189,192]. In patients with refractory ascites evaluated for TIPS placement,

an unusually high prevalence of POPH of 16% has been reported [193].

Natural history

The diagnosis of POPH carries a dreadful prognosis [194]. No cases of spontaneous resolution of POPH have been reported. A median survival as low as 6 months was noted in the pre-liver transplantation era [195]. In subsequent series, the overall 3- to 5-year probability of survival (irrespective of the medical management, including liver transplantation) was approximately 30%–50% [196–198]. The natural history of POPH is not well defined, however, and predicting survival in individual patients is a difficult task [189].

Complications of liver disease and those directly related to POPH (right-sided heart failure, sudden death) account for a similar proportion of deaths in patients with POPH. A low cardiac index is a strong predictor of mortality in these patients, particularly for death resulting from cardiopulmonary complications [189,197]. Increased plasma levels of brain natriuretic peptide reflect right ventricular stress and have been associated with poor prognosis in idiopathic PAH [199]. Limited data suggest that vasodilator therapy and liver transplantation influence the course of POPH, but the extent to which these interventions may reverse the condition or improve survival is unknown.

Pathophysiology
Pathology

The pathology of POPH is indistinguishable from that observed in idiopathic PAH, and is characterized by vasoconstriction and structural changes in the pulmonary arterial tree that result in the obstruction of pulmonary blood flow [190,200]. The main changes affect small pulmonary arteries and arterioles, and consist of hypertrophy of medial smooth muscle, with proliferation or fibrosis of endothelium and adventitia. Thrombosis with recanalization may develop in situ in these vessels. The plexiform lesion, characteristic of idiopathic PAH, can also be observed in POPH. It consists of small branches of pulmonary arteries dilated close to their origin that present thinning of medial smooth muscle, and an intralumenal plexus of endothelial cells and narrow slit-like channels.

Pathogenesis

Knowledge of the pathogenesis of POPH is limited, due to the rarity of the condition and the lack of adequate animal models. The mechanistic connection between portal and pulmonary hypertension is not completely understood, but some pathogenetic factors postulated for idiopathic PAH may be enhanced in patients with portal hypertension [201]. Two major features of portal hypertension may affect the pulmonary circulation [187,188]. First, the hyperdynamic circulation with increased cardiac output increases shear stress in the pulmonary vasculature and may lead to altered endothelial expression of genes involved in regulation of vascular tone and angiogenesis. Second, portosystemic shunting and defective liver metabolism expose the pulmonary vasculature to blood that has not been processed by the liver, which presumably causes an imbalance between vasodilator–vasoconstrictor and antiproliferative–growth-promoting mediators in the pulmonary circulation. This may include the elevation of levels of potent vasoconstrictors involved in the pathogenesis of idiopathic PAH, such as endothelin-1 (through ETA receptors) and 5-HT_2, and others such as prostaglandin $F_{2\alpha}$, thromboxane B_2 or angiotensin I. By contrast, the expression of prostacyclin synthase, the enzyme that produces the vasodilator prostacyclin, is decreased in small pulmonary arteries of patients with POPH [202]. Portosystemic shunting of bacterial products translocated from the intestines may lead to macrophage sequestration and secretion of cytokines in the pulmonary vasculature, which may contribute to the pathological process. The coagulopathy of patients with cirrhosis may also influence the development of in situ thrombosis in the affected vessels, causing further resistance to blood flow.

Many patients with portal hypertension are likely to present the above factors, but it is unclear why only a small subset of them develops POPH. An autoimmune origin of POHP has been postulated in some patients based on a high prevalence of autoimmune antibodies [197], but this finding is not conclusive. A genetic predisposition may also be a factor, but genetic variations linked to idiopathic PAH affecting bone morphogenetic protein receptor II, activin-like kinase type-1 or the 5-HT transporter have not been confirmed in patients with POPH [109,187].

Diagnosis
Clinical manifestations
Patients with POPH usually have a previous diagnosis of portal hypertension. Many patients may be asymptomatic [189], underscoring the need for screening patients with liver disease who will undergo surgical procedures, particularly liver transplantation. The diagnosis of POPH may be delayed more than 1 year after the onset of symptoms [189], with dyspnea on exertion being the most common complaint [195]. Patients can also present with progressive fatigue and orthopnea. The presence of chest discomfort and syncope indicates advanced disease. In addition to signs of liver disease and portal hypertension, patients with POPH will present signs derived from progressive right-sided heart dysfunction, which include jugular venous ingurgitation, cardiac auscultation with increase of the P_2 pulmonic valve component and tricuspid regurgitation murmur, right ventricular heave, and edema of lower extremities.

The differential diagnosis of dyspnea in liver disease is broad (Table 24.5), and reaching a diagnosis of POPH may require an extensive diagnostic workup [187,188]. Arterial blood gases in patients with POPH usually reveal an increase

Table 24.5 Differential diagnosis of cardiopulmonary dysfunction in liver disease

Intrinsic cardiopulmonary conditions
Obstructive lung diseases
  Chronic obstructive pulmonary disease
  Asthma
  Others, including emphysema
Diseases of lung parenchyma
  Pneumonia
  Interstitial lung disease
  Others, including atelectasis
Pulmonary vascular diseases
  Pulmonary embolism
  Secondary pulmonary hypertension (due to heart/lung disease or others)
Disorders of the heart and circulatory system
  Congestive heart failure
  Valvular heart disease
  Cardiomyopathy
  Others (including arrhythmias, coronary artery disease)

Conditions related to liver disease and portal hypertension
Associated with specific liver diseases
  α_1-Antitrypsin deficiency: emphysema
  Primary biliary cirrhosis: fibrosing alveolitis, pulmonary granulomas
  Sarcoidosis: lung restrictive disease, nonnecrotizing granulomas, cardiomyopathy
  Hemochromatosis: cardiomyopathy, arrhythmias
  Cystic fibrosis: bronchiectasis, pneumonia
General complications of liver disease and portal hypertension
  Ascites
  Hepatic hydrothorax
  Muscular wasting
Pulmonary vascular abnormalities
  Hepatopulmonary syndrome
  Portopulmonary hypertension

of the alveolar–arterial oxygen gradient, hypocapnia, and, less frequently, a mild degree of hypoxemia, even in the setting of moderate-to-severe POPH [203]. In moderate-advanced POPH, a chest radiograph may show a prominent main pulmonary artery and cardiomegaly without any parenchymal alterations. An electrocardiogram indicating right atrial enlargement, right ventricular hypertrophy, or right bundle branch block should increase the suspicion of POPH. Lung function tests are important to exclude significant air flow obstruction and other lung diseases, and frequently reveal a reduced diffusing capacity for carbon monoxide in patients with POPH. Ventilation/perfusion lung scanning may show a "mosaic" pattern in patients with POPH; segmental defects would instead suggest pulmonary embolism. Compared with the pulmonary angiographic pattern of idiopathic PAH, POPH presents a lesser degree of sparse arborization and tapering of peripheral arteries, and a dilation instead of narrowing of proximal pulmonary arteries [204].

Transthoracic echocardiography

Transthoracic Doppler echocardiography is the most important noninvasive test for screening POPH (Fig. 24.5). It may exclude valvulopathies and other cardiac causes of elevated MPAP, and also screens for HPS. Most patients with POPH (~ 80%–90%) present a tricuspid regurgitant jet, which allows estimation of the right ventricular systolic pressure (RVSP). The echocardiographic findings reflect the cardiac consequences of progressive resistance to pulmonary blood flow, including pulmonic valve insufficiency, right atrial dilation, right ventricular hypertrophy and dilation, interventricular septal wall thickening, and paradoxical septal motion.

The estimated RVSP is a useful screening parameter for POPH, but there is no consensus regarding which value should be used [205]. Most studies use estimated RVSP cutoff values of 40–50 mmHg, which have a sensitivity of almost 100% for detecting POPH [206]. The correlation between the RVSP values estimated by echocardiography and those directly measured during right heart catheterization is weak [192,207]. Furthermore, echocardiography cannot evaluate PVR. For these reasons, approximately 30%–40% of patients satisfying the previous estimated RVSP thresholds will have normal PVR measured during right heart catheterization and they will not be diagnosed with POPH [191,192]. Another echocardiographic parameter proposed for screening POPH is a pulmonary acceleration time > 100 ms [208], which may have better diagnostic accuracy and can be used in patients in whom RVSP cannot be estimated [192]. In addition to screening, transthoracic echocardiography is useful for following up patients with a diagnosis of POPH.

Hemodynamic assessment

Diagnosing POPH requires the performance of right heart catheterization (Fig. 24.5). This test allows the direct measurement of MPAP, PCW, and cardiac output, and the calculation of PVR and systemic vascular resistance (SVR). An increase of MPAP alone is not diagnostic of POPH in patients with portal hypertension. Hemodynamic parameters distinguish three origins of increased MPAP in these patients [109,206]:

1 *Hyperdynamic circulatory state.* This hemodynamic pattern is the most common in patients with liver disease. It is characterized by a significant increase of cardiac output and decreased SVR, with a normal PCW and normal or low PVR. MPAP may be mildly elevated as a result of increased cardiac output.

2 *Increased pulmonary venous volume.* In this case, MPAP is mildly or moderately elevated in the setting of an increased PCW, reflecting the presence of volume overload or left ventricular dysfunction. RVP is normal or mildly elevated.

3 *Pulmonary vascular obstruction.* This pattern must be present to diagnose POPH. It is distinguished by the significant increase of PVR, leading to elevations of MPAP that may be severe. PCW is normal or mildly decreased. In contrast to idiopathic PAH, cardiac output is usually increased in patients with POPH. A decrease of cardiac output in POPH indicates advanced right-sided heart failure, and is a sign of poor prognosis [189,197].

Hyperdynamic circulation and volume overload are common in patients with liver disease. According to traditional criteria, the diagnosis of POPH would be missed in these patients if PCWP is greater than 15 mmHg. To avoid this situation, use of the transpulmonary pressure gradient (TPG = MPAP – PCW) has been proposed [109]. A TGP > 12 mmHg indicates obstruction to flow, independent of the value of PCW [192].

The value of MPAP obtained during right heart catheterization is used to stage the severity of POPH into mild (> 25 and < 35 mmHg), moderate (≥ 35 and < 45 mmHg) and severe (≥ 45 mmHg) grades, which provides important prognostic information [109].

If POPH is diagnosed, an acute vasodilator testing should be performed during right heart catheterization, generally using epoprostenol i.v. or inhaled NO. A vasodilatory response is significant when MPAP and PVR decrease by more than 20% from baseline values without a decrease of cardiac output [109]. This test reflects to what extent the hypertensive state is caused by reversible vasoconstriction, helping to characterize the severity of the disease and the therapeutic expectations. In a small study of 14 patients with moderate-to-severe POPH, 6 (43%) presented a significant vasodilatory response to i.v. epoprostenol [209]. In these patients, epoprostenol i.v. induces greater increases of cardiac output than inhaled NO [210], and has been suggested to detect a higher proportion of responders [109].

Treatment
General medical treatment

The general management of patients with POPH consists in avoiding circumstances that may worsen portal hypertension, pulmonary vasoconstriction, or stress to the heart. Surgery should be indicated with caution in patients with POPH, even in those with mild disease, and it would require special anesthetic care [211]. TIPS is not recommended in patients with POPH, because the increase in cardiac output may worsen pulmonary hypertension and precipitate right-sided heart failure. Patients with POPH and hypoxemia may benefit from oxygen therapy to avoid hypoxic pulmonary vasoconstriction. Diuretics (furosemide, spirolonolactone) may be used in patients with volume overload. Withdrawal of β-blocker treatment in patients with POPH has been associated with improvements in exercise capacity and pulmonary hemodynamics [212]. Alternative methods for preventing variceal bleeding, therefore, may be desirable. Oral anticoagulation and calcium channel blockers, medications used for idiopathic PAH, are not recommended in patients with portal hypertension because they may increase the risk or severity of bleeding and the hepatic venous pressure gradient, respectively [213].

Specific vasodilator therapy

Specific vasodilator therapy improves symptoms, pulmonary hemodynamics, and survival in large clinical studies of idiopathic PAH [201]. In patients with POPH, however, the experience is limited to case reports and small, uncontrolled studies, impeding the establishment of conclusive guidelines. In general, this therapy is not offered to asymptomatic patients with mild POPH (MPAP < 35 mmHg), who should undergo only periodic follow-up with transthoracic echocardiography. Patients with moderate-to-severe POPH (MPAP > 35 mmHg) and a significant vasodilatory response may benefit from this therapy, especially if combined with liver transplantation. The duration of the effect of vasodilator therapy and its impact on POPH survival, however, are unknown.

Prostacyclin analogues

Epoprostenol, a potent pulmonary vasodilator with anti-proliferative and anti-platelet aggregating properties, is the best-studied agent. Because of the short half-life (3–5 min) of epoprostenol, treatment requires long-term catheterization of a central vein for continuous i.v. administration. In series totalling more than 45 cases, both the acute and long-term administration of epoprostenol significantly decreased MPAP and PVR and increased cardiac output in patients with POPH [209,214–217]. Common side effects include headache, flushing, diarrhea, nausea, muscle pain, and hypotension [201]. Development of splenomegaly with leukothrombocytopenia was reported in four patients [218]. The potential complications arising from long-term venous access, such as infection or thrombosis, are the major limitations for this therapy. Moreover, accidental interruption of the perfusion may cause life-threatening sudden pulmonary vasoconstriction. More stable prostacyclin analogues, such as iloprost and treprostinil (approved for idiopathic PAH by the US Food and Drug Administration [201]), and a variety of routes of administration (inhalation, oral, subcutaneous, i.v.) have been investigated. The experience with these agents in POPH, however, is still limited to anecdotal reports [219,220].

Endothelin receptor antagonists

Bosentan is a dual ETA and ETB receptor antagonist that can be administered orally. A dose-dependent increase of liver enzymes, however, occurred in approximately 11% of patients treated with this agent in clinical trials of idiopathic PAH [201]. In preliminary reports comprising a total of 13 patients with POPH and well-compensated cirrhosis, treatment with low-to-medium doses of bosentan for more than 1 year resulted in improvement of exercise capacity and pulmonary hemodynamics without notable adverse effects, except systemic arterial hypotension in one patient [221–223].

Phosphodiesterase inhibitors

Sildenafil is an oral medication also approved for idiopathic PAH. Sildenafil inhibits the degradation of NO by phospho-diesterase-5, promoting vasodilation. Preliminary reports have communicated variable improvements of exercise capacity or pulmonary hemodynamics in a total of 17 patients with advanced cirrhosis and severe POPH treated with sildenafil alone or in combination [224–227]. The administration of sildenafil, however, may exacerbate portal hypertension and hyperdynamic circulation [228], and variceal bleeding during treatment with sildenafil has been reported [229].

Other agents

It has been reported that MPAP and PVR were decreased by isosorbide-5-mononitrate [230] in one patient, and by inhaled NO in five out of six patients with POPH [231].

Liver transplantation

It is unclear how liver transplantation influences the natural history of POPH. Normalization, improvement, no change, and worsening of POPH have all been reported in patients undergoing liver transplantation [109,205]. In favorable cases, POPH may take months to years to resolve. De novo development of POPH, transition from HPS to POPH, and recurrence of POPH in cases of graft failure have also been noted after liver transplantation [187]. For these reasons, in contrast to HPS, POPH is not an indication for liver transplantation.

Impact of POPH on liver transplantation outcomes

The presence of POPH is associated with increased morbidity and mortality in patients undergoing liver transplantation. A transplant hospitalization mortality of 36% has been reported in these patients, with 40% of the deaths occurring intraoperatively [232]. Screening of POPH in liver transplant candidates and adequate staging by right heart catheterization are critical for assessing the risk of complications [233]. Despite adequate screening, a few patients may be diagnosed in the operating room [191,232]. The rate of mortality in patients with POPH undergoing liver transplantation increases from 0% if MPAP < 35 mmHg or TPG < 15 mmHg, to 50% if MPAP is between 35 and 50 mmHg and PVR ≥ 250 dyn·s·cm^5 (3.125 mmHg/L/min), to 100% if MPAP ≥ 50 mmHg [233]. Based on this and other studies, a MPAP ≥ 50 mmHg is usually considered an absolute contraindication for liver transplantation [109]. Successful liver transplantation of these patients, however, has been occasionally reported [234]. Eligible candidates with mild POPH (MPAP < 35 mmHg) could benefit from expedited liver transplantation before POPH progresses, but the provision of additional MELD points is controversial [205].

The risk of complications in patients with POPH undergoing liver transplantation is maximal during the induction of anesthesia, before and after graft reperfusion, and in the immediate postoperative period [235]. Increases of MPAP during reperfusion of the graft may cause right-sided heart failure [109], the main cause of intraoperative and perioperative mortality in these patients [232]. Dobutamine stress echocardiography with volume challenge may improve the prediction of this complication [236]. Circumstances that impair heart function, such as hypoxia, hypothermia, hyperkalemia, metabolic acidosis, or hypercarbia, should be prevented. Anesthesia with isofluorane and intraoperative use of vasodilators may help to control increases of MPAP in these patients [109,235]. Combined liver, heart, and lung transplantation has been reported in highly selected patients but remains experimental [237].

Specific vasodilator therapy for rescuing candidates for liver transplantation

Patients with moderate-to-severe POPH (MPAP > 35 mmHg) who do not have contraindications for liver transplantation are the most likely to benefit from vasodilator therapy. Using this approach, up to 75% of them may achieve reductions of MPAP below 35 mmHg and PVR below 400 dyn·s·cm^5 (5.0 mmHg/L/min) and can be successfully bridged to liver transplantation [187]. Preliminary data suggest that this combination provides a survival advantage to these patients [205,217]. Vasodilator therapy should continue during and after liver transplantation, but withdrawal has been safely achieved within 1 year in many patients [209,216,217]. Despite the evidence supporting the use of vasodilator therapy, a prospective collection of data from 1996 to 2001 in 10 liver transplant centers of the United States showed that vasodilator therapy is not commonly offered to these patients [232].

References

1. Ferenci P, Lockwood A, Mullen K, et al. Hepatic encephalopathy – definition, nomenclature, diagnosis, and quantification: final report of the working party at the 11th World Congresses of Gastroenterology, Vienna, 1998. Hepatology 2002;35:716.
2. Blei AT, Cordoba J. Hepatic encephalopathy. Am J Gastroenterol 2001;96:1968.
3. Conn HO, Leevy CM, Vlahcevic ZR, et al. Comparison of lactulose and neomycin in the treatment of chronic portal-systemic encephalopathy. A double blind controlled trial. Gastroenterology 1977;72:573.
4. Weissenborn K, Ennen JC, Schomerus H, et al. Neuropsychological characterization of hepatic encephalopathy. J Hepatol 2001;34:768.
5. Kullmann F, Hollerbach S, Holstege A, Scholmerich J. Subclinical hepatic encephalopathy: the diagnostic value of evoked potentials. J Hepatol 1995;22:101.
6. Kircheis G, Wettstein M, Timmermann L, et al. Critical flicker frequency for quantification of low-grade hepatic encephalopathy. Hepatology 2002;35:357.
7. Norenberg MD. The role of astrocytes in hepatic encephalopathy. Neurochem Pathol 1987;6:13.
8. Adams RD, Foley JM. The neurological disorder associated with liver disease. In: Merritt HH, Hare CC (eds). Metabolic and Toxic Diseases of the Nervous System. Baltimore: Williams and Wilkins, 1953:198.
9. Butterworth RF, Giguere JF, Michaud J, et al. Ammonia: key factor in the pathogenesis of hepatic encephalopathy. Neurochem Pathol 1987;6:1.
10. Mossakowski MJ, Renkawek K, Krasnicka Z, et al. Morphology and histochemistry of Wilsonian and hepatogenic gliopathy in tissue culture. Acta Neuropathol (Berl) 1970;16:1.
11. Butterworth RF. Neuronal cell death in hepatic encephalopathy. Metab Brain Dis 2007;22:309.
12. Cordoba J, Raguer N, Flavia M, et al. T2 hyperintensity along the cortico-spinal tract in cirrhosis relates to functional abnormalities. Hepatology 2003;38:1026.
13. Lockwood AH, Yap EW, Wong WH. Cerebral ammonia metabolism in patients with severe liver disease and minimal hepatic encephalopathy. J Cereb Blood Flow Metab 1991;11:337.
14. Keiding S, Sorensen M, Bender D, et al. Brain metabolism of 13N-ammonia during acute hepatic encephalopathy in cirrhosis measured by positron emission tomography. Hepatology 2006;43:42.
15. Chatauret N, Butterworth RF. Effects of liver failure on inter-organ trafficking of ammonia: implications for the treatment of encephalopathy. J Gastroenterol Hepatol 2004;19:S219.
16. Olde Damink SW, Deutz NE, Dejong CH, et al. Interorgan ammonia metabolism in liver failure. Neurochem Int 2002;41:177.
17. Ganda OP, Ruderman NB. Muscle nitrogen metabolism in chronic hepatic insufficiency. Metabolism 1976;25:427.
18. Desjardins P, Rao KV, Michalak A, et al. Effect of portacaval anastomosis on glutamine synthetase protein and gene expression in brain, liver and skeletal muscle. Metab Brain Dis 1999;14:273.
19. Lavoie J, Giguere JF, Layrargues GP, Butterworth RF. Activities of neuronal and astrocytic marker enzymes in autopsied brain tissue from patients with hepatic encephalopathy. Metab Brain Dis 1987;2:283.
20. Schliess F, Gorg B, Fischer R, et al. Ammonia induces MK-801-sensitive nitration and phosphorylation of protein tyrosine residues in rat astrocytes. FASEB J 2002;16:739.
21. Zwingmann C, Chatauret N, Leibfritz D, Butterworth RF. Selective increase of brain lactate synthesis in experimental acute liver failure: results of a [H-C] nuclear magnetic resonance study. Hepatology 2003;37:420.
22. Devenyi AG, Barron TF, Mamourian AC. Dystonia, hyperintense basal ganglia, and high whole blood manganese levels in Alagille's syndrome. Gastroenterology 1994;106:1068.
23. Mirowitz SA, Westrich TJ, Hirsch JD. Hyperintense basal ganglia on T1-weighted MR images in patients receiving parenteral nutrition. Radiology 1991;181:117.
24. Pomier-Layrargues G, Spahr L, Butterworth RF. Increased manganese concentrations in pallidum of cirrhotic patients. Lancet 1995;345:735.
25. Rose C, Butterworth RF, Zayed J, et al. Manganese deposition in basal ganglia structures results from both portal-systemic shunting and liver dysfunction. Gastroenterology 1999;117:640.
26. Lockwood AH, Weissenborn K, Bokemeyer M, et al. Correlations between cerebral glucose metabolism and neuropsychological test performance in nonalcoholic cirrhotics. Metab Brain Dis 2002;17:29.
27. Lockwood AH, Weissenborn K, Butterworth RF. An image of the brain in patients with liver disease. Curr Opin Neurol 1997;10:525.
28. Hindfelt B, Plum F, Duffy TE. Effect of acute ammonia intoxication on cerebral metabolism in rats with portacaval shunts. J Clin Invest 1977;59:386.
29. Yao H, Sadoshima S, Fujii K, et al. Cerebrospinal fluid lactate in patients with hepatic encephalopathy. Eur Neurol 1987;27:182.
30. Larsen FS, Gottstein J, Blei AT. Cerebral hyperemia and nitric oxide synthase in rats with ammonia-induced brain edema. J Hepatol 2001;34:548.
31. Schmidt W, Wolf G, Grungreiff K, et al. Hepatic encephalopathy influences high-affinity uptake of transmitter glutamate and aspartate into the hippocampal formation. Metab Brain Dis 1990;5:19.
32. Mena EE, Cotman CW. Pathologic concentrations of ammonium ions block L-glutamate uptake. Exp Neurol 1985;89:259.
33. Bender AS, Norenberg MD. Effects of ammonia on L-glutamate uptake in cultured astrocytes. Neurochem Res 1996;21:567.
34. Peterson C, Giguere JF, Cotman CW, Butterworth RF. Selective loss of N-methyl-D-aspartate-sensitive L-[^{3}H]glutamate binding sites in rat brain following portacaval anastomosis. J Neurochem 1990;55:386.
35. Maddison JE, Watson WE, Dodd PR, Johnston GA. Alterations in cortical [3H]kainate and alpha-[3H]amino-3-hydroxy-5-methyl-4-

isoxazolepropionic acid binding in a spontaneous canine model of chronic hepatic encephalopathy. J Neurochem 1991;56:1881.

36. Young SN, Lal S, Sourkes TL, et al. Relationships between tryptophan in serum and CSF, and 5-hydroxyindoleacetic acid in CSF of man: effect of cirrhosis of liver and probenecid administration. J Neurol Neurosurg Psychiatry 1975;38:322.

37. Huet PM, Pomier-Layrargues G, Duguay L, du Souich P. Blood-brain transport of tryptophan and phenylalanine: effect of portacaval shunt in dogs. Am J Physiol 1981;241:G163.

38. Bergeron M, Reader TA, Layrargues GP, Butterworth RF. Monoamines and metabolites in autopsied brain tissue from cirrhotic patients with hepatic encephalopathy. Neurochem Res 1989;14:853.

39. Bergeron M, Swain MS, Reader TA, et al. Effect of ammonia on brain serotonin metabolism in relation to function in the portacaval shunted rat. J Neurochem 1990;55:222.

40. Bengtsson F, Bugge M, Johansen KH, Butterworth RF. Brain tryptophan hydroxylation in the portacaval shunted rat: a hypothesis for the regulation of serotonin turnover in vivo. J Neurochem 1991; 56:1069.

41. Lozeva V, Montgomery JA, Tuomisto L, et al. Increased brain serotonin turnover correlates with the degree of shunting and hyperammonemia in rats following variable portal vein stenosis. J Hepatol 2004;40:742.

42. Mousseau DD, Baker GB, Butterworth RF. Increased density of catalytic sites and expression of brain monoamine oxidase A in humans with hepatic encephalopathy. J Neurochem 1997;68:1200.

43. Rao VL, Butterworth RF. Alterations of [3H]8-OH-DPAT and [3H]ketanserin binding sites in autopsied brain tissue from cirrhotic patients with hepatic encephalopathy. Neurosci Lett 1994;182:69.

44. Schafer DF, Jones EA. Hepatic encephalopathy and the gamma-aminobutyric-acid neurotransmitter system. Lancet 1982;1:18.

45. Butterworth RF, Giguere JF. Cerebral aminoacids in portal-systemic encephalopathy: lack of evidence for altered gamma-aminobutyric acid (GABA) function. Metab Brain Dis 1986;1:221.

46. Roy S, Pomier-Layrargues G, Butterworth RF, Huet PM. Hepatic encephalopathy in cirrhotic and portacaval shunted dogs: lack of changes in brain GABA uptake, brain GABA levels, brain glutamic acid decarboxylase activity and brain postsynaptic GABA receptors. Hepatology 1988;8:845.

47. Mans AM, Kukulka KM, McAvoy KJ, Rokosz NC. Regional distribution and kinetics of three sites on the GABAA receptor: lack of effect of portacaval shunting. J Cereb Blood Flow Metab 1992;12:334.

48. Mans AM, DeJoseph MR, Hawkins RA. Metabolic abnormalities and grade of encephalopathy in acute hepatic failure. J Neurochem 1994;63:1829.

49. Lavoie J, Giguere JF, Layrargues GP, Butterworth RF. Amino acid changes in autopsied brain tissue from cirrhotic patients with hepatic encephalopathy. J Neurochem 1987;49:692.

50. Butterworth RF, Lavoie J, Giguere JF, Pomier-Layrargues G. Affinities and densities of high-affinity [3H]muscimol (GABA-A) binding sites and of central benzodiazepine receptors are unchanged in autopsied brain tissue from cirrhotic patients with hepatic encephalopathy. Hepatology 1988;8:1084.

51. Pomier-Layrargues G, Giguere JF, Lavoie J, et al. Flumazenil in cirrhotic patients in hepatic coma: a randomized double-blind placebo-controlled crossover trial. Hepatology 1994;19:32.

52. Gyr K, Meier R, Haussler J, et al. Evaluation of the efficacy and safety of flumazenil in the treatment of portal systemic encephalopathy: a double blind, randomised, placebo controlled multicentre study. Gut 1996;39:319.

53. Mullen KD, Szauter KM, Kaminsky-Russ K. "Endogenous" benzodiazepine activity in body fluids of patients with hepatic encephalopathy. Lancet 1990;336:81.

54. Olasmaa M, Rothstein JD, Guidotti A, et al. Endogenous benzodiazepine receptor ligands in human and animal hepatic encephalopathy. J Neurochem 1990;55:2015.

55. Lavoie J, Layrargues GP, Butterworth RF. Increased densities of peripheral-type benzodiazepine receptors in brain autopsy samples from cirrhotic patients with hepatic encephalopathy. Hepatology 1990;11:874.

56. Giguere JF, Hamel E, Butterworth RF. Increased densities of binding sites for the 'peripheral-type' benzodiazepine receptor ligand [3H]PK 11195 in rat brain following portacaval anastomosis. Brain Res 1992;585:295.

57. Desjardins P, Bandeira P, Raghavendra Rao VL, et al. Increased expression of the peripheral-type benzodiazepine receptor-isoquinoline carboxamide binding protein mRNA in brain following portacaval anastomosis. Brain Res 1997;758:255.

58. Rothstein JD, McKhann G, Guarneri P, et al. Cerebrospinal fluid content of diazepam binding inhibitor in chronic hepatic encephalopathy. Ann Neurol 1989;26:57.

59. Butterworth RF, Tonon MC, Desy L, et al. Increased brain content of the endogenous benzodiazepine receptor ligand, octadecaneuropeptide (ODN), following portacaval anastomosis in the rat. Peptides 1991;12:119.

60. Shiraishi T, Black KL, Ikezaki K, Becker DP. Peripheral benzodiazepine induces morphological changes and proliferation of mitochondria in glioma cells. J Neurosci Res 1991;30:463.

61. Ahboucha S, Layrargues GP, Mamer O, Butterworth RF. Increased brain concentrations of a neuroinhibitory steroid in human hepatic encephalopathy. Ann Neurol 2005;58:169.

62. Lozeva-Thomas V, Ahonen P, Chatauret N, et al. Brain histamine in experimental acute liver failure: effects of L-histidine loading. Inflamm Res 2004;53(Suppl. 1):S55.

63. Jacobs EH, Yamatodani A, Timmerman H. Is histamine the final neurotransmitter in the entrainment of circadian rhythms in mammals? Trends Pharmacol Sci 2000;21:293.

64. Tasaka K. New Advances in Histamine Research. Tokyo: Spinger Verlag, 1994.

65. Cordoba J, Cabrera J, Lataif L, et al. High prevalence of sleep disturbance in cirrhosis. Hepatology 1998;27:339.

66. Lozeva V, Valjakka A, Lecklin A, et al. Effects of the histamine H(1) receptor blocker, pyrilamine, on spontaneous locomotor activity of rats with long-term portacaval anastomosis. Hepatology 2000;31: 336.

67. Bergeron M, Swain MS, Reader TA, Butterworth RF. Regional alterations of dopamine and its metabolites in rat brain following portacaval anastomosis. Neurochem Res 1995;20:79.

68. Mousseau DD, Perney P, Layrargues GP, Butterworth RF. Selective loss of pallidal dopamine D2 receptor density in hepatic encephalopathy. Neurosci Lett 1993;162:192.

69. Kato A, Watanabe Y, Sawara K, et al. Regional cerebral dopamine receptor binding activities in patients with liver cirrhosis: Results on positron emission tomography using [11C]-methylspiperone. Hepatology 2006;44:441A.

70. Thornton JR, Losowsky MS. Plasma methionine enkephalin concentration and prognosis in primary biliary cirrhosis. BMJ 1988;297: 1241.

71. Panerai AE, Salerno F, Baldissera F, et al. Brain beta-endorphin concentrations in experimental chronic liver disease. Brain Res 1982;247: 188.

72. de Waele JP, Audet RM, Leong DK, Butterworth RF. Portacaval anastomosis induces region-selective alterations of the endogenous opioid system in the rat brain. Hepatology 1996;24:895.

73. de Waele JP, Audet RM, Rose C, Butterworth RF. The portacaval-shunted rat: a new model for the study of the mechanisms controlling voluntary ethanol consumption and ethanol preference? Alcohol Clin Exp Res 1997;21:305.

74. Rao VL, Audet RM, Butterworth RF. Increased neuronal nitric oxide synthase expression in brain following portacaval anastomosis. Brain Res 1997;765:169.

75. Blei AT. Infection, inflammation and hepatic encephalopathy, synergism redefined. J Hepatol 2004;40:327.

76. Genesca J, Gonzalez A, Segura R, et al. Interleukin-6, nitric oxide, and the clinical and hemodynamic alterations of patients with liver cirrhosis. Am J Gastroenterol 1999;94:169.

77. Shawcross DL, Davies NA, Williams R, Jalan R. Systemic inflammatory response exacerbates the neuropsychological effects of induced hyperammonemia in cirrhosis. J Hepatol 2004;40:247.

78. Cordoba J, Lopez-Hellin J, Planas M, et al. Normal protein diet for episodic hepatic encephalopathy: results of a randomized study. J Hepatol 2004;41:38.

79. Marchesini G, Dioguardi FS, Bianchi GP, et al. Long-term oral branched-chain amino acid treatment in chronic hepatic encephalopathy. A randomized double-blind casein-controlled trial. The Italian Multicenter Study Group. J Hepatol 1990;11:92.

80. Gentile S, Guarino G, Romano M, et al. A randomized controlled trial of acarbose in hepatic encephalopathy. Clin Gastroenterol Hepatol 2005;3:184.

81. Liu Q, Duan ZP, Ha DK, et al. Symbiotic modulation of gut flora: effect on minimal hepatic encephalopathy in patients with cirrhosis. Hepatology 2004;39:1441.

82. Kircheis G, Nilius R, Held C, et al. Therapeutic efficacy of L-ornithine-L-aspartate infusions in patients with cirrhosis and hepatic encephalopathy: results of a placebo-controlled, double-blind study. Hepatology 1997;25:1351.

83. Rose C, Michalak A, Pannunzio P, et al. L-ornithine-L-aspartate in experimental portal-systemic encephalopathy: therapeutic efficacy and mechanism of action. Metab Brain Dis 1998;13:147.

84. Sushma S, Dasarathy S, Tandon RK, et al. Sodium benzoate in the treatment of acute hepatic encephalopathy: a double-blind randomized trial. Hepatology 1992;16:138.

85. Therrien G, Rose C, Butterworth J, Butterworth RF. Protective effect of L-carnitine in ammonia-precipitated encephalopathy in the portacaval shunted rat. Hepatology 1997;25:551.

86. Malaguarnera M, Pistone G, Elvira R, et al. Effects of L-carnitine in patients with hepatic encephalopathy. World J Gastroenterol 2005;11:7197.

87. Haefely WE. Allosteric modulation of the $GABA_A$ receptor channel: a mechanism for interaction with a multitude of central nervous system function. In: Möhler H, Da Prada M (eds). The Challenge of Neuropharmacology. Basel: Hoffman-La Roche, 1994:15.

88. Yurdaydin C, Gu ZQ, Nowak G, et al. Benzodiazepine receptor ligands are elevated in an animal model of hepatic encephalopathy: relationship between brain concentration and severity of encephalopathy. J Pharmacol Exp Ther 1993;265:565.

89. Bosman DK, van den Buijs CA, de Haan JG, et al. The effects of benzodiazepine-receptor antagonists and partial inverse agonists on acute hepatic encephalopathy in the rat. Gastroenterology 1991;101:772.

90. Ahboucha S, Coyne L, Hirakawa R, et al. An interaction between benzodiazepines and neuroactive steroids at GABA A receptors in cultured hippocampal neurons. Neurochem Int 2006;48:703.

91. Spahr L, Coeytaux A, Giostra E, et al. Histamine H1 blocker hydroxyzine improves sleep in patients with cirrhosis and minimal hepatic encephalopathy: a randomized controlled pilot trial. Am J Gastroenterol 2007;102:744.

92. Kjaergard LL, Liu J, Als-Nielsen B, Gluud C. Artificial and bioartificial support systems for acute and acute-on-chronic liver failure: a systematic review. JAMA 2003;289:217.

93. Heemann U, Treichel U, Loock J, et al. Albumin dialysis in cirrhosis with superimposed acute liver injury: a prospective, controlled study. Hepatology 2002;36:949.

94. Hassanein T, Tofteng F, Brown RS, Jr., et al. Randomized controlled study of extracorporeal albumin dialysis for hepatic encephalopathy in advanced cirrhosis. Hepatology 2007;46:1853.

95. Bustamante J, Rimola A, Ventura PJ, et al. Prognostic significance of hepatic encephalopathy in patients with cirrhosis. J Hepatol 1999;30:890.

96. Oppong KN, Al-Mardini H, Thick M, Record CO. Oral glutamine challenge in cirrhotics pre- and post-liver transplantation: a psychometric and analyzed EEG study. Hepatology 1997;26:870.

97. Cordoba J, Alonso J, Rovira A, et al. The development of low-grade cerebral edema in cirrhosis is supported by the evolution of (1)H-magnetic resonance abnormalities after liver transplantation. J Hepatol 2001;35:598.

98. Dam M, Burra P, Tedeschi U, et al. Regional cerebral blood flow changes in patients with cirrhosis assessed with 99mTc-HM-PAO single-photon emission computed tomography: effect of liver transplantation. J Hepatol 1998;29:78.

99. Burra P, Dam M, Chierichetti F, et al. 18F-fluorodeoxyglucose positron emission tomography study of brain metabolism in cirrhosis: effect of liver transplantation. Transplant Proc 1999;31:418.

100. Cordoba J, Sanpedro F, Alonso J, Rovira A. 1H magnetic resonance in the study of hepatic encephalopathy in humans. Metab Brain Dis 2002;17:415.

101. Pujol A, Graus F, Rimola A, et al. Predictive factors of in-hospital CNS complications following liver transplantation. Neurology 1994;44:1226.

102. Blanco R, De Girolami U, Jenkins RL, Khettry U. Neuropathology of liver transplantation. Clin Neuropathol 1995;14:109.

103. Mueller AR, Platz KP, Bechstein WO, et al. Neurotoxicity after orthotopic liver transplantation. A comparison between cyclosporine and FK506. Transplantation 1994;58:155.

104. Butterworth RF. Pathophysiology of alcoholic brain damage: synergistic effects of ethanol, thiamine deficiency and alcoholic liver disease. Metab Brain Dis 1995;10:1.

105. Forton DM, Allsop JM, Main J, et al. Evidence for a cerebral effect of the hepatitis C virus. Lancet 2001;358:38.

106. Fluckiger M. Vorkommen von trommelschagel formigen fingerendphalangen ohne chronische veranderungen an der lungen oder am herzen. Wien Klin Wochenschr 1884;34:1457.

107. Rodriguez-Roisin R, Agusti AG, Roca J. The hepatopulmonary syndrome: new name, old complexities. Thorax 1992;47:897.

108. Kennedy TC, Knudson RJ. Exercise-aggravated hypoxemia and orthodeoxia in cirrhosis. Chest 1977;72:305.

109. Rodriguez-Roisin R, Krowka MJ, Herve P, Fallon MB. Pulmonary-hepatic vascular disorders (PHD). Eur Respir J 2004;24:861.

110. Palma DT, Fallon MB. The hepatopulmonary syndrome. J Hepatol 2006;45:617.

111. Martinez GP, Barbera JA, Visa J, et al. Hepatopulmonary syndrome in candidates for liver transplantation. J Hepatol 2001;34:651.

112. Schenk P, Fuhrmann V, Madl C, et al. Hepatopulmonary syndrome: prevalence and predictive value of various cut offs for arterial oxygenation and their clinical consequences. Gut 2002;51:853.

113. Abrams GA, Sanders MK, Fallon MB. Utility of pulse oximetry in the detection of arterial hypoxemia in liver transplant candidates. Liver Transpl 2002;8:391.

114. Arguedas MR, Drake BB, Kapoor A, Fallon MB. Carboxyhemoglobin levels in cirrhotic patients with and without hepatopulmonary syndrome. Gastroenterology 2005;128:328.

115. Schenk P, Schoniger-Hekele M, Fuhrmann V, et al. Prognostic significance of the hepatopulmonary syndrome in patients with cirrhosis. Gastroenterology 2003;125:1042.

116. Abrams GA, Jaffe CC, Hoffer PB, et al. Diagnostic utility of contrast echocardiography and lung perfusion scan in patients with hepatopulmonary syndrome. Gastroenterology 1995;109:1283.

117. Rolla G, Brussino L, Colagrande P, et al. Exhaled nitric oxide and oxygenation abnormalities in hepatic cirrhosis. Hepatology 1997;26:842.

118. Aller R, Moya JL, Moreira V, et al. Diagnosis of hepatopulmonary syndrome with contrast transesophageal echocardiography: advantages over contrast transthoracic echocardiography. Dig Dis Sci 1999;44:1243.

119. Aller R, Moya JL, Moreira V, et al. Diagnosis and grading of intrapulmonary vascular dilatation in cirrhotic patients with contrast transesophageal echocardiography. J Hepatol 1999;31:1044.

120. Gupta D, Vijaya DR, Gupta R, et al. Prevalence of hepatopulmonary syndrome in cirrhosis and extrahepatic portal venous obstruction. Am J Gastroenterol 2001;96:3395.

121. Fuhrmann V, Madl C, Mueller C, et al. Hepatopulmonary syndrome in patients with hypoxic hepatitis. Gastroenterology 2006;131:69.

122. Williams A, Trewby P, Williams R, Reid L. Structural alterations to the pulmonary circulation in fulminant hepatic failure. Thorax 1979;34:447.

123. Saunders KB, Fernando SS, Dalton HR, Joseph A. Spontaneous improvement in a patient with the hepatopulmonary syndrome assessed by serial exercise tests. Thorax 1994;49:725.

124. Krowka MJ, Dickson ER, Cortese DA. Hepatopulmonary syndrome. Clinical observations and lack of therapeutic response to somatostatin analogue. Chest 1993;104:515.

125. Swanson KL, Wiesner RH, Krowka MJ. Natural history of hepatopulmonary syndrome: Impact of liver transplantation. Hepatology 2005;41:1122.

126. Hoffbauer FW, Rydell R. Multiple pulmonary arteriovenous fistulas in juvenile cirrhosis. Am J Med 1956;21:450.

127. Berthelot P, Walker JG, Sherlock S, Reid L. Arterial changes in the lungs in cirrhosis of the liver – lung spider nevi. N Engl J Med 1966;274:291.

128. Stanley NN, Williams AJ, Dewar CA, et al. Hypoxia and hydrothoraces in a case of liver cirrhosis: correlation of physiological, radiographic, scintigraphic, and pathological findings. Thorax 1977;32:457.

129. Davis HH, 2nd, Schwartz DJ, Lefrak SS, et al. Alveolar-capillary oxygen disequilibrium in hepatic cirrhosis. Chest 1978;73:507.

130. Hales MR. Multiple small arteriovenous fistulae of the lungs. Am J Pathol 1956;32:927.

131. Calabresi P, Abelmann WH. Porto-caval and porto-pulmonary anastomoses in Laennec's cirrhosis and in heart failure. J Clin Invest 1957;36:1257.

132. Massumi RA, Rios JC, Ticktin HE. Hemodynamic abnormalities and venous admixture in portal cirrhosis. Am J Med Sci 1965;250:275.

133. Agusti AG, Roca J, Rodriguez-Roisin R. Mechanisms of gas exchange impairment in patients with liver cirrhosis. Clin Chest Med 1996;17:49.

134. Rodriguez-Roisin R, Barbera JA. Hepatopulmonary syndrome: is NO the right answer? Gastroenterology 1997;113:682.

135. Rodriguez-Roisin R, Roca J, Agusti AG, et al. Gas exchange and pulmonary vascular reactivity in patients with liver cirrhosis. Am Rev Respir Dis 1987;135:1085.

136. Melot C, Naeije R, Dechamps P, et al. Pulmonary and extrapulmonary contributors to hypoxemia in liver cirrhosis. Am Rev Respir Dis 1989;139:632.

137. Hourani JM, Bellamy PE, Tashkin DP, et al. Pulmonary dysfunction in advanced liver disease: frequent occurrence of an abnormal diffusing capacity. Am J Med 1991;90:693.

138. Mohamed R, Freeman JW, Guest PJ, et al. Pulmonary gas exchange abnormalities in liver transplant candidates. Liver Transpl 2002;8:802.

139. Krowka MJ, Dickson ER, Wiesner RH, et al. A prospective study of pulmonary function and gas exchange following liver transplantation. Chest 1992;102:1161.

140. Abrams GA, Nanda NC, Dubovsky EV, et al. Use of macroaggregated albumin lung perfusion scan to diagnose hepatopulmonary syndrome: a new approach. Gastroenterology 1998;114:305.

141. Krowka MJ, Cortese DA. Hepatopulmonary syndrome: an evolving perspective in the era of liver transplantation. Hepatology 1990;11:138.

142. Krowka MJ. Caveats concerning hepatopulmonary syndrome. J Hepatol 2001;34:756.

143. Poterucha JJ, Krowka MJ, Dickson ER, et al. Failure of hepatopulmonary syndrome to resolve after liver transplantation and successful treatment with embolotherapy. Hepatology 1995;21:96.

144. Katsuta Y, Honma H, Zhang XJ, et al. Pulmonary blood transit time and impaired arterial oxygenation in patients with chronic liver disease. J Gastroenterol 2005;40:57.

145. Srivastava D, Preminger T, Lock JE, et al. Hepatic venous blood and the development of pulmonary arteriovenous malformations in congenital heart disease. Circulation 1995;92:1217.

146. Fallon MB. Hepatopulmonary syndrome: more than just a matter of tone? Hepatology 2006;43:912.

147. Chang SW, Ohara N. Pulmonary circulatory dysfunction in rats with biliary cirrhosis. An animal model of the hepatopulmonary syndrome. Am Rev Respir Dis 1992;145:798.

148. Fallon MB, Abrams GA, McGrath JW, et al. Common bile duct ligation in the rat: a model of intrapulmonary vasodilatation and hepatopulmonary syndrome. Am J Physiol 1997;272:G779.

149. Luo B, Liu L, Tang L, et al. ET-1 and TNF-alpha in HPS: analysis in prehepatic portal hypertension and biliary and nonbiliary cirrhosis in rats. Am J Physiol Gastrointest Liver Physiol 2004;286:G294.

150. Fallon MB. Mechanisms of pulmonary vascular complications of liver disease: hepatopulmonary syndrome. J Clin Gastroenterol 2005;39:S138.

151. Rolla G. Is nitric oxide the ultimate mediator in hepatopulmonary syndrome? J Hepatol 2003;38:668.

152. Rolla G, Bucca C, Brussino L. Methylene blue in the hepatopulmonary syndrome. N Engl J Med 1994;331:1098.

153. Schenk P, Madl C, Rezaie-Majd S, et al. Methylene blue improves the hepatopulmonary syndrome. Ann Intern Med 2000;133:701.

154. Brussino L, Bucca C, Morello M, et al. Effect on dyspnoea and hypoxaemia of inhaled N(G)-nitro-L-arginine methyl ester in hepatopulmonary syndrome. Lancet 2003;362:43.

155. Zhang XJ, Katsuta Y, Akimoto T, et al. Intrapulmonary vascular dilatation and nitric oxide in hypoxemic rats with chronic bile duct ligation. J Hepatol 2003;39:724.

156. Nunes H, Lebrec D, Mazmanian M, et al. Role of nitric oxide in hepatopulmonary syndrome in cirrhotic rats. Am J Respir Crit Care Med 2001;164:879.

157. Fallon MB, Abrams GA, Luo B, et al. The role of endothelial nitric oxide synthase in the pathogenesis of a rat model of hepatopulmonary syndrome. Gastroenterology 1997;113:606.

158. Zhang J, Ling Y, Luo B, et al. Analysis of pulmonary heme oxygenase-1 and nitric oxide synthase alterations in experimental hepatopulmonary syndrome. Gastroenterology 2003;125:1441.

159. Ling Y, Zhang J, Luo B, et al. The role of endothelin-1 and the endothelin B receptor in the pathogenesis of hepatopulmonary syndrome in the rat. Hepatology 2004;39:1593.

160. Rabiller A, Nunes H, Lebrec D, et al. Prevention of gram-negative translocation reduces the severity of hepatopulmonary syndrome. Am J Respir Crit Care Med 2002;166:514.

161. Carter EP, Hartsfield CL, Miyazono M, et al. Regulation of heme oxygenase-1 by nitric oxide during hepatopulmonary syndrome. Am J Physiol Lung Cell Mol Physiol 2002;283:L346.

162. Sztrymf B, Libert JM, Mougeot C, et al. Cirrhotic rats with bacterial translocation have higher incidence and severity of hepatopulmonary syndrome. J Gastroenterol Hepatol 2005;20:1538.

163. Sztrymf B, Rabiller A, Nunes H, et al. Prevention of hepatopulmonary syndrome and hyperdynamic state by pentoxifylline in cirrhotic rats. Eur Respir J 2004;23:752.

164. Fallon MB, Abrams GA. Pulmonary dysfunction in chronic liver disease. Hepatology 2000;32:859.

165. Gomez FP, Martinez-Palli G, Barbera JA, et al. Gas exchange mechanism of orthodeoxia in hepatopulmonary syndrome. Hepatology 2004;40:660.

166. Martinez G, Barbera JA, Navasa M, et al. Hepatopulmonary syndrome associated with cardiorespiratory disease. J Hepatol 1999;30:882.

167. Krowka MJ, Wiseman GA, Burnett OL, et al. Hepatopulmonary syndrome: a prospective study of relationships between severity of liver disease, PaO(2) response to 100% oxygen, and brain uptake after (99m)Tc MAA lung scanning. Chest 2000;118:615.

168. Krowka MJ. Hepatopulmonary syndrome: what are we learning from interventional radiology, liver transplantation, and other disorders? Gastroenterology 1995;109:1009.

169. Koksal D, Kacar S, Koksal AS, et al. Evaluation of intrapulmonary vascular dilatations with high-resolution computed thorax tomography in patients with hepatopulmonary syndrome. J Clin Gastroenterol 2006;40:77.

170. Lee KN, Lee HJ, Shin WW, Webb WR. Hypoxemia and liver cirrhosis (hepatopulmonary syndrome) in eight patients: comparison of the central and peripheral pulmonary vasculature. Radiology 1999;211: 549.

171. Fallon MB, Mulligan DC, Gish RG, Krowka MJ. Model for end-stage liver disease (MELD) exception for hepatopulmonary syndrome. Liver Transpl 2006;12(Suppl. 3):S105.

172. Arguedas MR, Abrams GA, Krowka MJ, Fallon MB. Prospective evaluation of outcomes and predictors of mortality in patients with hepatopulmonary syndrome undergoing liver transplantation. Hepatology 2003;37:192.

173. Roberts DN, Arguedas MR, Fallon MB. Cost-effectiveness of screening for hepatopulmonary syndrome in liver transplant candidates. Liver Transpl 2007;13:206.

174. Corpechot C, Barbu V, Wendum D, et al. Hypoxia-induced VEGF and collagen I expressions are associated with angiogenesis and fibrogenesis in experimental cirrhosis. Hepatology 2002;35:1010.

175. Fukushima KY, Yatsuhashi H, Kinoshita A, et al. Two cases of hepatopulmonary syndrome with improved liver function following long-term oxygen therapy. J Gastroenterol 2007;42:176.

176. Gomez FP, Barbera JA, Roca J, et al. Effects of nebulized N(G)-nitro-L-arginine methyl ester in patients with hepatopulmonary syndrome. Hepatology 2006;43:1084.

177. Almeida JA, Riordan SM, Liu J, et al. Deleterious effect of nitric oxide inhibition in chronic hepatopulmonary syndrome. Eur J Gastroenterol Hepatol 2007;19:341.

178. Abrams GA, Fallon MB. Treatment of hepatopulmonary syndrome with Allium sativum L. (garlic): a pilot trial. J Clin Gastroenterol 1998;27:232.

179. Akyuz F, Kaymakoglu S, Demir K, et al. Is there any medical therapeutic option in hepatopulmonary syndrome? A case report. Eur J Intern Med 2005;16:126.

180. Caldwell SH, Jeffers LJ, Narula OS, et al. Ancient remedies revisited: does Allium sativum (garlic) palliate the hepatopulmonary syndrome? J Clin Gastroenterol 1992;15:248.

181. Chan CC, Wu HC, Wu CH, Hsu CY. Hepatopulmonary syndrome in liver cirrhosis: report of a case. J Formos Med Assoc 1995;94:185.

182. Najafi Sani M, Kianifar HR, Kianee A, Khatami G. Effect of oral garlic on arterial oxygen pressure in children with hepatopulmonary syndrome. World J Gastroenterol 2006;12:2427.

183. Krowka MJ, Porayko MK, Plevak DJ, et al. Hepatopulmonary syndrome with progressive hypoxemia as an indication for liver transplantation: case reports and literature review. Mayo Clin Proc 1997;72:44.

184. Abrams GA, Rose K, Fallon MB, et al. Hepatopulmonary syndrome and venous emboli causing intracerebral hemorrhages after liver transplantation: a case report. Transplantation 1999;68:1809.

185. Martinez-Palli G, Barbera JA, Taura P, et al. Severe portopulmonary hypertension after liver transplantation in a patient with preexisting hepatopulmonary syndrome. J Hepatol 1999;31:1075.

186. Mantz FA, Jr., Craige E. Portal axis thrombosis with spontaneous portacaval shunt and resultant cor pulmonale. AMA Arch Pathol 1951;52:91.

187. Golbin JM, Krowka MJ. Portopulmonary hypertension. Clin Chest Med 2007;28:203.

188. Budhiraja R, Hassoun PM. Portopulmonary hypertension: a tale of two circulations. Chest 2003;123:562.

189. Hadengue A, Benhayoun MK, Lebrec D, Benhamou JP. Pulmonary hypertension complicating portal hypertension: prevalence and relation to splanchnic hemodynamics. Gastroenterology 1991;100: 520.

190. McDonnell PJ, Toye PA, Hutchins GM. Primary pulmonary hypertension and cirrhosis: are they related? Am Rev Respir Dis 1983;127: 437.

191. Colle IO, Moreau R, Godinho E, et al. Diagnosis of portopulmonary hypertension in candidates for liver transplantation: a prospective study. Hepatology 2003;37:401.

192. Krowka MJ, Swanson KL, Frantz RP, et al. Portopulmonary hypertension: Results from a 10-year screening algorithm. Hepatology 2006;44:1502.

193. Benjaminov FS, Prentice M, Sniderman KW, et al. Portopulmonary hypertension in decompensated cirrhosis with refractory ascites. Gut 2003;52:1355.

194. Krowka MJ. Portopulmonary hypertension and the issue of survival. Liver Transpl 2005;11:1026.

195. Robalino BD, Moodie DS. Association between primary pulmonary hypertension and portal hypertension: analysis of its pathophysiology and clinical, laboratory and hemodynamic manifestations. J Am Coll Cardiol 1991;17:492.

196. Kawut SM, Taichman DB, Ahya VN, et al. Hemodynamics and survival of patients with portopulmonary hypertension. Liver Transpl 2005;11:1107.

197. Herve P, Lebrec D, Brenot F, et al. Pulmonary vascular disorders in portal hypertension. Eur Respir J 1998;11:1153.

198. Swanson KL, Wiesner RH, Krowka M. Survival in portopulmonary hypertension and orthotopic liver transplantation. Liver Transpl 2005;11:c71.

199. Nagaya N, Nishikimi T, Uematsu M, et al. Plasma brain natriuretic peptide as a prognostic indicator in patients with primary pulmonary hypertension. Circulation 2000;102:865.

200. Schraufnagel DE, Kay JM. Structural and pathologic changes in the lung vasculature in chronic liver disease. Clin Chest Med 1996;17:1.

201. McLaughlin VV, McGoon MD. Pulmonary arterial hypertension. Circulation 2006;114:1417.

202. Tuder RM, Cool CD, Geraci MW, et al. Prostacyclin synthase expression is decreased in lungs from patients with severe pulmonary hypertension. Am J Respir Crit Care Med 1999;159:1925.

203. Swanson KL, Krowka MJ. Arterial oxygenation associated with portopulmonary hypertension. Chest 2002;121:1869.

204. Sakuma M, Souma S, Kitamukai O, et al. Portopulmonary hypertension: hemodynamics, pulmonary angiography, and configuration of the heart. Circ J 2005;69:1386.

205. Krowka MJ. Evolving dilemmas and management of portopulmonary hypertension. Semin Liver Dis 2006;26:265.

206. Passarella M, Fallon MB, Kawut SM. Portopulmonary hypertension. Clin Liver Dis 2006;10:653.

207. Cotton CL, Gandhi S, Vaitkus PT, et al. Role of echocardiography in detecting portopulmonary hypertension in liver transplant candidates. Liver Transpl 2002;8:1051.

208. Torregrosa M, Genesca J, Gonzalez A, et al. Role of Doppler echocardiography in the assessment of portopulmonary hypertension in liver transplantation candidates. Transplantation 2001;71:572.

209. Krowka MJ, Frantz RP, McGoon MD, et al. Improvement in pulmonary hemodynamics during intravenous epoprostenol (prostacyclin): A study of 15 patients with moderate to severe portopulmonary hypertension. Hepatology 1999;30:641.

210. Sitbon O, Brenot F, Denjean A, et al. Inhaled nitric oxide as a screening vasodilator agent in primary pulmonary hypertension. A dose-response study and comparison with prostacyclin. Am J Respir Crit Care Med 1995;151:384.

211. Blaise G, Langleben D, Hubert B. Pulmonary arterial hypertension: pathophysiology and anesthetic approach. Anesthesiology 2003;99: 1415.

212. Provencher S, Herve P, Jais X, et al. Deleterious effects of beta-blockers on exercise capacity and hemodynamics in patients with portopulmonary hypertension. Gastroenterology 2006;130:120.

213. Ota K, Shijo H, Kokawa H, et al. Effects of nifedipine on hepatic venous pressure gradient and portal vein blood flow in patients with cirrhosis. J Gastroenterol Hepatol 1995;10:198.

214. Kuo PC, Johnson LB, Plotkin JS, et al. Continuous intravenous infusion of epoprostenol for the treatment of portopulmonary hypertension. Transplantation 1997;63:604.

215. McLaughlin VV, Genthner DE, Panella MM, et al. Compassionate use of continuous prostacyclin in the management of secondary pulmonary hypertension: a case series. Ann Intern Med 1999;130: 740.

216. Sussman N, Kaza V, Barshes N, et al. Successful liver transplantation following medical management of portopulmonary hypertension: a single-center series. Am J Transplant 2006;6:2177.

217. Ashfaq M, Chinnakotla S, Rogers L, et al. The impact of treatment of portopulmonary hypertension on survival following liver transplantation. Am J Transplant 2007;7:1258.

218. Findlay JY, Plevak DJ, Krowka MJ, et al. Progressive splenomegaly after epoprostenol therapy in portopulmonary hypertension. Liver Transpl Surg 1999;5:362.

219. Minder S, Fischler M, Muellhaupt B, et al. Intravenous iloprost bridging to orthotopic liver transplantation in portopulmonary hypertension. Eur Respir J 2004;24:703.

220. Halank M, Marx C, Miehlke S, Hoeffken G. Use of aerosolized inhaled iloprost in the treatment of portopulmonary hypertension. J Gastroenterol 2004;39:1222.

221. Kuntzen C, Gulberg V, Gerbes AL. Use of a mixed endothelin receptor antagonist in portopulmonary hypertension: a safe and effective therapy? Gastroenterology 2005;128:164.

222. Hoeper MM, Halank M, Marx C, et al. Bosentan therapy for portopulmonary hypertension. Eur Respir J 2005;25:502.

223. Stahler G, von Hunnius P. Successful treatment of portopulmonary hypertension with bosentan: case report. Eur J Clin Invest 2006; 36(Suppl. 3):62.

224. Callejas Rubio JL, Salmeron Escobar J, Gonzalez-Calvin J, Ortego Centeno N. Successful treatment of severe portopulmonary hypertension in a patient with Child C cirrhosis by sildenafil. Liver Transpl 2006;12:690.

225. Chua R, Keogh A, Miyashita M. Novel use of sildenafil in the treatment of portopulmonary hypertension. J Heart Lung Transplant 2005;24:498.

226. Makisalo H, Koivusalo A, Vakkuri A, Hockerstedt K. Sildenafil for portopulmonary hypertension in a patient undergoing liver transplantation. Liver Transpl 2004;10:945.

227. Reichenberger F, Voswinckel R, Steveling E, et al. Sildenafil treatment for portopulmonary hypertension. Eur Respir J 2006;28:563.

228. Wang YW, Lin HC, Yang YY, et al. Sildenafil decreased pulmonary arterial pressure but may have exacerbated portal hypertension in a patient with cirrhosis and portopulmonary hypertension. J Gastroenterol 2006;41:593.

229. Finley DS, Lugo B, Ridgway J, et al. Fatal variceal rupture after sildenafil use: report of a case. Curr Surg 2005;62:55.

230. Ribas J, Angrill J, Barbera JA, et al. Isosorbide-5-mononitrate in the treatment of pulmonary hypertension associated with portal hypertension. Eur Respir J 1999;13:210.

231. Findlay JY, Harrison BA, Plevak DJ, Krowka MJ. Inhaled nitric oxide reduces pulmonary artery pressures in portopulmonary hypertension. Liver Transpl Surg 1999;5:381.

232. Krowka MJ, Mandell MS, Ramsay MA, et al. Hepatopulmonary syndrome and portopulmonary hypertension: a report of the multicenter liver transplant database. Liver Transpl 2004;10:174.

233. Krowka MJ, Plevak DJ, Findlay JY, et al. Pulmonary hemodynamics and perioperative cardiopulmonary-related mortality in patients with portopulmonary hypertension undergoing liver transplantation. Liver Transpl 2000;6:443.

234. Saner FH, Nadalin S, Pavlakovic G, et al. Portopulmonary hypertension in the early phase following liver transplantation. Transplantation 2006;82:887.

235. Csete M. Intraoperative management of liver transplant patients with pulmonary hypertension. Liver Transpl Surg 1997;3:454.

236. Kuo PC, Plotkin JS, Gaine S, et al. Portopulmonary hypertension and the liver transplant candidate. Transplantation 1999;67:1087.

237. Pirenne J, Verleden G, Nevens F, et al. Combined liver and (heart-)lung transplantation in liver transplant candidates with refractory portopulmonary hypertension. Transplantation 2002;73:140.

238. Riordan SM, Williams R. Treatment of hepatic encephalopathy. N Engl J Med 1997;337:473.

Definitions, 492
Incidence and demographics, 493
Etiology, 495
Clinical presentation and complications, 501
Prognosis in acute liver failure, 503
Management of acute liver failure, 505
Liver transplantation, 509
Investigational surgical approaches, 509
Artificial and bioartificial liver devices, 510

Acute liver failure (ALF), or fulminant hepatic failure, is a potentially life-threatening illness that is notoriously unpredictable and difficult to manage [1]. Clinically, ALF is defined by a rapid deterioration in hepatic function with progressive encephalopathy and coagulopathy developing within 26 weeks of symptom onset in an individual without preexisting liver disease [2,3]. Infectious, hemodynamic, and neurological complications may rapidly evolve into multisystem organ failure and death within a few days. Acute liver failure is a rare disease in the general population but can arise from a multitude of etiologies that vary substantially in their relative incidence and their likelihood for spontaneous recovery [4,5]. In the United States, the estimated annual incidence of ALF is 2300–2800 cases per year, with acetaminophen (paracetamol) hepatotoxicity and idiosyncratic drug reactions most commonly identified [3,6,7]. Optimal care of ALF patients requires a rapid assessment for treatable etiologies (Table 25.1) and coordinated intensive care provided by an experienced team of gastroenterology/hepatology specialists, intensivists, and transplant surgeons [1]. Although outcomes

with emergency liver transplantation continue to improve, less than 10% of patients with ALF are transplanted annually [6,7]. The aim of this chapter is to provide an organized approach to the diagnosis, treatment, and management of adult patients with ALF.

Definitions

Acute liver failure is defined as the rapid deterioration of hepatic function resulting in altered mentation and coagulopathy in an individual without preexisting liver disease [2,3]. Amongst infants and children it can be difficult to determine the presence and severity of encephalopathy, and alternative diagnostic criteria for ALF have been proposed [8]. Given the variation in symptom duration amongst adults, subcategories of ALF have been proposed, including: hyperacute liver failure (e.g., < 7 days from illness onset to ALF); acute liver failure (e.g., ALF onset within 7–21 days); and subacute liver failure (e.g., ALF developing 3–26 weeks after symptom onset) [9]. Although duration of illness has been regarded as an independent predictor of outcome, analyses suggest that the etiology of ALF may be a more important predictor of outcome [3,7,9]. This chapter will refer to ALF patients as those presenting with new-onset coagulopathy and encephalopathy within 26 weeks of symptom onset.

Principles of Clinical Gastroenterology. Edited by Tadataka Yamada, David H. Alpers, Anthony N. Kalloo, Neil Kaplowitz, Chung Owyang, and Don W. Powell. © 2008 Blackwell Publishing. ISBN 978-1-4051-69103

Table 25.1 Treatable causes of acute liver failure

	Etiology	Evaluation	Treatment
Viruses	Hepatitis B (HBV)	HBsAg, anti-HBc IgM, HBV-DNA by PCR	Lamivudine, entecavir
	Hepatitis D (HDV)	HDV-RNA, anti-HDV IgM, HDV antigen	Lamivudine, entecavir
	Cytomegalovirus (CMV)	CMV-DNA PCR, CMV-IgM, biopsy	Ganciclovir, valganciclovir
	Epstein–Barr virus (EBV)	EBV-DNA PCR, serology, biopsy	Steroids, acyclovir
	Herpes simplex virus (HSV)	HSV-DNA PCR, anti-HSV IgM, biopsy	Acyclovir
Metabolic	Wilson disease	Ceruloplasmin, urinary and hepatic copper, slit-lamp examination	Chelating agents ?Plasmapheresis
	Acute fatty liver of pregnancy, HELLP syndrome	Preeclampsia findings (hypertension, edema, proteinuria)	Emergency delivery of infant
	Ischemic hepatitis	Systemic hypotension (cardiogenic shock, pulmonary embolism, hypovolemia)	Reversal of hypotension, inotropes
	Autoimmune hepatitis	ANA, ASMA, IgG, IgM, IgA Liver biopsy	Steroids
Infiltrative	Metastatic malignancy	Imaging, liver biopsy	Chemotherapy
	Acute leukemia/lymphoma	Bone marrow aspiration, liver biopsy	Chemotherapy
Toxins	Acetaminophen toxicity	Medication history, serum APAP level ?APAP–cysteine adducts	N-acetylcysteine
	Idiosyncratic drug reaction	Temporal relationship	Withdraw suspect medication
	Amanita poisoning	Recent mushroom ingestion, severe gastrointestinal symptoms	Gastric lavage, charcoal, penicillin G, silymarin, hemodialysis
Other	Budd–Chiari syndrome	Liver ultrasound with Doppler, angiogram	Heparin, low-molecular-weight heparin

ANA, antinuclear antibody; APAP, acetaminophen; ASMA, anti-smooth muscle antibody; HBc, hepatitis B core antigen; HBsAg, hepatitis B surface antigen; HELLP, hemolysis, elevated liver enzymes, and low platelet count; PCR, polymerase chain reaction.

Incidence and demographics

Acute liver failure can develop in patients of all ages but the dominant etiologies differ markedly in adults compared with infants and children [7,8]. Multiple studies have demonstrated an unexplained predominance of adult females with ALF in nearly all etiological subgroups [7,10–13]. The estimated annual incidence of ALF varies from 1 per 10 000 in developing nations to 1 per 100 000 in Western countries [4,14]. In the United States there are an estimated 2300–2800 cases of ALF each year but prospective population-based studies to provide a more precise estimate of ALF incidence are not available [15]. In addition, retrospective studies of medical record databases are problematic because of the lack of specific ICD-9 (International Classification of Diseases, ninth revision) codes for ALF. The etiology of ALF varies worldwide, with acute hepatitis B virus (HBV) and hepatitis E virus (HEV) infection dominating in tropical and Asian countries, whereas drug-induced ALF is more commonly identified in Europe and the United States (Table 25.2) [7,14,16–18]. Patient outcomes also differ substantially throughout the

world, presumably because of the variable availability of intensive care unit (ICU) care and access to emergency liver transplantation.

The US Acute Liver Failure Study Group (ALFSG) has been prospectively tracking the etiology and outcome of adults with ALF at 23 participating centers since 1998. Analysis revealed that 73% of 838 ALF patients were women and their median age was 38 years (Table 25.3). Acetaminophen toxicity was the single most common cause of ALF, identified in 39% of the population (Fig. 25.1), and 48% of these patients reported unintentional acetaminophen overdose. Idiosyncratic drug reactions resulting from a multitude of prescription medications and herbal products were the second most common etiology (13%), with hepatitis B (7%), hepatitis A (3%), and ischemic hepatitis (4%) identified in fewer subjects. Indeterminate ALF, defined by the absence of an identifiable etiology, was noted in 17%. Overall survival was 67% at 3 weeks, with a 44% spontaneous recovery rate and 26% of the patients requiring emergency liver transplantation (Fig. 25.2). The mean time to transplantation was 2.5 days (range: 0–19 days) and 22% of the listed patients died while awaiting transplantation.

Table 25.2 Etiologies of acute liver failure in different parts of the world

	UK 1987–93	US 1998–2001	France 1986	India 1992–98	Japan 1998	Korea 1999–2004
n	941	308	330	458	93	114
% HBV/HDV	9	7	47	11	44	16
% HAV	9	4	4	4	4	4
% HEV	0	0	0	29	0	0
% Drugs[a]	60	52	17	5	0	32
% Indeterminate	17	17	22	47	41	33
% Other	5	20	10	4	11	15

a Drugs include acetaminophen and idiosyncratic drug toxicity.

HAV, hepatitis A virus; HBV, hepatitis B virus; HDV, hepatitis D virus; HEV, hepatitis E virus.

Data adapted from refs 43, 7, 126, 14, 52, and 219, respectively.

Table 25.3 Clinical features of 838 consecutive US adults with acute liver failure, 1998–2005

	APAP n = 374	Drug n = 99	Indeterminate n = 121	HAV n = 29	HBV n = 62	Others n = 153
Mean age (years)	36	40	38	48	41	41
% Female	74	68	56	48	50	76
Jaundice (days)	0	8.0	6.0	3.0	5.5	5.0
Median serum ALT (IU/L)	4200	571	899	2622	1500	649
Median bilirubin (mg/dL)	4.6	21.9	22.8	11.8	20.2	16.6
Outcomes at 3 weeks:						
Transplant (%)	9	45	41	31	47	35
Spontaneous survival (%)	63	22	26	55	26	31
Overall survival (%)	71	64	64	83	65	61

ALT, alanine aminotransferase; APAP, acetaminophen; HAV, hepatitis A virus; HBV, hepatitis B virus.

Data provided by Dr W.M. Lee, and the US Acute Liver Failure Study Group, December 2005.

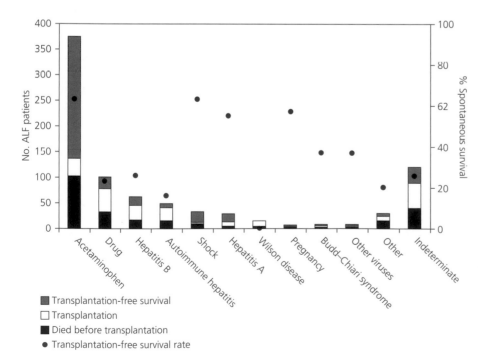

■ Transplantation-free survival
□ Transplantation
■ Died before transplantation
● Transplantation-free survival rate

Figure 25.1 Etiology and outcome in 838 consecutive adult acute liver failure (ALF) patients in the United States. Adult ALF patients were prospectively enrolled at 23 sites comprising the Acute Liver Failure Study Group from January 1998 through September 2005. Patients with acetaminophen overdose and severe acute hepatitis A virus (HAV) infection had the highest transplant-free survival rates of 63% and 55%, respectively, whereas subjects with idiosyncratic drug toxicity and indeterminate ALF had low spontaneous survival rates of 23% and 26%, respectively (W.M. Lee, personal communication, December 2005).

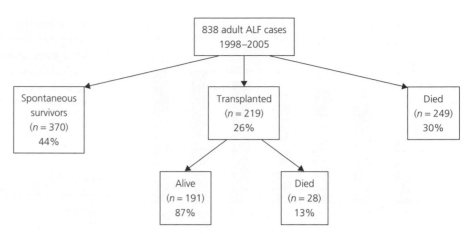

Figure 25.2 Overall outcome of 838 adult acute liver failure (ALF) patients enrolled in the US Acute Liver Failure Study Group (ALFSG). Overall patient survival was 67%, with 44% of the patients recovering with general supportive care and 26% undergoing emergency liver transplantation. Despite rapid listing and supportive care, 22% of the transplant candidates died pretransplant and the survival of the transplant recipients was 87% at 3 weeks of follow-up. The mean time from listing to transplantation was 2.5 days (range: 0–19 days) (W.M. Lee, personal communication, December 2005).

Etiology

Acetaminophen hepatotoxicity
Epidemiology and risk factors

Acetaminophen overdose is the most commonly identified cause of ALF in Western countries [7,16]. The frequency of acetaminophen-induced ALF in the United States appears to be increasing when compared with historical series (Table 25.4) [10,12,19,20]. This may, in part, be due to the prospective nature of the ALFSG study, with inclusion of nontransplant patients, compared with previous retrospective studies. In addition, the incidence of acetaminophen hepatotoxicity appears to be increasing within the US over the past 7 years [19] (Fig. 25.3). The rising incidence of acetaminophen-induced ALF, with a large proportion of unintentional overdose cases may, in part, relate to a shift from aspirin- to acetaminophen-based products for acute febrile illnesses in children and adults because of concerns about Reye syndrome.

Acetaminophen is a known direct hepatotoxin that can lead to severe acute hepatocellular liver injury in a dose-dependent manner. Acetaminophen hepatotoxicity occurs when high levels of the reactive intermediate metabolite, NAPQI (*N*-acetyl-*p*-benzoquinone imine), are formed by cytochrome P450-mediated oxidative metabolism [21]. When production of NAPQI exceeds detoxification capacity, hepatocyte damage can occur with binding of NAPQI to intracellular proteins. Chronic alcohol consumption, which induces CYP2E1 enzyme activity, may result in more NAPQI generation and also lead to hepatic glutathione depletion [22,23]. In addition, ingestion of other cytochrome P450 inducers, such as dilantin and isoniazid, have been implicated in lowering the threshold for acetaminophen hepatotoxicity [24]. Short-term fasting and poor nutritional status have also been implicated as clinical cofactors in patients with acetaminophen overdose [25]. Hepatotoxicity from acetaminophen is usually encountered when doses exceeding 10 g/day are ingested either intentionally or unintentionally. However, there are increasing reports of severe acetaminophen hepatotoxicity with ingestion of as little as 4 g/day and mild hepatotoxicity in healthy volunteers [26–28].

The annual mortality in the United States from acetaminophen toxicity is estimated at 500 deaths per year and as many as 20% of these deaths may be due to unintentional overdoses [29]. The majority of the reported 60 000 intentional

Table 25.4 Etiologies of acute liver failure (ALF) in the United States reported in published studies

	Ritt et al. 1958–68 (31)	Rakela et al. 1975–78 (64)	Rakela et al. 1974–82 (34)	Shakil et al. 1983–95 (177)	Schiodt et al. 1994–96 (295)	Ostapowicz et al. 1998–2001 (308)
% HAV	42	2	0	7	7	4
% HBV	32	34	18	19	10	7
% Idiosyncratic drug	23	17	18	12	12	13
% APAP	0	0	0	19	20	39
% Indeterminate	0	34	44	28	15	17
% Other	3	13	21	15	36	20

APAP, acetaminophen; HAV, hepatitis A virus; HBV, hepatitis B virus. Numbers in parentheses refer to number of patients.
Data adapted from refs 20, 12, 123, 11, 10, and 7, respectively.

Total ALF cases:

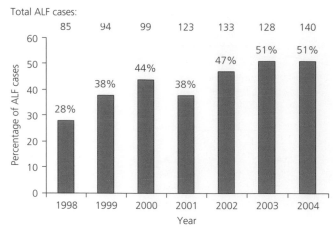

Figure 25.3 Annual incidence of acute liver failure (ALF) due to acetaminophen overdose as reported by the US Acute Liver Failure Study Group (ALFSG). There is a trend toward an increasing incidence of ALF caused by acetaminophen amongst consecutive patients enrolled in the US ALFSG between 1998 and 2004 and when compared with historical cohorts [19,20].

acetaminophen overdose cases occur in women, and not surprisingly women are also overrepresented in studies of acetaminophen induced ALF [13,30,31]. The incidence of unintentional acetaminophen overdose in general practice is not known, but nearly 50% of the acetaminophen-related ALF cases in the US ALFSG were unintentional [19]. In addition to the dose-dependent hepatotoxicity of acetaminophen, there are multiple reports demonstrating the nephrotoxicity of acetaminophen and potential cardiotoxicity that may account for rare deaths in the absence of overt cerebral edema [32].

Diagnosis and management

The hallmark of acetaminophen hepatotoxicity is the presence of towering transaminases, up to more than 400 times normal, with concomitant hypoprothrombinemia, metabolic acidosis, and renal failure. Most patients have a normal or only minimally elevated serum bilirubin at presentation because of the acuity of the liver injury. Serum acetaminophen levels are useful in assessing the risk of hepatotoxicity in subjects with a single time-point ingestion if a reliable history can be obtained [33]. However, the Rumack nomogram is not intended for patients presenting late or for subjects taking excessive doses of acetaminophen over several days [27]. In addition, serum bilirubin levels exceeding 10–15 mg/dL have been associated with false-positive serum acetaminophen levels in some colorometric assays [34]. Given these limitations, the detection of serum acetaminophen–cysteine adducts released from damaged hepatocytes may prove to be a more sensitive and specific biomarker for acetaminophen hepatotoxicity [35–37]. This assay may prove particularly useful in cases of diagnostic uncertainty when patients present with altered mental status or have a history of ingesting multiple acetaminophen-containing products [38]. In addition, the assay may prove useful when acetaminophen is a suspected cofactor in patients with severe acute hepatitis A virus (HAV) or HBV infection who self-medicate with acetaminophen during their viral prodrome [39,40]. However, the serum acetaminophen–cysteine adduct assay is not commercially available and requires further validation to determine its role in clinical practice.

Table 25.5 Diagnosis and management of acetaminophen overdose

Diagnosis

Ingestion of toxic dose of acetaminophen-containing product(s)
1 Review intake of all over-the-counter and prescription medications
2 More than 4 g acetaminophen in 24 h (usually > 10 g)
Consider diagnosis in all patients with unexplained serum ALT > 1000 IU/mL
1 Serum acetaminophen level (Rumack nomogram) if single dose ingestion
2 Check urine toxicology screen for other toxins or illicit substances
3 Bilirubin > 10 mg/dL may lead to false-positive serum acetaminophen levels

Management and treatment

Ipecac syrup/nasogastric lavage if within 4 h of ingestion
Activated charcoal 1 g/kg if within 4 h of ingestion
Admit to hospital if potential hepatotoxicity, coagulopathy, or altered mentation
Admit to ICU if encephalopathy
Liver biochemistries, electrolyte, arterial blood gas and lactate, PT/INR, and factor V levels at admission and q 12 h
Early transfer to transplant center if grade 2 encephalopathy or other adverse prognostic criteria[a]
Oral N-acetylcysteine (NAC):
  Loading dose: 140 mg/kg
  Maintenance dose: 70 mg/kg every 4 h for 17 doses or until INR < 1.5
  Mixing NAC with carbonated beverage can improve GI tolerance
  Nausea and vomiting in 20%, rare urticaria or bronchospasm
Intravenous N-acetylcysteine:
  Acetadote (Cumberland Phamaceuticals, Nashville, TN) is FDA approved for i.v. administration in acetaminophen overdose
  Telemetry monitoring recommended for infusion
  Indications: GI intolerance of oral NAC, ileus, pancreatitis or bowel obstruction, short gut syndrome, pregnancy
  Contraindications: known sulfa allergy
  Loading dose: 150 mg/kg in 250 mL D_5 over 1 h
  Maintenance dose: 50 mg/kg in 500 mL D_5 over 4 h then 125 mg/kg in 1000 mL D_5 over 19 h; 100 mg/kg in 1000 mL D_5 over 24 h × 2 days or until INR < 1.5
  Side effects: hypersensitivity or anaphylactoid reactions in 3%
  If mild hypersensitivity reaction, reduce infusion rate by 50% and consider i.v. diphenhydramine or steroids

a See text for further details.
ALT, alanine aminotransferase; D_5, 5% dextrose; FDA, US Food and Drug Administration; GI, gastrointestinal; ICU, intensive care unit; INR, international normalized ratio; PT, prothrombin time.

Standard medical therapy for acute acetaminophen overdose consists of induction of emesis by ipecac syrup, gastric lavage of pill fragments, and administration of activated charcoal to reduce acetaminophen absorbtion [3,41] (Table 25.5). The likelihood of subsequent hepatotoxicity can be estimated in subjects with a single time-point ingestion by measuring the initial serum acetaminophen level (i.e., the Rumack nomogram) [33]. However, it is important to identify all potential sources of acetaminophen-containing products ingested, such as over-the-counter analgesics and allergy, sinus, and sleep remedies that contain varying amounts of acetaminophen (Table 25.6). Because many prescription narcotic congeners also contain varying quantities

of acetaminophen, it is also important to review all prescription medications ingested (Table 25.7). Subjects with known or suspected intentional acetaminophen overdose should be hospitalized and assessed for their suicidal risk. Subjects at risk for hepatotoxicity based on their serum acetaminophen level, elevated serum aminotransferase levels, or prolonged prothrombin time should be administered oral N-acetylcysteine (NAC) as quickly as possible because delays in NAC administration have been associated with poorer outcomes [42,43]. Oral NAC is given as a loading dose of 140 mg/kg followed by 70 mg/kg every 4 h for up to 72 h. Most patients can tolerate oral NAC with the co-administration of antiemetics. However, an intravenous formulation of NAC

Table 25.6 Over-the-counter products that contain acetaminophen

Trade name	Active ingredients[a]	Amount of APAP per tablet or dose
Actifed products	Varies + APAP	325–500 mg
Alka-Seltzer products	Calcium carbonate + citric acid + potassium bicarbonate + sodium bicarbonate + APAP	250–325 mg
Allerest products	Varies + APAP	325–500 mg
Anacin, Anacin-3	Varies + APAP	80–500 mg, 100 mg/mL, 160 mg/5 mL
Arthritis Foundation Aspirin-Free	Varies + APAP	500 mg
Benadryl Allergy/Cold Tablets	Varies + APAP	500 mg
Children's Tylenol products	Varies + APAP	80–160 mg, 160 mg/5 mL
Comtrex products	Varies + APAP	325–1000 mg, 500 mg/5 mL, 500 mg/15 mL, 650 mg/oz, 1000 mg/oz, 1000 mg/5 mL
Datril Extra Strength	APAP	325–500 mg, 130 mg/5 mL
Drixoral products	Varies + APAP	325–500 mg
Excedrin migraine products	Aspirin + caffeine + APAP	250–500 mg
Goody's Extra Strength Headache Powder	Aspirin + caffeine + APAP	130–500 mg, 260 mg per powder paper
Liquiprin	APAP	80 mg/0.8 mL, 80 mg/1.66 mL, 80 mg/2.5 mL
Midrin	Isometheptene + dichloralphenazone + APAP	325 mg
NyQuil	Varies + APAP	250 mg, 167 mg/5 mL, 1000 mg/packet, 1000 mg/30 mL
Pamprin	Pamabrom + pyrilamine + diphenhydramine + APAP	250–500 mg, 650 mg/packet
Panadol	Caffeine + APAP	80–500 mg, 60 mg/0.6 ml, 80 mg/0.5 mL
Percogesic	Phenyltoloxamine + diphenhydramine + APAP	325–500 mg
Sine-Aid sinus medicine	Pseudoephedrine + APAP	500 mg
Sinutab products	Pseudoephedrine + APAP	325–500 mg, 1000 mg/oz
Sominex Pain Relief Formula	Diphenhydramine + APAP	500 mg
St. Joseph's Aspirin-free products	Phenylpropanolamine + APAP	80–500 mg, 60 mg/0.6 mL, 80 mg/0.8 mL, 80 mg/2.5 mL, 120 mg/5 mL, 160 mg/5 mL
Sudafed sinus products	Varies + APAP	325–500 mg
Tempra products	APAP	80, 160 mg/5 mL
TheraFlu products	Varies + APAP	325–650 mg, 650–1000 mg/packet
Tylenol products	Varies + APAP	325–650 mg, 250 mg/5 mL, 650 mg/30 mL, 650–1000 mg/packet, 1000 mg/30 mL
Vanquish products	Aspirin + caffeine + APAP	194 mg

a Contact Poison Control Center for exact dosage of constituents. This table is not an exhaustive list of all over-the-counter products that may contain acetaminophen.
APAP, acetaminophen.

Table 25.7 Prescription narcotic analgesics that contain acetaminophen

Trade name	Active ingredients[a]	Amount of APAP per tablet or dose
Anexsia	Hydrocodone + APAP	325–660 mg
Capital with Codeine Suspension	Codeine + APAP	120 mg/5 mL
Darvocet-N50	Propoxyphene + APAP	325 mg
Darvocet-N100	Propoxyphene + APAP	650 mg
Darvocet-A500	Propoxyphene + APAP	500 mg
Endocet	Oxycodone + APAP	325–650 mg
Esgic Plus	Butalbital + caffeine + APAP	500 mg
Fioricet	Butalbital + caffeine + APAP	325 mg
Fioricet with Codeine	Butalbital + caffeine + codeine + APAP	325 mg
Lorcet	Hydrocodone + APAP	325–750 mg, 500 mg/15 mL
Lortab	Hydrocodone + APAP	325–500 mg, 500 mg/15 mL
Maxidone	Hydrocodone + APAP	750 mg
Norco	Hydrocodone + APAP	325 mg
Panadol #3 and #4	Codeine + APAP	300 mg
Percocet/Oxycet	Oxycodone + APAP	325–650 mg
Phenaphen with Codeine	Codeine + APAP	325–650 mg
Roxicet	Oxycodone + APAP	325–500 mg, 325 mg/5 mL
Sedapap	Butalbital + APAP	650 mg
Talacen	Pentazocine + APAP	650 mg
Tylenol #2, #3, and #4	Codeine + APAP	300 mg
Tylox	Oxycodone + APAP	500 mg
Ultracet	Tramadol + APAP	325 mg
Vicodin	Hydrocodone + APAP	500 mg
Vicodin ES	Hydrocodone + APAP	750 mg
Vicodin HP	Hydrocodone + APAP	660 mg
Wygesic	Propoxyphene + APAP	650 mg
Zydone	Hydrocodone + APAP	400 mg

a Contact Poison Control Center or equivalent national poisons information service for exact dosage of constituents.
APAP, acetaminophen.

(Acetadote, Cumberland Pharmaceuticals, Nashville, TN) has been approved for use in overdose patients who are unable to tolerate oral NAC [44]. Most experts recommend a 72-h infusion of intravenous NAC, and use of this formulation in pregnant women with hepatotoxicity [45]. Because up to 3% of patients receiving i.v. NAC may develop a hypersensitivity reaction, the drug should only be administered in a monitored setting [44]. Because NAC is a sulfa derivative, it should not be administered to patients with known sulfa allergy or previous hypersensitivity reactions. Patients with mild to moderate intravenous infusion reactions should have the infusion rate decreased by 50% and receive antihistamines or corticosteroids as clinically indicated.

Unintentional acetaminophen overdose

A report from the US ALFSG demonstrated that nearly 50% of acetaminophen-related ALF occurs in patients without overt suicidal intent [19]. In the majority of these patients the total dose of acetaminophen ingested was excessive, and multiple acetaminophen-containing products were taken by 38% (Table 25.8). However, 50% of the unintentional patients reported ingesting only 4–10 g of acetaminophen-containing products per day. Contrary to previous reports, these subjects were no more likely to be receiving antidepressants nor to have a history of alcohol abuse than subjects with intentional acetaminophen overdose (Table 25.8). However, unintentional acetaminophen overdose patients had more advanced grades of hepatic encephalopathy at presentation, presumably due to the concomitant ingestion of narcotics. In addition, they also had lower serum aminotransferase and acetaminophen levels compared with intentional overdose patients. Fortunately, the majority of patients received NAC and the spontaneous survival rate was similar in both patient groups. The role of genetic or environmental cofactors in subjects with unintentional acetaminophen overdose is hotly debated but requires further study [45,46].

Table 25.8 Acetaminophen-related acute liver failure patients enrolled in the US Acute Liver Failure Study Group (1998–2003)

	Intentional APAP overdose ($n = 122$)	Unintentional APAP overdose ($n = 131$)
Presenting features		
Female	74%	73%
Pain	0	82%[a]
APAP (g) per day	29	10*
Total APAP ingested (g)	29	34
≥ 2 APAP formulations	5%	38%[a]
Alcohol	59%	53%
Antidepressants	38%	37%
Narcotic–APAP congener	18%	63%[a]
Serum ALT (IU/L)	5326	3319[a]
Serum APAP (mg/dL)	95	42
Outcomes		
King's College criteria	7%	20%
Listed	25%	27%
Transplanted	7%	9%
Overall survival	71%	72%

a $P < 0.05$, adapted from Larson et al. [19].
ALT, alanine aminotransferase; APAP, acetaminophen.

Table 25.9 Morbidity and mortality caused by acetaminophen overdose in the United Kingdom before and after regulatory actions in 1998

	1 year prior to legislation	3 years after legislation	P
APAP sales (10^6 tablets/year)	520	580	NS
APAP overdose cases	1733	1686	< 0.001
Liver transplant referrals	329	217	< 0.001
Liver transplant listings	42	35	0.06
Liver transplants done	31	24	0.07
APAP-related deaths	192	127	< 0.001

In 1998, regulatory changes involving the dispensing, packaging, and labeling of acetaminophen (APAP)-containing products were introduced in the United Kingdom. Data adapted from Hawton et al. [48].

Because acetaminophen hepatotoxicity is a leading cause of ALF and yet completely avoidable, some experts have called for restrictions regarding the quantity of acetaminophen dispensed and changes to the packaging and labeling of acetaminophen-containing products [38,46]. In the United Kingdom, limitations on the number of acetaminophen tablets available for single purchase, blister packaging, and other labeling changes were introduced in 1998 [47]. Following these measures, the number of patients with intentional acetaminophen overdose and those referred for liver transplantation have both been significantly reduced (Table 25.9) [48]. In addition, the mean quantity of acetaminophen ingested has been reduced while overall sales have remained unchanged [48]. In the United States, further education of practicing physicians, health-care providers, and patients regarding the presence of acetaminophen in multiple over-the-counter and prescription medications appears warranted in light of the high proportion of unintentional acetaminophen overdose cases leading to ALF. The US Food and Drug Administration (FDA) has proposed a series of changes in the labeling of all over-the-counter products that contain acetaminophen or nonsteroidal antiinflammatory drugs (NSAIDs) [49].

Additional limitations on the dispensing of prescription acetaminophen-narcotic congeners or reduction or elimination of the acetaminophen content of these products may prove worthwhile [46].

Hepatotropic viruses

Severe acute HAV, HBV, and HEV infection may lead to ALF in a minority of afflicted individuals. Establishing a diagnosis of HAV-related ALF relies on the detection of anti-HAV immunoglobulin M (IgM) (Table 25.1). Although young children, subjects over 50, and individuals with underlying liver disease may be more prone to develop severe acute HAV, the overall incidence of ALF due to acute HAV infection is less than 1% and appears to be declining [7,40]. An analysis of the United Network for Organ Sharing (UNOS) transplant database and the ALFSG confirmed a significant decline in the incidence of fulminant HAV in the United States between 1998 and 2005 [50].

Fulminant HBV infection is diagnosed by the presence of detectable hepatitis B surface antigen (HBsAg) or IgM antibody to hepatits B core antigen (anti-HBc). However, some patients with chronic HBV may have transiently detectable anti-HBc IgM during a spontaneous disease flare [51,52]. In addition, a minority of patients with fulminant HBV may have hepatitis delta virus (HDV) coinfection or superinfection, which can be confirmed by detection of anti-HDV antibodies. Although early studies suggested that pre-core and core-promoter variants of HBV may be associated with ALF, subsequent studies have failed to demonstrate this association [51,52]. The role of HBV genotypes and other host factors in HBV-related ALF is unclear but these patients have a low likelihood of spontaneous survival [51,53]. Because the pathogenesis of fulminant HBV is believed to be an overwhelming immune response to infected hepatocytes, the role of oral antiviral agents such as lamivudine or entecavir remains unclear but uncontrolled studies suggest that they are safe and potentially beneficial [54].

Severe acute HEV infection, which is a leading cause of ALF in tropical areas worldwide, occurs most commonly in pregnant women for unexplained reasons [55,56]. This diagnosis is established by detection of anti-HEV IgM antibody, and treatment is supportive. Severe acute HCV infection has also been reported to lead to ALF in some patients but this has not been confirmed in other large series [7,57]. Other nonhepatotropic viruses, including Epstein–Barr virus (EBV), cytomegalovirus (CMV), herpes simplex virus (HSV), varicella zoster virus, human herpes virus-6 (HHV-6), and parvovirus B-19, can all rarely present as ALF [58–60]. Whether these rare causes of ALF are due to unique viral variants or aberrant host immune responses is unclear. Making a diagnosis of ALF as a result of one of these nonhepatotropic viruses is frequently difficult and often requires histological confirmation. However, severe acute EBV, CMV, or HSV should be considered early on because they can be treated with antivirals (Table 25.1) [59].

Idiosyncratic drug reactions

Prescription and over-the-counter medications and herbal products are increasingly being recognized as common causes of severe acute hepatitis and ALF [61]. Furthermore, drug-induced liver injury (DILI) is a leading reason for the discontinuation of drugs in development and regulatory actions for previously approved drugs [62]. DILI is rare in the general population and felt to be the result of host metabolic idiosyncrasy. The majority of patients with severe DILI experience acute hepatocellular liver injury resulting in jaundice but some patients with severe cholestatic liver injury may also develop fatal ALF [61,63,64]. The incidence of severe idiosyncratic DILI varies greatly among drugs, ranging from 1 in 1000 patients receiving isoniazid to less than 1 in 1 000 000 patients treated with a beta-lactam antibiotic [65,66]. Multiple case series demonstrate that DILI, and progression to ALF, affect preponderantly women [13,63,64]. Whether women may be more susceptible to idiosyncratic drug-induced ALF because of differences in body weight, drug dosing, or metabolizing/detoxification enzyme activity requires further study.

Idiosyncratic drug reactions are characterized by a variable delay or latency period after initial ingestion but usually occur within the first 12 months of starting a new agent, except for unusual circumstances such as macrodantin hepatotoxicity [67]. Genetically determined variability in host toxification, detoxification, and regeneration pathways are implicated in the pathogenesis and outcome of these rare idiosyncratic events, but supportive human data are limited. In addition, the roles of medication dose, drug–drug interactions, alcohol consumption, and other environmental cofactors are largely unknown [68]. The Drug-Induced Liver Injury Network (http://dilin.dcri.duke.edu/) facilitates research into the etiologies and mechanisms of DILI, by prospectively collecting biological samples from well-phenotyped cases [68,69].

The primary treatment of drug-induced ALF is to discontinue the suspect agent, because subjects who continue to receive the offending agent may experience progressive liver injury [70]. An uncontrolled series suggested a potential role for steroids in some patients with severe DILI, but this approach remains controversial [71]. In addition, corticosteroids were found not to be beneficial in large, randomized controlled studies of ALF patients [12]. A diagnosis of DILI is notoriously difficult to establish because most patients have no immunoallergic features at presentation, many are taking multiple medications, and there is no objective confirmatory laboratory test. Liver histology in severe DILI is also of unclear benefit beyond excluding other treatable causes. Therefore, one has to exclude all competing causes and use imprecise causality assessment instruments to make a clinical diagnosis of DILI [72,73].

In addition to prescription drugs, a careful history of all herbal and complementary and alternative medicine consumption is needed in patients with unexplained ALF. Formulations of kava kava, ephedra, and various weight-loss agents have all been associated with ALF and subsequently withdrawn from the marketplace [7,74,75]. In one series, over 50% of the ALF cases seen at a single transplant center were believed to be caused by a herbal product [76]. Unfortunately, because herbal products are not closely regulated during the development, manufacturing, or marketing phases, it is nearly impossible to identify the specific hepatotoxic ingredient(s) in many of these mixtures.

Development of jaundice in combination with high serum aminotransferase levels in DILI patients has a reported mortality rate of 10% (i.e., the Hy rule) [62]. A retrospective review of 784 Swedish DILI cases confirmed that serum aspartate aminotransferase (AST) and bilirubin levels at presentation were the most important predictors of death or liver transplantation in patients with severe hepatocellular DILI [63]. A review of 95 Japanese DILI cases also identified serum bilirubin at presentation and a prolonged latency period to be significantly associated with death [77]. A review of the UNOS liver transplant database from 1990 to 2002 highlighted the etiologies and outcomes of 270 adult liver transplant recipients with drug-induced ALF [78]. A striking female predominance was reported (76%), the mean age was 35 years, and 49% were acetaminophen-related ALF patients. The most commonly implicated medications in the idiosyncratic DILI group included isoniazid (17.5%), propylthiouracil (9.5%), phenytoin (7.3%), and valproic acid (7.3%) [78]. The 1-year patient and graft survival rates were 77% and 71%, respectively. In the US ALFSG, medications implicated in ALF include antituberculosis agents ($n = 12$), antibiotics ($n = 11$), hypolipidemics ($n = 6$), phenytoin ($n = 5$), bromfenac ($n = 4$), and troglitazone ($n = 4$) (A. Reuben, unpublished observations, December 2005). The majority of the ALFSG subjects were also female (68%), had high serum bilirubin levels (median 22 mg/dL), and symptoms for a mean of 8 days prior to presentation (Table 25.3). Overall, the idiosyncratic DILI ALF patients had a poor prognosis, with a spontaneous survival rate of only 25% at 3 weeks. Therefore, any subject with suspected DILI who develops jaundice with coagulopathy or encephalopathy should be urgently referred to a liver transplant center.

Other identifiable causes of acute liver failure

Autoimmune hepatitis can rarely present as fulminant liver failure [79]. Autoimmune serologies and liver biopsy can aid in the diagnosis but many of these patients may have low-titer or undetectable autoantibodies. The benefit of corticosteroids in fulminant autoimmune hepatitis remains unclear. However, early identification of ALF caused by autoimmune hepatitis is important for clinical management because of the low spontaneous survival rate (Fig. 25.1). Acute liver failure is a well-reported complication of several pregnancy-related liver diseases, including acute fatty liver of pregnancy (AFLP) and the syndrome of hemolysis, elevated liver enzyme levels, and low platelet count (HELLP) [80–82]. Treatment for these conditions is directed toward prompt delivery of the fetus. The hallmark of AFLP is the rapid development of microvesicular steatosis in the third trimester with resultant mitochondrial dysfunction, metabolic acidosis, and coagulopathy with only mild-to-moderate serum aminotransferase elevations. Mothers with long-chain fatty acid metabolic defects (i.e., LCHAD deficiency) are at increased risk of developing AFLP, and genetic testing is available but only 25% of AFLP mothers carry an identifiable mutation [83]. Although most women with AFLP or HELLP improve with rapid delivery, some may require emergency liver transplantation. Severe acute viral hepatitis and HSV hepatitis may also present with ALF, particularly in the third trimester of pregnancy and both conditions are associated with a poor prognosis.

Sudden onset of severe hepatic outflow obstruction caused by occlusion of all three hepatic veins (i.e., Budd–Chiari syndrome) is another rare but potentially treatable cause of ALF (Table 25.1) [84]. Most of these subjects present with new-onset abdominal pain, hepatomegaly, and ascites. Over 80% of patients with Budd–Chiari syndrome have an identifiable thrombophilia, which may be treated with anticoagulation, but many patients require transplantation [85,86]. Arterial hypoperfusion of the liver caused by cardiogenic shock or hypovolumia can also lead to ischemic hepatitis, with a subset of patients progressing to ALF [87]. The outcome in these patients is primarily determined by the underlying cardiopulmonary disease, and transplantation is rarely required or indicated. Another rare cause of ALF is poisoning by ingestion of the mushroom *Amanita phalloides*, which often presents with severe gastrointestinal symptoms and diarrhea. Although diagnostic assays for amanita toxin levels are not available, patients can be successfully treated with i.v. penicillin G, silymarin, and dialysis although many may require transplantation [88–90].

Wilson disease is a hereditary disorder of impaired biliary excretion of copper that can present as ALF in up to 25% of adolescent or young adult patients [91]. Clues to a diagnosis of fulminant Wilson disease include the presence of Kayser–Fleischer rings in up to 50% of cases, low serum alkaline phosphatase levels, hemolytic anemia with hyperbilirubinemia, and low serum ceruloplasmin levels (but normal in 15%) [91,92]. Elevated serum and urinary copper levels are often present, but testing for these may not be feasible because of the frequent presence of concomitant renal failure [93]. A transjugular liver biopsy can definitively establish a diagnosis of Wilson disease with elevated quantitative hepatic copper levels and advanced hepatic fibrosis, but is often not feasible. Because fulminant Wilson disease is associated with 100% mortality in the absence of liver transplantation, it is recommended that all of these patients be listed for transplantation as soon as possible (Fig. 25.1). Methods to stabilize the patient who is awaiting transplantation include plasmapheresis, exchange transfusion, and albumin dialysis to reduce serum free copper levels [91].

Acute Hodgkin and non-Hodgkin lymphoma, metastatic carcinoma (e.g., lung, breast, melanoma), and several variants of leukemia are rare infiltrative causes of ALF [94,95]. Although a diagnosis of fulminant malignancy may be suspected based on history, laboratory studies, or imaging, liver biopsy is frequently required for confirmation and treatment. Overall, these patients have a poor prognosis and are not candidates for liver transplantation [7].

Indeterminate acute liver failure

No specific etiology of ALF can be identified in up to 20% of adult ALF patients [4,96]. Studies have failed to demonstrate occult infection with HBV, HEV, parvovirus B-19, and SEN-V in US ALFSG patients with indeterminate ALF [53,97,98]. Other proposed etiologies include occult autoimmune hepatitis or misdiagnosed acetaminophen hepatotoxicity [37]. In the US ALFSG, 19% of the indeterminate ALF cases had detectable serum acetaminophen–cysteine adducts and those patients tended to have higher serum aminotransferase levels and lower bilirubin levels at presentation compared with adduct-negative indeterminate patients [37]. However, it remains unclear if acetaminophen was the primary cause of ALF or simply a cofactor in these cases. In any event, subjects with indeterminate ALF have a poor likelihood of spontaneous recovery and should be rapidly referred for liver transplantation evaluation.

Clinical presentation and complications

Patients with ALF frequently present with nonspecific symptoms of fatigue, nausea, abdominal pain, and jaundice prior to developing encephalopathy and coagulopathy. Other clinical conditions with a systemic inflammatory response and jaundice may initially be confused with ALF, such as malaria, dengue fever, and hemorrhagic viral infection [99]. Additionally, systemic sepsis with resultant disseminated intravascular coagulation, altered mentation, and intrahepatic cholestasis can also mimic ALF. Lastly, alcoholic hepatitis and flares of chronic HBV may occasionally be mistaken for ALF. Therefore, clinicians must carefully review all available laboratory and clinical information when seeing a patient with possible ALF.

Although towering transaminases are noted at presentation in many ALF patients, others may have more subtle laboratory abnormalities caused by progressive hepatic necrosis ("burnout") or differing mechanisms of liver dysfunction (e.g., mitochondrial toxicity). Hepatocyte death in ALF can occur through programmed cell death (apoptosis) or direct toxic effects (necrosis) [99]. Direct hepatocellular damage can lead to impaired gluconeogenesis, glycogenolysis, and energy production, which predisposes to hypoglycemia and lactic acidosis. In addition, impaired hepatic synthesis of clotting factors with short half-lives, such as factors I, II, V, VII, IX, and X, can lead to hypoprothrombinemia and coagulopathy. Intravascular coagulation with failure to clear the products of coagulation frequently leads to further elevation in fibrin split products and D-dimer levels in ALF patients. Finally, impaired urea cycle metabolism in the liver and peripherally can lead to accumulation of ammonia and other toxins which contribute to the development of cerebral edema and encephalopathy.

Hepatic encephalopathy and cerebral edema

Neurological manifestations are pivotal in the progression and prognosis of ALF. The West Haven encephalopathy criteria, which were developed for patients with chronic liver disease, are frequently used for ALF encephalopathy grading: grade 1 (slow mentation); grade 2 (agitation, presence of asterixis); grade 3 (permanent somnolence); and grade 4 (coma) [1,100]. Patients progressing to stage 3 or 4 encephalopathy have a poorer outcome than those with a maximal encephalopathy grade of 1 or 2 (grade I survival = 70%, grade IV survival = 20%) [4,101]. The Glasgow coma score may be a more reliable means of assessing changes in advanced encephalopathy, with scores ranging from 3 to 15, but prospective studies are lacking. Seizures, decorticate posturing, and hemodynamic instability may develop in ALF patients as a result of cerebral edema and increased intracranial pressure [102].

The altered mental status of ALF patients is believed to be largely the result of the development of cerebral edema in the setting of a rapidly failing liver rather than portosystemic shunting of toxins. Two main hypotheses have been proposed to explain the development of cerebral edema in ALF [100,103]. The "glutamine hypothesis" is based on the detoxification of ammonia by astrocytes in the brain by the conversion of glutamate to glutamine, which results in increased tissue osmolarity and resultant brain edema [100]. In support of this, elevated arterial ammonia levels have been associated with the presence and progression of cerebral edema in ALF patients [104]. An alternative hypothesis contends that cerebral edema may develop as a result of the loss of intracerebral vascular autoregulation with resulting increases in brain water and volume [100,103]. Physiological studies support a loss of intracerebral vascular tone in ALF patients with advanced encephalopathy and improvement with specific interventions [103,105].

Infection

An oral temperature exceeding 100°F (37.8°C) or less than 96°F (35.5°C) in an ALF patient may be due to the underlying hepatocellular necrosis and inflammation but infection must always be considered and addressed. Unfortunately, many critically ill ALF patients with active infection will not mount a fever or develop localizing symptoms of infection [106]. Infectious complications develop in ALF patients because of the rapid loss of reticuloendothelial cell function (i.e., Kupffer cells), changes in neutrophil function, and impaired complement activation and opsonization [107]. As many as 90% of ALF patients will develop a bacterial infection during their hospital course, with bacteremia noted in 26% [106,107]. Additionally, fungal infections are another significant cause of morbidity and mortality, with infection rates as high as 32% [108]. Common sources of infection include lines and catheters and the respiratory and urinary tract. Emerging evidence suggests that infection leading to increased systemic inflammatory response can hasten the progression of encephalopathy in ALF and lead to poorer outcomes [103,109,110]. Therefore, early recognition and treatment of potential infections is critical to optimize patient survival. Unfortunately, infections and cerebral edema remain the leading causes of death in ALF patients.

Coagulopathy

The multifactorial coagulopathy of ALF is a marker of progressive hepatic dysfunction and liver failure [111]. The inability to synthesize the rapidly consumed clotting factors made in the liver (i.e., factors V, VII, IX, and X) contributes to the hypoprothrombinemia and increases the risk for clinically significant bleeding, which develops in about 10% of ALF patients. Vitamin K deficiency resulting from preexisting nutritional deficiencies and use of broad-spectrum antibiotics is also commonly observed in ALF patients. Thrombocytopenia, which is seen in up to 50% of ALF patients, may develop because of impaired hepatic thrombopoietin synthesis, development of acute portal hypertension and splenomegaly, drug effects, and disseminated intravascular consumptive coagulopathy [112,113]. The international normalized ratio (INR), as calculated from a prothrombin time, is a useful and readily available laboratory parameter for monitoring liver synthetic function in ALF patients. Serial assessments of factor V and VII levels have also been shown to be useful prognostic markers in acute hepatitis and ALF [114–116].

Multiorgan failure

Given the liver's central role in overall body homeostasis, it is not surprising that rapid deterioration of hepatic function can lead to multiorgan failure and eventual death. Loss of actin-scavenging ability with reduced levels of serum Gc globulin has been associated with poorer outcomes in nonacetaminophen ALF, presumably because of greater tissue hypoxia [117]. Commonly encountered hemodynamic abnormalities in ALF include tachycardia, hypotension, increased cardiac output, and low peripheral vascular resistance [103]. In addition, there is emerging evidence that adrenal dysfunction is a common complication of ALF and may contribute to prognosis and outcome [118,119]. Because most patients with progressive encephalopathy require mechanical intubation for airway protection, it can be difficult to differentiate pneumonia from noncardiogenic pulmonary edema, which are both common in ALF patients [120]. Finally, acute renal failure develops in 40%–70% of ALF patients; this can further increase the rates of infection and portends a poor prognosis [121,122].

Prognosis in acute liver failure

Patient survival rates have dramatically improved with the advent of emergency liver transplantation for ALF patients. Before the use of transplantation, the reported survival rates were 3%–18% [12,20,123]. Later studies reported survival to be 14%–25% without liver transplantation and 41%–49% with liver transplantation [10,11]. Amongst ALF transplant recipients, 1-year patient survival varies between 60% and 80% [5]. The maximal severity of encephalopathy and coagulopathy correlate inversely with survival in ALF [124,125]. Numerous prognostic scales have been devised to accurately predict outcome so that patients in greatest need of liver transplantation can be rapidly identified and prioritized. Thus far, only patients with fulminant Wilson disease have a 100% fatality in the absence of emergency liver transplantation [7].

Clichy criteria
The Clichy criteria were developed in a cohort of 115 medically managed fulminant HBV patients from a single center in France. A combination of encephalopathy grade and age-adjusted factor V level were found to be the most important predictors of survival. Specifically, transplantation was recommended if grade 3 or 4 encephalopathy and a factor V level below 20% were present in patients under 30 years of age, or below 30% in patients over 30 years of age [126,127]. However, this prognostic scale has been criticized for its performance when tested in other patient populations and the inability to obtain factor V levels in referring hospitals [128]. Nonetheless, many centers use serial fctor V levels as a means of assessing short-term prognosis.

King's College criteria
The King's College criteria are used by many liver transplant centers throughout the world [124,128]. The King's College criteria were developed from a retrospective cohort of 588 medically managed ALF patients and prospectively validated in an additional 175 ALF patients [129]. Readily obtained baseline and dynamic laboratory parameters were selected to enhance the usefulness of the criteria to clinicians. Separate criteria were developed for acetaminophen- and non-acetaminophen-related ALF. In the acetaminophen cohort, an arterial pH below 7.3 or INR greater than 6.5, serum creatinine greater than 3.4 mg/dL, and grade 3 or 4 encephalopathy had prognostic significance. In the nonacetaminophen cohort, an INR greater than 6.5 or three of the following were independent predictors of poor outcomes: unfavorable cause (non-A, non-B hepatitis, drug-induced etiology); jaundice for more than 7 days before encephalopathy; age under 10 years or greater than 40 years; INR greater than 3.5; and serum bilirubin greater than 17.5 mg/dL [129]. The positive predictive value of the King's criteria for death were 84% in the acetaminophen and 98% in the nonacetaminophen cohorts, respectively. By contrast, the negative predictive values were 86% and 82%, respectively [129]. These prognostic models have been tested in other patient cohorts with lower positive predictive value (PPV) and negative predictive value (NPV) values [11,130,131] (Table 25.10). The value of determining early arterial lactic acid levels in conjunction with the standard King's College criteria has been studied in patients with acetaminophen-induced ALF. A postresuscitation arterial lactate level exceeding 3.0 mmol/L, or an "early" value exceeding 3.5 mmol/L, had reported negative predictive values of 97% and 99%, respectively, but positive predictive values fell to 79% and 74%, respectively [99,132].

Other prognostic models
The Model for End-stage Liver Disease (MELD) was developed as a means to predict mortality for cirrhotic patients undergoing transjugular intrahepatic portosystemic shunt [133]. Simplification of the MELD equation to include only the objective parameters of serum creatinine, total bilirubin, and INR predicted 3-month survival better than the Child–Turcotte–Pugh score in liver transplant candidates [133]. As a result, the MELD score has become the means by which liver allografts are allocated to patients with chronic liver failure in the United States [133]. Interest has arisen in potentially using MELD scores to allocate livers to ALF patients [134,135]. Analysis revealed that patients with nonacetaminophen ALF had the poorest prognosis, which correlated with MELD scores, whereas the other patient groups had a high rate of spontaneous recovery, which was independent of MELD score [134].

Use of global assessment models has also been proposed further to prognosticate outcome in ALF patients [136,137]. Larson et al. showed that admission Acute Physiology and Chronic Health Evaluation (APACHE) II scores were superior to the King's College criteria and MELD scores in predicting outcomes in patients with acetaminophen-induced ALF [19]. Other potential prognostic laboratory markers

Table 25.10 Application of prognostic criteria to patients with acute liver failure

Prognostic scale	Positive predictive value (%)	Negative predictive value (%)	Predictive accuracy (%)
Acetaminophen hepatotoxicity			
King's College criteria (O'Grady et al., 1989 [129])			
Arterial pH < 7.3	95	78	81
INR > 6.5, Cr > 3.4 mg/dL, grade 3/4 HE	67	86	83
Overall	84	86	85
King's College criteria (Anand et al., 1997 [130])			
Arterial pH < 7.3	77	64	70
INR > 6.5, Cr > 3.4 mg/dL, grade 3/4 HE	79	72	73
Overall	73	71	72
King's College criteria (Shakil et al., 2000 [11])			
Arterial pH < 7.3	69	80	72
INR > 6.5, Cr > 3.4 mg/dL, grade 3/4 HE	100	79	86
King's College criteria and lactate (Bernal et al., 2002 [132])			
Overall	80	94	–
King's College criteria and phosphorus (Schmidt and Dalhoff, 2002 [139])			
Overall	80	93	92
Nonacetaminophen acute liver failure			
King's College criteria (O Grady et al., 1989 [129])			
INR > 6.5	100	26	46
Any three of five variables[a]	96	82	92
Overall	98	82	94
King's College criteria (Anand et al., 1997 [130])			
INR > 6.5	100	37	52
Any three of five variables[a]	65	17	52
Overall	68	25	61
King's College criteria (Shakil et al., 2000 [11])			
INR > 6.5	98	50	79
Any three of five variables[a]	91	42	74
Clichy criteria (Pauwels et al., 1993 [131])			
At admission	96	50	80
48 h prior to death	89	47	79

a INR > 3.5; jaundice to encephalopathy time > 7 days, non-A, non-B hepatitis or drug-induced etiology; age < 10 years or > 40 years; serum bilirubin > 17.5 mg/dL.
Adapted from Rakela et al. [123].
Cr, creatinine; HE, hepatic encephalopathy; INR, international normalized ratio.

include serum phosphate levels, which decline in patients who are able rapidly to regenerate [138–141]. Similarly, serum α-fetoprotein levels, which increase in patients undergoing rapid liver regeneration, have been positively associated with a greater likelihood of recovery [142,143]. However, these biochemical parameters will probably have inadequate predictive power by themselves and may prove more useful when combined with other prognostic variables [144].

Abdominal CT scanning to assess liver volume and hepatic histopathology have also been proposed, but both methods have substantial limitations in their sensitivity, specificity, and feasibility [145,146]. Because etiology appears to be an important and consistent predictor of outcome, disease-specific prognostic models may prove useful in the future for both nonacetaminophen- and acetaminophen-related ALF [7,56].

Management of acute liver failure

The clinical management of ALF patients has continued to improve, with advances in liver transplantation and critical care. A key principle in evaluating and caring for ALF patients is the rapidity and unpredictable manner in which they may deteriorate. Therefore, ALF patients should be managed in an intensive care unit to enable frequent neurological and hemodynamic monitoring and intervention [1,3]. Additionally, if the patient has a poor likelihood of recovery at presentation, early transfer to a liver transplant center is strongly recommended.

General measures

Rapid evaluation for treatable causes of ALF allows specific therapy aimed at the underlying disease process to be initiated (Table 25.1). However, with the exception of liver transplantation, there is no single medical intervention that has been shown to be beneficial to all ALF patients. Corticosteroids have failed to confer a morbidity or mortality benefit in three randomized controlled trials [12,147,148]. Similarly, intravenous prostaglandin E_1 infusions have not demonstrated any survival benefit despite promising pilot studies [149]. N-acetylcysteine (NAC) is of proven benefit in patients with acetaminophen hepatotoxicity [33,42]. There are also small pilot and physiological studies suggesting that NAC may be of benefit in nonacetaminophen ALF, possibly through an improvement in tissue oxygenation [150,151]. However, a systematic review of the literature failed to identify a survival benefit with NAC in nonacetaminophen ALF [152]. A multicenter, double-blind study of NAC in nonacetaminophen ALF has completed enrollment and will hopefully determine if this widely available agent may be of benefit. Additionally, studies of various extracorporeal bioartificial liver devices are underway. However, until these studies are completed, supportive ICU care to address the underlying pathophysiological abnormalities is recommended as the standard of care for ALF patients.

An experienced hepatologist and intensivist should be available to guide and direct the management of ALF patients. Consultation from transplant surgery, neurosurgery, and infectious diseases is also invaluable in patients with progressive disease or in need of liver transplantation. Placement of central venous access and arterial lines can assist with fluid resuscitation, infusion of medications, frequent laboratory monitoring, and titration of acid–base status. Routine laboratory tests, including serial lactate, factor V, INR, and liver biochemistries, should be obtained at least every 12 h to monitor for clinical changes. Glucose levels should be monitored hourly and supplemented as needed.

Neurological features

Continuous assessment of neurological status is crucial in the management of ALF patients (Table 25.11). Classical physical exam findings of intracranial hypertension, such as papilledema, loss of pupillary reflexes, and clonus, do not reliably correlate with intracranial pressure measurements or grade of encephalopathy. Similarly, head CT findings of cerebral edema are frequently a late occurrence and neither sensitive

---

Table 25.11 Management of cerebral edema in acute liver failure

Grade 1 or 2 encephalopathy

Grade 1: Mild changes in mood and speech, disordered sleep

Grade 2: Inappropriate behavior, mild irritability, agitation, or
  somnolence

Hyperreflexia, clonus, asterixis may or may not be present

Transfer to ICU for frequent monitoring and neurological checks:

1 Quiet environment with minimal stimuli

2 Avoid sedatives/hypnotics

D_{10} drip with hourly blood glucose monitoring

Lactulose may be of benefit in selected patients (see text)

Grade 3 or 4 encephalopathy

Grade 3: Somnolent but arousable to verbal command, marked
  confusion, incoherent speech

Grade 4: Unarousable to painful stimuli

Avoid medications with sedative properties (e.g., narcotics,
  benzodiazepines) unless intubated

Elevate head of bed to 30° from horizontal

  Avoid Valsalva maneuvers, vigorous straining, or suctioning

  Use cooling blankets to keep core temperature ≤ 37°C

Elective intubation if hypoxia, respiratory failure, or to protect airway

  If intubated, propofol or midazolam sedation preferred

Head CT to rule out intracranial hemorrhage

Consider ICP monitor placement

  Correct coagulopathy (INR < 1.5) with FFP or rFVIIa

  ICP catheter type should balance risk of procedure vs benefit of
    accurate data (e.g., epidural vs subdural vs parenchymal)

Measures for elevated ICP

Maintain CPP above 50 mmHg (CPP = MAP – ICP)

Hyperventilate to P_{CO_2} of ~ 28–30 mmHg

If ICP > 20 mmHg for > 5 min, mannitol 0.5–1.0 mg/kg bolus over 5 min

Monitor serum osmolarity and osmolar gap

If persistently elevated ICP, pentabarbitol infusion with 100–150-mg
  bolus over 15 min followed by continuous infusion at 1–3 mg/kg/h

  May need pressors if pentobarbital used or CPP < 50 mmHg

  Dopamine or levophed drips preferred

  Avoid vasopressin because of adverse effect on cerebral bloodflow[a]

  Moderate hypothermia (33°C–35°C) is investigational for refractory
    cerebral edema in ALF[a]

  Paralytic agent (atracurium) or propofol to prevent shivering

  Protocol for rewarming not established

Brain perfusion scan if prolonged increases in ICP to exclude brain death

---

a See text for discussion.

ALF, acute liver failure; CPP, cerebral perfusion pressure; CT, computed tomography; D_{10}, 10% dextrose; FFP, fresh frozen plasma; ICP, intracranial pressure; ICU, intensive care unit; INR, international normalized ratio; MAP, mean arterial pressure; rFVIIa, recombinant factor VIIa.

nor reliable enough to detect intracranial hypertension [153–155]. Although conventional MRI scanning and magnetic resonance spectroscopy may provide more accurate information, the scanning time and transportation logistics are usually prohibitive for critically ill ALF patients [156,157].

Intracranial pressure (ICP) monitoring is the most reliable, albeit invasive, means to follow changes in intracranial pressure in ALF patients [158]. Information gained from the ICP monitor can help guide management decisions regarding the use of mannitol and paralytic agents. However, controversy exists about whether ICP monitoring should be used in every patient with grade 3 or 4 encephalopathy or only in liver transplant candidates [158]. Sedation should be stopped for at least 2–4 h in intubated ALF patients being considered for ICP monitor placement to assess brain function, and a preoperative head CT is recommended to exclude spontaneous hemorrhage. Although parenchymal catheters are associated with a greater risk of bleeding, they also appear to provide more reliable pressure tracings [158,159]. ICP measurements can help intensivists maintain an adequate cerebral perfusion pressure (CPP) (i.e., > 50 mmHg) by the introduction of pressors to raise the mean arterial pressure (MAP) or other maneuvers to lower an elevated ICP (i.e., CPP = MAP – ICP).

Exacerbation of cerebral edema is prevented by placing the head of the bed at more than 30° from horizontal in all ALF patients [160]. Vigorous suctioning or other Valsalva maneuvers should be avoided to prevent surges in ICP. In addition, mechanical ventilation with high levels of positive end-expiratory pressure should be avoided because of potential worsening of cerebral edema. Cooling blankets can be used to keep the patient's core temperature below 37.0°C. Medications with sedative properties (especially long-acting benzodiazepines, narcotics, and diphenhydramine) should be avoided in nonintubated patients because they can obscure neurological changes. If sedation is required for patient comfort and safety, agents with a short half-life, such as midazolam and propofol, are preferred.

If a patient has evidence of clinical progression or an ICP exceeding 20 mmHg for more than 5–10 min, several measures can and should be undertaken [103]. Initially, hyperventilation of intubated patients to a P_{CO_2} of 28–30 mmHg is recommended to induce cerebral vasoconstriction, although this should not be used for extended periods [103,161]. Lactulose can help lower systemic ammonia levels in cirrhotic patients by its osmotic activity and acidification of the stool, but lactulose has not been prospectively tested in ALF patients [162]. In addition, there are concerns for free water depletion and potential abdominal distention with associated bowel ischemia. Nonetheless, many centers use lactulose, particularly in patients with subacute liver failure who may have more evidence of portosystemic shunting [1,3,162].

Mannitol at a dose of 0.5–1.0 g/kg is a first-line therapy for management of ICP surges exceeding 20 mmHg that do not respond to hyperventilation [163]. Mannitol works by draw-ing fluid into the intravascular space and reducing intracranial volume. Mannitol infusions should be withheld in patients with renal failure or fluid overload until renal replacement therapy has been initiated. In addition, monitoring of serum osmolarity is recommended to avoid a hyperosmolar state. Data have also suggested a potential benefit of hypertonic saline infusion to reduce the incidence and severity of intracranial hypertension [164]. In one study of 30 ALF patients, 30% hypertonic saline was infused at a rate of 5–20 mL/h to maintain serum sodium levels at 145–155 mmol/L. A significant decrease in intracranial hypertension was noted in the treated group compared with the untreated controls ($P = 0.003$). However, this treatment requires further study to establish its safety because of its narrow therapeutic window.

Thiopental and pentobarbital are centrally acting hypnotics that reduce brain oxygen utilization, which can be employed as second-line therapy for severe intracranial hypertension [165]. Pentobarbital is administered as a 100–150-mg bolus over 15 min followed by a continuous infusion at 1–3 mg/kg/h. Pentobarbital drug levels can be followed every 8 h with a therapeutic goal of 20–35 mg/L. Because barbiturate infusions can lead to systemic hypotension, dopamine may be required to maintain an adequate CPP. The use of propofol to reduce ICP has also been reported; this may be advantageous because of its lower risk of systemic hemodynamic effects [166].

Moderate hypothermia has been reported to reduce cerebral hyperemia and lower elevated intracranial pressure in ALF patients who are refractory to medical therapy [167–170]. By reducing the core body temperature to 33°C–35°C, cerebral oxygen utilization and blood flow are reduced, which can lower ICP. Whole-body hypothermia can be achieved by external cooling blankets, intravascular cooling devices, and body suits. Core body temperatures should be monitored using a rectal or intravascular thermometer. Sedation with a paralytic agent such as atracurium may be needed to prevent reflexive shivering, but some authors report that propofol or deep sedation are also effective [170]. The optimal means to safely rewarm hypothermic ALF patients has not been established. Because of the additional potential risks of hypothermia, including cardiac arrhythmias, worsening coagulopathy, hypotension, and impaired liver regeneration, randomized controlled trials of therapeutic and prophylactic hypothermia with ICP monitoring are needed before this investigational therapy can be recommended for routine use [171].

Seizures in ALF patients may be difficult to detect, particularly in patients receiving deep sedation or barbiturates. In one study of 42 intubated ALF patients, 31% had subclinical seizure activity, but the incidence was lower in patients who received prophylactic phenytoin [102]. As a result, continuous or intermittent electroencephalogram (EEG) monitoring is recommended by some experts for ALF patients with grade 3 or 4 coma, but this practice has not been widely adopted and other investigators have failed to demonstrate a survival benefit with prophylactic phenytoin [172]. Hypoglycemia and electrolyte disturbances should be excluded as precipitating factors for seizure development and aggressively treated if detected. Phenytoin can be intravenously administered as an 18 mg/kg loading dose over 30 min followed by 100 mg every 8 h [102]. Pentobarbital (3 mg/kg) may also be useful for refractory seizures.

Infectious aspects

Infectious complications are common in ALF patients and a leading cause of death (Table 25.12). Daily cultures of blood, urine, and sputum are recommended following admission to the ICU [107]. A diagnostic paracentesis should be performed on all patients with ascites at presentation or an unexplained fever or leukocytosis. Patients with ALF are commonly infected with staphylococcal species, streptococcal species, and gram-negative rods [1,107]. Coverage with a broad-spectrum antibiotic should be initiated if the patient develops fever, leukocytosis, or unexplained deterioration in clinical status [106,107]. A quinolone or third-generation cephalosporin is frequently used, and vancomycin can be added for patients with suspected line infection or further deterioration. Enteral decontamination with poorly absorbed antibiotics does not

---

Table 25.12 Management of infection in acute liver failure (ALF)

Sources

Bacterial infections in 80%–90% of patients with ALF
Bacteremia in ~ 25% of patients with ALF:
   Staphylococcal species
   Streptococcal species
   Gram-negative rods
Fungal infections in ~ 30% of patients with ALF:
   Candida albicans
   Aspergillus
Respiratory, urinary, and gastrointestinal sources most common:
   Invasive procedures and monitoring devices increase risk of infection

Diagnosis

High index of suspicion with low threshold to begin broad-spectrum
   antibiotics
   Suspect infection if fever, leukocytosis, left shift, or unexplained
     hypotension/acidemia/encephalopathy progression
Daily surveillance blood, urine, and sputum cultures recommended
Daily inspection of indwelling catheter sites and integument
Chest radiography as clinically indicated
Diagnostic paracentesis with cell count and culture at admission and as
   clinically indicated

Treatment

Broad-spectrum antibiotics if infection suspected
   Third-generation cephalosporin or quinolone and vancomycin
   Avoid aminoglycosides because of nephrotoxicity
Culture-guided selection of antibiotics when possible
If evidence of ongoing fever, leukocytosis, hypotension, or other sign of
   sepsis consider empirical antifungal therapy:
   Fluconazole
   Amphotericin

---

appear to alter the outcome of ALF patients who receive parenteral antibiotics [173]. If fungal infection is suspected or proven, fluconazole or amphotericin can be added.

Renal failure and fluid management

Acute renal failure in ALF is usually multifactorial, with components of acute tubular necrosis (ATN), hypovolemia, and even hepatorenal syndrome. Renal failure is particularly common in patients with acetaminophen toxicity and portends a poorer prognosis [174]. In addition to monitoring central pressures, a urinalysis and urine electrolyte determination can help distinguish ATN from hepatorenal and pre-renal causes of renal failure. Metabolic acidosis is a common complication of ALF that can be worsened by hypovolemia, infection, and poor perfusion pressures. In addition to serial arterial blood gas measurements, assessment of arterial lactate levels may prove useful in assessing fluid resuscitation, particularly in patients with acetaminophen hepatotoxicity [132]. Normal saline or other colloids may be helpful for management of hypovolemia. Avoidance of nephrotoxic agents is vitally important in ALF patients, especially the use of aminoglycosides, nonsteroidal antiinflammatory drugs and intravenous contrast dye. Nutritional therapy is also important, with enteral feeding preferred over parenteral nutrition given the high rate of infectious and metabolic complications with the latter. Hyponatremia is a poor prognostic sign in ALF, and serum sodium values less than 125 mmol/L should be avoided because hyponatremia can exacerbate cerebral edema [103].

If progressive renal failure ensues with oliguria, azotemia, or fluid overload, renal replacement therapy should be instituted. Continuous venovenous hemofiltration (CVVH) is preferred over standard hemodialysis as there are less dramatic fluid shifts, higher perfusion pressures, and less difficulty with hypotension in ALF patients [103,175]. Citrate anticoagulation may be preferred to heparin in patients with liver disease, but randomized controlled trials have not been completed.

Hemodynamic monitoring and inotropes

Acute liver failure is characterized by a hyperdynamic circulation with high cardiac output, low mean arterial pressure, and low systemic vascular resistance [103]. Following fluid resuscitation, dopamine and norepinephrine (noradrenaline) may be utilized to maintain an adequate MAP and CPP greater than 50 mmHg [1,3,103]. Vasopressin and its analogue terlipressin should not be used because of concerns for cerebral vasodilation and increased cerebral blood flow leading to worsening intracranial hypertension [176]. Placement of a Swan–Ganz catheter is helpful when inotropes or ICP monitors are utilized. Surges in systemic hypertension and bradycardia (Cushing reflex) may be a forerunner of impending uncal herniation. In terminal ALF, patients can become refractory to inotropes and die from circulatory failure. An albumin-technetium-99 (^{99}Tc) scan may be required to document the absence of blood flow in ALF patients with refractory cerebral edema. Acute liver failure patients that are declared brain dead may be suitable donors of extrahepatic organs.

Coagulopathy and bleeding

Serial INR and factor V levels provide useful prognostic information in ALF patients (Table 25.13). Therefore, routine correction of elevated INR levels with fresh frozen plasma (FFP) is not recommended unless there is evidence of active bleeding or an invasive procedure is planned. A trial of vitamin K, 10 mg subcutaneously for three consecutive days, is recommended because many ALF patients may be deficient at presentation. Before an invasive procedure such as central line placement, ICP monitoring, or liver biopsy, FFP can be infused in an attempt to decrease the INR below 1.5. However, the volume of FFP infused needs to be carefully monitored because of potential worsening of fluid overload and cerebral edema. Similarly, platelets should be maintained above 50 000 cells/mL, by platelet infusions, before invasive procedures [177]. Cryoprecipitate can be administered if the fibrinogen is less than 100 mg/dL. Acid suppression with a proton pump inhibitor should be used to prevent stress-related upper gastrointestinal bleeding and particularly in intubated ALF patients [178]. There is no efficacy or safety advantage to using sucralfate over a histamine-2 receptor blocker in critically ill patients [179].

Recombinant activated factor VII (rFVIIa; NovoSeven, NovoNordisk, Copenhagen) has been used before invasive procedures, including in ALF patients, to treat severe coagulopathy but it is not FDA approved for this indication [180,181]. The goal of rFVIIa infusion is to develop localized clot formation in areas of tissue factor release. Because of its high cost and risk of complications, most centers reserve rFVIIa infusion for patients with an INR greater than 1.5 despite infusion of at least 4 units of FFP and other depleted clotting factors. Typically a single, rapidly infused dose of 80 μg/kg enhances clot formation and normalizes the INR for 2–12 h. Contraindications to use of rFVIIa include Budd–Chiari syndrome, known or suspected malignancy, history of deep venous thrombosis/pulmonary embolism/thrombophilia, pregnancy, and hypersensitivity to vitamin K. The medication is administered as a bolus over 2–5 min immediately before invasive procedures; repeating coagulation parameters immediately thereafter is not recommended because of its short half-life. It remains unclear if additional doses or continuous infusions of rFVIIa will prevent spontaneous bleeding in ALF patients or reduce transfusion requirements during liver transplantation.

Table 25.13 Management of coagulopathy in acute liver failure (ALF)

Multifactorial etiology
Hypoprothrombinemia caused by reduced hepatic synthesis of coagulation factors and DIC/hypofibrinogenemia
Thrombocytopenia caused by reduced hepatic thrombopoietin production, consumption, acute portal hypertension, and reduced marrow production
  (e.g., aplastic anemia, acute viral illness)
Vitamin K deficiency resulting from poor oral intake and jaundice/cholestasis

Assessment
PT/INR, PTT, CBC + platelet count, and fibrinogen q 12 h
  Serial INR and factor V levels have prognostic value
Clinically significant bleeding in ~ 10% of ALF patients
  Mucocutaneous hemorrhage, GI bleeding, and bleeding at insertion sites

Management
GI bleeding prophylaxis recommended in all patients with proton pump inhibitor or H₂ blocker
Vitamin K 10 mg subcutaneously for 3 days recommended for all patients
Prophylactic FFP infusions are NOT RECOMMENDED in absence of active bleeding
  Concerns of volume overload/worsening cerebral edema
  Lose prognostic value of INR
If active bleeding or planned procedure:
  FFP to keep INR < 1.5
  Platelet infusion to keep platelet count > 50 000 cells/mL
  Cryoprecipitate to keep fibrinogen > 100 mg/dL
Consider rFVIIa only if contemplating invasive procedure such as ICP monitor placement and INR > 1.5 after 4 units of FFPᵃ
  Mechanism: enhances clot formation at areas of tissue factor release
  Contraindications: Budd–Chiari syndrome, malignancy, history of DVT/PE, pregnancy, thrombophilia
  Dose: administer as bolus rFVIIa at 80 μg/kg i.v. over 2–5 min
  Therapeutic window: half-life is 2–12 h for interventions

a Not approved by the US Food and Drug Administration for use in this setting.
CBC, complete blood count; DIC, disseminated intravascular coagulopathy; DVT, deep vein thrombosis; FFP, fresh frozen plasma; GI, gastrointestinal; INR, international normalized ratio; PE, pulmonary embolism; PT, prothrombin time; PTT, partial thromboplastin time; rFVIIa, recombinant factor VIIa.

Liver transplantation

Emergency liver transplantation is the only intervention with known survival benefit in ALF patients with a poor prognosis for recovery [182]. The outcomes with liver transplantation in ALF patients are closely linked to the severity of pretransplant illness and the nature of the graft utilized [183]. One-year survival of ALF patients undergoing liver transplantation is generally lower compared with other patients transplanted for chronic liver failure (70% vs 85%). This is probably the result of the emergent nature of the surgery, concomitant organ failure, and higher incidence of immunologically mediated graft dysfunction [5]. A rapid medical and surgical evaluation is required in all ALF transplant candidates before listing to exclude significant cardiopulmonary disease, malignancy, or other conditions that may negatively impact outcomes [1,5]. In addition, a comprehensive psychosocial evaluation to assess patient compliance, family support, and substance abuse issues is particularly important in subjects with acetaminophen overdose. More importantly, a dynamic assessment of the need and suitability of listed ALF patients for transplantation is required because of the unstable nature of this patient population and potential development of contraindications. In addition, the frequent delay in identifying a suitable organ for transplantation makes medical decision-making complex and difficult. Most centers consider the development of refractory hypotension, refractory intracranial hypertension, uncontrolled sepsis, or progressive multiorgan failure as contraindications to transplantation.

To facilitate the rapid distribution of organs to patients in need of a life-saving liver transplant, a specialized designation (i.e., status 1) was developed by UNOS for patients with a high risk of death in the next 7 days. Subjects eligible for status 1 designation include ALF patients with illness onset in the past 8 weeks, fulminant Wilson disease patients, and transplant recipients with primary graft nonfunction (PNF)

and early hepatic artery thromboses (HAT). Status 1 patients move ahead of all other listed patients with chronic liver failure and grafts are allocated to status 1 patients based on blood type, geography, and waiting time [134,184] (Table 25.14). In August 2005, modifications to the status 1 category were made including specific clinical and laboratory criteria for fulminant hepatic failure (FHF), HAT, and PNF. Livers are offered initially to status 1A adults or children whereas a status 1B category was developed for pediatric patients with chronic liver disease requiring intensive care, non-metastatic hepatoblastoma, and metabolic disease [185]. In calendar years 2004 and 2005, the Scientific Registry of Transplant Recipients (SRTR) reported that 1529 patients had been listed as status 1 [185]. Outcomes at 15 days after listing included 54.2% of patients having undergone transplantation, 16.1% dying or being too sick to transplant, 11.9% having recovered, 8.7% still listed for transplantation, and 9.1% delisted [185]. Extrapolating these data to the overall population indicates that less than 10% of the 2800 ALF patients receive a liver transplant each year in the United States.

Investigational surgical approaches

Total hepatectomy has been proposed as a means to stabilize ALF patients awaiting transplantation [186–188]. Theoretically, removal of the necrotic liver should reduce the release of proinflammatory cytokines and other toxic substances that may contribute to cerebral edema. However, the safety and efficacy of this radical intervention has not been established, and a hepatectomy should only be performed close to the time of planned liver transplantation. Auxiliary partial orthotopic liver transplantation (APOLT) involves the placement of a partial liver graft either heterotopically below the native liver or orthotopically following partial resection of the native liver [189,190]. Graft function is maintained posttransplant by standard immunosuppression. After recovery of

Table 25.14 Outcome of 720 UNOS status 1 patients listed between September 1999 and March 2002

	ALF Non-APAP	ALF APAP	PNF	HAT
n	312	76	268	67
Age (years)	39	32	50	48
Female	67%	80%	37%	30%
Lab MELD at listing	36	37	30	20
Outcomes				
Transplanted	60%	32%	56%	69%
Died on list	23%	22%	11%	6%
Survived without transplant	16%	46%	33%	25%

ALF, acute liver failure; APAP, acetaminophen; HAT, hepatic artery thromboses; MELD, Model for End-stage Liver Disease; PNF, primary nonfunction; UNOS, United Network for Organ Sharing.
Adapted from Wiesner [184].

the native liver has been confirmed radiographically and histologically, immunosuppression can be withdrawn, which will lead to immunological involution of the graft. Although 40% of APOLT recipients were able to be successfully weaned from immunosuppression, initial reports described high rates of surgical complications and retransplantation because of PNF [189]. Therefore, APOLT is not a recommended treatment for ALF patients outside clinical trials.

Living donor liver transplantation has also been reported for ALF patients given the critical shortage of suitable donor organs [191–194]. However, the requirement for rapid assessment and mobilization of the appropriate teams for living donor transplantation has raised concerns for donor safety and potential coercion. Nonetheless, in parts of the world where cadaveric organ donation is uncommon, living donor liver transplantation has been used in both adult and pediatric ALF patients, with outcomes inferior to whole cadaveric transplants because of higher rates of biliary and vascular complications, and PNF. In addition, the potential for delayed graft function with "small-for-size" grafts that are less than 0.8% of the recipient's body weight is of concern [192]. Therefore, living donor liver transplantation is not advisable for adult ALF patients if a whole cadaveric liver is available.

The intravascular or transsplenic transplantation of human hepatocytes has also been investigated in patients with ALF or metabolic defects [195–197]. Early experience appeared promising but complications from shunting of transplanted hepatocytes to extraabdominal vascular beds and limited survival of the hepatocytes in the liver or spleen has been reported [198]. A further hurdle is the large mass of human hepatocytes required to replace a whole human liver, besides difficulties with cell viability, immunological tolerance, and engraftment. Nonetheless, further work in this area utilizing hepatic stem cells may prove worthwhile if the signals of cellular differentiation and engraftment can be unraveled [199].

Artificial and bioartificial liver devices

Both artificial and bioartificial liver support devices are under active development for patients with acute and acute-on-chronic liver failure [200–202] (Table 25.15). Patients with ALF are an ideal population to consider studying liver replacement devices in an effort to bridge them to spontaneous recovery through native liver regeneration. However, clinical trial design is difficult because of variation in spontaneous recovery rates and the availability of liver transplantation. The ideal liver replacement device would perform normal hepatocyte functions, including detoxification, metabolism, and synthesis of crucial proteins. Early attempts at providing replacement of liver detoxification included hemodialysis, hemofiltration, exchange transfusion, plasma exchange, and

Table 25.15 Liver support systems under development

Device	Mechanism	Considerations	Outcomes
Artificial devices			
Charcoal hemoperfusion [203]	Blood perfused through activated charcoal column	Only provides filtration function; risk of thrombocytopenia and coagulopathy	Large RCT in ALF did not show any survival benefit
BioLogic-DT (formerly HemoTherapies, San Diego, CA) [219]	Hemodiabsorption with powdered activated charcoal	FDA approved for toxin overdose: limited use in US centers	Small controlled trials; no survival benefit
Molecular Absorbent Recycling System (MARS) (Gambro, Lakewood, CO) [205–207]	Albumin dialysis in series with hemodialyzer; removes water-soluble and albumin-bound toxins	Requires heparin; ?continuous or intermittent use; 50-kDa cutoff	Small ALF series showed improved hemodynamics; large RCT in France ongoing
Prometheus (Fresenius, Bad Homburg, Germany) [208,209]	Albumin dialysis with fractionated plasma separation and absorption with high-flux hemodialysis	Wide application for albumin-based dialysis devices; 300-kDa cutoff	11 acute-on-chronic liver failure patients; 10 hepatorenal patients
Bioartificial devices			
Hepatix ELAD (Extracorporeal Liver Assist Device) (Vitagen, San Diego, CA) [211]	Immortalized human hepatoblastoma cells in extracorporeal bioreactor	?Anticoagulation, bleeding; risk of transmitting transformed cells; intermittent vs continuous perfusion	Pilot study with 24 ALF patients; minimal survival benefit
HepatAssist device (Arbios Systems, Pasadena, CA) [212,217]	100 g of cryopreserved porcine hepatocytes in dialysis cartridge	Concern of zoonoses, xenoantibodies, and cell migration; requires plasmapheresis and anticoagulation	RCT with 171 ALF patients – no improvement in 30-day survival compared with controls

ALF, acute liver failure; FDA, US Food and Drug Administration; RCT, randomized controlled trial.

resin hemoperfusion, but none of these interventions led to improved outcomes [203,204]. Newer artificial detoxification devices, such as the BioLogic-DT and Molecular Absorbent Recirculating System (MARS), utilize charcoal or other adherent particles in an extracorporeal circuit [205–207]. The MARS device employs a combination of charcoal filters with albumin dialysis to remove water-soluble and albumin-bound toxins less than 50 kDa in size. Prometheus is another device that utilizes fractionated plasma separation and albumin dialysis, with a higher molecular weight cutoff of 300 kDa, which may lead to improved clearance of toxins [208,209]. However, all of these artificial devices only provide filtration function. In addition, there is a concern for complications related to the need for arterial and venous cannulation, anticoagulation, and other consequences of extracorporeal perfusion [201]. With the sorbent-based extracorporeal systems, improvement in hepatic encephalopathy has been reported but overall improvement in hepatic function or long-term benefit has not been shown [4,202]. A metaanalysis of the various artificial and bioartificial liver support devices demonstrated no overall reduction in mortality in ALF patients (RR = 0.95, 95% CI 0.71–1.29) but a possible mortality benefit in acute-on-chronic liver failure (RR = 0.67, 95% CI 0.51–0.90) suggesting the need for more studies with improved devices [210].

Bioartificial liver support devices utilize either human or other mammalian-derived hepatocytes in an extracorporeal circuit [211,212]. An advantage of these systems is that they can theoretically synthesize proteins and metabolize xenobiotics in addition to standard filtration and detoxification. However, maintaining viable and sterile hepatocytes for continuous extracorporeal use is a formidable challenge. In addition, there are concerns about transmission of hepatocytes to the host and activation of the clotting cascade. The use of porcine or other mammalian tissues can also lead to additional immunological problems, with development of xenoantibodies and potential infections including zoonoses [201,213]. Ex vivo whole pig-liver perfusion has been described in a small number of ALF patients as a bridge to transplant [214,215]. However, the development of xenoantibodies and the short duration of liver support provided has limited the application of this technique. Xenotransplantation of whole primate livers has also been reported but the development of rejection through xenoantibodies has precluded further attempts [216].

The largest randomized, controlled trial to assess the safety and efficacy of a bioartificial liver device in ALF patients to date has been reported [217,218]. The HepatAssist device, which contains 100 g of porcine hepatocytes loaded in a dialysis cartridge in series with charcoal filters, was utilized in this study of 171 patients. Patients with fulminant or subfulminant liver failure and those with PNF following liver transplantation were randomized to receive a daily 6-h treatment with the HepatAssist device or standard care. Although 30-day survival was found to be similar in both treatment groups (71% HepatAssist vs 62% control, $P = 0.26$), subgroup

analysis revealed a significantly higher survival rate in patients with hyperacute liver failure treated with the HepatAssist device (risk ratio 0.56; $P = 0.048$). This landmark study highlighted the difficulties of performing clinical trials in ALF and the need for adequate patient inclusion criteria and clinically relevant end points. In summary, neither artificial nor bioartificial liver devices are established treatment modalities for ALF patients. Further refinements of device components, perfusion circuitry, and understanding of liver regeneration are needed to help determine the potential therapeutic role of these devices in the future management of ALF patients.

References

1. Sass DA, Shakil AO. Fulminant hepatic failure. Liver Transplant 2005;11:594.
2. Trey C, Davidson CS. The management of fulminant hepatic failure. In: Popper H, Schaffner F (eds). Progress in Liver Disease. New York: Grune & Stratton, 1970:282.
3. Polson JP, Lee WM. AASLD position paper: The management of acute liver failure. Hepatology 2005;41:1179.
4. Lee WM. Acute liver failure in the United States. Semin Liver Dis 2003;23:217.
5. Higgins PD, Fontana RJ. Liver transplantation in acute liver failure. Panminerva Med 2002; 52:93.
6. Hoofnagle JH, Carithers RL, Shapiro C, et al. Fulminant hepatic failure: Summary of a workshop. Hepatology 1995;21:240.
7. Ostapowicz GA, Fontana RJ, Schiodt FV, et al. Results of a prospective study of acute liver failure at 17 tertiary care centers in the United States. Ann Intern Med 2002;137:947.
8. Squires RH, Shneider BL, Bucuvalas J, et al. Acute liver failure in children: the first 348 patients in the pediatric acute liver failure study group. J Pediatr 2006;148:652.
9. O'Grady JG, Schalm SW, Williams R. Acute liver failure: Redefining the syndromes. Lancet 1993;342:273.
10. Schiodt RV, Atillasoy E, Shakil A, et al. Etiology and outcome for 295 patients with acute liver failure in the United States. Liver Transpl Surg 1999;5:29.
11. Shakil A, Kramer D, Mazariegos G, et al. Acute liver failure: Clinical features, outcome analysis, and applicability of prognostic criteria. Liver Transplant 2000;6:163.
12. Rakela J, Mosley JW, Edwards VM, et al. A double-blinded randomized trial of hydrocortisone in acute hepatic failure. Dig Dis Sci 1991;36:1223.
13. Schiodt FV, Davern TA, Shakil O, et al. Viral hepatitis-related acute liver failure. Am J Gastroenterol 2003;98:448.
14. Acharya SK, Panda SK, Saxena A, et al. Acute hepatic failure in India: A perspective from the East. J Gastroenterol Hepatol 2000;15:473.
15. Kim WR, Brown RS, Terrault NA, et al. Burden of liver disease in the United States: Summary of a workshop. Hepatology 2002;36:227.
16. Bernal W. Changing patterns of causation and the use of transplantation in the United Kingdom. Semin Liver Dis 2003;23:227.
17. Jalan R. Acute liver failure: Current management and future prospects. J Hepatol 2005;42:S115.
18. Cheng VC, Lo CM, Lau GK. Current issues and treatment of fulminant hepatic failure including transplantation in Hong Kong and the Far East. Semin Liver Dis 2003;23:239.
19. Larson AM, Polson J, Fontana RJ, et al. Acetaminophen-induced acute liver failure: Results of a United States multicenter, prospective study. Hepatology 2005;42:1364.
20. Ritt DJ, Whelan G, Werner DJ, et al. Acute hepatic necrosis with stupor or coma. An analysis of 31 patients. Medicine 1969;48:151.
21. James LP, Mayeux PR, Hinson JA. Acetaminophen-induced hepatotoxicity. Drug Metab Dispos 2003;31:1499.

22. Slattery JT, Nelson SD, Thummel KE. The complex interaction between ethanol and acetaminophen. Clin Pharmacol Ther 1996;60:241.

23. Schmidt LE, Dalhoff K, Poulsen HE. Acute versus chronic alcohol consumption in acetaminophen-induced hepatotoxicity. Hepatology 2002;35:876.

24. Nolan CM, Sandblom RE, Thummel KE, et al. Hepatotoxicity associated with acetaminophen usage in patients receiving multiple drug therapy for tuberculosis. Chest 1994;105:408.

25. Whitcomb DC, Block GD. Association of acetaminophen hepatotoxicity with fasting and alcohol use. JAMA 1994;272:1845.

26. Schiodt FV, Rochling FA, Casey DL, et al. Acetaminophen toxicity in an urban county hospital. N Engl J Med 1997;337:1112.

27. Zimmerman HJ, Maddrey WC. Acetaminophen hepatotoxicity with regular intake of alcohol: Analysis of instances of therapeutic misadventure. Hepatology 1995;22:767.

28. Watkins PB, Kaplowitz N, Slattery JT, et al. Aminotransferase elevations in healthy adults receiving 4 grams of acetaminophen daily. JAMA 2006;296:87.

29. Nourjah P, Ahmad SR, Karowski C, et al. Estimates of acetaminophen (paracetamol)-associated overdoses in the United States. Pharmacoepidem Dr S 2006;15:398.

30. Lovitz TL, Klein-Schwartz W, White S, et al. 2000 annual report of the American Association of Poison Control centers toxic exposure surveillance system. Am J Emerg Med 2001;19:337.

31. Bond Gr, Hite LK. Population based incidence and outcome of acetaminophen poisoning by type of ingestion. Acad Emerg Med 1999;6:1115.

32. McCormick PA, Treanor D, McCormack, et al. Early death from paracetamol (acetaminophen) induced fulminant hepatic failure without cerebral oedema. J Hepatol 2003;39:547.

33. Rumack BH. Acetaminophen hepatotoxicity: The first 35 years. J Toxicol Clin Toxicol 2002;40:3.

34. Polson J, Orsulak PJ, Wians F, et al. Elevated bilirubin may cause false positive acetaminophen levels in hepatitis patients. Hepatology 2004;40:496A [abstract].

35. James LP, Farrar HC, Sullivan JE, et al. Measurement of acetaminophen-protein adducts in children and adolescents with acetaminophen overdoses. J Clin Phamacol 2001;41:846.

36. James LP, Alonso EM, Hynan LS, et al. Detection of acetaminophen protein adducts in children with acute liver failure of indeterminate cause. Pediatrics 2006;118:676.

37. Davern TJ, James LP, Hinson J, et al. Measurement of serum acetaminophen-protein adducts in patients with acute liver failure. Gastroenterology 2006;130:687.

38. Lee WM. Acetaminophen and the U.S. Acute Liver Failure Study Group: Lowering the risks of hepatic failure. Hepatology 2004;40:6.

39. Polson J, Ocama P, Larson AM, et al. Role of acetaminophen in acute liver failure due to viral hepatitis. Hepatology 2003;34:544A [abstract].

40. Rezende G, Roque-Afonso AM, Samuel D, et al. Viral and clinical factors associated with the fulminant course of hepatitis A infection. Hepatology 2003;38:613.

41. Sato RL, Wong JJ, Sumida SM, et al. Efficacy of superactivated charcoal administration late (3 hours) after acetaminophen overdose. Am J Emerg Med 2003;21:189.

42. Smilkstein MJ, Knapp GL, Kulig KW, et al. Efficacy of oral N-acetylcysteine in the treatment of acetaminophen overdose. N Engl J Med 1988;319:1557.

43. Makin AJ, Wendon J, Williams R. A 7-year experience of severe acetaminophen-induced hepatotoxicity (1987–1993). Gastroenterology 1995;109:1907.

44. Kao LW, Kirk MA, Furbee RB, et al. What is the rate of adverse events after oral N-acetylcysteine administered by the intravenous route to patients with suspected acetaminophen poisoning? Ann Emerg Med 2003;42:741.

45. Rumack BH. Acetaminophen misconceptions. Hepatology 2004;40:10.

46. Kaplowitz N. Acetaminophen hepatotoxicity: What do we know, what we don't know, and what do we do next? Hepatology 2004; 40:24.

47. Hawton K, Townsend E, Deeks J, et al. Effects of legislation restricting pack sizes of paracetamol and salicylate on self poisoning in the United Kingdom: Before and after study. BMJ 2001;322:1.

48. Hawton K, Simkin S, Deeks J, et al. UK legislation in analgesic packs: Before and after study of long term effect on poisonings. BMJ 2004; 329:1076.

49. Food and Drug Administration, 21 CRF Parts 201 and 343. Internal analgesic, antipyretic, and antirheumatic drug products for over the counter human use: proposed amendment of the tentative final monograph, Required warnings and other labeling. Federal Register Parts 201 and 343 (12/26/06).

50. Taylor RM, Davern T, Munoz S, et al. Fulminant hepatitis A virus in the United States: Incidence, prognosis, and outcomes. Hepatology 2006;44:1589.

51. Wai CT, Fontana RJ, Polson J, et al. Clinical outcome and virological characteristics of hepatitis B related acute liver failure in the United States. J Viral Hepat 2005;12:192.

52. Fujiwara K, Mochida S. Indications and criteria for liver transplantation for fulminant hepatic failure. J Gastroenterol 2001;37:74.

53. Teo EK, Ostapowicz G, Hussain M, et al. Hepatitis B infection in patients with acute liver failure in the United States. Hepatology 2001;33:972.

54. Schmilovitz-Weiss H, Ben-Ari Z, Sikular E, et al. Lamivudine treatment for acute severe hepatitis B: A pilot study. Liver Int 2004;24: 547.

55. Kharoo MS, Kamili S. Aetiology and prognostic factors in acute liver failure in India. J Viral Hepat 2003;10:224.

56. Pal R, Aggarwal R, Naik SR, et al. Immunological alterations in pregnant women with acute hepatitis E. J Gastroenterol Hepatol 2005; 20:1094.

57. Farci P, Alter HJ, Shimoda A, et al. Hepatitis C virus associated fulminant hepatic failure. N Engl J Med 199;335:631.

58. Kang AH, Graves CR. Herpes simplex hepatitis in pregnancy: A case report and review of the literature. Obstet Gynecol Surg 1999;54:463.

59. Peters DJ, Greene WH, Ruggiero F, et al. Herpes simplex induced fulminant hepatitis in adults: a call for empiric therapy. Dig Dis Sci 2000;45:2399.

60. Dits H, Frans E, Wilmer A, et al. Varicella-zoster virus infection associated with acute liver failure. Clin Infect Dis 1998;27:209.

61. Sgro C, Clinard F, Ouazir L, et al. Incidence of drug-induced hepatic injuries: A French population-based study. Hepatology 2002;36:451.

62. Lee WM, Senior JR. Recognizing drug induced liver injury: current problems, possible solutions. Toxicol Pathol 2005;33:155.

63. Bjornsson E, Olsson R. Outcome and prognostic markers in severe drug-induced liver disease. Hepatology 2005;42:481.

64. Andrade RJ, Lucena MI, Fernandez MC, et al. Drug-induced liver injury: An análisis of 461 incidences submitted to the Spanish registry over a 10-year period. Gastroenterology 2005;129:512.

65. Lee WM. Drug-induced hepatotoxicity. N Engl J Med 2003;349:474.

66. Fontana RJ, Shakil AO, Greenson JK, et al. Acute liver failure due to amoxicillin and amoxicillin/clavulanate. Dig Dis Sci 2005;50:1785.

67. Sharp JR, Ishak KG, Zimmerman HJ. Chronic active hepatitis and severe hepatic necrosis associated with nitrofurantoin. Ann Intern Med 1980;92:14.

68. Verma A, Lilienfeld DE. The need for a population-based surveillance system for liver disease in the United States. Pharmacoepidem Dr S 2004;13:821.

69. Watkins PB, Seeff LB. Drug Induced Liver Injury: Summary of a Single Topic Clinical Research Conference. Hepatology 2006;43:618.

70. Aithal PG, Day CP. The natural history of histologically proved drug induced liver disease. Gut 1999;44:731.

71. Dechene A, Treichel U, Gerken G, et al. Effectiveness of a steroid and ursodeoxycholic acid combination therapy with drug induced subactue liver failure. Hepatology 2005;42:358A [abstract].

72. Danan G, Benichou C. Causality assessment of adverse reactions – A novel method based on conclusions of international consensus meetings: Application to drug-induced liver injuries. J Clin Epidemiol 1993;46:1223.

73. Lucena MI, Camargo R, Andrade RJ, et al. Comparison of two clinical scales for causality assessment in hepatotoxicity. Hepatology 2001;33:123.

74. Sticke F, Baumuller HM, Seitz K, et al. Hepatitis induced by kava. J Hepatology 2003;39:62.

75. Favreau JT, Fyu ML, Braunstein G, et al. Severe hepatotoxicity associated with the dietary supplement lipokinetix. Ann Intern Med 2002;136:590.

76. Estes JD, Stolpman D, Olyaei, et al. High prevalence of potentially hepatotoxic herbal supplement use in patients with fulminant hepatic failure. Arch Surg 2003;138:852.

77. Ohmori S, Shiraki K, Inoue H, et al. Clinical characteristics and prognostic indicators of drug induced fulminant hepatic failure. Hepato-Gastroenterology 2003;50:1531.

78. Russo MW, Galanko JA, Shrestha R, et al. Liver transplantation for acute liver failure from drug induced liver injury in the United States. Liver Transpl 2004;10:1018.

79. Schiodt FV, Fontana RJ, Larson AM, et al. Autoimmune hepatitis-induced acute liver failure in the United States. Gastroenterology 2002;6:M1638.

80. Rolfes DB, Ishak KG. Acute fatty liver of pregnancy: a clinicopathologic study of 35 cases. Hepatology 1985;5:1149.

81. Weinstein L. Syndrome of hemolysis, elevated liver enzymes, and low platelet count: a severe consequence of hypertension in pregnancy. Am J Obstet Gynecol 1982;142:159.

82. Pereira SP, O'Donohue J, Wendon J, et al. Maternal and perinatal outcome in severe pregnancy-related liver disease. Hepatology 1997;26:1258.

83. Ibdah JA, Bennett MJ, Rinaldo P, et al. A fetal fatty-acid oxidation disorder as a cause of liver disease in pregnant women. N Engl J Med 1999;340:1723.

84. Fickert P, Ramschak H, Kenner L, et al. Acute Budd–Chiari syndrome with fulminant hepatic failure in a pregnant woman with factor V Leiden mutation. Gastroenterology 1996;111:1670.

85. Min AD, Atillasoy EO, Schwartz ME, et al. Reassessing the role of medical therapy in the management of hepatic vein thrombosis. Liver Transplant 1997;3:423.

86. Olzinski AT, Sanyal AJ. Treating Budd–Chiari syndrome: Making rational choices from a myriad of options. J Clin Gastroenterol 2000;30:155.

87. Taylor RM, Fontana RJ, Shakil AO, et al. Acute liver failure due to ischemic hepatitis: Natural history and predictors of outcome in a prospective, multi-center U.S. study. Gastroenterology 2005;128(4 Suppl. 2):A-706 [abstract].

88. Klein AS, Hart J, Brems JJ, et al. Amanita poisoning: treatment and the role of liver transplantation. Am J Med 1989;86:187.

89. Bartolini SO, Giannine A, Botti P, et al. Amanita poisoning: a clinical histopathological study of 64 cases of intoxication. Hepatogastroenterology 1985;32:299.

90. Broussard CN, Aggarwal A, Lacey SR, et al. Mushroom poisoning – from diarrhea to liver transplantation. Am J Gastroenterol 2001;96:3195.

91. Roberts EA, Schilsky ML. AASLD Practice guidelines: A practice guideline on Wilson disease. Hepatology 2003;37:1475.

92. Nazer H, Ede RJ, Mowat AP, et al. Wilson's disease: clinical presentation and use of prognostic index. Gut 1986;27:1377.

93. Korman JS, Volenberg I, Balko J, et al. Screening for Wilson disease in acute liver failure by serum testing: A comparison of currently used tests. Gastroenterology 2004;126:706A.

94. Woolf GM, Petrovic LM, Rojter SE, et al. Acute liver failure due to lymphoma. A diagnostic concern when considering liver transplantation. Dig Dis Sci 1994;391:1351.

95. Shehab TM, Kaminski MS, Lok ASF. Case report: acute liver failure due to hepatic involvement by hematologic malignancy. Dig Dis Sci 1997;42:1400.

96. Wigg AJ, Gunson BK, Mutimer DJ. Outcomes following liver transplantation for seronegative acute liver failure: Experience during a 12-year period with more than 100 patients. Liver Transplant 2005;11:27.

97. Lee WM, Brown KE, Young NS, et al. Brief report: No evidence of parvovirus B19 or hepatitis E virus as causes of acute liver failure. Dig Dis Sci 2006;51:1712.

98. Umemura T, Tanaka E, Ostapowicz G, et al. Investigation of SEN virus infection in patients with cryptogenic acute liver failure, hepatitis-associated aplastic anemia, or acute and chronic non-A-E hepatitis. J Inf Dis 2003;188:1545.

99. Riordan SM, Williams R. Mechanisms of hepatocyte injury, multi-organ failure, and prognostic criteria in acute liver failure. Semin Liver Dis 2003;23:203.

100. Blei AT. The pathophysiology of brain edema in acute liver failure. Neurochem Int 2005;47:71.

101. Vaquero J, Chung C, Cahill ME, et al. Pathogenesis of hepatic encephalopathy in acute liver failure. Semin Liver Dis 2003;23:259.

102. Ellis AJ, Wendon JA, Williams R. Subclinical seizure activity and prophylactic phenytoin infusion in acute liver failure: A controlled clinical trial. Hepatology 2000;32:536.

103. Jalan R. Pathophysiological basis of therapy of raised intracranial pressure in acute liver failure. Neurochem Int 2005;47:78.

104. Clemmesen JO, Larsen FS, Kondrup J, et al. Cerebral herniation in patients with acute liver failure is correlated with arterial ammonia concentration. Hepatology 1999;29:648.

105. Larsen FS, Ejlersen E, Hansen BA, et al. Functional loss of cerebral blood flow autoregulation in patient with fulminant hepatic failure. J Hepatol 1995;23:212.

106. Rolando N, Harvey F, Brahm J, et al. Prospective study of bacterial infection in acute liver failure: An analysis of fifty patients. Hepatology 1990;11:49.

107. Wade J, Rolando N, Philpott-Howard J, et al. Timing and etiology of bacterial infections in a liver intensive care unit J Hosp Infect 2003;53:144.

108. Rolando N, Harvey F, Brahm J, et al. Fungal infection: A common, unrecognized complication of acute liver failure. J Hepatol 1991;12:1.

109. Vaquero J, Polson J, Chung C, et al. Infection and the progression of encephalopathy in acute liver failure. Gastroenterology 2003;125:755.

110. Rolando N, Wade J, Davalos M, et al. The systemic inflammatory response syndrome in acute liver failure. Hepatology 2000;32:734.

111. Pereira SP, Langley PG, Williams R. The management of abnormalities of hemostasis in acute liver failure. Semin Liver Dis 1996;16:403.

112. Schiodt FV, Balko J, Schilsky M, et al. Thrombopoietin in acute liver failure. Hepatology 2003;37:558.

113. Pernambuco JR, Langley PG, Hughes RD, et al. Activation of the fibrinolytic system in patients with fulminant liver failure. Hepatology 1993;18:1350.

114. Pereira LM, Langley PG, Hayllar KM, et al. Coagulation factor V and VII/V ratio as predictors of outcome in paracetamol induced fulminant hepatic failure: relation to other prognostic indicators. Gut 1992;33:98.

115. Izumi S, Langley PG, Wendon J, et al. Coagulation factor V levels as a prognostic indicator in fulminant hepatic failure. Hepatology 1996;23:1507.

116. Elinav E, Ben-Dov I, Hai-Am E, et al. The predictive value of admission and follow up factor V and VII levels in patients with acute hepatitis and coagulopathy. J Hepatol 2005;42:82.

117. Schiodt FV, Rossaro L, Stravitz RT, et al. Gc-globulin and prognosis in acute liver failure. Liver Transplant 2005;11:1223.

118. Harry R, Auzinger G, Wendon J. The clinical importance of adrenal insufficiency in acute hepatic dysfunction. Hepatology 2002;36:395.

119. Marik PE, Gayowski T, Starzl TE, for the Hepatic Cortisol Research and Adrenal Pathophysiology Study Group. The hepatoadrenal syndrome: A common yet unrecognized clinical condition. Crit Care Med 2005;33:1254.

120. Baudouin SV, Howdle P, O'Grady JG, et al. Acute lung injury in fulminant hepatic failure following paracetamol poisoning. Thorax 1995;50:399.

121. Bihari DJ, Gimson AE, Williams R. Cardiovascular, pulmonary, and renal complications of fulminant hepatic failure. Semin Liver Dis 1986;6:119.

122. Ring-Larsen H, Palazzo U. Renal failure in fulminant hepatic failure and terminal cirrhosis: a comparison between incidence, types, and prognosis. Gut 1981;22:585.

123. Rakela J, Lange SM, Ludwig J, et al. Fulminant hepatitis: Mayo Clinic experience with 34 cases. Mayo Clin Proc 1985;60:289.

124. Neuberger J. Prediction of survival for patients with fulminant hepatic failure. Hepatology 2005;41:19.

125. O'Grady J. Attempting to predict the unpredictable in acute liver injury. J Hepatol 2005;42:5.

126. Bernuau J, Goudau A, Poynard T, et al. Multivariate analysis of prognostic factors in fulminant hepatitis B. Hepatology 1986;6:648.

127. Bismuth H, Samuel D, Castaing D, et al. Orthotopic liver transplantation in fulminant and subfulminant hepatitis. The Paul Brousse experience. Ann Surg 1995;222:109.

128. Riordan SM, Williams R. Use and validation of selection criteria for liver transplantation in acute liver failure [editorial]. Liver Transplant 2000;6:170.

129. O'Grady JG, Alexander GJ, Hayllar KM, et al. Early indicators of prognosis in fulminant hepatic failure. Gastroenterology 1989;97:439.

130. Anand AC, Nightingale P, Neuberger JM. Early indicators of prognosis in fulminant hepatic failure: an assessment of the King's criteria. J Hepatol 1997;26:62.

131. Pauwels A, Mostefa-Kara N, Florent C, et al. Emergency liver transplantation for acute liver failure: Evaluation of London and Clichy criteria. J Hepatol 1993;17:124.

132. Bernal W, Donaldson N, Wyncoll D, et al. Blood lactate as an early predictor of outcome in paracetamol-induced acute liver failure: a cohort study. Lancet 2002;359:558.

133. Weisner R, Edwards E, Freeman R, et al. Model for end-stage liver disease (MELD) and allocation of donor livers. Gastroenterology 2003;124:91.

134. Kremers WK, Ijperen MV, Kim WR, et al. MELD score as a predictor of pretransplant and posttransplant survival in OPTN/UNOS status 1 patients. Hepatology 2004;39:764.

135. Aydin C, Berk B, Fung JJ, et al. Applicability of MELD scoring system to predict prognosis in patients with acute liver failure. Hepatology 2003;38:554A [abstract].

136. Mitchell I, Bihari D, Chang R, et al. Earlier identification of patients at risk from acetaminophen-induced acute liver failure. Crit Care Med 1998;26:279.

137. Bernal W, Wendon J, Rela M, et al. Use and outcome of liver transplantation in acetaminophen-induced acute liver failure. Hepatology 1998;27:1050.

138. Davern TJ, Polson J, Lalani E, et al. Serum phosphate levels as a predictor of clinical outcome in acetaminophen induced acute liver failure. Hepatology 2003; AASLD meeting abstract.

139. Schmidt LE, Dalhoff K. Serum phosphate is an early predictor of outcome in severe acetaminophen-induced hepatotoxicity. Hepatology 2002;36:659.

140. Baquerizo A, Anselmo D, Shackleton C, et al. Phosphorus as an early predictive factor in patients with acute liver failure. Transplantation 2003;75:2007.

141. Chung PY, Sitrin MD, Te HS. Serum phosphorus levels predict clinical outcome in fulminant hepatic failure. Liver Transplant 2003;9:248.

142. Schiodt FV, Ostapowicz G, Murray N, et al. Alpha-fetoprotein and prognosis in acute liver failure. Liver Transplant 2006;12:1776.

143. Schmidt LE, Dalhoff K. Alpha-fetoprotein is a predictor of outcome in acetaminophen-induced liver injury. Hepatology 2005;41:26.

144. Dabos KJ, Newsome PN, Parkinson JA, et al. Biochemical prognostic markers of outcome in non-paracetamol-induced fulminant hepatic failure. Transplantation 2004;77:200.

145. Shakil AO, Jones BC, Lee RG, et al. Prognostic value of abdominal CT scanning and hepatic histopathology in patients with acute liver failure. Dig Dis Sci 2000;45:334.

146. Hanau C, Munoz SJ, Rubin R. Histopathological heterogeneity in fulminant hepatic failure. Hepatology 1995;21:345.

147. Ware AJ, Jones RE, Shorey JW, et al. A controlled trial of steroid therapy in massive hepatic necrosis. Am J Gastroenterol 1974;62:1303.

148. EASL study group. Randomised trial of steroid therapy in acute liver failure. Gut 1979;20:620.

149. Sterling RK, Luketic VA, Sanyal AJ, et al. Treatment of fulminant hepatic failure with intravenous prostaglandin E1. Liver Transpl Surg 1998;4:424.

150. Walsh TS, Hopton P, Philips BJ, et al. The effect of N-acetylcysteine on oxygen transport and uptake in patients with fulminant hepatic failure. Hepatology 1998;27:1332.

151. Harrison PM, Wendon JA, Gimson ES, et al. Improvement by acetylcysteine of hemodynamics and oxygen transport in fulminant hepatic failure. N Engl J Med 1991;324:1852.

152. Sklar GE, Subramaniam M. Acetylcysteine treatment for non-acetaminophen-induced acute liver failure. Ann Pharmacother 2004;38:498.

153. Munoz SJ, Robinson M, Northrup B, et al. Elevated intracranial pressure and computed tomography of the brain in fulminant hepatocellular failure. Hepatology 1991;13:209.

154. Wijdicks EFM, Plevak DJ, Rakela J, et al. Clinical and radiologic features of cerebral edema in fulminant hepatic failure. Mayo Clin Proc 1995;70:119.

155. Itai Y, Sekiyama K, Ahmadi T, et al. Fulminant hepatic failure: observation with serial CT. Radiology 1997;202:379.

156. Butterworth RF. Pathogenesis of hepatic encephalopathy: new insights from neuroimaging and molecular studies. J Hepatol 2003;39:278.

157. McConnell JR, Antonson DL, Ong CS, et al. Proton spectroscopy of brain glutamine in acute liver failure. Hepatology 1995;22:69.

158. Vaquero J, Fontana RJ, Larson AM, et al. Complications and use of intracranial pressure monitoring in patients with acute liver failure and severe encephalopathy. Liver Transplant 2005;11:1581.

159. Blei AT, Olafsson S, Webster S, et al. Complications of intracranial pressure monitoring in fulminant hepatic failure. Lancet 1993;341:157.

160. Durward QJ, Amacher AL, Del Maestro RF, et al. Cerebral and cardiovascular responses to changes in head elevation in patients with intracranial hypertension. J Neurosurg 1983;59:938.

161. Strauss G, Hansen BA, Knudsen GM, et al. Hyperventilation restores cerebral blood flow autoregulation in patients with acute liver failure. J Hepatol 1998;28:199.

162. Alba L, Hay JE, Angulo P, et al. Lactulose therapy in acute liver failure. J Hepatol 2002;36:33A.

163. Canalese J, Gimson AE, Davis C, et al. Controlled trial of dexamethasone and mannitol for the cerebral oedema of fulminant hepatic failure. Gut 1982;23:625.

164. Murphy N, Auzinger G, Bernal W, et al. The effect of hypertonic sodium chloride on intracranial pressure in patients with acute liver failure. Hepatology 2004;39:464.

165. Forbes A, Alexander GJ, O'Grady JG, et al. Thiopental infusion in the treatment of intracranial hypertension complicating fulminant hepatic failure. Hepatology 1989;10:306.

166. Wijkicks EF, Nyberg SL. Propofol to control intracranial pressure in fulminant hepatic failure. Transplant Proc 2002;34:1220.

167. Jalan R, Olde Damink SW, Deutz NE, et al. Moderate hypothermia for uncontrolled intracranial hypertension in acute liver failure. Lancet 1999;354:1164.

168. Jalan R, Olde Damink SW, Deutz NE, et al. Restoration of cerebral blood flow autoregulation and reactivity to carbon dioxide in acute liver failure by moderate hypothermia. Hepatology 2001;34:50.

169. Jalan R, Olde Damink SW, Deutz NE, et al. Moderate hypothermia prevents cerebral hyperemia and increase in intracranial pressure in patients undergoing liver transplantation for acute liver failure. Transplantation 2003;75:2034.

170. Jalan R, Olde Damink SW, Deutz NE, et al. Moderate hypothermia in patients with acute liver failure and uncontrolled intracranial hypertension. Gastroenterology 2004;127:1338.

171. Vaquero J, Blei AT. Cooling the patient with acute liver failure. Gastroenterology 2004;127:1626.

172. Bhatia V, Batra Y, Acharya SK. Prophylactic phenytoin does not improve cerebral edema or survival in acute liver failure. A controlled clinical trial. J Hepatol 2004;42:89.

173. Rolando N, Gimson A, Wade J, et al. Prospective controlled trial of selective parenteral and enteral antimicrobial regimen in fulminant liver failure. Hepatology 1993;17:196.

174. Cobden I, Record CO, Ward MK, et al. Paracetamol-induced acute renal failure in the absence of fulminant liver damage. BMJ 1982;284:21.

175. Davenport A, Will EJ, Davidson AM. Improved cardiovascular stability during continuous modes of renal replacement therapy in critically ill patients with acute hepatic and renal failure. Crit Care Med 1993;21:328.

176. Shawcross DL, Davies NA, Mookerjee RP, et al. Worsening of cerebral hyperemia by the administration of terlipressin in acute liver failure with severe encephalopathy. Hepatology 2004;39:471.

177. Drews R, Weinberger S. Thrombocytopenic disorders in critically ill patients. Am J Respir Crit Care Med 2000;162:347.

178. Martin LF, Booth FV, Karlstadt RG, et al. Continuous intravenous cimetidine decreases stress-related upper gastrointestinal hemorrhage without promoting pneumonia. Crit Care Med 1993;21:19.

179. Cook D, Guyatt G, Marshall J, et al. A comparison of sucralfate and ranitidine for the prevention of upper gastrointestinal bleeding in patients requiring mechanical ventilation. N Engl J Med 1998;338:l791.

180. Shami VM, Caldwell SH, Hespenheide EE, et al. Recombinant activated factor VII for coagulopathy in fulminant hepatic failure compared with conventional therapy. Liver Transpl 2003;9:138.

181. Caldwell SH, Chang C, Macik BG. Recombinant activated factor VII as a hemostatic agent in liver disease: A break from convention in need of controlled trials. Hepatology 2004;39:592.

182. Bernal W, Wendon J. Liver transplantation in adults with acute liver failure. J Hepatol 2004;40:192.

183. Devlin J, Wendon J, Heaton N, et al. Pretransplantation clinical status and outcome of emergency transplantation for acute liver failure. Hepatology 1995;21:1018.

184. Wiesner RH. MELD/PELD and the allocation of deceased donor livers for status 1 recipients with acute fulminant hepatic failure, primary nonfunction, hepatic artery thrombosis, and acute Wilson's disease. Liver Transplant 2004;10:S17.

185. 2006 OPTN/SRTR Annual Report, Table 9.2a. URL http://www.optn.org/AR2006/902a_li.htm [accessed on 15 February 2007].

186. Guirl MJ, Weinstein JS, Goldstein RM, et al. Two stage total hepatectomy and liver transplant for acute deterioration of chronic liver disease: a new bridge to transplantation. Liver Transpl 2004;10:564.

187. Jalan R, Pollok A, Shah S, et al. Liver derived pro-inflammatory cytokines may be important in producing intracranial hypertension in acute liver failure. J Hepatol 2002;37:356.

188. Ringe B, Lubbe N, Kuse E, et al. Management of emergencies before and after liver transplantation by early total hepatectomy. Transplant Proc 1993;25:1090.

189. Van Hoek B, de Boer J, Boudjema K, et al. Auxiliary versus orthotopic liver transplantation for acute liver failure. J Hepatol 1999;30:699.

190. Chenard-Neu MP, Boudjema K, Bernuau J, et al. Auxiliary liver transplantation: Regeneration of the native liver and outcome in 30 patients with fulminant hepatic failure – a multicentre European study. Hepatology 1996;23:1119.

191. Miwa S, Hasikura Y, Mita A, et al. Living-related liver transplantation for patients with fulminant and subfulminant hepatic failure. Hepatology 1999;30:1521.

192. Uemoto S, Inomata Y, Sakurai T, et al. Living donor liver transplantation for fulminant hepatic failure. Transplantation 2000;70:152.

193. Liu CL, Fan ST, Lo M, et al. Right lobe live donor liver transplantation improves survival of patients with acute liver failure. Br J Surg 2002;89:317.

194. Shiffman ML, Brown R Jr, Olthoff KM, et al. Living donor liver transplantation: Summary of a conference at the National Institutes of Health. Liver Transplant 2002;8:174.

195. Habibullah CM, Syed IH, Qamar A, et al. Human fetal hepatocyte transplantation in patients with fulminant hepatic failure. Transplantation 1994;58:951.

196. Mito M, Kusano M, Kawaura Y. Hepatocyte transplantation in man. Transplantation Proc 1992;24:3052.

197. Bilir B, Guinette D, Karrer F, et al. Hepatocyte transplantation in acute liver failure. Liver Transplant 2000;6:32.

198. Fox I, Chowdhury J, Kaufman S, et al. Treatment of the Crigler-Najar syndrome type I with hepatocyte transplantation. N Engl J Med 1998;338:1422.

199. Petersen BE, Bowen WC, Patrene KD, et al. Bone marrow as a potential source of hepatic oval cells. Science 1999;284:1168.

200. Allen JW, Hassanein T, Bhatia SN. Advances in bioartificial liver devices. Hepatology 2001;34:447.

201. Sen S, Williams R. New liver support devices in acute liver failure: A critical evaluation. Semin Liver Dis 2003;23:283.

202. Sen S, Williams R, Jalan R. Emerging indications for albumin dialysis. Am J Gastroenterol 2005;100:468.

203. O'Grady JG, Gimson AE, O'Brien CJ, et al. Controlled trials of charcoal hemoperfusion and prognostic factors in fulminant hepatic failure. Gastroenterology 1988;94:1186.

204. Redeker AG, Yamahiro HS. Controlled trial of exchange-transfusion therapy in fulminant hepatitis Lancet 1973;i:3.

205. Mitzner SR, Stange J, Klammt S, et al. Improvement of hepatorenal syndrome with extracorporeal albumin dialysis MARS: Results of a prospective, randomized, controlled clinical trial. Liver Transplant 2000;6:277.

206. Stange J, Mitzner SR, Risler T, et al. Molecular adsorbent recycling system (MARS): Clinical results of a new membrane based blood purification system for bioartificial liver support. Artif Organs 1999;23:319.

207. Schmidt LE, Wang LP, Hansen BA, Larsen FS. Systemic hemodynamic effects of treatment with the molecular adsorbents recirculating system in patients with hyperacute liver failure: A prospective controlled trial. Liver Transplant 2003;9:290.

208. Rifai K, Ernst T, Kretschmer U, et al. Prometheus – a new extracorporeal system for the treatment of liver failure. J Hepatol 2003;39:984.

209. Rifai K, Ernst T, Kretschmer U, et al. The Prometheus device for extracorporeal support of combined liver and renal failure. Blood Purif 2005;23:298.

210. Kjaergard LL, Liu J, Adilo Neilson B, et al. Artificial and bioartificial liver support systems for acute and acute-on-chronic liver failure. JAMA 2003;289:217.

211. Ellis AJ, Hughers RD, Wendon JA, et al. Pilot controlled trial of extracorporeal liver assist device in acute liver failure. Hepatology 1996;24:1446.

212. Watanabe FD, Mullon CJ, Hewitt WR, et al. Clinical experience with a bioartifical liver in the treatment of severe acute liver failure. A phase I clinical trial. Ann Surg 1997;225:484.

213. Baquerizo A, Kirilova V, Williamson I, et al. Acute liver failure patients treated with bioartifical porcine liver: Analysis of the humoral immune response against pig hepatocytes. Gastroenterology 2004;S1634 [abstract].

214. Chari RS, Collins BH, Magee JC, et al. Brief report: Treatment of hepatic failure with ex vivo pig-liver perfusion followed by liver transplantation. N Eng J Med 1994;331:234.

215. Horslen SP, Hammel JM, Fristoe LW, et al. Extracorporeal liver perfusion using human and pig livers for acute liver failure. Transplantation 2000;70:1472.

216. Starzl TE, Valdivia LA, Murase N, et al. The biological basis of and strategies for clinical xenotransplantation. Immunol Rev 1994;141:213.

217. Demetriou AA, Brown RS, Jr, Busuttil RW, et al. Prospective, randomized, multicenter controlled trial of a bioartificial liver in treating acute liver failure. Ann Surg 2004;239:660.

218. Demetriou AA. Hepatic assist devices. Panminerva Med 2005;47:31.

219. Lim YS, Kim KM, Lee HC, et al. Etiology and outcome of fulminant hepatic failure managed at a Korean liver transplant unit. Hepatology 2005;42:364A [abstract].

Approach to the patient with chronic viral hepatitis B or C

Sammy Saab, Hugo Rosen

Hepatitis B, 516
Hepatitis C, 520

Understanding laboratory serological tests for viral hepatitis is essential for differentiating current infection from immunity, and acute from chronic infection. As with most cases of liver disease, definitive diagnosis requires the use of laboratory tests. History, symptoms, and signs do not necessarily point to a specific cause [1]. Laboratory tests exist in different levels of specificity, with biochemical tests being the least specific and molecular tests the most specific.

Hepatitis B

Diagnosis

The presence of hepatitis B surface antigen (HBsAg) is required to define current hepatitis B infection. HBsAg is detected in both acute and chronic infection. The presence of IgM antibodies against hepatitis B core antigen (anti-HBc IgM) helps to differentiate between acute and chronic infection, with anti-HBc IgM present during acute infection. However, these antibodies may occasionally be found in the setting of chronic hepatitis B with reactivation. The presence of immunoglobulin G (IgG) antibodies against hepatitis B core antigen (anti-HBc IgG) is found in both acute and chronic infections. Antibodies against hepatitis B surface antigen (anti-HBs) indicate resolution of HBV infection, and protective immunity. Thus, the presence of HBsAg implies current infection, and the presence of anti-HBs indicates immunity (Table 26.1).

Occasionally, patients may have an isolated anti-HBc IgG, with no HBsAg and anti-HBs detected. There are four possible explanations for this finding including:

- resolution of chronic infection with waning anti-HBs titers
- "window period" infection in which a patient is infected but HBsAg titers have decreased and the anti-HBs is not yet detectable; these patients have increased anti-HBc IgM
- a false-positive anti-HBc (not infrequent in patients who have hepatitis C virus infection)
- active infection with waning HBsAg (undetectable) levels (Fig. 26.1).

Most cases of isolated anti-HBc IgG reflect prior resolved infection, and confirmation is not generally required. There are several possible tests that can be used to confirm its significance. Markers of viral replication such as hepatitis B virus E antigen (HBeAg) and HBV DNA would suggest active infection. Similarly, measuring anti-HBs after immunization is a way of confirming prior infection with resolution. If the patient had waning anti-HBs titers, the titers will increase after a single immunization.

Another set of serological tests can assess viral replication in patients with hepatitis B infection (i.e., HBsAg positive). HBeAg is found in the blood of patients with hepatitis B infection when there is active viral replication; antibodies to HBeAg (anti-HBe) indicate a lack of viral replication. However, this distinction is becoming blurred with the increasing appreciation of precore and core mutant hepatitis B viruses being associated with low levels of viral replication, yet with anti-HBe detected.

Molecular tests

Molecular tests are the most accurate method for assessing viral hepatitis. A number of assays are used to check the viral load, and they differ in their sensitivity. If an insensitive assay is used, false-negative results will occur. The viral load can be quantified using different units. For instance, earlier studies in hepatitis B used milliequivalents (mEq) and copies to express viral load. International Units (IU) is the standard method to describe the viral load [2,3].

Principles of Clinical Gastroenterology. Edited by Tadataka Yamada, David H. Alpers, Anthony N. Kalloo, Neil Kaplowitz, Chung Owyang, and Don W. Powell. © 2008 Blackwell Publishing. ISBN 978-1-4051-69103

Table 26.1 Interpretation of serological tests for hepatitis B

Serological tests				
HBsAg	HBc IgM	HBc IgG	Anti-HBs	Interpretation
+	+	+	−	Acute hepatitis B infection or reactivation
+	−	+	−	Chronic hepatitis B infection
−	−	+	+	Past exposure with resolution and immunity
−	−	−	+	Immunity from vaccination
−	+	+	−	Window period of acute hepatitis B
−	−	+	−	(i) Remote hepatitis B infection, anti-HBs no longer detectable; or (ii) recent recovery from acute infection; or (iii) undetectable level of HBsAg in infected patient; or (iv) false positive

Anti-HBs, antibody against hepatitis B surface antigen; HBc, hepatitis B virus core antigen; HBc IgM, immunoglobulin M against hepatitis B core antigen; HBc IgG, immunoglobulin G against hepatitis B core antigen; HBsAg, hepatitis B virus surface antigen; IgM, immunoglobulin M.

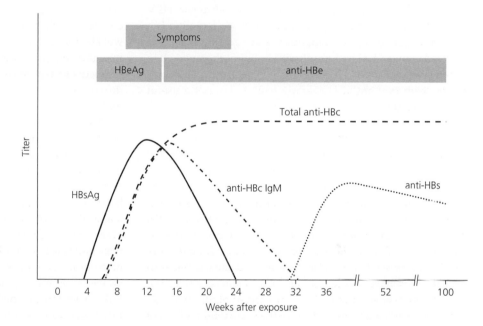

Figure 26.1 Typical course of resolved hepatitis B infection. Anti-HBs, antibody against hepatitis B surface antigen; anti-HBC, antibody against hepatitis B virus core antigen; anti-HBe, antibody against hepatitis B virus E antigen; HBeAg, hepatitis B virus E antigen; HBsAg, hepatitis B virus surface antigen; IgM, immunoglobulin M.

The viral load has replaced the HBeAg test for defining the presence of viral replication. This is particularly true because patients with precore and core mutants can have active viral replication despite not having HBeAg present. The viral load is also used to monitor treatment efficacy. One of the goals of antiviral therapy is to suppress viral replication. The assumption is that by decreasing the viral load, clinical outcome should also improve. This is particularly relevant because high viral load has been correlated with risks of cirrhosis and hepatocellular carcinoma [4,5].

Another molecular test is the genotype. There are eight (A–H) genotypes recognized with particular geographical regions [6,7]. Certain genotypes may be more associated with advanced liver disease and hepatocellular carcinoma, and others with response to therapy. The role of obtaining a genotype in clinical practice is controversial [2,3].

Histology

Indications for antiviral therapy in HBV generally rely on laboratory results. Patients with elevated liver enzymes, who have surpassed a particular viral threshold, are considered viable candidates for antiviral therapy. When there is a discrepancy between the liver enzymes and viral load, a liver biopsy is often performed to rule out underlying liver disease not apparent in the liver enzymes. If there is evidence of liver damage on the liver biopsy, then therapy should be considered. The threshold for starting therapy in patients with normal liver enzymes and an elevated viral load is at least moderate inflammation or significant fibrosis [3].

Treatment
Goals
The goal for all patients is normalization of liver enzymes, undetectable hepatitis B viral load, improvement of liver histology, and decreased risk of disease progression and development of hepatocellular carcinoma. With eradication of circulating HBV DNA, the other goals of liver enzyme elevation and histological improvement will follow. Patients who, after 6 months of treatment, do not have at least a 2 log drop in the serum HBV DNA should be considered for alternative therapy [3]. Another goal of therapy in HBeAg-positive patients, is e antigen loss and seroconversion to anti-HBe. Hepatitis B e antigen seroconversion, achievable in 16%–32% of patients in the first year of treatment [3,8], is an important end point because it suggests a more likely sustained HBV DNA loss with therapy. In patients who are hepatitis B e antigen negative, loss of hepatitis B e antigen is not an end point. Another ideal end point with antiviral therapy is loss or seroconversion of HBs antigen. As this occurs uncommonly with oral antiviral therapy (< 2%), it is not a useful clinical goal [8].

Indication
The threshold of when to start antiviral therapy is somewhat controversial, and two different guidelines are often followed. Both guidelines recommend antiviral therapy for patients with elevated HBV viral loads and serum aminotransferases. However, the guidelines differ as to the exact level of the viral load and aminotransferase elevation that is necessary to start therapy. For instance, the American Association for the Study of Liver Diseases (AASLD) guidelines indicate treatment in patients who have a viral load of greater than 20 000 IU/mL with liver enzymes greater than twice the upper limit of normal. In patients with less than twice the normal upper limit of liver enzyme elevation, a liver biopsy should be considered. The AASLD guidelines recognize that HBeAg-negative patients may have lower HBV DNA levels. By contrast, the Keeffe guidelines recommend that patients who are e antigen positive should have a minimum viral load of at least 20 000 IU/mL before starting therapy. However, a threshold of only 2000 IU/mL is appropriate in a patient who is hepatitis e antigen negative. Besides the viral threshold for starting therapy, another difference resides in the definition of abnormal liver enzymes. The AASLD guidelines indicate that an abnormal elevation requiring antiviral therapy is twice the upper limit of normal. However, the Keeffe guidelines define abnormal aminotransferases requiring antiviral therapy as greater than 19 IU/mL in a woman and 30 IU/mL in a man [2]. Furthermore, the Keeffe guidelines indicate than a liver biopsy should be considered in patients when there is a discrepancy between the viral load and the aminotransferases. In other words, in patients where the viral level is elevated but the aminotransferse level is normal, a liver biopsy should be performed and treatment offered if there is significant disease.

Options
There are six medications approved by the US Food and Drug Administration (FDA) to treat hepatitis B, including four oral medications. Comparing the relative efficacies of the different therapies can be difficult because of diverse populations studied and different viral assays used. Moreover, unlike interferon, which has defined treatment duration, there are no real temporal end points for oral antiviral therapy. Generally, treatment may be discontinued 6–12 months after HBeAg seroconversion [2]. HBeAg seroconversion implies a robust antiviral response to therapy. In HBeAg-negative patients, treatment duration is unclear because relapse is common.

The first medication approved for the treatment of chronic hepatitis B was interferon. Interferon is administered subcutaneously 5 million units daily or 10 million units thrice weekly for 12–24 weeks. In HBeAg-positive patients, the loss of HBeAg and the loss of HBV DNA was 33% and 37%, respectively, 6 months after therapy cessation [9]. There is a difference of 18% in seroconversion between patients treated with interferon and placebo. The durability of HBeAg seroconversion in patients treated with interferon is between 80% and 90% in patients followed for over 4 years. However, many of the patients continue to have low levels of HBV DNA detected. In HBeAg-negative patients, the loss of HBV DNA was 60%–70%. In HBeAg-negative patients treated with interferon, the durability of HBV DNA loss is 10%–20%. In some studies, the loss of HBsAg has been reported to be as high as 10% [10,11]. The introduction of pegylated interferon was associated with improved compliance and greater rates of response. However, treatment duration is longer with 48 weeks. Using pegylated interferon, the sustained loss of HBeAg, the rate of HBeAg seroconversion, and the loss of HBV DNA was 30%–34%, 27%–32%, and 25% in HBeAg-positive patients, respectively [12–14]. In HBeAg-negative patients, the loss of HBV DNA was 63% [15]. Interferon is associated with a number of adverse effects, including flu-like symptoms, psychiatric disturbances, and bone marrow toxicities. The predictors of response to interferon include liver enzymes twice the upper limit of normal and low HBV DNA levels [16–18]. Interferon is contraindicated in patients with cirrhosis [2,3].

The advantages of interferon over oral medications include a defined period of therapy, best probability of HBsAg loss, and no associated resistance. Thus, no cross-resistance should occur, which would impact future therapies. Interferon may be best for patients who are motivated, young, have no cirrhosis, have elevated liver enzymes, have a low HBV viral load, and are infected with genotype A or B.

Unlike interferon, oral medications have few associated

adverse effects, and consequently are gaining popularity in clinical practice. However, the duration of treatment is not temporary and treatment is discontinued only after the viral replication is halted. The oral medications are stratified along their chemical structure as either nucleoside and nucleotide analogues. The dosages of these medications need to be adjusted according to creatinine clearance.

Lamivudine, a nucleoside analogue, was the first oral drug approved by the FDA, in 1995. After one year of therapy in HBeAg-positive patients, the loss of HBeAg, the rate of HBeAg seroconversion, and the loss of HBV DNA was 17%–32%, 16%–21%, and 40%–44%, respectively [19–21]. In HBeAg-negative patients, the loss of HBV DNA was 60%–73% [22–25]. Durability of HBV DNA loss in HBeAg-negative patients is less than 10%, whereas in HBeAg-positive patients (who experienced e antigen loss) it ranges between 50% and 80%. The major limitation of lamivudine is the development of resistance, which occurs in 14%–32% of treated individuals after the first year [19–21]; as a result, the use of lamivudine as a first-line agent has been questioned. Resistance flares are associated with viral rebound, hepatic decompensation, and reversion of histological improvement, although in many patients there is no change in clinical status. It is recommended that for patients who develop resistance, a nucleotide analogue be added, and lamivudine continued because it is probably suppressing the wild-type virus. Another concern arising from lamivudine resistance is potential cross-resistance. For instance, patients with resistance to lamivudine are at risk of developing resistance to other drugs such as entecavir and telbivudine [26]. Patients treated with lamivudine resistance may also be at increased subsequent risk of adefovir resistance [27]. The predictors of response to lamivudine include elevated alanine aminotransferase (ALT) levels [28].

Because of associated resistance rates, lamivudine is no longer considered a first-line treatment. Significant mortality can be seen in patients with cirrhosis treated with lamivudine monotherapy who develop flares associated with resistance. Nevertheless, one role of lamivudine in clinical practice may be in patients undergoing chemotherapy [29–31].

Another nucleoside analogue is entecavir. In both HBeAg- and HBeAg-positive patients, entecavir has been shown to suppress viral load more effectively than lamivudine, but is similar in HBeAg loss and HBeAg seroconversion in HBeAg-positive patients. In HBeAg-positive patients the loss of HBeAg, HBeAg seroconversion, and the loss of HBV DNA was 22%, 21%, and 67%, respectively [32] at the end of treatment at week 48. In HBeAg-negative patients the loss of HBV DNA was observed in 90% at week 48 [33]. HBeAg seroconversion appears to be correlated with aminotransferase elevation. The greater the level of ALT, the more likely is HBeAg seroconversion. The durability of response after HBeAg seroconversion is over 70%. For HBV DNA load, the durability is approximately 40%. The durability of viral response in HBeAg-negative patients is unclear. In lamivudine-naive pati-

ents, resistance is rare [34]. In lamivudine-experienced patients, the use of entecavir resulted in 55% of treated patients achieving a composite end point of ALT less than 1.25 × upper limit of normal and HBV DNA less than 0.7 mEq/mL compared with 28% of patients continued on lamivudine and the end of treatment [35]. However, genotypic resistance was found in 10 patients, and 2 of 144 patients had viral rebound. The adverse effects of lamivudine and entecavir are similar.

The effectiveness and lack of resistance associated with entecavir make it a reasonable first-line option in patients with compensated and decompensated liver disease who are lamivudine-naive. Although entecavir is effective in lamivudine-experienced patients, cross-resistance may limit its use in this population.

Adefovir is a nucleotide analogue (unlike lamivudine and entecavir) with activity against hepatitis B. The advantages of adefovir are its long-term safety profile and low rate of resistance. However, its efficacy is slightly less than lamivudine and entecavir. Undetectable HBV DNA levels at 48 weeks of treatment were achieved in 21% and 51% of HBeAg-positive and HBeAg-negative patients, respectively [36,37]. In HBeAg-negative patients who completed one year of therapy, viral loss durability was less than 10%. HBeAg loss and seroconversion were seen in 24% and 12% of treated patients, respectively [36]. In HBeAg-positive patients durability of response after HBeAg seroconversion is approximately 90%. The main toxicity of adevofir is renal. Thus, the dose needs to be adjusted accordingly in patients with renal insufficiency. Studies have demonstrated the efficacy of adding adefovir to the treatment of patients with lamivudine resistance [38,39]. Furthermore, it appears that the sooner adefovir is added, the greater the likelihood of achieving a viral response to the medication. Adding adefovir appears to be a better option than replacing lamivudine completely. Long-term therapy with adefovir is associated with cumulative viral suppression, and infrequent viral resistance [40]. Despite prolonged therapy, relapse can occur with discontinuation.

The decrease in viral load with adefovir appears to be slower than with lamivudine and entecavir, but adefovir has been associated with lower resistance rates than lamivudine. The low resistance rates make adefovir particularly attractive in HBeAg-negative patients who require long-term therapy.

Telbivudine is a nucleoside analogue, and the latest oral medication to be approved by the FDA. Telbivudine has been demonstrated to be more efficacious than lamivudine at achieving HBV DNA suppression. Undetectable HBV DNA levels were achieved in 60% and 88% of HBeAg-positive and HBeAg-negative patients, respectively. HBeAg loss and seroconversion were seen in 26% and 22% of treated patients, respectively [41]. Viral breakthrough was seen in 15.8% of patients treated with lamivudine, compared with 4.5% of those receiving telbivudine. Although telbivudine is efficacious in suppressing viral replication, its associated viral breakthrough will limit its use in the clinical setting as monotherapy.

The role of combination therapy using telbivudine with nucleotide analogues requires investigation.

Hepatitis C

Diagnosis

Liver enzymes are commonly used to screen for hepatitis. Elevated levels indicate liver damage, and prompt investigation for the etiology. However, liver enzymes are an insensitive marker of liver damage in patients with hepatitis C. The degree of liver enzyme elevation does not correlate with the degree of liver damage. Approximately 20% of patients with hepatitis C and normal liver enzymes have histological damage that warrants antiviral therapy. In fact it is possible to have established cirrhosis despite normal liver enzymes [42,43].

In patients with risk factors for hepatitis or unexplained elevated liver enzymes, the laboratory test should be checking for hepatitis C antibodies [44,45]. The most common antibody test is the enzyme-linked immunosorbent assay (ELISA). Most laboratories use the third generation of ELISA, which is over 95% sensitive and 95% specific. False-negative results can be seen in immunocompromised individuals (including those on dialysis) and during an acute hepatitis C infection.

Another serological test for hepatitis C is the recombinant immunoblot assay (RIBA), which tests for similar antibodies as the ELISA. Before the advent of molecular tests for hepatitis C, RIBA was often used in clinical practice to confirm a positive ELISA tests. However, the RIBA confirms the presence of antibodies to hepatitis C, and not current infection. The current role of HCV RIBA is to confirm if the results of an ELISA are a true positive or a false positive, when HCV viral load is undetectable. If both the ELISA and RIBA are positive, and the HCV RNA is undetectable, then the patient probably has cleared the hepatitis C infection and does not have evidence of viral replication. However, it is important to note that HCV RNA may be below the level of detection. If the ELISA is positive, the RIBA is negative, and the HCV RNA undetectable, then the ELISA is probably a false positive and no further testing is required.

Molecular tests are used to confirm ongoing HCV replication and current infection [46]. The detection of HCV viral load is the gold standard for defining infection [47]. The viral load can be expressed in different units, including IU/mL, copies, mEq, and Eq, but the generally accepted unit is the IU [48].

Unlike viral loads for many other disease states, including hepatitis B and human immunodeficiency virus (HIV), the hepatitis C viral load does not correlate with liver disease severity or help predict severity. A higher viral load does not necessarily mean more advanced disease, nor does a lower viral load necessarily indicate mild disease.

The definition of what constitutes a low or high viral load is controversial. Because the viral load does not correlate with disease severity or prognosis, the definition relies on which viral load is associated with greater responses to antiviral therapy. A lower viral load has a better response than a higher viral load. Values of less than 800 000, 600 000, and 200 000 IU/mL have been considered as "low" in a variety of studies. A study found that a viral load of 400 000 IU/mL should be considered the "low" threshold value based on treated patients' response to antiviral therapy [49]. The viral load has varied uses in clinical practice including confirmation of active viral replication and infection, predicting response to antiviral therapy, and assessing antiviral therapy.

Besides HCV RNA, another molecular test is the HCV genotype. Like HCV RNA, HCV genotype is not associated with disease severity or prognosis. The role of genotype is to estimate the likelihood of achieving a sustained virological response and the duration of antiviral therapy [50–52]. For instance, the sustained virological response with genotype 1 is approximately 40%–45% with 48 weeks of therapy. In contrast, genotypes 2 and 3 are associated with a sustained virological response of between 65% and 75%, and patients require only 24 weeks of therapy.

Histology

A liver biopsy is essential for the assessment of patients infected with hepatitis C. It is helpful in assessing the degree of liver damage and determining the need for antiviral therapy, and for prognosis [53–55]. The biopsy should be interpreted by an experienced hepatopathologist, and a sufficient biopsy specimen should be at least 1.5 cm in length to minimize sampling error and ensure accuracy of interpretation. The biopsy is considered a relatively safe procedure, with the mortality risk ranging from 1/10 000 to 1/12 000 [56–58].

The liver biopsy is interpreted according to the degree of activity, fibrosis, and steatosis; the most important of these factors is the degree of fibrosis [53–55]. A common scoring system for the degree of fibrosis uses a scale of 0 to 4: 0 – no fibrosis; 1 – fibrosis limited to portal tracts; 2 – periportal or portal to portal tracts; 3 – fibrosis with distorted structure but no obvious cirrhosis; and 4 – probable or definitive cirrhosis [59,60]. Alcohol consumption, gender, HIV and HBV coinfection, and immunosuppression can affect the rate of fibrosis progression. Some patients can progress from minimal fibrosis to cirrhosis in one to two decades, whereas others may take longer, or never progress.

Because of the shorter duration and greater effectiveness of therapy with HCV genotypes 2 and 3, a liver biopsy may be optional in individuals with these genotypes. However, biopsy should be considered because patients with cirrhosis still require screening for complications such as hepatocellular carcinoma even if they achieve a sustained virological response [61].

Patients with minimal disease who are not felt to require therapy, should be considered for a repeat liver biopsy. The exact interval is controversial, depending on the degree of liver damage, but ranges between 2 and 5 years. As therapy becomes more effective and better tolerated, the threshold for treating will probably be lowered; eventually therapy with fewer side effects will be offered routinely even to patients with mild disease [62].

Treatment

Antiviral therapy has primary and secondary goals. The primary goal is to achieve a sustained virological response, that is, a nondetectable viral level 6 months after completing therapy. The secondary goals include normalization of liver enzymes, reversal of liver fibrosis, and prevention of hepatic decompensation. The efficacy of antiviral therapy has increased, with longer-acting interferons and the use of combination therapy with ribavirin. However, therapy can be associated with serious side effects, so the indications must be clearly defined.

Indications

Before beginning antiviral therapy, the risks and benefits need to be considered. The overall goal of therapy is to increase life expectancy and survival. In some patients, hepatitis C may be associated with symptoms of fatigue and depressed mood. Thus, interferon therapy may improve quality of life.

Antiviral therapy with pegylated interferon and ribavirin is associated with a sustained virological response in approximately 40% of patients. However, as described below, adverse effects can occur. Thus, the risks and benefits of therapy must be explored, and discussed with potential patients. A liver biopsy is usually performed to assess the degree of liver damage and need for antiviral therapy. The decision to recommend therapy depends on a number of factors, including the efficacy of available therapy, the presence of comorbid conditions, the duration of infection, the degree of liver damage, and the patient's age.

Viral responses

The viral response is used to assess outcome because it predicts the likelihood of achieving a long-term response, also called a sustained virological response (SVR). An undetectable viral level 4 weeks after starting therapy is considered a rapid virological response (RVR). At least a 2 log drop in viral level at week 12 indicates an early virological response (EVR). However, data suggest that a nondetectable viral level at week 12 is associated with a greater probability of achieving a sustained virological response than a 2 log reduction to a still detectable viral level. The viral load at the completion of treatment is known as the end-of-treatment response (ETR). The SVR is defined by a nondetectable viral load 6 months after completing therapy (Fig. 26.2).

Treatment strategies

Antiviral therapy with pegylated interferon and ribavirin
Since the mid-1980s there have been considerable advances in the treatment of chronic HCV as reflected by response rates,

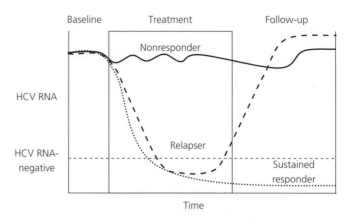

Figure 26.2 Viral response during hepatitis C (HCV) therapy.

which have increased from less than 10% with interferon monotherapy to approximately 50% with standard combination therapy. Pegylated forms of interferon (alfa-2a, Hoffman La-Roche; alfa-2b, Schering-Plough) are used once weekly in combination with daily oral ribavirin [62,63].

In a study of 1530 patients, Manns and colleagues [64] reported that patients with genotype 1 and treated with peginterferon alfa-2b and ribavirin had an SVR of 42% compared with 33% for patients treated with thrice weekly interferon and ribavirin. Patients with genotypes 2 or 3 had SVR rates of approximately 80% regardless of the treatment regimen. Similarly, Fried and colleagues [65] found SVR rates were significantly higher in patients treated with the combination of peginterferon alfa-2a and ribavirin (56%) compared with standard thrice weekly interferon and ribavirin (44%) Genotype 1-infected patients who received peginterferon achieved a SVR 46% of the time (vs 36% in those who received the standard interferon combination). Considerable experience has been garnered since the publication of these two seminal studies. Recommendations are that patients with genotype 1 exhibiting an early virological response should receive 48 weeks of peginterferon therapy with standard doses of ribavirin (1000–1200 mg/day), whereas patients with genotype 2 or 3 will need no more than 24 weeks (possibly shorter duration as discussed below) of therapy using a lower dose of ribavirin (800 mg/day) [62]. The factors consistently shown to be predictive of SVR are outlined in Table 26.2, and the expected response rates according to genotype are shown in Table 26.3. The majority of patients in the United States have genotype 1 and approximately half have high viral loads.

Management of side effects of antiviral therapy

The side effects from combination therapy with pegylated interferon and ribavirin are frequent and can lead to dose reduction or premature discontinuation (reviewed in refs [62,63] and outlined in Table 26.4). In particular, reduction of

Table 26.2 Factors associated with a sustained virological response to therapy for hepatitis C virus infection [49,62,63]

Non-genotype 1
Low viral load (< 400 000 IU/mL)[a]
Lack of bridging fibrosis/cirrhosis
Young age (< 45 years)
Female gender
Weight < 75 kg
Caucasian race
Adherence (> 80% of the prescribed treatment)

a The threshold viral load defining a low level is evolving. Previously, it was believed to be 800 000 IU/mL.

Table 26.3 Sustained virological response rates to standard therapy for chronic hepatitis C infection according to genotype [64,65,67,73,74]

Genotype 1	46%–52%
Genotype 2	76%–93%
Genotype 3	76%–79%
Genotype 4	60%–70%
Genotype 5	64%–71%
Genotype 6	40%

Table 26.4 Adverse events related to pegylated interferon and ribavirin in patients with chronic HCV infection

Related to interferon
Flu-like symptoms
Bone marrow suppression (especially leukopenia and thrombocytopenia)
Emotional effects (irritability, difficulty concentrating, memory disturbances, depression)
Autoimmune disorders (especially thyroiditis)
Hair loss
Rash
Visual disorders (rarely retinal hemorrhages, especially in diabetic patients and hypertensive patients)
Weight loss
Seizures
Hearing loss
Pancreatitis
Interstitial pneumonitis
Injection site reactions

Related to ribavirin
Hemolytic anemia
Chest congestion, dry cough, and dyspnea
Pruritus
Sinus disorders
Rash
Gout
Nausea
Diarrhea
Teratogenicity

Compiled from Dienstag & McHutchinson [62].

ribavirin dosing in the first 20 weeks appears to be associated with significantly diminished SVR rates [66]. Influenza-like symptoms (fever, myalgia, and rigors) occur in 42%–64% and can be managed with acetaminophen (paracetamol) or nonsteroidal antiinflammatory drugs; depression occurs in 22%–31%. Dose reductions (temporary or permanent) of either peginterferon for any adverse event occur in 32%–42% of patients [63–65,67]. Laboratory abnormalities such as neutropenia, anemia, and thrombocytopenia warrant frequent monitoring, and represent the most frequent indications for dose reduction. Data suggest that aggressive management of side effects improves quality of life and therefore patient adherence to therapy [68]. The use of antidepressant or anxiolytic medications and hemopoietic stem cell growth factors is increasing in the management of HCV therapy. Although these therapies may prevent dose reductions and increase the number of patients completing therapy, there are no data available to demonstrate definitively that such tactics translate into improved SVR rates in individual patients [69].

Duration of antiviral therapy

Because of the costs and side effects associated with antiviral therapy, it is critically important to identify clinically useful measures that could predict success or failure earlier in the course of treatment [63]. Moreover, as new therapies emerge, prediction of failure of interferon-based therapies might prompt consideration of a switch to these newer agents. Early virological response (EVR) was defined by Fried and colleagues [65] as a decrease of HCV RNA of at least 2 logs at treatment week 12 from pretreatment values (e.g., 10^4 IU/mL dropping from 10^6 IU/mL). Among those patients who failed to achieve EVR, only 3% went on to SVR, yielding a negative predictive value of 97%. In a similar analysis of patients receiving peginterferon alfa-2b and ribavirin, none of the patients who failed to achieve EVR went on to attain SVR [70]. Thus, the failure to achieve EVR accurately predicts the absence of SVR. It is critically important to compare HCV RNA from baseline and week 12 using the same assay. Measurement of HCV RNA at week 12 in patients with genotype 2 or 3 is not recommended because EVR is achieved in 97% of these patients (compared with 81% of those with genotype 1) [71].

It is important to recognize that EVR, developed initially as a guide to discontinue treatment in those likely to fail antiviral therapy, may not apply to special treatment groups, including African Americans [72], patients with recurrent HCV after liver transplantation, and patients with extrahepatic manifestations (e.g., vasculitis) where the end points of therapy may not be limited to SVR [54]. For the majority of patients, however, it is a useful management tool (Fig. 26.3).

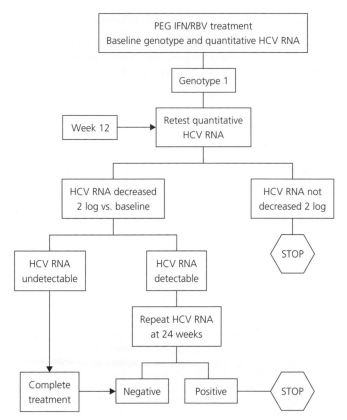

Figure 26.3 Application of early virological response for patients with genotype 1. HCV, hepatitis C virus; PEG IFN, pegylated interferon; RBV, ribavirin. From Fried & Hadziyannis [63], with permission from Thieme.

The dogma that genotypes 2 and 3 patients necessarily should receive 24 weeks of antiviral therapy and genotype 1-infected patients should receive 48 weeks of therapy has been challenged. Sixteen weeks of therapy with peginterferon alfa-2a plus weight-based ribavirin is sufficient for patients chronically infected with HCV genotype 2 (independent from pretreatment viremia) or genotype 3 (and a pretreatment HCV RNA level equal to or below 800 000 IU/mL) [73] who achieve a rapid virological response at week 4. Importantly, patients treated for 16 weeks also tended to report adverse events less frequently than patients treated for 24 weeks. In another study [74], the proportion of genotype 2 and 3 patients with relapse was higher among those treated for 12 weeks than those treated for the standard 24 weeks. However, 90% of patients with a relapse after 12 weeks of treatment subsequently had a response after an additional 24-week course of therapy. Therefore, even taking into consideration the rate of relapse, treatment for 12 or 16 weeks rather than 24 weeks appears to be appropriate for genotype 2 and 3 patients with an early response [73,74]. One randomized controlled trial has shown that in genotype 1-infected patients with detectable viremia at 4 weeks, extension of pegylated interferon and ribavirin from 48 to 72 weeks increases SVR rates from 28% to 44%, respectively ($P = 0.003$), without increasing the rate of adverse events [75].

Patients with HCV who fail to respond to pegylated interferon plus ribavirin represent a highly resistant group of patients who need more effective treatment strategies, preferably with multidrug combinations. In patients who have not responded to an initial course of pegylated interferon plus ribavirin, retreatment of these patients with another course of pegylated interferon plus ribavirin appears to be of marginal benefit.

Promising new agents

The small molecule BILN-2061 was the first specific inhibitor of the NS3/4A protease to demonstrate clinical antiviral activity in reducing HCV RNA [76]. Although BILN-2061 was effective, serious adverse effects precluded further

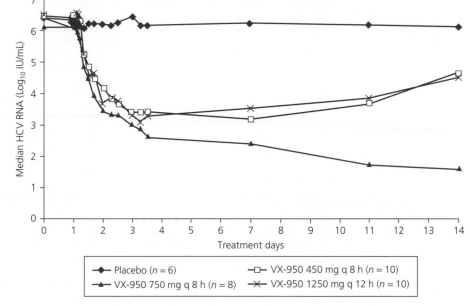

Figure 26.4 VX-950 treatment leads to decreases in hepatitis C virus (HCV) RNA. Dosing with VX-950 or placebo started on day 1 and ended on the evening of day 14. The day 0, or baseline, value is the median of all predose values. Median HCV RNA levels of patients in each treatment regimen are shown. Plasma HCV RNA concentrations were determined using the Roche COBAS TaqMan HCV assay. From Reesink et al. [77], with permission from Elsevier.

study. VX-950, a peptidomimetic inhibitor of NS3/4A, shown to demonstrate potent antiviral activity in HCV replicon assays, was tested in 28 patients, most of whom had previously failed interferon-based therapy [77]. Fourteen days of VX-950 treatment resulted in rapid and substantial viral decline: all patients treated with VX-950 had at least a 2 $\log_{10}$ decrease from baseline in HCV RNA, and two patients achieved undetectable levels of virus (Fig. 26.4). In addition, median ALT and aspartate aminotransferase (AST) levels, which were elevated at baseline, decreased during 14 days of dosing in all VX-950-dose groups, with a median decrease from baseline of 25–30 U/L for ALT and 12–22 U/L for AST. The fact there was evidence of clinical viral breakthrough related to selection of viral variants with decreased sensitivity to VX-950 suggests that these new agents will probably be used in conjunction with pegylated interferon and ribavirin.

References

1. Saab S, Martin P. Tests for acute and chronic viral hepatitis. Finding your way through the alphabet soup of infection and superinfection. Postgrad Med 2000;107:123,129.
2. Keeffe EB, Dieterich DT, Han SH, et al. A treatment algorithm for the management of chronic hepatitis B virus infection in the United States: an update. Clin Gastroenterol Hepatol 2006;4:936.
3. Lok AS, McMahon BJ. Chronic hepatitis B. Hepatology 2007;45:507.
4. Iloeje UH, Yang HI, Su J, et al., Risk Evaluation of Viral Load Elevation and Associated Liver Disease/Cancer-In HBV (the REVEAL-HBV) Study Group. Predicting cirrhosis risk based on the level of circulating hepatitis B viral load. Gastroenterology 2006;130:678.
5. Chen CJ, Yang HI, Su J, et al., REVEAL-HBV Study Group. Risk of hepatocellular carcinoma across a biological gradient of serum hepatitis B virus DNA level. JAMA. 2006;295:65.
6. Kidd-Ljunggren K, Miyakawa Y, Kidd AH. Genetic variability in hepatitis B virus. J Gen Virology 2002;83:1267.
7. Kramvis A, Kew MC. Relationship of genotypes of hepatitis B virus to mutations, disease progression and response to antiviral therapy. J Viral Hepatology 2005;12:456.
8. Hoofnagle JH. Hepatitis B – preventable and now treatable. N Engl J Med 2006;354:1074.
9. Wong DK, Cheung Am, O'Rourke K, et al. Effect of alpha-interferon treatment in patients with hepatitis B e antigen-positive chronic hepatitis B. A meta-analysis. Ann Intern Med 1993;119:312.
10. Fattovich G, Giustina G, Sanchez-Tapias J, et al. Delayed clearance of serum HBsAg in compensated cirrhosis B: relation to interferon alpha therapy and disease prognosis. European Concerted Action on Viral Hepatitis (EUROHEP). Am J Gastroenterol 1998;93:896.
11. Niederau C, Heintges T, Lange S. Long-term follow-up of HBeAg-positive patients treated with interferon alfa for chronic hepatitis B. N Engl J Med 1996;334:1422.
12. Cooksley WG, Piratvisuth T, Lee SD, et al. Peginterferon alpha-2a (40 kDa): an advance in the treatment of hepatitis B e antigen-positive chronic hepatitis B. J Viral Hepat 2003;10:298.
13. Chan HL, Leung NW, Hui Ay, et al. A randomized, controlled trial of combination therapy for chronic hepatitis B: comparing pegylated interferon-alpha2b and lamivudine with lamivudine alone. Ann Intern Med 2005;142:240.
14. Lau Gk, Piravsisuth T, Luo KX, et al. Peginterferon alfa-2a, lamivudine, and the combination for HBeAg-positive chronic hepatitis B. N Engl J Med 2005;352:2682.
15. Marcellin P, Lau GK, Bonino F, et al. Peginterferon alfa-2a alone, lamivudine alone, and the two in combination in patients with HBeAg-negative chronic hepatitis B. N Engl J Med. 2004;351:1206.
16. Brook MG, Karayiannis P, Thomas HC. Which patients with chronic hepatitis B virus infection will respond to alpha-interferon therapy? A statistical analysis of predictive factors. Hepatology 1989;10:761.
17. Perrillo RP. Factors influencing response to interferon in chronic hepatitis B: implications for Asian and western populations. Hepatology 1990;12:1433.
18. Lok AS, Wu PC, Lai CL, et al. A controlled trial of interferon with or without prednisone priming for chronic hepatitis B. Gastroenterology 1992;102:2091.
19. Dienstag JL, Schiff ER, Wright TL, et al. Lamivudine as initial treatment for chronic hepatitis B in the United States. N Engl J Med. 1999;341:1256.
20. Lai CL, Chien RN, Leug NW, et al. A one-year trial of lamivudine for chronic hepatitis B. Asia Hepatitis Lamivudine Study Group. N Engl J Med 1998;339:61.
21. Schalm SW, Heathcote J, Heathcote J, et al. Lamivudine and alpha interferon combination treatment of patients with chronic hepatitis B infection: a randomised trial. Gut 2000;46:562.
22. Lok AS, Hussain M, Cursano C, et al. Evolution of hepatitis B virus polymerase gene mutations in hepatitis B e antigen-negative patients receiving lamivudine therapy. Hepatology 2000;32:1145.
23. Hadziyannis SJ, Papatheodoridis GV, Dimou E, et al. Efficacy of long-term lamivudine monotherapy in patients with hepatitis B e antigen-negative chronic hepatitis B. Hepatology 2000;32:847.
24. Rizzetto M, Volpes R, Smedile A. Response of pre-core mutant chronic hepatitis B infection to lamivudine. J Med Virol 2000;61:398.
25. Papatheodoridis GV, Dimou E, Laras A, et al. Course of virologic breakthroughs under long-term lamivudine in HBeAg-negative precore mutant HBV liver disease. Hepatology 2002;36:219.
26. Yang H, Oi X, Sabogal A, et al. Cross-resistance testing of next-generation nucleoside and nucleotide analogues against lamivudine-resistant HBV. Antivir Ther 2005;10:625.
27. Fung SK, Chae HB, Fontana RJ, et al. Virologic response and resistance to adefovir in patients with chronic hepatitis B. Hepatology 2006;44:283.
28. Perrillo RP, Lai CL, Liaw YF, et al. Predictors of HBeAg loss after lamivudine treatment for chronic hepatitis B. Hepatology 2002;36:186.
29. Yeo W, Johnson PJ. Diagnosis, prevention and management of hepatitis B virus reactivation during anticancer therapy. Hepatology 2006;43:209.
30. Saab S, Dong M, Joseph T, Tong M. Hepatitis B prophylaxis in patients undergoing chemotherapy for lymphoma: a decision analysis model. Hepatology 2007;46:1049.
31. Martyak LA, Taqavi E, Saab S. Lamivudine prophylaxis is effective in reducing hepatitis B reactivation and reactivation-related mortality in chemotherapy patients: a metaanalysis. Liver Int 2007 (in press).
32. Chang TT, Gish R, de Man R, et al. A comparison of entecavir and lamivudine for HBeAg-positive chronic hepatitis B. N Engl J Med 2006;354:1001.
33. Chang TT, Gish R, Hadziyannis SJ, et al. A dose-ranging study of the efficacy and tolerability of entecavir in lamivudine-refractory chronic hepatitis B patients. Gastroenterology 2005;129:1198.
34. Colonno RJ, Rose R, Baldick CJ, et al. Entecavir resistance is rare in nucleoside naive patients with hepatitis B. Hepatology 2006;44:1656.
35. Sherman M, Yurdaydin C, Sollano J, et al. Entecavir for treatment of lamivudine-refractory, HBeAg-positive chronic hepatitis B. Gastroenterology 2006;130:2039.
36. Marcellin P, Chang TT, Lim SG, et al. Adefovir dipivoxil for the treatment of hepatitis B e antigen-positive chronic hepatitis B. N Engl J Med 2003;348:808.
37. Hadziyannis SJ, Tassopulos NC, Heathcote EJ, et al. Adefovir dipivoxil for the treatment of hepatitis B e antigen-negative chronic hepatitis B. N Engl J Med 2003;348:800.

38. Peters M, Hann HwH, Martin P, et al. Adefovir dipivoxil alone or in combination with lamivudine in patients with lamivudine-resistant chronic hepatitis B. Gastroenterology 2004;126:91.

39. Perillo R, Hann HW, Mutimer D, et al. Adefovir dipivoxil added to ongoing lamivudine in chronic hepatitis B with YMDD mutant hepatitis B virus. Gastroenterology 2004;126:81.

40. Hadziyannis SJ, Tassopoulos NC, Heathcote EJ, et al. Long-term therapy with adefovir dipivoxil for HBeAg-negative chronic hepatitis B for up to 5 years. Gastroenterology 2006;131:1743.

41. Lai CL, Leung N, Teo EK, et al. A 1-year trial of telbivudine, lamivudine, and the combination in patients with hepatitis B e antigen-positive chronic hepatitis B. Gastroenterology. 2005;129:528.

42. Pradat P, Alberti A, Poynard T, et al. Predictive value of ALT levels for histologic findings in chronic hepatitis C: a European collaborative study. Hepatology 2002;36:973.

43. Hui CK, Belaye T, Montegrande K, Wright TL. A comparison in the progression of liver fibrosis in chronic hepatitis C between persistently normal and elevated transaminase. J Hepatol 2003;38:511.

44. McHutchison JG, Gordon SC, Schiff ER, et al. Interferon alfa-2b alone or in combination with ribavirin as initial treatment for chronic hepatitis C. Hepatitis Interventional Therapy Group. N Engl J Med 1998;339:1485.

45. Kim AI, Saab S. Treatment of hepatitis C. Am J Med 2005;118:808.

46. Strader DB, Wright T, Thomas DL, Seeff LM, American Association for the Study of Liver Diseases. Diagnosis, management, and treatment of hepatitis C. Hepatology. 2004;39:1147.

47. Scott JD, Gretch DR. Molecular diagnostics of hepatitis C virus infection: a systematic review. JAMA 2007;297:724.

48. Saldanha J, Lelie N, Heath A. Establishment of the first international standard for nucleic acid amplification technology (NAT) assays for HCV RNA. WHO Collaborative Study Group. Vox Sang 1999;76:149.

49. Zehnter E, Mauss S, John C, et al. Better prediction of SVR in patients with HCV genotype 1(G1) with peginterferon alfa-2a (PEGASYS) plus ribavirin: Improving differentiation between low (LVL) and high baseline viral load (HVL). Hepatology 2006;368:958.

50. Manns MP, McHutchison JG, Gordon SC, et al. Peginterferon alfa-2b plus ribavirin compared with interferon alfa-2b plus ribavirin for initial treatment of chronic hepatitis C: a randomised trial. Lancet 2001;358:958.

51. Fried MW, Shiffman ML, Reddy KR, et al. Peginterferon alfa-2a plus ribavirin for chronic hepatitis C virus infection. N Engl J Med 2002;347:975.

52. Hadziyannis SJ, Sette H, Jr, Morgan TR, et al., PEGASYS International Study Group. Peginterferon-alpha2a and ribavirin combination therapy in chronic hepatitis C: a randomized study of treatment duration and ribavirin dose. Ann Intern Med 2004;140:346.

53. Yano M, Kumada H, Kage M, et al. The long-term pathological evolution of chronic hepatitis C. Hepatology 1996;23:1334.

54. Fontaine H, Nalpas B, Poulet B, et al. Hepatitis activity index is a key factor in determining the natural history of chronic hepatitis C. Hum Pathol 2001;32:904.

55. Marcellin P, Asselah T, Boyer N. Fibrosis and disease progression in hepatitis C. Hepatology 2002;36:S47.

56. Bravo AA, Sheth SG, Chopra S. Liver biopsy. N Engl J Med 2001;344:495.

57. McGill DB, Rakela J, Zinsmeister AR, Ott BJ. A 21-year old experience with major hemorrhage after percutaneous liver biopsy. Gastroenterology 1990;99:47.

58. Van Thiel DH, Avaler JS, Wright H, Tzakis A. Liver biopsy: its safety and complications as seen at a liver transplant center. Transplantation 1993;55:1087.

59. Bedossa P, Poynard T. An algorithm for the grading of activity in chronic hepatitis C. The METAVIR Cooperative Study Group. Hepatology 1996;24:289.

60. Scheuer PJ. Classification of chronic viral hepatitis: a need for reassessment. J Hepatol 1991;13:372.

61. Wong JB, Koff RS. Watchful waiting with periodic liver biopsy versus immediate empirical therapy for histologically mild chronic hepatitis C. A cost-effectiveness analysis. Ann Intern Med 2000;133:665.

62. Dienstag JL, McHutchinson JG. American Gastroenterological Association technical review on the management of hepatitis C. Gastroenterology 2006;130:231.

63. Fried MW, Hadziyannis SJ. Treatment of chronic hepatitis C infection with peginterferons plus ribavirin. Semin Liver Dis 2004;24(Suppl. 2):47.

64. Manns MP, McHutchinson JG, Gordon SC, et al. Peginterferon alfa-2b plus ribavirin compared with interferon alfa-2b plus ribavirin for initial treatment of chronic hepatitis C: a randomized trial. Lancet 2001;358:958.

65. Fried MW, Shiffman ML, Reddy KR, et al. Combination of peginterferon alfa-2a plus ribavirin in patients with chronic hepatitis C infection. N Engl J Med 2002;347:975.

66. Shiffman ML, Di Bisceglie AM, Lindsay KL, et al., Hepatitis C Antiviral Long-Term Treatment Against Cirrhosis Trial Group. Peginterferon alfa-2a and ribavirin in patients with chronic hepatitis C who have failed prior treatment. Gastroenterology 2004;126:1015.

67. Poynard T, McHutchison J, Manns M, et al. Impact of pegylated interferon alfa-2b and ribavirin on liver fibrosis in patients with chronic hepatitis C. Gastroenterology 2002;122:1303.

68. Russo MW, Fried MW. Side effects of therapy for chronic hepatitis C. Gastroenterology 2003;124:1711.

69. Curry MP, Afdhal NH. Use of growth factors with antiviral therapy for chronic hepatitis C. Clin Liver Dis 2005;9:439.

70. Davis GL, Wong JB, McHutchinson JG, et al. Early virologic response to treatment with peginterferon alfa-2b plus ribavirin in patients with chronic hepatitis C. Hepatology 2003;38:645.

71. Davis GL. Monitoring of viral levels during therapy of hepatitis C. Hepatology 2002;36:S145.

72. Conjeevaram HS, Fried MW, Jeffers LJ, et al. Peginterferon and ribavirin treatment in African American and Caucasian American patients with hepatitis C genotype 1. Gastroenterology 2006;131:470.

73. von Wagner M, Huber M, Berg T, et al. Peginterferon-alpha-2a (40KD) and ribavirin for 16 or 24 weeks in patients with genotype 2 or 3 chronic hepatitis C. Gastroenterology 2005;129:522.

74. Mangia A, Santoro R, Minerva N, et al. Peginterferon alfa-2b and ribavirin for 12 vs. 24 weeks in HCV genotype 2 or 3. N Engl J Med 2005;352:2609.

75. Sanchez-Tapias J, Diago M, Escartìn P, et al. Peginterferon-alfa2a plus ribavirin for 48 versus 72 weeks in patients with detectable hepatitis C virus RNA at week 4 of treatment. Gastroenterology 2006;131:451.

76. Hinrichsen H, Benhamou Y, Wedemeyer H, et al. Short-term antiviral efficacy of BILN 2061, a hepatitis C virus serine protease inhibitor, in hepatitis C genotype 1 patients. Gastroenterology 2004;127:1347.

77. Reesink HW, Zeuzem S, Weegink CJ, et al. Rapid decline of viral RNA in hepatitis C patients treated with VX-950: a phase Ib, placebo-controlled, randomized study. Gastroenterology 2006;131:997.

27 Approach to the patient with a liver mass

John A. Donovan, Edward G. Grant

Basic approach to the liver mass, 526
Hepatic hemangioma, 527
Focal nodular hyperplasia, 528
Hepatic adenoma, 529
Nodular regenerative hyperplasia, 530
Biliary cystadenoma, 531
Focal fatty change, 531
Regenerative and dysplastic nodules, 531
Summary, 532

Discovery of a mass in the liver is cause for immediate concern and urgency. The involved gastroenterologist or consulting hepatologist is most often responsible for further evaluations and for the rendering of a correct diagnosis. Evaluation of the hepatic mass requires knowledge of both benign and malignant lesions affecting the liver. Understanding the relative importance and natural history of specific hepatic lesions enables a systematic evaluation of the patient with a hepatic mass that should lead to a proper diagnosis. A correct diagnosis directs subsequent recommendations for additional study, indicates appropriate treatments, and guides future management. Conversely, an incorrect diagnosis may subject the patient to unnecessary medical therapies, expenses, risks, or poor outcomes.

Basic approach to the liver mass

Masses in the liver are usually detected by abdominal imaging performed for the evaluation of right upper quadrant pain, the screening of the patient at risk for hepatocellular carcinoma (HCC) and other malignancies, or by incidental

Principles of Clinical Gastroenterology. Edited by Tadataka Yamada, David H. Alpers, Anthony N. Kalloo, Neil Kaplowitz, Chung Owyang, and Don W. Powell. © 2008 Blackwell Publishing. ISBN 978-1-4051-69103

discovery during the investigation of other medical or surgical conditions. Differentiation of the discovered liver mass as a benign or malignant lesion of the liver is of paramount importance. Confirmation of a benign hepatic lesion usually confers an excellent prognosis and relieves the anxious patient.

Evaluation of the patient with a liver mass begins with a complete history, physical examination, and laboratory evaluation. A diagnosis of HCC is more likely in persons with chronic liver disease and cirrhosis, although HCC in individuals with noncirrhotic liver diseases, such as chronic hepatitis B and hemochromatosis, is not exceptional. Cholangiocarcinoma may complicate primary sclerosing cholangitis and is sometimes detected by screening laboratory tests, carcinoembryonic antigen (CEA), the CA19-9 tumor marker, or by biliary tract imaging performed during the evaluation of the jaundiced patient. Metastatic liver disease from lung, breast, pancreas, or colon may be suspected because of the known presence of a primary malignancy. HCC will not be discussed here; it is suspected in the setting of chronic liver disease or viral hepatitis. Also, cystic disease and hepatic abscess will not be considered here as these are identified by routine imaging.

In the adult, benign lesions of the liver include hemangiomas, hepatic adenomas, focal nodular hyperplasia, and a variety of other less common lesions including bile duct adenomas, nodular regenerative hyperplasia, and focal fatty change. Hepatic biochemistries are seldom of diagnostic importance or assistance. Characteristic radiographic findings,

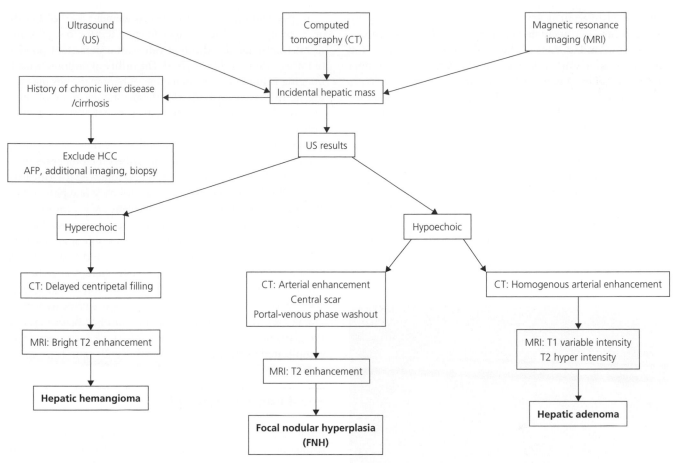

Figure 27.1 Suggested approach to the patient with a discovered liver mass. AFP, α-fetoprotein; HCC, hepatocellular carcinoma.

a confirmatory biopsy, or both most often enable the accurate diagnosis of a benign liver lesion. A recommended approach to the patient with a liver mass is outlined by the algorithm depicted in Fig. 27.1. The remainder of this chapter will discuss the more common and important benign neoplasms of the liver.

Hepatic hemangioma

Hepatic hemangioma is the most common benign liver tumor in men and women. Hepatic hemangiomas may range in size from less than 1 cm to greater than 20 cm in diameter and are more commonly located in the right hepatic lobe. Larger lesions are more common in women. Those measuring greater than 5 cm in diameter are classified as giant hemangiomas. The embryogenesis of the hemangioma is not completely understood but this lesion is more likely to occur in women than in men (5–6:1) [1]. This gender difference in incidence suggests a pathogenesis related to hormonal influences although this explanation is controversial. Enlargement of hepatic

hemangiomas has been described in pregnant women and in women taking oral contraceptives [2,3]. Others have reported that hepatic hemangiomas are not more prevalent in women taking birth control medications and that hemangiomas do not change in size with pregnancy [4].

Hemangiomas in the liver are sometimes associated with other medical conditions, including the Osler–Weber–Rendu and von Hippel–Lindau syndromes, type Ia glycogen storage disease, and systemic lupus erythematosus. Hepatic hemangiomas may precipitate the Kasabach–Merritt syndrome characterized by a consumptive thrombocytopenia and caused by local disseminated intravascular coagulation (DIC) within an involved hemangioma. The degree of thrombocytopenia in this rare condition, also known as thrombocytopenia–hemangioma syndrome, may be extreme and be associated with spontaneous bleeding, other morbidity, and mortality [1].

Most hepatic hemangiomas are incidentally discovered at the time of abdominal imaging performed for the evaluation of abdominal symptoms. Right upper quadrant pain and abdominal discomfort, when present, are most often caused by giant hemangiomas that retract the Glisson capsule and impinge on adjacent abdominal structures and viscera, or by exophytic and pedunculated hemangiomas that torse. Rarely, more acute and diffuse abdominal pain results from the spontaneous or traumatic rupture of a larger hemangioma and the resulting hemoperitoneum [5]. The typical hepatic hemangioma, because it is small, is not the cause of symptoms. Olivier and colleagues reported the results of 14 ablative therapies (resection 8, embolization 5, and hepatic artery ligation 1) for the management of intractable abdominal pain attributed to hepatic hemangiomas. Seven of the 14 patients had residual pain after the definitive therapy [6].

Hepatic hemangiomas usually demonstrate characteristic appearances on ultrasound, computed tomography (CT), magnetic resonance imaging (MRI), and nuclear medicine scintigraphy examinations. Ultrasound typically shows a hyperechoic lesion; CT a hypointense mass with delayed centripetal filling after contrast enhancement (Fig. 27.2); MRI an intense T2-weighted enhancement ("lightbulb sign"); and technetium-tagged red blood cell scan a persistent pooling of tracer within the lesion [7–9]. The utility of radionucleotide imaging is limited to the detection of hemangiomas measuring more than 3 cm [10]. The diagnostic accuracy of these noninvasive studies usually makes hepatic arteriography unnecessary.

The natural history of the hepatic hemangioma is usually benign. Okano and colleagues described the outcomes of 64 cavernous hemangiomas in 50 patients followed for a mean of 19 months. None increased in size and only one patient had abdominal pain [11]. Surgical intervention is almost never required except when spontaneous rupture occurs. Surgical excision, when indicated, is by local resection or enucleation [12]. Irradiation, radiofrequency ablation, and hepatic artery embolization can be utilized if ablative therapy is indicated [13–15]. There is report of portal hypertension resulting from pressure on the extrahepatic portal vein by a cavernous hemangioma [16]. Rarely, liver transplantation has been required for giant hemangiomas that are too large for resection or complicated by the Kasabach–Merritt syndrome [17].

Focal nodular hyperplasia

Focal nodular hyperplasia (FNH) is the second most common benign liver mass. The usual patient with FNH is a woman in her third to fifth decade with this incidental finding. FNH is more often solitary and typically measures less than 5 cm in the greatest dimension although multiple and larger lesions may occasionally occur. The usual FNH lesion does not cause symptoms. Rarely, enlargement may be the cause for abdominal pain. The hepatic mass represented by FNH must be differentiated from hepatic adenoma, HCC and hypervascular metastatic tumors, which may be mimicked by similar radiographic appearances.

The pathophysiology of FNH, like that for the hepatic hemangioma, is not completely understood. Most likely, FNH is caused by a nonspecific reaction to vascular injury caused by intrahepatic arteriovenous malformations. A nodular morphology and a rich arterial vascular supply suggest this etiology [18]. Earlier reports of a causative role for oral contraceptive pills have been discounted [19].

FNH lesions are characterized by "classical" or "atypical" histologies. Classical FNH is lobulated with a central scar and fibrous septa that radiate between nodules of proliferating hepatocytes. Atypical FNH is classified as telangiectatic, by cytological atypia, or as a mixed hyperplastic and adenomatous type. Regardless of FNH type, bile duct and Kupffer cell elements are present. The FNH lesion does not have a capsule but appears well circumscribed because of the compression of adjacent liver cords [20].

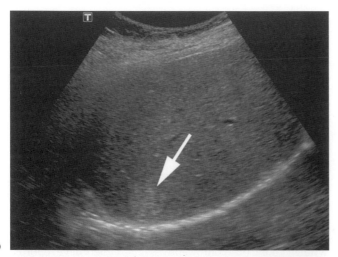
(a)

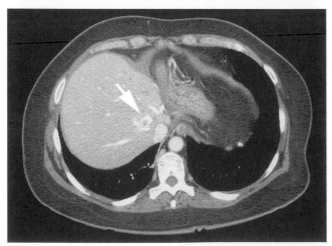
(b)

Figure 27.2 Hepatic hemangioma. **(a)** Longitudinal ultrasound imaging showing typical hyperechoic appearance (arrow). **(b)** Delayed computed tomography imaging shows almost complete centripetal enhancement and accentuation of peripheral nodularity (arrow).

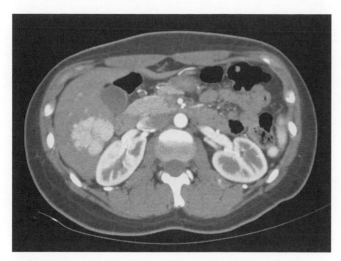

Figure 27.3 Focal nodular hyperplasia. Arterial phase computed tomography imaging shows an intensely enhancing nodular mass with a nonenhancing central scar.

FNH lesions are not well defined by ultrasound examination and are best imaged by CT or MRI studies. Unenhanced CT and T1-weighted MRI studies image an isodense or hypodense lesion. The low-attenuation central scar of FNH rapidly enhances on the arterial phase of contrast-enhanced CT and MRI studies (Fig. 27.3). Arterial enhancement is followed by a rapid washout on the portal venous phase. Fat, calcium, the absence of a central scar, or presence of a pseudocapsule may cause atypical appearances [21–24].

The incidental finding of FNH should not be an indication for therapeutic intervention. Rare enlargement or rupture causing symptomatic pain can be addressed by arterial embolization or resection [25–27].

Hepatic adenoma

Hepatic adenomas are benign hepatic lesions composed of normal-appearing hepatocytes. Portal structures and Kupffer cells, components of the normal hepatic architecture, are characteristically absent. Most hepatic adenomas are encapsulated by a fibrous capsule and are well demarcated. Some 70%–80% are solitary and two-thirds are located in the right lobe of the liver. The presence of multiple adenomas (more than 10) in a bilobar distribution defines a small subset of patients with hepatic adenomatosis [27]. Clinically, hepatic adenomas are important because of the potential risks for intratumoral hemorrhage, rupture, and transformation to HCC.

Hepatic adenomas are associated with glycogen storage disease types I and III. Males with these diagnoses are affected as often as females and for both there is a disproportionate incidence of multiple adenomas, or hepatic adenomatosis. Hepatic adenomas have more rarely been described in patients with Fanconi, Hurler, and combined immunodeficiency syndromes [29,30].

Women have hepatic adenomas more frequently than men (4:1). A promoting effect of oral contraceptive medications and estrogens is well established. Fifty percent of benign liver tumors in women taking oral contraceptives are hepatic adenomas. Among women who take an oral birth control agent the incidence of hepatic adenoma is 34/1 000 000 compared with an incidence of less than 2/1 000 000 in women not taking these medications [31]. The risk of developing a hepatic adenoma while taking oral contraceptives is further increased by patient age greater than 30 years, the estrogen content of the medication, the estrogen mestranol, a duration of use exceeding 6–12 months, and smoking. A variable reduction in the size of hepatic adenomas after withdrawal of oral contraception is possible but complete involution is rare [32,33].

Most individuals with hepatic adenomas are asymptomatic. Approximately one-third of patients with hepatic adenomas will have a variable amount of associated bleeding. The occasional patient may have indolent abdominal pain because of hemorrhage into the tumor. More unusual presentations may include the acute abdomen and shock because of frank rupture and hemoperitoneum. Acute hemorrhage from a ruptured hepatic adenoma is best managed by observation alone in the stable patient. Emergent resection or transcatheter embolization are reserved for treatment of the patient with hemodynamic instability caused by continuing hemorrhage [34–36].

The diagnosis of hepatic adenoma is usually established by hepatic imaging studies. Ultrasound appearance is usually of a hypoechoic mass. Mixed echogenicity may be present when intratumoral hemorrhage has occurred. A hyperechoic ultrasound appearance indicates fatty metamorphosis [37]. Ichikawa and colleagues described the CT characteristics of 44 adenomas in 25 patients. Unenhanced images outlined low-attenuation lesions in 86% of the cases that were typical of central necrosis, bleeding, or fat deposits in the tumor. Increased attenuation was present after more recent hemorrhage into the adenoma, and calcification was associated with more remote bleeding. All the adenomas showed homogeneous arterial phase enhancement followed by an isointense appearance of most (82%) in the portal venous phase (Fig. 27.4). Most had a defined margin (86%) and smooth contours (95%) [38]. Hepatic adenomas display bright or variable intensity on T1-weighted and hyperintensity on T2-weighted MRI examinations [39].

In individual cases, differentiating a hepatic adenoma from FNH may be difficult. Neither lesion is likely to be the cause of symptoms. When abdominal pain does occur it is

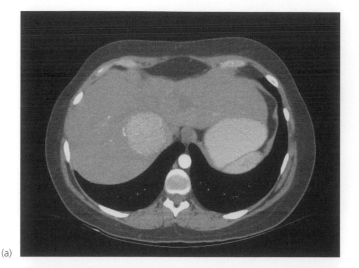

(a)

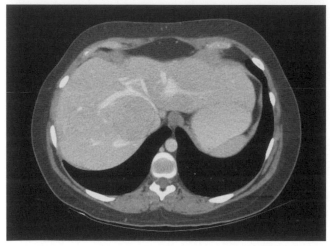

(b)

Figure 27.4 Hepatic adenoma. **(a)** Arterial phase computed tomography (CT) imaging demonstrates a homogeneous, well-defined, intensely enhancing hepatic adenoma. **(b)** During the portal venous phase of CT examination the adenoma becomes isodense to the normal liver. The middle hepatic vein is displaced anteriorly.

most often caused by hemorrhage into an adenoma. Contrast-enhanced ultrasonography may help in differentiating hepatic adenomas from FNH [40]. Hepatic adenomas display a homogeneous arterial enhancement whereas with FNH the enhancement is also seen in the portal phase of examination. Both hepatic adenomas and FNH demonstrate early arterial enhancement on contrast-enhanced CT and MRI examinations [41]. Grazioli and colleagues used MRI to study early and delayed contrast-enhanced patterns in 27 persons with hepatic adenomas (8 with hepatic adenomatosis) and 73 with FNH. In this study, early enhancement did not discriminate adenomas from FNH whereas a hypointense appearance on 1- to 3-h delayed images was characteristic of the hepatic

adenomas but not FNH [41]. Nuclear medicine scintigraphy does not highlight hepatic adenomas because of an absence of Kupffer cells responsible for the hepatic uptake of technetium. The result is a "cold spot" on obtained images.

The intrinsic concern with hepatic adenomas is the recognized potential for their malignant transformation to HCC. The hepatic adenoma-to-HCC sequence is well established. HCC may arise in an adenoma, during the use or after the therapeutic withdrawal of oral birth control medications, or following involution of an adenoma [42–44]. This potential for malignant transformation supports a policy of preemptive surgical resection unless otherwise contraindicated.

Nodular regenerative hyperplasia

Nodular regenerative hyperplasia (NRH) is characterized by diffuse, or occasionally focal, nodules of regenerating hepatocytes in the noncirrhotic liver. NRH occurs equally in men and women and is more prevalent with increasing age. Nodules of regenerating hepatocytes are generally less than 4 mm. in size but can coalesce to form larger nodules measuring up to 4 cm in diameter [45]. NRH is not related to hepatic inflammation or fibrosis. NRH is postulated to evolve from a microvascular insult to a hepatic acinus followed by involution, compensatory regeneration of adjacent hepatocytes, and nodule formation [46]. The participation of antiphospholipid and anticardiolipin antibodies in the development of NRH has been reported. NRH has been associated with a variety of autoimmune type disorders including rheumatoid arthritis with or without Felty syndrome, systemic lupus erythematosus, systemic sclerosis, polyarteritis nodosa, celiac sprue, and mixed connective tissue disorders. Myeloproliferative and lymphoproliferative disorders have also been implicated [47,48]. Even toxic effects of certain medications may play a role in the genesis of NRH. Geller and colleagues reported that 53% of the liver biopsies from 38 patients with inflammatory bowel diseases treated with 6-thioguanine showed NRH and implicated drug-induced microvascular injury as the cause [49].

An association between NRH and HCC has also been suggested. Nzeako and colleagues investigated this association and identified 23 cases (6.7%) of NRH in 342 noncirrhotic livers with coexisting HCC. Liver cell dysplasia was more prevalent in the patients with NRH. These authors noted that it could not be determined whether NRH developed as a consequence of portal vein invasion by HCC or if de novo HCC arose from dysplastic foci found in NRH [50].

NRH should be suspected in the patient without evidence of chronic liver disease or cirrhosis who presents with unexplained portal hypertension. Like cirrhosis, NRH can obstruct sinusoidal blood flow and alter portal hemodynamics. NRH is a recognized cause of noncirrhotic portal hypertension and the ensuing complications of encephalopathy, varices, hypersplenism, and, less often, ascites [51,52]. Nonspecific elevations of serum bilirubin, alkaline phosphatase, and, less frequently, the serum aminotransferases (AST and ALT) may be evident. Importantly, hepatic synthetic functions are characteristically preserved. Radiographic imaging in patients with NRH is usually precipitated by the findings of portal hypertension. Ultrasound, CT, and MRI studies may show hepatomegaly and a nodular liver surface as well as the radiographic manifestations of portal hypertension, which include splenomegaly, varices, and ascites. The relative small size of the characteristic lesion limits the sensitivity and specificity of diagnostic imaging in the diagnosis of NRH. Larger NRH nodules may appear hypoechoic by ultrasound, slightly enhanced by contrast CT, and slightly hypointense or hyperintense by nonenhanced T1- and T2-weighted MRI examinations. MRI contrast administration results in delayed phase enhancement [53]. Common to ultrasound, CT, and MRI studies is a hypoattenuating rim caused by the compression of adjacent hepatic sinusoids and parenchyma resulting in a "nodule within a nodule" appearance.

The diagnosis of NRH is more often dependent on the results of a diagnostic liver biopsy than on imaging. Pathologically, the appearance of NRH may be subtle. The pathology of NRH can be missed when a needle biopsy specimen is small or when nodule formation is focal. Diagnosis may be difficult to establish with use of hematoxylin–eosin stain but is made easier by the use of a reticulum stain. The absence of hepatic fibrosis and distorting septa distinguishes this condition from cirrhosis.

Management of NRH involves the control of symptoms caused by resulting portal hypertension. On occasion, the portal hypertensive complications of NRH indicate orthotopic liver transplantation [54].

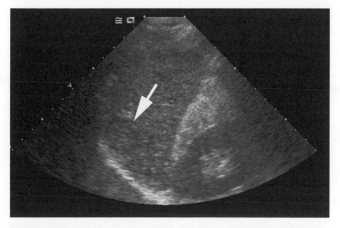

Figure 27.5 Regenerating nodule (arrow). Longitudinal ultrasound image of a regenerating nodule that is isoechoic to the surrounding liver.

Biliary cystadenoma

Biliary cystadenoma involving intrahepatic or extrahepatic bile ducts is a rare cystic neoplasm of mesenchymal and Meyenburg complex origins that accounts for less than 5% of hepatobiliary tumors. Predominantly seen in women in their fifth decade of life, this tumor may present with abdominal pain or biliary obstruction. Ultrasound or CT imaging defines a thick-walled, multiloculated, cystic mass with internal septations [55]. Endoscopic retrograde cholangiopancreatography (ERCP) may demonstrate bile duct obstruction [56]. Cyst aspiration characteristically yields a mucinous fluid. CEA or CA19-9 may be elevated in the serum or found in the cyst fluid [57]. Biliary cystadenoma is a premalignant lesion. Percutaneous ablation or incomplete surgical resection are associated with recurrence. Treatment, and differentiation from biliary cystadenocarcinoma, is by complete surgical resection [58].

Focal fatty change

Focal fatty change describes the localized and geometric deposit of macrovesicular fat in the liver. Focal fatty deposits are most often seen in the anteromedial portion of the medial segment of the left lobe (Couinaud segment IV) and adjacent to the falciform ligament. Location near the gallbladder and porta hepatis has also been reported. The subcapsular position of these lesions may result from local hyperperfusion that promotes the local accumulation of triglyceride in affected hepatocytes. Focal fatty lesions appear hyperechogenic on ultrasound images [59]. Contrast-enhanced CT study shows low-attenuation lesions traversed by vascular structures that betray a true mass effect. CT portography is not often necessary but demonstrates perfusion by portal blood flow that is not seen in true hepatic tumors [60]. More specific MR studies show a hypodense lesion on T1- and T2-weighted images with a diagnostically useful drop in intensity during out-of-phase sequence images [61].

Regenerative and dysplastic nodules

The discovery of regenerative or dysplastic lesions within the cirrhotic liver is of concern because of the association of liver cell dysplasia with HCC. Regenerative nodules can occur in both the noncirrhotic and cirrhotic liver but those with associated dysplasia are unique to the cirrhotic liver.

Characteristic imaging appearances of dysplastic nodules include mixed echogenicity by ultrasound (Fig. 27.5), arterial enhancement by contrast CT, and high-intensity T1-weighted and low-intensity T2-weighted enhancement by MRI [62].

Unfortunately, each of these imaging modalities is insensitive and of limited efficacy in the diagnosis of the dysplastic nodule. In a study by Kim and colleagues, preoperative ultrasound examinations failed to detect any of 20 dysplastic nodules present in explanted livers. Preoperative, triple-phase CT studies of cirrhotic livers identified only 8 of 76 (10%) dysplastic nodules present in 21 resection and 20 explant specimens [63]. In another study, triphasic CT examination before liver transplantation correctly identified only 9 of 23 (sensitivity 39%) dysplastic nodules that ranged in size from 0.7 to 2.0 cm (mean 1.0 cm) [64]. Krinsky and colleagues highlighted the similar limitations of MRI in detecting dysplastic nodules. Contrast-enhanced T1- and T2-weighted studies performed within 90 days of liver transplantation indicated a dysplastic nodule in only 3 of 18 (17%) livers with dysplastic nodules and depicted only 9 of 59 (15%) of nodules identified by explant pathology [65].

Hepatocarcinogenesis describes the sequenced progression of genetic, cellular, and clinicopathological changes that characterize the evolution of HCC from preneoplastic lesions in the cirrhotic liver. Microscopic foci of small-cell dysplasia, characterized by nuclear crowding, nuclear polymorphism, and an increased nucleocytoplasmic ratio precede the development of low-grade and high-grade dysplastic nodules. Seki and colleagues described the outcomes of 33 dysplastic nodules measuring less than 20 mm detected by ultrasound examinations. Eighty-eight percent disappeared or remained the same size for up to 70 months but four (12%) became HCC. Small-cell dysplasia and a hyperechoic appearance predicted malignant transformation [66]. The importance of the high-grade dysplastic nodule in hepatocarcinogenesis is also well established. Borzio and colleagues analyzed the outcomes of 90 consecutive dysplastic nodules detected by ultrasound examinations of cirrhotic livers. During a period of follow-up (mean 33 months) 28 of these nodules evolved to biopsy-proven HCC [67]. The presence of high-grade dysplasia in the original dysplastic nodule was an independent predictor of eventual hepatocellular malignancy [68].

Summary

Benign hepatic neoplasms are commonly discovered during the evaluation of conditions unrelated to disorders of the liver. Efficient and expeditious evaluation of the newly identified liver mass, differentiation of the lesion from a hepatic malignancy, and establishment of a correct and reassuring diagnosis is of exceptional importance. Absence of factors that identify the patient at risk for malignancy, a knowledge of the more common benign hepatic neoplasms, and the characteristic properties of benign liver masses defined by selected diagnostics enable the gastroenterologist or hepatologist to meet the associated diagnostic challenges and responsibilities.

References

1. Choi B, Nguyen M. The diagnosis and management of benign liver tumors. J Clin Gastroenterol 2005;39:401.
2. Seagusa T, Ito K, Oba N. Enlargement of multiple cavernous hemangiomas of the liver in association with pregnancy. Intern Med 1995; 34:207.
3. Gemer O, Moscovici O, Ben-Horin C, et al. Oral contraceptives and liver hemangioma: a case control study. Acta Obstet Gynecol Scand 2004;83:1199.
4. Cobey F, Salem R. A review of liver masses in pregnancy and a proposed algorithm for their diagnosis and management. Am J Surg 2004;182:181.
5. Hotokezaka M, Masayuki K, Nakamura K, et al. Traumatic rupture of hepatic hemangioma. J Clin Gastroenterol 1996;23:69.
6. Olivier Farges O, Daradkeh S, Bismuth H. Cavernous hemangiomas of the liver: Are there any indications for resection. World J Surg 1995;19:19.
7. Takahashi T, Katoh H, Okushiba S. Giant hepatic hemangioma with secondary portal hypertension: A case report of successful surgical treatment. Hepatogastroenterology 1997;44:1212.
8. Lee J, Choi B, Han J, et al. Improved sonographic imaging of hepatic hemangioma with contrast enhanced coded harmonic angiography: comparison with MR imaging. Ultrasound Med Biol 2002;28: 287.
9. Jang H, Kim T, Lim H, et al. Hepatic hemangioma: Atypical appearances on CT, MR imaging, and sonography. AJR Am J Roentgenol 2003;180:135.
10. Middleton M. Scintigraphic evaluation of hepatic mass lesions: emphasis on hemangioma detection. Semin Nuc Med 1996;26:4.
11. Okano H, Shiraki K, Inoue H, et al. Natural course of cavernous hepatic hemangioma. Oncol Report 2001;8:411.
12. Yoon S, Charny C, Fong Y, et al. Diagnosis, management, and outcomes of 115 patients with hepatic hemangioma. J Am Col Surg 2003;197:392.
13. Biswell B, Sandhu M, Lal P, Bal C. Role of radiotherapy in cavernous hemangioma of the liver. Indian J Gastroenterol 1995;14:95.
14. Zagoria R, Roth T, Levine E, Kavanagh P. Technical innovation. Radiofrequency ablation of a symptomatic hepatic cavernous hemangioma. AJR Am J Roentgenol 2004;182: 210.
15. Deeeutsc G, Yeh K, Bates W, Tannahill W. Embolization for management of hepatic hemangiomas. Amer Surg 2001;67:159.
16. Ferraz A, Sette M, Maia M, et al. Liver transplant for the treatment of giant hepatic hemangioma. Liver Transpl 2004;10:1436.
17. Kumashiro Y, Kasahara M, Nomoto K, et al. Living donor liver transplantation for giant hepatic hemangioma with Kasabach-Merritt syndrome with a posterior segment graft. Liver Transpl 2002;8:72.
18. Wanless I. The pathogenesis of focal nodular hyperplasia. J Gastroenterol Hepatol 2004;19:s342.
19. Mathieu D, Kobeiter H, Maison P, et al. Oral contraceptive use and focal nodular hyperplasia of the liver. Gastroenterology 2000;118:560.
20. Ngyuen B, Flejou J, Terris B, et al. Focal nodular hyperplasia of the liver: a comprehensive pathologic study of 305 lesions and recognition of new forms. Amer J Surg Path 1999;23:1441.
21. Hassain S, Terkivatan T, Zondervan P, et al. Focal nodular hyperplasia; findings at state of the art MR imaging, US, CT, and pathologic analysis. Radiographics 2004;24:3.
22. Mortele K, Praet M, Van Vlierberghe H, et al. CT and MR imaging findings in focal nodular hyperplasia of the liver. AJR Am J Roentgenol 2000;175.
23. Carlson S, Johnson C, Bender C, Welch T. CT of focal nodular hyperplasia of the liver. AJR Am J Roentgenol 2000;174:705.
24. Choi, C, Freeny P. Triphasic helical CT of hepatic focal nodular hyperplasia; incidence of atypical findings. AJR Am J Roentgenol 1998;170:391.
25. Vogl T, Own A, Hammersting R, et al. Transarterial embolization as a

therapeutic option for focal nodular hyperplasia in four patients. Eur Radiol 2006;16:670.

26. Koch N, Gintzburger D, Seelentag W, et al. Rupture of hepatic focal nodular hyperplasia. About two cases. Ann Surg 2006;131:279.

27. Arsenault T, Johnson D, Gormaan B, Burgart L. Hepatic adenomatosis. Mayo Clin Proc 1996;71:478.

28. Hwang N, Choi M, Lee J, et al. Clinical features of surgically resected focal nodular hyperplasia of the liver. Korean J Hepatol 2004;10:135.

29. Resnick M, Kozakewich H, Perez-Atayde A. Hepatic adenoma in the pediatric age group. Clinicopathological observations and assessment of cell proliferative activity. Am J Surg Path 1995;19:1181.

30. Gokhale R, Whitington P. Hepatic adenomatosis in an adolescent. J Pediatr Gastroenterol Nutr 1996:23:482.

31. Reddy K, Karnam U. Approach to the patient with a liver mass. In: Yamada T (ed.). Textbook of Gastroenterology. Philadelphia: Lippincott, Williams & Wilkins, 2003:967.

32. Kolb A. Benign liver tumors and oral contraceptives. Acta Chir Scand 1982;148:89.

33. Aseni P, Sansalone C, Vicenzo C, et al. Rapid disappearance of hepatic adenoma after contraception withdrawal. J Clin Gastroenterol 2001;33:234.

34. Terkavatan T, de Wilt J, de Man R, et al. Treatment of ruptured hepatic adenoma. Br J Surg 2002;88:207.

35. Chen M. Hepatic resection for benign tumours of the liver. J Gastroenterol Hepatol 2000;15:587.

36. Ault G, Wren S, Rall P, et al. Selective management of hepatic adenomas. Am Surg 1996;62:825.

37. Hung C, Changchien C, Lu S, et al. Sonographic features of hepatic adenomas with clinicopathologic correlation. Abdom Imaging 2000; 26:500.

38. Ichikawa T, Federle M, Grazioli L, Nalesnik M. Hepatocellular adenoma: multiphasic CT and histopathologic findings in 25 patients. Radiology 2000;214:861.

39. Grazioli L, Federle M, Brancatelli G, et al. Hepatic adenomas: imaging and pathologic findings. Radiographics 2001;21:887.

40. Dietrich C, Schuessler M, Trojan J, et al. Differentiation of focal nodular hyperplasia and hepatocellular adenoma by contrast-enhanced ultrasound. Br J Radiol 2005;78:704.

41. Graziola L, Morana G, Kirchin M, Schneider G. Accurate differentiation of focal nodular hyperplasia from hepatic adenoma at dimeglumine-enhanced MR imaging: prospective study. Radiology 2005;236:166.

42. Tesluk H, Lawrie J. Hepatocellular carcinoma. Its transformation to carcinoma in a user of oral contraceptives. Arch Pathol Lab Med 1981;105:296.

43. Korula J, Yellin A, Kanel G, et al. Hepatocellular carcinoma coexisting with hepatic adenoma. Incidental discovery after long-term oral contraceptive use. West J Med 1991;155:416.

44. Gordon S, Reddy K, Livingstone A, et al. Resolution of a contraceptive-steroid-induced hepatic adenoma with subsequent evolution into hepatocellular carcinoma. Ann Int Med 1986;105:547.

45. Nagorney D. Benign hepatic tumors: focal nodular hyperplasia and hepatocellular adenoma. World J Surg 1995;19:13.

46. Wanles I. The pathogenesis of focal nodular hyperplasia of the liver. J Gastroenterol Hepatol 2004;19(s7):S342.

47. Abraham S, Begum S, Isenberg D. Hepatic manifestations of autoimmune rheumatic diseases. Ann Rheum Dis 2004;63:123.

48. Riestra S, Dominguez F, Rodrigo L. Nodular regenerative hyperplasia in a patient with celiac disease. J Clin Gastroenterol 2001;34:323.

49. Geller S, Dubinsky M, Poordad F, et al. Early hepatic nodular hyperplasia and submicroscopic fibrosis associated with 6-thioguanine therapy in inflammatory bowel disease. Am J Surg Path 2004;28:1204.

50. Nzeako U, Goodman Z, Ishak Z. Hepatocellular carcinoma and nodular regenerative hyperplasia; possible pathogenetic relationship. Am J Gastroenterol 1996;91:879.

51. Gent-Pena E, Marin-Lorente JL, Echevarrai-Iturbe C, et al. Sinusoidal portal hypertension secondary to nodular regenerative hyperplasia of the liver. Gastroenterol Hepatol 1999;22:183.

52. Naber AH, Van Haelst U, Yap SH. Nodular regenerative hyperplasia of the liver: an important cause of portal hypertension in non-cirrhotic patients. J Hepatol 1991;12:94.

53. Casillas C, Marti-Bonmat L, Galant J. Pseudotumoral presentation of nodular regenerative hyperplasia of the liver: imaging in five patients including MR imaging. Eur Radiol 2004;7:654.

54. Radomski J, Chojnackii K, Moritz M, et al. Results of liver transplantation for nodular regenerative hyperplasia. Am Surg 200;66:1067.

55. Daniels J, Coad J, Payne W, et al. Biliary cystadenomas: hormone receptor expression and clinical management. Dig Dis Sci 2006;51: 623.

56. Van Steenbergen W, Ponette E, Marchal G, et al. Cystadenoma of the bile duct demonstrated by endoscopic retrograde cholangiography: an uncommon cause of extrahepatic obstruction. Am J Gastroenterol 1979;79:466.

57. Pinto M, Kaye A. Fine needle aspiration of cystic liver lesions. Cytologic examination and carcinoembryonic antigen assay of cyst contents. Acta Cytol 1989;33:852.

58. Thomas K, Welch D, Trueblood A, et al. Effective treatment of biliary cystadenoma. Ann Surg 2005;241:769.

59. Brawer M, Ausin G, Lewin K. Focal fatty change in the liver: a hitherto poorly recognized entity. Gastroenterology 1980;78:247.

60. Kammen B, Pacharn P, Thoeni R, et al. Focal fatty infiltration of the liver; analysis of presence and CT findings in children and young adults. AJR Am J Roentgenol 2001;177:1035.

61. Basaran C, Karcaaltincaba M, Akata D, et al. Fat containing lesions of the liver: cross-sectional imaging findings with emphasis on MRI. AJR Am J Roentgenol 2005;184:1103.

62. Choi B, Han J, Hong S, et al. Dysplastic nodules of the liver: imaging findings. Abdomin Imaging 1999;24:250.

63. Kim J, Lim H, Lee W. Detection of hepatocellular carcinoma and dysplastic nodules in cirrhotic liver: accuracy of ultrasound in transplant patients. J Ultrasound Med 2001;20:99.

64. Lim J, Kim M, Park C, et al. Dysplastic nodules in liver cirrhosis: detection with triple phase helical dynamic CT. Brit J Radiol 2004;77: 911.

65. Krinsky G, Lee V, Theise N, et al. Hepatocellular carcinoma and dysplastic nodules in patients with cirrhosis; prospective diagnosis with MR imaging and explantation correlation. Radiology 2001;219:445.

66. Seki S, Hiroki S, Takuya K, et al. Outcomes of dysplastic nodules in human cirrhotic liver: a clinicopathologic study. Clin Cancer Research 2000;6:3469.

67. Borzio M, Fargion S, Borzio F, et al. Impact of large regenerative, low grade and high grade dysplastic nodules in hepatocellular carcinoma development. J Hepatol 2003;39:208.

68. Libbrecht L, Craninx M, Nevens F, et al. Predictive value of liver cell dysplasia for development of hepatocellular carcinoma in patients with non-cirrhotic and cirrhotic chronic viral hepatitis. Histopathology 2001;39:66.

Common gastrointestinal complaints in pregnancy, 534
Chronic gastrointestinal diseases in pregnancy, 540
Gastrointestinal endoscopy during pregnancy, 544
Hepatobiliary diseases during pregnancy, 545
Infectious hepatitis and pregnancy, 550

The gastroenterologist plays an important role in the care of the pregnant patient with gastrointestinal or liver diseases. Thus, it is essential to have a thorough understanding of the presentation and management of common gastrointestinal diseases in the pregnant patient, such as gastroesophageal reflux disease and constipation, and diseases that are unique to pregnancy, such as hyperemesis gravidarum and acute fatty liver of pregnancy. The gastroenterologist should be closely involved in the management of the young female patient with chronic gastrointestinal diseases, such as inflammatory bowel disease, who wishes to conceive a healthy fetus and carry to term. There are also special considerations for pregnant patients undergoing endoscopic interventions for gastrointestinal complaints. The use of any drug during pregnancy or in women of childbearing potential requires that the potential benefits of the drug be weighed against possible hazards to the mother and fetus. Food and Drug Administration Pregnancy Categories for drugs are summarized in Table 28.1.

Common gastrointestinal complaints in pregnancy

Gastroesophageal reflux disease

Gastroesophageal reflux disease (GERD) is a condition in which reflux of acidic stomach contents into the esophagus provokes symptoms such as heartburn [1]. GERD affects both genders, with a slight predilection for men [2]. In a cross-sectional study of 543 adults, the prevalence of symptomatic GERD was similar for men and women, but fewer women harbored Barrett esophagus. However, the severity of symptoms in women was significantly higher than in men, and it was speculated that this may contribute to earlier disease recognition and therapy in women [3].

Heartburn occurs in approximately two-thirds of pregnant women [4]. The pathogenesis of GERD during pregnancy remains poorly understood but several mechanisms have been implicated. First, there is evidence from both human and animal studies that the increase in plasma progesterone alone or in combination with estrogens during pregnancy is responsible for the reduction of lower esophageal sphincter pressure [5–9]. Second, there is evidence from human studies that intragastric pressure is increased secondary to gastric compression by the enlarged uterus [10]. Whether this increase in intragastric pressure affects the lower esophageal sphincter pressure is less clear. In fact, it has been shown that the resting lower esophageal sphincter pressure will increase in response to increased abdominal pressure [8]. Third, there is evidence from human studies that esophageal peristalsis may be less effective during pregnancy, thus allowing for decreased acid clearance [11].

The diagnosis of GERD in pregnancy is based on symptoms. Conservative antireflux measures, such as the avoidance of late-night snacks, carbonated, caffeinated, and alcoholic drinks, juices, spicy food, and positional changes (such as elevation of the head of the bed by 15 cm) should be recommended to all patients (Fig. 28.1).

Antacids

First-line therapy for the treatment of GERD in pregnancy are calcium- or magnesium-containing antacids or a cytoprotect-

Principles of Clinical Gastroenterology. Edited by Tadataka Yamada, David H. Alpers, Anthony N. Kalloo, Neil Kaplowitz, Chung Owyang, and Don W. Powell. © 2008 Blackwell Publishing. ISBN 978-1-4051-69103

Table 28.1 US Food and Drug Administration pregnancy categories for drugs

Category	Interpretation
A	Adequate, well-controlled studies in pregnant women have not shown an increased risk of fetal abnormalities in any trimester of pregnancy
B	Animal studies have revealed no evidence of harm to the fetus; however, there are no adequate, well-controlled studies in pregnant women **OR** Animal studies have shown an adverse effect, but adequate and well-controlled studies in pregnant women have failed to demonstrate a risk to the fetus in any trimester
C	Animal studies have shown an adverse effect and there are no adequate and well-controlled studies in pregnant women **OR** No animal studies have been conducted and there are no adequate and well-controlled studies in pregnant women
D	Adequate well-controlled or observational studies in pregnant women have demonstrated a risk to the fetus. However, the benefits of therapy may outweigh the potential risk. For example, the drug may be acceptable if needed in a life-threatening situation or serious disease for which safer drugs cannot be used or are ineffective
X	Adequate well-controlled or observational studies in animals or pregnant women have demonstrated positive evidence of fetal abnormalities or risks. The use of the product is contraindicated in women who are or may become pregnant

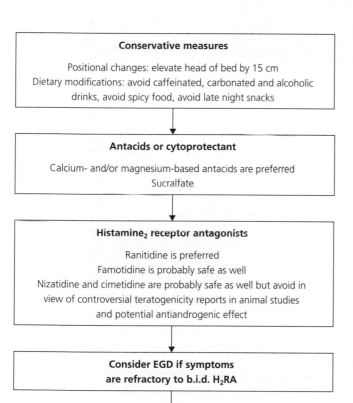

Figure 28.1 Management of gastroesophageal reflux disease (GERD) in pregnancy. b.i.d., twice a day; EGD, esophagogastroduodenoscopy; H₂RA, histamine H₂ receptor antagonist.

ive agent such as sucralfate (Table 28.2). This was reaffirmed at a consensus meeting on the management of GERD in pregnancy [12]. Calcium may have the added benefit of reducing hypertension and preeclampsia [13]. Magnesium sulfate has been shown to halve the risk of eclampsia and reduce the risk of maternal death in a randomized, placebo-controlled trial [14]. Antacids provide quick relief of symptoms and have been shown to be effective therapy, with an 80% improvement in symptoms (odds ratio [OR] 0.2; confidence interval [CI] 0.1–0.4) [12]. Sucralfate is a polysaccharide complex that contains aluminum oxide. Although fetal toxicity has been described with the parenteral use of aluminum in laboratory animals, the absorption of aluminum from orally administered sucralfate is minimal [15]. The safety and efficacy of sucralfate in pregnancy has been confirmed by several studies, including a randomized controlled study of 66 patients with heartburn and regurgitation [16,17].

Histamine H₂ receptor antagonists

Second-line therapy includes the use of histamine H₂ receptor antagonists (H₂RAs) [12]. All four H₂RAs given in Table 28.2 are available over the counter. All these agents cross the human placenta and all have been rated pregnancy category B. Exposure to H₂RAs during the first trimester does not present a major teratogenic risk. A prospective cohort study of 178 women who contacted a Teratology Information Service about gestational H₂RA use showed no increase in major malformations following first-trimester exposure (2.1% vs 3.5% for controls) [18].

When recommending H₂RA therapy to the pregnant patient, the following should be kept in mind. First, although none of the H₂RAs has been associated with teratogenicity in humans, there are conflicting reports of animal studies on the effect of

Table 28.2 Acid-suppressive medication during pregnancy

Drug class/name	FDA category[a]	Excreted in breast milk	Comments
Antacids (containing)		Antacids may pass into breast	
Aluminum	B	milk; not reported to cause	Avoid
Magnesium hydroxide	B	problems in nursing babies	Preferred
Calcium carbonate (Tums)	C		Preferred
H$_2$RAs			
Cimetidine (Tagamet)	B	Yes	Avoid
Ranitidine (Zantac)	B	Yes	Preferred
Nizatidine (Axid)	B	Yes	Avoid
Famotidine (Pepcid)	B	Yes	
Proton pump inhibitors			
Omeprazole (Prilosec)	C	Unknown	
Esomeprazole (Nexium)	C	Unknown	
Lansoprazole (Prevacid)	B	Yes	Preferred
Rabeprazole (Aciphex)	B	Unknown	
Pantoprazole (Protonix)	B	Unknown	
Cytoprotective agents			
Sucralfate (Carafate)	B	Minimal	

a See Table 28.1.
H$_2$RAs, histamine H$_2$ receptor antagonists.

nizatidine on the rate of spontaneous abortion and birth-weights [19–21]. Second, cimetidine is the only H$_2$RA that has been associated with a weak antiandrogenic effect in animals and in humans. Furthermore, there is a possible association of cimetidine use with the development of neonatal hepatitis, although this finding has not been confirmed [19,22]. Third, ranitidine is the only H$_2$RA that has been demonstrated to be both efficacious and safe in a double-blind, placebo-controlled, triple crossover trial in pregnant women with GERD symptoms refractory to conservative antireflux measures and antacids [23]. Twenty patients were randomized to receive the following three weekly regimens: ranitidine 150 mg twice daily; placebo in the morning and ranitidine 150 mg in the evening; or placebo twice daily. The average reduction of heartburn severity using twice-daily ranitidine was 55.6% compared with baseline (CI 34.8%–76.5%) and was 44.2% when compared with placebo (CI 15.4%–72.9%). No adverse fetal outcomes were reported. Thus, ranitidine is the H$_2$RA of choice for acid suppressive therapy during pregnancy.

Proton pump inhibitors

Third-line therapy includes the use of proton pump inhibitors. Although physicians are reluctant to prescribe proton pump inhibitors for the pregnant patient in view of the relatively short experience of the use of this category of drugs in comparison with acid-neutralizing agents and H$_2$RAs, more data have emerged describing its safety in pregnancy. One case report from the 1990s identified potential teratogenic effects of

omeprazole in two patients [24]. However, both pregnancies were conceived by artificial insemination followed by reimplantation. These procedures carry a higher risk for congenital malformations than normal pregnancies [16,25]. Since then several studies have confirmed the safety of proton pump inhibitors during pregnancy. A metaanalysis of five cohort studies with almost 600 exposed pregnancies found no major teratogenic risk when proton pump inhibitors (mainly omeprazole) were used in the recommended doses (relative risk [RR] 1.18, CI 0.72–1.94) [26]. A multicenter prospective controlled study by the European Network of Teratology Information Services of 295 pregnancies exposed to omeprazole (233 in the first trimester), 62 to lansoprazole (55 in first trimester), and 53 to pantoprazole (47 in first trimester), found no increased risk for congenital abnormalities in exposed vs control groups [27].

Few studies have reported on the effect of pregnancy on antireflux surgery. The theoretical concern has been that the increased abdominal pressure in addition to nausea and vomiting of pregnancy, may predispose to wrap disruption or herniation. In a retrospective, questionnaire-based study of 95 patients with a mean follow-up of 4.9 years, subsequent pregnancy did not adversely affect outcomes after antireflux surgery [28].

Peptic ulcer disease

Several epidemiological studies have reported a decreased incidence of peptic ulcer disease during pregnancy [19].

However, peptic ulcer disease during pregnancy may be underdiagnosed because diagnostic endoscopy and radiological studies are avoided for fetal safety. Moreover, peptic ulcer disease may be underdiagnosed because symptoms overlap with typical pregnancy-associated GERD-like symptoms with subsequent empirical use of acid suppressive therapy.

The risk factors for peptic ulcer disease during pregnancy are no different from the general population, and include smoking and use of nonsteroidal antiinflammatory drugs (NSAIDs). The role of *Helicobacter pylori* in the etiology of *H. pylori*-associated peptic ulcer disease during pregnancy remains unknown. The symptoms of peptic ulcer disease during pregnancy are also no different from the general population. Finally, the treatment for peptic ulcer disease is similar to that for GERD symptoms.

Role of *Helicobacter pylori* in gastrointestinal symptoms during pregnancy

H. pylori does not play a role in the pathogenesis of gastrointestinal symptoms in pregnancy. In a study of 416 pregnant patients, *H. pylori* seropositivity was determined at 10–14 weeks' gestation. Dyspeptic symptoms were recorded at 10–14 weeks' gestation and at 30–32 weeks' gestation by means of a questionnaire. Patients infected with *H. pylori* were no more likely than controls to experience dyspepsia, and *H. pylori* infection was not associated with preterm delivery, or maternal or neonatal morbidity [29]. In a study of 898 pregnant patients, 23% had *H. pylori* infection as determined by urea breath testing. Although gastrointestinal symptoms such as nausea, vomiting, and heartburn were common in this population, there was no association with *H. pylori* infection [30]. Finally, in a hospital-based cross-sectional study of 54 women in the first 16 gestational weeks, *H. pylori* seropositivity did not correlate with clinical symptoms. Moreover, no specific patterns of gastrointestinal symptoms were uncovered in the *H. pylori*-infected patients [31].

Diarrhea

The pathogenesis of diarrhea occurring during pregnancy is no different from the nonpregnant patient. As most episodes are self-limited, extensive evaluation is usually unnecessary. Nonsystemic medications should be tried first. Bulk agents may be useful because of their ability to absorb water. Systemic therapies for diarrhea during pregnancy are limited by safety concerns (Table 28.3).

Antidiarrheals

Bismuth subsalicylate (Pepto-Bismol)
Use of bismuth subsalicylate can result in absorption of salicylate and should be avoided during pregnancy. Salicylates are teratogenic and have been associated with low birthweight, neonatal hemorrhage, and increased perinatal mortality [32].

Kaolin and pectin (Kaopectate)
Kaolin and pectin preparations are not absorbed and were therefore considered the treatment of choice for diarrhea until 2003, when Kaopectate was reformulated to contain bismuth subsalicylate [33–35]. It should be avoided in pregnancy.

Diphenoxylate hydrochloride with atropine sulfate (Lomotil)
Diphenoxylate is a piperidine derivative with structural similarities to meperidine. Lomotil is teratogenic in animals [36]. The effects of Lomotil during pregnancy have not been adequately studied, but first-trimester use of Lomotil has been associated with malformations in a small number of children [37]. Lomotil is listed as a pregnancy category C drug and should be avoided during pregnancy. Because atropine crosses the placenta, caution is recommended when it is used during pregnancy. Diphenoxylic acid, the active metabolite of diphenoxylate, and atropine sulfate appear in human breast milk; infants of nursing mothers taking Lomotil may therefore exhibit some effects of the drugs.

Loperamide (Imodium)
Loperamide is a synthetic piperidine derivative used for the treatment of both acute and chronic diarrhea. Human data on its safety and risk in pregnancy are limited. No association between loperamide and congenital malformations was noted in a study of 108 newborns that had been exposed in utero to loperamide during the first trimester [38]. Similarly, in another study of 105 women exposed to loperamide in pregnancy, 84.7% with first-trimester exposure, there was no increase in major malformations between the study group and the control group. Thus, loperamide does not appear to represent a major teratogenic risk in humans when used for short-term courses at the recommended doses and has become the drug of choice for the treatment of diarrhea in pregnancy.

Constipation

The prevalence of constipation in pregnancy is as high as 11%–38% [39–41]. Constipation may occur de novo, or preexisting constipation may worsen during pregnancy. Studies on gastrointestinal transit in humans have been limited out of concern for fetal safety. Multiple factors play a role in the constipation of pregnancy, including delayed gastrointestinal motility resulting from hormonal changes, decreased physical activity, mechanical compression because of the enlarging gravid uterus, the presence of internal hemorrhoids, and iron supplementation [42]. Circulating progesterone may be the cause of slower gastrointestinal movement in mid- and late pregnancy. Animal studies have shown that progesterone exerts an inhibitory effect on colonic smooth muscle [40]. In addition, colonic transit was delayed in pregnant rats and in ovariectomized rats treated with estrogen and progesterone [43]. Two studies described prolonged orocecal transit in women in their second or third trimester of pregnancy compared with postpartum transit [42,44].

Table 28.3 Antidiarrheals and laxatives during pregnancy

Drug	FDA pregnancy category[a]	Excreted in breast milk	Comments
Antidiarrheals	1st/2nd/3rd		
Nonsystemic			
Kaolin and pectin	C/C/C	Yes	Avoid
Bulk-forming agents (see below)		Unknown	Preferred
Systemic			
Atropine/diphenoxylate	C/C/C	Yes	Not recommended
Loperamide	B/B/B	Yes	Preferred
Bismuth subsalicylate	C/C/D	Yes	Contraindicated
Bulk-forming agents			Bulk-forming agents should be taken with
Psyllium	B	Unknown	sufficient amounts of fluid
Methylcellulose	B	Unknown	
Polycarbophil	B	Unknown	
Osmotic laxatives			
PEG-based			
Polyethylene glycol	C	Unknown	Agent of choice
Saccharated			
Lactulose	B	Unknown	Preferred
Sorbitol (70%)	B	Unknown	Preferred
Glycerine	C	Unknown	Avoid
Magnesium- or sodium-based agents			
Magnesium oxide	B	Unknown	Preferred
Magnesium hydroxide	B	Unknown	Preferred
Sodium phosphate	C	Unknown	Avoid
Stimulant laxatives			
Anthraquinones			
Senna	C	Yes	Proven efficacy in randomized trial
Cascara sagrada	X	Yes	Only available as herbal supplement
Diphenylmethanes			
Bisacodyl	C	Unknown	
Stool softener			
Docusate	C	Unknown	Questionable efficacy in chronic constipation; report of neonatal hypomagnesemia
Serotonin agonist			
Tegaserod	B	Unknown	

a See Table 28.1.
PEG, polyethylene glycol.

Extensive investigation of new-onset constipation during pregnancy is seldom warranted. Routine evaluation begins with a history and determination of the patient's definition of constipation. Calcium or iron supplementation may contribute to the constipation of pregnancy. A digital rectal examination may be performed to rule out fecal impaction and to test for fecal occult blood. Routine blood work, including thyroid function tests, can be useful. Anoscopy or flexible sigmoidoscopy can be helpful when anorectal lesions are suspected or when bleeding accompanies constipation [45].

There is a substantial lack of controlled studies on the safety of laxatives during pregnancy. In the Cochrane Database of Systematic Reviews on interventions for treating constipation in pregnancy (last updated in 2004) only two randomized trial studies were identified as suitable for review [39,46,47].

The treatment of constipation during pregnancy should start with education on normal bowel function and behavioral modification, including increased physical activity and scheduled defecation in the morning and after meals to take advantage of the gastrocolic reflex (Fig. 28.2). Dietary changes,

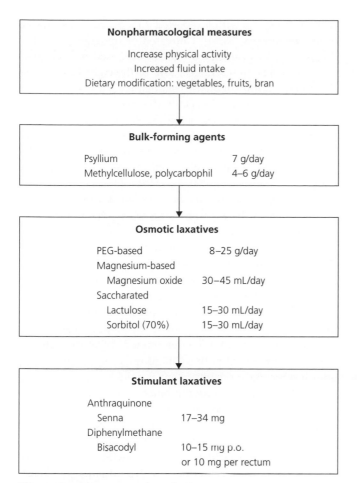

Nonpharmacological measures

Increase physical activity
Increased fluid intake
Dietary modification: vegetables, fruits, bran

Bulk-forming agents

Psyllium	7 g/day
Methylcellulose, polycarbophil	4–6 g/day

Osmotic laxatives

PEG-based	8–25 g/day
Magnesium-based	
Magnesium oxide	30–45 mL/day
Saccharated	
Lactulose	15–30 mL/day
Sorbitol (70%)	15–30 mL/day

Stimulant laxatives

Anthraquinone	
Senna	17–34 mg
Diphenylmethane	
Bisacodyl	10–15 mg p.o.
	or 10 mg per rectum

Figure 28.2 Management of constipation in pregnancy. PEG, polyethylene glycol; p.o., orally.

including increased fluid and fiber intake, may be helpful. Patients with poor dietary habits may add 2–6 tablespoons of bran to each meal [41,42].

Wheat- or corn-based fiber supplementation increased stool frequency in a dose-dependent manner in pregnant women with constipation in a 2-week placebo-controlled trial (OR 0.18, CI 0.05–0.670) [46,47]. Fiber supplementation may take up to one week to affect stool output. Patients should be encouraged to consume adequate amounts of fluid. Women who have difficulty increasing their dietary fiber intake may benefit from the addition of bulk-forming agents (e.g., psyllium, methylcellulose, or polycarbophil). Bulk-forming agents are safe because there is no systemic absorption.

If bulk-forming agents do not achieve a satisfactory response, osmotic laxatives can be added (Table 28.3). Although there are no randomized controlled studies to ensure their efficacy and safety during pregnancy, they are commonly used. Osmotic laxatives can be divided into polyethylene glycol (PEG)-based solutions, saccharated osmotics, and saline osmotics. PEG is considered the laxative of choice in pregnancy [34,35]. Only

1%–4% of PEG is absorbed. However, it is not metabolized or biotransformed and animal studies have not demonstrated a teratogenic effect. It is therefore unlikely to have a teratogenic effect in humans [12]. In an open label study of PEG-4000 in 40 pregnant women from 6 to 38 weeks' gestation, treatment with PEG-4000 significantly increased the number of bowel movements per week (from 1.66 ± 0.48 to 3.16 ± 1.05; $P < 0.01$) and constipation resolved in 73% of women [48]. Sorbitol and lactulose are classified as pregnancy category B. These saccharated osmotics are poorly absorbed and have been associated with abdominal bloating and discomfort. The saline osmotics are generally considered safe for temporary use during pregnancy. Electrolyte abnormalities such as hypermagnesemia may occur, although this is uncommon in the healthy pregnant woman [41]. The sodium-based osmotic laxative Phospho-soda should be avoided during pregnancy as it promotes sodium and water retention.

Stimulant laxatives (anthraquinones and diphenylmethanes) should only be considered as a second-line laxative option. Stimulant laxatives may cause diarrhea or abdominal pain. Electrolyte disturbances are mostly seen with chronic use or the use of unusually high doses. Of the anthraquinone laxatives, senna has been shown to be safe during pregnancy. In one study of pregnant women randomized to senna, dioctyl sodium succinate, sterculia plus frangula, or sterculia, the stimulant laxative senna was more effective than bulk-forming agents (OR 0.30, CI 0.14–0.61) [39,47]. Cascara sagrada (Spanish missionaries noticed its use among the natives and called it "sacred bark," hence the Spanish name) is only available as a herbal supplement. It should be avoided during pregnancy. The only diphenylmethane laxative available for over-the-counter use is bisacodyl. Bisacodyl is classified as pregnancy category C. The safety of bisacodyl during pregnancy has not been established, but there is no evidence of adverse effects.

Stool softeners are not effective in treating existing chronic constipation, but may be useful in patients who need to avoid straining. Neonatal hypomagnesemia has been associated with maternal use of docusate [49].

Tegaserod, a serotonin (5-hydroxytryptamine type 4 receptor [5-HT$_4$]) agonist, has not been studied in pregnant woman.

Hemorrhoids

Hemorrhoids are common during pregnancy. They most frequently appear during the third trimester. The symptoms of internal hemorrhoids include itching, bleeding, and prolapse. External hemorrhoids only become symptomatic when thrombosed. Multiple factors have been implicated in the development of hemorrhoids during pregnancy. These include an increase in hemorrhoidal size because of increased venous dilation and engorgement in combination with increased pressure from the growing fetus on the rectum and the perineum. It is most important to prevent the development of hemorrhoids during pregnancy by adequate management of constipation (as described above). Pregnant woman should avoid heavy lifting and prolonged periods of standing.

Conservative recommendations for treatment of hemorrhoids include 10-min sitz baths several times a day. For those patients who do not have a bath, small plastic tubs can be purchased for placement over the toilet. Some women find comfort with an ice pack (wrapped in a towel to prevent direct contact with the skin) or cold compresses whereas others prefer a heating pad. Topical therapy includes the use of nonprescription products varying from local anesthetics and astringents to hydrocortisone cream. However, data supporting the use of topical agents are lacking. Creams containing the vasoconstricting agents epinephrine (adrenaline) or phenylephrine (such as the popular over-the-counter drug Preparation H) should be avoided during pregnancy especially in women with hypertension, diabetes, or fluid overload [42].

Rubber band ligation and infrared coagulation have not been been studied for safety and efficacy during pregnancy. Injection sclerotherapy for first- and second-degree hemorrhoids has been described as safe and effective during pregnancy, with rare recurrences [42,50]. Excisional hemorrhoidectomy appears to be safe in selected pregnant patients. In a study of 25 pregnant women undergoing closed hemorrhoidectomy for intractable pain under local anesthesia, all patients experienced relief of pain the day after surgery, except for one patient who required hemostatic packing during the postoperative period [51]. There were no other maternal or fetal complications. Vaginal delivery may be contraindicated in patients with severe prolapsing or thrombosed hemorrhoids or following surgical intervention for hemorrhoids late in pregnancy. As hemorrhoids are likely to recur with a subsequent pregnancy, a more definitive therapy may be indicated prior to conception.

Chronic gastrointestinal diseases in pregnancy

Celiac disease

Celiac disease, also referred to as nontropical sprue or gluten-sensitive enteropathy, is an immune-mediated disorder induced by dietary wheat gliadin and related proteins in genetically susceptible individuals. It is characterized by chronic inflammation of the small intestinal mucosa. Intestinal symptoms include diarrhea, abdominal discomfort, and weight loss. Nongastrointestinal manifestations include osteoporosis, cancer, and infertility. As many as 3 million US citizens (approximately 1% of the US population) may be affected [52].

Fertility

Women with symptomatic untreated celiac disease have shortened reproductive periods with delayed menarche and early menopause, with a reported 40% of women suffering from amenorrhea [53,54]. Untreated or undiagnosed celiac disease has been associated with an increased risk for infertility, recurrent miscarriages, low birthweight babies, and shortened duration of breast-feeding [54–57]. These risks are reduced when celiac disease is diagnosed and effectively treated with a gluten-free diet [54,55,58–60]. The mechanism for reduced fertility remains unknown. Fertility problems are also more common in men with celiac disease due to gonadal dysfunction [54]. Hyperprolactinemia is seen in 25% of celiac patients and causes impotence and loss of libido.

Studies have focused on the risks for adverse outcomes of pregnancy in the asymptomatic celiac patient. In a large population-based study of asymptomatic individuals in Italy, celiac disease was not associated with an excess risk of abortion, premature delivery, low birthweight, or intrauterine growth retardation [61]. In contrast, Gasbarrini et al. [62] demonstrated that women having recurrent miscarriages or intrauterine growth retardation could have subclinical celiac disease. Thus, the risks of latent or subclinical celiac disease for pregnancy remain to be determined. Whether a gluten-free diet is of benefit to this subgroup is controversial. This issue has become more important as epidemiological studies suggest that atypical or asymptomatic celiac disease is more widespread than previously realized.

Screening for celiac disease should be considered as part of the diagnostic workup of infertile women. Furthermore, celiac disease should be considered in women with recurrent spontaneous abortions, intrauterine growth retardation, or persistent hematological or gastrointestinal abnormalities during pregnancy. Women with celiac disease who wish to get pregnant should maintain a gluten-free diet to optimize their chances of an uncomplicated pregnancy. In addition, folic acid, calcium, iron, and vitamin B supplementation is necessary. The recommended dose of oral folate is at least 5 mg daily [53]. Vitamin K malabsorption may occur, and the prothrombin ratio should be determined prior to delivery [53].

Inflammatory bowel disease

Inflammatory bowel disease (IBD) includes ulcerative colitis and Crohn's disease. IBD affects both genders nearly equally [63]. Crohn's disease is more common in women of childbearing age [53].

Fertility

Fertility of women with ulcerative colitis and inactive Crohn's disease is usually no different from women in the general population. However, active Crohn's disease, particularly in the ileum, can impair fertility because of scarring of the fallopian tubes and ovaries [64]. A case-controlled, survey-based study investigated fertility and pregnancy outcomes in 275 women with Crohn's disease and in age-matched controls [65]. Women with Crohn's disease more frequently failed to become pregnant compared with controls (42% vs

28%). However, this study did not control for other factors such as lack of sexual intimacy and disease activity. Other studies have demonstrated that women with ulcerative colitis and women with quiescent Crohn's disease had normal fertility when compared with the general population [66,67].

Infertility is more frequently observed in women with a history of abdominal surgery [66,67]. The preferred surgical intervention for ulcerative colitis is the ileal pouch anal anastomosis, which offers intestinal continuity and fecal continence. Although an ileal pouch anal anastomosis does not affect menstrual function, fertility may be adversely affected, possibly as a result of pelvic adhesions [66,67]. Women with ulcerative colitis who are planning to conceive should therefore, if possible, defer a colectomy until they have established their family. For those women who do have an ileal pouch anal anastomosis, pregnancy is safe and there are no contraindications to vaginal delivery [68]. Fecal incontinence may occur, usually during the third trimester, but pouch function returns to prepregnancy status in most females [68–70].

The majority of medications used in the treatment of IBD do not adversely affect fertility. However, men taking sulfasalazine develop oligospermia, reduced sperm motility, and abnormal sperm morphology, which are fully reversible within several weeks of discontinuation of the drug [71].

Effect of pregnancy on inflammatory bowel disease

As a general rule, women with active IBD at the time of conception will experience active disease throughout the pregnancy, whereas women with inactive disease will continue to do well. Approximately one-third of patients with inactive IBD will relapse during gestation [37,72]. Conversely, if conception occurs at a time when IBD is active, remission will occur in one-third of patients [73]. No data exist on the optimal duration of remission before conception.

Patients with ulcerative colitis can expect a normal vaginal delivery. Patients with Crohn's disease and active perineal involvement should plan for a cesarian section. If patients with Crohn's disease do undergo a vaginal delivery, episiotomy should be avoided. High rates of perineal involvement follow vaginal delivery with episiotomy in patients with Crohn's disease, including those without preexisting perirectal complications [73,74].

Effect of inflammatory bowel disease on pregnancy

Women with active IBD, especially with Crohn's disease, are at risk of having low-birthweight and premature babies [75–78]. A historical registry-based case-controlled study investigated birthweight and frequency of preterm delivery in women with Crohn's disease [79]. Children born to patients with Crohn's disease averaged 105–142 g less in birthweight compared with children born to mothers without Crohn's disease. The risk of low birthweight (< 2500 g) was increased (OR 2.4; CI 1.1–2.3), as was the risk of preterm delivery (OR 1.6; CI 1.1–2.3).

No data have been published showing an increased risk for congenital abnormalities in inactive Crohn's disease. However, women with ulcerative colitis may be at increased risk for giving birth to children with congenital abnormalities. A large, population-based cross-sectional retrospective study reported a fourfold increase in congenital malformations in children born to mothers with ulcerative colitis compared with controls (7.9% vs 1.7%, $P < 0.001$) [75]. A second large, population-based study found a selective increase of some congenital abnormalities such as limb deficiencies, obstructive urinary congenital abnormalities, and multiple congenital abnormalities (OR 6.2, CI 2.9–13; OR 3.3, CI 1.1–9.5; and OR 2.6, CI 1.3–5.4, respectively) [80]. It remains to be determined whether the association between maternal ulcerative colitis and an increased risk of certain congenital abnormalities is causal.

Drug treatment during pregnancy

Medical treatment of IBD generally does not affect fertility and has proved to be safe during pregnancy. Active disease during pregnancy should be treated, as the risks of not treating are greater than the risks of treating. 5-Aminosalicylic acid (5-ASA) preparations are considered first-line therapy in IBD (Table 28.4). They have been used for many years and their safety has been demonstrated in several large clinical trials. Immunomodulators may be useful in patients with chronically active disease who are dependent on these drugs to maintain remission. Short courses of the most frequently used antibiotics in IBD, metronidazole and ciprofloxacin, are probably safe during pregnancy but data on long-term treatment are not available.

Aminosalicylates

Sulfasalazine

About 30% of an oral dose of sulfasalazine is absorbed in the small intestine; the rest passes into the colon where bacterial azoreductases cleave it into 5-aminosalicylic acid and sulfapyridine. Sulfasalazine interferes with normal folate metabolism by displacing folate from the enzyme dihydrofolate reductase, thereby blocking the conversion of folate to its more active metabolites. Women are advised to take daily supplemental folate (at least 2 mg daily) prior to conception to decrease the risk of neural tube defects and continue folate supplementation for the remainder of the pregnancy. A few reports from the early 1980s suggested a possible teratogenic effect of sulfasalazine [81–83]. However, larger studies have not confirmed these findings [77,84–86]. Sulfasalazine and sulfapyridine cross the placenta and are present in fetal serum in concentrations similar to those found in maternal serum [87–89]. A negligible amount of sulfasalazine is found in the milk of lactating women taking therapeutic amounts of the drug, but the concentration of sulfapyridine is 45% that in maternal serum [90]. At therapeutic concentrations, neither sulfasalazine nor sulfapyridine cause significant displacement

Table 28.4 Pharmacotherapy in inflammatory bowel disease (IBD) during pregnancy

Drug	Pregnancy category[a]	Excreted in breast milk	Comments
5-Aminosalicyclic acid			
Sulfasalazine	B	Yes	Avoid in men prior to conception Folate supplementation indicated prior to conception and during pregnancy
Mesalamine	B		Generally considered safe
Asacol		Yes	
Pentasa		Yes	
Rowasa		Unknown	
Olsalazine	C	Yes	Avoid
Dipentum			
Balsalazide	B	Unknown	Considered safe but no human data
Colazide			
Corticosteroids			
Prednisone	B	Yes	Avoid (esp. in first trimester)
Solu-Medrol	B	Yes	Avoid
Budesonide	C	Yes	Limited data
Purine analogues			
Azathioprine	D	Yes	Generally considered safe
Mercaptopurine	D	Yes	Generally considered safe
Anti-tumor necrosis factor			
Infliximab	B	Unknown	Limited data on safety
Antibiotics			
Metronidazole	B	Yes	Probably safe for short-term therapy
Quinolones	C	Unknown	Probably safe for short-term therapy
Immunosuppressants			
Cyclosporine	C	Yes	Avoid
Antimetabolites			
Methotrexate	X	Yes	Contraindicated

a See Table 28.1.

of bilirubin from albumin and the risk of kernicterus does not appear to be increased by treatment of the mother with sulfasalazine during pregnancy or lactation [87–90].

Mesalamine

About 25% of administered mesalamine is absorbed from the colon. In a prospective study of 165 women exposed to mesalamine during pregnancy, there was no increase in major malformations (0.8% for mesalamine vs 3.8% for non-teratogenic controls; $P = 0.23$). There was an increase in the rate of preterm deliveries (13.0% vs 4.7%; $P = 0.02$) and a decrease in the mean birthweight (3253 ± 546 g vs 3461 ± 542 g; $P = 0.0005$). Thus, mesalamine does not represent a major teratogenic risk in humans when given in the recommended

doses and its use in pregnancy is generally considered safe [91–94].

Olsalazine

Large doses of olsalazine cause birth defects in animals. Olsalazine should be avoided in pregnancy [37].

Topical 5-aminosalicylic acid (5-ASA) appears safe, effective, and well tolerated in the management of pregnant patients with distal colitis [95].

Corticosteroids

Corticosteroids are indicated in severe IBD exacerbations. Corticosteroids cross the placental barrier and are rapidly converted to less active metabolites by placental 11-hydroxygenase resulting in low fetal blood levels [64]. Thus, adrenal insufficiency is rarely seen in neonates. Although most studies have not found an association with major congenital abnormalities [85,96], a metaanalysis of epidemiological studies published in 2000 did report a 3.4-fold increase in the risk of oral cleft with steroid exposure in the first trimester, which is consistent with existing animal studies [97]. Corticosteroids should be avoided in the first trimester. Rectal preparations may be used until the third trimester unless miscarriage or premature delivery is a concern [37].

Budesonide is a synthetic glucocorticoid. It is released in the small bowel and is indicated for the treatment of Crohn's disease involving the ileocecal area. It acts topically and has a high first-pass metabolism resulting in low plasma levels. To date there are no studies on the use of oral budesonide during pregnancy. Budesonide is listed as a pregnancy category C drug for its teratogenic and embryocidal effect in rabbits and rats when given subcutaneously in doses up to 0.5 times the recommended human dose on a body surface area basis [64].

Azathioprine and 6-mercaptopurine

Azathioprine and 6-mercaptopurine (6-MP) are immunomodulators used in the treatment of steroid-resistant or steroid-dependent IBD. Azathioprine is metabolized to 6-MP, which interacts in purine metabolism and is therefore considered to have mutagenic potential. Azathioprine has no effect on semen quality and male fertility [98]. 6-Mercaptopurine can cross the placenta. Early in pregnancy, the fetal liver is unable to metabolize 6-MP as it does not make the necessary enzyme.

Physicians have been reluctant to use immunomodulators in the pregnant patient with IBD for several reasons. First, there was evidence for teratogenicity in animal studies from the 1960s [99,100]. Secondly, there were relatively few retrospective studies on the safety of immunomodulators in the pregnant patient with IBD, most of which reported an increased risk for congenital malformations [101]. Similarly, an increased risk for congenital malformations was found in some studies of children fathered by men treated with azathioprine or 6-MP [102–104], whereas other studies did not find this [98]. Most studies were limited by the retrospective nature of the data collection, the small sample size, and the lack of information regarding disease activity in the fathers and comorbidity in the mothers [105].

A clearer picture emerged following a retrospective cohort study of 155 patients who had conceived at least one child while exposed to 6-MP. Patients had taken 6-MP either remotely, in the 2 months before conception, or throughout pregnancy. IBD patients who had their pregnancies before taking 6-MP were used as controls. There was no statistical difference in conception failures (defined as a spontaneous abortion), abortion secondary to a birth defect, major congenital malformations, perinatal neoplasia, or perinatal infections among male or female patients taking 6-MP compared with controls (RR = 0.85 [CI: 0.47–1.55], $P = 0.59$) [106]. A second retrospective

study confirmed that azathioprine at a dose of 100 mg/day and 6-MP at a dose of 75 mg/day is probably safe for pregnant patients [94].

In a position statement from the Italian Group for Inflammatory Bowel Disease on the appropriateness of immunosuppressive drugs as assessed by the RAND method (a combination of evidence from the literature and experts' opinions), the use of azathioprine or 6-MP was rated appropriate in late pregnancy and during nursing in patients with active disease under treatment [107]. The group deemed it inappropriate to start immunosuppressive therapy before conception and in early pregnancy. Finally, the group recommended that both male and female patients with chronically active disease, who depend on immunomodulators to maintain remission, do not stop their medication 6 to 18 months prior to conception. In fact, discontinuation of 6-MP may increase the chance of fetal loss (29.2% vs 14.3% in women with no history of 6-MP exposure) according to one study [108].

Cyclosporine

Cyclosporine (ciclosporin) is an inhibitor of calcineurin that suppresses proinflammatory transcription factors. Cyclosporine crosses the placenta. It is only used in the treatment of severe refractory ulcerative colitis in an attempt to avoid urgent surgery. Most of the experience with cyclosporine during pregnancy comes from the transplant literature. A metaanalysis of 15 studies (total patients 410) did not achieve statistical significance for malformations (OR 3.83; CI 0.75–19.6) [109]. The overall prevalence rate of prematurity was 56.3%, although it did not reach statistical significance (OR 1.52; CI 1.00–2.32). Thus, cyclosporine does not appear to be a major human teratogen but it may be associated with increased rates of prematurity. Only a few case reports have been published on its use in pregnant patients with IBD, with favorable fetal outcomes [110,111].

Methotrexate

Methotrexate is mutagenic and teratogenic and has been associated with a high rate of spontaneous abortions. If conception occurs, there is a high risk for craniofacial and limb defects and central nervous system abnormalities. It is contraindicated in pregnancy or in anyone considering conception [37].

Anti-tumor necrosis factor antibodies

Infliximab, a chimeric monoclonal antibody to tumor necrosis factor-α, is effective for the induction and maintenance of remission in patients with Crohn's disease. To maintain remission, infliximab needs to be administered every 8 weeks. Infliximab crosses the placenta but may not be excreted in breast milk [112].

Results from the 2004 Infliximab Safety Database identified 146 pregnancies with *unintentional* infliximab exposure before or after confirmed pregnancy [113]. One hundred and thirty-one patients were exposed directly to infliximab and 15 partners were indirectly exposed to the drug. Pregnancy outcome data were available for 96/131 directly exposed and 10/15 indirectly exposed patients. Live births occurred in 67% (64/96), miscarriages in 15% (14/96), and therapeutic termination in 19% (18/96) of the pregnancies directly exposed to infliximab. Miscarriage occurred in 10% (1/10) of the indirect exposures. These results do not differ from those expected in the general pregnant population or pregnant women with Crohn's disease not exposed to infliximab. The first data on the *intentional* use of infliximab during pregnancy are derived from a retrospective multicenter chart review of women with Crohn's disease [114]. Eight women intentionally received maintenance infliximab infusions throughout their pregnancy, and two women intentionally received their first infliximab infusions. All pregnancies ended with live births and none of the infants had congenital malformations, intrauterine growth retardation, or were small for their gestational age. Although the data are limited, it appears that the use of infliximab during pregnancy is safe.

Antibiotics

Metronidazole

No data exist on the use of metronidazole for the treatment of IBD during pregnancy. However, metronidazole does not represent a major teratogenic risk when used short-term for the treatment of infection during pregnancy. Two metaanalyses and one prospective study failed to show a relationship between birth defects and metronidazole exposure for the treatment of infections during the first trimester [115,116].

Ciprofloxacin

Ciprofloxacin has been associated with musculoskeletal abnormalities in immature animals [117]. No data exist on the use of ciprofloxacin for the treatment of IBD during pregnancy, but quinolone exposure for the treatment of infections during the first trimester of pregnancy does not appear to be associated with an increased risk of malformations or musculoskeletal problems [94,118,119].

Although metronidazole and ciprofloxacin may not represent a major teratogenic risk when used for short-term courses at the recommended doses, they should not be used in the chronic treatment of IBD as safer alternatives exist.

Colorectal cancer

Colorectal cancer is the third leading type of cancer in the United States and the second leading cause of cancer-related deaths [120]. The incidence of colon cancer during pregnancy has been estimated at 1 in 13 000.

Colon cancer during pregnancy

Colorectal cancer in the pregnant population is likely to be associated with genetic syndromes or strong risk factors. Cancer in young females is more common in the rectum than in the colon [121]. The presenting symptoms are no different from other patients and include abdominal pain, rectal bleeding, altered bowel habits, and involuntary weight loss. However, pregnant patients usually present with advanced colon cancer as a result of delayed diagnosis. Common pitfalls in the diagnosis include the lack of consideration of colorectal cancer in the differential diagnosis in the young female pregnant patient, and the attribution of clinical symptoms such as nausea, vomiting, and rectal bleeding to the pregnancy [121]. Abnormal blood findings, such as iron deficiency anemia, hypoalbuminemia, and elevated alkaline phosphatase, may be attributed to the pregnancy as well, and iron deficiency from blood loss and hepatic metastases may be missed [121]. Colon cancer has not been associated with metastases to the fetus. Carcinoembryonic antigen (CEA) levels are unaffected by pregnancy and, if elevated, support a diagnosis of colon cancer [121]. Computed tomography (CT) scan and colonoscopy are contraindicated during pregnancy but sigmoidoscopy is not. Primary therapy is surgery; chemotherapy and radiotherapy are generally contraindicated during pregnancy. If the cancer is detected during the first half of the pregnancy, surgery can be performed with minimal risk to the fetus. However, if the cancer is detected in the second half of the pregnancy, surgery should be delayed until after the delivery, which should be initiated at the earliest time of fetal viability [121].

Physicians should consider colon cancer in the differential diagnosis in the pregnant patient with gastrointestinal symptoms, as earlier diagnosis will improve the prognosis.

Colorectal cancer screening in the female patient

Colonoscopy is one of the recommended colorectal cancer screening modalities. Studies have demonstrated a female preference for women endoscopists, with as many as 5% of women stating that they would not undergo a colonoscopy unless guaranteed a woman endoscopist [122–124]. The most common reason for this gender preference was embarrassment.

Physicians recommending endoscopic colorectal cancer screening should therefore consider gender preference for an endoscopist in the female population as this may improve participation of female patients in colorectal cancer screening.

Gastrointestinal endoscopy during pregnancy

Endoscopy during pregnancy raises concerns for fetal safety because of the risk for induction of premature labor, drug-induced teratogenesis, scope-related placental abruption or fetal trauma, cardiac arrhythmias, systemic hypotension or hypertension, and hypoxia [125]. There are few published studies on endoscopy during pregnancy. One case-controlled study of 83 upper endoscopies did not detect any fetal risk from the procedure [125]. Similarly, a retrospective study involving 46 patients undergoing 48 sigmoidoscopies and 8

Table 28.5 Drugs for conscious sedation during pregnancy

Drug	Pregnancy category[a]	Comments
Meperidine	B	Preferred
Fentanyl	C	Avoid
Midazolam	D	Preferred
Diazepam	D	Avoid; possible association with oral cleft
Propofol	B	Requires administration by anesthesiologist; considered relatively safe during pregnancy
Simethicone	C	Avoid
Glucagon	B	Avoid
Naloxone	B	No data on fetal safety
Flumazenil	C	No data on fetal safety

a See Table 28.1.

patients undergoing 8 colonoscopies during pregnancy did not detect any fetal risks [125].

Conscious sedation in pregnancy

Careful attention should be paid to the medications used for conscious sedation (Table 28.5). Diazepam and midazolam should be avoided because of a possible association with teratogenicity. Midazolam may cause drowsiness, bradycardia, or breathing difficulty in the newborn infant when administered during the last few days before delivery. Fentanyl may not be teratogenic, but was found to be embryocidal in rats. Fentanyl can decrease fetal heart rate variability [125] and has been associated with neonatal respiratory depression. Although meperidine can also produce respiratory depression, it is the medication of choice for conscious sedation during pregnancy in view of its better-documented fetal safety profile. Two large studies demonstrated no teratogenicity from meperidine infusion during the first trimester [125]. To avoid fetal oversedation, no more than 75 mg meperidine should be used [121]. Propofol is considered safe during pregnancy, but data on fetal safety during the first trimester are lacking [125].

Clinical indication for endoscopy during pregnancy

Esophagogastroduodenoscopy (EGD) is indicated in pregnant patients with significant upper gastrointestinal bleeding. In patients with preexisting portal hypertension, gestation may be associated with an increase in portal venous pressure and an increase in size of esophageal varices. Elevation in portal venous pressure is related to a 40%–50% increase in plasma volume [126,127]. Variceal bleeding usually occurs in the second or third trimester. Despite a paucity of controlled trials, both sclerotherapy and band ligation have been reported to be efficacious and safe. EGD is rarely indicated or useful in the evaluation of nausea, vomiting, or uncomplicated gastroesophageal reflux disease.

Sigmoidoscopy is indicated in pregnant patients with lower gastrointestinal bleeding, a sigmoid or rectal mass or stricture, and for severe refractory diarrhea. Sigmoidoscopy is rarely indicated for lower abdominal pain or a change in bowel habits [125].

Colonoscopy may be indicated in pregnant patients for suspected colon cancer and for uncontrolled colonic hemorrhage.

Endoscopic retrograde cholangiopancreatography (ERCP) is indicated in pregnant patients with cholelithiasis complicated by persistent cholestasis, suspected choledocholithiasis, pancreatitis, or cholangitis [125]. Special attention should be paid to minimizing fetal radiation exposure. This can be achieved by lead shielding, limiting fluoroscopy time, and avoidance of spot radiographs. Some authors advocate placing a radiation dosimetry badge on the maternal abdomen over the uterine fundus.

Percutaneous endoscopic gastrostomy (PEG) may be indicated in a pregnant patient. A few case reports have documented successful PEG placement in pregnant patients who were unable to keep up with their nutritional requirements for a healthy pregnancy for a variety of reasons. The greatest concern during PEG placement is the potential risk for uterine puncture and fetal damage with the transabdominal needle. Ultrasonographic marking of the superior aspect of the uterus may aid the choosing of a safe location [128]. Attention should be paid to the effect of the growing uterus on the tension of the bumper in the stomach so as to avoid pressure necrosis [128].

Hepatobiliary diseases during pregnancy

The liver diseases of pregnancy can be divided into four categories: hyperemesis gravidarum, intrahepatic cholestasis of pregnancy, acute fatty liver of pregnancy, and the syndrome of hemolysis, elevated liver enzymes, and low platelet count (HELLP syndrome).

Hyperemesis gravidarum and the treatment of nausea and vomiting in pregnancy

Hyperemesis gravidarum is the most severe form of nausea and vomiting of pregnancy. It usually starts in the first trimester. Unlike the milder and commonplace nausea and vomiting of pregnancy, hyperemesis gravidarum causes dehydration, electrolyte disturbances, weight loss, and nutritional deficiencies. Hyperemesis gravidarum is reported in 0.5%–2% of all pregnancies. It is more common during first pregnancies and in multiple pregnancies, and is likely to recur with future pregnancies. Liver involvement occurs in approximately 50% of patients and typically consists of mild elevation in serum aminotransferases.

The pathogenesis of hyperemesis remains largely unknown, although many factors have been implicated, such as pregnancy-related hormones and various other hormones

Table 28.6 Pharmacological therapy for nausea and vomiting of pregnancy

Medication	Pregnancy category[a]	Dose
Pyridoxine (vitamin B-6)	A	25 mg t.i.d., p.o.
Antiemetics		
Chlorpromazine	C	10–25 mg b.i.d.–q.i.d., p.o.
Prochlorperazine	C	5–10 mg t.i.d.–q.i.d., p.o.
Promethazine	C	12.5–25 mg every 4–6 h p.o.
Trimethobenzamide	C	250 mg t.i.d.–q.i.d., p.o.
Ondansetron	B	8 mg b.i.d.–t.i.d., p.o.
Droperidol	C	0.5–2 mg i.v. or i.m. every 3–4 h
Antihistamines		
Diphenhydramine	B	25–50 mg every 4–8 h p.o.
Meclizine	B	25 mg every 4–6 h p.o.
Dimenhydrinate	B	50–100 mg every 4–6 h p.o.
Doxylamine	A	25 mg q.d. p.o.
Prokinetics		
Metoclopramide	B	5–10 mg t.i.d. p.o.

a See Table 28.1.

b.i.d., twice a day; i.m., intramuscularly; i.v., intravenously; p.o., orally; q.d., once a day; q.i.d., four times a day; t.i.d., three times a day.

including leptin, placental growth hormone, prolactin, and thyroid and adrenal cortical hormones [129,130]. In addition, infectious, immunological, psychological, metabolic, and anatomical causes for hyperemesis gravidarum have been reported [129,130].

The management of nausea and vomiting of pregnancy depends on the severity of the symptoms. Treatment starts with conservative dietary changes (frequent, bland-tasting, small meals; avoidance of smells and food textures) and non-pharmacological therapy [131]. If these conservative measures fail, pharmacological therapy with antiemetic medications is indicated (Table 28.6). In severe cases, hospitalization, total parenteral nutrition, or percutanous feeding-tube placement may be necessary.

Nonpharmacological therapy

Ginger is a popular alternative treatment for morning sickness. A review of six double-blind randomized controlled trials on the efficacy and safety of ginger showed superiority of ginger over placebo in four of six trials. The other two trials found ginger to be as effective as the reference drug vitamin B-6 [132].

Acupressure on the Chinese acupuncture point P6 (Neiguan), located on the anteromedial aspect of the forearm, at a three-fingers' distance above the wrist, may be useful in some patients, although its efficacy is controversial [133–136].

Pharmacological therapy

In the Cochrane Database of Systematic Reviews on interventions for nausea and vomiting in pregnancy (last updated in 2003), 27 randomized trial studies were identified as suitable for review [137]. For milder degrees of nausea and vomiting (21 trials) antinausea treatments included different antihistamine medications, vitamin B-6 (pyridoxine), the combination tablet Bendectin (a combination of pyridoxine and doxylamine), acupressure, and ginger. For hyperemesis gravidarum (seven trials) antinausea treatments included oral ginger root extract, oral or injected corticosteroids or injected adrenocorticotropic hormone (ACTH), intravenous diazepam, and acupuncture. There was an overall reduction in nausea from antiemetic medication (OR 0.16; CI 0.08–0.33). No trials of treatments for hyperemesis gravidarum show any evidence of benefit. There is little information on effects on fetal outcomes from randomized controlled trials, but observational studies suggest no increased risk for teratogenicity from any of these treatments.

Pyridoxine and doxylamine (Bendectin)

Bendectin was the drug of choice for treatment of nausea and vomiting during pregnancy in the United States until the early 1980s [138]. By 1980, one-fourth to one-third of pregnant women in the United States were using Bendectin during their pregnancy. It was withdrawn from the market after public allegations of teratogenic effects. However, meta-analyses of many epidemiological cohort and case–control studies found no evidence for such a teratogenic effect. Furthermore, an ecological investigation found no decrease in the incidence of birth defects following the decrease and subsequent cessation of Bendectin use in the United States, further supporting the lack of an association. At the same time, the National Hospital Discharge Survey data demonstrated that the US hospitalization rate for nausea and vomiting of pregnancy doubled after the reduction and subsequent cessation of Bendectin use. Bendectin is available in Canada under the tradename Diclectin (pyridoxine 10 mg and doxylamine 10 mg). A prospective, open-label, controlled, interventional study showed preemptive treatment with Diclectin to be effective in preventing severe nausea and vomiting in women with a history of severe nausea and vomiting during a previous pregnancy [139]. In a randomized, double-blind, placebo-controlled study, pyridoxine by itself (25 mg three times a day) significantly reduced nausea scores in patients with severe nausea but not in patients with mild to moderate nausea [140].

Phenothiazines

Although there is an overall paucity of data on the efficacy and safety of prochlorperazine and promethazine during pregnancy, they are considered first-line antiemetics. If there is no response, trimethobenzamide can be tried. A slight increase in severe congenital anomalies has been suggested [141].

Antihistamines

Antihistamines are generally considered safe for use in pregnancy. Doxylamine is a histamine H_1 receptor antagonist (H_1RA) used in Diclectin. Doxylamine and meclizine were not found to be associated with teratogenicity in a large, prospective, observational study of pregnancy and child development [141].

Butyrophenones

Droperidol, a butyrophenone with dopamine antagonist activity, has been reported as safe but insufficient data exist [142,143]. Droperidol has been associated with Q–T prolongation and cardiac arrhythmias.

5-HT₃ receptor antagonist

The 5-HT_3 antagonist ondansetron has not been studied in double-blind, placebo-controlled trials to assess its efficacy and safety for the treatment of nausea and vomiting. A prospective comparative observational study found no increased risk for major malformations in 169 women exposed to ondansetron during pregnancy [144]. Granisetron and dolasetron have not been studied in pregnant women.

Prokinetics

Metoclopramide, a partial 5-HT_3 antagonist and 5-HT_4 agonist, has been successfully used in the treatment of nausea and vomiting as well as in hyperemesis gravidarum [145]. It has not been associated with teratogenic effects but preterm delivery has been reported [145–147].

Corticosteroids

The role of corticosteroids in the treatment of hyperemesis gravidarum is controversial. Although initial studies suggested a beneficial effect, later studies have not been able to confirm this [148–151]. In addition, a 3.4-fold increased risk of oral cleft has been associated with steroid use in the first trimester [97].

Summary

Thus, phenothiazines and H_1RAs are safe and effective for the treatment of nausea and vomiting. Metoclopramide, droperidol, and ondansetron may be effective, but safety data are insufficient to recommend them as first-line agents.

Intrahepatic cholestasis of pregnancy

Intrahepatic cholestasis of pregnancy (ICP) is the most common liver condition in pregnancy. It usually presents in the third trimester and is characterized by pruritus with or without jaundice, which resolves after delivery [152]. Pruritus is often nocturnal and is most pronounced on the palms and soles. The main laboratory characteristics are increased serum alanine aminotransferase (ALT) activities and elevated serum bile acid concentrations [152–154]. Serum γ-glutamyltransferase (GGT) activity remains within normal limits or is increased [153,155]. The risk for premature delivery or intrauterine fetal death is increased with ICP [152–154,156,157], and ICP frequently recurs with subsequent pregnancies [153]. There is a familial component to the disease, with parous sisters of affected patients having a 12-fold increased risk of developing ICP (OR 12.6; CI 5.6–28.1) [158]. The pathogenesis of ICP remains unknown. However, clinical and epidemiological studies suggest mainly hormonal and genetic factors. It is increasingly recognized that genetically determined functional changes in hepatobiliary transport systems are important risk factors for the development of ICP. One of these transporters is the class III multidrug resistance 3 (MDR3) P-glycoprotein, which mediates the translocation of phosphatidylcholine across the canalicular membrane of the hepatocyte [159]. Homozygous mutations in the human MDR3 gene have been associated with progressive familial intrahepatic cholestasis, whereas heterozygous mutations have been detected in women affected by ICP [159–164]. The gene encoding the bile salt export pump (BSEP) has been presented as another possible susceptibility gene for ICP [165,166]. However, other studies do not support a strong role for BSEP in the pathogenesis of ICP [167,168].

Intrauterine fetal death in ICP mainly occurs after 37 weeks [169]. The pathogenesis of uterine fetal death in ICP remains unclear [170]. A Swedish prospective cohort study of 45 485 pregnancies found a 1.5% incidence of ICP based on an elevated fasting serum bile acid level greater than 10 μmol/L [171]. The probability of fetal complications increased by 1%–2% per additional μmol/L increment in serum bile acids. No increase of adverse fetal outcomes in ICP was detected with bile acid levels less than 40 μmol/L. The authors concluded that women with bile acid levels below 40 μmol/L should be managed expectantly, whereas women with higher bile acid levels might be candidates for more aggressive therapy. This recommendation is controversial but deserves further evaluation with randomized studies comparing outcomes of active and expectant management [172].

The medical management of ICP centers on adequate suppression of pruritus. In a clinical trial of 84 women with ICP, patients were randomized to receive ursodeoxycholic acid (8–10 mg/kg bodyweight daily; $n = 42$) or cholestyramine (8 g daily; $n = 42$) for 14 days [173]. Pruritus was more effectively reduced by ursodeoxycholic acid than cholestyramine (66.6% vs 19.0%, respectively; $P < 0.005$). Babies were delivered significantly closer to term by patients treated with ursodeoxycholic acid than by those treated with cholestyramine (38.7 ± 1.7 vs 37.4 ± 1.5 weeks, respectively, $P < 0.05$). Serum alanine aminotransferase (ALT) and aspartate aminotransferase (AST) activities were markedly reduced, by 78.5% and 73.8%, respectively, after ursodeoxycholic acid, but by only 21.4% each after cholestyramine therapy ($P < 0.01$ vs ursodeoxycholic acid). Endogenous serum bile acid levels decreased by 59.5% and 19.0%, respectively ($P < 0.02$).

Ursodeoxycholic acid, but not cholestyramine, was free of adverse effects [173].

In a clinical trial of 46 women with intrahepatic cholestasis of pregnancy randomized to oral S-adenosyl-L-methionine 500 mg twice daily or oral ursodeoxycholic acid 300 mg twice daily, ursodeoxycholic acid was more effective than S-adenosyl-L-methionine at improving the concentration of serum bile acids and other parameters of liver function, whereas both therapies improved symptoms in approximately 60% of cases [174]. Other studies have also confirmed the efficacy of ursodeoxycholic acid use in ICP [175].

The role of dexamethasone in the treatment of ICP will most likely be limited. One small, observational study of 10 women found decreased bile acid levels and improved pruritus in all women treated with 12 mg oral dexamethasone daily for 7 days [176]. However, a double-blind, placebo-controlled trial of 130 women with ICP, comparing the effect of ursodeoxycholic acid (1 g/day for 3 weeks), dexamethasone (12 mg/day for 1 week and placebo during weeks 2 and 3), and placebo (3 weeks) on pruritus and biochemical markers of cholestasis [177], did not confirm such an effect. Dexamethasone yielded no alleviation of pruritus or reduction of ALT, whereas ursodeoxycholic acid improved pruritus and reduced serum bile acids in patients with severe ICP (serum bile acids ≥ 40 µmol/L) only [177].

In summary, delivery at the earliest time of fetal maturity is the treatment of choice in patients with ICP. Ursodeoxycholic acid and cholestyramine are first-line therapy in the medical treatment of pruritus. Dexamethasone should be considered in the individual patient. Plasmapheresis may present an alternative approach in patients with severe, refractory symptoms [178].

Acute fatty liver of pregnancy

Acute fatty liver of pregnancy (AFP) affects women of all ages, races, and ethnic backgrounds but is uncommon; the incidence ranges from 1 in 6000 to 1 in 13 000 pregnancies [179]. AFP usually presents in the third trimester with a sudden onset of nonspecific symptoms such as malaise, fatigue, and headache. As the disease progresses nausea, vomiting, and abdominal pain as well as jaundice, symptoms of encephalopathy, hypoglycemia, and coagulopathy may develop. Laboratory findings include elevated liver aminotransferases, increased direct bilirubin and ammonia levels, increased white blood cell count, and anemia. Disease progression may lead to renal failure and clotting disorders as a result of decreased antithrombin III activity, decreased fibrinogen, thrombocytopenia, and prolongation of prothrombin time and partial thromboplastin time [180].

Hepatic histopathology shows pericentral microvesicular fat with minimal inflammation or necrosis. Liver biopsy is usually not indicated for diagnosis.

Acute fatty liver of pregnancy has been associated with a recessively inherited disorder of mitochondrial fatty acid oxidation [179–181]. Fatty acid oxidation is the principal pathway for the catabolism of fatty acids, which happens within the mitochondria of the cell through the β-oxidation pathway, and is essential for energy production during periods of fasting and stress. This metabolic pathway is critical for the neonate, who has limited glycogen reserve and a high metabolic rate. β-Oxidation is mediated by a variety of enzymes including mitochondrial trifunctional protein (MTP) [179–181]. MTP is a complex protein that catalyzes the last three steps of long-chain fatty acid oxidation (Fig. 28.3). It includes the enzyme long-chain 3-hydroxyacyl-CoA

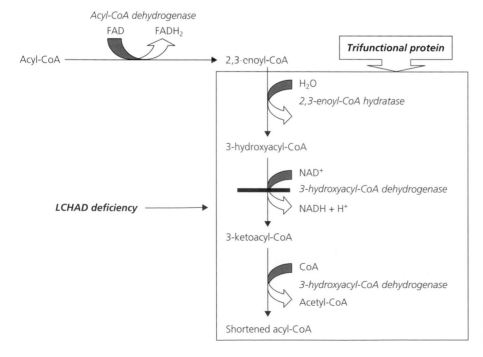

Figure 28.3 Mitochondrial fatty acid oxidation. LCHAD, long-chain 3-hydroxyacyl-CoA dehydrogenase.

dehydrogenase (LCHAD). Both MTP and LCHAD deficiency in the fetus have been associated with maternal preeclampsia, HELLP syndrome, and AFP [181–186].

Pregnancy with an LCHAD- or MTP-deficient fetus often becomes complicated in the third trimester by liver disease, when the metabolic demands of pregnancy increase. It has been speculated that increasing levels of plasma fatty acids may overwhelm the heterozygous mother's capacity for effective metabolism of long-chain fatty acids, leading to an accumulation of potentially toxic fatty acid metabolites in the maternal circulation with subsequent damage to the maternal liver [179,187]. It is not known why some women with an LCHAD- or MTP-deficient fetus develop AFP and others do not. In addition, AFP is not always associated with MTP or LCHAD deficiency, consistent with the existence of other genetic abnormalities associated with AFP.

The treatment of AFP is delivery. Patients usually improve promptly following delivery. Early institution of a high-carbohydrate, low-fat formula is essential for the neonate and fasting episodes lasting more than 4 h should be avoided. The mother should be screened and counseled regarding carrier status and risks for subsequent pregnancies. Women at risk for AFP should be monitored closely during pregnancy and instructed to maintain a high-carbohydrate, low-fat diet. Medications that can interfere with fatty acid oxidation such as NSAIDs, salicylates, tetracycline, and valproic acid should be avoided.

The clinical manifestations of fatty acid oxidation disorders in children vary and can include metabolic acidosis, hypoglycemia with absent ketone production, hyperammonemia, liver failure, severe cardiac and skeletal myopathy, neuropathy, retinopathy, and sudden death [188,189]. Fetal fatty acid oxidation disorders are frequently diagnosed in the perinatal period. In fact, some US states have instituted routine screening for fatty acid oxidation disorders and universal newborn screening may be implemented in the future [188].

HELLP syndrome
HELLP syndrome is characterized by microangiopathic hemolytic anemia, elevated liver enzymes, and thrombocytopenia. HELLP usually presents in the third trimester with symptoms similar to those seen in AFP, such as nausea, vomiting, and abdominal pain. HELLP can develop postpartum as well. Hypertension is frequently present. Laboratory findings include elevated liver enzymes, renal failure, proteinuria, and, in advanced cases, disseminated intravascular coagulation. The classic hepatic lesion associated with HELLP syndrome is periportal or focal parenchymal necrosis in which hyaline deposits of fibrin-like material can be seen in the sinusoids. HELLP has been associated with intrauterine growth retardation, sudden fetal death, and perinatal instability [190–192]. Maternal mortality is low.

The pathogenesis of HELLP remains largely unknown. In a multicenter retrospective study of 88 infants born to women with HELLP syndrome, neither fetal LCHAD deficiency nor fatty acid β-oxidation defects were present [193].

Treatment of choice is immediate delivery. Some experts have advocated the use of steroids with the intention of improving neonatal outcomes by lowering the incidence of such complications as respiratory distress syndrome and intraventricular hemorrhage and to reduce maternal morbidity [194]. In the Cochrane Database of Systematic Reviews on interventions for treating HELLP syndrome, five studies were reviewed of which three were conducted antepartum and two postpartum [195]. The reviewers concluded that there is insufficient evidence to determine whether adjunctive steroid use in HELLP syndrome decreases maternal and perinatal mortality or major morbidity.

Cholelithiasis and cholecystitis
Both the frequency and number of pregnancies are major risk factors for cholesterol gallstones [196–199]. In a prospective study of 3254 women concerning the incidence, natural history, and risk factors for biliary sludge and stones, sludge or stones were found in 5.1% by the second trimester, 7.9% by the third trimester, and 10.2% by 4–6 weeks postpartum [200]. Regression of sludge and stones was common, such that overall 4.2% had new sludge or stones postpartum. Most women with gallbladder disease were asymptomatic but 0.8% underwent cholecystectomy in the first year postpartum. Obesity (body mass index greater than 30) was a strong independent risk factor for pregnancy-associated gallbladder disease (OR 4.45; CI 2.59–7.64) as well as serum leptin levels (OR per 1 ng/dL increase 1.05; CI 1.01–1.11).

Several factors enhance cholesterol gallstone formation during pregnancy. First, progesterone has an inhibitory effect on the contractility of gastrointestinal smooth muscle, including the gallbladder. Thus, biliary stasis may develop during pregnancy, characterized by an increase in the fasting and residual volumes and by a decrease in emptying capacity [201,202]. Second, the lithogenic or cholesterol saturation index of fasting hepatic and gallbladder bile is increased during the second and third trimesters as well as cholesterol secretion [203].

Symptoms of cholelithiasis and cholecystitis are similar in pregnant and nonpregnant patients [204]. Patients with cholecystitis typically present with leukocytosis, and mild elevation of aminotransferases and bilirubin levels. The alkaline phosphatase level progressively increases during normal pregnancy and is unhelpful in distinguishing hepatobiliary disease. A liver ultrasound scan is indicated in all pregnant patients in whom cholelithiasis or cholecystitis is suspected, although ultrasound examination may be more difficult in the third trimester because of gallbladder displacement. Computed tomography (CT) is accurate but exposes the fetus to ionizing radiation. Magnetic resonance imaging (MRI) provides excellent anatomical resolution and tissue characterization without ionizing radiation and diagnosis frequently requires no contrast administration; it should be reserved for those patients in whom ultrasound results are inconclusive and patient care depends on further imaging [205,206].

Management of symptomatic cholelithiasis is similar in pregnant and nonpregnant patients [207,208]. First-line therapy consists of adequate pain control, intravenous fluids, and antibiotics. In certain patients, ERCP may be indicated [209,210].

Open cholecystectomy can be safely accomplished in the first or second trimester [211]. Laparoscopic cholecystectomy also has been described as safe during the first or second trimester [208,212–214]. Furthermore, laparoscopic surgery has been associated with early return of bowel function, early ambulation, rapid return to normal activity, low rate of wound infection and hernia, less pain after the operation, less fetal depression as a result of reduced narcotic use in the postoperative period, reduction in hospitalization days, and minimal manipulation of the uterus while obtaining adequate exposure. The latter leads to less uterine irritability, and a reduction in spontaneous abortion, preterm labor, and premature delivery [212,215]. However, adverse complications, such as puncture of the gravid uterus and pneumoamnion, have been reported with laparoscopic appendectomy, leading some experts to advocate laparotomy after 16 weeks of gestation [216]. A prospective study comparing open vs laparoscopic cholecystectomy in pregnancy is needed to determine fully the effects on maternal and fetal safety.

Infectious hepatitis and pregnancy

Hepatitis A
Hepatitis A virus (HAV) is an RNA virus in the Picornaviridae family. It is transmitted by the fecal–oral route, usually as a result of contaminated food or water, or from person to person through exposure to blood or other contaminated body fluids. Pregnant woman are at risk for acute HAV if they are exposed to an infected household member or if they work in a setting in which poor sanitary habits are common (i.e., a day-care facility). Acute infection is confirmed by the presence of HAV immunoglobulin M (IgM) antibodies. Maternal–fetal transmission has not been established, most likely because of the short viremic phase and the absence of a chronic carrier state [217,218]. However, HAV infection during pregnancy can cause the woman to be at increased risk for severe systemic infection, spontaneous abortion, and premature delivery [217,218]. Post-HAV exposure prophylaxis is therefore recommended for the HAV immunoglobulin G (IgG) antibody-negative pregnant woman, in the form of immunoglobulin and HAV vaccine [218]. Although formal studies of hepatitis A vaccine in pregnancy have not been conducted, the vaccine has been used extensively in pregnancy without adverse outcomes. HAV vaccination is not contraindicated in breast-feeding. Newborn infants of hepatitis A-infected mothers whose symptoms first manifested

between 2 weeks before and 9 weeks after delivery should receive immunoglobulin.

Hepatitis B
Hepatitis B virus (HBV) is a double-stranded DNA virus in the Hepadnaviridae family. Infection with HBV during pregnancy can result in severe maternal disease, fetal loss, and vertical transmission of infection from the mother to the fetus [218]. Testing for HBV surface antigen (HBsAg) is recommended for all pregnant women at the first prenatal visit [219]. Those women at high risk for HBV infection, such as heterosexual adults with multiple sexual partners, persons with a recently acquired sexually transmitted disease, intravenous drug users, sexual or household contacts of HbsAg-positive persons, or persons with an occupational risk for exposure to blood or blood-contaminated body fluids, should be vaccinated. HBV vaccination can be safely administered during pregnancy and breast-feeding [218].

The concern of maternal HBV infection is transmission to the fetus. Vertical transmission can occur in the setting of maternal chronic hepatitis and maternal acute hepatitis. Transmission can occur in utero, at birth, and postnatally. At-birth transmission is the principal route of vertical transmission. The risk of HBV vertical transmission is 10% in HBsAg-positive mothers who are HBV e antigen (HBeAg) negative, antibody to HBV surface antigen (HBsAg) positive, and have undetectable HBV DNA levels. However, the risk can be as high as 90% in HBsAg-positive mothers who are HBeAg positive and have detectable HBV DNA levels [220,221]. Furthermore, vertical transmission rates correlate with maternal HBV DNA levels before delivery [222–224]. The vertical transmission rate significantly increased with HBV DNA levels $= 10^8$ copies/mL [222].

In cases of acute HBV infection complicating pregnancy, the prevalence of neonatal infection depends on the time during gestation that maternal infection occurs [225]. Neonatal HBV infection is rare if maternal infection takes place in the first trimester but has been reported as high as 67% if maternal infection takes place in the third trimester, and in virtually all of those infected in the immediate postpartum period [225–227].

Chronic HBV carriers can safely initiate breast-feeding as long as the child receives appropriate immunoprophylaxis at birth [228,229].

Children born to HBsAg-positive mothers should receive HBV immunoglobulin and HBV vaccine at 1 week, 1 month and 6 months after birth [227]. These interventions reduce the risk of perinatal transmission of HBV to less than 3% [222,226]. Maternal HBsAg carriers have an increased risk of gestational diabetes mellitus, antepartum hemorrhage, and threatened preterm labor [230].

Infants of women who are HBsAg positive should receive HBV immunoglobulin 200 IU intramuscularly when the mother is positive for HBeAg, or 100 IU if the mother is negative for

HBeAg. Hepatitis B virus vaccine should be administered at the same time at another site within 12 h of birth. It is recommended that the infant is administered the dose in the anterolateral muscle of the thigh. Protective efficacy is more than 95% [217]. The child will receive a second close of HBV vaccine at 1 month with the second dose of HBV immunoglobulin, and a third vaccine at 6 months of age [227].

There is no evidence to support the use of cesarian delivery to reduce vertical transmission of HBV. The pharmacological approach to the treatment of chronic HBV includes the use of immune modulators (recombinant interferon alfa-2b) and direct inhibitors of HBV replication (lamivudine). Interferon has been described as toxic in some animal studies and should be avoided during pregnancy. Lamivudine has been administered during the last month of pregnancy and may reduce the residual risk of perinatal transmission when used in combination with postdelivery immunoprophylaxis [231]. This approach presents a valuable strategy to minimize viral load at the time of delivery.

Hepatitis C

Only women with risk factors for hepatitis C virus (HCV) infection should be considered for prenatal testing [232,233]. These risk factors include past or present intravenous drug use; blood transfusion before the introduction of anti-HCV screening of blood units; patients requiring ongoing transfusion support; patients with abnormal aminotransferase levels; and patients who have undergone organ or tissue transplantation from unscreened donors. Systematic prenatal screening of all women for HCV infection is not indicated in view of the lack of effective therapy for preventing vertical transmission.

The reported rates of HCV vertical transmission vary from 3% to 12% [234,235]. High maternal viral load has been associated with an increased risk of vertical transmission, and this might explain the higher transmission rates found in HIV coinfected women, in whom the immunosuppression status may facilitate HCV replication [235,236]. However, the amounts of viral load overlap in transmitting and nontransmitting mothers in most studies, and no threshold values have been identified to predict or exclude transmission [235]. The presence of serum HCV RNA immediately after birth in the neonate has a high diagnostic and prognostic value in identifying those neonates who will develop chronic HCV [237]. No data are available to determine whether interferon therapy can reduce the risk of vertical transmission of HCV infection. Some studies suggest that cesarian delivery may reduce vertical transmission of HCV [236,238] but this is not routinely recommended as these findings have not been confirmed in large, randomized controlled trials.

Diagnosis of infection in the neonate can be established by antibody testing after 18 months of age, as maternal antibodies may persist for up to 18 months after birth. If diagnosis is desired prior to 18 months of age, testing for HCV RNA can be performed. All neonates born to HCV-infected mothers should receive HBV immunoprophylaxis as they may be at high risk for a superimposed HBV infection and because superimposed HBV infection may be more severe in those with preexisting underlying liver disease. There is no evidence that breast-feeding spreads HCV. Mothers who are HCV positive should consider abstaining from breast-feeding if their nipples are cracked or bleeding [239].

Hepatitis E

Hepatitis E virus (HEV) is a hepatotropic virus with small, nonenveloped virions. Infection spreads by the fecal–oral route, usually through contaminated water. It has been suggested that the infection may also be transmitted through blood transfusions [240,241]. Acute infection is confirmed by the presence of HEV IgM antibodies; HEV IgG antibodies persist for at least a few years. Infection with HEV is endemic in southeast and central Asia. Pregnancy increases the severity of HEV infection but the underlying pathogenesis for this observation remains unknown. The outbreaks are characterized by a high attack rate and mortality (up to 25%) among pregnant women. Vertical transmission from the infected mother to the baby commonly occurs, with significant perinatal morbidity and mortality [240–242]. There is no specific treatment available for HEV infection.

Summary

In summary, the course of acute hepatitis is generally unaffected by pregnancy, except in patients with hepatitis E. Chronic hepatitis B or C infections may be transmitted to neonates; however, HBV transmission is effectively prevented with perinatal HBV vaccination and prophylaxis with HBV immunoglobulin. The risk of transmission of hepatitis C to the infant has been associated with the mother's viral RNA load.

References

1. Locke GR, 3rd, Talley NJ, Fett SL, et al. Prevalence and clinical spectrum of gastroesophageal reflux: a population-based study in Olmsted County, Minnesota. Gastroenterology 1997;112:1448.
2. Mold JW, Rankin RA. Symptomatic gastroesophageal reflux in the elderly. J Am Geriatr Soc 1987;35:649.
3. Lin M, Gerson LB, Lascar R, et al. Features of gastroesophageal reflux disease in women. Am J Gastroenterol 2004;99:1442.
4. Richter JE. Gastroesophageal reflux disease during pregnancy. Gastroenterol Clin North Am 2003;32:235.
5. Fisher RS, Roberts GS, Grabowski CJ, Cohen S. Inhibition of lower esophageal sphincter circular muscle by female sex hormones. Am J Physiol 1978;234:E243.
6. Fisher RS, Roberts GS, Grabowski CJ, Cohen S. Altered lower esophageal sphincter function during early pregnancy. Gastroenterology 1978;74:1233.
7. Schulze K, Christensen J. Lower sphincter of the opossum esophagus in pseudopregnancy. Gastroenterology 1977;73:1082.
8. Van Thiel DH, Wald A. Evidence refuting a role for increased abdominal pressure in the pathogenesis of the heartburn associated with pregnancy. Am J Obstet Gynecol 1981;140:420.

9. Van Thiel DH, Gavaler JS, Joshi SN, et al. Heartburn of pregnancy. Gastroenterology 1977;72:666.

10. Spence AA, Moir DD, Finlay WE. Observations on intragastric pressure. Anaesthesia 1967;22:249.

11. Ulmsten U, Sundstrom G. Esophageal manometry in pregnant and nonpregnant women. Am J Obstet Gynecol 1978;132:260.

12. Tytgat GN, Heading RC, Muller-Lissner S, et al. Contemporary understanding and management of reflux and constipation in the general population and pregnancy: a consensus meeting. Aliment Pharmacol Ther 2003;18:291.

13. Villar J, Belizan JM. Same nutrient, different hypotheses: disparities in trials of calcium supplementation during pregnancy. Am J Clin Nutr 2000;71(Suppl.):1375S.

14. Altman D, Carroli G, Duley L, et al. Do women with pre-eclampsia, and their babies, benefit from magnesium sulphate? The Magpie Trial: a randomised placebo-controlled trial. Lancet 2002;359:1877.

15. Lione A. Aluminum toxicology and the aluminum-containing medications. Pharmacol Ther 1985;29:255.

16. Broussard CN, Richter JE. Treating gastro-oesophageal reflux disease during pregnancy and lactation: what are the safest therapy options? Drug Saf 1998;19:325.

17. Ranchet G, Gangemi O, Petrone M. Sucralfate in the treatment of gravidic pyrosis. G Ital Ostet Ginecol 1990;12:1.

18. Magee LA, Inocencion G, Kamboj L, et al. Safety of first trimester exposure to histamine H2 blockers. A prospective cohort study. Dig Dis Sci 1996;41:1145.

19. Cappell MS. Gastric and duodenal ulcers during pregnancy. Gastroenterol Clin North Am 2003;32:263.

20. Morton DM. Pharmacology and toxicology of nizatidine. Scand J Gastroenterol Suppl 1987;136:1.

21. Neubauer BL, Goode RL, Best KL, et al. Endocrine effects of a new histamine H2-receptor antagonist, nizatidine (LY139037), in the male rat. Toxicol Appl Pharmacol 1990;102:219.

22. Glade G, Saccar CL, Pereira GR. Cimetidine in pregnancy: apparent transient liver impairment in the newborn. Am J Dis Child 1980;134:87.

23. Larson JD, Patatanian E, Miner PB, Jr., et al. Double-blind, placebo-controlled study of ranitidine for gastroesophageal reflux symptoms during pregnancy. Obstet Gynecol 1997;90:83.

24. Tsirigotis M, Yazdani N, Craft I. Potential effects of omeprazole in pregnancy. Hum Reprod 1995;10:2177.

25. Kurinczuk JJ, Bower C. Birth defects in infants conceived by intracytoplasmic sperm injection: an alternative interpretation. BMJ 1997;315:1260; discussion 5.

26. Nikfar S, Abdollahi M, Moretti ME, et al. Use of proton pump inhibitors during pregnancy and rates of major malformations: a meta-analysis. Dig Dis Sci 2002;47:1526.

27. Diav-Citrin O, Arnon J, Shechtman S, et al. The safety of proton pump inhibitors in pregnancy: a multicentre prospective controlled study. Aliment Pharmacol Ther 2005;21:269.

28. Gonzalez R, Bowers SP, Swafford V, Smith CD. Pregnancy and delivery after antireflux surgery. Am J Surg 2004;188:34.

29. McKenna D, Watson P, Dornan J. *Helicobacter pylori* infection and dyspepsia in pregnancy. Obstet Gynecol 2003;102:845.

30. Weyermann M, Brenner H, Adler G, et al. *Helicobacter pylori* infection and the occurrence and severity of gastrointestinal symptoms during pregnancy. Am J Obstet Gynecol 2003;189:526.

31. Wu CY, Tseng JJ, Chou MM, et al. Correlation between *Helicobacter pylori* infection and gastrointestinal symptoms in pregnancy. Adv Ther 2000;17:152.

32. Collins E. Maternal and fetal effects of acetaminophen and salicylates in pregnancy. Obstet Gynecol 1981;58:57S.

33. Black RA, Hill DA. Over-the-counter medications in pregnancy. Am Fam Physician 2003;67:2517.

34. Mahadevan U, Kane S. American Gastroenterological Association Institute technical review on the use of gastrointestinal medications in pregnancy. Gastroenterology 2006;131:283.

35. Mahadevan U, Kane S. American Gastroenterological Association Institute medical position statement on the use of gastrointestinal medications in pregnancy. Gastroenterology 2006;131:278.

36. Steinlauf AF, Present DH. Medical management of the pregnant patient with inflammatory bowel disease. Gastroenterol Clin North Am 2004;33:361.

37. Ferrero S, Ragni N. Inflammatory bowel disease: management issues during pregnancy. Arch Gynecol Obstet 2004;270:79.

38. Briggs GG, Freeman RK, Yaffe SJ. Drugs in Pregnancy and Lacatation: a Reference Guide to Fetal and Neonatal Risk, 4th edn. Baltimore: Williams & Wilkins, 1994:501.

39. Greenhalf JO, Leonard HS. Laxatives in the treatment of constipation in pregnant and breast-feeding mothers. Practitioner 1973;210:259.

40. Levy N, Lemberg E, Sharf M. Bowel habit in pregnancy. Digestion 1971;4:216.

41. Prather CM. Pregnancy-related constipation. Curr Gastroenterol Rep 2004;6:402.

42. Wald A. Constipation, diarrhea, and symptomatic hemorrhoids during pregnancy. Gastroenterol Clin North Am 2003;32:309.

43. Ryan JP, Bhojwani A. Colonic transit in rats: effect of ovariectomy, sex steroid hormones, and pregnancy. Am J Physiol 1986;251:G46.

44. Lawson M, Kern F, Jr., Everson GT. Gastrointestinal transit time in human pregnancy: prolongation in the second and third trimesters followed by postpartum normalization. Gastroenterology 1985;89:996.

45. Bonapace ES, Jr., Fisher RS. Constipation and diarrhea in pregnancy. Gastroenterol Clin North Am 1998;27:197.

46. Anderson AS, Whichelow MJ. Constipation during pregnancy: dietary fibre intake and the effect of fibre supplementation. Hum Nutr Appl Nutr 1985;39:202.

47. Jewell DJ, Young G. Interventions for treating constipation in pregnancy. Cochrane Database Syst Rev. 2001:CD001142.

48. Neri I, Blasi I, Castro P, et al. Polyethylene glycol electrolyte solution (Isocolan) for constipation during pregnancy: an observational open-label study. J Midwifery Womens Health 2004;49:355.

49. Schindler AM. Isolated neonatal hypomagnesaemia associated with maternal overuse of stool softener. Lancet 1984;2:822.

50. Medich DS, Fazio VW. Hemorrhoids, anal fissure, and carcinoma of the colon, rectum, and anus during pregnancy. Surg Clin North Am 1995;75:77.

51. Saleeby RG, Jr., Rosen L, Stasik JJ, et al. Hemorrhoidectomy during pregnancy: risk or relief? Dis Colon Rectum 1991;34:260.

52. James SP. This month at the NIH: Final statement of NIH Consensus Conference on celiac disease. Gastroenterology 2005;128:6.

53. De Carolis S, Botta A, Fatigante G, et al. Celiac disease and inflammatory bowel disease in pregnancy. Lupus 2004;13:653.

54. Sher KS, Jayanthi V, Probert CS, et al. Infertility, obstetric and gynaecological problems in coeliac sprue. Dig Dis 1994;12:186.

55. Ciacci C, Cirillo M, Auriemma G, et al. Celiac disease and pregnancy outcome. Am J Gastroenterol 1996;91:718.

56. Collin P, Vilska S, Heinonen PK, et al. Infertility and coeliac disease. Gut 1996;39:382.

57. Molteni N, Bardella MT, Bianchi PA. Obstetric and gynecological problems in women with untreated celiac sprue. J Clin Gastroenterol 1990;12:37.

58. Ferguson R, Holmes GK, Cooke WT. Coeliac disease, fertility, and pregnancy. Scand J Gastroenterol 1982;17:65.

59. Ludvigsson JF, Montgomery SM, Ekbom A. Celiac disease and risk of adverse fetal outcome: a population-based cohort study. Gastroenterology 2005;129:454.

60. Sher KS, Mayberry JF. Female fertility, obstetric and gynaecological history in coeliac disease: a case control study. Acta Paediatr Suppl 1996;412:76.

61. Greco L, Veneziano A, Di Donato L, et al. Undiagnosed coeliac disease does not appear to be associated with unfavourable outcome of pregnancy. Gut 2004;53:149.

62. Gasbarrini A, Torre ES, Trivellini C, et al. Recurrent spontaneous abortion and intrauterine fetal growth retardation as symptoms of coeliac disease. Lancet 2000;356:399.

63. Bradley RJ, Rosen MP. Subfertility and gastrointestinal disease: "unexplained" is often undiagnosed. Obstet Gynecol Surv 2004;59:108.

64. Kane S. Inflammatory bowel disease in pregnancy. Gastroenterol Clin North Am 2003;32:323.

65. Trachter AB, Rogers AI, Leiblum SR. Inflammatory bowel disease in women: impact on relationship and sexual health. Inflamm Bowel Dis 2002;8:413.

66. Hudson M, Flett G, Sinclair TS, et al. Fertility and pregnancy in inflammatory bowel disease. Int J Gynaecol Obstet 1997;58:229.

67. Ording Olsen K, Juul S, Berndtsson I, et al. Ulcerative colitis: female fecundity before diagnosis, during disease, and after surgery compared with a population sample. Gastroenterology 2002;122:15.

68. Kitayama T, Funayama Y, Fukushima K, et al. Anal function during pregnancy and postpartum after ileal pouch anal anastomosis for ulcerative colitis. Surg Today 2005;35:211.

69. Farouk R, Pemberton JH, Wolff BG, et al. Functional outcomes after ileal pouch-anal anastomosis for chronic ulcerative colitis. Ann Surg 2000;231:919.

70. Ravid A, Richard CS, Spencer LM, et al. Pregnancy, delivery, and pouch function after ileal pouch-anal anastomosis for ulcerative colitis. Dis Colon Rectum 2002;45:1283.

71. O'Morain C, Smethurst P, Dore CJ, Levi AJ. Reversible male infertility due to sulphasalazine: studies in man and rat. Gut 1984;25:1078.

72. Katz JA. Pregnancy and inflammatory bowel disease. Curr Opin Gastroenterol 2004;20:328.

73. Korelitz BI. Inflammatory bowel disease and pregnancy. Gastroenterol Clin North Am 1998;27:213.

74. Brandt LJ, Estabrook SG, Reinus JF. Results of a survey to evaluate whether vaginal delivery and episiotomy lead to perineal involvement in women with Crohn's disease. Am J Gastroenterol 1995;90:1918.

75. Dominitz JA, Young JC, Boyko EJ. Outcomes of infants born to mothers with inflammatory bowel disease: a population-based cohort study. Am J Gastroenterol 2002;97:641.

76. Elbaz G, Fich A, Levy A, et al. Inflammatory bowel disease and preterm delivery. Int J Gynaecol Obstet 2005;90:193.

77. Kornfeld D, Cnattingius S, Ekbom A. Pregnancy outcomes in women with inflammatory bowel disease – a population-based cohort study. Am J Obstet Gynecol 1997;177:942.

78. Moser MA, Okun NB, Mayes DC, Bailey RJ. Crohn's disease, pregnancy, and birth weight. Am J Gastroenterol 2000;95:1021.

79. Fonager K, Sorensen HT, Olsen J, et al. Pregnancy outcome for women with Crohn's disease: a follow-up study based on linkage between national registries. Am J Gastroenterol 1998;93:2426.

80. Norgard B, Fonager K, Sorensen HT, Olsen J. Birth outcomes of women with ulcerative colitis: a nationwide Danish cohort study. Am J Gastroenterol 2000;95:3165.

81. Craxi A, Pagliarello F. Possible embryotoxicity of sulfasalazine. Arch Intern Med 1980;140:1674.

82. Hoo JJ, Hadro TA, Von Behren P. Possible teratogenicity of sulfasalazine. N Engl J Med 1988;318:1128.

83. Newman NM, Correy JF. Possible teratogenicity of sulphasalazine. Med J Aust 1983;28:528.

84. Khosla R, Willoughby CP, Jewell DP. Crohn's disease and pregnancy. Gut 1984;25:52.

85. Mogadam M, Dobbins WO, 3rd, Korelitz BI, Ahmed SW. Pregnancy in inflammatory bowel disease: effect of sulfasalazine and corticosteroids on fetal outcome. Gastroenterology 1981;80:72.

86. Willoughby CP, Truelove SC. Ulcerative colitis and pregnancy. Gut 1980;21:469.

87. Jarnerot G, Andersen S, Esbjorner E, et al. Albumin reserve for binding of bilirubin in maternal and cord serum under treatment with sulphasalazine. Scand J Gastroenterol 1981;16:1049.

88. Jarnerot G, Into-Malmberg MB. Sulphasalazine treatment during breast feeding. Scand J Gastroenterol 1979;14:869.

89. Jarnerot G, Into-Malmberg MB, Esbjorner E. Placental transfer of sulphasalazine and sulphapyridine and some of its metabolites. Scand J Gastroenterol 1981;16:693.

90. Esbjorner E, Jarnerot G, Wranne L. Sulphasalazine and sulphapyridine serum levels in children to mothers treated with sulphasalazine during pregnancy and lactation. Acta Paediatr Scand 1987;76:137.

91. Diav-Citrin O, Park YH, Veerasuntharam G, et al. The safety of mesalamine in human pregnancy: a prospective controlled cohort study. Gastroenterology 1998;114:23.

92. Habal FM, Hui G, Greenberg GR. Oral 5-aminosalicylic acid for inflammatory bowel disease in pregnancy: safety and clinical course. Gastroenterology 1993;105:1057.

93. Marteau P, Tennenbaum R, Elefant E, et al. Foetal outcome in women with inflammatory bowel disease treated during pregnancy with oral mesalazine microgranules. Aliment Pharmacol Ther 1998;12:1101.

94. Moskovitz DN, Bodian C, Chapman ML, et al. The effect on the fetus of medications used to treat pregnant inflammatory bowel-disease patients. Am J Gastroenterol 2004;99:656.

95. Bell CM, Habal FM. Safety of topical 5-aminosalicylic acid in pregnancy. Am J Gastroenterol 1997;92:2201.

96. Koren G, Pastuszak A, Ito S. Drugs in pregnancy. N Engl J Med 1998;338:1128.

97. Park-Wyllie L, Mazzotta P, Pastuszak A, et al. Birth defects after maternal exposure to corticosteroids: prospective cohort study and meta-analysis of epidemiological studies. Teratology 2000;62:385.

98. Dejaco C, Mittermaier C, Reinisch W, et al. Azathioprine treatment and male fertility in inflammatory bowel disease. Gastroenterology 2001;121:1048.

99. Tuchmann-Duplessis H, Mercier-Parot L. Production in rabbits of malformations of the extremities by administration of azathioprine and 6-mercaptopurine. C R Seances Soc Biol Fil 1966;160:501.

100. Rosenkrantz JG, Githens JH, Cox SM, Kellum DL. Azathioprine (Imuran) and pregnancy. Am J Obstet Gynecol 1967;97:387.

101. Norgard B, Pedersen L, Fonager K, et al. Azathioprine, mercaptopurine and birth outcome: a population-based cohort study. Aliment Pharmacol Ther 2003;17:827.

102. Korelitz BI, Rajapakse RO. Further evidence that 6-MP taken by the father with IBD provides risk of congenital anomaly to the pregnancy. Am J Gastroenterol 2001;96:252.

103. Norgard B, Pedersen L, Jacobsen J, et al. The risk of congenital abnormalities in children fathered by men treated with azathioprine or mercaptopurine before conception. Aliment Pharmacol Ther 2004;19:679.

104. Rajapakse RO, Korelitz BI, Zlatanic J, et al. Outcome of pregnancies when fathers are treated with 6-mercaptopurine for inflammatory bowel disease. Am J Gastroenterol 2000;95:684.

105. Kane SV. What's good for the goose should be good for the gander – 6-MP use in fathers with inflammatory bowel disease. Am J Gastroenterol 2000;95:581.

106. Francella A, Dyan A, Bodian C, et al. The safety of 6-mercaptopurine for childbearing patients with inflammatory bowel disease: a retrospective cohort study. Gastroenterology 2003;124:9.

107. Caprilli R, Angelucci E, Cocco A, et al. Appropriateness of immunosuppressive drugs in inflammatory bowel diseases assessed by RAND method: Italian Group for IBD (IG-IBD) position statement. Dig Liver Dis 2005;37:407.

108. Zlatanic J, Korelitz BI, Rajapakse R, et al. Complications of pregnancy and child development after cessation of treatment with 6-mercaptopurine for inflammatory bowel disease. J Clin Gastroenterol 2003;36:303.

109. Bar Oz B, Hackman R, Einarson T, Koren G. Pregnancy outcome after cyclosporine therapy during pregnancy: a meta-analysis. Transplantation 2001;71:1051.

110. Bertschinger P, Himmelmann A, Risti B, Follath F. Cyclosporine treatment of severe ulcerative colitis during pregnancy. Am J Gastroenterol 1995;90:330.

111. Jayaprakash A, Gould S, Lim AG, Shehata HA. Use of cyclosporin in pregnancy. Gut 2004;53:1386.

112. Vasiliauskas EA, Church JA, Silverman N, et al. Case report: evidence for transplacental transfer of maternally administered infliximab to the newborn. Clin Gastroenterol Hepatol 2006;4:1255.

113. Katz JA, Antoni C, Keenan GF, et al. Outcome of pregnancy in women receiving infliximab for the treatment of Crohn's disease and rheumatoid arthritis. Am J Gastroenterol 2004;99:2385.

114. Mahadevan U, Kane S, Sandborn WJ, et al. Intentional infliximab use during pregnancy for induction or maintenance of remission in Crohn's disease. Aliment Pharmacol Ther 2005;21:733–8.

115. Burtin P, Taddio A, Ariburnu O, et al. Safety of metronidazole in pregnancy: a meta-analysis. Am J Obstet Gynecol 1995;172:525.

116. Caro-Paton T, Carvajal A, Martin de Diego I, et al. Is metronidazole teratogenic? A meta-analysis. Br J Clin Pharmacol 1997;44:179.

117. Linseman DA, Hampton LA, Branstetter DG. Quinolone-induced arthropathy in the neonatal mouse. Morphological analysis of articular lesions produced by pipemidic acid and ciprofloxacin. Fundam Appl Toxicol 1995;28:59.

118. Berkovitch M, Pastuszak A, Gazarian M, et al. Safety of the new quinolones in pregnancy. Obstet Gynecol 1994;84:535.

119. Loebstein R, Addis A, Ho E, et al. Pregnancy outcome following gestational exposure to fluoroquinolones: a multicenter prospective controlled study. Antimicrob Agents Chemother 1998;42:1336.

120. Jemal A, Murray T, Ward E, et al. Cancer statistics, 2005. CA Cancer J Clin 2005;55:10.

121. Cappell MS. Colon cancer during pregnancy. Gastroenterol Clin North Am 2003;32:341.

122. Fidler H, Hartnett A, Cheng Man K, et al. Sex and familiarity of colonoscopists: patient preferences. Endoscopy 2000;32:481.

123. Menees SB, Inadomi JM, Korsnes S, Elta GH. Women patients' preference for women physicians is a barrier to colon cancer screening. Gastrointest Endosc 2005;62:219.

124. Varadarajulu S, Petruff C, Ramsey WH. Patient preferences for gender of endoscopists. Gastrointest Endosc 2002;56:170.

125. Cappell MS. The fetal safety and clinical efficacy of gastrointestinal endoscopy during pregnancy. Gastroenterol Clin North Am 2003; 32:123.

126. Schreyer P, Caspi E, El-Hindi JM, Eshchar J. Cirrhosis – pregnancy and delivery: a review. Obstet Gynecol Surv 1982;37:304.

127. Starkel P, Horsmans Y, Geubel A. Endoscopic band ligation: a safe technique to control bleeding esophageal varices in pregnancy. Gastrointest Endosc 1998;48:212.

128. Shaheen NJ, Crosby MA, Grimm IS, Isaacs K. The use of percutaneous endoscopic gastrostomy in pregnancy. Gastrointest Endosc 1997;46:564.

129. Koch KL, Frissora CL. Nausea and vomiting during pregnancy. Gastroenterol Clin North Am 2003;32:201,vi.

130. Verberg MF, Gillott DJ, Al-Fardan N, Grudzinskas JG. Hyperemesis gravidarum, a literature review. Hum Reprod Update 2005;11:527.

131. Quinlan JD, Hill DA. Nausea and vomiting of pregnancy. Am Fam Physician 2003;68:121.

132. Borrelli F, Capasso R, Izzo AA. Effectiveness and safety of ginger in the treatment of pregnancy-induced nausea and vomiting. Obstet Gynecol 2005;106:640.

133. de Aloysio D, Penacchioni P. Morning sickness control in early pregnancy by Neiguan point acupressure. Obstet Gynecol 1992;80:852.

134. Norheim AJ, Pedersen EJ, Fonnebo V, Berge L. Acupressure treatment of morning sickness in pregnancy. A randomised, double-blind, placebo-controlled study. Scand J Prim Health Care 2001;19:43.

135. O'Brien B, Relyea MJ, Taerum T. Efficacy of P6 acupressure in the treatment of nausea and vomiting during pregnancy. Am J Obstet Gynecol 1996;174:708.

136. Werntoft E, Dykes AK. Effect of acupressure on nausea and vomiting during pregnancy. A randomised, placebo-controlled, pilot study. J Reprod Med 2001;46:835.

137. Jewell D, Young G. Interventions for nausea and vomiting in early pregnancy. Cochrane Database Syst Rev 2003:CD000145.

138. Kutcher JS, Engle A, Firth J, Lamm SH. Bendectin and birth defects. II: Ecological analyses. Birth Defects Res A Clin Mol Teratol 2003;67:88.

139. Koren G, Maltepe C. Pre-emptive therapy for severe nausea and vomiting of pregnancy and hyperemesis gravidarum. J Obstet Gynaecol 2004;24:530.

140. Sahakian V, Rouse D, Sipes S, et al. Vitamin B6 is effective therapy for nausea and vomiting of pregnancy: a randomized, double-blind placebo-controlled study. Obstet Gynecol 1991;78:33.

141. Miklovich L, van den Berg BJ. An evaluation of the teratogenicity of certain antinauseant drugs. Am J Obstet Gynecol 1976;125:244.

142. Magee LA, Mazzotta P, Koren G. Evidence-based view of safety and effectiveness of pharmacologic therapy for nausea and vomiting of pregnancy (NVP). Am J Obstet Gynecol 2002;186:S256.

143. Nageotte MP, Briggs GG, Towers CV, Asrat T. Droperidol and diphenhydramine in the management of hyperemesis gravidarum. Am J Obstet Gynecol 1996;174:1801; discussion 5.

144. Einarson A, Maltepe C, Navioz Y, et al. The safety of ondansetron for nausea and vomiting of pregnancy: a prospective comparative study. BJOG 2004;111:940.

145. Berkovitch M, Mazzota P, Greenberg R, et al. Metoclopramide for nausea and vomiting of pregnancy: a prospective multicenter international study. Am J Perinatol 2002;19:311.

146. Berkovitch M, Elbirt D, Addis A, et al. Fetal effects of metoclopramide therapy for nausea and vomiting of pregnancy. N Engl J Med 2000;343:445.

147. Sorensen HT, Nielsen GL, Christensen K, et al. Birth outcome following maternal use of metoclopramide. The Euromap study group. Br J Clin Pharmacol 2000;49:264.

148. Nelson-Piercy C, Fayers P, de Swiet M. Randomised, double-blind, placebo-controlled trial of corticosteroids for the treatment of hyperemesis gravidarum. BJOG 2001;108:9.

149. Safari HR, Fassett MJ, Souter IC, et al. The efficacy of methylprednisolone in the treatment of hyperemesis gravidarum: a randomized, double-blind, controlled study. Am J Obstet Gynecol 1998;179: 921.

150. Whittaker R. Randomised, double-blind, placebo-controlled trial of corticosteroids for the treatment of hyperemesis gravidarum. BJOG 2003;110:88.

151. Yost NP, McIntire DD, Wians FH, Jr., et al. A randomized, placebo-controlled trial of corticosteroids for hyperemesis due to pregnancy. Obstet Gynecol 2003;102:1250.

152. Reyes H. The spectrum of liver and gastrointestinal disease seen in cholestasis of pregnancy. Gastroenterol Clin North Am 1992;21:905.

153. Bacq Y, Sapey T, Brechot MC, et al. Intrahepatic cholestasis of pregnancy: a French prospective study. Hepatology 1997;26:358.

154. Fagan EA. Intrahepatic cholestasis of pregnancy. Clin Liver Dis 1999;3:603.

155. Serrano MA, Brites D, Larena MG, et al. Beneficial effect of ursodeoxycholic acid on alterations induced by cholestasis of pregnancy in bile acid transport across the human placenta. J Hepatol 1998;28:829.

156. Milkiewicz P, Elias E, Williamson C, Weaver J. Obstetric cholestasis. BMJ 2002;324:123.

157. Reyes H. Review: intrahepatic cholestasis. A puzzling disorder of pregnancy. J Gastroenterol Hepatol 1997;12:211.

158. Eloranta ML, Heinonen S, Mononen T, Saarikoski S. Risk of obstetric cholestasis in sisters of index patients. Clin Genet 2001;60:42.

159. de Vree JM, Jacquemin E, Sturm E, et al. Mutations in the MDR3 gene cause progressive familial intrahepatic cholestasis. Proc Natl Acad Sci U S A 1998;95:282.

160. Dixon PH, Weerasekera N, Linton KJ, et al. Heterozygous MDR3 missense mutation associated with intrahepatic cholestasis of pregnancy: evidence for a defect in protein trafficking. Hum Mol Genet 2000;9:1209.

161. Gendrot C, Bacq Y, Brechot MC, et al. A second heterozygous MDR3 nonsense mutation associated with intrahepatic cholestasis of pregnancy. J Med Genet 2003;40:e32.

162. Jacquemin E, Cresteil D, Manouvrier S, et al. Heterozygous nonsense mutation of the MDR3 gene in familial intrahepatic cholestasis of pregnancy. Lancet 1999;353:210.

163. Jacquemin E, De Vree JM, Cresteil D, et al. The wide spectrum of multidrug resistance 3 deficiency: from neonatal cholestasis to cirrhosis of adulthood. Gastroenterology 2001;120:1448.

164. Rosmorduc O, Hermelin B, Poupon R. MDR3 gene defect in adults with symptomatic intrahepatic and gallbladder cholesterol cholelithiasis. Gastroenterology 2001;120:1459.

165. Eloranta ML, Hakli T, Hiltunen M, et al. Association of single nucleotide polymorphisms of the bile salt export pump gene with intrahepatic cholestasis of pregnancy. Scand J Gastroenterol 2003;38:648.

166. Mullenbach R, Bennett A, Tetlow N, et al. ATP8B1 mutations in British cases with intrahepatic cholestasis of pregnancy. Gut 2005;54:829.

167. Painter JN, Savander M, Sistonen P, et al. A known polymorphism in the bile salt export pump gene is not a risk allele for intrahepatic cholestasis of pregnancy. Scand J Gastroenterol 2004;39:694.

168. Pauli-Magnus C, Lang T, Meier Y, et al. Sequence analysis of bile salt export pump (ABCB11) and multidrug resistance p-glycoprotein 3 (ABCB4, MDR3) in patients with intrahepatic cholestasis of pregnancy. Pharmacogenetics 2004;14:91.

169. Williamson C, Hems LM, Goulis DG, et al. Clinical outcome in a series of cases of obstetric cholestasis identified via a patient support group. BJOG 2004;111:676.

170. Lammert F, Marschall HU, Glantz A, Matern S. Intrahepatic cholestasis of pregnancy: molecular pathogenesis, diagnosis and management. J Hepatol 2000;33:1012.

171. Glantz A, Marschall HU, Mattsson LA. Intrahepatic cholestasis of pregnancy: Relationships between bile acid levels and fetal complication rates. Hepatology 2004;40:467.

172. Sentilhes L, Verspyck E, Roman H, Marpeau L. Intrahepatic cholestasis of pregnancy and bile acid levels. Hepatology 2005;42:737; author reply 8.

173. Kondrackiene J, Beuers U, Kupcinskas L. Efficacy and safety of ursodeoxycholic acid versus cholestyramine in intrahepatic cholestasis of pregnancy. Gastroenterology 2005;129:894.

174. Roncaglia N, Locatelli A, Arreghini A, et al. A randomised controlled trial of ursodeoxycholic acid and S-adenosyl-L-methionine in the treatment of gestational cholestasis. BJOG 2004 ;111:17–21.

175. Zapata R, Sandoval L, Palma J, et al. Ursodeoxycholic acid in the treatment of intrahepatic cholestasis of pregnancy. A 12-year experience. Liver Int 2005;25:548.

176. Hirvioja ML, Tuimala R, Vuori J. The treatment of intrahepatic cholestasis of pregnancy by dexamethasone. Br J Obstet Gynaecol 1992;99:109.

177. Glantz A, Marschall HU, Lammert F, Mattsson LA. Intrahepatic cholestasis of pregnancy: a randomized controlled trial comparing dexamethasone and ursodeoxycholic acid. Hepatology 2005;42:1399.

178. Warren JE, Blaylock RC, Silver RM. Plasmapheresis for the treatment of intrahepatic cholestasis of pregnancy refractory to medical treatment. Am J Obstet Gynecol 2005;192:2088.

179. Jamerson PA. The association between acute fatty liver of pregnancy and fatty acid oxidation disorders. J Obstet Gynecol Neonatal Nurs 2005;34:87.

180. Treem WR. Mitochondrial fatty acid oxidation and acute fatty liver of pregnancy. Semin Gastrointest Dis 2002;13:55.

181. Ibdah JA, Bennett MJ, Rinaldo P, et al. A fetal fatty-acid oxidation disorder as a cause of liver disease in pregnant women. N Engl J Med 1999;340:1723.

182. Isaacs JD, Jr., Sims HF, Powell CK, et al. Maternal acute fatty liver of pregnancy associated with fetal trifunctional protein deficiency: molecular characterization of a novel maternal mutant allele. Pediatr Res 1996;40:393.

183. Sims HF, Brackett JC, Powell CK, et al. The molecular basis of pediatric long chain 3-hydroxyacyl-CoA dehydrogenase deficiency associated with maternal acute fatty liver of pregnancy. Proc Natl Acad Sci USA 1995;92:841.

184. Treem WR, Shoup ME, Hale DE, et al. Acute fatty liver of pregnancy, hemolysis, elevated liver enzymes, and low platelets syndrome, and long chain 3-hydroxyacyl-coenzyme A dehydrogenase deficiency. Am J Gastroenterol 1996;91:2293.

185. Wilcken B, Leung KC, Hammond J, et al. Pregnancy and fetal long-chain 3-hydroxyacyl coenzyme A dehydrogenase deficiency. Lancet 1993;341:407.

186. Yang Z, Zhao Y, Bennett MJ, et al. Fetal genotypes and pregnancy outcomes in 35 families with mitochondrial trifunctional protein mutations. Am J Obstet Gynecol 2002;187:715.

187. Blish KR, Ibdah JA. Maternal heterozygosity for a mitochondrial trifunctional protein mutation as a cause for liver disease in pregnancy. Med Hypotheses 2005;64:96.

188. Shekhawat PS, Matern D, Strauss AW. Fetal fatty acid oxidation disorders, their effect on maternal health and neonatal outcome: impact of expanded newborn screening on their diagnosis and management. Pediatr Res 2005;57:78R.

189. Strauss AW, Powell CK, Hale DE, et al. Molecular basis of human mitochondrial very-long-chain acyl-CoA dehydrogenase deficiency causing cardiomyopathy and sudden death in childhood. Proc Natl Acad Sci USA 1995;92:10496.

190. Raval DS, Co S, Reid MA, Pildes R. Maternal and neonatal outcome of pregnancies complicated with maternal HELLP syndrome. J Perinatol 1997;17:266.

191. Roberts JM. Preeclampsia: what we know and what we do not know. Semin Perinatol 2000;24:24.

192. Roberts JM, Cooper DW. Pathogenesis and genetics of pre-eclampsia. Lancet 2001;357:53.

193. Holub M, Bodamer OA, Item C, et al. Lack of correlation between fatty acid oxidation disorders and haemolysis, elevated liver enzymes, low platelets (HELLP) syndrome? Acta Paediatr 2005;94:48.

194. O'Brien JM, Barton JR. Controversies with the diagnosis and management of HELLP syndrome. Clin Obstet Gynecol 2005;48:460.

195. Matchaba P, Moodley J. Corticosteroids for HELLP syndrome in pregnancy. Cochrane Database Syst Rev 2004:CD002076.

196. Everhart JE, Khare M, Hill M, Maurer KR. Prevalence and ethnic differences in gallbladder disease in the United States. Gastroenterology 1999;117:632.

197. Friedman GD, Kannel WB, Dawber TR. The epidemiology of gallbladder disease: observations in the Framingham Study. J Chronic Dis 1966;19:273.

198. Stampfer MJ, Maclure KM, Colditz GA, et al. Risk of symptomatic gallstones in women with severe obesity. Am J Clin Nutr 1992;55:652.

199. Thijs C, Knipschild P, Leffers P. Pregnancy and gallstone disease: an empiric demonstration of the importance of specification of risk periods. Am J Epidemiol 1991;134:186.

200. Ko CW, Beresford SA, Schulte SJ, et al. Incidence, natural history, and risk factors for biliary sludge and stones during pregnancy. Hepatology 2005;41:359.

201. Daignault PG, Fazekas AG, Rosenthall L, Fried GM. Relationship between gallbladder contraction and progesterone receptors in patients with gallstones. Am J Surg 1988;155:147.

202. Kline LW, Karpinski E. Progesterone inhibits gallbladder motility through multiple signaling pathways. Steroids 2005;70:673.

203. Kern F, Jr., Everson GT, DeMark B, et al. Biliary lipids, bile acids, and gallbladder function in the human female. Effects of pregnancy and the ovulatory cycle. J Clin Invest 1981;68:1229.

204. Fallon WF, Jr., Newman JS, Fallon GL, Malangoni MA. The surgical management of intra-abdominal inflammatory conditions during pregnancy. Surg Clin North Am 1995;75:15.

205. Brown MA, Birchard KR, Semelka RC. Magnetic resonance evaluation of pregnant patients with acute abdominal pain. Semin Ultrasound CT MR 2005;26:206.

206. Leyendecker JR, Gorengaut V, Brown JJ. MR imaging of maternal diseases of the abdomen and pelvis during pregnancy and the immediate postpartum period. Radiographics 2004;24:1301.

207. Lu EJ, Curet MJ, El-Sayed YY, Kirkwood KS. Medical versus surgical management of biliary tract disease in pregnancy. Am J Surg 2004;188:755.

208. Rollins MD, Chan KJ, Price RR. Laparoscopy for appendicitis and cholelithiasis during pregnancy: a new standard of care. Surg Endosc 2004;18:237.

209. Kahaleh M, Hartwell GD, Arseneau KO, et al. Safety and efficacy of ERCP in pregnancy. Gastrointest Endosc 2004;60:287.

210. Tham TC, Vandervoort J, Wong RC, et al. Safety of ERCP during pregnancy. Am J Gastroenterol 2003;98:308.

211. Hill LM, Johnson CE, Lee RA. Cholecystectomy in pregnancy. Obstet Gynecol 1975;46:291.

212. Al-Fozan H, Tulandi T. Safety and risks of laparoscopy in pregnancy. Curr Opin Obstet Gynecol 2002;14:375.

213. Patel SG, Veverka TJ. Laparoscopic cholecystectomy in pregnancy. Curr Surg 2002;59:74.

214. Rizzo AG. Laparoscopic surgery in pregnancy: long-term follow-up. J Laparoendosc Adv Surg Tech A 2003;13:11.

215. Curet MJ. Special problems in laparoscopic surgery. Previous abdominal surgery, obesity, and pregnancy. Surg Clin North Am 2000;80:1093.

216. Friedman JD, Ramsey PS, Ramin KD, Berry C. Pneumoamnion and pregnancy loss after second-trimester laparoscopic surgery. Obstet Gynecol 2002;99:512.

217. Gall SA. Maternal immunization. Obstet Gynecol Clin North Am 2003;30:623.

218. Gall SA. Expanding the use of hepatitis vaccines in obstetrics and gynecology. Am J Med 2005;118:96S.

219. Kirkham C, Harris S, Grzybowski S. Evidence-based prenatal care: part II. Third-trimester care and prevention of infectious diseases. Am Fam Physician 2005;71:1555.

220. Mishra L, Seeff LB. Viral hepatitis, A through E, complicating pregnancy. Gastroenterol Clin North Am 1992;21:873.

221. Samuels P, Cohen AW. Pregnancies complicated by liver disease and liver dysfunction. Obstet Gynecol Clin North Am 1992;19:745.

222. Li XM, Shi MF, Yang YB, et al. Effect of hepatitis B immunoglobulin on interruption of HBV intrauterine infection. World J Gastroenterol 2004;10:3215.

223. Ngui SL, Andrews NJ, Underhill GS, et al. Failed postnatal immunoprophylaxis for hepatitis B: characteristics of maternal hepatitis B virus as risk factors. Clin Infect Dis 1998;27:100.

224. Wang Z, Zhang J, Yang H, et al. Quantitative analysis of HBV DNA level and HBeAg titer in hepatitis B surface antigen positive mothers and their babies: HBeAg passage through the placenta and the rate of decay in babies. J Med Virol 2003;71:360.

225. Tong MJ, Thursby M, Rakela J, et al. Studies on the maternal-infant transmission of the viruses which cause acute hepatitis. Gastroenterology 1981;80:999.

226. Hunt CM, Sharara AI. Liver disease in pregnancy. Am Fam Physician 1999;59:829.

227. Ranger-Rogez S, Denis F. Hepatitis B mother-to-child transmission. Expert Rev Anti Infect Ther 2004;2:133.

228. Hill JB, Sheffield JS, Kim MJ, et al. Risk of hepatitis B transmission in breast-fed infants of chronic hepatitis B carriers. Obstet Gynecol 2002;99:1049.

229. Wang JS, Zhu QR, Wang XH. Breastfeeding does not pose any additional risk of immunoprophylaxis failure on infants of HBV carrier mothers. Int J Clin Pract 2003;57:100.

230. Tse KY, Ho LF, Lao T. The impact of maternal HBsAg carrier status on pregnancy outcomes: A case-control study. J Hepatol 2005;43:771.

231. van Zonneveld M, van Nunen AB, Niesters HG, et al. Lamivudine treatment during pregnancy to prevent perinatal transmission of hepatitis B virus infection. J Viral Hepat 2003;10:294.

232. Plunkett BA, Grobman WA. Routine hepatitis C virus screening in pregnancy: a cost-effectiveness analysis. Am J Obstet Gynecol 2005;192:1153.

233. Su GL. Hepatitis C in pregnancy. Curr Gastroenterol Rep 2005;7:45.

234. Syriopoulou V, Nikolopoulou G, Daikos GL, et al. Mother to child transmission of hepatitis C virus: rate of infection and risk factors. Scand J Infect Dis 2005;37:350.

235. Tovo PA, Lazier L, Versace A. Hepatitis B virus and hepatitis C virus infections in children. Curr Opin Infect Dis 2005;18:261.

236. Steininger C, Kundi M, Jatzko G, et al. Increased risk of mother-to-infant transmission of hepatitis C virus by intrapartum infantile exposure to maternal blood. J Infect Dis 2003;187:345.

237. Saez A, Losa M, Lo Iacono O, et al. Diagnostic and prognostic value of virologic tests in vertical transmission of hepatitis C virus infection: results of a large prospective study in pregnant women. Hepatogastroenterology 2004;51:1104.

238. Gibb DM, Goodall RL, Dunn DT, et al. Mother-to-child transmission of hepatitis C virus: evidence for preventable peripartum transmission. Lancet 2000;356:904.

239. Mast EE. Mother-to-infant hepatitis C virus transmission and breastfeeding. Adv Exp Med Biol 2004;554:211.

240. Khuroo MS, Kamili S, Jameel S. Vertical transmission of hepatitis E virus. Lancet 1995;345:1025.

241. Khuroo MS, Kamili S, Yattoo GN. Hepatitis E virus infection may be transmitted through blood transfusions in an endemic area. J Gastroenterol Hepatol 2004;19:778.

242. Kumar A, Beniwal M, Kar P, et al. Hepatitis E in pregnancy. Int J Gynaecol Obstet 2004;85:240.

29 General nutritional principles

David H. Alpers, Beth Taylor, Samuel Klein

Basic nutritional principles, 557
Altered nutritional states, 580

Basic nutritional principles

Body composition

The human body consists of 35 components that are organized into five levels of increasing complexity: atomic (e.g., nitrogen, potassium), molecular (e.g., water, protein), cellular (e.g., body cell mass, intra- and extracellular fluid), tissue (e.g., skeletal muscle, adipose tissue), and whole body (e.g., weight, height). A healthy, lean man is composed of 55%–60% water, 15%–20% fat, 15%–20% protein (one-half in skeletal muscle), 1% glycogen (four-fifths in muscle, one-fifth in liver), and 4% minerals [1]. Although sophisticated techniques are available to measure each body component, the definitions of some commonly used terms can be confusing. *Fat mass* represents all body triglycerides, which are present in adipose tissue, muscle, and liver. *Adipose tissue* is about 83% fat (e.g., triglyceride), 15% water, and 2% protein. *Fat-free mass* refers to total body mass minus total fat mass. *Lean body mass* is defined as total body mass minus adipose tissue. The body also can be divided into cellular and extracellular mass. *Body cell mass* is defined as the cellular components of all tissues (35%–45% of the body weight in healthy men, 30%–40% in women) and can be measured by total exchangeable potassium [2]. *Extracellular mass* is defined as the heterogeneous group of tissues and fluids supporting the body cell mass.

Diet for healthy people

Many guidelines have been developed over the years for general use by the US population for health maintenance and disease prevention. Although these have been published at different times and represent the input of a large number of experts with diverse interests, all expert panels have reported remarkably simple and consistent recommendations for healthy adults. Two of these sets of guidelines are widely disseminated.

The 2005 *Dietary Guidelines for Americans*, developed by the US Department of Health and Human Services and the US Department of Agriculture, provides guidelines for a healthy diet and body weight [3] (Table 29.1). These guidelines are similar to those recommended by the American Heart Association [4]. Both reports recommend the following:
- consume a variety of fruits, vegetables, and whole-grain products
- balance energy intake with energy needs and prevent gradual weight gain over time by making small decreases in energy intake while increasing physical activity
- limit intake of foods that contain high levels of saturated fatty acids, and keep consumption of *trans* fatty acid as low as possible
- limit dietary salt intake and alcohol consumption
- engage in regular physical activity.

Although the recommendations listed in Table 29.1 are generalized for all Americans, special considerations may be needed for African Americans and other minority groups.

In the last 25 years, the prevalence of obesity has increased markedly throughout the world. The World Health Organization [5] and the National Institutes of Health (NIH) [6,7] have proposed guidelines for classifying weight status by body mass index (BMI) (Table 29.2).

It is often helpful to estimate a patient's energy requirement when making recommendations of calorie intake. The Harris–Benedict equation is a useful tool for estimating resting energy requirements (Table 29.3). For estimates of overall energy use, the *recommended daily allowance* (RDA) figures are simple and useful (Table 29.4).

Most guidelines suggest an *adequate intake* (AI) of calcium (1300 mg/day for adolescents, 1000 mg/day for adult men and nonpregnant women aged 19–50, and 1200 mg/day for adults older than 50 years) [8]. Milk contains the highest concentration of calcium – 280–300 mg/225-g (8-oz) cup. There is as yet no convincing evidence that additional protection against osteopenia is achieved by ingesting calcium over the

Principles of Clinical Gastroenterology. Edited by Tadataka Yamada, David H. Alpers, Anthony N. Kalloo, Neil Kaplowitz, Chung Owyang, and Don W. Powell. © 2008 Blackwell Publishing. ISBN 978-1-4051-69103

Table 29.1 Dietary guidelines for adult Americans, 2005

Theme	Guideline	Practical recommendations
Aim for fitness	Do not become obese	Maintain body mass index between 18.5 and 24.9 kg/m^2
	Be physically active on a daily basis	To reduce risks of chronic disease, engage in 30 min of moderate exercise (e.g., brisk walking) daily. To help manage body weight, engage in 60 min of moderate exercise daily
Build a healthy base	Enjoy a wide variety of foods	Increase intake of low-energy, nutrient-dense foods (e.g., fruits, vegetables)
	Consume a variety of fruits, vegetables, and grains daily. Eat more dark-green and orange vegetables. Eat at least 85 g (3 oz) of whole-grain cereals, breads, crackers, rice, or pasta	Consume 2 cups of fruit, 2½ cups of vegetables, 170 g (6 oz) of grains daily 28 g (1 oz) ≈ 1 slice bread, 1 cup breakfast cereal, or ½ cup cooked rice, cereal, or pasta
	Maintain calcium intake	Consume lactose-free products or other calcium sources, such as fortified foods and beverages, if you are unable to ingest milk or milk products
	Maintain moderate protein intake	Consume 150 g (5½ oz) daily of low-fat lean meats and poultry Vary your protein sources by choosing fish, beans, peas, nuts, and seeds
Choose sensibly	Choose a diet low in saturated fats and cholesterol	Keep total fat intake between 20% and 35%, and combined saturated and *trans* fatty acids to < 10% of total calories. Limit cholesterol intake to < 300 mg/day
	Moderation in salt intake	Consume < 2300 mg (~ 1 tsp salt) sodium per day. Persons with hypertension, African Americans, and middle-aged and older adults should consume ≤ 1500 mg/day
	Choose and prepare foods and beverages with little added sugars or intense sweetners	
	Do not smoke	
	Drink alcoholic beverages in moderation, if at all	Limit drinks to one or two per day
Food safety	Avoid microbial foodborne illness	Clean hands and surfaces prior to contact with food. Cook foods to a safe temperature. Chill perishable food promptly. Avoid unpasteurized milk or milk products, raw or partially cooked eggs, and raw or undercooked meat and poultry

Amounts are based on a daily intake of 8350 kJ (2000 kcal).
Adapted from US Department of Health and Human Services, US Department of Agriculture [3] and Krauss et al. [4].

Table 29.2 Disease risk associated with body mass index

	Obesity class	BMI (kg/m^2)	Disease risk
Underweight		< 18.5	Increased
Normal		18.5–24.9	Normal
Overweight		25.0–29.9	Increased
Obesity	I	30.0–34.9	High
	II	35.0–39.9	Very high
Extreme obesity	III	≥ 40.0	Extremely high

Additional risks: (i) waist circumference > 100 cm (40 in) in men and > 90 cm (35 in) in women; and (ii) poor aerobic fitness.
BMI, body mass index.
Adapted from National Institutes of Health, National Heart, Lung, and Blood Institute [7].

recommended AI. Salt (NaCl) should be limited to 6 g/day or less, and alcohol to 28 g (1 oz) of pure alcohol per day (28 g is the equivalent of two cans of beer, two small glasses of wine, or two average cocktails).

The implementation of the published recommendations depends on two other federally supported guidelines. The RDA [9–13] is the level judged to be high enough to ensure an adequate intake for the majority of the normal population, not the minimal intake necessary to avoid negative balance. The values for the RDA vary with age and gender. These values should not be confused with the US RDAs, standards set by the US Food and Drug Administration in 1973 for the purposes of food labeling for the entire population. The term "US RDA" has been replaced by *reference daily intake* (RDI) and *daily reference value* (DRV). The latter provides for total and saturated fat, cholesterol, total carbohydrates, dietary fiber,

Table 29.3 Formulas for estimating resting energy expenditure

Harris–Benedict equation [41]
Men = 66 + (13.7 x W) + (5 x H) − (6.8 x A)
Women = 665 + (9.6 x W) + (1.8 x H) − (4.7 x A)

Owen et al. [43]
Men = 879 + (10.2 x W)
Women = 795 + (7.18 x W)

World Health Organization [56]

Age (years)	Male	Female
0–3	(60.9 × W) − 54	(61.0 × W) − 51
3–10	(22.7 × W) − 495	(22.5 × W) + 499
10–18	(17.5 × W) + 651	(12.2 × W) + 746
18–30	(15.3 × W) + 679	(14.7 × W) + 996
30–60	(11.2 × W) + 879	(8.7 × W) + 829
> 60	(13.5 × W) + 987	(10.5 × W) + 596

A, age (years); H, height (cm); W, weight (kg).

Table 29.4 Calculation of energy requirement

Level of activity	Activity factor (x REE)	Average energy expenditure[a] (kcal/kg per day)
Very light		
Men	1.3	31
Women	1.3	30
Light		
Men	1.6	38
Women	1.5	35
Moderate		
Men	1.7	41
Women	1.6	37
Heavy		
Men	2.1	50
Women	1.9	44

a Estimated from World Health Organization equations for median weights of persons aged 19–74 years; activity factor 1.0 = 100.4 kJ/kg (24.0 kcal/kg) for males, 97 kJ/kg (23.2 kcal/kg) for females.
REE, resting energy expenditure.
Adapted from Standing Committee on the Scientific Evaluation of Dietary Reference Intakes, Food and Nutrition Board, Institute of Medicine [13].

sodium, potassium, and protein – nutrients for which no US RDA was available [12,13]. The RDI and DRV are the basis for the daily values that appear on all food labels in the United States, and reflect DRVs and RDIs for a 2000-calorie reference diet. The new recommended dietary intake levels are called *dietary reference intakes* (DRIs), a collective term that includes the *estimated average requirement* (EAR), the RDA, the AI, and the *tolerable upper intake level* (UL) (Table 29.5) [8–13]. These terms were developed by the Institute of Medicine in the United States along with Health Canada. The EAR is the daily nutrient intake value estimated to meet the requirements of half of an age- and gender-specific group. It often is derived from balance studies and is used in setting the RDA, the intake level sufficient to meet the nutrient needs of most people within a given life-stage and gender group. The RDA also includes a factor to account for variation within the group, usually estimated at 10% (i.e., coefficient of variation, or CV). If insufficient data are available to calculate an EAR, AI is used, based on observed intake consistent with good health. The UL is the maximum amount of a nutrient that can be ingested without posing a health threat and was included because so many nutrients are ingested at levels far exceeding those possible from the diet.

These guidelines account for group, and in some cases individual, variability, but they are not meant for use in patients with either acute or chronic diseases. Rather, they should be used as baseline estimates for planning individual nutrient intake. Such adjustments are particularly important in diseases characterized by malabsorption or catabolism, in contrast to simple lack of intake. Confirmation of sufficient nutrient provision can then be monitored by tests specific for each macro- or micronutrient.

MyPyramid is a food guide that incorporates recommendations from the 2005 *Dietary Guidelines for Americans* and is available on the US Department of Agriculture (USDA) website (www.mypyramid.gov). MyPyramid is part of an overall food guidance system designed to meet the need for a more individualized approach to improving diet and lifestyle. Five basic food groups are emphasized: grains, vegetables, fruits, low-fat milk and milk products, and meat and beans. The concept assumes that meals are built on a basis of grains, fruits, and vegetables, and supplemented with low-fat milk products and other protein sources in the meat group. MyPyramid comes with a warning to use fats and sweets sparingly and advocates a sensible balance between food and physical activity.

Glycemic index

The glycemic index of a food represents the relative increase in blood glucose that occurs over 2 h after consuming that food compared with either glucose or white bread [14]. Glycemic load is defined as the product of the glycemic index of a food and the amount of carbohydrate in a serving. Diets of foods with a low glycemic index and low glycemic load have been proposed to improve glycemic control in diabetes and to enhance weight loss in obesity. Glycemic control is better in subjects who have type 2 diabetes if a portion of carbohydrate intake is replaced by fat [15]. A study of

Table 29.5 Dietary reference intakes: recommended intakes for individuals

Life-stage group	Calcium (mg/day)	Phosphorus (mg/day)	Magnesium (mg/day)	Vitamin D (μg/day)[a,b]	Fluoride (mg/day)	Thiamin (mg/day)	Riboflavin (mg/day)	Niacin (mg/day)[c]	Vitamin B-6 (mg/day)	Folate (μg/day)[d]	Vitamin B-12 (μg/day)	Pantothenic acid (mg/day)
Infants												
0–6 months	210*	100*	30*	5*	0.01*	0.2*	0.3*	2*	0.1*	65*	0.4*	1.7*
7–12 months	270*	275*	75*	5*	0.5*	0.3*	0.4*	4*	0.3*	80*	0.5*	1.8*
Children												
1–3 years	500*	**460**	**80**	5*	0.7*	**0.5**	**0.5**	**6**	**0.5**	**150**	0.9	2*
4–8 years	800*	**500**	**130**	5*	1*	**0.6**	**0.6**	**8**	**0.6**	**200**	1.2	3*
Males												
9–13 years	1300*	**1250**	**240**	5*	2*	0.9	0.9	12	1.0	**300**	1.8	4*
14–18 years	1300*	**1250**	**410**	5*	3*	1.2	1.3	16	1.3	**400**	2.4	5*
19–30 years	1000*	**700**	**400**	5*	4*	1.2	1.3	16	1.3	**400**	2.4	5*
31–50 years	1000*	**700**	**420**	5*	4*	1.2	1.3	16	1.3	**400**	2.4	5*
51–70 years	1200*	**700**	**420**	10*	4*	1.2	1.3	16	1.7	**400**	2.4[g]	5*
> 70 years	1200*	**700**	**420**	15*	4*	1.2	1.3	16	1.7	**400**	2.4[g]	5*
Females												
9–13 years	1300*	**1250**	**240**	5*	2*	0.9	0.9	12	1.0	**300**	1.8	4*
14–18 years	1300*	**1250**	**360**	5*	3*	1.0	1.0	14	1.2	**400**[h]	2.4	5*
19–30 years	1000*	**700**	**310**	5*	3*	1.1	1.1	14	1.3	**400**[h]	2.4	5*
31–50 years	1000*	**700**	**320**	5*	3*	1.1	1.1	14	1.3	**400**[h]	2.4	5*
51–70 years	1200*	**700**	**320**	10*	3*	1.1	1.1	14	1.5	**400**	2.4[g]	5*
> 70 years	1200*	**700**	**320**	15*	3*	1.1	1.1	14	1.5	**400**	2.4[g]	5*
Pregnancy												
≤ 18 years	1300*	**1250**	**400**	5*	3*	1.4	1.4	18	1.9	**600**[i]	2.6	6*
19–30 years	1000*	**700**	**350**	5*	3*	1.4	1.4	18	1.9	**600**[i]	2.6	6*
31–50 years	1000*	**700**	**360**	5*	3*	1.4	1.4	18	1.9	**600**[i]	2.6	6*
Lactation												
≤ 18 years	1300*	**1250**	**360**	5*	3*	1.4	1.6	17	2.0	**500**	2.8	7*
19–30 years	1000*	**700**	**310**	5*	3*	1.4	1.6	17	2.0	**500**	2.8	7*
31–50 years	1000*	**700**	**320**	5*	3*	1.4	1.6	17	2.0	**500**	2.8	7*

This table presents Recommended Dietary Allowances (RDAs) in **bold type** and Adequate Intakes (AIs) in ordinary type followed by an asterisk (*). RDAs and AIs may both be used as goals for individual intake. RDAs are set to meet the needs of almost all (97%–98%) individuals in a group. For healthy breast-fed infants, the AI is the mean intake. The AI for other life-stage and gender groups is believed to cover the needs of all individuals in the group, but lack of data or uncertainty in the data prevent specification with confidence of either percentage of individuals covered by this intake.

a As cholecalciferol. 1 μg cholecalciferol = 40 IU vitamin D.

b In the absence of adequate exposure to sunlight.

c As niacin equivalents (NE). 1 mg of niacin = 60 mg tryptophan; 0–6 months = preformed niacin (not NE).

d As dietary folate equivalents (DFE). 1 DFE = 1 μg food folate = 0.6 μg folic acid from fortified food or as a supplement consumed with food = 0.5 μg of a supplement taken on an empty stomach.

e Although AIs have been set for choline, there are few data to assess whether a dietary supply of choline is needed at all stages of the life cycle, and it may be that the choline requirement can be met by endogenous synthesis at some of these stages.

overweight adolescents showed that altering dietary glycemic load by reducing both total carbohydrate content (45%–50% of energy intake) and consuming foods with a low glycemic index resulted in greater weight loss compared with a conventional low-fat (25%–30%) diet [16]. However, additional research is needed to clarify the long-term efficacy of diets with a low glycemic load for patients with diabetes or obesity.

Chemoprevention of gastrointestinal cancers

One of the special applications of dietary recommendations for healthy people is to prevent gastrointestinal cancers. The general recommendations for such diets are similar to those that support health in the entire population. However, it has been estimated that about one-third of all cancers are related to diet, and that most colorectal cancer in the United States

Table 29.5 continued

Biotin (µg/day)	Choline[e] (mg/day)	Vitamin C (mg/day)	Vitamin E[f] (mg/day)	Selenium (µg/day)	Vitamin A[i] (µg)	Vitamin K (µg/day)	Chromium (µg/day)	Copper (µg/day)	Iodine (µg/day)	Iron (mg/day)	Manganese (mg/day)	Molybdenum (µg/day)	Zinc (mg/day)
5*	125*	40*	4*	15*	400*	2.0*	0.2*	200*	110*	0.27*	0.003*	2*	2*
6*	150*	50*	5*	20*	500*	2.5*	5.5*	200*	130*	11	0.6*	3*	3
8*	200*	15	6	20	300	30*	11*	340	90	7	1.2*	17	3
12*	250*	25	7	30	400	55*	15*	440	90	10	1.5*	22	5
20*	375*	45	11	40	600	60*	25*	700	120	8	1.9*	34	8
25*	550*	75	15	55	900	75*	35*	890	150	11	2.2*	43	11
30*	550*	90	15	55	900	120*	35*	900	150	8	2.3*	45	11
30*	550*	90	15	55	900	120*	35*	900	150	8	2.3*	45	11
30*	550*	90	15	55	900	120*	30*	900	150	8	2.3*	45	11
30*	550*	90	15	55	900	120*	30*	900	150	8	2.3*	45	11
20*	375*	45	11	40	600	60*	21*	700	120	8	1.6*	34	8
25*	400*	65	15	55	700	75*	24*	890	150	15	1.6*	43	9
30*	425*	75	15	55	700	90*	25*	900	150	18	1.8*	45	8
30*	425*	75	15	55	700	90*	25*	900	150	18	1.8*	45	8
30*	425*	75	15	55	700	90*	20*	900	150	8	1.8*	45	8
30*	425*	75	15	55	700	90*	20*	900	150	8	1.8*	45	8
30*	450*	80	15	60	750	75*	29*	1000	220	27	2.0*	50	12
30*	450*	85	15	60	770	90*	30*	1000	220	27	2.0*	50	11
30*	450*	85	15	60	770	90*	30*	1000	220	27	2.0*	50	11
35*	550*	115	19	70	1200	75*	44*	1300	290	10	2.6*	50	13
35*	550*	120	19	70	1300	90*	45*	1300	290	9	2.6*	50	12
35*	550*	120	19	70	1300	90*	45*	1300	290	9	2.6	50	12

f As α-tocopherol. α-Tocopherol includes *RRR*-α-tocopherol, the only form of α-tocopherol that occurs naturally in foods, and the 2*R*-stereoisomeric forms of α-tocopherol (*RRR*-, *RSR*-, *RRS*-, and *RSS*-α-tocopherol) that occur in fortified foods and supplements. It does not include the 2*S*-stereoisomeric forms of α-tocopherol (*SRR*-, *SSR*-, *SRS*-, and *SSS*-α-tocopherol), also found in fortified foods and supplements.

g Because 10%–30% of older people may malabsorb foodbound vitamin B-12, it is advisable for those older than 50 years to meet their RDA mainly by consuming foods fortified with vitamin B-12 or a supplement containing vitamin B-12.

h In view of evidence linking folate intake with neural tube defects in the fetus, it is recommended that all women capable of becoming pregnant consume 400 µg from supplements or fortified foods in addition to food folate from a varied diet.

i It is assumed that women will continue consuming 400 µg from supplements or fortified food until their pregnancy is confirmed and they enter prenatal care, which ordinarily occurs after the end of the periconceptional period – the critical time for formation of the neural tube.

j As retinol activity equivalents (RE). 1 RE = 1 µg all-*trans*-retinal, 12 µg β-carotene, 24 µg α-carotene, or 24 µg β-cryptoxanthin.

Data are compiled from the Standing Committee on the Scientific Evaluation of Dietary Reference Intakes, Food and Nutrition Board, Institute of Medicine [9–11].

might be prevented by dietary alterations [17]. Although epidemiological data have suggested associations between overall diets or environment and the risk for cancer incidence or mortality, it has proved difficult to identify the dietary components that might influence such risks, and to demonstrate their benefit in a prospective fashion [18–20]. Table 29.6 summarizes many of the data associating risks for colorectal cancer with dietary components. Few of the reported associations have been convincing. When dietary components have been identified and tested prospectively, the data, in general, are negative, even when premalignant end points are examined, such as colorectal polyps [21].

Epidemiological evidence (case–control and cohort studies) has suggested that people with cancer have a lower intake of

Table 29.6 Epidemiological evidence on dietary factors and colorectal cancer risk

Factor	Correlational studies	Case control studies	Prospective studies
Dietary fiber	1	1	2
Vegetables	3	3	2
Fruits	3	2	1
Cholesterol	1	1	0
Red meat	2	2	1
Antioxidant vitamins	1	1	1
Folate	1	3	3
Alcohol	2	2	2
Calcium	2	2	1
Vitamin D	1	1	1
Selenium	1	1	1

3 = convincing, 2 = probable, 1 = possible, 0 = insufficient.
Adapted from Forman et al. [26].

raw, fresh, leafy green, or cruciferous vegetables, as well as raw or fresh fruits, especially citrus fruits, but a prospective analysis of 285 526 women showed no association between total or specific vegetable consumption and the risk of breast cancer [22]. Similar findings were noted in a prospective study of risk for colorectal cancer [23]. Although the ingestion of such foods has increased in the United States, the average intake is less than 0.7 servings of vegetables or fruits per day. Moreover, a large cohort study (Iowa Women's Health Study of more than 40 000 women) showed no protective effect of vegetables or fruits on colorectal carcinoma incidence, except for garlic [21]. The antioxidant vitamins A, C, and E are among those compounds thought to be responsible for the possible effects of vegetables and fruits on carcinogenesis. A meta-analysis of 14 randomized trials of antioxidant supplements found no evidence that these could prevent gastrointestinal cancer [24]. In fact, the supplements seemed to increase overall mortality, an effect that may be related to high-dose vitamin E supplementation [25]. Other studies have tested the addition of individual or combinations of vitamins (or β-carotene) on the incidence of colorectal adenoma formation, but have found little prophylactic efficacy [17,26]. Epidemiological studies have provided positive associations between current vitamin use and decreased cancer risk. However, the past use of supplements (including multivitamins) may modestly reduce the risk of colorectal cancer, and blunt the effects of added supplements in controlled trials [27].

The other dietary component that has been most extensively studied is fiber. Two extensive reviews have examined the descriptive and case control studies of the association of dietary fiber with colorectal cancer [28,29]. Most studies showed some inverse correlation, suggesting a protective effect of fiber. In the Health Professionals Follow-up Study involving men, a 64% reduction in cancer was noted in those with the highest quintile of fiber intake (> 28.3 g/day) compared with those on the lowest intake (< 16.6 g/day) [30]. Results from two large studies of women, the Nurses Health Study [31] and the Iowa Women's Study [32], showed no effect. However, two large prospective epidemiological studies reported protection against colorectal cancer [33] and colonic adenomas [34] in subjects with high fiber intake. Prospective studies suggest that an effect of fiber may occur only in men. Interventional studies using fiber supplements often yield inconclusive results [17,28,29].

The data regarding the effect of other dietary components on the incidence of colorectal cancer or adenomas are too fragmentary or incomplete to permit strong recommendations [17]. Some evidence suggests an effect of folate, and its role is being tested in interventional studies. Alcohol (> 30 g/day) may increase the incidence of adenomas in the distal colon and rectum. Although many case control and cohort studies suggested that calcium protected against the development of colorectal cancer, other studies with larger cohorts showed no effect. The role of vitamin C has not been confirmed [35]. The results of interventional studies are conflicting, and the end point used has been colonic cell proliferation, not adenoma or carcinoma incidence.

Although numerous studies examining the role of nutrition in prevention of gastrointestinal cancer exist, the interventional studies do not support specific dietary recommendations, as most of the data only demonstrate associations between diet and cancer prevention. However, intake levels of fruits, vegetables, fiber, and calcium as outlined in the Dietary Guidelines for Americans should be given specific dietary recommendations, as most of the data only demonstrate associations between diet and cancer prevention. Intake levels of fruits, vegetables, fiber, and calcium, as outlined in the Dietary Guidelines for Americans, should be recommended.

Energy metabolism

The human body continuously consumes energy for the maintenance of ionic and osmotic gradients, cell transport, nerve conduction, intermediary metabolism, biosynthesis, heat generation, and the performance of involuntary and voluntary mechanical work. Energy is provided largely by the mitochondrial production of high-energy phosphate bonds generated by the oxidation of fat, carbohydrate, and protein. After the hydrolysis of carbohydrates to simple sugars, fats to fatty acids and glycerol, and proteins to amino acids, most of these small molecules are converted to the acetyl unit of acetyl coenzyme A (CoA), generating a small amount of ATP in the process. Acetyl-CoA is a common breakdown product of the three macronutrients. Acetyl-CoA, carrying most of the chemical energy of the original macronutrients, enters the citric acid cycle and undergoes oxidative phosphorylation, the final common pathways in the oxidation of food molecules

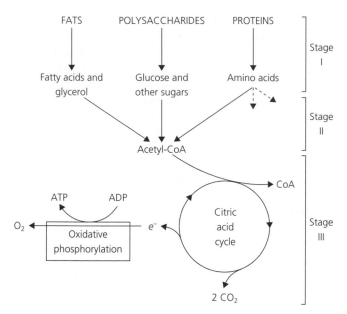

Figure 29.1 Stages in the extraction of energy from foodstuffs. CoA, coenzyme A. From Stryer L. Biochemistry, 3rd edn. New York: WH Freeman, 1988:325.

Table 29.7 Body energy stores

Tissue	Fuel	Energy
Adipose tissue	Triglyceride	585 000 kJ (140 000 kcal)
Muscle	Glycogen	8400 kJ (2000 kcal)
	Triglyceride	12 500 kJ (3000 kcal)
Liver	Glycogen	1250 kJ (300 kcal)
	Triglyceride	2100 kJ (500 kcal)

(Fig. 29.1). Many amino acids enter the citric acid cycle as α-ketoglutarate or oxaloacetate rather than as acetyl-CoA.

A portion of the energy released during substrate oxidation is not used to perform work and is dissipated as heat. Therefore, energy production is traditionally measured in terms of heat production. One kilocalorie (kcal), equal to 4.184 kilojoules (kJ), is the amount of heat required to raise the temperature of 1 kg of water by 1°C. Normally, body temperature is carefully maintained within narrow limits so that heat production equals heat loss. Energy production can be determined directly (direct calorimetry) by measuring the transfer of heat from the body to water circulating in specially designed chambers or suits. Energy production also can be measured indirectly (indirect calorimetry) by measuring carbon dioxide (CO_2) production and oxygen (O_2) consumption, because the amount of heat produced during substrate oxidation is proportional to the amount of CO_2 produced and O_2 consumed [36]. The relationship between CO_2 production and O_2 consumption can be used to estimate the relative oxidation of different substrates [37].

Dietary carbohydrates, fats, and proteins can be used as fuel soon after their ingestion, or they can be stored by the body for subsequent oxidation. Endogenous energy stores (Table 29.7), which are continuously being mobilized and oxidized, become a critical source of fuel during postabsorptive conditions and when energy intake is inadequate to meet energy demands. The largest source of endogenous energy is triglyceride in adipose tissue, which is uniquely designed to store fuel. Triglycerides have a high energy density and release 39.3 kJ/g (9.4 kcal/g) when oxidized. Adipose tissue is composed almost entirely of triglycerides in an oil form,

which constitute 85% of adipocyte weight. In comparison, glycogen, the other major source of endogenous fuel, generates only 17.2 kJ/g (4.1 kcal/g) on oxidation. Glycogen takes up a considerable amount of space because it is stored in liver and muscle tissue as a gel containing 2–4 g of water for every gram of glycogen [38]. The mobilization of adipose tissue yields 25–33 kJ/g (6–8 kcal/g), whereas the mobilization of glycogen yields only 4–8 kJ/g (1–2 kcal/g). The energy stored in the adipose tissue of a lean man can provide enough fuel for him to survive 2 months of total energy restriction [39], whereas the energy present as liver glycogen is consumed within 24 h of fasting. Certain cells and tissues, such as the brain, prefer glucose as a fuel, and others, such as bone marrow, erythrocytes, leukocytes, renal medulla, eye tissues, and peripheral nerve tissue, require glucose because they cannot oxidize fatty acids. None of the macronutrients is completely absorbed; some are excreted in the feces. Based on the average digestibility of fat (95%) and carbohydrate (97%), the digestible energy derived from fat is 37.6 kJ/g (9.0 kcal/g), and that from carbohydrate is 16.7 kJ/g (4.0 kcal/g).

Components of energy expenditure

Total energy requirements include the sum of *resting energy expenditure* (REE), the thermic effect of physical activity (TEPA), the thermic effect of feeding (TEF), and adaptive thermogenesis (AT). The resting energy expenditure is the energy consumed while lying quietly awake in the postabsorptive state. Normally, REE accounts for about 70% of total daily energy expenditure. Energy requirements of different tissues and organs are heterogeneous, however. Energy consumption by the body's most metabolically active organs – the brain, liver, kidney, and heart – accounts for 60% of REE; these constitute only 5% of total body mass (Table 29.8). By contrast, adipose tissue, which accounts for about 20% and 30% of body weight in lean men and women, respectively, consumes less than 5% of REE.

Across mammalian species, REE is related to body weight; REE is proportional to the three-fourths power of body weight (weight$^{0.75}$) [40]. Several equations have been used to estimate resting energy requirements in humans based on measurements of REE in healthy subjects (see Table 29.2) [41–44]. These equations generate values that are usually

Table 29.8 Postabsorptive energy requirements

Tissue	Mass		Energy expenditure	
	g	% Total	kJ/day (kcal/day)	% Total
Gut	2000	3	1250 (300)	13
Brain	1400	2	1675 (400)	18
Liver	1600	2.2	1840 (440)	19
Heart	300	0.4	985 (235)	10
Kidneys	300	0.5	835 (200)	10
Adipose tissue	14 000	20	290 (70)	4
Skeletal muscle	28 000	40	1675 (400)	18

within 10% of measured values in healthy volunteers but are less accurate in persons who are at the extremes of weight (i.e., extremely lean or obese) or who are ill. Starvation and severe hypocaloric feeding decrease the resting metabolic rate to values some 15%–20% below that expected for actual body size, whereas illness and injury can increase energy requirements.

Physical activity usually accounts for 15%–20% of total energy expenditure. The precise contribution of the TEPA to total energy expenditure depends on the intensity and duration of activities. At rest, skeletal muscle accounts for 20% of total energy requirements. However, during moderate- to high-intensity aerobic exercise, energy consumed by working muscles can increase more than 50-fold, causing a 15-fold increase in total energy expenditure.

The TEF represents the energy costs of digestion, absorption, transport, metabolism, and storage of nutrients, and it also may involve AT. Eating or infusing nutrients increases the metabolic rate by about 5%–10% of the ingested or infused calories and depends on the specific foods consumed. Normally, 12%–20% of the energy in ingested protein, 6%–12% of carbohydrate energy, and 2%–3% of fat energy is expended.

Adaptive thermogenesis is a proposed mechanism for wasting excess energy to maintain a constant body weight despite fluctuating amounts of energy intake, or for maintaining body heat during exposure to different environmental temperatures [45]. The concept of a "dual control" system for AT has been introduced [46]. In addition to a "rapid reaction" control system function as the attenuator of energy balance, under conditions of positive energy balance AT may be regarded as a "slow reaction" control system, functioning specifically as an accelerator for fat deposition [45]. It has been proposed that energy expenditure and heat production for AT and TEF involve brown adipose tissue, a specialized, highly vascularized, thermogenic tissue innervated by sympathetic nerves [47]. Brown adipose tissue is packed with large mitochondria possessing an uncoupling protein that uncouples ATP synthesis from respiration [48,49]. In this situation, the rate of substrate oxidization does not depend on the availability of ADP precursor, and the reaction can

continue at high rates, permitting even small quantities of brown adipose tissue to increase heat production markedly. Radioimmunoassays for the uncoupling protein have demonstrated the presence of brown adipose tissue in humans of all ages [49]; other studies suggest that uncoupling protein expression also can be induced in white adipose tissue [50]. The physiological importance of AT in energy metabolism in humans is not clear. In societies where food is plentiful and the level of daily physical activity is low, the variations in AT among individuals may be important in determining their trend toward weight maintenance or weight gain.

Proteins

Proteins are composed of amino acids joined together by peptide bonds. Twenty different amino acids are commonly found in human proteins. Differences in the sequences of amino acids in proteins permit diverse structures and functions; proteins serve as enzymes, carriers, receptors, hormones, and structural elements. The amino acid sequence determines the location of sites for covalent attachment of carbohydrate and ultimately determines the protein's three-dimensional configuration and specific function. Nitrogen also is present in the body in the form of free amino acids. Free amino acids are in a dynamic state, whether they are being incorporated into tissue proteins, undergoing catabolic reactions, or being used for the synthesis of other nitrogen-containing compounds [51].

Protein quality

Protein quality is related to the ability of the protein to support metabolic homeostasis and growth, which is determined by amino acid content and bioavailability. Some amino acids (histidine, isoleucine, leucine, lysine, methionine, phenylalanine, threonine, tryptophan, valine, and possibly arginine) are considered essential because their carbon skeletons cannot be synthesized by the body. These amino acids must be consumed in the diet for normal function and survival. Other amino acids (glycine, alanine, serine, cysteine, cystine, tyrosine, glutamine, glutamic acid, asparagine, and aspartic acid) are nonessential because their carbon skeletons can be produced endogenously. In general, the greater the ratio of essential to nonessential amino acids, the better the quality of protein.

The ability to digest protein and absorb its component amino acids also affects protein quality. True absorption ranges from 97%–99% for proteins in meat, milk, and eggs, to 75% for proteins in potatoes and navy beans [52,53]. Protein bioavailability also can be affected by food preparation. For example, some lysine is lost by heating in the presence of reducing sugars. By contrast, heating increases the bioavailability of soy protein by inactivating the trypsin inhibitor present in soybeans [54]. In general, the proteins of eggs, milk, fish, red meat, and poultry are high in biological value, and the protein in wheat gluten is low [52,53,55].

Nitrogen balance

Nitrogen balance is the difference between intake and output. Nitrogen is excreted primarily in the urine as urea, creatinine, porphyrins, ammonia, and uric acid. The relative proportions of these compounds can vary, but urea usually accounts for about 80% of urinary nitrogen. During fasting conditions, urinary nitrogen reaches a low level of about 2 mg/kcal of REE, or about 40 mg/kg of body weight. About 1–3 g of nitrogen is normally lost per day from fecal and other sources [13]. Fecal nitrogen losses reflect unabsorbed protein in the diet and in intestinal secretions and sloughed epithelial cells. The amount of endogenous protein that normally enters the intestinal lumen is about 50 g/day. Absorption of exogenous and endogenous protein is so efficient that fecal nitrogen is normally only 1–2 g/day. Minor amounts of nitrogen are lost through intact skin, nasal secretions, semen, menstrual fluid, and hair cuttings.

Nitrogen balance can be used to estimate protein balance because about 16% of protein consists of nitrogen, and it is assumed that almost all body nitrogen is incorporated into protein or amino acids. A positive balance (i.e., intake greater than losses) represents a net increase in total body protein, whereas a negative balance (i.e., losses greater than intake) demonstrates net protein catabolism. One gram of nitrogen represents about 6.25 g of protein, which is equivalent to 30 g of hydrated lean body mass.

Nitrogen balance is affected by protein intake and quality, energy intake, and nutritional status. Inadequate energy intake increases protein requirements. When protein intake is suboptimal, nitrogen balance can be improved by increasing energy intake. Therefore, nitrogen balance reflects both protein intake and energy balance. Most normal adults can maintain nitrogen equilibrium by ingesting 0.5 g of high-quality protein per kilogram of body weight per day. The range of recommended intake for adults is 0.5–0.8 g/kg/day [13,51,56,57], which provides a margin of safety to allow for decreased biological availability and increased requirements in subsets of the population. The average protein in a Western diet has only 75% of the biological value of egg protein [51,58]. Intravenously administered amino acids are as effective in promoting nitrogen balance as oral protein [59].

Infancy is a time of intense growth, and the protein requirements per unit of body weight for infants are higher than those for adults. The healthy infant also requires a higher proportion of essential to nonessential amino acids [60]. The growth spurt of adolescence, the only extrauterine period during which growth velocity increases, occurs between 10 and 13 years of age for US girls and between 12 and 15 years of age for US boys, and contributes about 15% of final adult height and 50% of adult weight [61]. The guidelines for protein and calorie needs in infancy, childhood, and adolescence are summarized in Table 29.9. The nutritional demands of a normal pregnancy average about 335 000 kJ (80 000 kcal) – that is, roughly 1250 kJ/day (300 kcal/day) – and 950 g of protein (i.e., 3.5 g/day). The Food and Nutrition Board of the Institute of Medicine has set the RDA for protein during pregnancy at 1.1 g/kg/day, an increase of 25 g/day over the RDA for nonpregnant women aged 25 years or older [13]. For lactating women over 25 years of age whose average daily output of milk is 850 mL, a protein intake of 1.3 g/kg/day, or 25 g/day of additional protein, is recommended by the Food and Nutrition Board [13].

Protein metabolism

Body proteins are in a state of constant flux, with protein synthesis and breakdown occurring simultaneously. Normal daily protein turnover is 1%–2% of total body protein and results largely from the degradation of muscle and hepatic proteins. Protein degradation involves the enzymatic hydrolysis of protein to its constituent amino acids. More than 75% of the amino acids released by protein breakdown are reused for the synthesis of new proteins; the remaining amino acids are oxidized. Proteases within cell lysosomes are responsible for most protein degradation [62–66]. However, proteases are also found in plasma membranes and in the cytosol. The carbon skeletons of amino acids can be oxidized for energy or used for the synthesis of glucose, ketone bodies, and fatty acids [2]. Nitrogen can be released as ammonia into the bloodstream and delivered to the liver, where it is converted to urea.

The metabolism of amino acids involves the transfer of nitrogen between organs from the periphery to the liver (Fig. 29.2). The liver is a workhorse for amino acid metabolism and is the site of synthesis for urea and plasma proteins. It is the main site of catabolism for the essential amino acids, with the exception of the branched-chain amino acids leucine, isoleucine, and valine, which are degraded in muscle and kidney.

Skeletal muscle preferentially takes up the branched-chain amino acids after each meal and is the primary site of metabolism for these amino acids. Although leucine, isoleucine, and valine constitute only 8% of dietary amino acids, they make up 60% of the amino acids in the systemic circulation [67,68]. When muscle proteins are catabolized, the branched-chain amino acids undergo transamination, yielding alanine, glutamine, and branched-chain keto acids. The keto acids are used by the muscle as fuel, and alanine and glutamine are exported and taken up predominantly by the liver and intestine, respectively [67]. These two amino acids account for more than 50% of the total amino acid nitrogen released from muscle [68–70]. The kidneys also take up glutamine, which is the major substrate for renal ammonia production [71].

Lipids

Lipids are a heterogeneous group of compounds that are soluble in organic solvents. Lipids include triglycerides (fat), sterols, glycolipids, phospholipids, and fat-soluble vitamins. These compounds serve as a source of energy, structural

Table 29.9 Dietary reference intake values for energy and protein in individuals by life-stage group

| Life-stage group | Energy EER[a], kJ/day (kcal/day) | | Protein[b] | | | | | |
| | M | F | AI or RDA (g/day) | | EAR (g/kg/day) | | RDA (g/kg/day) | |
			M	F	M	F	M	F
0–6 months	2385 (570)[c]	2218 (530)	9.1[k]	9.1				
7–12 months	3109 (743)[d]	2828 (676)	11	11	1.0	1.0	1.2	1.2
1–2 years	4376 (1046)[e]	4150 (992)						
1–3 years			13	13	0.87	0.87	1.05	1.05
3–8 years	7289 (1742)[f]	6870 (1642)						
4–8 years			19	19	0.76	0.76	0.95	0.95
9–13 years	9535 (2279)[g]	8665 (2071)	34	34	0.76	0.76	0.95	0.95
14–18 years	13 188 (3152)[h]	9908 (2368)	52	46	0.73	0.71	0.85	0.85
> 18 years	12 832 (3067)[i]	10 054 (2403)[j]	56	46	0.66	0.66	0.80	0.80

a Based on energy expenditure plus energy deposition for moderately active Americans and Canadians up to age 18, but only for energy expenditure < 18 years.
b Based on nitrogen equilibrium plus protein deposition, except for 0–6 years (average consumption of protein from human milk) and < 18 years (nitrogen equilibrium only).
c Total for a 3-month-old.
d Total for a 9-month-old.
e Total for a 24-month-old.
f Total for a 6-year-old.
g Total for an 11-year-old.
h Total for a 16-year-old.
i Total for a 19-year-old.
j For subjects older than 19 years subtract 42 kJ/day (10 kcal/day) for males and 29 kJ/day (7 kcal/day) for females.
k Based on AI only.
EER, estimated energy requirement; AI, adequate intake, the observed average or experimentally determined intake by a defined population or subgroup that appears to sustain a defined nutritional status. The AI is not equivalent to an RDA; EAR, estimated average requirement, the intake that meets the estimated nutrient need of half of the individuals in a group; RDA, recommended dietary allowance, the intake that meets the nutrient needs of almost all (97%–98%) individuals in a group. The EAR and RDA for protein for the first half of pregnancy are the same as those of a nonpregnant woman.
Adapted from Standing Committee on the Scientific Evaluation of Dietary Reference Intakes, Food and Nutrition Board, Institute of Medicine [13].

components of cell membranes, carriers of essential nutrients, and precursors for the synthesis of steroid hormones, prostaglandins, thromboxanes, and leukotrienes. Dietary lipids are composed mainly of triglycerides, which contain mostly saturated and unsaturated long-chain fatty acids with a 16- to 18-carbon chain length.

Lipid metabolism

The use of fat as a fuel requires the hydrolysis of triglyceride to free fatty acid and glycerol and the tissue uptake of free fatty acids for subsequent oxidation. Hormone-sensitive lipase within adipocytes hydrolyzes adipose tissue triglycerides and releases free fatty acids into the bloodstream, where they are bound to plasma proteins and delivered to other tissues. Lipoprotein lipase at the lumenal surface of the capillary endothelium hydrolyzes plasma triglycerides and releases free fatty acids for local tissue uptake. Fatty acids are transported across the cell membrane by passive diffusion, facilitated diffusion, and active transport. Membrane and cytosolic

fatty acid-binding proteins are important in transporting fatty acids across the cell membrane and in directing fatty acids from the cell membrane to different metabolic sites. This intracellular fatty acid transport system enhances fatty acid uptake by maintaining a fatty acid concentration gradient and prevents potentially toxic interactions between fatty acids and intracellular organelles. Long-chain fatty acids are delivered across the outer and inner mitochondrial membranes by a carnitine-dependent transport system. Inside the mitochondria, fatty acids are degraded by β-oxidation to acetyl-CoA, which enters the tricarboxylic acid cycle (see Fig. 29.2).

Ketone bodies are produced solely by the liver and are generated by the partial oxidation of fatty acids. Ketone body production increases when the rate of fatty acid production is much greater than the rate of fatty acid oxidation, such as during starvation or uncontrolled diabetes mellitus. In these conditions, ketone bodies become an important fuel and are released into the bloodstream for delivery to extrahepatic

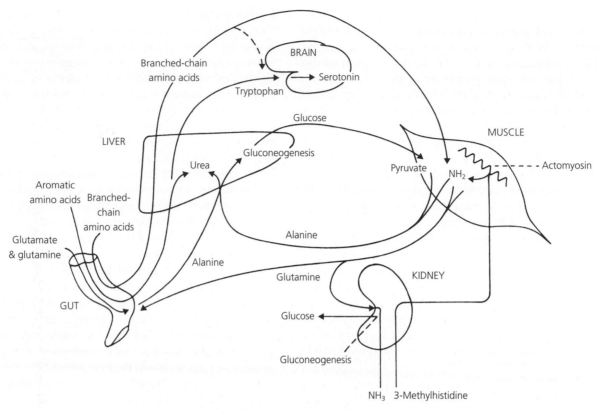

Figure 29.2 Interactions of organs in the metabolism of some major amino acids. Adapted from Munro HN. Interactions of the liver and muscle in the regulation of metabolism in response to nutritional and other factors. In: Arias IM, Popper H, Schachter D, et al. (eds). The Liver: Biology and Pathobiology. New York: Raven Press, 1982:681.

tissues. Ketone bodies represent a water-soluble fuel derived from water-insoluble fatty acids. Ketone bodies can cross the blood–brain barrier to replace glucose as the major fuel for the brain, sparing plasma glucose for consumption by other tissues [72].

The biosynthesis of fatty acids is mediated by fatty acid synthase, a multienzyme complex embodied in a single polypeptide chain. It elongates the molecule by sequential addition of two-carbon units and stops with the formation of palmitic acid, a 16-carbon fatty acid. The formation of malonyl-CoA from acetyl-CoA is the committed step in fatty acid biosynthesis and the most important step of regulation. The enzyme that catalyzes this step, acetyl-CoA carboxylase, is stimulated by citrate. Citrate is abundant when ATP and acetyl-CoA are abundant, a condition appropriate for fat synthesis. Palmitoyl-CoA, the end product of fatty acid synthesis, antagonizes the activation of acetyl-CoA carboxylase by citrate.

Essential fatty acids

Most fatty acids can be synthesized by the liver, but humans lack the desaturase enzyme needed to produce the n-3 double bond (between carbons 3 and 4, counted from the methyl end) and the n-6 double bond (between carbons 6 and 7) in the fatty acid series. Essential fatty acids are important constituents of cell membranes and precursors of the eicosanoids [73]. Arachidonic acid (C20:4, n-6), a precursor of eicosanoids, prostaglandins, leukotrienes, prostacyclins, and thromboxanes, is synthesized from linoleic acid [73,74]. Vegetable oils, such as corn, soybean, sunflower, peanut, and cottonseed oils, are rich sources of linoleic acid [73,74]. Linoleic acid (C18:2, n-6) should constitute at least 2%, and linolenic acid (C18:3, n-6, -9, -12) at least 0.5%, of the daily energy intake to prevent the occurrence of essential fatty acid deficiency, usually manifested as a specific alteration in the plasma fatty acid profile and a skin rash. An elevated ratio of triene to tetraene (> 0.4) is characteristic of essential fatty acid deficiency as a result of increased production of eicosatrienoic acid, a fatty acid containing three double bonds (i.e., triene) derived from oleic acid (C18:1), and of decreased arachidonic acid production, a tetraene derived from linoleic acid elongation [75,76]. Essential fatty acid deficiency is rare in adult humans because of sufficient essential fatty acids stored in adipose tissue. However, continuous infusion of lipid-free total parenteral nutrition (TPN) can cause abnormalities of the triene-to-tetraene ratio within 10 days because of increased plasma insulin concentrations, which inhibit lipolysis and the release of essential fatty acids [76].

Fish oils

Fish oils are ω-3 polyunsaturated fatty acids (PUFAs) found in marine animals, particularly fatty fish, such as herring, salmon, bluefish, and tuna [77,78]. Epidemiological studies suggest a possible protective effect of fish oils, especially eicosapentaenoic acid (EPA) and docosahexaenoic acid (DHA), against cardiovascular disease and breast cancer [79–82]. In sufficient doses, fish oil prolongs the bleeding time and decreases the production of the proaggregating substance thromboxane A$_2$ [83–86]. Animal models suggest that fish oils have an inhibitory effect on coronary atherosclerosis and intimal hyperplasia [77,83,84]. The significant hypotriglyceridemic effects of fish oils have been confirmed repeatedly in healthy persons and in persons with various degrees of hyperlipidemia [85–92]. In a study involving 11 323 patients with a recent myocardial infarction, a 45% reduction in sudden death was noted at 42 months. Interestingly, the reduction of sudden cardiac death started to be significant at 4 months. This suggests that the benefit of PUFAs may not be mediated only by antiatherosclerotic and antithrombotic effects, but may also involve antiarrhythmic effects [77,81,83,84]. The effects on serum cholesterol and low-density lipoprotein (LDL) levels have varied [77,92,93]. The ω-3 fatty acids generally suppress cellular inflammatory responses by changing the end products of eicosanoid synthesis [77,90,94–96]. Dietary supplementation with fish oil suppresses the production by monocytes of the polypeptide cytokines interleukin-1 (IL-1) and tumor necrosis factor (TNF), suggesting an additional mechanism by which fish oils may exert an antiinflammatory effect [94,97]. Successful outcomes of numerous randomized trials led the American Heart Association to release the following guidelines in 2002:

• all adults should eat fish, especially fatty fish, at least two times per week
• patients with documented coronary heart disease should consume about 1 g of EPA and DHA (combined) per day
• an EPA and DHA supplement may be beneficial for patients with hypertriglyceridemia [98].

Structured triglycerides

Structured triglycerides are lipids that have been chemically or enzymatically altered. They are used in nutritional admixtures and generally are prepared with reesterification of a long-chain fatty acid in the *sn*-2 position and medium-chain fatty acids in the *sn*-1 or -3 position of the glycerol molecule. Studies conducted in different animal models of burn injury, endotoxic shock, trauma, and ischemia/reperfusion injury have shown that the use of structured triglycerides improves protein and energy metabolism and increases intestinal absorption, compared with physical mixtures of long-chain and medium-chain fatty acids [99–105]. A study of patients with cancer of the upper gastrointestinal tract found that structured triglycerides reduce gastrointestinal complications and improve hepatic and renal function [106].

Carbohydrates

Carbohydrates, which constitute most of the earth's organic matter, are important sources of metabolic fuel. In the United States, carbohydrates normally account for about 50% of ingested calories; about 60% is complex carbohydrate, primarily starch, and most of the remainder is sucrose and lactose [107]. About 10–20 g of indigestible carbohydrate (i.e., soluble and insoluble fibers) are consumed daily. They all undergo hydrolysis in the colon to yield glucose, other simple sugars, and short-chain fatty acids. Some cells and tissues, such as erythrocytes, leukocytes, renal medulla, eye tissues, and peripheral nerve tissue, do not have the capacity for citric acid cycle activity and require glucose as a fuel for anaerobic glycolysis. The brain prefers glucose as a fuel. Daily glucose requirements include 40 g/day for anaerobic tissues and 140 g/day for the brain [108].

Absorbed glucose that is not directly oxidized can be stored as energy in the form of glycogen or fat, which requires about 5% and 25%, respectively, of the original substrate oxidative energy potential. Glycogen is a branching, long-chain polymer of glucose molecules that has water and electrolytes between the chains. It is found in most tissues but significant amounts are stored only in the liver and skeletal muscle. The primary function of hepatic glycogen, amounting to about 100 g in a healthy adult, is to maintain blood glucose levels. Plasma glucose is an essential fuel for glucose-dependent tissues. Glycogen in skeletal muscle serves to supply glucose to the muscle itself during physical activity.

Glycolysis

The conversion of glucose to pyruvate in the cytosol of cells is known as glycolysis, a process that results in the generation of ATP but does not require oxygen. Pyruvate represents a major metabolic junction; it can be reduced to lactate, transaminated to form alanine, or enter the mitochondria and undergo carboxylation to oxaloacetate or oxidative decarboxylation to acetyl-CoA (Fig. 29.3).

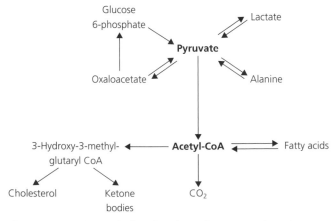

Figure 29.3 Major metabolic end products of pyruvate and acetyl-coenzyme A in mammals. From Stryer L. Biochemistry, 3rd edn. New York: WH Freeman, 1988:633.

Citric acid cycle and oxidative phosphorylation

The citric acid cycle (i.e., tricarboxylic acid cycle, or Krebs cycle) represents a series of reactions that occur in mitochondria. Carbohydrates, lipids, and amino acids enter the cycle after being metabolized to acetyl-CoA, and are completely oxidized to CO_2 and water. Vital biosynthetic intermediates are produced by the cycle, which plays a major role in gluconeogenesis, lipogenesis, and amino acid transamination and deamination. As acetyl-CoA is oxidized, reduced nicotinamide adenine dinucleotide (NADH) and reduced flavin adenine dinucleotide ($FADH_2$) are formed, which transfer the electrons to the respiratory chain in the inner mitochondrial membrane. In the mitochondria, the transfer of high-energy electrons from NADH or $FADH_2$ down the electron transport chain is coupled to the generation of ATP, a process known as *oxidative phosphorylation*. Glycolysis (i.e., anaerobic respiration) yields a net of only 2 ATPs per molecule of glucose, whereas aerobic metabolism (i.e., citric acid cycle and oxidative phosphorylation) yields 36 ATPs for each molecule of glucose oxidized.

Glucose production

Hepatic glycogenolysis is responsible for most of the glucose produced endogenously in the fed and postabsorptive states. Other mechanisms for glucose production are active and become critically important when hepatic glycogen is depleted, such as during prolonged starvation and endurance exercise. Gluconeogenesis is the process by which glucose is synthesized from noncarbohydrate precursors, lactate, glycerol, and most amino acids (principally alanine). Gluconeogenesis occurs primarily in the liver, but the kidneys also produce glucose, especially during prolonged fasting.

The Cori and glucose–alanine cycles provide mechanisms for generating plasma glucose for glucose-dependent tissues from 3-carbon intermediates released from peripheral tissues [109]. The *Cori cycle* (or lactic acid cycle) resynthesizes glucose that has been partially metabolized to lactate by peripheral tissues. Lactate produced principally by muscle, erythrocytes, and adipose tissue is transported to the liver and kidneys, where it is converted to glucose (gluconeogenesis) and released into the bloodstream. The *glucose–alanine cycle* shuttles glucose from the liver to muscle and alanine from muscle to liver. In this cycle, pyruvate is transaminated to alanine, which is transported to the liver and converted to glucose, which is then returned to muscle through the bloodstream.

Fiber

The accepted definition of dietary fiber is plant cell-wall components, both polysaccharides and noncarbohydrate components, that resist digestion by enzymes of the small intestine. The polysaccharide compounds in dietary fiber, which are the structural and matrix components of plant cell walls, consist primarily of cellulose, hemicelluloses, and pectins [110], as well as fructooligosaccharides and resistant starches.

Examples of foods with high cellulose content include wheat bran, apple and pear skin, and strawberries; foods with notable hemicellulose content include whole grains; and foods with high levels of pectins include bananas, apples, and oranges. Cellulose is a β1-4-linked polymer of glucose and the main structural component of plant cell walls. Hemicellulose consists of branched polymers of pentose and hexose sugars. Other noncellulose polysaccharides include pectins, which are complex mixtures of colloidal polysaccharides, and several polysaccharides not associated with the cell wall, including mucilages and gums. These compounds are branched polymers containing many uronic acids that hold water and form gels. They are highly branched in growing plants and become less branched as the support structure develops. They act as adhesives and are insoluble in the unripe fruit, becoming soluble only as the fruit matures. Undigested oligosaccharides, such as those associated with flatus (e.g., stachyose and raffinose), are soluble and not included in the definition of fiber.

Fructooligosaccharides are mixtures of β2-1-linked β-D-fructose monomers. These molecules include inulin-type fructans (linear polymers) and levans (branched fructans) and are present in many edible plants, such as wheat grains and members of the onion family. The daily consumption of oligofructoses by North American populations is estimated at 1–12 g, slightly more in Western Europe [111]. The β-C2 linkage makes these polymers resistant to hydrolysis by human digestive enzymes, and they are fermented and metabolized in the colon to short-chain fatty acids. This colonic fermentation produces a change in the microflora, enhancing bifidobacteria and decreasing *Bacteroides* organisms, clostridia, and other anaerobes. Fructooligosaccharides are the best studied of the prebiotics, defined as "a nondigestible food ingredient that beneficially affects the host by selectively stimulating the growth or the activity of one or a limited number of bacteria in the colon and thus improves host health" [112].

Resistant starches (RSs) are defined as starches that enter the colon: RS1 is physically inaccessible starch because of the particle size or entrapment in food; RS2 and RS3 are resistant to amylase action because of their compact (unbranched) structure, by being either unbranched (RS2) or made retrograde (RS3) – that is, altered during food processing [113]. Most resistant starches are produced during food preparation. Intake of such starches with a typical Western diet is estimated to be 5–10 g/day.

Other components of dietary fiber include polyphenols (especially flavonoids) and other cell wall-associated non-polysaccharide substances. Polyphenols are products of plant metabolism and range from single-ring phenols to highly polymerized compounds, such as tannins and lignins. Only lignins are included in the determination of dietary fiber, although they constitute about 12% of plant organic compounds. Lignins include a group of phenylpropane polymers of varying sizes, because they are continually polymerized as the plant ages. They reinforce the cellulose support structure and inhibit microbial cell wall digestion. Lignins are thus resistant to all anaerobic digestion systems and are not partially metabolized in the colon, as are the cell wall polysaccharides. They represent only a small part of the human diet (~ 0.2%).

Phenolic acids and aldehydes, such as vanillin, are common, but the most common of the plant phenolics are flavonoids, consisting of two aromatic rings linked through three carbons that form an oxygenated heterocyclic ring [114]. Flavonoids and other polyphenols are ubiquitous in plants and beverages. They contribute to the bitterness of tea and other beverages [9]. Polyphenols usually account for less than 1% of the dry matter of plants, but they can reach concentrations of 4000–7000 mg/mL in red wines and fruit juices [114]. The typical adult dietary intake of polyphenols in the United States is 1–1.1 g/day, with flavonoids accounting for about 4% of the total. Like other fiber components, polyphenols are degraded and their metabolites are absorbed in the colon, but the effect of these compounds on short-chain fatty acid production and microflora depends on the type of compound and the microorganisms present. Polyphenols bind proteins and precipitate them in the intestinal lumen, and they can decrease the absorption of nitrogen, fat, and some minerals, including iron.

Interest in polyphenols generally has focused on their antioxidant properties, particularly in relation to carcinogens and LDL oxidation. Some evidence suggests that moderate consumption of tea, a rich source of flavonoids, may protect against several forms of cancer, cardiovascular diseases, and kidney stone formation [115]. The blacker the tea, the more the polyphenols have been oxidized, lowering the possible effective role of these compounds. Herbal teas are not true teas (which derive from the shrub *Camellia sinensis*) and have a much lower flavonoid content. Tea contributes more than 60% of dietary flavonoids, onions about 13%, and grapes, apples, red wine, and dairy products most of the rest. The consumption of 1–2 cups of tea a day has been associated with health benefits in epidemiological studies [116], including 50% decreased mortality from stroke in men and 20%–40% decreased from cancer of the mouth, pancreas, colon, esophagus, skin, lung, prostate, and bladder. These data show only associations, not causation, and the results must be confirmed by prospective intervention studies. However, phenolics can, under some conditions, act as prooxidants [116], so the consumption of large amounts of phenolics as foods or supplements cannot be recommended until more data are available.

The heterogeneity of dietary fiber has inspired numerous classification schemes, including those based on source, chemistry, structure, water solubility, detergent solubility, physicochemical properties, and physiological actions. *Crude fiber* was a term commonly used until the early 1970s. It refers to the residue of plant material that remains when food is extracted by dilute acids and alkalis. Although crude fiber is the measurement still referred to in most food tables, it underestimates by 80%–90% the amount of material in foods that is undigestible by human digestive enzymes [13,117].

The physiological effects of dietary fiber on gastrointestinal function are complex because of their heterogeneity and the changes in the lumenal environment along the gastrointestinal tract. Combinations of fibers may have effects that differ from those of individual purified preparations, and the same purified fiber can have different effects depending on how finely or coarsely it is ground. The quantitative measurements of the fiber content of foods alone do not always allow prediction of their biological action.

Many physical properties of dietary fiber are physiologically important, including hydratability, viscosity, ion-exchange properties, and adsorptive capacity. Hydratability relates to the ability of a fiber to form viscous gels. It is a function of the physical and chemical composition of the fiber, including particle size, the age of the plant, and the chemical properties of the surrounding solvent. Some dietary fibers, such as lignins and pectins, have a significant capacity to bind and exchange ions, particularly calcium, iron, magnesium, zinc, and phosphorus, and to adsorb materials such as bile salts, proteins, and bacterial cells [13].

Fermentation of fiber by colonic bacteria generates volatile short-chain fatty acids, acetate, propionate, and butyrate, which serve as a systemic fuel and as the preferred energy substrate of colonocytes [118]. In general, water-insoluble fibers (e.g., wheat bran, bagasse) are less subject to fermentation and hold more water than do the water-soluble fibers (e.g., vegetable fiber, pectins, gums). Therefore, water-insoluble fibers have a greater effect on stool mass than water-soluble fibers. However, the ingestion of degradable fiber stimulates bacterial growth and generates a fecal mass composed largely of bacteria. Although the total number of bacteria can be affected by diet, there is no convincing evidence that dietary changes produce major changes in the composition of colonic microflora [119].

The rate of gastric emptying and the rate of digestion and absorption are influenced by fiber components. Guar gum and pectins increase the viscosity of the chyme and slow gastric emptying, but particulate fibers (e.g., wheat bran) appear to promote more rapid gastric emptying [117]. Fiber can decrease or increase mouth-to-anus transit time depending on fiber type, particle size, and bulk-forming capacity [120]. Intestinal transit time and stool bulk are inversely related. A large particle size (e.g., coarse wheat bran) produces a greater increase in stool bulk and a greater decrease in transit time than does a small particle size (e.g., finely ground bran). The mechanism by which fiber decreases colonic transit time is unknown but may be related to an increase in colonic peristalsis secondary to increased fecal mass [120].

If dietary fiber prevents colon carcinoma (see "Chemoprevention of gastrointestinal cancers" above), it might do so by several mechanisms: a decrease in colonic transit time, so that the time that colonic mucosa is exposed to carcinogens is shortened; adsorption of carcinogenic sterols or other carcinogens; dilution of potential carcinogens by increasing stool volume; and alteration of the relative number of anaerobic and aerobic bacteria in the colon [121]. The treatment of irritable bowel syndrome with a high-fiber diet (especially a diet that includes wheat bran and commercial fiber supplements) has produced conflicting results, but overall no benefit has yet been demonstrated [122]. Several studies have shown that bran and other fiber supplements are effective in preventing constipation, but the side effects include flatulence, distention, and bloating, perhaps related to a long colonic residence time and bacterial fermentation [123].

Fiber may prevent and treat hemorrhoids by decreasing straining during defecation. Straining causes engorgement of the vascular cushion lining the distal rectum and anal canal, making it more vulnerable to shearing stress. The passage of hard fecal masses through the anal canal exacerbates these shearing forces and displaces the vascular cushion caudally, where it may be trapped temporarily by contraction of the anal sphincter [124]. A trial of fiber is a reasonable initial therapeutic approach for many patients who have hemorrhoids.

Micronutrients: minerals and vitamins

The RDAs and AIs are based on the amount of a nutrient needed for an individual to avoid deficiency, or on the average daily amount that populations must consume to prevent deficiency (see Table 29.5). Statistically, the RDA is set as two standard deviations above the mean requirement, so that 97% of healthy persons are covered. The RDAs thus exceed the needs of many healthy persons. They are established only for healthy persons and were never intended as guidelines for therapy. For some nutrients (e.g., sodium, chloride, potassium), the evidence suggests that daily requirements are much lower than the content of the average diet in the United States. The Food and Nutrition Board has provided an estimated minimal requirement for these nutrients (Table 29.10). The RDIs and DRVs were established in 1993 for the purposes of food labeling and are derived from the 1989 RDAs for micronutrients [125]. What appears on food labels are neither DRVs nor RDIs but daily values, reflecting the recommendations for a 2000-calorie reference diet.

Minerals

Sodium [12]

Sodium, the principal cation in extracellular fluid, is necessary for maintenance of intravascular fluid volume and membrane potentials [125–127]. Total body sodium ranges from 48 to 60 mEq/g and is dependent on body size. The range for intake is 0.2–10.3 g/day. A 70-kg man has about 83–97 g of sodium in his body, about one-fourth of which is in the skeleton and cannot be exchanged. The kidney regulates sodium excretion by aldosterone action in the distal tubule in

Table 29.10 Adequate intakes for healthy persons for sodium, chloride, and potassium

Age	Sodium (mg/day)	Chloride (mg/day)	Potassium (mg/day)
0–6 months	0.12	0.18	0.4
7–12 months	0.37	0.57	0.7
1–3 years	1.0	1.5	3.0
4–8 years	1.2	1.9	3.8
9–12 years	1.5	2.3	4.5
19–50 years	1.5	2.3	4.7
50–70 years	1.3	2.0	4.7
> 70 years	1.2	1.8	4.7

The adequate intake (AI) does not allow for prolonged losses by vomiting, diarrhea, or excessive dieting. The AI is not equivalent to the recommended dietary allowance (RDA).

Adapted from Standing Committee on the Scientific Evaluation of Dietary Reference Intakes, Food and Nutrition Board, Institute of Medicine [12].

response to intravascular volume. Obligatory sodium losses are small compared with body stores. The minimum requirement to replace sweat, fecal, and urinary losses per day is about 0.18 g (8 mmol). Because almost all sodium is absorbed in the intestine, renal regulation of excessive sodium absorption is crucial.

Sodium is abundant in foods, not only as the chloride salt but as the bicarbonate, glutamate, phosphate, caseinate, benzoate, nitrate, propionate, sulfate, and citrate salts, among others. It is also present in many condiments, such as catsup, meat tenderizer, prepared mustards, olives, pickles, sauces, butter, margarine, and salad dressings. Water softeners can increase the content of sodium in water. Medications may contain sodium, although only a few contain enough to cause a problem.

Deficiency from inadequate intake alone is rarely encountered. Increased losses from the gut (e.g., vomiting, diarrhea, or drainage) or kidney (e.g., diuresis, salt-wasting renal disease, adrenal insufficiency) or excessive perspiration are the usual causes. Approximate mean concentrations of sodium in various fluids (in mmol/L) are sweat, 30–70; saliva, 10–20; gastric juice, 70; bile, 145; pancreatic juice, 130; jejunal secretion, 115; ileal secretion, 100; and normal stool, 5.

Potassium [12]

Potassium is the primary cation in intracellular fluid, in which its concentration is 140–160 mEq/L [12,126–128]. The 2% of total body potassium present in the extracellular fluid is important in influencing resting membrane function, particularly in the cardiac muscle. The kidney is the major site of potassium excretion, which is normally regulated not by filtered load but by the action of aldosterone and systemic pH in the distal tubule. It is absorbed efficiently in the upper intestine but secreted in the colon, another aldosterone-sensitive tissue. Colonic secretion is aided by the electronegativity of the lumen. As with sodium, the amount lost in the stool is volume dependent. Most adults consume between 2 and 3.5 g daily. Abundant food sources (i.e., > 200 mg per portion) include meats and fish, vegetables (especially potatoes), nuts, fruits, and milk. In unprocessed foods, the usual anions are organic (e.g., citrate), whereas in processed foods with added potassium, the anion usually is chloride. Most salt substitutes use potassium chloride to replace sodium chloride, and contain about 2000 mg potassium per teaspoon. Moderate potassium deficiency occurs usually without hypokalemia, and is characterized by increased blood pressure in response to salt intake, increased risk of kidney stones, and increases in bone turnover. Hyperkalemia causes cardiac arrhythmias, muscle weakness, and glucose intolerance.

Calcium [8]

Calcium is the most abundant cation in the body. About 99% resides in bone; the other 1% is a crucial mediator for neural transmission, myocardial function, excitation and contraction of muscle, coagulation, cell division, maintenance of intercellular tight junctions, and enzyme function [8,129–132]. Many factors affect the intestinal absorption of calcium: lumenal pH, lumenal binders, transit time, the presence in the diet of the few foods that are rich in calcium, and vitamin D status [8,131]. The process is inefficient in that only about 33% of the daily calcium requirement is absorbed by the intestine, in part due to an obligatory loss of calcium each day from the intestine and kidney. During periods of growth or new bone formation, the calcium requirement increases. The risk for a negative calcium balance is great, especially during childhood, adolescence, pregnancy, or lactation. The RDA for adults is 1000 mg/day (see Table 29.5), but typical diets in the United States provide only about 750 mg/day [8]. Unlike many of the other RDAs, these recommendations are meant not as nutrient requirements for individuals, but as an average requirement for nearly all healthy persons in a particular life-stage or gender group. The debate continues regarding the need for calcium guidelines based on the relationship between calcium intake and bone health [133]. The RDA was raised for adolescents to 1300 mg/day, based on increased bone growth during this life stage. The increased recommendation in older persons to 1200 mg/day is based on decreased calcium absorption in that group. Milk and dairy products are the richest source of calcium (providing about 60% of dietary calcium), and it is most bioavailable in those sources in the form of calcium citrate, but, there is little evidence for its superiority in promoting bone mineralization [134]. Each 225-g (8-oz) cup of milk contains about 280–300 mg of calcium. Green leafy vegetables are a good source, but the bioavailability is more irregular than that in milk products because the calcium is present as the phytate, oxalate, or other organic anion salt. These salts are poorly ionized and absorbed. The single universal requirement for calcium intake at each life-stage without reference to intake of protein, sodium, or phytate has been challenged, based on the observation that calcium intakes are low in parts of the world where fracture rates are low, but protein intake also is low, whereas phytate intake is high [135]. Other rich dietary sources are fish with edible bones, such as sardines and salmon.

Lumenal calcium is most actively transported in the duodenum, but in humans most calcium is absorbed in the ileum [129]. About 150–300 mg is secreted into the lumen each day. After glomerular filtration, about 98% of calcium is reabsorbed by the renal tubules [132]. Normal levels of serum calcium are tightly regulated by the action of parathyroid hormone and vitamin D and are not related to total body stores, except when deficiency is severe. Bone density is not a sensitive indicator of calcium deficiency, but it is a measure of body stores, and its determination can detect decreases in bone mass exceeding 1%–2% [136]. Ionized serum calcium is a measure of the hormonally regulated calcium concentration. Half of serum calcium is protein bound, 10% is complexed with anions, and 40% is ionized and physiologically active. Under most circumstances, ionized serum calcium reflects body stores, but when acutely altered, its concentration may be low in the presence of normal total body calcium [137].

Magnesium [8]

Magnesium is the second most abundant intracellular cation. About 70% of the total is in bone, and the rest is in soft tissues. Less than 1% is in extracellular fluids, where 20%–30% is bound to protein. Serum magnesium levels do not closely mimic body stores. The magnesium concentration in cells is high, like that of potassium, but magnesium leaves the cells less readily. Magnesium is important for neuromuscular transmission, and it is an essential cofactor in many enzyme reactions, including oxidative phosphorylation and nucleic acid synthesis. It also plays a role in wound healing, myocardial contractility, membrane stability, and coagulation [138–141].

The RDA averages about 350 mg (29 mEq) for adults: 400–420 mg for men and 310–320 mg for women. The typical adult diet in the United States provides 20–40 mEq/day. Food sources are well distributed, but nuts, cereals, seafood, meats, legumes, and green vegetables are rich food sources [138,139]. Like that of calcium, the intestinal absorption of magnesium is relatively inefficient (i.e., 30%–40%), and most absorption occurs in the ileum. However, magnesium differs from calcium in that there is little obligatory intestinal loss, so magnesium balance is maintained even with a low dietary intake if no abnormal losses occur. Loss from the body occurs in regulated function, mostly through the kidney (2%–3% of the filtered load) [138–141]. Serum magnesium is the standard for assessing body stores, but it is falsely elevated by hemolysis and does not always reflect either intracellular stores or active extracellular ionized magnesium [125,137].

Phosphorus [8]

Phosphorus is the major intracellular anion (100 mmol/L) [141–143]. It is essential for normal membrane function, regulation of enzyme systems, and generation and storage of energy. It affects the delivery of oxygen to tissue by regulating the concentration of 2,3-diphosphoglycerate in red blood cells. However, 80%–85% of total body phosphorus resides in bone.

The requirements for phosphorus parallel those of calcium. The new RDA is only 700 mg/day for adults, somewhat below the DRI for calcium, although daily intakes in the United States range from 1000 to 1500 mg. Like magnesium, urinary phosphorus excretion does not reflect a low dietary intake, so balance studies are misleading. Moreover, the efficiency of phosphorus absorption varies with the food source and the dietary calcium-to-phosphorus ratio. In general, if protein intake is adequate, so is phosphorus intake [8]. Phosphorus is a constituent of all cells and is abundant in most foods, especially meats, dairy products, and carbonated beverages. The amount of phosphorus in food additives is increasing, a change that can lead to decreased bone mass [144]. Phosphorus is a component of some gut lavage preparations (e.g., Fleet, Accu-Prep, Visicol, Fleet Phospho-soda). The absorption of phosphorus requires hydrolysis of the organic phosphates in food by intestinal alkaline phosphatase and is promoted by the action of 1,25-dihydroxyvitamin D-3. Five sodium-dependent phosphate cotransporters (NPT) have been identified [143]. It is the NPT2b form, expressed in the small intestine, that mediates phosphate absorption. Net absorption is 60%–80% of ingested phosphorus. The kidney adjusts phosphate excretion over a wide range, mostly using NPT2a but also NPT2c and NPT3, so deficiency from low intake or malabsorption is rare. In fact, reabsorption can increase to 99.8% if the dietary intake of phosphorus is low [141].

Iron [11]

The body stores of iron are not regulated by increased or decreased excretion, but rather by control of the rate of intestinal absorption, which is increased during deficiency. Daily losses normally occur from the gastrointestinal tract, skin, and urine. Fecal losses predominate, ranging from 6 to 16 mg/day, most of which is unabsorbed dietary iron. About 1 mg of endogenous iron is lost in the stool per day. Additional losses occur from the uterus in women, amounting to 0.5–1.0 mg/day averaged over a whole month. The requirements for iron per kilogram of body weight are highest during infancy (because of low body stores), periods of rapid growth (adolescence and pregnancy), and periods of excessive loss (menstruation).

The RDA assigned by the 2001 DRI Committee for all age groups of men and postmenopausal women is 8 mg/day; the RDA for premenopausal women is 18 mg/day [11]. The recommended intake during pregnancy is 27 mg/day. At birth, even the child of an iron-deficient mother has normal stores because the fetus has priority for available iron. Milk is a poor dietary source of iron, but the AI for infants aged 0–6 months has been set at 0.27 mg/day, based on the daily amount of iron in ingested milk (~ 0.35 mg/L). It is assumed that milk intake and requirements correlate with body size. Therefore, this AI may not be sufficient for infants with a lower milk intake. Three months after birth, the requirement for iron increases because of growth, and the RDA of 11 mg/day for infants aged 7–12 months assumes that feedings complementary to milk are in place. It is during this period that the infant is most at risk for iron deficiency. During adolescence, the hemoglobin level rises 0.5–1.0 mg/dL per year, requiring 50–100 mg of iron per year, and 300 mg during adolescence.

Food iron is available in a variety of red meats, nuts, seeds, and egg yolks. Milk products, potatoes, and fresh fruit are poor sources. Iron availability can vary by as much as 10-fold between meals with similar iron content [145]. Iron in vegetables varies according to growth conditions of the plant. Heme iron in vegetables is not so readily available for absorption as that in meat. Heme iron requires reduction to the ferrous state (by ascorbic acid) for maximal absorption. Heme iron accounts for less than 40% of dietary iron in the United States. The iron content of some foods (e.g., bread flour) is increased by fortification. Iron supplements can decrease absorption efficiency of dietary iron. Vegetarians are at risk for dietary iron deficiency because of the more limited absorption of nonheme iron. Iron is involved in many reactions as a cofactor for enzymes (heme or otherwise) and as a major constituent of heme as an oxygen-carrying cofactor.

Iron is absorbed primarily in the duodenum and upper jejunum. The absorption of inorganic iron is enhanced by gastric acid, ascorbic acid, and other organic acids, including the amino acids histidine, lysine, and cysteine, which form iron chelates [11,146]. Absorption is decreased when iron forms an insoluble complex in the lumen with dietary phytates or phosphates, or with antacids or other medications. In the duodenal lumen, dietary iron is reduced to the ferrous state by ferric reductase (Dcytb, duodenal cytochrome b), transported into the cell by the divalent metal transporter, DMT1, and released by way of ferroportin into the circulation [147]. Hephaestin is another protein that facilitates iron release from the enterocyte. Hepatocytes take up iron, either free or bound to transferrin (Tf), by Tf receptor 1 or 2. The TfR2 receptor is the major sensor of circulating Tf–iron complexes and influences the expression of hepcidin, the protein that downregulates ferroportin-mediated iron release from enterocytes, macrophages, and hepatocytes [148]. Hepcidin levels are inappropriately low in hereditary hemochromatosis, and are increased in patients with inflammatory conditions. Hepcidin appears to be the major gatekeeper for iron absorption. Normally about 10% of iron is absorbed, but in iron deficiency states this can increase to 30%. After absorption, iron is stored as ferritin in the liver, spleen, and bone marrow. The functional compartment of iron (hemoglobin, myoglobin) accounts for most of the total body iron, ranging from about 2180 to 2750 mg for the average woman and man, respectively.

Zinc [11]

The body contains 1.5–2.5 g of zinc, so that it is the second most abundant trace mineral after iron. Although the turnover of isotopic zinc in adults is 6 mg/day, balance studies show that 12.5 mg of dietary zinc is needed to maintain positive balance [11]. The daily loss of 2.5 mg/day is mostly in feces, and absorption ranges from 20% to 40% of dietary zinc, depending on the fiber content of the diet (inversely related). Zinc bioavailability from a vegetarian diet is moderate (30%–35% is absorbed) with phytate:zinc ratios of 5:15. More zinc may be needed in diets that are high in legumes, whole grains, seeds, and nuts, because in those diets the phytate:zinc ratio may approach 15. The 2001 DRI Committee report set the RDA at 9 and 8 mg/day for girls and boys aged 9 to 13 years, respectively, and at 8 and 11 mg/day for adult women and men, respectively [11]. The RDA for pregnancy is 13 mg for adolescents and 11 mg for women older than 18 years. During lactation, the RDA is increased by 1 mg/day.

Like other divalent cations, zinc is absorbed inefficiently along the entire length of the small intestine. A series of zinc transporters have been identified in humans. Zinc transporters have a binding domain that is rich in histidine residues. These transporters are thought to be important in absorption, and include: ZnT1, which is expressed in duodenal and jejunal villi; DCT1, which directs the influx of iron, zinc, copper, cadmium, and manganese; and ZnT1 and ZnT2, which mediate the efflux of the same minerals [149]. Zinc absorption is decreased by lumenal binders (phosphate and others), as is the absorption of calcium and magnesium [150]. Inorganic iron, especially when ingested as a supplement, impairs inorganic zinc absorption [151]. Absorption can be enhanced, however, by animal proteins and sulfur-containing amino acids, and by hydroxy acids [152]. Zinc absorption may be increased during states that increase demand for the mineral, including infancy, pregnancy, and lactation.

Zinc plays a critical role in the growth and function of cells. It is a cofactor for many enzymes that participate in the metabolism of carbohydrate, fat, and protein [11]. It is necessary for cell growth and proliferation, sexual maturation, reproduction, and dark adaptation and night vision, and it may play a role in wound healing and immune defenses. Finally, it may activate or inhibit enzymes, modify membrane functions, or bind to DNA transcription factors.

Copper [11]

Copper is an essential trace mineral for humans. Estimates of copper requirements are based on balance studies, fecal and other losses, and absorption at each life stage [11]. Obligatory losses for adults are about 580 µg/day, and absorption averages about 25% of dietary copper intake. Most absorbed copper is excreted in bile, although some biliary copper is reabsorbed by way of an enterohepatic circulation [153]. When intestinal and biliary losses occur, the copper requirement increases. The AI for infants is based on intake of milk (120 µg/L) and is set at 200 µg/day for infants aged 0–6 months and 220 µg/day for infants aged 7–12 months. The RDA is 900 µg/day for men and women aged 19 years or older [11].

The body contains about 100 mg of copper, 30 mg of which is bound to proteins and enzymes. The liver contains about one-third of the body stores of copper, mostly in enzymes, including ceruloplasmin, cytochrome oxidase, superoxide dismutase, tyrosinase, lysyl oxidase, and histaminase [154]. Copper is important for normal skeletal and nervous system development, erythropoiesis, leukopoiesis, and iron absorption, and as an antioxidant.

Copper absorption is efficient (35%–70%) compared with the absorption of other trace elements, but the efficiency is reduced in the elderly. Copper absorption and intracellular metabolism are complex processes [155]. A high-affinity copper transport protein, hCtr1, may transport copper across the apical enterocyte membrane by endocytosis. There is no free copper in the cell because it is bound to chaperones (e.g., to CCS, the chaperone for copper and zinc, and to metallothioneins 1 and 2) [155]. The Menkes disease protein, ATP7A, is a membrane-associated P-type ATPase that is required for copper secretion into the portal vein. Hephaestin is a multicopper oxidase that is a membrane-bound analogue of ceruloplasmin required for iron (but not copper) secretion from the intestine [156]. Absorbed copper is transferred in plasma to ceruloplasmin and albumin, and it is taken up by the liver by hCtr1-mediated transport. It is distributed to various cellular compartments by a series of small cytoplasmic copper chaperones [155]. In all tissues apart from the liver, ATP7A mediates copper efflux in the Golgi apparatus and subsequently in the plasma membrane, as the protein moves to the plasma membrane. In the liver, copper is guided to ATP7B, a copper-transporting ATPase, by the Wilson disease protein, ATOX1, a metal chaperone [157]. Copper is then bound to glutathione and metallothionein. The multicanalicular organic anion transporter, cMOAT, transports the copper–glutathione complexes into bile. When intracellular levels of copper increase, ATP7B is redistributed to exocytic vesicles for delivery to bile, similar to the process for the Menkes gene protein ATP7A in nonhepatic cells.

Other trace minerals

Selenium is essential to the antioxidant system, being a component of more than 20 selenoproteins, including six glutathione peroxidases [10,158]. Thus, its function is linked with that of vitamin E. Chromium potentiates the action of insulin at the cell receptor level and plays a role as a cofactor for insulin [159]. Manganese is a cofactor for many enzymes with widely varying functions, from superoxide dismutase to hydrolases and kinases, but a deficiency state in humans has not been identified [11]. Iodine is an essential component of the thyroid hormones and is thus integral to their function [11,125]. Iodine is transported by the sodium/glucose co-transport family solute carrier SLC5 [160]. Fluoride is concentrated in bones and teeth and is required for normal growth. The major source of fluoride is fluoridated water. Although deficiency of most of these minerals occurs in humans, the occurrence of such deficiency is unusual in developed countries. For this reason, they are used in clinical practice primarily as TPN supplements.

Vanadium, nickel, cobalt, tin, and silicon are considered essential in mammals because deficiencies have been produced experimentally, but human deficiencies have not been reported [11]. Other elements, including cadmium, lead, boron, aluminum, arsenic, mercury, strontium, and lithium, have not yet been proved essential. Most of these elements, with the exception of boron, are probably present in sufficient quantities as contaminants in TPN solutions [161].

Vitamins

Thiamin (vitamin B-1) [9]

Thiamin is essential for the function of many enzyme systems and plays a major role in energy production. Thiamin pyro-phosphate is a coenzyme in the oxidative decarboxylation of α-ketoacids to aldehydes, and it catalyzes transketolase activity in the pentose phosphate cycle. It is important for nucleotide synthesis and provides cofactors for fatty acid synthesis. Blood pyruvate levels increase with thiamin deficiency. The requirement usually is related to the intake of energy, especially carbohydrate. The RDA for adults is 0.5 mg thiamin for every 4184 kJ (1000 kcal) in the diet [9]. Allowances are based on the effects of varying dietary thiamin and the relationship with signs of clinical deficiency or with urinary excretion of thiamin or serum transketolase activity. Thiamin is synthesized by many plants. It is abundant in all foods and is added to many commercial baked products and cereals. Because thiamin is lost easily in the cooking and processing of food, its content in food varies according to preparation. Thiamin is transported into cells by the SLC19 folate/thiamin transporter family; specifically, the A2 and A3 types [162]. In polarized cells, such as enterocytes, thiamin is found at the apical and basolateral membranes (Table 29.11).

Riboflavin (vitamin B-2) [9]

Riboflavin is a major component of two essential coenzymes: flavin adenine dinucleotide (FAD) and flavin mononucleotide (FMN). It forms the active portion of these coenzymes, which are involved in biological oxidations. Riboflavin requirements

Table 29.11 Mechanisms of absorption of water-soluble vitamins

Vitamin	Source of ingested vitamin	Transporter	Extent documented	Intracellular regulation
Thiamin (B-1)	Diet, bacteria	Human thiamin transporters 1 and 2 SLC19A2 and SLC19A3 genes	Small bowel? colon, apical < basolateral	Ca^{2+}/calmodulin
Riboflavin (B-2)	Diet	Na-independent carrier-mediated	Small bowel, colonocytes	PKA, Ca^{2+}/calmodulin
Niacin (B-3)	Diet, metabolism (from tryptophan)	Na-independent, acid-dependent	Small bowel	Tyrosine kinase
Pyridoxine (B-6)	Diet	Na-independent		PKA-mediated
Biotin	Diet, bacteria	Na-dependent multivitamin transporter (SMVT)	Small bowel	PKC, Ca^{2+}/calmodulin, biotin (extracellular)
Pantothenic acid	Diet, bacteria	SMVT	Small bowel, colonocytes	
Folate	Diet, bacteria	Reduced folate carrier	Small bowel, pancreas, apical > basolateral	Tyrosine kinase, cAMP, pH-dependent
Cobalamin (B-12)	Diet	Cubilin–amnionless complex	Small bowel, proximal renal tubule, choroid plexus, apical	Development
Ascorbate (C)	Diet	Na-dependent vitamin C transporter SVCT1 (SLC23A1 gene), facilitated glucose transporters GLUT1, GLUT3, and GLUT4 for dehydro-L-ascorbate	Small bowel, apical SVCT2 basolateral	PKC-mediated Ascorbic acid (extracellular)

cAMP, cyclic adenosine monophosphate; PKA, protein kinase A; PKC, protein kinase C.

are linked with metabolic function, like those for thiamin. However, unlike the requirements for thiamin, those for riboflavin are unrelated to food energy intake. The RDA is set at 1.1 mg/day and 1.3 mg/day for adult women and men, respectively [9]. Requirements have been assessed by measuring urinary excretion and by observing signs of deficiency. Riboflavin is available in all leafy vegetables, in meats and fish, and in milk and eggs. The average Western diet contains about 2.7 mg/day. The vitamin can be lost during food processing and by the action of ultraviolet light. Absorption is efficient and occurs by an active carrier-mediated process in the small intestine. Riboflavin enters the plasma as free flavin mononucleotide (FMN) or riboflavin, and after dephosphorylation of flavin adenine dinucleotide (FAD) and FMN, is reformed into FAD and FMN inside the enterocyte. The vitamin is rephosphorylated to permit transport across the basolateral membrane, and is excreted from the kidney unmetabolized [163].

Niacin (vitamin B-3) [9]

The term "niacin" encompasses nicotinic acid and its amide form, nicotinamide. It is a component of two coenzymes, nicotinamide adenine dinucleotide (NAD) and nicotinamide adenine dinucleotide phosphate (NADP), which participate in more than 50 metabolic reactions. Humans can synthesize about 1 mg of niacin from 60 mg of the amino acid tryptophan. Deficiency depends on the limited availability of niacin and tryptophan [164]. The RDA is reported in niacin equivalents (NEs) (1 NE = 1 mg of niacin = 60 mg of tryptophan). The RDA has been estimated at 14 mg and 16 mg NE daily for women and men aged 14 years or older, respectively [9]. Average Western diets provide 16–24 NE/day. Nicotinic acid is present in most foods, except fats and oils. Meat, fish, and grain products are good dietary sources. Much is lost during grain processing, but it is added as fortification to the finished products. Niacin is well absorbed in the small intestine by a sodium-independent, acid-sensitive process.

Pyridoxine (vitamin B-6) [9]

The term "vitamin B-6" refers to three naturally occurring pyridines: pyridoxine, pyridoxal, and pyridoxamine. All forms function similarly. Vitamin B-6 is essential for the function of many aminotransferases and amino acid decarboxylases. It is involved in the metabolism of all amino acids and in the synthesis of acetylcholine, porphyrin, arachidonic acid, dopamine, serotonin, and bile acids. Requirements are increased with a higher protein intake. The RDA for adults aged 19–50 years is 1.3 mg/day for average protein intake. Low levels of all three forms are present in all foods, with meats, fish, and grains being good sources. The vitamin B-6 allowance has been estimated by using a ratio of 0.016 mg of vitamin per gram of protein ingested. Because energy and protein intakes are lower in the older population, RDAs are increased for persons older than 50 years, and the estimates for women

(i.e., 1.5 mg/day) are lower than those for men (i.e., 1.7 mg/day) [9]. Vitamin B-6 is synthesized by microorganisms in the intestine, primarily in the colon, where the vitamin is not absorbed. Vitamin B-6 is rapidly absorbed in the small intestine by a sodium-independent transporter, and is excreted in the urine as the metabolized product, 4-pyridoxic acid. Certain drugs are pyridoxine antagonists (e.g., isoniazid, hydralazine, penicillamine). A deficiency of vitamin B-6 and other B vitamins can occur in chronic alcoholics.

Folate (folacin, folic acid) [9]

"Folacin" is a generic term for compounds that have a structure and function similar to that of folic acid, that is, pteroylglutamic acid (PGA). The many forms differ in the degree of reduction of the double bonds in the ring structure (e.g., tetrahydrofolate), the presence of 1-carbon groups (e.g., methyltetrahydrofolate), and the number of glutamyl residues in the peptide chain (e.g., folate pentaglutamate). Folate functions as a carrier of 1-carbon groups from donor to recipient molecules and is necessary for the synthesis of nucleic acids, the initiation of protein synthesis, and the synthesis of acetylcholine and methionine. Three other vitamins – cobalamin, ascorbic acid, and niacin – are involved in converting folate to its active coenzyme forms [9,165]. Pteroylglutamic acid is the form of folate used commercially, and it is a relatively poor substrate for dihydrofolate reductase. As a result, tissue utilization is poorer for PGA than for natural methylated or reduced folates found in food. However, folate requirements have been based on replacement with PGA.

The RDA for folate has been modified dramatically from the 1989 estimate of 200 μg/day for adults to 400 μg [9]. This change was the result of recognition of the role of folate in reducing the incidence of neural defects [166], and the role of elevated serum homocysteine concentrations as a cardiovascular risk factor [167]. Dietary folate is reported in folate equivalents, in recognition of the greater bioavailability of synthetic folic acid compared with natural folate. The RDA for women aged 14–50 years is 400 μg/day, and should comprise synthetic folic acid plus dietary folate. During pregnancy, the amount of synthetic folic acid is specified at 400 μg/day [9].

The vitamin is abundant in citrus juices, enriched cereals and breads, legumes, liver, nuts, and green leafy vegetables. To prevent neural defects, the US Food and Drug Administration (FDA) has, since 1998, required that all cereal grains are fortified with 140 μg of folate/100 g of grain [168]. It is estimated that this supplements the average daily dietary intake (50–500 μg) by 215–240 μg, and the incidence of neural defects has decreased by about 25%. Folate occurs in food largely in the polyglutamate form, and its bioavailability generally is high. However, boiling, steaming, or frying can lead to significant losses. Folate is absorbed in the proximal small intestine through active transport mediated by the reduced folate carrier, the apical SLC19A1 sodium/folate cotransporter [162]. It is converted in the liver and other tissues to the

5-methyltetrahydrofolate form and is stored as polyglutamate [169]. Total body stores are relatively small and can be depleted in a few months if dietary intake is negligible. Folate can enter the serum or the bile and be reabsorbed, undergoing an enterohepatic circulation amounting to about 100 μg/day. In diseases that cause malabsorption, body stores of folate are lost more rapidly than in simple dietary deficiency.

Cobalamin (vitamin B-12) [9]

Cobalamin contains a cobalt atom to which are bound active groups, including hydroxy-, methyl, and nitro- moieties. The vitamin functions as a carrier for methyl and hydrogen groups. It is required for reactions catalyzed by two enzymes, methionine synthase and methylmalonic acid mutase, and thus participates in methionine and succinyl-CoA synthesis. The total body content of cobalamin is 2–2.5 mg, most of which is in the liver, and the half-life is 1.5–3.5 years. Thus, daily losses average about 1.3 μg/day. The RDA was set at 2 μg/day for adults, based on 70% absorption efficiency [9]. However, because 10%–30% of adults older than 51 years may have protein-bound cobalamin malabsorption, the new RDA has been set at 2.4 μg/day [9]. Although this malabsorption probably is caused by reduced pepsin and gastric acid secretion, most elderly persons have some intrinsic factor. Thus, it is recommended by some experts that most intake in older persons be in the form of a dietary supplement, to ensure its adequacy [170]. The vitamin is synthesized only by bacteria and enters animal tissues after the ingestion of contaminated foods or production in the gut lumen. It is found only in animal products, including meat, fish, eggs, and milk. The average Western diet contains 5–15 μg/day. Cobalamin is relatively stable during cooking and processing.

The absorption of cobalamin is complex [171]. In food, it is bound to enzymes from which it is released by gastric proteases. It is bound to haptocorrin in the stomach, released from haptocorrin by the action of pancreatic enzymes, and then bound to intrinsic factor, with which it is absorbed in the ileum by the process of receptor-mediated endocytosis. The receptor for the intrinsic factor–cobalamin complex, cubilin, is a large, multifunctional protein that also binds apolipoproteins [172]. Studies of the mutations in Imerslund–Grasbeck syndrome (congenital vitamin B-12 malabsorption) have uncovered a 45–50-kDa transmembrane protein that colocalizes with cubilin, called amnionless (AMN) [173]. The amino-terminal portion of AMN directs endocytosis, and is essential for cobalamin absorption, whereas the carboxy terminal is necessary for embryonic development. In the enterocyte, the vitamin is released from intrinsic factor, bound to transcobalamin II, and delivered to the tissues complexed to that protein. It is released into the bile bound again to haptocorrin, and 5–10 μg/day undergoes an enterohepatic circulation. As with folate, body stores are lost more rapidly if malabsorption is present because endogenous as well as dietary cobalamin is lost.

Ascorbic acid (vitamin C) [10]

Ascorbic acid is an essential cofactor for several hydroxylation reactions and plays a key role in the synthesis of collagen. It may also function as an antioxidant for vitamins A and E, and is involved in the formation of norepinephrine (noradrenaline) and serotonin. This role in neurotransmitter synthesis may explain the fatigue and weakness seen in scurvy [174]. A daily intake of 10 mg of ascorbic acid cures clinical signs of scurvy but does not maintain body stores. The previous RDA of 60 mg/day produced wide fluctuations in plasma levels. The ascorbic acid requirement is also compounded by its possible chemoprotective value in some disorders (e.g., colon cancer, heart diseases, cataracts), at doses far in excess of those needed to prevent scurvy. Intake of 200 mg of ascorbic acid per day is needed to begin to saturate tissues, an intake that approximates the vitamin C content of diets (~ 225 mg/day) that allow maximal protective effects of the vitamin [175]. The new DRI values represent a compromise between the old RDA value and those needed for chemoprevention, and are set at 75 mg/day and 90 mg/day for adult women and men, respectively [10]. During pregnancy and lactation, the RDA should be increased by 10 mg/day and 45 mg/day, respectively. The vitamin is especially concentrated in green vegetables and citrus fruits, although it is widespread in foods. The vitamin C content of food depends on the state of ripeness and on the method of preparation because ascorbic acid is sensitive to heating and oxidation. It is well absorbed in the small intestine by two sodium-dependent cotransporters (SVCT1 and SVCT2) at intakes of up to 180 mg/day [176]. Over that amount, the proportion appearing in the stool increases, and at high doses (> 3–4 g/day), diarrhea can result.

Biotin [9]

Biotin is a coenzyme for various carboxylases and is important in the metabolism of carbohydrate, protein, and fat [177]. It is produced by colonic bacteria and absorbed in the small bowel and colon by facilitated diffusion. Because of this endogenous production, an RDA has not been determined, but the AI for adults has been estimated at a DRI of 30 μg/day [9]. Absorption of the vitamin is mediated by a sodium-dependent multivitamin transporter (SMVT) [178].

Pantothenic acid [9]

Pantothenic acid is a precursor of CoA, which is essential for the metabolism of fats, carbohydrates, and proteins and for the synthesis of steroids and porphyrins [9,179]. It is widely distributed in foods, especially animal tissues, whole-grain cereals, and legumes. Microflora may produce some pantothenic acid, but the data in humans are not clear. Although an RDA has not been established, the estimated AI for older adolescents and for adults is 5 mg/day. Pantothenic acid is well absorbed in the intestine by means of SMVT, and is excreted unchanged in the urine.

Vitamin A [11]

Vitamin A is the collective term for vitamin A alcohol (retinol) and its related biologically active forms. It is essential for growth and development, the maintenance of epithelial cells, the stability of cell membranes, reproduction, and vision in dim light [11,180]. The β-carotenes are precursors of vitamin A and appear to have additional beneficial functions, probably as antioxidants [181]. The DRI allowance for vitamin A is based on many nutritional studies and amounts to 900 µg of retinol per day for men and 700 µg/day for women [11]. The recommendations for β-carotene are even more complex because no reproducible biological activities are available to establish adequate intake. Some epidemiological studies show correlations between low serum levels (still in the normal range) and protection from cancer, but intervention studies have not been positive [182]. Moreover, some carotenoids (e.g., lutein) are accumulated in the retina preferentially, whereas others (e.g., lycopene) lack provitamin A function but exhibit other biological activity. The data were judged by the DRI Committee to be insufficient to make a recommendation on the required percentage of dietary vitamin A that must be derived from provitamin A carotenoids [11].

Vitamin A synthesis is limited to plants and microorganisms. Its activity in foods usually is expressed in international units (IUs) and an equivalent value established with retinol activity, accounting for both vitamin A and provitamin compounds in the diet. The previously accepted 6:1 equivalence of β-carotene to vitamin A has been questioned because of the inefficient bioconversion of plant carotenoids. Thus, the new conversions are 1 retinol equivalent (RE) = 1 µg of all-*trans*-retinal, or 12 µg of β-carotene, or 24 µg of mixed carotenes. One RE is also equivalent to 3.3 IU of retinol activity or 10 IU of β-carotene activity. This means that older food tables have overestimated the vitamin A activity in foods. This change may be of special importance in less-developed countries that rely mostly on vegetable products for their vitamin A. Animal products are rich sources, including liver, kidney, dairy products, and eggs. Carotenoids, especially β-carotene, are found in green and yellow vegetables. There are more than 400 carotenoids in foods, only about 60 of which have provitamin A activity. In the United States, dairy products and margarines are supplemented with retinyl esters, and these products are the major dietary source of the vitamin.

Vitamin A, ingested in the form of long-chain retinyl esters, is hydrolyzed to retinol by lipases and esterases in bile and pancreatic secretions or in milk. More than 80% of the vitamin is absorbed passively by an as yet unknown mechanism, reincorporated into retinyl esters, packaged into chylomicrons, transported in the lymphatic circulation, and stored in the liver, which controls release of the vitamin [11,183]. Carotene is absorbed passively, but less well than vitamin A (40%–60%). Most is hydrolyzed to retinol inside the enterocyte, and a small amount is absorbed intact. After vitamin A is released from the liver, it is transported in the plasma as a trimolecular complex with retinol-binding protein and transthyretin [183]. If stores are adequate, any excess vitamin A is excreted in bile. A small amount is excreted in urine along with other metabolites. About 10% of hepatic retinol is converted to retinoic acid, which in turn is conjugated with glucuronide and undergoes enterohepatic circulation. As in the case of folate, cobalamin, and 1,25-dihydroxyvitamin D, this enterohepatic circulation leads to the loss of endogenous as well as dietary vitamin A if malabsorption occurs.

Vitamin D [8]

Vitamin D is the designation for a group of sterols and their metabolites that have antirachitic activity [8]. Cholecalciferol (vitamin D-3) is formed in the skin from 7-dehydrocholesterol by the action of ultraviolet light, and about 100 IU/day (10 µg = 400 IU) is produced in persons living in the temperate zone [184]. Ergocalciferol (vitamin D-2) is present in plants. Vitamin D is a provitamin, with the active metabolite being 1,25-dihydroxyvitamin D. The active vitamin promotes the intestinal absorption of calcium and phosphorus, in conjunction with parathyroid hormone. The vitamin is necessary for normal bone formation and regulates calcium and phosphorus metabolism in bone and kidney [185]. Vitamin D may play an important role in the prevention of chronic diseases other than osteoporosis, such as cancer and diabetes [184], but more studies will be needed before it is known if providing additional vitamin D will alter the outcomes in these diseases.

A major problem in determining an estimated average requirement (EAR) for vitamin D is that the indicator for adequacy is not clear (Table 29.12) [186]. The potential indicators to identify insufficiency reflect the multiple actions of vitamin D. Because more than 90% of circulating 25-hydroxyvitamin D-3 is derived from skin and is endogenously produced, daily requirements have not been established [186]. The DRIs are based on AIs. Because vitamin D deficiency is more prevalent in older adults, the recommended AI for adults older than 50 years is twice that of younger adults (10 vs 5 µg/day, or 400 vs 200 IU), and for adults older than 70 years it is tripled (15 µg/day) [8]. However, some experts feel that the AI should be as high as 800 µg/day, based on the amount needed to achieve levels of 25(OH)$_2$-vitamin D sufficient to suppress parathormone levels [184].

Vitamin D occurs naturally in foods of animal origin, such as fish-liver oils, eggs, liver, and dairy products. Fortified foods supply the major dietary sources, although most vitamin D is made endogenously. Vitamin D is absorbed in the small intestine along with other lipids, but it requires bile salt micelle formation for efficient absorption. It is transported in the lymph with chylomicrons and other lipoproteins. The serum content of vitamin D is not limited by the content of the specific vitamin D-binding protein, and the ingestion of excessive doses can produce toxic levels of vitamin D or its metabolites in the serum. Vitamin D is stored in fat depots

Table 29.12 Potential candidates for functions/indicators of vitamin D sufficiency

Indicator	Vitamin D effect on function	Indicator of insufficiency
Serum (s) Ca^{2+}, P	Normal serum levels maintained	↓ [Ca]s, ↓ [P]s
Calcium absorption	Optimizes absorption	↓ % absorption of Ca^{2+}
Parathyroid hormone (PTH)	Active transport of Ca^{2+}, restores [PTH]s	↑ [PTH]s
Fracture risk	↓ PTH levels to normal, ↓ bone turnover	↑ Risk related to D status
Muscle strength	Active transport of PO$_4$, ↓ PTH, restores intracellular [PO$_4$]	↓ Muscle strength
Bone turnover	Normalizes turnover	↓ Turnover, ↑ resorption
Immunomodulation	Maturation of antigen-presenting cells	↑ T-cell proliferation, ↓ killer cells
Cell proliferation	↓ Proliferation	More cells in G1 vs G2 phase

(e.g., liver, adipose tissue) and muscle, and it is released slowly. The 25-hydroxyl group is added in the liver, and the 1-hydroxyl group in the kidney. 1,25-Dihydroxyvitamin D and other polar metabolites are excreted in the bile and undergo an enterohepatic circulation. Malabsorption disorders produce earlier deficiency because endogenous as well as exogenous vitamin is lost. Small amounts of the vitamin are excreted in the urine.

Vitamin E [10]

The term "vitamin E" refers to two groups of lipid-soluble compounds, tocopherols and tocotrienols, that are found in plants. α-Tocopherol is the most active and abundant of these compounds. These compounds function as fat-soluble antioxidants and free-radical scavengers, in conjunction with the selenium–glutathione peroxidase system. The natural form is complex, covering eight different structures produced by plants (tocopherols α, β, γ, and δ, plus corresponding tocotrienols) [187]. Tocopherols contain a phytyl tail with three places that could be in either L- or R- configuration. Commercial vitamin E is a mixture of tocopherols and tocotrienols. α-Tocopherol is all *RRR*-α-tocopherol. The bioavailability of these forms varies, but the capsule form of vitamin E may be relatively less readily available [188]. The RDA previously was based on the assumptions that the diet had no more than 0.1 ppm of selenium, average amounts of sulfur amino acids, a ratio of vitamin E to PUFAs of 0.4, and less than 1.5% linoleic acid in a diet containing 7500–12 500 kJ (1800–3000 kcal). Later recommendations also consider the possible role of vitamin E as an antioxidant in preventing disease, the increased intake of PUFAs in the United States, and the serum vitamin E values from NHANES III (Third National Health and Nutrition Examination Survey, 1998–1994) [10]. Thus, the new DRIs are set about 50% higher than the 1989 levels (15 mg/day for adults). The vitamin is abundant in the lipids of green leafy plants, in vegetable oils, and in seeds. Foods high in PUFAs also are excellent sources of vitamin E [10,187].

Vitamin E is absorbed passively from the small intestine with other lipids, and its absorption, like that of other fat-soluble vitamins, requires bile salt micelles. Only about 40% of an oral dose is absorbed. The natural form is an acetate ester; bile salt-dependent pancreatic esterase also is required for absorption. There is no specific serum carrier for vitamin E. Because it is bound to LDL and other lipoproteins, serum levels are proportional to total lipids. The vitamin is delivered to the liver after the action of lipoprotein lipase, and from the liver it is delivered in lipoproteins to adipose tissue, where it is stored. Tocopherol-associated proteins (TAPs) may be important in lipoprotein transfer. α-Tocopherol transfer protein (TTP) activity is mediated by the ABCA1 transporter. Both TTP and TAP belong to a family of hydrophobic ligand-binding proteins with a *cis*-retinal-binding motif sequence (CPAR-TRIO) shared with cellular retinol-binding protein, but the mechanism of hepatic secretion of vitamin E is unclear [189]. Excess vitamin E is excreted in bile or metabolized by β- or ω-oxidation by cytochrome P450-dependent hydroxylases [190]. Vitamin E destroys tissue peroxides that promote the oxidation of LDL [189] and prevents platelet adhesion by an antioxidant-independent mechanism [191]. These effects are the basis for the potential effect of the vitamin in preventing ischemic damage.

Vitamin K [11]

The term "vitamin K" designates naphthoquinone compounds with antihemorrhagic activity. They are crucial for the production of plasma clotting factors II (prothrombin), VII, IX, and X. Two forms occur naturally: vitamin K-1 (phylloquinones) in green plants and vitamin K-2 (menaquinones) in bacteria. Colonic bacterial synthesis provides an estimated 2 μg/kg of body weight, and absorption of that source presumably occurs by backwash into the terminal ileum. The RDAs of 1989 were based on the function of the vitamin for clotting proteins, but the requirement may be greater for the nonhepatic vitamin K-dependent proteins, especially those in bone [192]. Because of the lack of data on which to estimate an average requirement, the DRIs are based on AIs, set at 90 μg/day and 120 μg/day for adult women and men, respectively [11]. Therapeutic sources of vitamin K are synthetic compounds. Vitamin K (150 μg/day) is included in the new FDA recommended guidelines for adult parenteral multivitamins [193]. The best food sources are green leafy vegetables, and they are considered to be the major source of the vitamin despite some endogenous production.

Vitamin K is passively absorbed in the small intestine, a process that requires bile salt micelles and pancreatic enzymes. Unlike the other fat-soluble vitamins, vitamin K is not stored in large amounts in adipose tissue. The plasma form is carried on lipoproteins, but the storage form is primarily long-chain menaquinones. The vitamin is concentrated in the liver and is excreted in bile, stool, and urine [11,194]. Vitamin K acts by carboxylating selected glutamic acid residues of proteins to form α-carboxyglutamic acid (Gla), which binds calcium [194]. The coagulation function of the vitamin K-dependent hepatic proteins (e.g., prothrombin and factors VII, IX, and X) and the function of the bone proteins (e.g., osteocalcin, matrix Gla protein) are proportional to the degree of carboxylation. Dietary intake of 200–500 µg/day of vitamin K has been suggested as necessary for optimal γ-carboxylation of osteocalcin [195]. Other vitamin K-dependent proteins of unknown function are present in other tissues.

Conditionally essential nutrients
Choline
Choline can be synthesized in sufficient amounts to support normal metabolism of healthy animals and humans, and so was not considered an essential nutrient. However, in some pathological conditions this nutrient is conditionally essential; it is also essential for normal neonatal metabolism [196]. Choline is a precursor for acetylcholine, phospholipids, and the methyl donor betaine. It is absorbed from the intestine by transporter proteins, but it is not clear whether this process is mediated by the same high-affinity choline transporter, CHT1, that mediates endocytosis in neural tissue. Foods with high choline content include liver, eggs, peanut butter, and milk, and lower amounts occur in all raw foods. Human intake is estimated to be about 0.6–1.0 g/day. Gut flora degrade choline to many products, including betaine and methylamines. A choline deficiency syndrome has never been described in humans, but the Food and Drug Nutrition Board of the Institute of Medicine classifies choline as an essential nutrient [9], based on a study that showed lower plasma choline and phosphatidylcholine levels in subjects fed a choline-free diet for 3 weeks. In addition, some data suggest a partial reversal in hepatic abnormalities following choline supplementation [197]. The AI for infants is set at 17–18 mg/kg, and for adults at 550 mg/day for men, and 425 mg/day for women. A 20% lipid emulsion for TPN provides 11.6–132 mmol/L of phosphatidylcholine. The tolerable upper intake level (UL) for choline is 3.5 g/day, as higher amounts may cause hypotension and a fishy body odor from a metabolite, trimethylamine.

Carnitine
Carnitine is not an essential nutrient for adults, although it may be conditionally essential for neonates [196]. It functions

to transfer long-chain fatty acids into mitochondria, improves glucose disposal, and may reduce insulin resistance [198]. Carnitine is made in the liver and kidney, and ingested mostly in milk and meats. Various disease states can alter carnitine status, including renal tubular dysfunction (Fanconi syndrome), chronic renal failure and hemodialysis, and certain medications including zidovudine and valproic acid [198]. Levocarnitine (Carnitor) is approved for such deficiencies, and produces modest effects at 2 g/day when given to patients with anemia caused by renal failure, pain in chronic diabetic neuropathy, and cardiac ischemia.

Arginine
Arginine is not considered an essential amino acid by the Food and Drug Nutrition Board of the Institute of Medicine [13]. However, sepsis appears to produce a conditional deficiency [199]. Arginine is a precursor for nitric oxide, and its potential benefits are related to replacing nitric oxide (NO) in severe illness. It can be given safely, and although laboratory end points can improve, its clinical efficacy is still uncertain [200]. Most studies use arginine in therapy as a component of commercial products that also contain n-3 fatty acids, branched-chain fatty acids, and nucleotides. There is no reason to recommend arginine or other immunoactive substances to critically ill patients [201].

Glutamine
Glutamine, along with aspartate, is an important energy source for the small intestine, but it has not been classified as an essential amino acid [13]. A special role for glutamine has been suggested for the treatment of critically ill patients, because it is the most abundant extracellular amino acid – it is used at high rates by many tissues, including the central nervous system and immune cells, and its levels fall during critical illness [202]. Supplemental glutamine has been reported to improve some immunological markers and reduce rates of infectious complications in some studies [203]. Glutamine has also been used in the treatment of mucositis caused by chemotherapy or radiotherapy [204]. The problems with assessing the considerable literature on glutamine are many, and include the greatly different patient populations, the variety of end points tested, the relatively short follow-up, the lack of adequately powered studies, and the lack of reproducible improvement of significant clinical end points [205]. Further studies are needed before glutamine supplementation can be recommended for use in critically ill patients.

Altered nutritional states

Starvation
The metabolic response to starvation enhances survival by increasing the use of adipose tissue triglycerides as a source of fuel, preventing severe hypoglycemia, conserving lean

tissue, and decreasing the metabolic rate. The duration of survival during starvation depends on the amount of body fat and lean body mass. In lean men, death occurs after about 60 days of starvation [39], whereas obese persons can survive complete energy deprivation for more than 1 year without obvious adverse consequences [206].

Marked metabolic adaptations occur within the first 24 h of fasting. The mobilization of adipose tissue triglycerides, ketone body production, and the oxidation of plasma fatty acids increase, whereas hepatic glucose production and plasma glucose oxidation decrease [207].

The rate of lipolysis of adipose tissue triglycerides increases because of a decrease in circulating insulin, an increase in plasma epinephrine (adrenaline) concentration, and an increase in the lipolytic response to catecholamines [208–210]. After 3 days of fasting, lipolysis of adipose tissue triglycerides increases to more than double the values observed after an overnight (i.e., 12-h) fast. The increases in lipolysis and plasma fatty acid concentrations promote rates of fatty acid oxidation. The increased delivery of free fatty acids to the liver in conjunction with a decrease in the plasma ratio of insulin to glucagon stimulates hepatic ketone body production [211]. The rate of ketogenesis is maximal by 3 days of starvation; plasma ketone body concentration increases 75-fold by 7 days [212]. Ketone bodies are water soluble and able to cross the blood–brain barrier. As plasma ketone body concentrations increase, ketone body oxidation by the brain increases; by 7 days of starvation, ketone bodies provide 70% of the brain's energy needs [213]. The shift in fuel use by the brain helps spare the limited supply of plasma glucose for glucose-requiring tissues.

Whole-body glucose production decreases by more than half during the first few days of fasting because of a marked reduction in hepatic glucose output [214]. Only 15% of hepatic glycogen stores remain after 24 h of fasting [215]. Therefore, the contribution of gluconeogenesis from plasma precursors to total hepatic glucose output increases as the rate of hepatic glycogenolysis declines. As fasting continues, the conversion of glutamine to glucose in the kidney represents almost 50% of total glucose production.

Normally, about 70 g of amino acids is mobilized from protein stores and about 10 g of nitrogen is excreted in the urine [216]. During starvation, it is critical to slow down the rate of protein breakdown to prevent clinically significant protein losses. If protein breakdown proceeded at a normal rate throughout starvation, a potentially lethal amount of muscle protein would be catabolized in less than 3 weeks. The increase in ketone bodies [217] and starvation-induced inactivation of thyroid hormone – conversion of triiodothyronine (T_3) to reverse T_3 [218] – directly inhibit muscle protein breakdown.

Energy expenditure is conserved during fasting because of a decrease in physical activity caused by fatigue and a decrease in the resting metabolic rate, which decreases by 10%–15% at 7 days because of the diminished size and function of metabolically active tissues [219], increased conversion of active thyroid hormone to its inactive form [220], and suppressed sympathetic nervous system activity [221].

Maximum adaptation occurs as starvation continues. After 14 days of fasting, the rates of lipid, carbohydrate, and protein metabolism reach a plateau. Adipose tissue provides more than 90% of daily energy requirements. Muscle protein breakdown decreases to less than 30 g/day, causing a marked decrease in urea nitrogen production and excretion. Fluid requirements decrease because the diminished osmotic load from urea causes a decline in urine volume to 200 mL/day. Total glucose production decreases to about 75 g/day, providing fuel for glycolytic tissues (40 g/day) and the brain (35 g/day) while maintaining a constant plasma glucose concentration. Energy expenditure decreases by 20%–25% after 30 days of fasting [222] and remains relatively constant thereafter despite continued starvation.

During the terminal phase of starvation, body fat mass, muscle protein, and the size of most organs are markedly decreased. The weight and protein content of the brain remain relatively stable throughout starvation. In rodent models, when fat stores are depleted, the energy derived from body fat decreases and muscle protein catabolism increases. Death occurs when 30% of muscle protein is lost [223].

Metabolic response to illness and injury

The metabolic response to illness and injury is characterized by hypermetabolism, negative nitrogen balance, insulin resistance and hyperglycemia, and increased mobilization and oxidation of adipose tissue triglycerides. These events are produced by a complex cascade of endogenous mediators that cause a predictable physiological response. Increased production and secretion of the counterregulatory hormones (e.g., catecholamines, glucagon, and glucocorticoids) and cytokines are probably responsible for most of the observed responses to illness and injury.

In the 1930s, the classic work of Cutherbertson [224] on long-bone fractures provided the basis of our understanding of the metabolic response to injury. Cuthbertson demonstrated that the response to injury could be divided into two phases: the early ebb phase (12–24 h after trauma) and the subsequent flow phase. The ebb phase is characterized by decreases in blood pressure, oxygen consumption, cardiac output, and body temperature. The flow phase is characterized by hypermetabolism and increases in oxygen consumption, cardiac output, body temperature, and the urinary excretion of nitrogen, potassium, and phosphorus. Subsequently, Moore [225] divided the flow phase into the catabolic and anabolic phases. The restoration of tissue perfusion marks the beginning of the catabolic phase and lasts for days to weeks, depending on the severity of injury, medical intervention, and the premorbid health of the patient. This phase is characterized by catabolism, heat production, negative nitrogen balance, and hyperglycemia [224,225]. It ends after volume deficits are corrected, infection is controlled, pain is eliminated, and oxygenation is restored. At this point, net anabolism may occur, resulting in a slow reaccumulation of protein and body fat.

Hormone and cytokine mediators

During the flow phase, the secretion of several hormones is increased, and they act synergistically to generate alterations in intermediary metabolism. Catecholamines increase lipolysis and hepatic glucose production. Glucagon increases hepatic gluconeogenesis and glycogenolysis. Cortisol enhances protein breakdown and increases hepatic gluconeogenesis.

Cytokines, produced by macrophages, lymphocytes, Kupffer cells, and endothelial cells, are also critical mediators of the metabolic response. Tumor necrosis factor is believed to be the primary cytokine mediating many of the responses to infection and trauma, including fever, increased acute-phase protein synthesis, protein catabolism, hypotension, decreased lipoprotein lipase activity, and metabolic acidosis [226–230]. Interleukin-1 and TNF act synergistically in promoting tissue injury and stimulating the release of counterregulatory hormones [231]; IL-1 causes fever, hypotension, and increased insulin and glucagon secretion, and it affects the concentrations of plasma divalent cations. The liver is stimulated by IL-1 to synthesize metallothioneins, which sequester zinc, and IL-1 mediates the sequestration of iron in hemosiderin and ferritin, depriving invading organisms of these trace elements [228–235]. Other aspects of the acute-phase response stimulated by IL-1 include fibrinogen and C-reactive protein production by hepatocytes and the release of lactoferrin by neutrophils [232,233]. Interleukin-1 enhances immunoglobulin production by B lymphocytes and is a potent stimulus for the synthesis and release of IL-2 by T lymphocytes [232,233,236]. Interleukin-6 is also inducible by TNF and functions primarily as a stimulator of the hepatic acute-phase protein response and lymphocyte proliferation [231,236]. Interleukin-8 is inducible by TNF and IL-1 and is a potent neutrophil chemoattractant [236].

Energy metabolism

Increases in metabolic rate correlate directly with the severity of illness and injury [237]. For example, the REE increases after uncomplicated surgery by about 10%, after long-bone fractures by 20%, and after multiple trauma by 50%. The REE rarely exceeds twice the normal rate regardless of the extent of injury [223]. In fact, even patients with severe burns usually do not experience an increase in REE by more than 50% for any prolonged period [238]. In certain types of injury, a temporary resetting of the hypothalamic thermoregulatory set point is responsible for a 1–2°C elevation of body temperature known as *posttraumatic fever* [226,239]. The REE increases about 12% for each 1°C increase in core body temperature. Because the central temperature set point is higher, the com-

fort temperature for an injured patient is elevated, and elevating the ambient temperature decreases the energy requirement [223].

Protein metabolism

Illness or injury increases protein synthesis and protein breakdown. The increase in protein breakdown is greater than the increase in protein synthesis, resulting in negative nitrogen balance. Skeletal muscle is the major site of protein catabolism, but increased catabolism of extracellular proteins, including acute-phase reactants, coagulation system proteins, and complement system proteins, also occurs [232,240–242]. Considerable protein synthesis is directed toward host defense, including phagocyte activity, hormones, cytokines, intracellular proteins, immunoglobulins, complement, coagulation system proteins, and acute-phase reactant glycoproteins [232].

The composition of amino acids released by muscle does not reflect the composition of muscle proteins. The branched-chain amino acids of skeletal muscle are metabolized within the muscle cell for energy, and transamination generates glutamine and alanine. As a result, alanine and glutamine, which constitute only 12% of muscle protein, make up 50%–60% of the amino acids released into the plasma by muscle. Conversely, branched-chain amino acids make up 15% of the muscle protein but only 6% of the amino acids released [232,237]. Glutamine is taken up and metabolized by the kidneys at an accelerated rate, providing additional ammonium for excretion to help maintain acid–base balance in the face of the acidosis that frequently accompanies critical illness [237]. In addition to carrying amino groups from the periphery to the liver and kidney, glutamine serves as a major energy source for the lymphocytes, fibroblasts, and the gastrointestinal tract [243]. Alanine is captured by the liver for gluconeogenesis, and its nitrogen contributes to the increase in ureagenesis [244].

During severe illness, nitrogen losses may reach 20–40 g/day. This represents catabolism of 600–1200 g of lean body mass per day. Providing exogenous nitrogen and energy may [245] or may not [246] decrease the rate of catabolism, but it enhances protein synthesis and thereby decreases negative nitrogen balance [243,247].

Carbohydrate metabolism

The stress response is marked by hyperglycemia, in large part related to hepatic gluconeogenesis fueled by lactate, pyruvate, glycerol, alanine, and other glucogenic amino acids. Hepatic glucose production may exceed 500 g/day and is resistant to suppression by insulin [248]. Peripheral insulin resistance decreases skeletal muscle glucose uptake, which also contributes to hyperglycemia [226]. Glucose consumption by wounds and injured extremities is increased to provide fuel for inflammatory cells, such as fibroblasts, macrophages, and leukocytes. These cells metabolize glucose anaerobically and can release large quantities of lactate into the bloodstream, which is subsequently recycled to glucose by the liver.

Lipid metabolism

Fat is a major oxidative fuel in critically ill patients, even when exogenous carbohydrates are administered. The rate of lipolysis correlates directly with the severity of illness [249]. The increased delivery of fatty acids to the liver stimulates very-low-density lipoprotein (VLDL) production. However, the rate of VLDL secretion is not adequate to remove the excessive supply of fatty acids and thus contributes to hepatic fat accumulation. Hypertriglyceridemia can occur because of both increased VLDL production and decreased peripheral lipoprotein lipase activity and VLDL clearance.

References

1. Beddoe AH, Straet SJ, Hill GL. Evaluation of an in vivo prompt gamma neutron activation facility for body composition studies in critically ill intensive care patients: results on 41 normals. Metabolism 1984;33:270.
2. Moore FD, Olesen KH, McMurrey JD, et al. The Body Cell Mass and its Supporting Environment. Philadelphia: WB Saunders, 1963.
3. US Department of Health and Human Services, US Department of Agriculture. Nutrition and your health: dietary guidelines for Americans, 6th edn. Washington DC, 2005 (http://www.healthierus.gov/dietaryguidelines).
4. Krauss RM, Eckel RH, Howard B, et al. American Heart Association dietary guidelines revision 2000: a statement for healthcare professionals from the nutrition committee of the American Heart Association. Circulation 2000;102:2284.
5. World Health Organization. Obesity: preventing and managing the global epidemic. Report of a WHO Consultation on Obesity. Geneva: World Health Organization, 1998.
6. National Institute of Health, National Heart, Lung, and Blood Institute, North American Association for the study of Obesity. The practical guide: identification, evaluation and treatment of overweight and obesity in adults (http://www.nhlbi.nih.gov/guidelines/obesity/prctgd_c.pdf).
7. National Institutes of Health, National Heart, Lung, and Blood Institute. Clinical guidelines on the identification, evaluation, and treatment of overweight and obesity in adults – the evidence report. Obes Res 1998;6:54S.
8. Standing Committee on the Scientific Evaluation of Dietary Reference Intakes, Food and Nutrition Board, Institute of Medicine. Dietary Reference Intakes for Calcium, Phosphorus, Magnesium, Vitamin D, and Fluoride. Washington, DC: National Academy Press, 1997.
9. Standing Committee on the Scientific Evaluation of Dietary Reference Intakes, Food and Nutrition Board, Institute of Medicine. Dietary Reference Intakes for Thiamin, Riboflavin, Niacin, Vitamin B$_6$, Folate, Vitamin B$_{12}$, Pantothenic Acid, Biotin, and Choline. Washington, DC: National Academy Press, 2000.
10. Standing Committee on the Scientific Evaluation of Dietary Reference Intakes, Food and Nutrition Board, Institute of Medicine. Dietary Reference Intakes for Vitamin E, Vitamin C, Selenium, and Carotenoids. Washington, DC: National Academy Press, 2000.
11. Standing Committee on the Scientific Evaluation of Dietary Reference Intakes, Food and Nutrition Board, Institute of Medicine. Dietary Reference Intakes for Vitamin A, Vitamin K, Arsenic, Boron, Chromium, Copper, Iodine, Iron, Manganese, Molybdenum, Nickel, Silicon, Canadium, and Zinc. Washington, DC: National Academy Press, 2002.
12. Standing Committee on the Scientific Evaluation of Dietary Reference Intakes, Food and Nutrition Board, Institute of Medicine. Dietary Reference Intakes for Water, Potassium, Sodium, Chloride, and Sulfate. Washington DC: National Academy Press, 2004.
13. Standing Committee on the Scientific Evaluation of Dietary Reference Intakes, Food and Nutrition Board, Institute of Medicine. Dietary Reference Intakes for Energy, Carbohydrate, Fiber, Fat, Fatty Acids, Cholesterol, Protein, and Amino Acids. Washington DC: National Academy Press, 2005.
14. Jenkins DJ, Wolever TM, Taylor RH, et al. Glycemic index of foods: a physiological basis for carbohydrate exchange. Am J Clin Nutr 1981;34:362.
15. Garg A, Grundy SM, Unger RH. Comparison of effects of high and low carbohydrate diets on plasma lipoproteins and insulin sensitivity in patients with mild NIDDM. Diabetes 1992;41:1278.
16. Ebbeling CB, Leidig MM, Sinclair KB, et al. A reduced-glycemic load diet in the treatment of adolescent obesity. Arch Pediatr Adolesc Med 2003;157:773.
17. Kim Y-I, Mason JB. Nutrition chemoprevention of gastrointestinal cancers: a critical review. Nutr Rev 1996;54:259.
18. American Institute for Cancer Research. 11th Annual Research Conference on Diet, Nutrition, and Cancer. J Nutr 2001;131:3025S.
19. National Research Council, Commission on Life Sciences, Food and Nutrition Board, Committee on Diet and Health. Diet and Health Implications for Reducing Chronic Disease Risk. Washington, DC: National Academy Press, 1989.
20. Cummings JH, Bingham SA. Diet and the prevention of cancer. Br Med J 1998;317:1636.
21. Janne PA, Mayer RJ. Chemoprevention of colorectal cancer. N Engl J Med 2000;342:1960.
22. van Gils CH, Peeters PHM, Bueno-de-Mesquita HB, et al. Consumption of vegetables and fruits and risk of breast cancer. JAMA 2005;203:183.
23. McCullough ML, Robertson AS, Chao A, et al. A prospective study of whole grains, fruits, vegetables, and colon cancer risk. Cancer Causes Control 2003;14:959.
24. Bjelakovic G, Nikolova D, Simonetti RG, Gluud C. Antioxidant supplements for prevention of gastrointestinal cancers: a systematic review and meta-analysis. Lancet 2004;364:1219.
25. Miller EF, Pastor-Barriusco R, Dalal D, et al. Meta-analysis: high-dosage vitamin supplementation may increase all-cause mortality. Ann Intern Med 2005;142:37.
26. Forman MR, Hursting SD, Umer A, Barrett JC. Nutrition and cancer prevention: A multi-disciplinary perspective on human trials. Annu Rev Nutr 2004;24:223.
27. Jacobs EJ, Connell CJ, Chao A, et al. Multivitamin use and colorectal cancer incidence in a US cohort: does timing matter? Am J Epidemiol 2003;158:621.
28. AGA Clinical Practice Economics Committee. AGA technical review: impact of dietary fiber on colon cancer occurrence. Gastroenterology 2000;118:1235.
29. Hill MJ. Cereals, cereal fibre and colorectal cancer risk: a review of the epidemiological literature. Eur J Cancer Prev 1998;7(Suppl. 2):S5.
30. Giovannucci E, Stampfer MJ, Colditz G, et al. Relationship of diet to risk of colorectal cancer in men. J Natl Cancer Inst 1992;84:91.
31. Willet WC, Stampfer JM, Colditz GA, et al. Relation of meat, fat, and fiber intake to the risk of colon cancer in a prospective study among women. N Engl J Med 1990;323:1664.
32. Steinmetz KA, Kushi LH, Bostick RM, et al. Vegetables, fruit, and colon cancer in the Iowa Women's Health Study. Am J Epidemiol 1994;139:1.
33. Bingham SA, Day NE, Luben R, et al. Dietary fibre in food and protection against colorectal cancer in the European Prospective Investigation into Cancer and Nutrition (EPIC): an observational study. Lancet 2003;361:1496.
34. Peters U, Sinha R, Chatterjee N, et al. Dietary fibre and colorectal

adenoma in a colorectal cancer early detection programme. Lancet 2003;361:1491.

35. Lee KW, Lee HJ, Surh YJ, Lee CY. Vitamin C and cancer chemoprevention: reappraisal. Am J Clin Nutr 2003;78:1074.

36. Weir JB. New methods for calculating metabolic rate with special reference to protein metabolism. J Physiol 1949;109:1.

37. Frayn K. Calculation of substrate oxidation rates in vivo from gaseous exchange. J Appl Physiol 1983;55:628.

38. Fenn WO, Haege LF. The deposition of glycogen with water in the livers of cats. J Biol Chem 1940;136:87.

39. Leiter LA, Marliss B. Survival during fasting may depend on fat as well as protein stores. JAMA 1982;248:2306.

40. Kleiber M. The Fire of Life: an Introduction to Animal Energetics. New York: John Wiley and Sons, 1961.

41. Harris JA, Benedict FG. Standard basal metabolism constants for physiologists and clinicians. In: A Biometric Study of Basal Metabolism in Man. Publication 279, The Carnegie Institute of Washington. Philadelphia: JB Lippincott, 1919:223.

42. World Health Organization. Energy and protein requirements. Report of a joint FAO/WHO/UNU expert consultation. WHO technical report series No. 724. Geneva: World Health Organization, 1985.

43. Owen OE, Kavle E, Owen RS, et al. A reappraisal of caloric requirements in healthy women. Am J Clin Nutr 1986;44:1.

44. Ireton-Jones CS, Borman KR, Turner WW. Nutrition considerations in the management of ventilator-dependent patients. Nutr Clin Pract 1993;8:60.

45. Dulloo AG, Jacquet J, Montani JP. Pathways from weight fluctuations to metabolic diseases: focus on maladaptive thermogenesis during catch-up fat. Int J Obes Rel Metab Disord 2002;26:S46.

46. Dulloo AG, Seydoux J, Jacquet J. Adaptive thermogenesis and uncoupling proteins: a reappraisal of their roles in fat metabolism and energy balance. Physio Behav 2004;83:587.

47. Dulloo AG, Miller DS. Obesity: a disorder of the sympathetic nervous system. World Rev Nutr Diet 1987;50:1.

48. Stock MJ. Thermogenesis and brown fat: relevance to human obesity. Infusion Ther 1989;16:282.

49. Himms-Hagen J. Brown adipose tissue thermogenesis and obesity. Prog Lipid Res 1989;28:67.

50. Nagase I, Yoshida T, Kumamoto K, et al. Expression of uncoupling protein in skeletal muscle and white adipose tissue of obese mice treated with thermogenic β_3-adrenergic agonist. J Clin Invest 1996; 97:2898.

51. Munro HN, Crim MC. The proteins and amino acids. In: Shils ME, Young VR (eds). Modern Nutrition in Health and Disease, 7th edn. Philadelphia: Lea & Febiger, 1988:1.

52. Allison JB. Biological evaluation of proteins. Physiol Rev 1955;35:664.

53. Bressani R. Human assays and applications. In: Bodwell CE (ed.). Evaluation of Proteins for Humans. Westport, CT: AVI Publishing, 1977:81.

54. Foster GD, Know LS, Dempsey DT, Mullen JL. Caloric requirements in total parenteral nutrition. J Am Coll Nutr 1987;6:231.

55. Kakade ML, Hoffa DE, Liener IE. Contribution of trypsin inhibitors to the deleterious effects of unheated soybeans fed to rats. J Nutr 1973;103:1772.

56. World Health Organization. WHO/FAO/UNO report: energy and protein requirements. WHO technical report series No. 724. Geneva: World Health Organization, 1985.

57. Monsen ER. The 10th edition of the recommended dietary allowances: what's new in the 1989 RDAs? J Am Diet Assoc 1989;89:1748.

58. Callaway DH, Margen H. Variation in endogenous nitrogen excretion and dietary nitrogen utilization as determinants of human protein requirement. J Nutr 1971;101:204.

59. Anderson GH, Patel DG, Jeejeebhoy KN. Design and evaluation by nitrogen balance and blood aminograms of an amino acid mixture for total parenteral nutrition of adults with gastrointestinal disease. J Clin Invest 1974;53:904.

60. Heird WC, Cooper A. Nutrition in infants and children. In: Shils ME, Young VR (eds). Modern Nutrition in Health and Disease, 7th edn. Philadelphia: Lea & Febiger, 1988:944.

61. Gong EJ, Heald FP. Diet, nutrition and adolescence. In: Shils ME, Young VR (eds). Modern Nutrition in Health and Disease, 7th edn. Philadelphia: Lea & Febiger, 1988:969.

62. Mortimer GE. Intracellular protein catabolism and its control during nutrient deprivation and supply. Annu Rev Nutr 1987;7:539.

63. Bond JS, Butler PE. Intracellular proteases. Annu Rev Biochem 1987;56:333.

64. Horl WH, Wanner C, Schollmeyer P. Proteinases in catabolism and malnutrition. JPEN J Parenter Enteral Nutr 1987;11(Suppl.):98.

65. Katunuma N. New biological functions of intracellular proteases and their endogenous inhibitors as bioreactants. Adv Enzyme Regul 1990;30:377.

66. Beynon RJ, Bond JS. Catabolism of intracellular protein: molecular aspects. Am J Physiol 1986;20:C141.

67. Jeejeebhoy KN. Nutrient metabolism. In: Kinney JM, Jeejeebhoy KN, Hill GL, Owen OE (eds). Nutrition and Metabolism in Patient Care. Philadelphia: WB Saunders, 1988:60.

68. Elwyn DH, Parikh HC, Shoemaker WC. Amino acid movements between gut, liver, and periphery in unanesthetized dogs. Am J Physiol 1968;215:1260.

69. Rodwell VW. Catabolism of amino acid nitrogen. In: Murray RK, Granner DK, Mayes PA, Rodwell VW (eds). Harper's Biochemistry. Norwalk, CT: Appleton & Lange, 1988:271.

70. Wharen J, Felig P, Hagenfeldt TL. Effect of protein ingestion on splanchnic and leg metabolism in normal man and in patients with diabetes mellitus. J Clin Invest 1976;57:987.

71. Souba WW. Interorgan ammonia metabolism in health and disease: a surgeon's view. JPEN J Parenter Enteral Nutr 1987;11:569.

72. McGarry JD. Lipid metabolism. I: Utilization and storage of energy in lipid form. In: Devlin TM (ed.). Textbook of Biochemistry: With Clinical Correlations, 3rd edn. New York: Wiley-Liss, 1992:387.

73. Hariharan JK. Essential fatty acids. Indian Pediatr 1988;25:67.

74. Friedman Z. Essential fatty acids revisited. Am J Dis Child 1980; 134:406.

75. Holman RT. Essential fatty acid deficiency. In: Holman RT (ed.). Progress in the Chemistry of Fats and Other Lipids. Oxford: Pergamon Press, 1968:275.

76. Gottschlich MM. Selection of optimal lipid sources in enteral and parenteral nutrition. Nutr Clin Pract 1992;7:152.

77. Gorlin R. The biological actions and potential clinical significance of dietary omega-3 fatty acid. Arch Intern Med 1988;148:2043.

78. Uauy-Dagach R, Valenzuela A. Marine oils as a source of omega-3 fatty acids in the diet. How to optimize the health benefits. Prog Food Nutr Sci 1992;16:199.

79. Bang HO, Dyerberg J, Nielsen AB. Plasma lipid and lipoprotein pattern in Greenlandic west-coast Eskimos. Lancet 1971;2:1153.

80. GISSI-Prevenzione Investigators. Dietary supplementation with n-3 polyunsaturated fatty acids and vitamin E after myocardial infarction: results of the GISSI-Prevenzione trial. Lancet 1999;354: 447.

81. Marchioli R, Barzi F, Bomba E, et al. Early protection against sudden death by n-3 polyunsaturated fatty acids after myocardial infarction: time-course analysis of the results of the Gruppo Italiano per lo Studio della Sopravvivenza nell'Infarto Miocardico (GISSI)-Prevenzione. Circulation 2002;105:1897.

82. Singh R, Niaz M, Sharma J, et al. Randomized, double-blind, placebo-controlled trial of fish oil and mustard oil in patients with suspected acute myocardial infarction: the Indian experiment of infarct survival – 4. Cardiovasc Drugs Ther 1997;11:485.

83. Israel DH, Gorlin R. Fish oils in the prevention of atherosclerosis. J Am Coll Cardiol 1992;19:174.

84. Fitzgerald GA, Braden G, Fitzgerald DJ, Knapp HR. Fish oils in cardiovascular disease. J Intern Med 1989;225(Suppl. 1):25.

85. Dyerberg J, Bang HO, Stofferson E, et al. Eicosa-pentanoic acid and prevention of thrombosis and atherosclerosis. Lancet 1978;2:11.

86. Dyerberg J, Bang HO. Hemostatic function and platelet polyunsaturated fatty acids in Eskimos. Lancet 1979;2:433.

87. Fehily AM, Burr ML, Phillips KM, Deadman NM. The effect of fatty fish on plasma lipid and lipoprotein concentrations. Am J Clin Nutr 1983;38:349.

88. Bronsgeest-Schoute HC, Van Gent CM, Luten JB, Ruiter A. The effect of various intakes of ω3 fatty acids on the blood lipid composition in healthy human subjects. Am J Clin Nutr 1981;341:1752.

89. Phillipson BE, Rothrock DW, Connor WE, et al. Reduction of plasma lipids, lipoproteins, and apoproteins by dietary fish oils in patients with hypertriglyceridemia. N Engl J Med 1985;312:1210.

90. Schectman G, Kaul S, Cherayil GD, et al. Can the hypotriglyceridemic effect of fish oil concentrate be sustained? Ann Intern Med 1989;110:346.

91. Herzberg GR. The 1990 Borden Award lecture: dietary regulation of fatty acid and triglyceride metabolism. Can J Physiol Pharmacol 1991;69:1637.

92. Nestel PJ. Effects of n-3 fatty acids on lipid metabolism. Annu Rev Nutr 1990;10:149.

93. Harris WS, Dujovne CA, Zucker M, Johnson B. Effects of a low saturated fat, low cholesterol fish oil supplement in hypertriglyceridemic patients. Ann Intern Med 1988;109:465.

94. Katz DP, Schwartz S, Askanazi J. Biochemical and cellular basis for potential therapeutic value on n-3 fatty acids derived from fish oil. Nutrition 1993;9:113.

95. Yetiv JZ. Clinical applications of fish oil. JAMA 1988;260:665.

96. Lee TH, Hoover RL, Williams JD, et al. Effect of dietary enrichment with eicosapentanoic and docosahexanoic acids on in vitro neutrophil and monocyte leukotriene generation and neutrophil function. N Engl J Med 1985;312:1219.

97. Endres S, Ghorbani R, Kelley VE, et al. The effect of dietary supplementation with n-3 polyunsaturated fatty acids on the synthesis in interleukin-1 and tumor necrosis factor by mononuclear cells. N Engl J Med 1989;320:265.

98. Kris-Etherton PM, Harris WS, Appel LJ. AHA Scientific Statement: Fish consumption, fish oil, omega-3 fatty acids, and cardiovascular disease. Circulation 2002;106:2747.

99. DeMichele SJ, Karlstad MD, Babayan VK, et al. Enhanced skeletal muscle and liver protein synthesis with structured lipid in enterally fed burned rats. Metabolism. 1988;37:787.

100. DeMichele SJ, Karlstad MD, Bistrian BR, et al. Enteral nutrition with structured lipid: effect on protein metabolism in thermal injury. Am J Clin Nutr 1989;50:1295.

101. Maiz A, Yamazaki K, Sobrado J, et al. Protein metabolism during total parenteral nutrition (TPN) in injured rats using medium-chain triglycerides. Metabolism 1984;33:901.

102. Chan S, McCowen KC, Bistrian B. Medium-chain triglyceride and n-3 polyunsaturated fatty acid-containing emulsions in intravenous nutrition. Curr Opin Clin Nutr Metab Care 1998;1:163.

103. Teo TC, DeMichele SJ, Selleck, et al. Administration of structured lipid composed of MCT and fish oil reduces net protein catabolism in enterally fed burned rats. Ann Surg 1989;210:100.

104. Teo TC, Selleck KM, Wan JM, et al. Long-term feeding with structured lipid composed of medium-chain and n-3 fatty acids ameliorates endotoxic shock in guinea pigs. Metabolism 1991;40:1152.

105. Tso P, Lee T, DeMichele SJ. Randomized structured triglycerides increase lymphatic absorption of tocopherol and retinal compared with the equivalent physical mixture in a rat model of fat malabsorption. J Nutr 2001;131:2157.

106. Kenler AS, Swails WS, Driscoll DS, et al. Early enteral feeding in postsurgical cancer patients: fish oil structured lipid-based polymeric formula versus a standard polymeric formula. Ann Surg 1996;223:316.

107. Owen OE. Regulation of energy and metabolism. In: Kinney JM, Jeejeebhoy KN, Hill GL, Owen OE (eds). Nutrition and Metabolism in Patient Care. Philadelphia: WB Saunders, 1988:35.

108. McDonald I. Carbohydrates. In: Shils ME, Young VR (eds). Modern Nutrition in Health and Disease, 7th edn. Philadelphia: Lea & Febiger, 1988:38.

109. Harris RA. Carbohydrate metabolism. I. Major metabolic pathways and their control. In: Devlin TM (ed.). Textbook of Biochemistry: with Clinical Correlations, 3rd edn. New York: Wiley-Liss, 1992:291.

110. Gallagher DD, Schneeman BO. Dietary fiber. In: Bowman BA, Russell RM (eds). Present Knowledge in Nutrition, 8th edn. Washington, DC: ILSI Press, 2001:83.

111. Tokunaga T. Novel physiological function of fructo-oligosaccharides. Biofactors 2004;21:89.

112. Schrezenmeier J, de Vrese M. Probiotics, prebiotics, and synbiotics – approaching a definition. Am J Clin Nutr 2001;73:361S.

113. Kendall CWC, Emam A, Ausutin LS, Jenkins DJ. Resistant starches and health. J AOAC Int 2004;87:769.

114. Beecher GR. Overview of dietary flavonoids: nomenclature, occurrence and intake. J Nutr 2003;133:3248S.

115. Trevisanato SI, Kim Y-I. Tea and health. Nutr Rev 2000;58:1.

116. Sakihama Y, Cohen MY, Grace SC, Yamasaki H. Plant phenolic antioxidant and prooxidant activities: phenolics-induced oxidation damage mediated by metals in plants. Toxicology 2002;177:67.

117. Dietary fiber and health – a report by the Council on Scientific Affairs, American Medical Association. JAMA 1989;262:542.

118. Lim CC, Fergusoin LR, Tannock GW. Dietary fibres as 'prebiotics': implications for colorectal cancer. Mol Nutr Food Res 2005;49:609.

119. Salyers AA. Diet and the colonic environment: measuring the response of human colonic bacteria to changes in the host's diet. In: Valhouny GV, Kritchevsky D (eds). Dietary Fiber. New York: Plenum, 1986:119.

120. Read NW. Dietary fiber and bowel transit. In: Valhouny GV, Kritchevsky D (eds). Dietary Fiber. New York: Plenum, 1986:81.

121. Kritchevsky D. Dietary fiber. Annu Rev Nutr 1988;8:301.

122. Quartero AO, Meinecke-Schmidt V, Mures J, et al. Bulking agents, antispasmodic and antidepressant medication for the treatment of irritable bowel syndrome. Cochrane Database Syst Rev 2005: CD003460.

123. Scarlett Y. Medical management of fecal incontinence. Gastroenterology 2004;126:S55.

124. Gearhart SL. Symptomatic hemorrhoids. Adv Surg 2004;38:167.

125. Alpers DH, Stenson WF, Bier DM. Manual of Nutritional Therapeutics, 4th edn. Philadelphia: Lippincott Williams & Wilkins, 2001.

126. Preuss HG. Sodium, chloride, and potassium. In: Bowman BA, Russell RM (eds). Present Knowledge in Nutrition, 8th edn. Washington, DC: ILSI Press, 2001:302.

127. Adrogue HJ, Madias N. Hyponatremia. N Engl J Med 2000;342:1581.

128. Gennari FJ. Hypokalemia. N Engl J Med 1998;339:451.

129. Bushinsky DA, Monk RD. Calcium. Lancet 1998;352:306.

130. Weaver CM, Heaney RT. Allen LH, Wood RJ. Calcium. In: Shils ME, Shike M, Ross AC, et al. (eds). Modern Nutrition in Health and Disease, 10th edn. Philadelphia: Lippincott Williams & Wilkins, 2006:194.

131. Knochel JP. Phosphorus. In: Shils ME, Shike M, Ross AC, et al. Modern Nutrition in Health and Disease, 10th edn. Philadelphia: Lippincott Williams & Wilkins, 2006:211.

132. Weaver CM. Calcium. In: Bowman BA, Russell RM (eds). Present Knowledge in Nutrition, 8th edn. Washington, DC: ILSI Press, 2001:273.

133. Miller GD. Year 2000 dietary guidelines: new thoughts for a new millenium. Heaney RP. There should be a dietary guideline for calcium. Specker BL. Should there be a dietary guideline for calcium intake? No. Am J Clin Nutr 2000;71:657;658;661.

134. Lanon AJ, Berkow SE, Barnard ND. Calcium, dairy products, and bone health in children and young adults: a reevaluation of the evidence. Pediatrics 2005;115:736.

135. Nordin C. Calcium requirement is a sliding scale. Am J Clin Nutr 2000;71:1381.

136. Hodgson SF, Watts NB, Bilizikian J, et al. AACE medical guidelines for clinical practice for the prevention and treatment of postmenopausal osteoporosis: 2001 edition with selected updates for 2003. Endocr Pract 2003;2:544.

137. Sauberlich HE. Laboratory Tests for the Assessment of Nutritional Status, 2nd edn. Boca Raton, FL: CRC Press, 1999.

138. Shils ME. Magnesium. In: Shils ME, Shike M, Ross AC, et al. (eds). Modern Nutrition in Health and Disease, 10th edn. Philadelphia: Lippincott Williams & Wilkins 2006:223.

139. Fleet JC, Cashman KD. Magnesium. In: Bowman BA, Russell RM (eds). Present Knowledge in Nutrition, 8th edn. Washington, DC: ILSI Press, 2001:292.

140. Reinhart RA. Magnesium metabolism. A review with special reference to the relationship between intracellular content and serum levels. Arch Intern Med 1988;148:2415.

141. Weisinger JR. Magnesium and phosphorus. Lancet 1998;352:391.

142. LaRoche M. Phosphate, the renal tubule, and the musculoskeletal system. Joint Bone Spine 2001;68:211.

143. Takeda E, Yamamoto H, Nashiki K, et al. Inorganic phosphate homeostasis and the role of dietary phosphorus. J Cell Mol Med 2004;8:191.

144. Tucker KL, Troy L, Morita K, et al. Carbonated beverage consumption and bone mineral density. J Bone Miner Res 2003;18:S241.

145. Hunt JR. Bioavailability of iron, zinc, and other trace minerals from vegetarian diets. Am J Clin Nutr 2003;78:633S.

146. Yip R. Iron. In: Bowman BA, Russell RM (eds). Present Knowledge in Nutrition, 8th edn. Washington, DC: ILSI Press, 2001:311.

147. Fleming RE, Bacon BR. Orchestration of iron homeostasis. N Engl J Med 2005;352:1741.

148. Frazer DM, Anderson GJ. The orchestration of body iron intake: how and where do enterocytes receive their cues? Blood Cell Mol Dis 2003;30:288.

149. Harris ED. Cellular transporters for zinc. Nutr Rev 2002;60:121.

150. Kerbs NF. Overview of zinc absorption and excretion in the human gastrointestinal tract. J Nutr 2000;130:1374S.

151. Whittaker P. Iron and zinc interactions in humans. Am J Clin Nutr 1998;68:442S.

152. Lönnerdal B. Dietary factors influencing zinc absorption. J Nutr 2000;130:1378S.

153. Klevay LM, Medeiros DM. Deliberations and evaluations of the approaches, endpoints, and paradigms for dietary recommendations about copper. J Nutr 1996;126:2419S.

154. Hughes J, Buttriss J. An update on copper. Nutrition Bulletin 2000;25:271.

155. Prohaska JR, Gybina AA. Intracellular copper transport in mammals. J Nutr 2004;124:1003.

156. Eisenstein RS. Discovery of the ceruloplasmin homologue hephaestin: new insight into the copper/iron connection. Nutr Rev 2000;58:22.

157. Schilsky ML. Wilson disease: new insights into pathogenesis, diagnosis, and future therapy. Curr Gastroenterol Rep 2005;7:26.

158. Beckett GJ, Arthur JR. Selenium and endocrine systems. J Endocrinology 2005;184:455.

159. Jeejeebhoy KN. The role of chromium in nutrition and therapeutics and as a potential toxin. Nutr Rev 1999;57:329.

160. Wright EM, Turk E. The sodium/glucose cotransport family SLC5. Pflugers Arch-Eur J Physiol 2004;447:510.

161. Berner YN, Schuller TR, Nielsen FH, et al. Selected ultratrace elements in total parenteral nutrition solutions. Am J Clin Nutr 1989;50:1079.

162. Ganapathy V, Smith SB, Prasad PD. SLC19: the folate/thiamine transporter family. Pflugers Arch-Eur J Physiol 2004;447:641.

163. Powers HJ. Riboflavin (vitamin B-2) and health. Am J Clin Nutr 2003;77:1352.

164. Jacob RA. Niacin. In: Bowman BA, Russell RM (eds). Present Knowledge in Nutrition, 8th edn. Washington, DC: ILSI Press, 2001:199.

165. Bailey LB, Moyers S, Gregory JF. Folic acid. In: Bowman BA, Russell RM (eds). Present Knowledge in Nutrition, 8th edn. Washington, DC: ILSI Press, 2001:214.

166. Botto LD, Moore CA, Khoury MJ, Erickson JD. Neural tube defects. N Engl J Med 1999;341:1509.

167. Ueland PM, Refsum H, Beresford SAA, Vollset SE. The controversy over homocysteine and cardiovascular risk. Am J Clin Nutr 2000;72:324.

168. Anonymous. Folate supplementation to prevent neural tube defects. Med Letter 2004;46:17.

169. Said HM, Kumar C. Intestinal absorption of vitamins. Curr Opin Gastroenterol 1999;15:172.

170. Herbert V. Recommended dietary intakes (RDI) of folate in humans. Am J Clin Nutr 1987;45:661.

171. Seetharam B, Alpers DH. Cobalamin binding proteins and their receptors. In: Dakshinamurti K (ed). Vitamin Receptors: Vitamins as Ligands in Cell Communication. Cambridge, UK: Cambridge University Press, 1994:78.

172. Moestrup SK, Kozyraki R. Cubilin, a high-density lipoprotein receptor. Curr Opin Lipidol 2000;11:133.

173. Alpers DH. What is new in vitamin B12? Curr Opin Gastroenterol 2005;21:183.

174. Packer L, Fuchs J. Vitamin C in Health and Disease. New York: Marcel Dekker, 1997.

175. Levine M, Conry-Cantilena C, Wang Y, et al. Vitamin C pharmacokinetics in healthy volunteers: evidence for a recommended dietary allowance. Proc Natl Acad Sci U S A 1996;93:3704.

176. Wilson JX. Regulation of vitamin C transport. Annu Rev Nutr 2005;25:105.

177. Said HM. Biotin: the forgotten vitamin. Am J Clin Nutr 2002;75:179.

178. Said HM, Mohammed ZM. Intestinal absorption of water-soluble vitamins: an update. Curr Opin Gastroenterol 2006;22:140.

179. Miller JW, Rogers LM, Rucker RB. Pantothenic acid. In: Bowman BA, Russell RM (eds). Present Knowledge in Nutrition, 8th edn. Washington, DC: ILSI Press, 2001:253.

180. Ross AC. Vitamin A and retinoids. In: Shils ME, Shike M, Caballero B, Cousins RJ (eds). Modern Nutrition in Health and Disease, 10th edn. Philadelphia: Lippincott Williams & Wilkins 2006:351.

181. Pryor WA, Stahl W, Rock CL. Beta carotene: from biochemistry to clinical trials. Nutr Rev 2000;58:39.

182. Cooper DA, Eldridge AL, Peters JC. Dietary carotenoids and certain cancers, heart disease, and age-related macular degeneration: a review of recent research. Nutr Rev 1999;57:201.

183. Harrison EH. Mechanisms of digestion and absorption of dietary vitamin A. Annu Rev Nutr 2005;25:87.

184. Holick MF. Vitamin D: importance in the prevention of cancers, type I diabetes, heart disease, and osteoporosis. Am J Clin Nutr 2004;79:362.

185. Monday A, Wang Z, Dhar PK. Bone and the kidney: a systems biology approach to the molecular mechanisms of renal osteodystrophy. Curr Mol Med 2005;5:489.

186. Whiting SJ, Calvo MS. Dietary recommendations for vitamin D: a critical need for functional endpoints to establish an estimated average requirement. J Nutr 2005;135:304.

187. Brigelius-Flohe R, Kelly FJ, Salonen JT, et al. The European perspective on vitamin E: current knowledge and future research. Am J Clin Nutr 2002;76:703.

188. Leonard SW, Good CK, Gugger ET, Traber MG. Vitamin E bioavailability from fortified breakfast cereal is greater than that from encapsulated supplements. Am J Clin Nutr 2004;79:86.

189. Traber MG. Vitamin E regulation. Curr Opin Gastroenterol 2005;21:223.

190. Hacquebard M, Carpentier YA. Vitamin E: absorption, plasma transport and cell uptake. Curr Opin Clin Nutr Metab Care 2005;8:133.

191. Traber MG. Vitamin E. In: Shils ME, Shike M, Ross AC, et al. (eds). Modern Nutrition in Health and Disease, 10th edn. Philadelphia: Lippincott Williams & Wilkins, 2005:396.

192. Booth SL, Suttie JW. Dietary intake and adequacy of vitamin K. J Nutr 1998;128:785.

193. Helphingstine CJ, Bistrian BR. New Food and Drug Administration requirements for inclusion of vitamin K in adult parenteral vitamins. JPEN J Parenter Enteral Nutr 2003;27:220.

194. Ferland G. Vitamin K In: Bowman BA, Russell RM (eds). Present Knowledge in Nutrition, 8th edn. Washington, DC: ILSI Press, 2001:164.

195. Hodges S, Walter P, Ranbeck W, et al. Beyond deficiency: potential benefits of increased intake of vitamin K for bone and vascular health. Eur J Nutr 2004;43:325.

196. Garrow TA. Choline and carnitine. In: Bowman BA, Russell RM

197. Buchman AL, Ament ME, Sobel M, et al. Choline deficiency causes reversible hepatic abnormalities in patients receiving parenteral nutrition: proof of a human choline requirement: a placebo-controlled trial. JPEN J Parenter Enteral Nutr 2001;25:260

198. Anonymous. L-carnitine. Med Lett Drugs Ther 2004;46:95.

199. Luiking YC, Poeze M, Dejong CH, et al. Sepsis: an arginine deficiency state? Crit Care Med 2004;32:2135.

200. Arginine metabolism: enzymology, nutrition, and clinical significance. Proceedings of a symposium dedicated to the memory of Vernon R. Young. April 5–6, 2004, Bermuda. J Nutr 2004;134:2741S.

201. Heyland DK, Novak F, Drover JW, et al. Should immunonutrition become routine in critically ill patients? JAMA 2001;286:944.

202. Buchman AL. Glutamine: commercially essential or conditionally essential? A critical appraisal of the human data. Am J Clin Nutr 2001;74:25.

203. Novak F, Heyland DK, Avenell A, et al. Glutamine supplementation in serious illness: a systematic review of the evidence. Crit Care Med 2002;30:2022.

204. Savarese DMF, Savy G, Vahdat L, et al. Prevention of chemotherapy and radiation toxicity with glutamine. Cancer Treat Rev 2003;29:501.

205. Alpers DH. Glutamine: do the data support the cause for supplementation in humans? Gastroenterology 2006;130:S106.

206. Stewart W, Fleming LW. Features of a successful therapeutic fast of 382 days' duration. Postgrad Med J 1973;49:203.

207. Klein S, Sakurai Y, Romijn JA, Carroll RM. Progressive alterations in lipid and glucose metabolism during short-term fasting in humans. Am J Physiol 1993;265:E801.

208. Klein S, Holland OB, Wolfe RR. Importance of blood glucose concentration in regulating lipolysis during fasting in humans. Am J Physiol 1990;258:E32.

209. Klein S, Peters EJ, Holland OB, Wolfe RR. Effect of short- and long-term β-adrenergic blockade on lipolysis during fasting in humans. Am J Physiol 1989;257:E65.

210. Wolfe RR, Peters EJ, Klein S, et al. Effect of short-term fasting on lipolytic responsiveness in normal and obese human subjects. Am J Physiol 1987;252 (Endocrinol Metab 15):E189.

211. Foster DW. From glycogen to ketones and back. Diabetes 1984;33:1188.

212. Garber AJ, Menzel PH, Boden G, Owen OE. Hepatic ketogenesis and gluconeogenesis in humans. J Clin Invest 1974;54:981.

213. Owen OE, Morgan AP, Kemp HG, et al. Brain metabolism during fasting. J Clin Invest 1967;46:1589.

214. Jahoor F, Peters EJ, Wolfe RR. The relationship between gluconeogenic substrate supply and glucose production in humans. Am J Physiol 1990;258 (Endocrinol Metab 21):E288.

215. Nilsson LH, Hultman E. Liver glycogen in man – the effect of total starvation or a carbohydrate-poor diet followed by carbohydrate refeeding. Scand J Lab Clin Invest 1973;32:325.

216. Aoki TT. Metabolic adaptations to starvation, semistarvation, and carbohydrate restriction. In: Selvey N, White PL (eds) Nutrition in the 1980s: Constraints on Our Knowledge. New York: Alan R Liss, 1981:161.

217. Vignati L, Finley RJ, Haag S, Aoki TT. Protein conservation during prolonged fast: a function of triiodothyronine levels. Trans Assoc Am Physicians 1978;91:169.

218. Sherwin RS, Hendler RG, Felig P. Effect of ketone infusions on amino acid and nitrogen metabolism in man. J Clin Invest 1975;55:1382.

219. Keys A, Brozek J, Henschel A, et al. The Biology of Human Starvation. Minneapolis: University of Minnesota Press, 1950.

220. Vagenakis AG, Burger A, Portnary GI, et al. Diversion of peripheral thyroxine metabolism from activating to inactivating pathways during complete fasting. J Clin Endocrinol Metab 1975;41:191.

221. Young JB, Rosa RM, Landsberg L. Dissociation of sympathetic nervous system and adrenal medullary responses. Am J Physiol 1984;247:E35.

222. Benedict FG. A Study of Prolonged Fasting. Washington, DC: Carnegie Institute, 1915 (publication No. 203).

223. Hagan SN, Scow RO. Effect of fasting on muscle proteins and fat in young rats of different ages. Am J Physiol 1957;188:91.

224. Cuthbertson DP. Observations on the disturbance of metabolism produced by injury to the limbs. Q J Med 1932;1:233.

225. Moore FD. Bodily changes during surgical convalescence. Ann Surg 1959;137:289.

226. Fong Y, Lowry SF. Metabolic consequences of critical illness. In: Barie PS, Shires GT (eds). Surgical Intensive Care. Boston: Little, Brown and Company, 1993:893.

227. Pomposelli JJ, Flores BS, Bistrian BR. Role of biochemical mediators in clinical nutrition and surgical metabolism. JPEN J Parenter Enteral Nutr 1988;12:212.

228. Tracey KJ, Beuthea B, Lowry SF, et al. Shock and tissue injury induced by recombinant human cachectin. Science 1986;234:470.

229. Michie HR, Manogue KR, Spriggs DR. Detection of circulating tumor necrosis factor after endotoxin administration. N Engl J Med 1988;318:1481.

230. Beutler B. The presence of cachectin/tumor necrosis factor in human disease states. Am J Med 1988;85:287.

231. Barie PS, Jones WG. Multiple organ failure. In: Barie PS, Shires GT (eds). Surgical Intensive Care. Boston: Little, Brown and Company, 1993:147.

232. Beisel WR. Metabolic response to infection. In: Kinney JM, Jeejeebhoy KN, Hill GL, Owen OE (eds). Nutrition and Metabolism in Patient Care. Philadelphia: WB Saunders, 1988:605.

233. Dinarello CA. Cytokines as endogenous pyrogens. J Infect Dis 1999;179:S294.

234. Bron D, Meuleman N, Mascaux C. Biological basis of anemia. Semin Oncol 2001;28:S1.

235. Means RT Jr. Advances in the anemia of chronic disease. Int J Hematol 1999;70:7.

236. Fahey TJ, Tracey KJ. Cytokines, tumor necrosis factor, and other mediators of sepsis. In: Carlson RW, Geheb MA (eds). Principles and Practice of Medical Intensive care. Philadelphia: WB Saunders, 1993:311.

237. Souba WW, Wilmore DW. Diet and nutrition in the care of the patient with surgery, trauma, and sepsis. In: Shils ME, Young VR (eds). Modern Nutrition in Health and Disease, 7th edn. Philadelphia: Lea & Febiger, 1988:1306.

238. Allard JP, Jeejeebhoy KN, Whitwell J, et al. Factors influencing energy expenditure in patients with burns. J Trauma 1988;28:199.

239. Wilmore DW, Orcutt TW, Mason AD, Pruitt BA. Alterations in hypothalamic function following thermal injury. J Trauma 1975;15:697.

240. Douglas RG, Shaw JH. Metabolic response to sepsis and trauma. Br J Surg 1989;76:115.

241. Goldstein SA, Elwyn DH. The effects of injury and sepsis on fuel utilization. Annu Rev Nutr 1989;9:445.

242. Shaw JH, Wolfe RR. Energy and protein metabolism in sepsis and trauma. Aust N Z J Surg 1978;57:41.

243. Gann DS, Amaral JF, Caldwell MD. Metabolic response to injury, stress and starvation. In: Davis JH, Drucker WR, Foster RS, et al. (eds). Clinical Surgery. St Louis: CV Mosby, 1987:337.

244. Beisel WR, Wannemacher RW. Gluconeogenesis, ureagenesis, and ketogenesis during sepsis. JPEN J Parenter Enteral Nutr 1980;4:277.

245. Jahoor F, Shangraw RE, Miyoshi H, et al. Role of insulin and glucose oxidation in mediating the protein catabolism of burns and sepsis. Am J Physiol 1989;257:E323.

246. Sakurai Y, Aarsland S, Herndon DN, et al. Stimulation of muscle protein synthesis by long-term insulin infusion in severely burned patients. Ann Surg 1995;222:283.

247. Cuthbertson DP. The metabolic response to injury and its nutritional implications: retrospect and prospect. JPEN J Parenter Enteral Nutr 1979;3:108.

248. Long C, Kinney JM, Geiger JW. Nonsuppressibility of gluconeogenesis by glucose septic patients. Metabolism 1976;25:193.

249. Klein S, Peters EJ, Shangraw RE, Wolf RR. Lipolytic response to metabolic stress in patients with critical illness. Crit Care Med 1991;19:776.

30 Approach to the patient requiring nutritional supplementation

David H. Alpers, Beth Taylor, Samuel Klein

Nutritional assessment, 588
Choosing the route for nutritional support, 591
Enteral nutrition, 592
Parenteral nutrition, 596
Nutritional support in the hospitalized patient with gastrointestinal disease, 599
Micronutrient deficiency and treatment, 600

Nutritional assessment

Most methods used to evaluate nutritional status are aimed at identifying specific nutrient deficiencies or protein–energy malnutrition. The diagnoses and treatments of specific nutrient deficiencies are usually straightforward. For example, potassium deficiency can be identified by measuring the serum potassium concentration and can be corrected by oral or intravenous potassium supplementation. In contrast, the diagnosis of protein–energy malnutrition is more complicated. Commonly used indicators of nutritional status have been validated by linking nutritional indicators with clinical outcome; patients with abnormal indicators have a worse outcome than patients with normal indicators. However, all indicators are influenced by illness or injury, so it is difficult to separate the contribution of malnutrition from that of the illness itself. Therefore, if nutritional status is linked to the severity of disease, patients who are "malnourished" may have a poor outcome simply because they are sicker than patients who are "well nourished." Moreover, nutritional therapy may not improve outcome unless malnutrition is an independent contributor to adverse medical events.

Nutritional assessment techniques
Specific nutrient deficiency
A careful history and physical examination, routine blood tests, and selected laboratory tests based on the history and physical examination findings can be used to diagnose specific macronutrient, mineral, vitamin, and trace mineral deficiencies (Tables 30.1–30.3) [1].

Protein–energy malnutrition
Ideally, nutritional assessment is used to identify those patients who will benefit from nutritional support. However, the indicators used to assess protein–energy malnutrition have been validated by determining their relationship to clinical outcome rather than to the response of patients to nutritional therapy.

Body mass and composition
In general, unintentional weight loss is associated with an adverse clinical outcome [2]. However, the assessment of changes in body weight can be confounded by errors in recall and changes in body water. Anthropometry, the measurement of triceps and subscapular skinfold thickness, provides an index of body fat and muscle mass, which is compared with the values in standard tables. Although the interpretation of these data may be limited by differences in age and ethnicity between patients and the standard population, interrater variability, and hydration, markedly abnormal values (below the 5th percentile) usually predict a poor clinical outcome. Body muscle mass can also be assessed in the clinical setting by measuring the urinary creatinine excretion [3]. Patient values can be compared with those in tables indicating an expected amount of creatinine excretion in relationship to height in subjects consuming a meat-free diet [1]. The body mass index (BMI), which is obtained by dividing weight (kilograms) by the square of the height (meters squared), can help identify patients at increased risk for medical complications (Table 30.4).

Principles of Clinical Gastroenterology. Edited by Tadataka Yamada, David H. Alpers, Anthony N. Kalloo, Neil Kaplowitz, Chung Owyang, and Don W. Powell. © 2008 Blackwell Publishing. ISBN 978-1-4051-69103

Table 30.1 Some physical signs of nutritional deficiency

	Finding	Deficiency
Hair	Thin, sparse	Protein, zinc, biotin
	Flag sign (transverse depigmentation)	Protein, copper
	Easy pluckability	Protein
Nails	Spoon-shaped (koilonychia)	Iron
	No luster, transverse ridging	Protein–energy
Skin	Dry, scaling (xerosis)	Vitamin A, zinc
	Seborrheic dermatitis	Essential fatty acids (EFAs), zinc, pyridoxine, biotin
	Flaky paint dermatosis	Protein
	Follicular hyperkeratosis	Vitamin A, vitamin C, EFAs
	Nasolabial seborrhea	Niacin (B-1), pyridoxine (B-6), riboflavin (B-2)
	Petechiae, purpura	Vitamin C, vitamin K, vitamin A
	Pigmentation, desquamation	Niacin (pellagra)
	Pallor	Folate, iron, cobalamin, copper, biotin
Eyes	Angular palpebritis	Riboflavin
	Blepharitis	B vitamins
	Corneal vascularization	Riboflavin
	Dull, dry conjunctivae	Vitamin A
	Bitot spots	Vitamin A
	Keratomalacia	Vitamin A
	Fundal capillary microaneurysms	Vitamin C
	Ophthalmoplegia	Thiamin (Wernicke encephalopathy)
Mouth	Angular stomatitis	B vitamins, iron, protein
	Cheilosis	Riboflavin, niacin, pyridoxine, protein
	Atrophic lingual papillae	Niacin, iron, riboflavin, folate, cobalamin
	Glossitis (scarlet, raw)	Niacin, pyridoxine, riboflavin, folate, cobalamin
	Decreased sense of taste and smell	Vitamin A, ?zinc
	Swollen, bleeding gums	Vitamin C
Glands	Parotid enlargement	Protein
	"Sicca" syndrome	Ascorbic acid
	Thyroid enlargement	Iodine
Heart	Enlargement, tachycardia, high-output failure	Thiamin (wet beriberi)
	Small heart, decreased output	Protein–energy
	Cardiomyopathy	Selenium
	Cardiac arrhythmias	Magnesium, potassium
Extremities	Edema	Protein, thiamin
	Muscle weakness	Protein–energy, selenium
	Bone and joint tenderness (child)	Vitamin C, vitamin A
	Osteopenia, bone pain	Vitamin D, calcium, phosphorus, vitamin C
Neurological	Confabulation, disorientation	Thiamin (Korsakoff psychosis)
	Decreased positional and vibratory senses, ataxia	Cobalamin, thiamin
	Decreased tendon reflexes	Thiamin
	Weakness, paresthesia	Cobalamin, pyridoxine, thiamin
	Mental disorders	Cobalamin, niacin, thiamin, magnesium
Other	Delayed wound healing	Vitamin C, protein, ?zinc, ?EFAs
	Hypogonadism, delayed puberty	Zinc
	Glucose intolerance	Chromium

Table 30.2 Clinical laboratory tests for detection of vitamin deficiency

Vitamin	Test	Source	Reference range (units)[a]		Usefulness
			Marginal	Deficient	
B-1	Transketolase ratio	RBC	1.16–1.24	> 1.25	+ When severe
	Thiamin	Serum		< 12.7 (nmol/L)	Direct measure
	Thiamin	Urine		< 27 (μg/g creatinine)	
B-2	GSH-reductase ratio	Serum	1.20–1.40	> 1.40	Body stores
	Riboflavin	Urine	27–79	< 27 (μg/g creatinine)	Recent intake
B-6	AST activity ratio	RBC	1.70–1.85	> 1.85	Body stores
	Pyridoxal 5-PO$_4$	Plasma	20–30	< 20 (nmol/L)	Stores, sensitive
	4-Pyridoxic acid	Urine		< 3.0 (μmol/day)	Recent intake
	Total vitamin B-6	Urine		< 0.5 (μmol/day)	Recent intake
Niacin	N-methylnicotinamide	Urine	0.5–2.5	< 0.5 (mg/g creatinine)	Recent intake
	2-Pyridone	Urine	2.0–3.9	< 2.0 (mg/g creatinine)	Recent intake
Folate	Folic acid	Plasma	3.0–5.9	< 3.0 (ng/mL)	Stores + intake
	Folic acid	RBC	140–159	< 140 (ng/mL)	Body stores
Folate or B-12	Homocysteine	Plasma	12–15	> 15 (μmol/L)	Function
B-12	Cobalamin	Serum	150–200	< 150 (pg/mL)	Body stores
	Methylmalonic acid	Serum		> 376 (nmol/L)	Function
	Holotranscobalamin II	Serum	40–60	> 60 (pg/mL)	Function
C	Ascorbic acid	Serum	11–23	< 11 (μmol/L)	Recent intake
	Ascorbic acid	WBC	10–20	< 10 (μg/10^8 cells)	Stores
A	Retinol	Plasma	10–19	< 10 (μg/dL)	Stores + intake
	Retinol-binding protein	Plasma		< 50 (mg/L)	Function
D	25-OH vitamin D	Serum	12–25	< 12 (nmol/L)	Body stores
	1,25-dihydroxyvitamin D	Serum	48–65	< 48 (pmol/L)	Function
E	α-Tocopherol	Serum	5.0–7.0	< 5 (μg/mL)	Body stores
	α-Tocopherol/total lipid	Serum	0.8–1.0	< 0.8	Preferred
	H$_2$O$_2$ hemolysis	RBC	10–20	> 20 (%)	Function
K	Prothrombin time	Plasma	1.5–2.0	2.0 (s over control)	Function
	Phylloquinone			< 0.35 (nmol/L)	Recent intake

a Precise values may vary between laboratories.
AST, aspartate aminotransferase; GSH, reduced glutathione; RBC, red blood cells; WBC, white blood cells.
Adapted from Alpers et al. [1].

Serum protein concentrations

The concentrations of several plasma proteins, particularly albumin, correlate with clinical outcome: a low plasma albumin concentration is associated with an increased incidence of medical complications [4,5]. Illness or injury, however, rather than malnutrition per se, are responsible for hypoalbuminemia in sick patients [6]. Inflammation and injury decrease albumin synthesis, increase albumin degradation, and increase albumin transcapillary losses. Specific gastrointestinal, renal, and cardiac diseases can increase albumin losses through the gut or kidney. Wounds, burns, and peritonitis cause losses from surface tissues. Nutritional support itself

does not usually alter serum albumin levels [7]. Serum concentrations of transferrin, retinol-binding protein, and thyroxine-binding prealbumin are also affected by inflammation, so that they are unreliable as a measure of protein–energy malnutrition.

Immune system function

The total circulating lymphocyte count and delayed cutaneous hypersensitivity to skin test antigens have been used as clinical indicators of malnutrition. Although depression of circulating lymphocytes (< 200/mm^3) and anergy assessed by delayed cutaneous hypersensitivity are associated with a

Table 30.3 Laboratory detection of micronutrient mineral deficiency

Nutrient	Test	Source	Reference range (units)[a]	Usefulness
Iron	Iron	Serum	50–200 (µg/dL)	Poor measure of body stores
	Total iron-binding capacity	Serum	245–400 (µg/dL)	
	Iron-binding saturation		15–50 (%)	Insensitive for iron status
	Transferrin	Serum	200–400 (µg/dL)	Preferred over TIBC if available
	Ferritin	Serum	12–300 (ng/mL)	Measures body stores: high specificity when stores low, poor sensitivity
Zinc	Zinc	Plasma	20–130 (µg/dL)	Poor specificity for body stores
	Zinc tolerance test	Plasma	> Twofold increase over baseline at 2 h	For malabsorption
Copper	Copper	Serum	55–175 (µg/dL)	Insensitive for body stores
	Ceruloplasmin	Plasma	10–60 (mg/dL)	Independent of body stores
Selenium	Selenium	Serum	100–340 (ng/mL)	Insensitive for body stores
	Glutathione peroxidase	Plasma	455–800 (U/L)	More sensitive for body stores

a May vary in different laboratories.
TIBC, total iron-binding capacity.
Adapted from Alpers et al. [1].

Table 30.4 Body mass index (BMI) as a measure of associated disease risk

Weight category	BMI (kg/m²)	Risk
Extremely underweight	< 14.0	Extremely high
Underweight	14.1–18.4	Increased in smokers, chronic illness
Normal	18.5–24.9	Normal
Overweight	25–29.9	Increased
Obesity		
Class I	30.0–34.9	High
Class II	35.0–39.9	Very high
Class III	≥ 40.0	Extremely high

Adapted from National Institute of Diabetes and Digestive and Kidney Diseases. Clinical guidelines on the identification, evaluation, and treatment of overweight and obesity in adults – the evidence report. Obes Res 1998;6:S53.

poor clinical outcome, they are not specific for nutritional deficiency and are affected by specific diseases, injury, and certain drugs.

Subjective global assessment
The subjective global assessment involves a focused history and physical examination to determine the adequacy of nutrient intake and the possible effect of malnutrition on body composition and organ function (Fig. 30.1) [8,9]. In addition, it includes an analysis of the patient's future ability to ingest adequate nutrients. The findings of the history and physical examination are subjectively weighted to rank patients as well nourished, moderately malnourished, or severely malnourished. Patients who are judged to be severely malnourished are at high risk for medical complications and adverse outcome [8,10].

There is no "gold standard" for determining nutritional status. All current approaches are influenced by the severity of illness and have been validated by assessing clinical outcome rather than by nutrition-specific parameters. Therefore, current nutritional assessment techniques identify sick patients. Although it is often assumed that "malnourished" patients will benefit from nutritional support, this assumption has not been documented in prospective randomized clinical trials [11].

Choosing the route for nutritional support

The decision to initiate nonvolitional nutritional support is complex and involves a clinical assessment of the patient's nutrient intake, body fat and protein mass, protein and energy requirements, severity of illness, and anticipated duration of inadequate volitional intake. Once it has been decided that nonvolitional nutritional support is indicated, the route of nutritional support must be considered. The usual course is to choose the oral or enteral route when this approach can be used effectively and safely. There are several reasons for this choice. First, enteral nutrition may provide nutrients that are not available from parenteral nutrition. The best example of this principle is the provision of short-chain fatty acids to the colonic mucosa through the bacterial degradation of fiber

A History

1 Weight change

Overall loss in past 6 months: amount = _____ kg

Change in past week: _____ increase

_____ no change

_____ decrease

2 Dietary intake change (relative to normal)

_____ No change

_____ Change: duration = _____ weeks

type: _____ suboptimal solid diet _____ full liquid diet

_____ hypocaloric liquids _____ starvation

3 Gastrointestinal symptoms (that persisted > 2 weeks)

_____ none _____ anorexia _____ nausea _____ vomiting _____ diarrhea

4 Functional capacity

_____ No dysfunction (e.g., full capacity)

_____ Dysfunction: duration = _____ weeks

_____ working suboptimally

_____ ambulatory

_____ bedridden

5 Disease and its relation to nutritional requirements

Primary diagnosis (specify) _____

Metabolic demand (stress) _____ none _____ low _____ moderate _____ high

B Physical (for each trait specify: 0 = normal, 1+ = mild, 2+ = moderate, 3+ = severe)

_____ loss of subcutaneous fat (triceps, chest)

_____ muscle wasting (quadriceps, deltoids, temporals)

_____ ankle edema, sacral edema

_____ ascites

_____ tongue or skin lesions suggesting nutrient deficiency

C SGA rating (select one)

_____ A = Well nourished (minimal or no restriction of food intake or absorption, minimal change in function, weight stable or increasing)

_____ B = Moderately malnourished (food restriction, some function changes, little or no change in body mass)

_____ C = Severely malnourished (definitely decreased intake, function, and body mass)

Figure 30.1 Subjective global assessment (SGA) of nutritional status. Adapted from Klein et al. [11].

or unabsorbed carbohydrate. The provision of this important colonic energy source may maintain colonic function [12]. Second, it is felt that lumenal nutrients may prevent atrophy in the small intestinal mucosa. Atrophy occurs in rats fed by parenteral nutrition, but the importance of this phenomenon in humans is still uncertain [13]. Finally, enteral feeding may be safer than parenteral nutrition [14–16].

If oral or enteral feeding is chosen, intestinal motility and the absorptive surface must be adequate. Other disorders that interfere with enteral feeding include severe diarrheal illnesses, extensive inflammatory bowel disease, acute gastrointestinal bleeding, conditions that will require abdominal surgery in the near future, obstructing small bowel or colonic lesions, and acute inflammation of the pancreas or biliary tract. Guidelines have been developed that provide useful and practical information for the clinician [17,18]. The guidelines for use in specific disorders, such as AIDS, are practical modifications of the generalized guidelines, with special emphasis on the problems of feeding patients with that disorder [19]. However, the clinician should not rely on a set pattern of guidelines for decisions regarding nutritional support. The published guidelines should be used as resource material to aid in the clinical judgment required for each patient.

Enteral nutrition

The availability of so many different types of nutritionally complete diets and defined formulas makes it possible for many hospitalized patients to receive adequate nutrient intake by oral or enteral tube feedings.

Whole-food diets include a regular hospital diet and diets modified in either consistency (e.g., clear-liquid, full-liquid, pureed, and soft diets) or nutrient content (e.g., low-residue, low-fat, low-sodium, low-protein, and high-fiber diets). In many cases, nutrient intake can be increased by encouraging the ingestion of ordinary food and by avoiding missed meals and unpalatable diets. Many patients eat more if they are given assistance at mealtimes and provided with desired foods, and if some food is supplied by relatives and friends is allowed.

Table 30.5 Classification of commercially available enteral nutrition products

Modular type	Indication	Examples
Intact protein	Standard	Boost, Ensure, Isosource, Nutren 1.0, Osmolite, Petpinex 1.0, Peptinex 1.5, Peptinex DT, Resource
	Volume-restricted	Boost Plus, Ensure Plus, Isosource 1.5, Jevity 1.5, Nutren 1.5, Nutren 2.0, Resource 2.0
	High-protein	Boost High Protein, Isosource HN, Nutren Replete, Osmolite 1, Osmolite 1.5, Promote
	Disease-specific	Boost Diabetic, Diabetisource AC, Ensure Plus, Glucerna, Juven, Nepro, Novasource Pulmonary, Novasource Renal, Nutren Glytrol, Nutren Pulmonary, NutriHep, Oxepa, Pulmocare, Renalcal, Suplena
	Immunonutrition	Crucial, Impact, Impact Advanced Recovery, Impact Glutamine, Impact with Fiber, Perative, Pivot 1.5, TraumaCal
	Fiber supplement	Ensure Fiber, Fibersource, Jevity 1, Nutren 1.0 Fiber, Nutren ProBalance, Nutren Replete Fiber, Promote With Fiber, Resource Benefiber
	Milk-based	Carnation Instant, Carnation Instant No Sugar Added, Resource Instant Breakfast, Resource Milkshake
Elemental	Digestion-impaired	Crucial, Peptamen, Vivonex TEN, Vital HN, Optimental, Peptinex, FAA free amino acid diet
Protein-limited	Protein supplement	Additions (526 kcal/100 g), Resource Beneprotein (357 kcal/100 g)
CHO-limited	CHO supplement	Resource Benecalorie (800 kcal/100 g), Polycose liquid (10 kcal/5 mL), Polycose powder (380 kcal/100 g)
Fat-limited	Fat supplement	MCT oil (830 kcal/100 g)

Note: caloric density ranges from 1.0 to 1.5 kcal/mL for the intact protein and elemental products, except for the volume-restricted products, in which the caloric density is 1.5–2.0 kcal/mL and is often identified in the product name by number.
CHO, carbohydrate.

Defined formulas are commercially made products with a known "defined" nutrient composition (Table 30.5). These formulas can be divided into five categories: feeding modules, monomeric formulas, oligomeric formulas, polymeric formulas, and disease-specific formulas. Feeding modules consist of single nutrients, such as protein (intact protein, hydrolyzed protein, or crystalline amino acids), carbohydrate (glucose polymers), or fat (long-chain or medium-chain triglycerides), that can be used to supplement a specific diet or be part of a modular enteral system composed of several nutrient modules.

Monomeric (elemental) formulas contain nitrogen in the form of free amino acids and usually only small amounts of fat (< 5% of total calories). Therefore, these formulas can be useful in patients who require an extremely low-fat diet. However, monomeric formulas are hyperosmolar, unpalatable, and more expensive than polymeric formulas, and in the absence of pancreatic insufficiency, they are absorbed no better than oligomeric or polymeric formulas [20].

Oligomeric (semielemental) formulas contain hydrolyzed protein in the form of small peptides and sometimes free amino acids. Fat represents 5%–40% of energy content as either long-chain triglycerides or a combination of long-chain and medium-chain triglycerides. Data from several studies suggest that oligomeric diets can reduce diarrhea and other gastrointestinal side effects in critically ill patients [21] and in patients receiving abdominal irradiation and chemotherapy [22]. However, the purported clinical benefits of oligomeric formulas require confirmation in large prospect-

ive clinical trials before precise recommendations regarding their use can be made.

Polymeric formulas contain nitrogen in the form of whole proteins. These formulas can be categorized into three groups: blenderized food formulas, milk-based formulas, and lactose-free formulas. Milk-based formulas usually contain milk as a source of protein and fat and tend to be more palatable than other defined diets. Although milk-based formulas can be problematic for lactose-intolerant patients, they are often tolerated when infused continuously to decrease the load of lactose delivered to the intestine at any one time. Lactose-free formulas are the most commonly used polymeric formulas in hospitalized patients, and many modifications in protein and fat content are available. Disease-specific formulas have been designed for patients who have specific illnesses, including hepatic insufficiency, renal insufficiency, pulmonary insufficiency, diabetes, and severe metabolic stress. In general, the clinical superiority of these formulas over less expensive, standard polymeric enteral formulas remains controversial. However, branched-chain amino acid-enriched formulas may permit greater nitrogen intake in selected patients with chronic protein-intolerant hepatic encephalopathy (see "Nutritional support in the hospitalized patient with gastrointestinal disease"), and renal failure formulas contain much smaller amounts of sodium, potassium, phosphorus, and magnesium than standard formulas.

Over the last 10 years more than 500 articles have been published addressing the benefits and risks of immunonutrition. Immunonutrition formulas are supplemented with one or a combination of immune stimulants, such as arginine, glutamine, omega-3 fatty acids, and nucleotides (Table 30.5). A metaanalysis of randomized clinical trials comparing immunonutrition to standard products concluded there were no significant effects on mortality, infectious complications, length of stay, or time on the ventilator in critically ill patients [23]. A higher mortality rate has been observed in septic patients receiving immunonutrition when compared with similar patients receiving parenteral nutrition [24]. However, a significant reduction in infectious complications and length of stay was observed in elective surgery patients. Interpreting the data on immunonutrition is hampered by differing study populations, inconsistent use of blinding, the use of different control feeds, and small sample sizes.

A positive caloric balance is necessary to optimize and sometimes to achieve positive nitrogen balance, and to incorporate amino acids into new protein. To achieve this goal, the ingestion of about 25–35 kcal/g of protein (105–146 kJ/g) (~ 150–200 kcal/g [630–835 kJ/g] of nitrogen) is required. This ratio is based on the derivation of 10%–15% of caloric needs during catabolism from protein degradation.

Oral rehydration therapy

Patients with protracted vomiting or diarrhea can lose excessive amounts of fluid and electrolytes. Oral rehydration therapy enhances sodium and water absorption by stimulating sodium/glucose cotransport in the small intestine. Oral rehydration therapy has been demonstrated to have considerable clinical benefits in patients with severe gastrointestinal fluid and mineral losses, such as those with cholera-induced diarrhea, high-output ostomies, and short bowel syndrome [25–31].

A variety of oral rehydration solutions are available (Table 30.6). The World Health Organization developed a solution based on the results of studies in patients with cholera [30]. The glucose component of an oral rehydration solution should be provided at concentrations between 70 and 150 mmol/L. Higher concentrations of glucose can be deleterious because the increase in osmolality may reduce water absorption. Making the solution hypotonic by replacing glucose with rice solids or other polymeric forms can decrease stool output compared with isotonic solutions [26–29]. In patients with short bowel syndrome ending in a jejunostomy, net sodium and fluid balance is related to jejunal length. Patients with less than 100 cm of jejunum are usually net secretors, whereas those with more than 100 cm of jejunum are usually net absorbers [31]. The use of oral rehydration therapy can markedly decrease ostomy output and convert some patients from net secretors to net absorbers. In these patients, the consumption of electrolyte replacement drinks containing 60 mmol or less of sodium per liter causes a negative sodium and fluid balance, whereas the balance becomes positive after the ingestion of solutions containing 90 mEq/L and is maximal at concentrations of 120 to 160 mEq/L [32,33]. Sport drinks and commercially made defined liquid formula diets do not contain an adequate amount of sodium for maximal fluid absorption in patients with severe short bowel syndrome and a jejunostomy.

Tube feeding
General principles

Enteral tube feeding is useful in patients who have a functional gastrointestinal tract but who cannot or will not ingest adequate nutrients. Many approaches to tube feeding are possible (e.g., nasogastric, nasoduodenal, nasojejunal, gastrostomy, jejunostomy, pharyngostomy, esophagostomy tubes) and depend on physician experience, clinical prognosis, anticipated duration of feeding, patency and motility of the gut, risk for aspiration of gastric contents, and patient preference.

Table 30.6 Characteristics of selected oral rehydration solutions

Product	Na (mEq/L)	K (mEq/L)	Cl (mEq/L)	Citrate (mEq/L)	kcal/L	CHO (g/L)	mOsmol/kg
Equalyte	78	22	68	30	100	30	305
CeraLyte 70	70	20	98	30	165	40	235
CeraLyte 50	50	20	40	30	240	60	240
Pedialyte	45	20	35	30	100	20	300
Gatorade	20	3	N/A	N/A	210	45	330
WHO[a]	90	20	80	30	80	20	200
Washington University[b]	105	0	100	10	85	20	250

a WHO (World Health Organization) formula: mix 3/4 tsp (teaspoon) sodium chloride, 1/2 tsp sodium citrate, 1/4 tsp potassium chloride, and 4 tsp glucose (dextrose) in 1 L (4 1/4 cups) of distilled water.
b Washington University formula: mix 3/4 tsp sodium chloride, 1/2 tsp sodium citrate, and 3 tbsp (tablespoons) + 1 tsp Polycose powder in 1 L (4 1/4 cups) of distilled water.
CHO, carbohydrate.
Adapted from Klein S. Nutritional therapy. In: Ahya S, Flood K, Paranjothi S (eds). The Washington Manual of Medical Therapeutics, 30th edn. Philadelphia: Lippincott Williams & Wilkins, 2000:27.

Short-term feeding (< 6 weeks) can be achieved by the placement of a soft, small-bore nasogastric or nasoenteric feeding tube. These tubes are made of silicone or polyurethane and can be left in place without the tissue irritation or pressure necrosis caused by larger polyvinyl chloride tubes. Many patients are able to eat with the tube in place, which permits the use of tube feeding to supplement oral intake. Nasogastric feeding is usually the most appropriate route, but orogastric feeding can be used in cases of nasal injury or gross nasal deformity. Nasoduodenal or nasojejunal feeding is useful in patients with gastroparesis. In addition, by taking advantage of the barrier function of the pyloric and gastroesophageal sphincters, nasoenteric feeding may decrease the incidence of aspiration in high-risk patients. However, the prevention of aspiration by feeding beyond the pylorus has not been proved in clinical trials.

Most patients who require long-term tube feeding (> 6 weeks) should have a gastrostomy or jejunostomy tube placed. These tubes can be placed endoscopically, radiologically, or surgically, depending on the clinical situation and local expertise. Percutaneous endoscopic gastrostomy can be performed within 30 min and is successfully completed in more than 90% of attempts [34]. Gastrostomy tubes can be placed percutaneously without endoscopy by inserting the catheter directly into the stomach by a peel-away sheath introduced over a previously placed J-wire guide [35]. This approach is particularly useful in patients with an obstructing lesion of the esophagus or hypopharynx that prevents passage of an endoscope or a gastrostomy tube bumper. A summation of data from several large series suggests that percutaneous endoscopic gastrostomy tube placement is associated with mortality in 0.5%, major complications (peristomal leakage with peritonitis, necrotizing fasciitis of the anterior abdominal wall, gastric hemorrhage) in 1%, and minor complications (minor wound infections, stomal leaks, tube extrusion or migration, aspiration, gastrocolic fistula, ileus, fever) in 8% of patients [36]. Jejunal tube placement can be achieved by threading a tube through an existing gastrostomy or by percutaneous endoscopic jejunostomy in patients with previous partial or total gastrectomy [37–41].

Surgical gastrostomy is more expensive than percutaneous endoscopic gastrostomy unless the tube is placed during an operation performed for another reason. A jejunostomy tube may also be placed at the time of abdominal surgery and consists of a subserosal tunnel or needle catheter jejunostomy. Gastrostomy and jejunostomy tubes can also be placed by using laparoscopic techniques.

Administration of tube feeding

Patients with feeding tubes in their stomach can often tolerate intermittent gravity feedings, in which the total amount of daily formula is divided into four to six equal portions that are infused by gravity over 30–60 min. The patient's upper body should be elevated by more than 30° during and for at least 1 h after feeding. Intermittent feedings are useful for patients who cannot be positioned with the head of the bed continuously elevated or who require greater freedom from feeding. However, patients who experience nausea and early satiety with bolus gravity feedings may require continuous infusion at a slower rate. Patients who have gastroparesis often tolerate gastric tube feedings when they are started at a slow rate (e.g., 10 mL/h) and advanced by small increments (e.g., 10 mL/h every 8–12 h). However, patients with severe gastroparesis require passage of the feeding tube tip past the ligament of Treitz. Continuous infusion should always be used when feeding directly into the duodenum or jejunum to avoid distention, abdominal pain, and dumping syndrome.

Complications

Mechanical, metabolic, and gastrointestinal complications can occur in patients receiving tube feedings. Although the placement of nasogastric tubes is usually safe, tubes can be misplaced, particularly in unconscious patients. Intubation of the tracheobronchial tree has been reported in up to 15% of patients, and intracranial placement can occur in patients with skull fractures. Feeding tubes can cause nasopharyngeal erosions, pharyngitis, sinusitis, otitis media, pneumothorax, and gastrointestinal tract perforation.

Small-diameter nasogastric tubes (e.g., 8F or 9F) are usually used to lessen nasopharyngeal irritation. These small tubes often become occluded by inspissated feedings or pulverized medications given through the tube. Frequent flushing of the tube with 30–60 mL of water and avoiding the administration of pill fragments whenever possible help maintain patency. Many techniques for unclogging tubes have been published and include the gentle infusion of small quantities of carbonated beverage, pancreatic enzymes, and 95% ethyl alcohol into the tube. In addition, commercially made products can be obtained that either dissolve or mechanically remove the obstruction. Metabolic complications, such as hypokalemia, hyponatremia, hypophosphatemia, and hyperglycemia, can occur [40]. Patients should be monitored for metabolic abnormalities, particularly severely malnourished patients during the initial refeeding period.

Gastrointestinal side effects of tube feedings include nausea and vomiting, pulmonary aspiration, abdominal pain, and diarrhea. Diarrhea is the most common complication and occurs in 30%–50% of critically ill patients receiving tube feedings. Diarrhea is often caused by antibiotic use [41] and the use of liquid medications and elixirs that contain nonabsorbable carbohydrates, such as sorbitol [42]. Patients with normal gastrointestinal tract function can tolerate larger volumes of tube feedings. In one study, tube feeding did not cause diarrhea in healthy subjects until it was given at rates exceeding 200 mL/h [43]. Several case reports have also documented an association between small bowel necrosis and jejunal feedings in critically ill patients [44]. Most of these patients were receiving pressors to maintain an adequate blood pressure, suggesting that the increased oxygen requirements associated with feeding can cause ischemia in patients whose intestinal blood flow is unable to increase.

Parenteral nutrition

In some patients, enteral feedings are either contraindicated or cannot be provided in sufficient quantities to meet nutritional requirements. In these cases, parenteral nutritional support can be a valuable adjunctive and sometimes life-saving therapy. Certainly, patients who are unable to ingest "adequate" nutrients for a "prolonged" period of time require nutritional therapy to prevent the adverse effects of malnutrition. However, the precise definitions of "adequate" and "prolonged" are not clear and are likely to differ from patient to patient depending on the amount of body energy stores and lean body mass, the presence of preexisting medical illnesses, and the level of metabolic stress. The use of parenteral nutrition is often recommended if enteral intake has been, or is anticipated to be, inadequate for 5–10 days [45]. However, carefully performed, well-designed, prospective randomized clinical trials to support the efficacy of this approach for many clinical situations are few in number [46]. Therefore, the use of parenteral nutrition requires a careful integration of data from pertinent clinical trials, clinical expertise in the illness or injury being treated, a reasonable estimate of the anticipated duration of inadequate food intake, clinical expertise in nutritional therapy, and input from patients and their families.

Central parenteral nutrition
General principles
The ability to use a central vein to supply nutrient requirements for growth and maintenance was realized more than 30 years ago when catheters were inserted into the superior vena cava of beagle dogs to provide the sole source of nutrients for 72–256 days [47]. Today, the use of central parenteral nutrition (CPN), also known as *total parenteral nutrition* (TPN), is commonplace. Although percutaneous infraclavicular subclavian vein catheterization with advancement of the catheter tip to the junction of the superior vena cava and right atrium is the most commonly used technique for catheter placement, many other approaches have been successfully performed when the subclavian vein is not accessible, including internal jugular, basilic, saphenous, and femoral veins, and even thoracotomy with direct insertion into the right azygos vein [48] or the right atrial appendage [49]. In addition, peripherally inserted central venous catheters can be used to provide CPN. In this approach, insertion by a physician is not required, and the technique cannot cause pneumothorax or traumatic injury to arteries or nerves, but it is associated with an increased risk for thrombosis

if the catheter tip is placed proximal to the superior vena cava [50].

Parenteral nutrient solutions provide all the basic nutrient requirements, including fluids, proteins, carbohydrates, fats, minerals, trace elements, and vitamins (Table 30.7). The lipid component can be piggybacked to the primary nutrient mixture, or a total nutrient admixture can be prepared, which reduces handling costs and potential breaks in sterility. However, total nutrient admixtures prevent visible inspection for particulate matter. Invisible calcium and phosphorus precipitates have caused fatal pulmonary emboli in patients receiving parenteral nutrition [51]. Therefore, pharmacy standards regarding physicochemical compatibility should be closely followed in all patients receiving CPN, and in-line filters should be used with all parenteral nutrient solutions. Even a careful inspection of clear nutrient solutions cannot detect small microprecipitates, which can obstruct small pulmonary capillaries [52].

The specific formulation prescribed for a patient depends on the patient's estimated nutrient requirements and ability to tolerate specific nutrients without adverse effects. The patient's protein, energy, and fluid requirements are the most important initial considerations in designing the appropriate parenteral formulation. Protein requirements are met by infusing standard solutions composed of crystalline amino acids containing 40%–50% essential and 50%–60% non-essential amino acids, usually with little or no glutamine, glutamate, aspartate, asparagine, tyrosine, and cysteine. Most hospitalized patients require between 1.0 and 1.5 g of protein per kilogram body weight per day. Some amino acid solutions have been modified for specific disease states, such as those enriched in branched-chain amino acids (advocated for patients with hepatic encephalopathy) and those containing 67%–100% essential amino acids (advocated for patients with renal insufficiency). However, the clinical superiority of these formulations over standard amino acid solutions has not been well documented in clinical trials [53,54].

The major sources of energy are glucose and lipid. However, infused amino acids are also oxidized and should be included in the estimate of energy provided as part of the parenteral formulation. Glucose (dextrose) is usually the predominant energy source in CPN formulations and is the required fuel for erythrocytes, white blood cells, bone marrow, and renal medulla (~ 40 g/day) and the preferred fuel for the brain (~ 120 g/day). Each gram of hydrated dextrose provides 3.4 kcal (14.2 kJ) and is readily oxidized unless excessive amounts are infused. In stable postoperative patients, increasing the rate of glucose infusion up to, but not more than, 7 mg/kg/min increases the rate of glucose oxidation [55,56]. Lipid emulsions contain soybean oil or a combination of soybean and safflower oil triglycerides, egg yolk phospholipids as an emulsifying agent, and glycerin to maintain isosmolarity. These emulsions provide energy and are a source of essential fatty acids, linoleic and linolenic acids. Lipid

Table 30.7 Delivery of nutrients during total (central) parenteral nutrition

Nutrient	Formulation for delivery	Frequency, suggested dose
Water	Diluent in base solution	Daily, 2–3 L
Amino acids	3.5%–10% solutions of crystalline amino acids in base solution or 3:1 mixtures	Daily, 12%–24% of total kcal
Carbohydrate	20% dextrose in base solution or 3:1 mixtures	Daily, 55%–65% of total kcal
Phospholipid	10%–30% soybean/safflower oil emulsion in 3:1 mixtures (1.1–3.0 kcal/mL)	Daily to weekly, 20%–25% of total kcal
Essential fatty acids	3:1 mixtures i.v., corn oil orally (5–15 mL), or topical skin application	Daily to weekly, ~ 11 g/day (1%–2% of kcal/day)
Vitamins A, D, E, C, B complex	Multivitamin preparation in base solution	Daily or q.o.d., 10 mL
Vitamin B-12	Injection s.c. (1 mg/mL) or oral tablet	Monthly (1 mg s.c.) or daily (100 µg/day orally)
Vitamin K	Aqueous colloidal solution	Weekly, 10 mg s.c.
Sodium	Amino acid solutions and NaCl/acetate added	Daily, 60–120 mEq
Potassium	Amino acid solutions and KCl added	Daily, 30–80 mEq
Chloride	Amino acid solutions and Na/KCl added	Daily, 80–140 mEq
Calcium	Calcium gluconate added to base solution	Daily, 4.6–9.2 mEq
Magnesium	Amino acid solutions and $MgSO_4$	Daily, 8.1–24.3 mEq
Phosphorus	Na/K phosphate added to diluted base solution	Daily, 12–24 mmol
Iron	Iron dextran added separately to maintain stores	Monthly, titrated to needs
Trace minerals	Trace mineral solutions	Daily, 1 mL

Note: Each component of total parenteral nutrition can be ordered separately, according to patient need. The amino acid concentration is chosen according to the need for nitrogen. Lipid is not needed beyond the requirement for essential fatty acids but is often provided daily to restrict volume. i.v., intravenously; q.o.d., every other day; s.c., subcutaneously.

calories are as effective as additional glucose calories in conserving body nitrogen economy and supporting protein metabolism once absolute tissue requirements for glucose have been met [57,58]. The optimal percentage of calories that should be infused as fat is not known. At least 5% of total calories should be given as lipids to prevent essential fatty acid deficiency. The rate of lipid emulsion infusion should probably not exceed 0.7 kcal/kg/h because most complications associated with lipid emulsion infusions have been reported when more than 1.0 kcal/kg/h (0.11 g/kg/h) was provided [59]. Lipid emulsion infusion, containing ω-6 polyunsaturated fatty acids (PUFAs), can cause pulmonary dysfunction [60], hepatic phospholipidosis [61], impaired immune system function [62], pancreatitis [63], decreased platelet aggregation [64], fat overload syndrome [65], and hypersensitivity reactions [66–68]. Therefore, olive oil-based lipid emulsions and medium- and long-chain triglyceride lipid emulsions are being developed [69,70]. Together, carbohydrate and lipid should provide 25–35 kcal/g of protein to optimize incorporation of amino acids into new protein.

Complications

Mechanical, infectious, metabolic, and gastrointestinal complications are associated with the use of CPN. Administering CPN under the guidance of experienced teams decreases the incidence of most complications [71]. Percutaneous insertion of a central venous catheter can damage local structures and cause pneumothorax, brachial plexus injury, subclavian and carotid artery puncture, hemothorax, thoracic duct injury, and chylothorax. In addition, the catheter can be sheared off, become occluded, or cause subclavian vein or superior vena cava thrombosis [72–74].

Catheter-related sepsis is the most common serious complication in patients receiving CPN; even when meticulous care is provided, catheter-related sepsis occurs in up to 4% of hospitalized patients [75]. Multiple-lumen central catheters that are used for CPN are associated with an increased incidence of infections compared with single-lumen catheters [75]. Catheter-related sepsis should be considered in all patients in whom a fever or leukocytosis develops while they are receiving CPN. The catheter tunnel and exit site should be carefully inspected, and any exit site drainage should be cultured. Blood cultures should be obtained from the central line and a peripheral vein. The presence of subcutaneous infection along the catheter tunnel or clinical toxicity (e.g., hypotension) without another known source of infection is an indication for immediate catheter removal. If no evidence of tunnel infection or clinical toxicity is found, the catheter can remain in place, and empirical antibiotic therapy should be started through the central venous catheter. Blood cultures should be obtained again in 48–72 h to ensure clearance of bacteremia. The catheter should be removed from patients who have blood cultures that are positive for fungus or *Staphylococcus aureus*, polymicrobial infection, persistent or recurrent catheter-related bacteremia, or persistent fever without another suspected source of infection [76].

The metabolic complications observed in patients receiving parenteral nutrition are usually caused by inappropriate nutrient administration resulting in nutrient excesses or deficiencies or both. Parenteral nutrition has a propensity to cause hyperglycemia in hospitalized patients. Since 2001, there exists good evidence that even minor elevations in blood glucose (BG) levels in intensive are unit (ICU) patients lead to increased mortality when compared with true normoglycemia (BG 80–110 mg/dL) [77,78]. In the less stressed patient a BG goal of less than 150 mg/dL may be more appropriate as there have been no clinical trials published in this patient group. Blood glucose should be kept below a concentration of 120 mg/dL in pregnant patients to avoid the complications of gestational diabetes and large-for-gestational-age births. Metabolic bone disease, including osteopenia and osteomalacia, has been observed in patients receiving long-term (> 3 months) CPN [79].

Several hepatobiliary abnormalities have been observed in patients receiving CPN, and these are usually more severe and more frequent in infants than in adults [80]. Hepatic abnormalities include alterations in liver biochemistries, steatosis, steatohepatitis, lipidosis and phospholipidosis, cholestasis, fibrosis, and cirrhosis. Most hepatic abnormalities occur early and are transient, but in a small subset of patients receiving long-term (> 16 weeks) CPN, progressive and more serious liver disease develops [81]. Biliary abnormalities include acalculous cholecystitis, gallbladder sludge, and cholelithiasis, and these usually occur in patients receiving relatively prolonged (> 4 weeks) courses of CPN. Acalculous cholecystitis has been reported in about 5% [82], cholelithiasis in about 30%, and gallbladder sludge in up to 100% [83] of patients receiving prolonged CPN. The pathogenesis of acalculous cholecystitis is unclear. Gallbladder stasis is an important contributing factor in the pathogenesis of gallbladder sludge and stones.

Maintaining regular gallbladder contractions by either enteral feedings or cholecystokinin injections prevents gallbladder sludge and gallstone formation [84,85].

Peripheral parenteral nutrition

Peripheral parenteral nutrition (PPN) consists of a mixture of nutrients containing a final concentration of 5%–10% dextrose, 2%–5% amino acids, electrolytes, and vitamins and minerals. This crystalloid solution is mixed with a 10% or 20% lipid emulsion as an all-in-one admixture, or the lipid emulsion can be piggybacked to the distal port of the intravenous infusion line. To ensure that adequate calories can be given in a reasonable volume, the lipid component usually provides approximately half of the total calories.

The use of a peripheral vein to provide nutritional support avoids many of the mechanical and infectious complications of CPN but is associated with a high risk for thrombophlebitis, which occurs in up to 94% of patients [86]. However, the use of PPN has become possible in many patients since the development of safe isotonic lipid emulsions and a better understanding of the causes of PPN-induced thrombophlebitis.

Several factors are important in the pathogenesis of thrombophlebitis in patients receiving PPN [87,88]:
• the osmolality, pH, and lipid content of the PPN solution, and the presence of particulate matter
• the diameter, length, and composition of the catheter
• the duration, rate, and volume of the infusion
• the diameter and anatomical position of the vein
• the insertion technique.

Adherence to the following principles can increase the life of a single infusion site to more than 10 days in many patients:
• provide at least 50% of total energy as a lipid emulsion, add 500–1000 U of heparin and 5 mg of hydrocortisone per liter of solution, and add sodium hydroxide if needed to achieve a pH of 7.4
• insert a fine-bore 22- or 23-gauge polyvinyl pyrrolidine-coated polyurethane catheter in as large a vein as possible in the proximal forearm with use of a sterile technique
• place a 5-mg glyceryl trinitrate ointment patch over the infusion site
• infuse the PPN solution with a volumetric pump and keep the total infused volume below 3500 mL
• filter the solution with an in-line 1.2-μm filter.

Home parenteral nutrition

The ability to provide parenteral nutrition at home was first demonstrated in 1970 [89]. In 1992, approximately 40 000 patients (120 per million residents) received home parenteral nutrition (HPN) in the United States [90], a tenfold higher rate than that in Europe (1–12 per million residents) [90–92]. Patients with benign diseases have a much better outcome than those with terminal illnesses. Patients with benign gastrointestinal disease and receiving HPN have a better outcome and decreased HPN days spent in the hospital than those with terminal illnesses. In addition, it has been reported that patients with benign disease and receiving HPN had a 5% 1-year mortality compared with 80% of their counterparts with terminal illnesses [93].

HPN is usually given through an implantable subcutaneous port or a catheter inserted in the subclavian vein and tunneled subcutaneously to exit on the anterior chest. Nutrient formulations are infused for 8 to 12 h overnight to allow patients to be active during the day. Intravenous lipids may not be necessary for patients who eat and are able to absorb adequate amounts of fat, whereas others may receive 20%–30% of their calories as a lipid emulsion. The development of multichamber bags with an extended shelf life allows the delivery of more CPN bags to home patients at one time [94]. The most serious common complication is catheter-related sepsis, most often caused by *S. aureus* or *Staphylococcus epidermidis*. However, a 5-year review of HTPN patients demonstrated a 50% decline in the incidence of catheter-related sepsis from 1997 to 2001 [95]. Nonetheless, venous thrombosis, chronic liver disease, cholelithiasis, and metabolic bone disease are all associated with the prolonged use of HPN.

Nutritional support in the hospitalized patient with gastrointestinal disease

The major purpose of nutritional therapy is to prevent or correct specific nutrient deficiencies and to prevent the adverse effects of protein–energy malnutrition. Nutritional support has also been proposed as a primary therapy for patients with certain gastrointestinal diseases, such as inflammatory bowel disease and hepatic encephalopathy. In this section, we review the available data evaluating the clinical efficacy of nutritional support in patients with gastrointestinal diseases. Whenever possible, only the data from prospective randomized clinical trials are considered because this approach is the most reliable technique for evaluating the usefulness of therapy.

Short bowel syndrome
Patients who have undergone massive intestinal resection often require nutritional support for optimal function and survival. The length of the remaining jejunum, the presence of the ileocecal valve, and whether the colon is intact are critical determinants of the need for nutritional support [96]. In general, patients with a jejunostomy and less than 90 cm of jejunum, or those with a colon in continuity but less than 50 cm of jejunum, are likely to require parenteral nutrition. Providing nutrients with continuous nighttime tube feedings [97] or fluid and electrolytes with oral rehydration therapy [32] (see "Oral rehydration therapy" above) can sometimes decrease or eliminate the need for parenteral therapy.

Inflammatory bowel disease
Enteral nutrition
Three metaanalyses of published prospective randomized clinical trials concluded that enteral nutrition is not as effective as corticosteroids. In addition, no benefit of elemental over nonelemental formulas was noted [98–100]. The true clinical efficacy of enteral nutritional therapy has not been evaluated because no study has compared patients receiving dietary therapy with an untreated control group. However, the overall remission rate reported with enteral nutrition therapy is about 60% [98,99], which is higher than the range of 20%–40% reported for placebo-treated patients with moderate disease [101,102].

Parenteral nutrition
Data from several prospective randomized clinical trials found that "bowel rest" is not necessary to achieve clinical remission in patients with active Crohn's disease; patients who received TPN plus bowel rest fared no better than those receiving TPN plus oral/enteral feeding [103,104]. A beneficial effect of TPN in patients with Crohn's disease or ulcerative colitis has not been demonstrated in prospective randomized clinical trials. No significant differences in clinical response rates were found in hospitalized patients with severe disease exacerbations who were randomized to receive TPN and steroid therapy or an oral/enteral diet and steroid therapy [105–107]. Nonetheless, TPN may be useful in patients with severe inflammatory bowel disease who cannot eat because of prolonged ileus or who might benefit from bowel rest because of severe diarrhea or anticipated surgery.

Specific nutrient therapy
Fish oil supplementation may produce a modest decrease in the activity of ulcerative colitis [108,109], may help to lower the steroid dose, and may prevent early but not late relapse [110], but it is not effective by itself. Two prospective randomized clinical trials of maintaining clinical remission in patients with Crohn's disease have shown both success [111] and failure [112]. Short-chain fatty acids have not been shown to be effective for rectal disease in ulcerative colitis [113].

Gastrointestinal fistulae
No prospective randomized clinical trials have evaluated the efficacy of TPN, but "bowel rest" may improve the clinical outcome of selected patients with fistulae. Before the use of TPN, mortality in patients with gastrointestinal fistulae was caused by malnutrition, fluid losses, and peritonitis. A retrospective analysis of patients with small bowel fistulae showed an improved outcome for those who received nutritional support [114]. Anastomotic fistulae at sites of recent resection in Crohn's disease may close permanently with TPN and bowel rest, although octreotide therapy may also be necessary for success in some patients [115]. However, fistula

closure is not well maintained after an oral diet is reinstituted in patients with active disease at the origin of the fistula, or with postfistula obstruction.

Growth failure in children

Total parenteral nutrition or oral/enteral supplemental feedings can initiate catch-up growth, resulting in marked increases in height and weight, in children with inflammatory bowel disease and growth failure [116–119]. In fact, even intermittent enteral feeding can improve growth [120,121].

Acute pancreatitis

Most patients with acute pancreatitis are unable to eat because oral feeding can cause abdominal pain and increase serum amylase and lipase concentrations. Nonetheless, nutritional support is not useful in patients with mild or moderate pancreatitis because of the rapid resolution of symptoms and ability to begin oral feeding within several days. In addition, no benefit of parenteral nutrition compared with enteral nutrition has been demonstrated in patients with mild or moderate pancreatitis [122], and in one study, the use of TPN was associated with a higher prevalence of catheter-related sepsis and insulin requirements [123]. However, nutritional support may be necessary in about 10%–20% of patients with pancreatitis who have severe and complicated disease when a prolonged period of starvation is anticipated.

It has been shown that it is possible to provide enteral feeding to patients who have mild to moderate [122] or severe [124–126] pancreatitis, without causing an exacerbation of symptoms, when feeding is delivered distal to the ligament of Treitz into the upper jejunum. Moreover, in prospective randomized clinical trials that compared enteral with parenteral nutritional therapy in patients with severe pancreatitis, those who were randomized to receive enteral nutrition showed a greater reduction in acute-phase-response proteins, a greater improvement in disease severity scores, and fewer medical complications than those given parenteral nutrition [124]. These findings led to the recommendation by an international consensus conference to provide nutrition support by jejunostomy feedings rather than CPN in patients with severe acute pancreatitis [127]. However, it is not known whether enteral feeding was beneficial or whether parenteral feeding was harmful because no study included an unfed control group.

Providing a portion of total calories as lipid can help prevent hyperglycemia in glucose-intolerant patients with pancreatitis. However, it is important to ensure adequate triglyceride clearance because hypertriglyceridemia induced by infusion of fat emulsions can cause a relapse of pancreatitis [63].

Liver disease
Alcoholic hepatitis
One prospective randomized clinical trial compared PPN with an anabolic steroid, oxandrolone, or the combination for 21 days and found no change in mortality but improved Child–Pugh scores in those receiving PPN plus oxandrolone [128,129]. In another study, nutritional therapy improved liver function and reduced early mortality (1- and 6-month) in a subgroup with moderate "malnutrition" or liver disease [130]. No improvement was noted in the group with severe disease. It is clear that these markers correlate with the severity of liver disease and with clinical outcome [131].

Alcoholic cirrhosis
Several prospective randomized clinical trials showed that enteral nutrition in patients hospitalized for complications of cirrhosis led to an improved clinical status [132–134]. A single study showed that enteral feeding of a branched-chain amino acid formula reduced mortality [135]. However, the ad lib diet group ingested only about half the calories of the enterally fed group, and the control group had an unusually high mortality rate (47%).

Hepatic encephalopathy
In a metaanalysis of nine prospective randomized clinical trials evaluating the use of TPN enriched with branched-chain amino acids in patients with acute encephalopathy [53], recovery from encephalopathy was improved during short-term (7–14 days) treatment. However, the variability in mortality rates was so great that no conclusion could be reached regarding that outcome measure. No benefit of branched-chain amino acid therapy was detected in the one study that compared a group that received branched-chain amino acid-enriched TPN with a control group that received standard amino acids. Studies of the use of enteral solutions containing branched-chain amino acids in patients with chronic encephalopathy have yielded conflicting results. However, the studies with the largest number of patients showed clinical benefits in protein-intolerant patients [136].

Micronutrient deficiency and treatment

Tissues that proliferate rapidly (skin, oral and gastrointestinal mucosa, hair, bone marrow) or in which metabolic rates are high (muscle, gastrointestinal mucosa) are at greatest risk for signs of deficiency at an early stage. Clues regarding deficiency come from a history of reduced intake or increased losses (or of conditions that make those situations more likely), physical examination findings, and results of laboratory tests that ideally determine body stores of the nutrient. The signs and symptoms of nutritional deficiency in adult patients are listed in Table 30.1. The laboratory values for the major vitamins and minerals are listed in Tables 30.2 and 30.3. A more detailed discussion of these nutrients and the assessment of their status can be found in general references [1,137,138].

Sodium (Na+)

Deficiency

Sodium depletion usually presents with symptoms of dehydration because of concomitant water loss. Severe depletion presents with nausea, vomiting, exhaustion, cramps, seizures, and ultimately cardiovascular collapse. On the physical examination, mucosal xerosis, sunken eyeballs, and mental confusion can be present, but none of these are specific findings. In older patients, other explanations are often present for all these signs [139]. Orthostatic hypotension is often used to estimate the intravascular volume and is defined as a systolic blood pressure below 20 mmHg or a diastolic blood pressure below 10 mmHg within 3 min after standing, with or without a rise in the heart rate of 5 to 10 beats/min [140]. The signs of total body sodium excess are weight gain and edema. The presence of either of these would not reflect sodium deficiency. If sodium deficiency is the result of increased gastrointestinal or cutaneous losses, the urine osmolality is increased and the urine sodium concentration is less than 10 mEq/L. If sodium deficiency is the result of diuretic therapy, the urine osmolality is decreased and the urine sodium concentration is more than 10 mEq/L.

Assessment

The serum sodium concentration primarily reflects water, not sodium, balance. Thus, any serum concentration is possible when deficiency is present, depending on the relative deficits of water and sodium. If hyponatremia is present but the cause is not apparent, the serum osmolality should be measured. In hospitalized patients, hyponatremia is most often the result of dilution by excess free water, not depletion of sodium. The free water excess is usually caused by cardiac, hepatic, or renal insufficiency or by overly enthusiastic fluid administration and is accompanied by edema and weight gain. When normovolemia is present, the hyponatremia may be caused either by inappropriate secretion of antidiuretic hormone or by displacement of sodium osmoles with elevated glucose or urea as osmoles.

Treatment

When signs of volume depletion are present, at least a 10% reduction in extracellular fluid volume has occurred [141]. The sodium deficit can be estimated as follows: Na deficit (mEq) = ([Na desired] – [Na observed]) × 0.6 × weight (kg). Sodium is usually replaced with NaCl (1 g = 17 mEq Na), either orally, enterally, or parenterally. Symptomatic hyponatremia (e.g., seizures, lethargy) is treated with intravenous 0.9% NaCl or occasionally with hypertonic (3% or 5%) NaCl. Sodium infusion should be designed to increase the serum concentration by 1 mEq/h until it reaches 120 mEq/L. Too rapid restoration has been associated with permanent neurological deficits resulting from central pontine myelinolysis. When sodium depletion is accompanied by hypernatremia or normonatremia, the appropriate amount of water should be supplied along with the sodium to achieve or maintain a normal serum sodium concentration. Chronic losses from diarrhea, vomiting, or ileostomy should be treated in adults with an oral rehydration solution that provides a carbohydrate source along with adequate sodium, so that Na/solute-coupled cotransport can occur and maximize the rate of sodium repletion. These solutions are discussed in the section "Enteral nutrition" above. Sodium toxicity can result from excessive administration of NaCl. Symptoms of toxicity include vomiting, diarrhea, peripheral vascular collapse, respiratory depression, and death.

Potassium (K+)

Deficiency

Hypokalemia (< 3.5 mEq/L) rarely is caused by decreased intake but can result from shifts between the extra- and intracellular compartments of the body occurring while the total body potassium remains normal. This shift can be caused by alkalosis and the administration of glucose or insulin. Alternatively, decreased body stores result from increased renal excretion or intestinal losses, with subsequent shift of potassium from extra- to intracellular compartments. Loss of gastric contents by vomiting produces hypovolemia and metabolic acidosis, leading to increased renal K^+ loss. Increased K^+ loss from diarrhea produces hypovolemia, but with metabolic acidosis, yet can still produce hypokalemia from Na^+–K^+ exchange in the colon. Other causes of renal losses include mineralocorticoid excess, some antibiotics, and, rarely, renal tubular acidosis. In pure deficiency states, each decrease of 1 mEq/L corresponds to a loss of 200–300 mEq of body potassium. The loss of 5%–10% of body stores is usually tolerated without symptoms, but when serum levels fall below 3.0 mEq/L, weakness, paresthesias, confusion, cramps, myalgias, and cardiovascular abnormalities can occur [142].

Assessment

The normal serum level of potassium is 3.5–4.5 mEq/L and reflects both body stores and the availability of glucose as an energy source. Red blood cell hemolysis or extreme leukocytosis without hemolysis can result in spurious hyperkalemia. Total body potassium deficit cannot be estimated accurately especially by urinary K^+([K^+]u), as that merely reflects the renal response to circulating volume, pH, or plasma K^+ ([K^+]p) (Table 30.8). The transtubular K^+ concentration gradient (TTKG) is a simple calculation that can provide a semiquantitative measure of K^+ secretion in the cortical collecting duct (CCD) [143]: [K^+]ccd = [K^+]u/(Osm_u/Osm_p), the urine–plasma osmolality ratio. If the urine osmolality exceeds that of plasma, then TTKG = [K^+]ccd/[K^+]p, and it can be used to assist in the differential diagnosis of hypokalemia. TTKG is correlated with plasma aldosterone levels in hypokalemic patients.

Treatment

Treatment should be provided if symptoms are attributed to the hypokalemia, or if other conditions, such as chronic liver

Table 30.8 Expected values for tests that are helpful in the differential diagnosis of hypo- or hyperkalemia

Test	Normal	Hypokalemia	Hyperkalemia
24-h K+ excretion	60–80 mmol/day 6–8 mmol/mmol creatinine	< 10 mmol/day < 1–1.5 mmol/mmol creatinine	> 150 mmol/day > 10–15 mmol/mmol creatinine
Urinary Na+/K+	2.3–2.7	GI loss 2.5–2.6 Diuretics 2.6	Aldosteronism 1.4
Spot urine K+	Variable due to K+ secretion and water reabsorption	Diarrhea < 20 Renal > 20	Variable
TTKG	2–5	Diarrhea < 2 Diuretics 5–10 Vomiting 2–5	Aldosteronism > 10

GI, gastrointestinal; TTKG, transtubular potassium concentration gradient.

disease, are present that would exacerbate the hypokalemia. Alkalosis tends to lower the serum potassium concentration, whereas acidosis raises it. Thus, alkalosis can be treated first before the addition of potassium salts, but the same should not be done when acidosis is present. Oral replacement should be used if possible because this allows the serum potassium concentration to rise slowly in equilibrium with the intracellular compartment. Either food or supplement (Table 30.9) sources should be used. Foods rich in K+ (> 400 mg/serving)

include cantaloupe, potato, dried fruits, avocado, skim milk, banana, fruit juices, and many fruits. The administration of 20–40 mEq at a time up to four times a day is safe. The chloride salt is preferred when renal or gastric losses account for the hypokalemia. When hypokalemia is secondary to diarrhea, one of the alkalinizing salts (e.g., citrate, acetate, bicarbonate) is preferred. The slow-release, matrix, and microencapsulated forms are better tolerated than liquid preparations. The slow-release forms have reduced the risk of small bowel

Table 30.9 Oral potassium products comparison chart

Dosage forms	Potassium salt(s)	Brand names	Potassium content	Comments
Liquid	Potassium chloride	Various	10, 15, 20, 30, 40 mEq/15 mL	Rapid absorption, low frequency of gastrointestinal ulceration, unpleasant taste
	Mixture of potassium acetate/biocarbonate/citrate	Trikates, Tri-K	45 mEq/15 mL	Preferred forms in patients with delayed gastrointestinal transit time, avoid nonchloride salts in metabolic alkalosis
Powder	Potassium gluconate	Kaon	20 mEq/15 mL	Must be dissolved in water before use, avoid nonchloride salts in metabolic alkalosis
	Potassium chloride	Various	15, 20, 25 mEq/packet	
	Mixture of potassium bicarbonate/citrate	Various	25, 50 mEq/packet	
Effervescent tablets	Potassium chloride	Various	25, 50 mEq/tablet	
Sustained-release capsules, tablets	Potassium chloride	Various	8, 10, 20 mEq/capsule	Wax matrix or polymer-coated crystals in gelatin capsule, bioequivalent to liquid forms, avoid in patients with delayed gastrointestinal transit time, poorly effective in short bowel syndrome
Salt substitutes	Potassium chloride	Adolph's, Morton's, Nu-Salt, No Salt, various	Powder 50–70 mEq/tsp	Inexpensive dietary source, prescribe specific amount to avoid hyperkalemia; contraindicated in oliguria, severe renal disease

Adapted from Knoben JE, Anderson PO. Handbook of Clinical Drug Data, 7th edn. Hamilton, IL: Drug Intelligence Publications, 1993:663; Olin BR (ed.) Facts and Comparisons. St. Louis: Facts and Comparisons, 1992:16; and Stanaszek WF, Romankiewicz JA. Current approaches to management of potassium deficiency. Drug Int Pharm 1985;19:176.

ulcers and strictures but may not be useful for patients with short bowel syndrome. For intravenous therapy, the infusion rate should not exceed 20 mEq/h unless cardiac monitoring is included. The chloride salt is usually best for intravenous therapy, except when phosphate is used for treating the associated hypophosphatemia of diabetic ketoacidosis. In the presence of acidosis, potassium acetate is the best choice. Hyperkalemia should be avoided during therapy because levels above 8.0 mEq/L carry a severe risk for cardiac dysfunction, including bradycardia, asystole, and ventricular fibrillation. Skeletal muscle weakness, areflexia or hyperreflexia, paralysis, and fatigue may also occur at these high levels.

Calcium

Deficiency

The conditions that cause hypocalcemia requiring calcium supplementation include vitamin D deficiency, failure of vitamin D synthesis or action, hypoparathyroidism, hypomagnesemia, severe acute pancreatitis, malabsorption syndromes, neoplasms with osteoblastic metastases, and medications, including aminoglycosides, cisplatin, calcitonin, furosemide, mithramycin, phosphates, and anticonvulsants [144]. Acute manifestations include tetany, altered myocardial function and arrhythmias, hyperreflexia, paresthesias, seizures, mental status changes, and choreoathetotic movements. The electrocardiogram shows prolonged Q–T intervals with normal QRS complexes. Chronic deficiency may not be associated with hypocalcemia. With a total body content of 1000 g and a net daily loss of 100 mg/day, a 20% decrease in body stores (which could be easily detected) would take 2000 days, or about 6 years, to develop. Osteopenia usually presents with fractures or bone pain. However, patients identified as being at high risk for the development of osteopenia should begin treatment well before this occurs. Risk factors include cigarette smoking, family history of osteoporosis, sedentary lifestyle, long-term glucocorticoid therapy, long-term anticonvulsant therapy, early surgical or natural menopause (< 50 years), and testicular failure (secondary to drug therapy or disease).

Assessment

Recent intake or absorption is assessed by 24-h urinary calcium [137]. At levels of absorption above 2 mg/kg (corresponding to an intake of 6 mg/kg), urinary calcium equals absorbed calcium. When absorption is low, urinary calcium levels do not decline proportionally, unlike the levels of sodium, potassium, magnesium, and phosphorus, all of which are better absorbed with better-regulated urinary excretion. Urinary calcium is used primarily to determine that absorption is low and to follow the patient after oral replacement is begun, to ensure that absorption becomes normal and that hypercalciuria does not ensue. Urinary calcium excretion of more than 300 mg/day is an indication to reduce the dose of calcium (or vitamin D). Serum calcium is tightly regulated and only falls below normal when severe deficiency occurs.

Pseudohypocalcemia can be caused by hypoalbuminemia and by gadolinium administration, a treatment that precipitates calcium [145]. Body stores of calcium are assessed by bone densitometry, with many centers using dualenergy x-ray absorptiometry. The accuracy of this method is equal to that of quantitative computed tomography and is sensitive to changes of 9%–12% in bone mass [146]. Results must be compared with those of age- and gender-matched controls and are useful for diagnosis and following the response to therapy. Bone densitometry should be used to screen all patients at high risk for the development of osteopenia and to guide treatment decisions for selected postmenopausal women, but it is not recommended for routine screening. Serum calcium and alkaline phosphatase levels do not become abnormal until total body calcium depletion is severe.

Treatment

Treatment of acute symptomatic hypocalcemia is required immediately to prevent laryngospasm, seizures, and cardiac arrhythmias. A total of 200–300 mg of elemental calcium should be given intravenously over 5 min as 1 g of calcium chloride or 2–3 g of calcium gluconate (10 mL of 10% calcium gluconate = 1 g of calcium). This should be followed by an infusion of calcium of 0.5–2.0 mg/kg/h [144,147]. The serum calcium should normalize in 6–12 h while the vital signs and electrocardiographic activity are monitored. Patients with chronic hypocalcemia or osteopenia on the basis of poor intake or absorption should be treated with oral supplements of up to 2.5–3.0 g/day given in divided doses. The best dietary source of calcium is milk, and this can be used if clinically tolerated. Otherwise, a number of oral calcium salts are available that vary in elemental calcium content (Table 30.10) [148]. Calcium carbonate is used most often because of the high percentage of elemental calcium, but it is rather insoluble. If the urinary calcium does not increase with calcium carbonate, another, more soluble salt (e.g., calcium gluconate) may be tried, with or without the addition of vitamin D. People who take calcium supplements may be at risk for ingesting lead, although the amount of lead in bone meal has dropped as a consequence of a decrease in the levels of environmental lead from gasoline and paint. When tested by the Natural Resources Defense Council, many of the 20 major brands of calcium supplements marketed in California contained enough lead to increase the average intake of 5–10 μg by 50% [149]. The supplements tested that were lowest in lead content (< 0.5 μg per dose) were Children's Mylanta, Posture-D High Potency Calcium with Vitamin D, and Tums 500 Calcium Supplement.

When malabsorption is present, the doses of vitamin D used are large (25 000–50 000 IU given from once a week to daily). Alternatively, the more soluble forms of vitamin D, especially 1,25-dihydroxyvitamin D, may be effective. Treatment programs must be individualized and monitored closely. Thiazides can decrease the urinary loss of calcium (thereby

Table 30.10 Selected oral calcium supplements

Salt in mineral supplements	Percentage of elemental calcium	Tablet size (mg)	Amount of calcium per tablet (mg)
Calcium carbonate	40		
Caltrate + D (200 IU)		1500	600
Os-Cal 500 + D (200 IU)		1250	500
Tums Ultra		1000	400
Viactin (100 IU D)		1250	500
Calcium phosphate	38		
Posture + D		1600	600
Calcium acetate	25	1000	250
Calcium citrate	21		
Citracal + D (200 IU)		1200	315
Calcium citrate 1000			250
Calcium lactate	13	650	85
Calcium gluconate	9	500	45
Calcium glubionate	6.5	1800/5 mL	115/5 mL

Foods	Serving	Amount/serving (mg)
Skim milk/yogurt	1 cup	302
Cheese, hard	1 oz	~ 250
Cheese, soft	1 oz	~ 175
Tofu	½ cup	~ 250
Broccoli, boiled	½ cup	36
Kale, cooked	½ cup	47

D, vitamin D; 1 cup = 8 fl oz (240 mL); 1 oz = 28 g.

rendering the urinary determination less meaningful) but also increase the urinary loss of magnesium. Thus, their use in patients with osteopenia must be carefully considered. Supplemental calcium may predispose some individuals to kidney stones but decreases the risk for oxalate stones in patients with short bowel syndrome. The development of calcium toxicity in patients with malabsorption is rare but can occur in patients with osteopenia and normal absorption, especially if they are also receiving supplemental vitamin D. Hypercalcemia can cause anorexia, nausea, constipation, polyuria, fatigue, weakness, confusion, lethargy, decreased deep tendon reflexes, shortened Q–T and prolonged P–R interval and QRS complex duration, and cardiac arrest [147].

Magnesium
Deficiency
Symptomatic magnesium deficiency is usually the result of decreased absorption or increased losses in the urine or from the gastrointestinal tract, especially in patients with extensive small bowel resection [150]. Excessive urinary loss, usually caused by decreased tubular reabsorption, occurs in a variety of circumstances [151]. Medications that promote renal loss include diuretics, aminoglycosides, cyclosporine (ciclosporin), amphotericin B, cisplatin, and digitalis [152]. Increased renal losses also occur in hypercalcemia, volume expansion, tubular

dysfunction, acute and chronic alcoholism, diabetes mellitus, hyperparathyroidism, and hypophosphatemia. Magnesium deficiency may occur in type 2 diabetes mellitus and precede the diabetes. Added magnesium may improve diabetic control if the serum levels are low initially [153]. Hypomagnesemia caused by a shift of magnesium from the extracellular to the intracellular compartment may result from feeding, treatment of diabetic ketoacidosis, parathyroidectomy, acute pancreatitis, and correction of acidosis in renal failure. Hypomagnesemia is often associated with and can be a cause of hypocalcemia, hypokalemia, and hypophosphatemia [153]. Hypomagnesemia can present as tremor, myoclonic jerks, ataxia, tetany, ventricular dysrhythmias, tachycardia, hypotension, cardiac arrest, apathy, depression, delirium, hallucinations, and psychosis [154]. The signs and symptoms of hypomagnesemia are often a consequence of the hypocalcemia resulting from the same condition (e.g., malabsorption) or of the decreased parathyroid hormone secretion that occurs when hypomagnesemia is severe.

Assessment
In the absence of excess fecal or renal losses, urinary excretion reflects intake and absorption of magnesium [138]. When the serum magnesium is low in patients with short bowel syndrome, the urinary magnesium excretion may also be low

and perhaps more sensitive than the serum magnesium [155]. Serum magnesium concentrations do not correlate well with total body stores, but it is reasonable to assume that depletion is present when the serum concentration is less than 1.0 mg/dL [152]. Because magnesium is primarily an intracellular ion, the best indicator of depletion may be a measurement of the content in white cells, although only a few studies have compared this value with those in other tissue pools [138]. A load test for magnesium depletion has been described, but its usefulness has not been satisfactorily documented.

Treatment

Moderate to severe deficiency should be treated parenterally, especially if tetany or ventricular arrhythmias are present. An intravenous loading dose of 4 to 8 mmol should be given first, followed by 25 mmol/day thereafter until the plasma magnesium is above 0.4 mmol/L [156]. If hypocalcemia or hypokalemia is present, magnesium should be replaced first. Repletion is best achieved with slow, continuous infusions to avoid rapid increases in urinary excretion. Replacement should be monitored closely with serial serum concentrations and evaluation of deep tendon reflexes. Hypermagnesemia

(> 3.0 mg/dL) should be avoided because vasodilation, nausea, vomiting, drowsiness, lethargy, hypotension, bradycardia, depressed deep tendon reflexes, and a prolonged P–R interval can develop.

Patients with mild deficiency or ongoing magnesium losses should receive foods rich in magnesium or an oral supplement. A variety of magnesium salts are available, but many of them, especially the oxide and hydroxide, are virtually insoluble (Table 30.11). Because magnesium is poorly absorbed, it is best to give it in frequent small doses. Potassium-sparing diuretics such as spironolactone decrease urinary magnesium losses and may be useful, especially in patients who are also hypokalemic. However, some patients will require parenteral supplements. Outpatients unresponsive to oral therapy can be treated with intramuscular injections of 2.0 mL of 50% magnesium sulfate solution (8.1 mEq) in each buttock at intervals as needed.

Phosphorus
Deficiency

Most patients in whom clinical evidence of hypophosphatemia develops have an underlying wasting condition [157,158],

Table 30.11 Magnesium products comparison chart

Product	Dosage forms[a]	Magnesium content (mEq/g)[b]	Comments
Magnesium carbonate	Tablet, 250 mg	23.7	Poorly soluble, low absorption
Magnesium, chelated	Tablet, 500 mg	8.2	Amino acid chelate; sodium-free, oral use only
Magnesium chloride	Solution, 200 mg/mL	9.8	Used i.v. or orally as a 5% solution; alternative to parenteral $MgSO_4$
	Enteric-coated tablet, 535 mg		Sold as Slo-Mag
Magnesium citrate	Solution, 60 mg/mL	4.4	Oral use only
Magnesium gluconate	Tablet, 500 mg, 1000 mg/5 mL	4.8	Very soluble, well absorbed
Magnesium hydroxide	Suspension, 40–80 mg/mL	34.0	Readily available in combination antacid formulations; start with 5-mL suspension or 1 tablet, increase as tolerated to four times daily; may require gastric acid to be absorbed; inexpensive
	Tablet, 600 mg		
Magnesium lactate	Sustained-release tablet, 700 mg	9.8	Sold as Mag-Tab SR
Magnesium oxide	Capsule, 140 mg Tablet, 250 mg, 400 mg, 420 mg, 500 mg	49.6	Poorly soluble; net absorption low, especially in malabsorption
Magnesium sulfate	Solution, 10%, 12.5%, 50%	8.1	Use i.v., i.m., or p.o.

a Magnesium products exhibit variable absorption; increase dose incrementally until no further rise in serum magnesium occurs or until diarrhea ensues. Oral magnesium alleviates diarrhea in some patients with malabsorption.

b 1 mEq = 12 mg = 0.5 mmol Mg.

i.m., intramuscularly; i.v., intravenously; p.o., orally.

Adapted from Knoben JE, Anderson PO. Handbook of Clinical Drug Data, 7th edn. Hamilton, IL: Drug Intelligence Publications, 1993:657; Olin BR (ed.) Facts and Comparisons. St. Louis: Facts and Comparisons, 1992;14a; and Fink EB. Magnesium deficiency: etiology and clinical spectrum. Acta Med Scand Suppl 1981;647:125.

such as malabsorption, malnutrition of any cause, cancer, or chronic alcoholism. Causes of hypophosphatemia include increased urinary losses, shifts of serum phosphorus into the intracellular compartment, and reduced absorption. Absorption is decreased with the use of phosphate-binding antacids, vitamin D deficiency, and parathyroid hormone deficiency. Renal loss is increased in metabolic alkalosis, diuretic therapy, renal tubular dysfunction, osmotic diuresis, hyperparathyroidism, and long-term corticosteroid therapy [156]. When carbohydrate is administered or when phosphate-rich lean tissue is restored and insufficient phosphorus is available, serum levels can fall [156]. Signs and symptoms of hypophosphatemia include hemolytic anemia (serum phosphorus concentration < 0.5 mg/dL), rhabdomyolysis (< 1.0 mg/dL), and other complications that occur with lesser degrees of depletion, including platelet dysfunction, metabolic acidosis, peripheral neuropathy, central nervous system dysfunction, metabolic encephalopathy, and cardiac failure. Most cases of hypophosphatemia appear to be associated with intercompartmental shifts of phosphorus rather than with decreases in the total body pool, although this distinction is not easy to make.

Assessment

The normal serum phosphorus concentration is 2.5–4.5 mg/dL. Levels lower than 1.0 mg/dL usually cause symptoms [156,157].

Treatment

If hypophosphatemia is the result of therapy with phosphate-binding medications (antacids, sucralfate), stopping the medication is sufficient. If oral or enteral intake is possible, supplementation for other causes of a serum phosphate level below 2.5 mg/dL can be provided with milk (1000 mg or 32 mmol/quart (0.9 L) of skim milk) or with other oral preparations in doses of 2–3 g/day (e.g., Neutra-Phos K or Uro-KP Neutral with 250 mg or 8.0 mmol per capsule or dose of powder). Most of the oral preparations, however, cause diarrhea (secondary to lactose intolerance in the case of milk and the phosphate content in the others), which may limit their use in patients with malabsorption. Intravenous supplementation should be limited to those who cannot take oral preparations or who have severe hypophosphatemia (< 1.0 mg/dL). The exact amount needed to restore serum phosphorus cannot be predicted because severe hypophosphatemia may occur with normal body stores of phosphorus. The dose of intravenous phosphate can be adjusted to serum phosphorus levels and to body weight (Table 30.12). When hypocalcemia or renal failure is present, great caution should be used in administering phosphate by any route, but especially intravenously. Too rapid administration can cause calcium phosphate precipitation in renal tubules and other tissues.

Table 30.12 Intravenous phosphorus repletion protocol according to body weight

| | Single phosphorus dose (mmol) | | |
| | Body weight (kg) | | |
Serum [P] (mg/dL)	40–66	61–80	81–120
< 1.0	30	40	50
1.0–1.7	20	30	40
1.8–2.2	10	15	20

A single dose restores serum [P] to normal within 24 h in 76% of patients.
From Taylor BE, Huey WY, Buchman TG, et al. Treatment of hypophosphatemia using a protocol based on patient weight and serum phosphorus levels in a surgical intensive care unit. J Am Coll Surg 2004;198:198.

Iron
Deficiency [158,159]

For clinicians, the sequelae of the last stage of iron deficiency, when stores are depleted and anemia occurs, are equated with iron deficiency. However, the role of delivering oxygen to the tissues is dependent not only on hemoglobin concentration but also on the ability of iron-containing proteins in mitochondria to process the oxygen. Such changes may account for the symptoms more prevalent in children (i.e., anorexia, decreased resistance to infection, and reversible protein-losing enteropathy) and for other features not easily explained by anemia, such as angular stomatitis, atrophic lingual papillae, koilonychia, and behavioral or cognitive changes [160]. Cognitive changes have been correlated with low hemoglobin levels in dieting adults, although it is not clear whether the iron was causative [161]. When anemia develops, weakness and pallor predominate. Iron supplements can decrease fatigue in women who are not anemic (mean ferritin concentration 10.5 μg/L), showing that iron deficiency can be recognized and treated preclinically [162].

Assessment

The hemoglobin and hematocrit are the initial and best screening tests [163], but the results should be interpreted with caution. The patient's age and gender have to be considered in assessing the iron status of any individual. Moreover, hemoglobin concentrations can be altered by dehydration or overhydration, chronic inflammation or infection, protein–calorie malnutrition, cobalamin or folate deficiency, hemoglobinopathies, and pregnancy. Thus, hemoglobin is at best an indirect index of the iron status. The ferritin levels in serum are directly proportional to marrow iron stores and inversely proportional to transferrin levels, with each milligram per liter representing 10 mg of storage iron. Low levels of serum ferritin (< 15 ng/mL) in the presence of anemia nearly always reflect decreased iron stores, and values up to 35 ng/mL are suggestive [1]. However, ferritin levels can be elevated in cases of acute and chronic inflammation, cobalamin or folate deficiency, leukemia or lymphoma or other tumors, alcohol intake, and hyperthyroidism. Thus, values between 15 and 100 ng/mL can be seen in patients with iron deficiency. Serum iron levels alone are not a good measure of the iron status because they do not reflect a stable body pool. About 35 mg is turned over in the plasma each day, and levels can change rapidly in response to acute inflammation. In iron deficiency, serum transferrin levels rise whereas iron levels fall, so that the percentage of saturation falls below 15%. When chronic inflammation, infection, or liver disease is present, serum transferrin levels fall. Transferrin synthesis is downregulated by iron status at the level of translation, so that transferrin levels are elevated in iron deficiency. Thus, a low percentage of saturation in the presence of low transferrin levels does not reflect iron deficiency but rather the anemia of chronic inflammation. Table 30.13 outlines the predictive value of the usual tests in iron deficiency compared with anemia of chronic inflammation [163].

How to proceed when ferritin values are above 35 ng/mL is not clear, and transferrin receptors have been suggested as a possible aid [164]. The amount of uptake of transferrin into cells is regulated by alterations in the number of soluble transferrin receptors (sTfR) on the surface of cells and is most dependent on marrow erythropoiesis activity [164], although intracellular concentration of iron is also important. The highest concentration of transferrin receptors is on cells with the greatest need for iron, such as reticulocytes. A truncated form of the receptor is found in human plasma bound to transferrin, and its content is elevated in iron deficiency, even if mild and of recent onset. The levels of transferrin receptor are not affected by inflammation or liver disease, because cytokines and other factors suppress erythropoiesis through inhibition of erythropoietin production. Thus, the levels of

transferrin receptor can be used to distinguish iron deficiency from the anemia of chronic disease. Normal sTfR levels average 5.0 ± 1.0 mg/L, but the lack of an international standard makes comparison of laboratory values difficult. Receptor levels are also increased when erythropoiesis is stimulated by hemolysis or ineffective erythropoiesis.

Treatment

Oral iron is available in a wide variety of preparations as a single nutrient or in combination with other vitamins and minerals. The amount used is not important so long as it is adequate to replenish body stores, with an assumption of 20% absorption at the start of treatment for iron deficiency. The approximate percentages of the preparations as elemental iron are as follows: sulfate anhydrous, 30%; sulfate $7H_2O$ hydrated, 20%; fumarate, 33%; and gluconate, 11.6%. The dose should be calculated based on the elemental iron content. A standard dosing schedule is ferrous sulfate (65 mg of elemental iron) two to three times a day between meals. Side effects include nausea, indigestion, diarrhea, and abdominal cramping and can limit the amount that can be ingested. Side effects may be less common when slow-release forms are used, but the iron may be made less available by delaying release to beyond the duodenum, the site of maximal absorption. The total iron deficit can be determined roughly by calculating the amount needed to replenish hemoglobin, with an additional gram for repleting tissue stores: iron deficit (mg) in males = body weight (lb) × (15 – hemoglobin [g/dL]) + 1000. A hemoglobin value of 12 or 13 g/dL can be used for females, 14 or 15 g/dL for males. If 10% absorption throughout therapy is assumed, the total dose required can be calculated. Once the daily tolerable supplement is determined for a patient, the length of treatment necessary to replete the stores can be calculated. Oral preparations should be continued for 1–3 months after the hemoglobin level is restored to allow for restoration of other tissue stores. Parenteral iron is used only when oral iron is not tolerated or effective. Iron dextran (50 mg/mL) is available for intramuscular or intravenous use. The total dose required to replete stores is based on the patient's weight and hemoglobin level:

$$\text{Total iron (mg)} = 0.3 \times \text{body weight (lb)} \times 100$$

$$- \frac{\text{hemoglobin (g/dL)} \times 100}{14.8}$$

The intravenous route is safe when the iron is diluted in normal saline solution and administered over 2–3 h [165] (Table 30.14). A test dose of 25 mg of iron dextran should be given initially, and the daily dose should not exceed 100 mg if one wishes to minimize the risk for side effects. A test dose is not required for the other parenteral iron preparations. However, medium-dose (100–400 mg) or high-dose (500–1000 mg

Table 30.13 Serum tests that differentiate anemia of chronic inflammation (ACI) from iron deficiency anemia (FeD)

Serum test	ACI	FeD	Both
Iron	↓	↓	↓
Transferrin	↓ or NL	↑	↓
Transferrin saturation	↓	↓	↓
Ferritin	↑	↓	↓ to NL
Soluble transferrin receptor (sTfR)	↓	↑	NL to ↑
sTfR/log ferritin	< 1	> 2	> 2
Cytokine levels	↑	NL	↑

NL, normal.
Adapted from Weiss & Goodnough [163].

Table 30.14 Parenteral iron therapy

Parameter	Iron dextran	Sodium ferric gluconate	Iron sucrose
Product	INFeD (100 mg/2 mL) DexFerrum (100 mg/2 mL) Desferal (500 mg/vial)	Ferrlecit (62.5 mg/5 mL)	Venofer (100 mg/5 mL)
Test dose	Required	Not required	Not required
Recommended dose	100 mg/day to repletion	125 mg/dialysis session × 8 doses May repeat p.r.n. for ferritin < 100 ng/mL and Tf saturation < 26%	100 mg 1–3 times/week × 10 doses – repeat p.r.n.
Maximal dose	May give to full replacement	10 mL (25 mg)	5 mL (100 mg)
Method	Diluted in 250–1 L over 4–6 h	Undiluted 12.5 mg/min Diluted in 100 mL NS over 60 min	Undiluted up to 20 mg/min, or diluted in 100 mL NS over > 15 min
TPN compatible	Nonlipid solutions	Not studied	Not studied

Limitations	Stop oral iron
	Do not exceed calculated dose
		↓ Dose by 50% for ferritin
		  > 100 ng/mL, or Tf saturation
		  > 35%
		Hold dose for ferritin
		  > 500 ng/mL or Tf saturation
		  > 50%
			Same as Fe gluconate

NS, normal saline; p.r.n., as required; Tf, transferrin; TPN, total parenteral nutrition.
Adapted from Kumpf [165] and Aronoff [167].

up to full replacement) regimens of iron dextran can be used safely and more conveniently, provided adequate precautions are taken and the patient is observed during the infusion [165]. Anaphylaxis is extremely rare when iron dextran is given in this way. However, the patient should be closely supervised and parenteral iron given with caution to anyone with asthma or allergy. Epinephrine (adrenaline) should be available for acute hypersensitivity reactions, and antihistaminics can be given for symptoms of urticaria, rashes, sweating, dizziness, headache, nausea, and fever. Ferric gluconate is the preparation preferred by some experts [166]. All parenteral iron preparations are fairly safe, with the incidence of serious adverse events ranging from 0.4% to 2.5% [167]. Most patients with Crohn's disease who require parenteral iron will respond, but erythropoietin can enhance the response [168].

Zinc
Deficiency
Zinc deficiency is difficult to identify, because plasma zinc is an insensitive predictor of zinc status; thus, deficiency is probably underdiagnosed. Overt deficiency in otherwise healthy individuals is not reported in the United States, but the growth of children can be limited by inadequate dietary zinc [169]. Patients with gastrointestinal disease (Crohn's disease, short bowel syndrome), cystic fibrosis, pancreatic insufficiency, or chronic diarrhea from any cause are at increased

risk for zinc deficiency because of increased losses in the stool and decreased intake [170]. Diarrheal stool contains about 17 mEq of zinc per liter, in excess of the recommended dietary allowance (RDA). Other conditions predisposing to zinc deficiency include cirrhosis, sickle cell anemia, pregnancy, pica, and penicillamine treatment [171]. Clinical manifestations include growth retardation (in children), skin lesions on the face and limbs (which can vary from moist and pustular to seborrheic and acneiform), alopecia, diarrhea, apathy, night blindness, and possibly poor wound healing and loss of taste. However, the single double-blinded study of the effect of zinc supplements on taste and smell dysfunction did not support a role for zinc [171].

Assessment
None of the available methods reliably reflects either recent intake or absorption or body stores. The fasting plasma concentration is most often used, but it correlates poorly with total body zinc except when the patient is severely deficient. Most zinc in blood is in red cells, so that even small amounts of hemolysis can alter plasma zinc. Most plasma zinc is bound tightly to α_2-macroglobulins or loosely to albumin. Thus, hypoproteinemia can lower zinc levels. The plasma level may be falsely low because it can be decreased by many other factors, such as stress, infection, polypharmacy (displacing zinc from albumin), and corticosteroids [1,138]. Levels below 50 µg/mL are often associated with some symptoms,

and patients with levels below 30 µg/mL nearly always have some manifestation of deficiency. Metallothionein is a zinc/copper-binding protein that is reduced in zinc deficiency, and its red cell content has been low when zinc plasma levels were normal, perhaps reflecting a functional zinc pool [172]. At present, however, if zinc deficiency is suspected, it is best diagnosed by the symptomatic response to zinc therapy.

Treatment

Zinc is available as a single nutrient and as a component of many multivitamin and mineral preparations. Zinc supplementation should be provided to persons at risk for the development of deficiency, as well as to those with symptomatic deficiency [173]. Zinc sulfate (67 mg or 220 mg) contains 15 or 50 mg of elemental zinc. Thus, unlike a single dose of other minerals, a single dose of zinc exceeds the RDA, and oral therapy is usually sufficient although absorption is only about 20%. Parenteral zinc therapy is also available as the sulfate or chloride. Zinc is safe to use; the minimum oral toxic dose is 500 mg/day [1]. Long-term ingestion of high doses (450 g/day) can induce copper deficiency [174]. Zinc supplements have reduced the incidence, prevalence, duration, and severity of diarrhea and pneumonia in children from developing nations, presumably because the availability of dietary zinc in such regions is limited [175]. Because of its effect in diarrhea of children, zinc has been added to some oral rehydration solutions. Zinc does not appear to help in treatment of the common cold [176]. Supplemental zinc decreases measures of iron status in patients with low iron reserves [177]. Although zinc is not usually considered a toxic metal, a familial syndrome of hyperzincemia is associated with recurrent infections, hepatosplenomegaly, inflammatory skin lesions, arthritis, and anemia [178].

Copper
Deficiency

Copper deficiency in adults is rare. It can occur in patients receiving TPN without copper supplementation and in patients treated with chelating agents, such as D-penicillamine, with or without large doses of zinc [179]. Premature infants, malnourished or malabsorbing patients, and persons with Menkes syndrome, an inherited defect in copper absorption, are at higher risk for the development of deficiency [180]. Neutropenia, anemia, diarrhea, and scurvy-like bone changes can occur, but detection of early deficiency can be difficult [181]. A clinical myelopathy similar to subacute combined degeneration is being increasingly reported with severe copper deficiency [182]. Copper supplementation should also be considered for patients with increased gastrointestinal fluid losses, especially from chronic biliary tract fistulae, because biliary secretion is the major excretory route for copper [179].

Assessment

Laboratory assessment of copper status is difficult because serum concentrations do not correlate well with tissue levels.

Because 80% of copper is bound to ceruloplasmin (each milligram binds 3.3 µg of copper) and the rest to other proteins, the level does not correlate with intake [183]. However, tissue copper levels are relatively stable and change slowly. Thus, when deficiency occurs, the plasma level often falls earlier than the tissue levels. Normal levels are increased by estrogens or oral contraceptives, pregnancy, and acute and chronic infections. Levels are decreased in nephrosis, Wilson disease, and any cause of protein malnutrition. Free copper levels are more instructive than total levels and can be estimated by calculating bound copper (bound copper = ceruloplasmin [µg/dL] × 3) and subtracting it from the total. Values below 25 µg/dL are normal [184]. This calculation is more sensitive in detecting elevated copper levels (as in Wilson disease) than in detecting copper deficiency.

Treatment

Oral supplementation can be provided by the copper sulfate in multivitamin and mineral preparations, which contain 0.4 mg of elemental copper per milligram of copper sulfate. The daily dose of 2–3 mg is adequate to treat deficiency in adults. The suggested maintenance intravenous dose is 0.3–1.5 mg/day, but the dose should be reduced to 0.15 mg/day for patients with cholestasis [185]. To treat deficiency, 2 to 3 mg/day has been given intravenously, repeated thrice weekly until the ceruloplasmin level normalizes, usually in about 10 days. There is a large margin of safety in using copper supplements, but acute oral ingestion of more than 15 mg of elemental copper produces nausea, vomiting, diarrhea, abdominal cramps, and mucosal ulceration. At larger doses, hemolysis, gastrointestinal bleeding, azotemia, and jaundice can occur. The treatment of toxicity includes gastric lavage and 1 g of D-penicillamine per day [186].

Thiamin (vitamin B-1)
Deficiency

Deficiency of thiamin may be caused by decreased intake or increased tissue utilization, or by a combination of factors. Thus, the usual clinical settings include pregnancy, chronic alcoholism, malabsorption syndromes, chronic nausea and vomiting, prolonged febrile illnesses, and chronic renal dialysis. The total requirement is usually more than 1 mg/day in adults, and the total stores are only about 30 mg, so deficiency can develop fairly rapidly. In parts of the world where polished rice is the staple cereal in the diet, beriberi (weakness, paresthesias, high-output cardiac failure) is seen. In the United States, where food thiamin is abundant, the deficiency syndrome is often seen in conjunction with deficiency of other B vitamins. Symptoms and signs include peripheral neuropathy, limb weakness, cerebellar dysfunction, subacute necrotizing encephalomyelopathy, and Wernicke encephalopathy (apathy, confusion, ataxia, photophobia, nystagmus, paralysis of upward gaze). Signs of deficiency may worsen if glucose is given without thiamin. If lactic acidosis is also present, signs of heart failure may develop [187]. Thiamin deficiency should be considered in the differential diagnosis of lactic acidosis.

Assessment

Recent intake or absorption, but not body stores, is correlated with urinary excretion. The amount excreted is greater during childhood, when growth is rapid, so the result (micrograms of thiamin per gram of creatinine) must be compared with the values in age-matched controls. Body stores are measured either directly in blood or serum by high-performance liquid chromatography or by the erythrocyte transketolase assay, which measures a thiamin-dependent enzyme activity. The activity coefficient of the enzyme is determined by the activity in the presence and absence of added thiamin. In deficiency states, more stimulation occurs, and the activity coefficient is above 1.25 [138].

Treatment

Thiamin hydrochloride is available as a single nutrient in oral and parenteral forms and as a constituent of almost all multivitamin preparations. Adults with mild deficiency should receive 10–20 mg intramuscularly or 25–50 mg orally twice daily for 1 week, followed by an oral maintenance dose of 2–5 mg/day. Benfotiamine (S-benzoylthiamine-O-monophosphate) is a lipid-soluble thiamin analogue that achieves plasma levels five times that of comparable doses of thiamin [188]. There is no clinical correlation with these higher plasma levels. Critically ill patients, especially those with central nervous system manifestations of deficiency, should receive doses of 50–100 mg twice daily intravenously for 3 days, followed by oral supplementation of 5–30 mg/day until a normal diet is resumed. The thiamin should be given before any carbohydrate is administered to avoid enhancing the deficiency. Because thiamin deficiency is often associated with deficiencies of other B vitamins, multiple vitamins should be given. Rare responses to parenteral thiamin include feelings of warmth, tingling, pruritus, nausea, sweating, and anaphylactic reaction [189]. It has been suggested that thiamin improves energy levels during exercise and in the elderly, and cognition in Alzheimer disease, but the few studies performed do not support these conclusions [190].

Riboflavin (vitamin B-2)
Deficiency

Riboflavin deficiency usually occurs along with deficiencies of other B vitamins, especially in patients with malabsorption and chronic alcoholism. Early symptoms relate to oral or eye lesions. Angular stomatitis (maceration and fissuring of the mucocutaneous junction at the angles of the mouth), cheilosis (inflammation of the lips), glossitis, geographic tongue, seborrhea-like dermatitis, pruritus, photophobia, corneal vascularization, and visual impairment may occur. The differential diagnosis of the lip lesions includes poorly fitting dentures with malocclusion, allergy (e.g., lipstick, toothpaste), and iron deficiency anemia. Other vitamin B deficiencies can cause the tongue lesions. Some of these symptoms occur in vitamin B-6 deficiency because the oxidase necessary to produce functional vitamin B-6 is riboflavin-dependent [191].

Assessment

Urinary excretion correlates well with intake because the vitamin is excreted unmetabolized. With fasting or prolonged bed rest, urinary excretion can be falsely elevated. Levels below 40 μ/g of creatinine signify extremely low intake in an adult. Body stores of riboflavin are assessed by measuring the riboflavin-dependent enzyme erythrocyte glutathione reductase in the blood. An activity coefficient above 1.2 (stimulated/control activity) signifies deficiency [138].

Treatment

Deficiency can be treated with 5–10 mg/day orally, along with other vitamins [192]. When malabsorption is present, a prophylactic dose of 3 mg/day is recommended, usually as part of a multivitamin preparation. Riboflavin may cause a yellow-orange appearance to the urine but is remarkably nontoxic.

Niacin (vitamin B-3)
Deficiency

Because of the niacin supplementation of grains and breads, the classical deficiency syndrome of pellagra (dermatitis, dementia, diarrhea) is rare in the United States. Deficiency is seen most often in patients on a diet of meat, cornmeal, and molasses, with chronic alcoholism, malabsorption syndromes, or carcinoid syndrome, in which a large amount of tryptophan (niacin precursor) is converted instead to serotonin. Pellagra rarely occurs in the carcinoid syndrome, and when it does it can be overcome with oral niacin. Hartnup disease is associated with a defect in tryptophan absorption and can also predispose to deficiency [193]. Isoniazid therapy can lead to deficiency because hydrazines form adducts with pyridoxal phosphate. The last enzyme in the conversion of tryptophan to nicotinic acid, kynureninase, requires pyridoxal, thereby linking the deficiency of these two vitamins. Moreover, isoniazid resembles nicotinic acid and acts as an inhibitor. In niacin deficiency, the dermatitis occurs over exposed areas and is scaly. Twenty percent of patients get dyssebacea, referring to plugs of inspissated sebum projecting from deleted orifices of sebaceous glands, appearing first along the alae nasi, spreading over the nose, and then the forehead, lips, and chin. It is not inflammatory, and is unrelated to sunlight, unlike the dermatitis, and can precede the dermatitis by weeks. Painful tongue and angular stomatitis are seen but may be caused in part by accompanying riboflavin deficiency. Diarrhea is probably caused by the direct effect of niacin deficiency on epithelial cell function. Central nervous system dysfunction includes irritability, headache, insomnia, psychosis, hallucinations, and seizures.

Assessment

The urine content of the niacin metabolite *N*-methylnicotinamide reflects intake and absorption and is less than 0.5 mg/g of creatinine in adults with deficient intake. No test is available for body stores of niacin, although the results of one study in young men suggested that an erythrocyte ratio of nicotinamide adenine dinucleotide (NAD) to nicotinamide adenine dinucleotide phosphate (NADP) below 1.0 might reflect deficiency [138].

Treatment

Isolated niacin deficiency is unusual in the United States, so treatment with other B vitamins often accompanies niacin replacement. Depending on their severity, the symptoms of pellagra respond to oral doses of 100–500 mg of niacin per day [193]. Mental, gastrointestinal, and oral symptoms clear rapidly, but the resolution of skin lesions may require weeks to months. Large doses of nicotinic acid (1–3 g/day) used to treat hypercholesterolemia can cause flushing, pruritus, burning sensations, nausea, vomiting, heartburn, diarrhea, dizziness, and tachycardia. Hyperglycemia and increased serum aminotransferase and bilirubin levels can occur at doses as low as 750 mg of nicotinic acid per day [194].

Pyridoxine (vitamin B-6)

Deficiency

Because vitamin B-6 is abundant in foods and is produced by colonic bacteria, dietary deficiency is rare. It is most often reported as a result of treatment with pyridoxine antagonists, especially isoniazid, hydralazine, oral contraceptives, dopamine, and D-penicillamine. Rarely, deficiency occurs in chronic alcoholism or malabsorption, usually in association with deficiencies of other B vitamins. The clinical manifestations include peripheral neuropathy, seborrheic dermatitis around the eyes and nasolabial folds, and oral lesions (angular stomatitis, cheilosis, glossitis), similar to those seen in riboflavin and niacin deficiencies. Seizures and sideroblastic anemia may also occur [195]. Hyperhomocystinuria has been identified as an independent risk factor for vascular disease and may be caused in part by a deficiency of cystathionine synthase, the vitamin B-6-dependent enzyme that catalyzes the conversion of homocysteine to cystathionine. Twelve large-scale randomized studies have examined the effect of B-vitamin supplementation on cardiovascular risk, and shown that homocysteine levels can be normalized, but any effect on clinical outcomes is still uncertain [196]. It is premature to recommend the use of these supplements to alter atherogenesis in this subset of patients with hyperhomocystinemia [197]. Low vitamin B-6 levels have been associated with an increased risk for first venous thrombosis in a single study [198], so it is not inconceivable that vitamin supplementation might carry some risk on its own.

Assessment

Recent intake is reflected by the urinary excretion of metabolites. A low intake correlates with excretion of less than 500 μg of 4-pyridoxic acid per day. Body stores are measured by the erythrocyte aminotransferase index, with a determination of enzyme activity in the presence and absence of pyridoxal phosphate. Deficiency is correlated with an erythrocyte aspartate aminotransferase (E-AST) index above 2.2. Alternatively, pyridoxal phosphate can be measured in whole blood (50–120 nmol/L) or plasma (> 30 nmol/L), although the levels associated with deficiency have not been precisely determined [138].

Treatment

Pyridoxal phosphate is available in both oral and parenteral forms. Suspected deficiency should be treated with 50–150 mg/day orally, especially when neuropathy is present. A multiple vitamin preparation containing 2–5 mg of pyridoxine should be added to provide the other B vitamins. Some experts suggest such a supplement for all patients on isoniazid and similar inhibitors, whereas others suggest supplements only for those patients at high risk for the development of neuropathy. Pyridoxine is used in large doses for isoniazid overdose, *Gyromitra* (monomethylhydrazine) mushroom poisoning, and hydrazine overexposure [199]. When pyridoxal phosphate is ingested in large amounts (2–6 g/day), a peripheral neuropathy may develop [200]. Pyridoxine antagonizes levodopa by stimulating the decarboxylation of dopa to dopamine. Therefore, patients taking levodopa should limit their pyridoxine intake to less than 5 mg/day [201].

Folate

Deficiency

Folate deficiency is associated with poor socioeconomic and dietary conditions, especially with chronic alcoholism (usually > 80 g/day) and malabsorption syndromes. Alcohol can increase urinary folate excretion [202]. Deficiency also results from competition for absorption (sulfasalazine), long-term anticonvulsant therapy (usually years), increased utilization (pregnancy, hemolytic anemia, leukemia, chronic myelofibrosis), and inhibition of dihydrofolate reductase (the enzyme that converts folate to the active coenzyme) by methotrexate, trimethoprim, and pyrimethamine [203]. A cerebral folate deficiency syndrome can be produced by folate receptor antibodies in infants, older children, and occasionally in adults, resulting from blocked folate transport into the brain [204]. Serum and erythrocyte folate levels and serum homocysteine are normal, but 5-methyltetrahydrofolate concentration in the cerebrospinal fluid is low and accounts for the developmental and neurological abnormalities. If folate stores are normal initially, symptoms will appear in about 4 months. The primary manifestation of classical folate deficiency is macrocytic anemia, often accompanied by thrombocytopenia and leukopenia. Other symptoms may include glossitis, diarrhea, fatigue, and possibly (but uncommonly) neurological signs.

Two other significant forms of folate deficiency occur in the absence of classical evidence of deficiency. Women consuming too little folic acid during early pregnancy are at increased risk for delivering children with neural tube defects. The Dietary Reference Intake Committee has confirmed the recommendation of the US Department of Health and Human Services that all women capable of becoming pregnant ingest 400 μg of synthetic folic acid daily [203]. Hyperhomocystinemia can be caused by folate deficiency if it is not accompanied by elevated methylmalonic acid levels. High levels of homocysteine are correlated with an increased risk for myocardial infarction in some studies, in about 10% of patients [197]. Although the folate levels are normal, the hyperhomocystinemia can be corrected by supplemental folate, but it is not clear that the risk for heart disease is altered. The epidemiological data implicating homocysteine as a factor in cardiovascular risk are strong, but data from some prospective interventional studies have been less consistent [197,205]. Although a low folate status is a strong determinant of elevated total homocysteine levels, the folate status was not associated with homocysteine levels [143], nor with an increased risk for coronary atherosclerosis [206]. These data are consistent with overrating of homocysteine as a risk factor for heart disease. Similarly, the importance of homocysteine and folate levels as risk factors for stroke is probably small [207].

Assessment
Because folate deficiency develops during decreased intake or absorption, the first laboratory abnormality to develop is a decrease in the serum folate (2–6 ng/mL), which is sensitive to changes in intake [138]. Values below 2 ng/mL are usually associated with megaloblastic anemia and decreased tissue reserves. Because about 50% of serum folate is bound to albumin, hypoalbuminemia can produce falsely low serum folate levels. Body stores of folate can be measured by red cell folate more accurately than by serum folate. Both red and white cells contain much more folate than serum does, so hemolysis or a leukemoid reaction can falsely elevate the serum folate. When both serum folate (< 2 ng/mL) and red cell folate (< 140 ng/mL) are low, folate deficiency is the cause. When cobalamin deficiency is present, folate may not be well utilized in 15%–25% of cases, so serum folate rises and red cell folate falls. Multilobed polymorphonuclear cells and macrocytic anemia develop after tissue folate levels fall [138]. Serum homocysteine levels above 30 μmol/L are consistent with folate deficiency if the methylmalonic acid levels are normal.

Treatment
Oral folate supplements are available in tablets up to 1 mg, but the unreduced pteroylglutamic acid is the form used.

Most of this form is excreted unchanged or after degradation, so the dose of this supplement cannot be compared with the true folate requirements. Folinic acid (5-formyltetrahydrofolate) is needed for treating the cerebral folate syndrome. The parenteral route is used only if oral therapy is not possible or malabsorption is severe. A reticulocyte response is seen in 3–5 days, and a peak response occurs in 5–10 days. The 400-μg dose found in multivitamin preparations is usually adequate as maintenance therapy for patients with malabsorption or alcoholism. For patients on sulfasalazine or with hemolytic anemia, a dose of 1 mg/day is suggested. Folate can lower plasma homocysteine, but the data do not yet support a preventive role for folate in cardiovascular disease, stroke, or other chronic diseases [205–208]. Betaine (trimethylglycine) is a methyl donor, approved by the US Food and Drug Administration (FDA) for the treatment of homocystinuria, that does lower plasma homocysteine, but not more so than folate [209]. Foltx (folic acid 2.5 mg, cyanocobalamin 1 mg, and pyridoxine 25 mg) is an over-the-counter preparation promoted for hyperhomocysteinemia, but its benefit compared with existing preparations is unknown. Folate is remarkably nontoxic. Large doses (> 100 times the RDA) can precipitate convulsions in patients treated with phenytoin [210]. Giving folate to a patient with cobalamin deficiency corrects the anemia but does not prevent irreversible neurological damage. The tolerable upper intake level (UL) for folate of 1000 μg/day has been challenged because all but eight cases of masking neurological progression (not just worsening anemia) in vitamin B-12 deficiency occurred in patients taking more than 5 mg of folate per day [211].

Cobalamin (vitamin B-12)
Deficiency
A dietary deficiency of cobalamin occurs only in lacto-ovo-vegetarians who do not consume any food of animal origin. The most common causes in adults are gastric lesions (especially the atrophic gastritis associated with pernicious anemia or gastrectomy), lesions or resection of the terminal ileum (especially in Crohn's disease), and bacterial overgrowth. Gastric pathology accounts for well over half the cases. An increasingly common cause of low serum cobalamin levels is AIDS. The significance of the low levels is not always clear, but some patients manifest subtle alterations in mental and cognitive abilities [212]. Reversible chorea and dystonia have been reported as a result of cobalamin deficiency [213]. Deficiency also occurs rarely in patients with severe chronic pancreatitis, congenital deficiency of the carrier protein transcobalamin II (TCII), or an inability to utilize food-bound cobalamin in the absence of other gastric pathology [214]. Symptoms are insidious and develop over 2–3 years, sooner if malabsorption is the cause. A sore tongue, paresthesias, anorexia, loss of taste, diarrhea, dyspepsia, hair loss, impotence, irritability, and psychiatric illness (e.g., depression) can

be present. Numbness and tingling, especially in the lower extremities, can progress to loss of vibratory sensation, loss of coordination, muscle weakness, and atrophy, and memory disturbances can develop [215]. Macrocytic anemia with megaloblastic bone marrow and multilobed nuclei in the polymorphonuclear leukocytes is frequently, but not alw ays, present. The macrocytic anemia must be differentiated from chronic liver disease and from hypothyroidism. Many patients, especially those who are elderly, present with neurological symptoms and signs in the absence of anemia assessment.

Assessment

The diagnosis of cobalamin deficiency is usually suspected on the basis of hematological findings [216]. The serum concentration of cobalamin usually correlates with body stores. Unlike the folate concentration, the cobalamin concentration in red cells is no higher than that in serum, so hemolysis is not a cause of falsely elevated values. In humans, only a small proportion of cobalamin is carried on TCII, the protein that delivers the vitamin to the tissues. Thus, there can be a stage at which the serum level is normal (cobalamin is bound to haptocorrin) but tissue levels are low. Falsely high levels can be seen in leukocytosis (release of haptocorrin, increasing the total serum binding capacity) and in acute liver disease (release of body stores). Conversely, serum levels can be low when body stores are normal. Protein deficiency can lower serum levels without affecting tissue delivery if the TCII levels are normal. Levels are low in pregnant women because of dilution and redistribution of binding proteins. Serum cobalamin levels below 150 pg/mL (110 pmol/mL) are always associated with deficiency if causes of falsely low levels are not present (folate or protein deficiency, pregnancy). Levels between 150 and 200 pg/mL should be considered suspect and should lead to further testing with methylmalonic acid

and homocysteine levels, correlation with abnormal hematological or neurological findings, or both. A subtle presentation of cobalamin deficiency is especially likely in elderly patients [217]. In doubtful cases, a therapeutic trial with cobalamin is safe, and reversal of the abnormal findings is diagnostic.

Biochemical tests for cobalamin deficiency can clarify cases in which the serum cobalamin levels combined with the clinical picture are not definitive. The workup should also include a careful neurological examination. The serum can be assayed for metabolites that increase when the function of the two cobalamin-dependent enzymes is impaired: methylmalonyl-CoA mutase (methylmalonic acid increased) and methionine synthase (homocysteine increased). Folate deficiency leads to an increase in homocysteine levels (> 20 μmol/L) but not in methylmalonic acid levels, whereas cobalamin deficiency increases methylmalonic acid (> 390 nmol/L) as well [218]. Methylmalonic acid levels can be elevated in the absence of cobalamin deficiency when renal insufficiency is present. Because TCII is the protein that delivers cobalamin to tissues but accounts for less than 10% of serum cobalamin binding, low holo-TCII concentrations have been reported as the earliest sign of negative cobalamin balance [89]. This test is not used routinely. The selection of the various tests for cobalamin deficiency depends on the stage of deficiency suspected (Table 30.15). Early sensory neuropathy can be linked to cobalamin deficiency by evidence of myelopathy obtained by spiral magnetic resonance imaging (MRI) [219].

Because abnormal serum measurements of cobalamin metabolism precede the late manifestations of tissue damage, it is recommended that populations at risk are screened. These include strict vegetarians, persons older than 65 years of age with decreased food intake, and patients with any of the following: unexplained neurological or psychiatric

Table 30.15 Laboratory tests in sequential stages of cobalamin deficiency

| Parameter | Stage of cobalamin deficiency | | | | |
	None	I	II	III	IV
Cbl balance	Normal	Negative balance of stores	Depletion (early)	Tissue damage (late)	
Serum holo-TCII	> 60 pg/mL	Low	Low	Low	Low
Serum Cbl	> 201 pg/mL	> 201 pg/mL	> 201 pg/mL	Low	Low
Serum MMA	< 376 nmol/L	< 376 nmol/L	< 376 nmol/L	High	High
Serum Hcy	< 15 μmol/L	< 15 μmol/L	< 15 μmol/L	High	High
RBC folate	> 160 pg/mL	> 160 pg/mL	> 160 pg/mL	> 140 pg/mL	> 100 pg/mL
Neurological symptoms	None	None	None	Sometimes	Frequent
MCV	Normal	Normal	Normal	Normal	High
Hemoglobin	Normal	Normal	Normal	Normal	Low

Cbl, cobalamin; Hcy, homocysteine; MCV, mean corpuscular volume; MMA, methylmalonic acid; RBC, red blood cell; TCII, transcobalamin II.
Adapted from Herbert VD. Round Table Series 66. London: Royal Society of Medicine Press, 1999.

symptoms or anemia, long-term use of proton pump inhibitors, autoimmune diseases, AIDS, previous gastric surgery, Crohn's disease of the ileum, and malabsorption from any cause. Screening should be done with serum holo-TCII measurements if available, either alone or in conjunction with serum cobalamin. If serum cobalamin alone is used and values below 350 pg/mL are obtained, metabolite assays should be performed if cobalamin deficiency is suspected clinically. The combination of a serum cobalamin value below 350 pmol/mL and an elevated methylmalonic acid concentration has a specificity of 98% for cobalamin deficiency [220].

Intake or absorption should be assessed only when clinically indicated. If gastric atrophy is demonstrated by biopsy, or if gastrectomy is known from the history or the radiographic findings, it is not usually necessary to confirm the absence of intrinsic factor by a Schilling test. Urinary excretion of less than 5% labeled cobalamin is diagnostic of malabsorption, whereas excretion of more than 10% labeled cobalamin is normal, but many results are indeterminate (5%–10%) [1,138]. This lack of sensitivity is also a factor in deciding whether to proceed with the test. The two major causes of a falsely normal Schilling test result are an erroneous value (intertest variability can be as high as 30%–50%) and malabsorption of food cobalamin, presumably because of an inability of gastric proteases to liberate the vitamin. The Schilling test must be performed with labeled food cobalamin (usually in liver or scrambled eggs) to make the diagnosis because the standard Schilling test uses free cobalamin. However, the commercially available versions of the test have not been uniformly standardized.

Treatment

If cobalamin deficiency is caused simply by decreased intake without malabsorption, 3–6 µg of oral cobalamin per day will suffice. However, if malabsorption is present, either because of lack of intrinsic factor or of intestinal disease, then losses of up to 10 µg/day must be allowed for. Deficiency is treated with 100 to 1000 µg/day for 5–10 days, followed by at least 300 µg/month, given by subcutaneous injection, indefinitely. Alternatively, oral or sublingual cobalamin can be given with equal efficacy (2 or 1 mg/day, respectively) to take advantage of the inefficient (~ 1%) absorption of the vitamin in the absence of intrinsic factor [221]. Nasal spray and nasal gel formulations of cyanocobalamin (Nascobal) are available, in the recommended dose of 500 µg once per week [222]. Although normal cobalamin levels can be restored by larger doses, no studies have documented equal efficacy with the much more expensive nasal preparation. Increased well-being is noted within 24 h of initiating treatment, painful glossitis improves in 48 h, and reticulocytosis begins in 5 to 7 days. Serum folate falls rapidly. The reversal of neurological signs may take 6 months or more. No significant toxicity has been reported with therapeutic doses of oral or parenteral cobalamin.

Ascorbic acid (vitamin C)

Deficiency

Scurvy develops in 2–3 months if the diet is deficient in ascorbic acid. It occurs in the United States only rarely, usually in cases of chronic alcoholism, malabsorption, or food faddism. Early symptoms are weakness, lassitude, irritability, aching joints and muscles, and weight loss. Later, perifollicular hyperkeratotic papules appear on the buttocks, thighs, and legs, followed by petechiae on the lower legs [223]. In advanced deficiency, the gums become swollen, red, and spongy and hemorrhaging occurs, especially from the gums and in the skin and muscles. Anemia is common. No deficiency syndrome other than scurvy has been reported.

Assessment

Plasma ascorbate levels reflect recent intake. Thus, a low serum concentration precedes clinical scurvy [138]. Low levels do not necessarily denote scurvy, however. Levels can be falsely low in patients with chronic inflammatory diseases, in cigarette smokers, after severe emotional stress, and in women taking oral contraceptives. Levels below 0.2 mg/dL (11 µmol/L) denote deficient intake or absorption; that level is reached in 3–5 months. Leukocyte ascorbate concentration is better correlated with body stores (< 150 µmol/L represents a high risk for deficiency), but the assay is technically difficult and requires large blood samples. Because the diagnosis of scurvy should be made quickly, plasma ascorbate is the initial test of choice.

Treatment

Scurvy may respond to as little as 10 mg of vitamin C per day, but doses between 60–100 mg/day and 250 mg four times daily are recommended to replenish body stores. Large doses of ascorbic acid (2–6 g/day) have been reported to cause diarrhea, promote the formation of renal oxalate stones, increase the excretion of basic drugs by acidifying the urine (e.g., tricyclic antidepressants), decrease the excretion of acidic drugs (e.g., aspirin), and interfere with many laboratory tests, including the fecal tests for occult blood that depend on oxidation of the substrate for a positive reaction. However, the reports of clinically adverse effects with supplemental vitamin C have largely not been substantiated in normal healthy populations [224]. However, despite small benefits regarding the duration and severity of rhinovirus infection in experimental settings, there is no evidence that vitamin C reduces the incidence or severity of the common cold in the general population [225]. Epidemiological studies have noted an inverse relationship between serum levels and coronary artery disease, hypertension, cataracts, and carcinomas, but no evidence for benefit from intervention has been found [226]. It is not indicated to recommend supplemental vitamin C for these conditions.

Biotin

A dietary deficiency of biotin is rare [203,227], but it can be caused by excessive consumption of raw egg white, which contains avidin, a biotin-binding glycoprotein. The serum assay is available, but is complex, involving high-performance liquid chromatography combined with avidin binding. The effects of deficiency include anorexia, nausea, dermatitis, alopecia, mental depression, and organic aciduria. Symptoms disappear with doses of 0.15 to 0.3 mg parenterally, or with 0.2–10 mg/day orally for a few days. No adverse effects of such treatment have been reported.

Pantothenic acid

Definite clinical deficiency has not been reported in humans, probably because the vitamin is so abundant in foods [203]. The "burning feet" syndrome seen in malnourished patients may respond to pantothenic acid, but it is unclear whether this represents a specific deficiency. If deficiency is suspected, 10 mg of calcium pantothenate can be used.

Vitamin A [228,229]
Deficiency

Vitamin A deficiency is usually the result of decreased intake or of fat malabsorption. Contributing factors include impaired conversion of carotenoids to vitamin A (in mucosal disease), decreased storage capacity (in liver disease), decreased levels of serum transport proteins (in liver disease or protein malnutrition), and increased urinary losses (in cancer, tuberculosis, or urinary tract infections) [228].

Inadequate intake is rare in the United States, but the number of new cases of corneal disease caused by vitamin A deficiency worldwide approaches 1 million each year [229]. It takes about 2 years to deplete hepatic stores. Symptoms of deficiency are night blindness, xerophthalmia, follicular hyperkeratosis, altered taste and smell, increased cerebrospinal fluid pressure, and increased infections [230]. When zinc deficiency is also present, the effect on visual adaptation may be magnified.

Assessment

The intake of both carotene and vitamin A is reflected in the serum levels. Decreased intake is reflected in serum vitamin A levels between 10 and 20 µg/dL [138]. A level below 10 µg/dL indicates deficiency. Low carotene levels are meaningful only if carotene is being ingested in the diet because there are no body stores of carotene. In severe liver disease and chronic infection, serum vitamin A levels may fall because retinol-binding protein is not produced in normal amounts. However, carotene levels tend to rise because less carotene is converted to vitamin A in these conditions. Vitamin A can be elevated with normal carotene levels in patients ingesting excess amounts of vitamin A or in patients on chronic hemodialysis because of a decreased conversion of retinol to retinoic acid. Elevated carotene levels with normal retinol are seen in persons ingesting excess amounts of carotene and also in patients with anorexia nervosa, hypothyroidism, hyperlipidemia, or the hypercholesterolemia of diabetes [138].

Treatment

Vitamin A is provided in the form of free retinol. Deficiency states respond to daily oral doses of the vitamin of between 5000 and 50 000 IU. Intramuscular delivery can also be used [1]. Because of their antioxidant properties, carotenoids have been implicated in many chronic diseases often linked with vitamins E and C, the other vitamin antioxidants [223]. However, no convincing evidence is yet available to support supplementation with any antioxidant vitamins, carotenoids, or preformed vitamin A to prevent malignancies or cataracts. Some data suggest that vitamin A may help children with infections to grow [231]. Doses of vitamin A suggested for patients with severe malabsorption are 50 000 IU/day for young infants (0–6 months), 100 000 IU for older infants (6–12 months), and 200 000 IU for children over 1 year of age. Doses of vitamin A above the RDA are contraindicated in pregnant women because of the potential for teratogenicity. The minimum daily dose that is toxic to patients without malabsorption is 25 000–50 000 IU. Toxicity is correlated with serum levels of vitamin A above 1000 µg/dL. Symptoms of chronic toxicity include dry mouth and mucous membranes, skeletal pain, increased cerebrospinal fluid pressure, alopecia, anorexia, irritability, hepatic dysfunction, exophthalmos, and hypercalcemia. Carotene cannot be converted to retinol fast enough for even large doses to produce retinol toxicity.

Vitamin D (cholecalciferol)
Deficiency

Vitamin D deficiency secondary to inadequate intake is rare in the United States, in part because milk products are fortified with the vitamin. Even persons who do not consume dairy products usually obtain adequate sunlight exposure to prevent vitamin D deficiency. However, in elderly persons with little exposure to sunlight, decreased vitamin D intake or synthesis along with inadequate calcium intake may contribute to a high incidence of bone fractures [232]. Deficiency should be considered in any patient with steatorrhea (malabsorption of dietary vitamin and polar metabolites by the enterohepatic circulation) or severe liver disease (decreased 25-hydroxylase activity) or kidney disease (lack of 1α-hydroxylase), as well as in patients with Crohn's disease or previous ileal resection [233]. Vitamin D deficiency causes hypocalcemia and hypophosphatemia, which result in increased parathyroid hormone secretion and bone demineralization. In time, this sequence leads to osteomalacia in adults and rickets in children and can be an unrecognized factor in acute hip fracture [234]. Tetany results from severe hypocalcemia, and muscle weakness is correlated with hypophosphatemia and depletion of muscle phosphate. Patients with risk factors for the development of osteopenia (cigarette smoking, family history, sedentary lifestyle, long-term glucocorticoid therapy, long-term anticonvulsant therapy, early menopause, testicular failure) should be followed even more carefully if they are at risk for vitamin D deficiency. Long-term alcohol abuse is also an overlooked cause of osteoporosis in men [235]. Risk factors for metabolic bone disease in patients with liver disease include female gender, Caucasian race, estrogen deficiency, low–normal BMI, corticosteroid use, and tobacco abuse [236].

Assessment

The 25-hydroxyvitamin D serum level is low when body stores, intake, or endogenous production of the vitamin are low [237]. Thus, this parameter is satisfactory for assessing vitamin D status with respect to deficiency and toxicity. However, the assay is variable: the competitive protein binding assay gives results some 20%–30% higher than the radioimmunoassay (RIA) [166]. Levels of 32 μg/L (80 nmol/L) have been advocated as the upper range of normal, based on the ability to restore plasma parathyroid hormone (PTH) concentrations to normal [238,239]. The production of 25-hydroxyvitamin D is not closely regulated and rises or falls as its substrate is made available. The concentration in serum is 5–10 times that in other tissues except for adipose tissue. It is bound in serum to a binding protein that is normally only 5% saturated, and the half-life is long (24 h). Thus, recent exposure to sunlight or increased oral intake are reflected in the serum level. Levels are low in dietary deficiency, decreased absorption, lack of sunlight, prematurity, and severe liver disease; low levels are also associated with drugs that alter the metabolism (e.g., anticonvulsants). High levels are seen in growing children, conditions in which parathyroid hormone levels are elevated, sarcoidosis, and some forms of idiopathic hypercalciuria.

Patients at risk for deficiency should be followed with periodic measurements of the serum 25-hydroxyvitamin D level, as well as bone density and 24-h urinary calcium measurements, to assess the status of calcium stores and intake (see "Calcium" above). 1,25-Dihydroxyvitamin D can also be measured in the serum. The production of this isoform is closely regulated, but by extracellular ionized calcium not by vitamin D stores, unless the latter are extremely low. The level of this vitamin correlates with vitamin D function more than with stores. Serum 1,25-dihydroxyvitamin D levels are low in profound vitamin D deficiency, chronic renal disease, hypoparathyroidism, vitamin D-resistant rickets type I, and osteolytic conditions not caused by increased PTH levels (cancer, hyperthyroidism). Primary hyperparathyroidism, vitamin D-resistant rickets type II, and pregnancy are conditions in which levels are elevated. Hypervitaminosis D elevates 25-hydroxyvitamin D levels markedly, but 1,25-dihydroxyvitamin D levels are little affected. Table 30.16 provides suggested guidelines for evaluating the vitamin D status.

Treatment

Oral vitamin D does not maintain the vitamin D status as well as endogenous vitamin D; the latter is released more constantly from the skin and is not converted so rapidly to other isomers by the liver, to which virtually all orally administered vitamin D is exposed following absorption. Nonetheless, oral supplements are needed sometimes, especially in patients with fat malabsorption, uremia, long-term corticosteroid use, and possibly postmenopausal osteoporosis, although the proper place of vitamin D supplementation in the management of osteoporosis is still uncertain. Adults with vitamin D deficiency should receive 0.1–0.2 mg (4000–8000 IU) of cholecalciferol daily by mouth. Much larger doses should be used if malabsorption is present, although the exact dose needed may vary widely. Theoretically, the more polar forms, 25-hydroxyvitamin D (calciferol) and 1,25-dihydroxyvitamin D (calcitriol), should be useful in patients with malabsorption [240,241], but the absorptive advantage is probably not sufficient to justify the great increase in cost. Analogues of vitamin D are available for use in chronic renal failure, being designed to decrease the hypercalcemic effect while restoring bone mass [242]. Paricalcitol (19-nor-1α-25-dihydroxyvitamin D-2) also improves survival from cardiovascular and infectious causes of death. The efficacy of treatment should be assessed by periodic measurement of the 25-hydroxyvitamin D level, with the dose adjusted to keep the serum level within the normal range. In patients with malabsorption, one should determine that the function of vitamin D has also been restored – that is, that

Table 30.16 Suggested guidelines for evaluating vitamin D status

Test	Deficient	Low	Acceptable	High
25-Hydroxyvitamin D				
(nmol/L)	≤ 30	< 60	≥ 80	> 200
(ng/mL)	≤ 12	< 24	≥ 32	> 80
1,25-Dihydroxyvitamin D				
(pmol/L)			48–100	
(pg/mL)		20–42		
24-h urinary calcium (mg/kg)	< 2		> 2	
Bone density (SD below mean)	> 2.5	> 2	1–1.5	

calcium absorption has been normalized – by bringing the 24-hour urinary calcium into the normal range. The risk for toxicity in patients with malabsorption is extremely slight. In other patients, hypercalcemia and hypercalciuria may develop. The estimated minimal toxic daily oral dose for healthy adults is 0.125 mg (5000 IU) [1,232]. Nausea, anorexia, itching, polyuria, abdominal pain, constipation, bone pain, metallic taste, and dehydration may be present early, followed by other manifestations of hypercalcemia. Vitamin D toxicity is reversible if renal damage is not severe.

Vitamin E
Deficiency
Deficiency of vitamin E is uncommon in humans. Persons at risk include newborns and premature infants, patients with fat malabsorption or biliary obstruction, and food faddists. Vitamin E does not cross the placenta well and is poorly absorbed in newborns. Severe fat malabsorption in cystic fibrosis, abetalipoproteinemia, short bowel syndrome, biliary obstruction, and excessive mineral oil ingestion can lead to deficiency [243]. Unsteady gait, tremor, weakness, ophthalmoplegia, pigmentary retinopathy, and proprioceptive impairment have been noted in adult malabsorptive syndromes, along with red cell hemolysis. A similar progressive neurological syndrome has been reported in children with cholestatic liver disease [244].

Assessment
Deficiency can be documented by a low serum α-tocopherol concentration (< 11.6 µmol/L or < 5.0 µg/mL) [89]. Because the vitamin is carried in serum by lipoproteins, the plasma concentration of vitamin E is low in any hypolipidemic state. Therefore, the ratio of α-tocopherol to total lipid (triglyceride + cholesterol) is a more accurate indicator of vitamin E status than is the vitamin level alone [245]. Ratios of more than 0.8 mg of α-tocopherol per gram of total lipid or more than 0.22 mg of α-tocopherol per gram of cholesterol are normal. Ethane and pentane are generated through the peroxidation of n-3 and n-6 fatty acids, respectively. Breath ethane has been used to evaluate the vitamin E status and follow therapy in children because the level rises with deficiency [246].

Treatment
Large oral doses of D-α-tocopherol acetate, up to 600 mg (800–900 IU) per day, are needed, especially in patients with malabsorption. A water-soluble form of the vitamin (D-α-tocopherol-PEG-1000 succinate) is available over the counter as Liqui-E [247]. This compound forms micelles when given in doses above 25 mg/kg/day and may assist in the absorption of other fat-soluble vitamins. The results of the use of vitamin E to treat chronic diseases have been mixed, but overall are negative for heart disease, either alone or in combination with other antioxidants [248]. The American Heart Association consensus statement does not recommend the routine use of vitamin E [249]. Data for protection by vitamin E in prostate and other cancers is still inconclusive [250]. No consistent ill effects are seen with up to 3200 IU (2112 mg) per day in healthy persons. At doses from 100 to 1100 mg/day, oxidation of vitamin K to its active form can be inhibited, and high-dose vitamin E may be problematic in patients with bleeding disorders. However, the use of 800–1200 IU/day had no effect on the prothrombin time of patients on warfarin therapy [190].

Vitamin K
Deficiency
Nutritional deficiency of vitamin K is uncommon in adults because of the large amount in foods and because bacteria synthesize the vitamin in the intestinal lumen. Deficiency is most commonly the result of fat malabsorption, often compounded by poor intake and diminished liver function or decreased bile excretion [251]. Inhibition of bacterial biosynthesis by broad-spectrum antibiotics can be important. Deficiency is manifested by easy bruising and clotting abnormalities.

Assessment
The most commonly used clinically applicable test for vitamin K deficiency is the one-stage prothrombin time. The clotting factors tested (II, V, VII, and IX) are all responsive to vitamin K except for factor V. Factor VII has the shortest half-life and is the usual rate-limiting factor. The prothrombin time does not test vitamin K stores and is abnormal when deficiency is present, when the synthesis of clotting factors is impaired by liver disease, or when factors are consumed in intravascular coagulation. Thus, the test is nonspecific. Response of the prothrombin time to 5–10 mg of parenteral vitamin K for 2 to 3 days confirms the presence of a deficiency state. Plasma phylloquinone reflects recent intake, but is not a good measure of body stores. Determination of the urinary α-carboxyglutamic acid (Gla) level may be even more sensitive because it tests a function of vitamin K, and the level can be low when blood coagulation is normal [252]. Plasma levels of Gla proteins may be useful in detecting deficiency of vitamin K but have not been widely used. These proteins include undercarboxylated prothrombin (PIVKA-II) and carboxylated/undercarboxylated osteocalcin [8].

Treatment
Long-term therapy with doses titrated to the prothrombin time (~ 2 mg daily or every other day) should be restricted to patients with malabsorption. Patients on anticoagulant therapy should eat a well-balanced diet with consistent intake of vitamin K, avoiding fluctuations of high-content foods (egg yolk, vegetable oils, green leafy vegetables). For anticoagulant overdose, 1–2.5 mg oral phytomenadione (vitamin K-1) will decrease the international normalized ratio (INR) from 5–9 to 1–5 in 24–48 h [253]. For an INR greater than 10, a 5-mg initial dose of vitamin K-1 is recommended. The vitamin is

available for subcutaneous or intramuscular injection at 2 or 10 mg/mL. Vitamin K is not a component of any multivitamin preparation and must be prescribed individually.

References

1. Alpers DH, Stenson WF, Bier DM. Manual of Nutritional Therapeutics, 4th edn. Philadelphia: Lippincott Williams & Wilkins, 2001.
2. DeWys WD, Begg C, Lavin PT, et al. Prognostic effect of weight loss prior to chemotherapy in cancer patients. Am J Med 1980;69:491.
3. Forbes GF, Bruining GJ. Urinary creatinine excretion and lean body mass. Am J Clin Nutr 1976;29:1359.
4. Anderson CF, Wochos DN. The utility of serum albumin values in the nutritional assessment of hospitalized patients. Mayo Clin Proc 1982;57:181.
5. Apelgren KN, Rombeau JL, Twomey PL, Miller RA. Comparison of nutritional indices and outcome in critically ill patients. Crit Care Med 1982;10:305.
6. Franch-Arcas G. The meaning of hypoalbuminaemia in clinical practice. Clin Nutr 2001;20:265.
7. Raguso CA, Dupertuis YM, Pichard C. The role of visceral proteins in the nutritional assessment of intensive care unit patients. Curr Opin Clin Nutr Metab Care 2003;6:211.
8. Baker JP, Detsky AS, Wesson DE, et al. Nutritional assessment: a comparison of clinical judgment and objective measurements. N Engl J Med 1982;306:969.
9. Detsky AS, McLaughlin JR, Baker JP, et al. What is subjective global assessment of nutritional status? JPEN J Parenter Enteral Nutr 1987;11:8.
10. Naber TH, Schermer T, De Bree A, et al. Prevalence of malnutrition in nonsurgical hospitalized patients and its association with disease complications. Am J Clin Nutr 1997;66:1232.
11. Klein S, Kinney J, Jeejeebhoy K, et al. Nutrition support in clinical practice: review of published data and recommendations for future research directions. JPEN J Parenter Enteral Nutr 1997;21:133.
12. Velazquez OC, Lederer HM, Rombeau JL. Butyrate and the colonocyte. Production, absorption, metabolism, and therapeutic implications. Adv Exp Med Biol 1997;427:123.
13. Alpers DH, Stenson WF. Does total parenteral nutrition-induced intestinal mucosal atrophy occur in humans and can it be affected by enteral supplements?. Curr Opin Gastroenterol 1996;12:169.
14. Suchner U, Senftleben U, Eckart T, et al. Enteral versus parenteral nutrition: effects on gastrointestinal function and metabolism. Nutrition 1996;12:13.
15. Scolapio JS. A review of the trends in the use of enteral and parenteral nutrition support. J Clin Gastroenterol 2004;38:403.
16. Braga M, Vignali A, Gianotti L, et al. Immune and nutritional effects of early enteral nutrition after major abdominal operations. Eur J Surg 1996;162:105.
17. ASPEN Board of Directors. Guidelines for the use of parenteral and enteral nutrition in adult and pediatric patients. JPEN J Parenter Enteral Nutr 1993;17(Suppl. 4):1SA.
18. American Gastroenterological Association Medical Position Statement: Guidelines for the use of enteral nutrition. Gastroenterology 1995;108:1280.
19. American Gastroenterological Association Medical Position Statement: Guidelines for the management of malnutrition and cachexia, chronic diarrhea, and hepatobiliary disease in patients with human immunodeficiency virus infection. Gastroenterology 1996;111:1722.
20. Grimble GK, Silk DBA. The nitrogen source of elemental diets – an unresolved issue. Nutr Clin Pract 1990;5:227.
21. Brinson RR, Kolts BE. Diarrhea associated with severe hypoalbuminemia: a comparison of a peptide-based chemically defined diet and a standard enteral alimentation. Crit Care Med 1988;16:130.
22. Bounous G, Gentile JM, Hugon J. Elemental diet in the management of the intestinal lesion produced by 5-fluorouracil in man. Can J Surg 1971;14:312.
23. Heyland DK, Novak F, Drover JW, et al. Should immunonutrition become routine in critically ill patients? A systematic review of the evidence. JAMA 2001;286:944.
24. Bertolini G, Iapichino G, Radrizzani D, et al. Early enteral immunonutrition in patients with severe sepsis: results of an interim analysis of a randomized multicenter clinical trial. Intensive Care Med 2003;29:834.
25. Nalin DR, Cash RA, Rafiqul I, et al. Oral maintenance therapy for cholera in adults. Lancet 1968;2:370.
26. Thillainayagam AV, Hunt JB, Farthing JG. Enhancing clinical efficacy of oral rehydration therapy: is low osmolality the key? Gastroenterology 1998;114:197.
27. Avery ME, Snyder JD. Oral therapy for acute diarrhea. N Engl J Med 1990;323:891.
28. Alam NH, Ahmed T, Khatun M, Molla AM. Effects of food with two oral rehydration therapies: a randomized controlled clinical trial. Gut 1992;33:560.
29. Hunt JB, Elliott EJ, Fairclough PD, et al. Water and solute absorption from hypotonic glucose-electrolyte solutions in human jejunum. Gut 1992;33:479.
30. Pizarro D, Posada G, Sandi L, Moran JR. Rice-based oral electrolyte solutions for the management of infantile diarrhea. N Engl J Med 1991;324:517.
31. Nightingale JMD, Lennard-Jones JE, Walker ER, Farthing MJG. Jejunal efflux in short bowel syndrome. Lancet 1990;336:765.
32. Lennard-Jones JE. Oral rehydration solutions in short bowel syndrome. Clin Ther 1990;12:129.
33. Nalin DR, Hirschhorn N, Greenough W, et al. Clinical concerns about reduced-osmolarity oral rehydration solution. JAMA 2004;291:2632.
34. Ponsky JL, Gauderer MWL, Stellato TA, Aszode A. Percutaneous approach to enteral alimentation. Am J Surg 1985;149:102.
35. Russell TR, Brotman M, Norris F. Percutaneous gastrostomy: a new, simplified, and cost-effective technique. Am J Surg 1984;184:132.
36. Klein S, Heare BR, Soloway RD. The "buried bumper" syndrome: a complication of percutaneous endoscopic gastrostomy. Am J Gastroenterol 1990;85:448.
37. Shike M, Schroy P, Ritchie MA, et al. Percutaneous endoscopic jejunostomy on cancer patients with previous gastric resection. Gastrointest Endosc 1987;33:372.
38. Ho C-S, Yeung EY. Percutaneous gastrostomy and transgastric jejunostomy. AJR Am J Roentgenol 1992;158:251.
39. Kirby DF, Clifton GL, Turner H, et al. Early enteral nutrition after brain injury by percutaneous endoscopic gastrojejunostomy. JPEN J Parenter Enteral Nutr 1991;15:298.
40. Vanlandingham S, Simpson S, Daniel P, Newmark SR. Metabolic abnormalities in patients supported with enteral tube feeding. JPEN J Parenter Enteral Nutr 1981;5:322.
41. Guenter PA, Settle RG, Perlmutter S, et al. Tube feeding-related diarrhea in acutely ill patients. JPEN J Parenter Enteral Nutr 1991;15:277.
42. Edes TE, Walk BE, Austin JL. Diarrhea in tube-fed patients: feeding formula not necessarily the cause. Am J Med 1990;88:91.
43. Kandil HE, Opper FH, Switzer BR, Heizer WD. Marked resistance of normal subjects to tube-feeding-induced diarrhea: the role of magnesium. Am Clin J Nutr 1993;57:73.
44. Marvin RG, McKinley BA, McQuiggan M, et al. Nonocclusive bowel necrosis occurring in critically ill trauma patients receiving enteral nutrition manifests no reliable clinical signs for early dectection. Am J Surg 2000;179:7.
45. Pillar B, Perry S. Evaluating total parenteral nutrition: final report and core statement of the technology assessment and practice guidelines forum. In: Program on Technology and Health Care, Department of Community and Family Medicine. Washington, DC: Georgetown University School of Medicine, 1990:29.
46. Koretz RL, Lipman TO, Klein S. American Gastroenterological

Association Technical Review: Parenteral nutrition. Gastroenterology 2001;121:970.

47. Dudrick SJ, Wilmore DW, Vars HM, Rhoads JE. Long-term total parenteral nutrition with growth, development, and positive nitrogen balance. Surgery 1968;64:134.

48. Malt RA, Kempster M. Direct azygos vein and superior vena cava cannulation for parenteral nutrition. JPEN J Parenter Enteral Nutr 1983;7:580.

49. Jensen GL, Bistrian BR. Techniques for administering total parenteral nutrition. J Crit Illness 1989;4:87.

50. Kearns PJ, Coleman S, Wehner JH. Complications of long-arm catheters: a randomized trial of central vs. peripheral tips location. JPEN J Parenter Enteral Nutr 1996;20:20.

51. Hill SE, Heldman LS, Goo EDH, et al. Case report. Fatal microvascular pulmonary emboli from precipitation of a total nutrient admixture solution. JPEN J Parenter Enteral Nutr 1996;20:81.

52. Driscoll DF. Total nutrient admixtures: theory and practice. Clin Nutr 1995;10:114.

53. Naylor CB, O'Rourke K, Detsky AS, Baker JP. Parenteral nutrition with branched-chain amino acids in hepatic encephalopathy: a meta-analysis. Gastroenterology 1989;97:1033.

54. Kopple JD. The nutrition management of the patient with acute renal failure. JPEN J Parenter Enteral Nutr 1996;20:3.

55. Wolfe RR, O'Donnell TF Jr, Stone MD, et al. Investigation of factors determining the optimal glucose infusion rate in total parenteral nutrition. Metabolism 1980;29:892.

56. Covelli HD, Black JW, Olsen MS, Beckman JF. Respiratory failure precipitated by high carbohydrate loads. Ann Intern Med 1981;95:579.

57. Smith RC, Burkinshaw L, Hill GL. Optimal energy and nitrogen intake for gastroenterological patients requiring intravenous nutrition. Gastroenterology 1982;82:445.

58. Jeejeebhoy KN, Anderson GH, Nakhooda AF. Metabolic studies in total parenteral nutrition with lipid in man. J Clin Invest 1976;57:125.

59. Miles JM. Intravenous fat emulsions in nutritional support. Curr Opin Gastroenterol 1991;7:306.

60. Skeie B, Askanazi J, Rothkopf MM, et al. Intravenous fat emulsions and lung function: a review. Crit Care Med 1988;16:183.

61. DeGott C, Messing B, Moreau D, et al. Liver phospholipids induced by parenteral nutrition: histologic, histochemical, and ultrasound investigation. Gastroenterology 1988;95:183.

62. Seidner DL, Mascioli EA, Istfan NW, et al. Effect of long-chain triglyceride emulsions on reticuloendothelial system function in humans. JPEN J Parenter Enteral Nutr 1989;13:614.

63. Lashner BA, Kirsner JB, Hanauer SB. Acute pancreatitis associated with high-concentration lipid emulsion during total parenteral nutrition therapy for Crohn's disease. Gastroenterology 1986;90:1039.

64. Aviram M, Deckelbaum RJ. Intralipid infusion into humans reduces in vitro platelet aggregation and alters platelet lipid composition. Metabolism 1989;38:343.

65. Belin RP, Bivins BA, Jona JZ, Young VL. Fat overload with a 10% soybean oil emulsion. Arch Surg 1976;111:1391.

66. Hiyama DT, Griggs B, Mittman RJ, et al. Hypersensitivity following lipid emulsion infusion in an adult patient. JPEN J Parenter Enteral Nutr 1989;13:318.

67. Grimm H, Tibell A, Norrlind B, et al. Immunoregulation by parenteral lipids: impact of the n-3 to n-6 fatty acids ratio. JPEN J Parenter Enteral Nutr 1994;18:417.

68. Furukawa K, Yamamori H, Takagi K, et al. Influences of soybean oil emulsion on stress response and cell-mediated immune function in moderately or severely stressed patients. Nutrition 2002;18:235.

69. Antebi H, Mansoor O, Ferrier C, et al. Liver function and plasma antioxidant status in intensive care unit patients requiring total parenteral nutrition: comparison of 2 fat emulsions. JPEN J Parenter Enteral Nutr 2004;28:142.

70. Garcia-de-Lorenzo A, Lopez-Martinez J, Planas M, et al. Safety and metabolic tolerance of a concentrated long-chain triglyceride lipid emulsion in critically ill septic and trauma patients. JPEN J Parenter Enteral Nutr 2003;27:208.

71. Nehme AB. Nutritional support of the hospitalized patient: the team concept. JAMA 1980;243:1906.

72. Bozzetti F, Scarpa D, Terno G, et al. Subclavian venous thrombosis due to indwelling catheters: a prospective study on 52 patients. JPEN J Parenter Enteral Nutr 1981;7:560.

73. Brismar B, Hardstedt C, Jacobson S, et al. Reduction of catheter-associated thrombosis in parenteral nutrition of intravenous heparin therapy. Arch Surg 1982;117:1196.

74. Bern MM, Lokich JJ, Wallach SR, et al. Very-low-dose warfarin can prevent thrombosis. A randomized prospective trial. Ann Intern Med 1990;112:423.

75. Clark-Christoff N, Watters VA, Sparks W, et al. Use of triple-lumen subclavian catheters for administration of total parenteral nutrition. JPEN J Parenter Enteral Nutr 1992;16:403.

76. Mermel LA, Farr BM, Sherertz RJ, et al. Guidelines for the management of intravascular catheter-related infections. Clin Infect Dis 2001;32:1249.

77. Van Den Berghe G, Wouters P, Weekers F, et al. Intensive insulin therapy in critically ill patients. N Engl J Med 2001;345:1359.

78. Krinsley JS. Effect of intensive glucose management protocol on the mortality of critically ill adult patients. Mayo Clin Proc 2004;79:992.

79. Klein GL, Coburn JW. Parenteral nutrition: effect on bone and mineral homeostasis. Annu Rev Nutr 1991;11:93.

80. Klein S. Total parenteral nutrition and the liver. In Schiff L, Schiff ER (eds). Diseases of the Liver, 6th edn. Philadelphia: Lippincott-Raven, 1993:1505.

81. Cavicchi M, Beau P, Crenn P, et al. Prevalence of liver disease and contributing factors in patients receiving home parenteral nutrition for permanent intestinal failure. Ann Intern Med 2000;132:525.

82. Roslyn JJ, Pitt HA, Mann LL, et al. Gallbladder disease in patients on long-term parenteral nutrition. Gastroenterology 1983;84:148.

83. Messing B, Bories C, Kunstlinger F, Bemier JJ. Does total parenteral nutrition induce gallbladder sludge formation and lithiasis? Gastroenterology 1983;84:1012.

84. Roslyn JJ, DenBesten L, Thompson JE, Jr. Effects of periodic emptying of gallbladder on gallbladder function and formation of cholesterol gallstones. Surg Forum 1979;30:403.

85. Sitzmann JV, Pitt HA, Steinborn PA, et al. Cholecystokinin prevents parenteral nutrition-induced biliary sludge in humans. Surg Gynecol Obstet 1990;170:25.

86. Khawaja HT, Williams JD, Weaver PC. Transdermal glyceryl trinitrate to allow peripheral total parenteral nutrition: a double-blind placebo-controlled feasibility study. J R Soc Med 1991;84:69.

87. Everitt NJ, McMahon MJ. Peripheral intravenous nutrition. Nutrition 1994;10:49.

88. Tighe MJ, Wong C, Martin IG, McMahon MJ. Do heparin, hydrocortisone, and glycerol trinitrate influence thrombophlebitis during full intravenous nutrition via a peripheral vein. JPEN J Parenter Enteral Nutr 1995;19:507.

89. Shils ME, Wright WL, Turnbull A, Brescia F. Long-term parenteral nutrition through an external arteriovenous shunt. N Engl J Med 1970;283:341.

90. Howard L, Ament M, Fleming CR, et al. Current use and clinical outcome of home parenteral and enteral nutrition therapies in the United States. Gastroenterology 1995;109:355.

91. Richards DM, Deeks JJ, Sheldon TA, Shaffer JL. Home parenteral nutrition: a systematic review. Health Technol Assess 1997;1:i,1.

92. Van Gossum A, Bakker H, Bozzetti F, et al. Home parenteral nutrition in adults: a European multicentre survey in 1997. Clin Nutr 1999;18:135.

93. Fleming CR. Comprehensive care of the patient with gut failure: present and future. Trans Am Clin Climatol Assoc 1986;98:197.

94. Muhlebach S. Practical aspects of multichamber bags for total parenteral nutrition. Surr Opin in Clin Nutr Metab Care 2005;8:291.

95. Ireton-Jones C, DeLegge M. Home parenteral nutrition registry: a five-year retrospective evaluation of outcomes of patients receiving home parenteral nutrition support. Nutrition 2005;21:156.

96. Gouttebel MC, Saint-Aubert B, Astre C, Joyeux H. Total parenteral nutrition needs in different types of short bowel syndrome. Dig Dis Sci 1986;31:718.

97. Heymsfield SB, Smith-Andrews JL, Hersh T. Home nasoenteric feeding for malabsorption and weight loss refractory to conventional therapy. Ann Intern Med 1983;98:168.

98. Griffiths AM, Ohlsson A, Sherman PM, et al. Meta-analysis of enteral nutrition as a primary treatment of active Crohn's disease. Gastroenterology 1995;108:1056.

99. Fernandez-Banares F, Cabre E, Esteve-Comas M, et al. Is enteral nutrition effective in inducing clinical remission in active Crohn's disease? A meta-analysis of the randomized clinical trials. JPEN J Parenter Enteral Nutr 1995;19:356.

100. Messori A, Trallori G, D'Albasio G, et al. Defined-formula diets versus steroids in the treatment of active Crohn's disease. A meta-analysis. Scand J Gastroenterol 1996;31:267.

101. Summers RW, Switz DM, Sessions JT, Jr, et al. National cooperative Crohn's disease study: results of drug treatment. Gastroenterology 1979;77:847.

102. Meyers S, Janowitz HD. "Natural history" of Crohn's disease. An analytic review of the placebo lesson. Gastroenterology 1984;87:1189.

103. Wright RA, Adler EC. Peripheral parenteral nutrition is no better than enteral nutrition in acute exacerbation of Crohn's disease: a prospective trial. J Clin Gastroenterol 1990;12:396.

104. Lochs H. Has total bowel rest been a beneficial effect in the treatment of Crohn's disease?. Clin Nutr 1983;2:61.

105. Dickinson RJ, Ashton MG, Axon AT, et al. Controlled trial of intravenous hyperalimentation and total bowel rest as an adjunct to the routine therapy of acute colitis. Gastroenterology 1980;79:1199.

106. McIntyre PB, Powell-Tuck J, Wood SR, et al. Controlled trial of bowel rest in the treatment of severe acute colitis. Gut 1986;27:481.

107. Gonzalez-Huix F, Fernandex-Banares F, Esteve-Comas M, et al. Enteral versus parenteral nutrition as adjunct therapy in acute ulcerative colitis. Am J Gastroenterol 1993;88:227.

108. Hawthorne AB, Daneshmend TK, Hawkey CJ, et al. Treatment of ulcerative colitis with fish oil supplementation: a prospective 12-month randomized controlled trial. Gut 1992;33:922.

109. Stenson WF, Cort D, Rodgers J, et al. Dietary supplementation with fish oils in ulcerative colitis. Ann Intern Med 1992;116:609.

110. Koeschke K, Ueberschaer B, Pietsch A, et al. n-3 fatty acids only delay early relapse of ulcerative colitis in remission. Dig Dis Sci 1996;41:2087.

111. Belluzzi A, Brignola C, Campieri M, et al. Effect of an enteric-coated fish-oil preparation on relapses in Crohn's disease. N Engl J Med 1996;334:1557.

112. Lorenz-Meyer H, Bauer P, Nicolay C, et al. Omega-3 fatty acids and low-carbohydrate diet for maintenance of remission in Crohn's disease. Scand J Gastroenterol 1996;31:778.

113. Weschmeyer P, Pemberton JH, Phillips SF. Chronic pouchitis after ileal pouch-anal anastomosis: responses to butyrate and glutamine suppositories in a pilot study. Mayo Clin Proc 1993;68:978.

114. Himal HS, Allard JR, Nadeau JE, et al. The importance of adequate nutrition in closure of small intestinal fistulas. Br J Surg 1974;61:724.

115. Leandros E, Antonakis PT, Albanopoulos K, et al. Somatostatin versus octreotide in the treatment of patients with gastrointestinal and pancreatic fistulas. Can J Gastroenterol 2004;18:303.

116. Kelts DG, Grand RJ, Davis-Kraft, et al. Nutritional basis of growth failure in children and adolescents with Crohn's disease. Gastroenterology 1978;76:720.

117. Polk DB, Hattner JT, Kerner JA. Improved growth and disease activity after intermittent administration of a defined formula diet in children with Crohn's disease. JPEN J Parenter Enteral Nutr 1992;16:499.

118. Kirschner BS, Klich JR, Kalman SS, et al. Reversal of growth retardation in Crohn's disease with therapy emphasizing oral nutritional restitution. Gastroenterology 1981;80:10.

119. Aiges H, Markowitz J, Rosa J, et al. Home nocturnal supplemental nasogastric feedings in growth-retarded adolescents with Crohn's disease. Gastroenterology 1989;97:905.

119. Sanderson IR, Udeen S, Davis PSW, et al. Remission induced by elemental diet in small bowel Crohn's disease. Arch Dis Child 1987; 61:123.

120. Belli DC, Seidman E, Bouthiller L. Chronic intermittent elemental diet improves growth failure in children with Crohn's disease. Gastroenterology 1988;94:603.

121. McClave SA, Greene LM, Snider HL, et al. Comparison of the safety of early enteral versus parenteral nutrition in mild acute pancreatitis. JPEN J Parenter Enteral Nutr 1997;21:14.

122. Sax HC, Warner BW, Talamini MA, et al. Early total parenteral nutrition in acute pancreatitis: lack of beneficial effects. Am J Surg 1987;153:117.

123. Kalfarentzos F, Kehagias J, Mead N, et al. Enteral nutrition is superior to parenteral nutrition in severe acute pancreatitis: results of a randomized prospective trial. Br J Surg 1997;84:1665.

124. Eatock FC, Chong PC, Menezes N, et al. Nasogastric feeding is a safe and practical alternative feeding in severe acute pancreatitis: a randomized controlled trial. Pancreatology 2001;1:A149.

125. Abou-Assi S, Craig K, O'Keefe SJ. Hypocaloric jejunal feeding is better than total parenteral nutrition in acute pancreatitis: results of a randomized comparative study. Am J Gastroenterol 2002;97:2255.

126. Gupta R, Patel K, Calder PC, et al. A randomized clinical trial to assess the effect of total enteral and total parenteral nutritional support on metabolic, inflammatory and oxidative markers in patients with predicted severe acute pancreatitis. Pancreatology 2003:3: 406.

127. Nathens AB, Curtis JR, Beale RJ, et al. Management of the critically ill patient with severe acute pancreatitis. Crit Care Med 2004;32:2524.

128. Bonkovsky HL, Fiellin DA, Smith DA, et al. A randomized, controlled trial of treatment of alcoholic hepatitis with parenteral nutrition and oxandrolone. I. Short-term effects on liver function. Am J Gastroenterol 1991;86:1200.

129. Bonkovsky HL, Singh RH, Jafri IH, et al. A randomized, controlled trial of treatment of alcoholic hepatitis with parenteral nutrition and oxandrolone. II. Short-term effects on nitrogen metabolism, metabolic balance, and nutrition. Am J Gastroenterol 1991;86:1209.

130. Mendenhall CL, Mortitz TE, Roselle GA, et al. A study of oral nutrition support with oxandrolone in malnourished patients with alcoholic hepatitis: results of a Department of Veterans Affairs cooperative study. Hepatology 1993;17:564.

131. Mendenhall C, Bongiovanni G, Goldberg S, et al. VA Cooperative Study on Alcoholic Hepatitis III: Changes in protein-calorie malnutrition associated with 30 days of hospitalization with and without enteral nutritional therapy. JPEN J Parenter Enteral Nutr 1985;9: 590.

132. Kearns PJ, Young H, Garcia G, et al. Accelerated improvement of alcoholic liver disease with enteral nutrition. Gastroenterology 1992; 102:200.

133. Hirsch S, Bunout D, de la Maza R, et al. Controlled trial on nutrition supplementation in outpatients with symptomatic alcoholic cirrhosis. JPEN J Parenter Enteral Nutr 1992;17:119.

134. Naveau S, Pelletier G, Poynard T, et al. A randomized clinical trial of supplementary parenteral nutrition in jaundiced alcoholic cirrhotic patients. Hepatology 1986;6:270.

135. Cabre E, Gonzalez-Huix FG, Abad-Lacruz A, et al. Effect of total enteral nutrition on the short-term outcome of severely malnourished cirrhotics. Gastroenterology 1990;98:715.

136. Marsano L, McClain CJ. Nutrition and alcoholic liver disease. JPEN J Parenter Enteral Nutr 1991;15:337.

137. Shils ME, Olson JA, Shike M, Ross AC. Modern Nutrition in Health and Disease, 9th edn. Philadelphia: Lea & Febiger, 1999.

138. Sauberlich HE. Laboratory Tests for the Assessment of Nutritional Status, 2nd edn. Boca Raton, FL: CRC Press, 1999.

139. McGee S, Abernethy WB, Simel DL. Is this patient hypovolemic?. JAMA 1999;281:1022.

140. Consensus statement on the definition of orthostatic hypotension, pure autonomic failure, and multiple system atrophy. Neurology 1996;46:1470.

141. Androgue HJ, Madias N. Hyponatremia. N Engl J Med 2000;342:1581.

142. Gennari FJ. Hypokalemia. N Engl J Med 1998;339:451.

143. Halperin ML, Kamel KS. Potassium. Lancet 1998;352:135.

144. Zaloga GD. Hypocalcemia in the critically ill. Crit Care Med 1992;20:251.

145. Karg HP, Scott MG, Joe BN, et al. Model for predicting the impact of gadolinium on plasma calcium measured by the o-cresolphthalein method. Clin Chem 2004;50:741.

146. Raisz LG. Clinical practice: screening for osteoporosis. N Eng J Med 2005;353:164.

147. Weaver CM. Calcium. Bowman BA, Russell RM (eds). Present Knowledge in Nutrition, 8th edn. Washington, DC: ILSI Press, 2001:273.

148. Anon. Calcium supplements. Med Lett 2000;42:29.

149. Anonymous. Calcium supplements: get the lead out. Consumer's Rep 1997;62:6.

150. Mouw DR, Latessa RA, Sullo EJ. What are the causes of hypomagnesemia? J Family Practice 2005;54:174.

151. Kelepouris E, Agus ZS. Hypomagnesemia: renal magnesium handling. Semin Nephrol 1998;18:58.

152. Rude RK, Shils ME. Magnesium. In: Shils M, Shike M, Ross AC, et al. (eds). Modern Nutrition in Health and Disease, 10th edn. Philadelphia: Lippincott Williams & Wilkins, 2006:223.

153. Rodriguez-Moran M, Guerrero-Romero F. Oral magnesium supplementation improves insulin sensitivity and metabolic control in type 2 diabetes subjects: a randomized double-blind controlled trial. Diabetes Care 2003;26:1147.

154. Reinhart RA. Magnesium metabolism. Arch Intern Med 1988;148:2415.

155. Fleming CR, George L, Stoner GL, et al. The importance of urinary magnesium values in patients with gut failure. Mayo Clin Proc 1996;71:21.

156. Weisinger JR. Magnesium and phosphorus. Lancet 1998;352:391.

157. LaRoche M. Phosphate, the renal tubule, and the musculoskeletal system. Joint Bone Spine 2001;68:211.

158. Anderson JE, Sell ML, Garner SC, Calvo MS. Phosphorus. In: Shils M, Shike M, Ross AC, et al. (eds). Modern Nutrition in Health and Disease, 10th edn. Philadelphia: Lippincott Williams & Wilkins, 2006:281.

159. Umbreit J. Iron deficiency: a concise review. Am J Hematol 2005;78:225.

160. Lozoff B, Jimenez E, Hagen J, et al. Poorer behavioral and developmental outcome more than 10 years after treatment for iron deficiency in infancy. Pediatrics 2000;105:E51.

161. Kretsch MJ, Fong AK, Green MW, Johnson HL. Cognitive function, iron status, and hemoglobin concentration in obese dieting women. Eur J Clin Nutr 1998;52:512.

162. Verdon F, Burnard B, Stubi CL, et al. Iron supplementation for unexplained fatigue in non-anaemic women: double blind randomized placebo controlled trial. BMJ 2003;326:1124.

163. Weiss G, Goodnough LT. Anemia of chronic disease. N Eng J Med 2005;352:1011.

164. Beguin Y. Soluble transferrin receptor for the evaluation of erythropoiesis and iron status. Clin Chim Acta 2003;329:9.

165. Kumpf VJ. Update on parenteral iron therapy. Nutrition in Clinical Practice 2003;18:318.

166. Eschbach JW. Iron requirements in erythropoietin therapy. Best Pract Res Cl Ha 2005;18:347.

167. Aronoff GR. Safety of intravenous iron in clinical practice: implications for anemia management protocols. J Am Soc Nephrol 2004;15:S99.

168. Christodoulou DK, Tsienos EV. Anemia in inflammatory bowel disease – the role of recombinant human erythropoietin. Eur J Intern Med 2000;11:222.

169. Fung ER, Kawcheak DA, Zernel DS, et al. Plasma zinc is an insensitive indicator of zinc status: the use of plasma zinc in children with sickle cell disease. Nutrition in Clinical Practice 2002;17:365.

170. Wapnir RA. Zinc deficiency: malnutrition and the gastrointestinal tract. J Nutr 2000;130:1388S.

171. Henkin RI, Schecter PJ, Friedewald WT, et al. A double-blind study of the effects of zinc sulfate on taste and smell dysfunction. Am J Med Sci 1976;272:285.

172. Wood RJ. Assessment of marginal zinc status in humans. J Nutr 2000;130:1350S.

173. Hambridge M. Human zinc deficiency. J Nutr 2000;130:1344S.

174. Fosmire GF. Zinc toxicity. Am J Clin Nutr 1990;51:225.

175. Walker CF, Black RE. Zinc and the risk of infectious disease. Annu Rev Nutr 2004;24:255.

176. Marshall I. Zinc for the common cold. Cochrane Database Syst Rev 2000:CD001364.

177. Donangelo CM, Woodhouse LR, King SM, et al. Supplemental zinc lowers measures of iron status in young women with low iron reserves. J Nutr 2002;132:1860.

178. Sampson B, Fagerol Mx, Sunderkotter C, et al. Hyperzincemia and hypercalprotectinemia: a new disorder of zinc metabolism. Lancet 2002;360:1742.

179. Turnlund JR. Copper. Shils M, et al. (eds). Modern Nutrition in Health and Disease, 10th edn. Philadelphia: Lippincott Williams & Wilkins, 2006.

180. Schilsky ML. Wilson disease: new insights into pathogenesis, diagnosis, and future therapy. Curr Gastroenterol Reports 2005;7:26.

181. Danks DM. Copper deficiency in humans. Annu Rev Nutr 1988;8:235.

182. Kumar N, Gross JD, Ahlskog JE. Copper deficiency myelopathy produces a clinical picture like subacute combined degeneration. Neurology 2004;63:33.

183. Linder MC, Hazegh-Azam M. Copper biochemistry and molecular biology. Am J Clin Nutr 1996;63:797S.

184. Pena MMO, Lee J, Thiele DJ. A delicate balance: homeostatic control of copper uptake and distribution. J Nutr 1999;129:1251.

185. Fleming CR. Trace element metabolism in adult patients requiring total parenteral. nutrition. Am J Clin Nutr 1989;49:573.

186. Bremner I. Manifestations of copper excess. Am J Clin Nutr 1998;67(Suppl. 5):S1069.

187. Campbell C. Lactic acidosis and thiamine deficiency [letter]. Lancet 1984;2:446.

188. Frank T, Bitsch R, Maiwald J, Stein G. High thiamine diphosphate concentrations in erythrocytes can be achieved by oral administration of benfotiamine. Eur J Clin Pharmacol 2000;26:251.

189. Alhadeff L, Gueltieri CT, Lipton M. Toxic effects of water-soluble vitamins. Nutr Rev 1984;42:33.

190. Fragakis AS. The Professional's Guide to Popular Dietary Supplements, 2nd edn. Hoboken, NJ: John Wiley & Sons, 2002.

191. Laforenza U, Patrini C, Alvisi C, et al. Thiamin uptake in human intestinal biopsy specimens, including observations from a patient with acute thiamine deficiency. Am J Clin Nutr 1997;66:320.

192. McCormick DB. Riboflavin. In: Shils M, Shike M, Ross AC, et al. (eds). Modern Nutrition in Health and Disease, 10th edn. Philadelphia: Lippincott Williams & Wilkins, 2006:434.

193. Bourgeois C, Cervantes-Laurean D, Moss J. Niacin. In: Shils M, Shike M, Ross AC, et al. (eds). Modern Nutrition in Health and Disease, 10th edn. Philadelphia: Lippincott Williams & Wilkins, 2006:442.

194. Rizkallah GS, Mertens MK, Brown ML. Should liver enzymes be checked in a patient taking niacin? J Fam Pract 2005;54:265.

195. Mackay AD, Davis SR, Gregory JF. Vitamin B_6. In: Shils M, Shike M, Ross AC, et al. (eds). Modern Nutrition in Health and Disease, 10th edn. Philadelphia: Lippincott Williams & Wilkins, 2006:452.

196. Clarke R. Homocysteine-lowering trials for prevention of heart disease and stroke. Sem Vasc Med 2005;5:215.

197. Cesari M, Rossi GP, Stichhi D, Pessina AC. Is homocysteine important as a risk factor for coronary artery disease? Nutr Metab Cardiovasc Dis 2005;15:140.

198. Eichinger S. Homocysteine, vitamin B6 and the risk of recurrent venous thromboembolism. Pathophysiol Haemost Thromb 2004;33:342.

199. Llereux P, Penaloza A, Gris M. Pyridoxine in clinical toxicology: a review. Eur J Emerg Med 2005;12:78.

200. Schaumberg H, Kaplan J, Windebank A, et al. Sensory neuropathy from pyridoxine abuse: a new megavitamin syndrome. N Engl J Med 1983;309:445.

201. Roe DA. Diet and Drug Interactions. New York: Van Nostrand Reinhold, 1989.

202. Weir DG, McGing PG, Scott JM. Folate metabolism, the enterohepatic circulation, and alcohol. Biochem Pharmacol 1985;34:1.

203. Standing Committee on Scientific Evaluation of Dietary Reference Intakes. Food and Nutrition Board, Institute of Medicine. Dietary reference intakes for thiamin, riboflavin, niacin, vitamin B_6, folate, vitamin B_{12}, pantothenic acid, biotin, and choline. Washington, DC: National Academy Press, 1999.

204. Ramaekers VT, Rothenberg SP, Sequira JM, et al. Autoantibodies to folate receptors in the cerebral folate deficiency syndrome. N Engl J Med 2005;352:1985.

205. Voutilainen S, Jirtanen JK, Rissanen TH, et al. Serum folate and homocysteine and the incidence of acute coronary events: the Kuopio Ischaemic Heart Disease Risk Factor Study. Am J Clin Nutr 2004;80:317.

206. Ganji V, Kafai MR. Demographic, health, lifestyle, and blood vitamin determinants of serum total homocysteine concentration in the Third National Health & Nutrition Survey 1988–1994. Am J Clin Nutr 2003;77:826.

207. Toole JF, Lalinow MR, Chambless LE, et al. Lowering homocysteine in patients with ischemic stroke to prevent recurrent stroke, myocardial infarction, and death. J Am Med Assoc 2004;29:565.

208. Schwammental Y, Tanne D. Homocysteine, B-vitamin supplementation and stroke prevention: from observational status to interventional trials. Lancet Neurol 2004;3:493.

209. Anonymous. Lowering plasma homocysteine. The Medical Letter 2003;45:85.

210. Herbert V. Recommended dietary intake (RDI) of folates in humans. Am J Clin Nutr 1987;45:661.

211. Lewis CJ, Crane NT, Wilson DB, Yetley EA. Estimated folate intakes: data updated to reflect food fortification, increased bioavailability, and dietary supplement use. Am J Clin Nutr 1999;70:198.

212. Beach RS, Morgan R, Wilkie F, et al. Plasma vitamin B_{12} levels as a potential cofactor in studies of human immunodeficiency virus type 1-related cognitive changes. Arch Neurol 1992;49:501.

213. Pacchetti C, Cristina S, Nappi G. Reversible chorea and focal dystonia in vitamin B12 deficiency [letter]. N Engl J Med 2002;347:295.

214. Miller A, Furlong D, Burrows BA, Slingerland DW. Bound vitamin B_{12} absorption in patients with low serum B_{12} levels. Am J Hematol 1992;40:163.

215. Healton EB, Savage DG, Brust JCM, et al. Neurologic aspects of cobalamin deficiency. Medicine 1991;70:229.

216. Amos RJ, Dawson DW, Fish DI, et al. Guidelines on the investigation and diagnosis of cobalamin and folate deficiencies: a publication of the British Committee for Standards in Haematology. Clin Lab Haematol 1994;16:101.

217. Stabler SP. Screening the older population for cobalamin (vitamin B_{12}) deficiency. J Am Geriatr Soc 1995;43:1290.

218. Allen RH, Stabler SP, Savage DG, Lindenbaum J. Metabolic abnormalities in cobalamin (vitamin B_{12}) and folate deficiency. FASEB J 1993;9:1344.

219. Fritschi J, Sturznegger M. Spiral MRI supporting myelopathic origin of early symptoms in unsuspected cobalamin deficiency. Eur Neurol 2003;49:146.

220. Lindenbaum J, Rosenberg IH, Wilson PW, et al. Prevalence of cobalamin deficiency in the Framingham elderly population. Am J Clin Nutr 1994;60:2.

221. Kuzminski AM, Del Giacco EJ, Allen RH, et al. Effective treatment of cobalamin deficiency with oral cobalamin. Blood 1998;92:1191.

222. Anonymous. Vitamin B12 nasal spray. The Medical Letter 2005;47:64.

223. Standing Committee on Scientific Evaluation of Dietary Reference Intakes. Food and Nutrition Board, Institute of Medicine. Dietary reference intakes for vitamin C, vitamin E, selenium, beta-carotene, and other carotenoids. Washington, DC: National Academy Press, 2000.

224. Johnston CS. Biomarkers for establishing a tolerable upper intake level for vitamin C. Nutr Rev 1999;10:128.

225. Douglas RM, Hemila H, D'Souza R, et al. Vitamin C for preventing and treating the common cold. Cochrane Database Syst Rev 2004;CD000980.

226. Padayatty SJ, Katz A, Wang Y, et al. Vitamin C as an antioxidant: evaluation of its role in disease prevention. J Am Coll Nutr 2003;22:18.

227. Said H. Biotin: the forgotten vitamin. Am J Clin Nutr 2002;75:179.

228. Standing Committee on Scientific Evaluation of Dietary Reference Intakes. Food and Nutrition Board, Institute of Medicine. Dietary reference intakes for vitamin A, vitamin K, arsenic, boron, chromium, copper, iodine, iron, manganese, molybdenum, nickel, silicon, vanadium, and zinc. Washington, DC: National Academy Press, 2001.

229. Villamor E, Mbisa R, Spiegelman D, et al. Vitamin A supplements ameliorate the adverse effect of HIV-1, malaria, and diarrheal infections on child growth. Pediatrics 2002;190:E6.

230. Ross DA. Recommendations for vitamin A supplementation. J Nutr 2002;131:2902S.

231. Ross CA. Vitamin A and carotenoids. In: Shils M, Shike M, Ross AC, et al. (eds). Modern Nutrition in Health and Disease, 10th edn. Philadelphia: Lippincott Williams & Wilkins, 2006:351.

232. Standing Committee on Scientific Evaluation of Dietary Reference Intakes. Food and Nutrition Board, Institute of Medicine. Dietary reference intakes for calcium, phosphorus, magnesium, vitamin D, and fluoride. Washington, DC: National Academy Press, 1997.

233. Looker AC, Gunter EW. Hypovitaminosis D in medical inpatients. N Engl J Med 1998;339:344.

234. LeBoff MS, Kohlmeier L, Hurwitz S, et al. Occult vitamin D deficiency in postmenopausal US women with acute hip fracture. JAMA 1999;281:1505.

235. Spencer H, Rubio N, Rubio E, et al. Chronic alcoholism. Frequently overlooked cause of osteoporosis in man. Am J Med 1986;80:393.

236. Carey E, Balan V. Metabolic bone disease in patients with liver disease. Curr Gastroenterol Rep 2003;5:71.

237. Binkley N, Krueger D, Cowgill CS, et al. Assay variation confounds the diagnosis of hypovitaminosis D: a call for standardization. J Clin Endocrinol Metab 2004;89:3152.

238. Hollis BW. Circulating 25-hydroxyvitamin D levels indicative of vitamin D insufficiency: implications for establishing a new dietary intake recommendation for vitamin D. J Nutr 2005;135:317.

239. Zitterman A. Vitamin D in preventive medicine: are we ignoring the evidence? Br J Nutr 2003;89:552.

240. Leichtmann GA, Bengoa JM, Bolt MJ, Sitrin MD. Intestinal absorption of cholecalciferol and 25-hydroxycholecalciferol in patients with Crohn's disease and intestinal resection. Am J Clin Nutr 1991;54:548.

241. Sitrin M, Bengoa JM. Intestinal absorption of cholecalciferol and 25-hydroxycholecalciferol in chronic cholestatic liver disease. Am J Clin Nutr 1987;46:1011.

242. Wu-Wong JR, Tian J, Goltzman D. Vitamin D analogs as therapeutic agents: a clinical study update. Curr Opin Investigational Drugs 2004;5:320.

243. Pryor WA. Vitamin E. In: Bowman BA, Russell RM (eds). Present Knowledge in Nutrition, 8th edn. Washington, DC: ILSI Press, 2001:156.

244. Rosenblum J, Keating JP, Prensky AL, Nelson JS. A progressive neurologic syndrome in children with chronic liver disease. N Engl J Med 1981;304:503.

245. Sokol RJ, Heubi JE, Iannaccone ST, et al. Vitamin E deficiency with normal serum vitamin E concentrations in children with chronic cholestasis. N Engl J Med 1984;310:1209.

246. Refat M, Moore JJ, Kanzui M, et al. Utility of breath ethane as a noninvasive biomarker of vitamin E status in children. Pediatr Res 1991;30:396.

247. Sokol RJ, Butler-Simon N, Conner C, et al. Multicenter trial of D-α-tocopherol polyethylene glycol 1000 succinate for treatment of vitamin E deficiency in children with chronic cholestasis. Gastroenterology 1993;104:1727.

248. Jialal I, Devaraj S. Scientific evidence to support a vitamin E and heart disease health claim: research needs. J Nutr 2005;135:348.

249. Tribble DL. Antioxidant consumption and risk of coronary heart disease: emphasis on vitamin C, vitamin E, and β-carotene: a statement for healthcare professionals from the American Heart Association. Circulation 1999;99:591.

250. Friedrich MJ. To "E" or not to "E", vitamin E's role in health and disease is the question. JAMA 2004;292:671.

251. Krasinski SD, Russell RM, Furie RC, et al. The prevalence of vitamin K deficiency in chronic gastrointestinal disorders. Am J Clin Nutr 1985;41:639.

252. Singh H, Duerksen DR. Vitamin K and nutrition support. Nutrition in Clinical Practice 2003;18:359.

253. Hanslick T, Prinseau J. The use of vitamin K in patients on anticoagulant therapy: a practical guide. Am J Cardiovasc Drugs 2004;4:43.

31 Genetic counseling for gastrointestinal patients

Cindy Solomon, Deborah W. Neklason, Angela Schwab, Randall W. Burt

Principles of genetics, 624
Genetic testing and counseling, 634
Genetic tools and technologies, 641
Summary and conclusions, 642

The science of genetics has quickly translated into new medical applications, including methods of disease screening, susceptibility testing, diagnostics, and therapeutics. The clinical application of genetic knowledge is expected to expand dramatically with the sequencing of the entire human genome. All this change requires the physician to have a thorough understanding of modern genetics. Only in this way can the application of the many genetic advances be realized in the clinic.

An important part of the clinical application of genetics is patient education by the health-care team. Many disease discussions must involve genetics. Patient education is particularly important when genetic testing is being considered. Both patient and physician must understand the impact of genetic testing on medical management, future health, and family members. Each of these issues must be addressed in making the decision to proceed with genetic testing. For many diseases, the incorporation of genetic counseling into the evaluation and treatment process is becoming a practical necessity.

This chapter reviews the basic and clinical genetics needed by the practicing gastroenterologist, both to understand emerging relevant genetic discoveries and to apply them in the clinical setting. The principles of genetic testing and counseling are then presented. Such knowledge will enable the practitioner to educate the patient in making informed clinical decisions. Many of the examples relate to genetic counseling and testing for inherited colorectal polyp and cancer conditions because much knowledge and experience have been accumulated in this area. However, with an increased understanding of other pediatric and adult conditions, such as celiac disease, irritable bowel disease, and pancreatitis, genetic counseling and testing for these conditions may soon become mainstream.

Principles of genetics

Types of genetic disorders

Genetic disorders can be categorized into four major groups. Knowledge of the types of genetic disorders is important for understanding the etiology, occurrence, and recurrence risks of inherited disorders.

Chromosomal disorders

Chromosomal disorders occur when the chromosomal number or structure differs from that normally expected. There are two types of chromosomes: sex chromosomes (X and Y) and autosomes (males and females have two copies of each autosome, which include chromosomes 1–22). A person with a chromosomal disorder may have an extra chromosome (e.g., Down syndrome, in which an individual has three copies of chromosome 21) or lack a chromosome (e.g., Turner syndrome, in which a female subject has one instead of two X chromosomes). Chromosomal disorders also include duplication, absence, or structural rearrangement of large segments of chromosomes (e.g., DiGeorge syndrome). Chromosomal disorders can be inherited; however, many chromosomal disorders result in impaired infertility thereby reducing transmission. Examples of chromosomal disorders and their gastrointestinal (GI) manifestations can be found in Table 31.1. If a chromosomal disorder is suspected, karyotype (examination of chromosome number and structure) or other analysis can be performed on blood lymphocytes, as described later in "Types of mutations."

Principles of Clinical Gastroenterology. Edited by Tadataka Yamada, David H. Alpers, Anthony N. Kalloo, Neil Kaplowitz, Chung Owyang, and Don W. Powell. © 2008 Blackwell Publishing. ISBN 978-1-4051-69103

Table 31.1 Examples of chromosomal disorders with associated congenital gastrointestinal manifestations

Chromosomal disorders	Gastrointestinal manifestations
Duplication of 3q	Umbilical hernia, omphalocele
Deletion of 9p	Inguinal or umbilical hernia, diaphragmatic hernia
Deletion of 11q	Pyloric stenosis, inguinal hernia
Microdeletion of 22q11.2 (DiGeorge syndrome)	Esophageal atresia, velopharyngeal insufficiency, imperforate anus, diaphragmatic hernia
Trisomy 13 (Patau syndrome)	Omphalocele, heterotopic pancreatic or splenic tissue, incomplete rotation of colon, Meckel diverticulum, enlarged gallbladder, diaphragmatic defect
Trisomy 18 (Edwards syndrome)	Inguinal or umbilical hernia, malposed or funnel-shaped anus, hypoplastic diaphragm, Meckel diverticulum, heterotopic pancreatic or splenic tissue, omphalocele, incomplete rotation of colon, pyloric stenosis, extrahepatic biliary atresia, hypoplastic gallbladder, gallstones, imperforate anus
Trisomy 21 (Down syndrome)	Tracheal stenosis with hourglass trachea and midtracheal absence of tracheal pars membranacea, tracheoesophageal fistula, duodenal atresia, omphalocele, pyloric stenosis, annular pancreas, Hirschsprung disease, imperforate anus

A rare situation called mosaicism occurs when one cell in embryonic development acquires a mutation. Any future cells derived from this one cell will contain the same mutation. Consequently, the individual will have both normal and abnormal cells, and is mosaic for the disorder. Mosaicism may or may not affect the phenotype of the individual or pose a risk to his or her offspring.

Mendelian disorders

Mendelian disorders are named after Gregor Mendel, an Austrian monk who lived in the mid-19th century and is considered to be the father of genetics. Mendelian disorders are caused by mutations in single genes and can be passed to offspring in an autosomal dominant, autosomal recessive, or sex-linked fashion. Although a mutant gene may cause the condition, the severity of the disease may be influenced by environmental factors. Examples of single-gene disorders affecting the GI tract are listed in Table 31.2. Table 31.3 lists inherited disorders known to cause a predisposition to GI tract cancers.

Mitochondrial disorders

Mitochondria, organelles found in the cytoplasm of a cell, have their own DNA molecules that carry genes encoding components that are important in energy metabolism of the cell. Mutations in the mitochondrial genes cause several genetic disorders, including mitochondrial neurogastrointestinal encephalopathy syndrome (MNGIE) (see Table 31.2). Mitochondrial genes are maternally inherited through the mitochondria in the cytoplasm of the egg. Sperm have few mitochondria; none of them enter the egg during fertilization and thus are not passed on to offspring. A female affected with a mitochondrial disorder will pass the disorder to all her offspring (100% transmission), whereas no offspring will inherit the disorder from an affected male (Fig. 31.1).

Multifactorial/complex disorders

Although much is understood about chromosomal, mendelian, and mitochondrial disorders, these conditions reflect only a small proportion of inherited disorders. Multifactorial/complex disorders are more common and currently less well understood. As their name implies, these disorders are caused by a combination of factors through gene–gene interactions or gene–environment interactions. Twin studies are useful to assess the quantitative impact of gene and environmental influences on disorders. One twin study, for example, estimated that approximately 35% of colon cancers arise from heritable factors [1]. The known inherited colorectal cancer predisposition syndromes constitute 5%–10% of the familial aggregation, implying that additional colon cancer susceptibilities are yet to be defined [2].

Many of the common gastrointestinal conditions, such as Hirschsprung, Crohn's, and other inflammatory bowel diseases, result as a combination of inherited and environmental factors [3–5]. Common and rare disorders and the genes implicated in their etiology are described on the website for Online Mendelian Inheritance in Man (www.ncbi.nlm.nih.gov/sites/entrez?db=OMIM).

Modes of inheritance

Mendelian (single-gene) disorders include those passed to offspring through autosomal dominant, autosomal recessive, and sex-linked forms of inheritance. Humans have two copies (alleles) of each gene located on the autosomes. If both alleles are the same, the individual is homozygous for that gene. If two different alleles are present, the individual is a heterozygote.

Table 31.2 Examples of monogenic (mendelian) disorders with congenital gastrointestinal manifestations

Syndrome	Gene (chromosome)	Inheritance mode	Gastrointestinal manifestations
Aarskog syndrome	*FGDY* (Xp)	X-linked recessive	Inguinal hernia, Hirschsprung disease, midgut malrotation
Alagille syndrome	*JAG1* (20p)	AD	Hepatic involvement presenting as cholestasis, jaundice, pruritus, and liver failure
Beckwith–Wiedemann syndrome	*BWS* (11p)	Several	Omphalocele or other umbilical anomaly, posterior diaphragmatic eventration, hepatomegaly, hepatoblastoma, hyperplastic bladder
Cystic fibrosis	*CFTR* (7q)	AR	Pancreatic insufficiency (80%), meconium ileus in neonates, biliary cirrhosis, distal intestinal obstruction syndrome, rectal prolapse, adenocarcinoma of the ileum
Familial lipoprotein lipase deficiency	*LPL* (8p)	AR	Hepatomegaly, splenomegaly, and abdominal pain resulting from pancreatitis or chylomicronemia
Hereditary hemochromatosis	*HFE* (6p)	AR	Hepatic fibrosis or cirrhosis; inappropriately high iron absorption in gastrointestinal mucosa, liver, pancreas
Hurler syndrome	*IDUA* (4p)	AR	Hepatosplenomegaly, inguinal or umbilical hernia
Marfan syndrome	*FBN1* (15q)	AD	Inguinal and diaphragmatic hernias, incomplete rotation of colon
Medium-chain acyl-coenzyme A dehydrogenase deficiency	*ACADM* (1p)	AR	Hepatomegaly and acute liver disease
Mitochondrial encephalomyopathy, lactic acidosis, and stroke-like episodes (MELAS)	Mitochondrial DNA	Mitochondrial	Recurrent vomiting, anorexia, gastrointestinal dysmotility
Mitochondrial neurogastrointestinal encephalopathy syndrome (MNGIE)	22q and mitochondrial DNA	AR, mitochondrial	Malabsorption, gastrointestinal dysmotility
Pearson marrow–pancreas syndrome	Mitochondrial DNA	Mitochondrial	Exocrine pancreatic dysfunction, malabsorption, pancreatic fibrosis, splenic atrophy
Simpson–Golabi–Behmel syndrome	*GPC3* (Xq)	X-linked recessive	Umbilical or inguinal hernia, diaphragmatic hernia, intestinal malrotation, pyloric ring, polysplenia, hepatosplenomegaly
von Hippel–Lindau syndrome	*VHL* (3p)	AD	Pancreatic lesions that are simply cysts that can occasionally cause biliary obstruction
Waardenburg syndrome type I	*PAX3* (2q)	AD	Hirschsprung aganglionosis, esophageal and anal atresia
Wilson disease	*ATP7B* (13q)	AR	Liver disease presenting as recurrent jaundice, simple acute self-limited hepatitis-like illness, autoimmune-type hepatitis, fulminant hepatic failure, or chronic liver disease

AD, autosomal dominant; AR, autosomal recessive.

Autosomal dominant

The basis of autosomal dominant inheritance is that an alteration in *one* of the two copies of the gene leads to disease. One allele has a mutation, and the corresponding allele on the other chromosome is normal. Figure 31.2 shows a typical autosomal dominant pedigree. The rules of autosomal dominant inheritance are as follows:

• An affected individual has a 50% chance of passing on the mutant gene and a 50% chance of passing on the normal gene to each offspring.

• The disorder appears to be transmitted vertically (i.e., an apparent transmission from grandparent to parent to child is present).

• Males and females are affected equally and can pass the disorder onto their offspring (i.e., male-to-male transmission occurs).

Table 31.3 Hereditary cancer syndromes predisposing to increased risk for gastrointestinal neoplasms

Syndrome	Gene (locus)	Inheritance mode	Gastrointestinal and other neoplasms
Familial adenomatous polyposis (FAP)	*APC* (5q)	AD	Colon, duodenal, pancreatic, thyroid, gastric, hepatoblastoma
MYH-associated polyposis (MAP)	*MUTYH* (1p)	AR	Colon, unknown
Familial gastric cancer	*CDH1* (16q)	AD	Gastric
Hereditary nonpolyposis colorectal cancer (HNPCC)	*MLH1* (3p), *MSH2* (2p), *MSH6* (2p), *PMS2* (7q)	AD	Colon, endometrial, ovarian, gastric, urinary tract, renal cell adenocarcinoma, biliary tract, gallbladder, small bowel
Turcot syndrome	*APC* (5q), *MLH1* (3p), *MSH2* (2p)	AD	Colon and brain cancers; two-thirds of cases variants of FAP and most often associated with medulloblastoma; one-third of cases a variant of HNPCC and associated with glioblastoma
Muir–Torre syndrome	*MLH1* (3p), *MSH2* (2p), *MSH6* (2p), *PMS2* (7q)	AD	Variant of HNPCC associated with sebaceous adenoma, epithelioma, or carcinoma
Peutz–Jeghers syndrome	*STK11* (19p)	AD	Colon, gastric, duodenal, small bowel, breast, pancreatic, endometrial, ovarian, adenoma malignum (cervix), sex cord tumor with annular tubules (females), Sertoli cell tumor (males)
Juvenile polyposis	*SMAD4/DPC4* (18q), *BMPR1A* (10q), (*PTEN*)[a]	AD	Colon, gastric, duodenal
Cowden syndrome	*PTEN* (10q)	AD	Colon, thyroid, breast, uterine, ovarian

a Some cases of juvenile polyposis have been reported to have mutations in the *PTEN* gene; however, these cases may have been clinically misdiagnosed and may have been Cowden syndrome [2].
AD, autosomal dominant; AR, autosomal recessive.

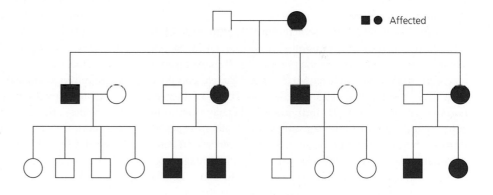

Figure 31.1 Typical pedigree showing mitochondrial inheritance. Males are represented by squares and females by circles. All offspring of an affected female will inherit the disorder, whereas none of the children of an affected male will.

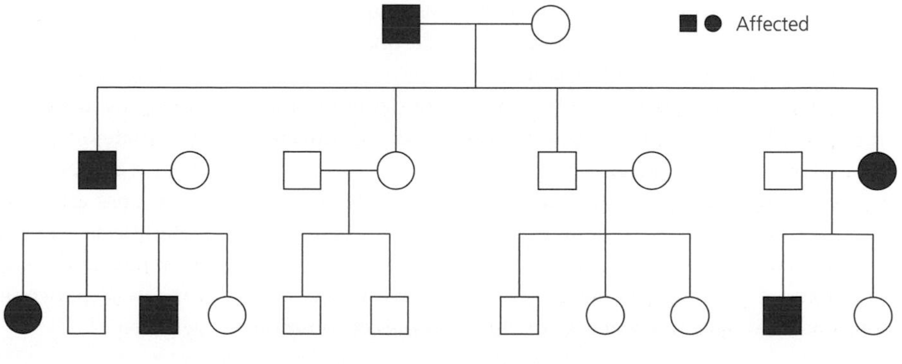

Figure 31.2 Typical pedigree showing autosomal dominant inheritance. Males are represented by squares and females by circles. Males and females are equally affected. Vertical transmission of the disorder is apparent.

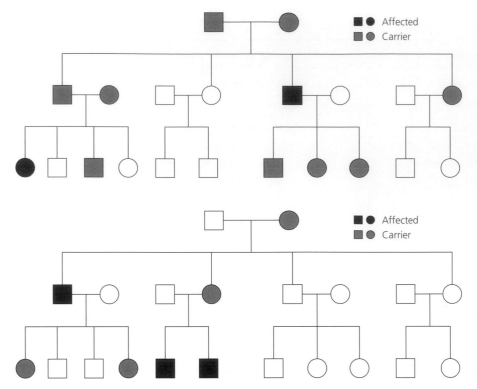

Figure 31.3 Typical pedigree showing autosomal recessive inheritance. Males are represented by squares and females by circles. Males and females are equally affected. An individual must inherit two copies of a mutant gene at a given locus to be affected.

Figure 31.4 Typical pedigree showing X-linked recessive inheritance. Males are represented by squares and females by circles. Males are more likely to be affected, whereas females are more likely to be carriers.

• An affected individual has an affected parent and generations are not skipped (exceptions are new mutation and incomplete penetrance).

Autosomal recessive

Autosomal recessive disorders require that an individual inherits two copies of a mutant gene at a given locus, one disease-causing allele from each parent (Fig. 31.3). Autosomal recessive disorders, such as MUTYH-associated polyposis (MAP), express themselves only when both copies of the gene harbor the mutation [6,7]. Individuals who have only one copy of the mutant gene typically do not manifest symptoms of the disorder and are referred to as *carriers*. In some disorders, carrier status affords a selective advantage (e.g., carriers of sickle cell anemia are resistant to malaria). The rules of autosomal recessive inheritance are as follows:

• A mating between two carrier parents results in a 25% chance that they will have an affected child, and a 75% chance that they will have a normal child. Of the phenotypically normal children, two-thirds will be carriers and one-third will have two normal copies of the gene.

• The disorder appears to be transmitted horizontally (i.e., multiple siblings can be affected without having affected parents or affected children).

• Males and females are affected equally.

Sex-linked

Sex-linked disorders involve the sex-determining X and Y chromosomes. The difference in sex chromosome composition between males and females is the basis for understanding X-linked disorders. Men who inherit an abnormal gene on the X chromosome (the X chromosome in males is always inherited from the mother) will be affected by the associated disorder. Because women have two X chromosomes, the inheritance is similar to that of autosomal dominant and recessive disorders. In X-linked dominant disorders, one mutant allele is sufficient to cause the disorder in females, whereas two mutant alleles are required to cause the disorder in X-linked recessive disorders in females. A typical pedigree showing X-linked recessive inheritance appears in Fig. 31.4. X-linked recessive disorders are more common than X-linked dominant disorders. The rules of X-linked recessive inheritance are as follows:

• Affected men are common, whereas affected women are not (unless an affected man and a carrier woman produce offspring).

• All the daughters of an affected male will be carriers. None of his sons will be affected or carriers because fathers pass on a Y chromosome to their sons, not an X chromosome (no male-to-male transmission).

• Male offspring of carrier women have a 50% chance of being affected and a 50% chance of being unaffected.

• Female offspring of carrier women have a 50% chance of being a carrier and a 50% chance of having two normal alleles.

• Because affected men have carrier daughters, who in turn have affected sons, the disorder appears to "skip" generations.

• Rarely with certain X-linked recessive disorders, female carriers display mild symptoms of the disorder (e.g., fragile X syndrome).

Other rules of genetics

Knowledge of the basic modes of inheritance is important in assessing occurrence and recurrence risks for patients. Other genetic concepts must also be applied to provide accurate education and risk assessment to individuals and their families.

Delayed age at onset

Hemochromatosis demonstrates the feature of delayed age at onset. Individuals born with the hemochromatosis genotype have two mutant copies of the *HFE* gene and typically do not exhibit any features related to iron overload until middle age [8]. Females usually express symptoms later than males because of their monthly menses (see Table 31.2). The presence of a deleterious genotype does not necessarily lead to a phenotypic expression from birth.

Penetrance

Penetrance refers to the likelihood of disease expression if the disease-causing gene is present. For example, individuals with familial adenomatous polyposis (FAP) are thought to have nearly a 100% chance of developing colon polyps and subsequent colon cancer if prophylactic colectomy is not performed, and therefore the penetrance of FAP is 100%. The likelihood of an individual with hereditary nonpolyposis colorectal cancer (HNPCC) developing colon cancer in his or her lifetime is close to 80%; therefore, the penetrance of colon cancer in HNPCC is 80%. Every clinical feature of a genetic disorder has a penetrance level.

Nonpenetrance

Fundamental to the interpretation of the family history is an awareness of nonpenetrance. Nonpenetrance is illustrated by the individual with a mutant genotype in whom the disease or condition never develops. Nonpenetrance may complicate the interpretation of the family history, especially in the case of disorders inherited in an autosomal dominant pattern, where the disorder may not be expressed in each generation, but will appear to skip a generation. Nonpenetrance is also illustrated by the individual who dies of other causes before the disorder develops, who undergoes prophylactic surgery, or who does not undergo testing to determine if they have the disorder. In certain instances, a family member can have children and several other relatives affected with the disorder and they personally do not manifest the disorder – this person is referred to as an obligate carrier.

New mutation

The clinician must also consider the possibility of a new mutation (i.e., neither parent has the disease-causing mutation). Mutations in human genes may occur randomly during gamete maturation or early in embryogenesis. A gamete mutation will be replicated and become a part of every cell in the body of the affected individual. Every genetic disorder has an associated new mutation rate. For example, although reports of new mutations in the genes associated with HNPCC are rare, 25% of individuals in whom FAP is newly diagnosed and do not have a previously known family history of FAP represent new mutations [9].

Pleiotropy

Many genes, including mutated *APC* genes that cause FAP, exhibit pleiotropy. Pleiotropy occurs when a mutated gene has more than one phenotypic effect on the body. For example, in an individual with FAP, colonic polyps, desmoid tumors, osteomas, or thyroid cancer can develop. Although colon cancer is the greatest risk, it is not the only phenotypic effect. The other findings are said to be pleiotropic manifestations of the mutant gene.

Variable expressivity

Variable expressivity is the concept that the same genetic disorder is expressed to a different extent in different individuals. In some individuals with hemochromatosis, for example, cirrhosis of the liver and heart disease may result, whereas only slightly elevated iron levels and no organ damage may develop in other individuals. Gene expression can be modified by intraallelic variation, other genes, environmental factors, and other unknown factors.

Genetic heterogeneity and locus heterogeneity

Critical to identifying the possible etiology of a clinical presentation is the awareness that similar phenotypes may have different genetic causes. For example, although pancreatitis is strongly associated with environmental factors such as alcohol use or gallstones, mutations in two genes have been shown to be associated with pancreatitis. These include the genes for cationic trypsinogen (*PRSS1*) and a trypsin inhibitor (*PST1* or *SPINK1*). The term *locus heterogeneity* indicates that mutations in any one of several related genes may result in the same genetic disorder. HNPCC is a disorder caused by mutations in any one of several DNA mismatch repair genes (*MLH1, MSH2, MSH6,* and *PMS2*). Knowledge of the genetic disorders that have locus heterogeneity is essential in ordering the proper genetic test or series of tests if the mutation is not found initially.

Allelic heterogeneity

One contribution to variable expressivity is allelic heterogeneity. The term simply means different mutations in the same gene. These different mutations may result in different and distinct phenotypes. A good example is FAP, in which some features are related to the location of the mutation in the *APC* gene. Mutations in the 5' or 3' (beginning or end) region of the *APC* gene are generally associated with an attenuated version of FAP (also called *attenuated adenomatous polyposis coli*). In this disorder, fewer polyps form at later ages than in typical FAP [10,11]. In contrast, mutations located between codons 1250 and 1464 are associated with a profuse (> 5000 polyps) phenotype [12]. An ongoing area of study involves the correlation of genotype to phenotype to establish the molecular and health impact of mutations in certain areas of the gene. As with the FAP example, AFAP has lower cancer risks and, thus, management is less aggressive.

Compound heterozygosity

Compound heterozygosity occurs when an individual has two different disease-causing alleles at a specific locus. Individuals with compound heterozygosity can be affected with an autosomal recessive disorder such as cystic fibrosis. The *CFTR* gene is responsible for cystic fibrosis when both alleles contain mutations. Seventy percent of all *CFTR* mutations are caused by deletion of three base pairs coding for a phenylalanine at amino acid 508, commonly called the ΔF508 mutation. Many individuals with cystic fibrosis have two ΔF508 mutations and are homozygotes. Individuals who have a ΔF508 mutation on one allele and a different mutation, such as R117H, on the second allele are compound heterozygotes. Different disease-causing mutations can affect the phenotype of an individual, as explained under "Allelic heterogeneity" above. For example, individuals with cystic fibrosis who have two ΔF508 mutations almost always have pancreatic insufficiency, whereas compound heterozygotes with one ΔF508 mutation and one R117H mutation are less likely to have pancreatic insufficiency.

Somatic vs germ-line mutations

In the field of cancer genetics, it is important to understand the concept of somatic vs germ-line mutations. Somatic mutations are acquired after embryogenesis. Only descendants of the somatically mutated cell carry the mutation. Somatic mutations are not found in cells in other parts of the body and cannot be passed on to offspring. Germ-line mutations are inherited mutations or those that occur at the beginning of embryogenesis, so that they are present in every cell of the body. An individual with a germ-line mutation can pass the mutation on to his or her offspring. Mutations of the *APC* gene, for example, may be germ-line or somatic. In FAP, the germ-line *APC* mutation is present in every cell of the body, so that colonic polyposis and FAP develop, and the disorder is passed to offspring. Interestingly, somatic *APC* mutations are present in most adenomatous polyps and colon cancers, and appear to be an early change in neoplastic development.

Basic concepts of molecular genetics
Structure of DNA and RNA

The most basic components of genetic material are the nucleotides that make up deoxyribonucleic acid (DNA) and ribonucleic acid (RNA), which in turn are the building blocks of the genome. Each *nucleotide* has a backbone composed of a 5-carbon sugar (deoxyribose for DNA and ribose for RNA), a phosphate, and one of several different nitrogen-containing rings known as *bases*. The bases are either pyrimidine or purine compounds. Pyrimidines include cytosine (C), thymine (T), and uracil (U), and purines include adenine (A) and guanine (G).

Nucleotides are joined together by a phosphodiester link between the 5′ and 3′ carbon atoms of the sugars to make a strand of DNA or RNA. Strands are described and schematically viewed in the 5′ to 3′ orientation because enzymes almost always work in that direction. DNA exists as a double-stranded helix in the nucleus of cells. Each DNA strand is oriented in complementary, but opposing, 5′ to 3′ directions. The strands are held together by noncovalent and specific interactions: adenine pairs only with thymine of the opposing strand and cytosine with guanine. The complementary pair of DNA nucleotide bases is referred to as a *base pair*. RNA, on the other hand, is generally single-stranded and is found in the nucleus *and* cytosol of the cell.

DNA replication

DNA is replicated for cell division, called *mitosis*, or for gamete (egg and sperm) formation, called *meiosis*. Replication proceeds by way of a protein complex referred to as *DNA polymerase*. Errors in DNA replication are monitored and repaired by mismatch repair (MMR) protein complexes, a function that maintains the integrity of the DNA. Two additional DNA repair pathways, base excision repair (BER) and nucleotide excision repair (NER), are important to repair DNA bases damaged between rounds of replication.

Transcription and translation

Whereas DNA carries the instructions in the form of genes, it is proteins that perform the actual functions in the body. RNA synthesis is the first step in protein production. The process of making RNA from DNA takes place in the nucleus and is called transcription. RNA is synthesized from a single strand of DNA, which serves as the template. Synthesis is accomplished by a complex of proteins called *RNA polymerase*. In RNA–DNA templating, the pairing of bases is slightly different, in that uracil pairs with adenine and cytosine with guanine. Although the primary function of RNA is to encode proteins, RNA itself is also a part of ribosomes, transfer RNAs, and small ribonucleoprotein particles. The primary RNA transcript contains three main types of component:

• regulatory elements, which are involved in controlling the protein synthetic process
• exons, which contain coding sequences that are translated into amino acids and eventually proteins
• introns, which are interspersed between the coding sequences but are themselves noncoding and thus not translated into amino acids (Fig. 31.5).

Before the RNA leaves the nucleus, enzymes remove all the introns, and the resulting messenger RNA (mRNA) molecule contains only the regulatory elements and a continuous stretch

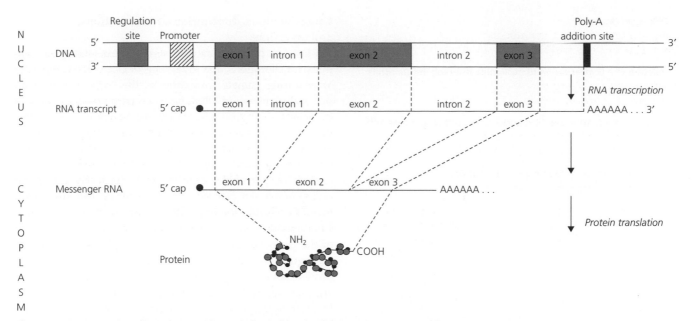

Figure 31.5 Organization of genetic material. DNA is the double-stranded molecule that contains the genetic code and includes coding (exons) and noncoding (introns) segments. In a multistep process, DNA is transcribed into RNA and spliced into messenger RNA (mRNA), which contains regulatory elements and exons but no introns. The mRNA is translated into a series of amino acids that combine to form a specific protein. Proteins are the molecules that function within cells.

of coding sequence to be translated into protein. In the cytosol, the mRNA strand is read in sets of three nucleotides, called *codons*, each of which is translated into a specific amino acid. The first codon, or *start codon*, is almost always an AUG, which is translated into a methionine. As reading proceeds, these amino acids are linked together as a polypeptide chain by the ribosome complex. In a manner analogous to the 5'-to-3' directionality of nucleic acids, amino acids are added to the carboxyl-terminal end of a growing polypeptide chain, resulting in an "amino" to "carboxyl" orientation. Each of the codons is translated into one of 20 amino acids or a stop codon. The stop codon tells the ribosome that it is at the end of the protein. The genetic code is precise but is also "degenerate," meaning that multiple codons can encode a single amino acid. For example, the genetic code for the amino acid valine can be GUU, GUC, GUA, or GUG.

Types of mutations

There are multiple types of genetic changes that can result in a defective protein or decreased protein expression and thereby cause a genetic disorder. Understanding the basis of the genetic change is important because it significantly influences the type of molecular diagnostic testing that should be considered. It is also important to recognize that many DNA changes do not result in disease, but are part of normal genetic variation. A DNA variant with a frequency of under 1% is regarded as a mutation (disease causing), whereas a variant seen with a frequency greater than 1% is typically considered a polymorphism (normal genetic variation). Polymorphisms can be completely inconsequential or

can have a phenotype with subtle consequences (e.g., differences in drug metabolism or minor variations in disease susceptibility). There are many variants that have an unknown effect on the individual. These are called *variants of unknown significance*. Familiarity with the different mutation types is important to understand the results, choices and the limitations of clinical genetic testing.

Amino acid changes (missense or nonsense mutations)

The first major class of mutations consists of amino acid changes in the coding sequence. Nucleotide errors can result in three categories of amino acid changes: silent, missense, and nonsense mutations. Mutations are said to be *silent* when the altered codon encodes the same amino acid as the normal nucleotide sequence. For example, if a GUU is changed or mutated to a GUC, it still encodes the amino acid valine. Mutations are called *missense* when the substitution results in a changed codon that encodes a different amino acid. As an example, if a GUA is changed to a CUA, the resulting amino acid is changed from a valine to a leucine. Finally, nucleotide changes are called *nonsense mutations* when the alteration results in a "stop" signal codon instead of an amino acid codon. Stop codons include the base triplets UAA, UAG, and UGA. In the wrong place, these codons result in a truncated or shortened protein.

Small deletions and insertions (frameshift mutations)

The second class of mutations includes small deletions and insertions. One or more nucleotide(s) are deleted from or added to the DNA sequence in this type of mutation. If the

Wild-type sequence
```
ATG GCA TTA CCA ACA CTA GCT GAC
Met Ala Leu Pro Thr Leu Ala Asp
```

Deletion of a G after the third nucleotide resulting in frameshift
```
ATG*CAT TAC CAA CAC TAG
Met His Tyr Gln His STOP
```

Insertion of a G after the third nucleotide resulting in frameshift
```
ATG GGC ATT ACC AAC ACT AGC TGA
Met Gly Ile Thr Asn Thr Ser STOP
```

In-frame insertion of three nucleotides (GGG)
```
ATG GGG GCA TTA CCA ACA CTA GCT GAC
Met Gly Ala Leu Pro Thr Leu Ala Asp
```

Figure 31.6 Nucleotide insertion and deletion mutations. Nucleotide insertions and deletions may cause in-frame or frameshift mutations. The deletion or insertion of nucleotides in multiples of other than three base pairs causes frameshift mutations that result in major alterations to the amino acid sequence. The insertion of nucleotides in multiples of three does not cause frameshift mutations but does cause alterations in the amino acid sequence.

changes are within the exons or coding portions of the DNA, they often result in a shift of the triplet reading frame and are thus called *frameshift mutations*. The triplet code "downstream" from the insertion or deletion (also said to be "3-prime" or "after" the insertion or deletion) is shifted out of phase or "out of frame" so that an incorrect triplet code results. Frameshift mutations are therefore also categorized as nonsense mutations (Fig. 31.6). Frameshift mutations result in erroneous amino acids and usually an accidental *stop codon* downstream from the mutation causing a shortened or truncated protein. Thus, deletions and insertions virtually always cause disease, unless they consist of a multiple of three codons, whereby the original triplet reading frame is maintained, with only the insertion or deletion of whole codons. In that case, only a single amino acid change occurs with potential results as described above.

Splice-site and regulatory mutations

Mutations also occur in the introns, between the coding sequences. Introns encode sequences, generally close to exons, that precisely specify their own excision. Changes that occur within 4–10 nucleotides of these sequences may constitute *splice-site mutations*, depending on the residual function of the altered sequence. When splice-site mutations occur, an exon is often skipped, and a partial protein with a deleted segment is the result. Additionally, frameshifts can occur when the exons combine improperly, as previously described. Mutations can also occur in the regulatory (e.g., promoter) segments of the DNA, although these are often difficult to identify. These types of regulatory mutations can result in a failure of proteins to be expressed at the correct levels, in the correct tissues, or at the correct time.

Large deletions, duplications, translocations, and inversions

The last class of mutations consists of large deletions, duplications, translocations, and inversions of DNA. These typically arise during gamete formation as the consequence of an unequal exchange of DNA between chromosomes and can be passed down through subsequent generations. A *deletion* involves loss of genetic material, and *duplication* occurs when one section of genetic information is repeated more than once. *Translocations* occur when a section of DNA moves to another location on the same chromosome or onto a different chromosome. An *inversion* results when a section of DNA inverts itself into the opposite orientation. In each of these situations, the genetic changes can result in loss of expression of the gene, expression of a mutated or truncated protein, misregulation of the gene, or generation of a novel hybrid protein. Some of these mutations can be detected by cytogenetic methods that look at chromosomes. Large alterations in DNA, for example, can be detected by examining the Giemsa banding patterns of metaphase chromosomes for correct number and size (karyotyping) or by probing chromosomes with fluorescent DNA markers (fluorescence in situ hybridization, or FISH). The more subtle changes can be detected by Southern blotting methods.

Specific techniques used in mutation detection

A number of laboratory methods are used to detect the various mutation types and determine whether they give rise to disease. It is important to know which methods are being used and what other methods are available if a suspected mutation is not initially found. Mutation detection rates vary based on the gene and the testing technique used. A genetic testing laboratory attempts to identify mutations within the scope of the molecular methods that they use, then distinguishes those genetic changes that are known to cause a disorder from harmless changes, and reports them. However, if the functional consequence of a mutation is not clear, the report will indicate "variation of uncertain significance." This type of result is uninformative and clinical management must then rely on clinical findings. In some situations, additional molecular tests can be employed to explore the functional consequence of these changes, but these types of exploration are often beyond the scope of genetic testing laboratories and require collaboration with a research laboratory. To provide the most information to the family, genetic testing should first be done on a family member who exhibits the disorder. If a mutation cannot be found in the index case, then all family members should be treated as potentially having the disease risk and undergo surveillance and testing for the disorder. Familiarity with the types of mutations that occur in specific disorders is also important and determines the specific test ordered. For example, site-specific mutation analysis for specific mutations or a panel of common mutations, is performed for hemochromatosis and cystic fibrosis, whereas complete gene sequencing is performed for familial adenomatous polyposis (FAP).

Sequencing

DNA sequencing is the gold standard for clinical genetic testing. It is the process of determining the order of nucleotide bases (A, C, G, and T) for all the coding regions and certain intronic regions of the gene of interest. If a mutation is not found by sequencing, other methods should be considered as described below. The limitations of sequencing include: high cost and failure to detect large genetic rearrangements and deletions, mutations in regulatory and intronic regions, and occasionally even single nucleotide changes in exon sequence.

Mutation screening methods

Heteroduplex analysis (also called confirmation-specific gel electrophoresis or CSGE), denaturing-gradient gel electrophoresis (DGGE), and single-strand conformation polymorphism (SSCP) represent screening methods that can be used to complement sequence analysis. Once one of these methods indicates a DNA variant, sequencing is required to confirm the change and determine if it is a normal variant in the human population or a disease-causing mutation. Each of these methods involves polymerase chain reaction (PCR) amplification of a specific region of DNA, typically the exons of the gene. Each method applies a slightly different experimental condition to distinguish a single nucleotide change out of a stretch of hundreds of nucleotides. In the past, these methods employed gel electrophoresis for detection of the DNA changes. Sophisticated instruments are available for detection based on both electrophoretic and liquid chromatography – e.g., denaturing high-performance liquid chromatography (HPLC) – technology. These instruments are increasingly being used by clinical testing labs to screen for DNA sequence variants and offer a higher sensitivity for mutation detection, lower cost and better time efficiency. Although new detection tools are available the basic concepts behind DNA analysis remain the same. Mutation detection rates vary depending on the gene, analysis method, and detection tool used, but are typically greater than 90%. SSCP has the greatest variability in mutation detection, ranging from 60% to 95%.

Protein truncation test (PTT)

The PTT is useful for disorders, such as FAP, where the gene is commonly truncated resulting in a shortened protein. With the PTT method, protein is synthesized in vitro from the DNA in question. Viable cells from the subject are required to generate a full-length complementary DNA (cDNA; a copy of the messenger RNA with the introns removed) of the gene. If a nonsense mutation is present (i.e., one that results in a stop codon and a shortened protein), two bands are observed on the electrophoresis gel, one for the normal protein and one for the shortened protein. PTT fails to detect changes in cases of a large deletion, or if the truncation is at the start or the end of the gene or gene segment. In the clinical setting, PTT is used to indicate the presence of a truncating mutation and it may be followed by sequencing to determine the exact mutation.

Methods for detecting large deletions, duplications, and rearrangements

Southern blotting is a commonly used method for the detection of large intragenic deletions or duplications that go undetected by sequencing (> 100 base pairs). Patient DNA is cut with one or several restriction enzymes and the resulting pieces are separated by size using gel electrophoresis. The exons of the gene are detected using oligonucleotides or cloned DNA. If a large deletion is present, there will be one or more different-sized bands. The DNA used for detection can provide an indication of which exons are present or absent.

A second and increasingly popular method to detect large intragenic deletions or duplications is quantitative PCR [13]. In this method, PCR is performed on sections of the gene, and increases or decreases in the PCR product amount are compared with appropriate controls. Multiplex ligation-dependent probe amplification (MLPA) is a robust modification of quantitative PCR that is being used by laboratories to detect exon deletions, exon duplications, and chromosomal trisomies [14].

Some deletions or duplications are sufficiently large that they can be detected in a cytogenetics laboratory with FISH (> 25 000 base pairs) or karyotype analysis (> 3 000 000 base pairs).

Linkage analysis

Linkage analysis can be used clinically if the gene location is known but a specific mutation has not been identified in the family using other detection methods. Linkage analysis investigates whether specific genetic markers segregate with a certain disease or characteristic in a family. In a dominant genetic disorder, one set of genetic markers near the gene responsible for the syndrome is passed from an affected parent to his or her offspring with a 50% probability. By following the unique pattern of genetic markers from affected parent to affected child, but not from affected parent to unaffected child, linkage between a locus and a genetic disorder can be established. In a recessive genetic disorder, the set of genetic markers is followed from both parents, and the combination of two sets of genetic markers in offspring segregates with the genetic disorder. In this case, both parents are usually clinically unaffected. A genetic marker within 5 centimorgans (cM, about 5 million base pairs of DNA) of a disease gene is considered useful for genetic counseling.

Site-specific mutation analysis

Once a specific mutation has been identified in an index case of a family, site-specific mutation analysis is used to examine the presence or absence of that particular mutation in other family members. A number of PCR-based methods are used, often specific to the mutation found in the family. The various techniques are not described here, but of note, these techniques are all highly accurate and much less expensive than original mutation identification testing in the index case of a family. In fact, accuracy is near 100% so that clinical screening and management of tested individuals can be based on the results.

Genetic testing and counseling

Definition of genetic testing

Genetic testing broadly refers to analysis of DNA, RNA, chromosomes, proteins, or certain metabolites to detect changes related to a genetic disorder. Genetic testing is standard of care for a number of GI conditions. The discoveries of the Human Genome Project will inevitably lead to an increasing array of genetic tests for the diagnosis of both unusual and common GI disorders. In addition to the above definition, genetic testing may also refer to the analysis of specific tissue to assess for acquired or somatic mutations. For example, genetic testing may be performed on cancer tissue. The information can be used better to characterize the molecular and biological nature of a particular disease so that treatment can be targeted – e.g., HER-2 testing in breast cancer, microsatellite instability (MSI) testing in colon cancer. Some types of somatic genetic testing can provide information on the likelihood that an underlying inherited mutation is present. For example, colon cancer tissue can be evaluated for MSI or loss of MLH1, MSH2, MSH6, or PMS2 proteins by immunohistochemistry, each a characteristic associated with HNPCC cancers.

Impact of genetic testing on clinical management

Genetic testing is useful to confirm a diagnosis of a suspected disorder, or to determine who is at risk presymptomatically or at risk of having offspring with a particular disorder. Precise screening and treatment recommendations are emerging for many genetic disorders, in part because of the ability to determine accurately who has the inherited disorder in question.

Genetic test results can significantly alter medical management regimens, as exemplified by HNPCC. Treatment for most cases of cecal cancer is a right hemicolectomy; however, a subtotal colectomy is recommended in individuals with cecal cancer found to have a mutation causing HNPCC [15]. Prophylactic colectomy is also being discussed in HNPCC, as is prophylactic gastrectomy for inherited gastric cancer that arises from mutations of the CDH1 gene [16]. Knowledge of HNPCC mutations in a family enables clinically unaffected at-risk family members to be genetically tested to determine if they are mutation carriers, and thus require more frequent cancer screening at younger ages than the general population.

Chemoprevention is an emerging approach that may be of great benefit to those at increased risk for colon cancer. The use of celecoxib (Celebrex), a cyclooxygenase-2 inhibitor, to induce the regression of adenomatous polyps in FAP patients who still have a rectum after colectomy has been approved by the US Food and Drug Administration (FDA) [17]. Aspirin, other nonsteroidal antiinflammatory drugs, folate, calcium, and estrogens have shown promise in decreasing the incidence of adenomatous polyps and colon cancer [18]. Genetic testing may well direct how such therapies are applied, by precisely defining an at-risk population that can gain the greatest benefit from chemoprevention.

Pharmacogenetics is the study of variations in drug uptake, binding, distribution, metabolism, and excretion based on inherited determinants. As information emerges, genetic testing may be a major factor in medication choice and dosing.

Classification of genetic testing

Genetic testing falls into several categories, discussed in the next sections. Although genetic testing is a powerful tool to guide the clinical care of the at-risk or affected individual, attention should be given to its current limitations. The main limitation of genetic testing is that the sensitivity and specificity of testing methodologies for most disorders are not 100%. One must also be aware that the common jargon of "GENE-X negative" usually means "GENE-X unknown," unless the test is for a specific mutation. A negative or indeterminate result in an individual without a prior identification of a family-specific mutation does not indicate the absence of a deleterious mutation for a suspected syndrome or the lack of a genetic etiology. *Such misinterpretations are potentially fatal when medical management ceases for an at-risk individual* [19]. If a mutation cannot be found in the index case, then all family members should be treated as potentially having the disease risk.

Diagnostic or initial genetic testing

Diagnostic testing is genetic testing performed in a person suspected of having an inherited disorder. An example would be a 40-year-old with ten adenomatous polyps but no known family history of polyposis. Finding a mutation of the APC gene confirms the diagnosis of FAP or attenuated FAP and allows the clinician to proceed with appropriate screening and therapy. Failure to identify a mutation in APC allows one to consider that the patient may have biallelic mutations in the MYH gene. If mutations in both the APC and MYH genes are not identified, the diagnosis remains unclear. In this situation, clinicians are left to use their best clinical judgment.

For many individuals, clinicians can make a disorder diagnosis based on clinical findings. In these situations, genetic testing enables identification of a disease-causing mutation so that family members not presenting with clinical symptoms may undergo testing to determine their genetic status.

Presymptomatic testing or testing when the disorder mutation is known

Knowledge of a specific disorder mutation in a family allows family members at risk for the disorder to undergo presymptomatic testing. Presymptomatic testing involves testing healthy family members for the presence or absence of a specific mutation previously identified in an affected family member. A positive test result in a presymptomatic family member indicates that the person being tested carries the mutation and therefore has a genetic diagnosis of the *predisposition* to the disorder in question. Appropriate screening and surveillance can then be planned. A negative test result (i.e., failure to find the mutation known to be segregating in the family) means that the person tested does not have the disorder that is present in the family and screening or management can be altered accordingly.

A note of caution here is that a positive genetic diagnosis is not equivalent to a clinical diagnosis. Many features of the disorder in question may or may not appear, depending on the observed penetrance of each of the features. This concept is frequently misunderstood by patients and requires careful attention. For example, a positive HNPCC genetic test result on an unaffected person does not mean that he or she currently has cancer. Instead it conveys a level of risk for that individual to develop cancer in the future. Accurate education and counseling are important at this stage. The patient must be educated about the likelihood of the development of certain disease features and should understand that appropriate management can prevent many of the consequences of the disorder. A genetic diagnosis of FAP, for example, implies a 100% risk for eventual polyposis, but colon cancer can virtually always be prevented with appropriate surveillance and surgery. A genetic diagnosis of HNPCC confers an 80% lifetime risk for colon cancer (not 100%), which likewise can almost always be prevented through appropriate surveillance.

Carrier testing

Carrier testing is performed for autosomal recessive and sex-linked disorders to discover if an individual is a heterozygous carrier of a gene mutation. Carrier testing may be appropriate for unaffected individuals with a relative who has an autosomal recessive or sex-linked disorder. Additionally, members of different ethnic groups may be more likely to be gene carriers because of increased carrier frequencies in specific populations, and carrier testing is routinely offered to these groups (see "General population screening" below). Often carrier testing is used prior to conception or early in pregnancy to determine the risks of having a child affected with a specific disorder.

Prenatal testing

In prenatal testing, the health status of a fetus is evaluated during pregnancy. This may be desired because of an abnormal result of a screening test, such as ultrasonography, or because of an increased risk associated with the family history or maternal age. Fetal cells are most commonly obtained through amniocentesis or chorionic villus sampling. Karyotyping to look for chromosomal disorders, or mutation analysis to look for a specific gene mutation known to be present in the family, may be applied to these cells.

Newborn screening

In newborn screening, a blood sample taken shortly after birth is used for genetic testing for specific genetic disorders whose consequences could be prevented or ameliorated by early treatment. All states in the United States require screening for several genetic disorders, most of which are metabolic.

General population screening

General population screening is commonly encountered in prenatal diagnosis or newborn screening because early medical intervention prevents disease or reduces its severity. A number of state-supported screening programs for genetic disorders with GI involvement are outlined in Table 31.4; the panel of screening tests varies by state.

Population-wide screening for most genetic disorders is not available or even indicated. Screening of the general population for a particular disease can be justified only in the case of a highly penetrant disorder for which effective medical treatments are available. Founder mutations or a high prevalence of disease carriers supports population genetic screening for certain disorders, such as sickle cell anemia, in certain

Table 31.4 Newborn and prenatal screening

Screening tests	Gastrointestinally related symptoms
Phenylketonuria	Neonatal vomiting
Galactosemia	Diarrhea, hepatomegaly, vomiting, progressive liver dysfunction leading to cirrhosis if untreated
Maple syrup urine disease	Pancreatitis, vomiting
Homocystinuria	Inguinal hernia, fatty changes in liver, pancreatitis
Sickle cell disease	Cholelithiasis, splenomegaly, splenic syndrome
Cystic fibrosis	Pancreatic insufficiency, meconium ileus in neonates, biliary cirrhosis, distal intestinal obstruction syndrome, rectal prolapse, adenocarcinoma of the ileum
Tyrosinemia (type I)	Hepatosplenomegaly, hepatic cirrhosis, hepatocellular carcinoma, pancreatic islet hypertrophy, ascites, jaundice, vomiting, paralytic ileus, diarrhea, melena

Table 31.5 Areas to be covered by genetic counseling

Collection of background information

Patient demographic data and relevant medical history

Family history with construction of a pedigree

Verification of family cancers, polyps, or other condition under
    evaluation

Patient's perception of risk

Psychological stability and concerns

Patient educational issues covered

Basic concepts of inheritance

Characteristics of the syndrome in question, including age-specific risks

Syndrome management, including recommended approaches for
    prevention, if available

Determinations made

Likelihood of syndrome diagnosis

Estimated risks for self and family members

Optimal screening and prevention strategies

Utility of possible genetic testing

Table 31.6 General indications for genetic consultation based on
needs of special populations

Fetuses, newborns, and young children

Known or suspected metabolic disorder

Known or suspected familial chromosomal abnormality

Family history of a child or children with multiple malformations or
    unusual appearance

Child with mental or developmental delays

Child with birth defect

**Population at increased risk for inherited gastrointestinal
conditions or cancers**

Multiple family members on same side of family with same condition or
    cancer type (e.g., gastric ulcer and hereditary hemochromatosis)

Clustering of conditions or cancers seen in a specific syndrome (e.g.,
    colon and endometrial cancers in hereditary nonpolyposis colorectal
    cancer)

Condition or cancer diagnosed at a younger age than is expected for
    that cancer or than is typically seen in the general population

Multifocal primary cancer occurrences in the same organ or different
    organs

Bilateral development of condition or cancer in paired organs

Presence of rare tumors (e.g., glioblastoma)

Excess cancer cases or condition in same side of family

Occurrence of condition or cancer in same individual with congenital
    anomalies or birth defects

Expectant parents or those planning a pregnancy

Maternal exposure to teratogens before or during pregnancy

Maternal diagnosis of gastrointestinal disease requiring medication
    before, during, and after pregnancy

Recurrent pregnancy losses/stillbirths

Couples of "advanced age" (women older than 35, men older than 55)

Consanguineous couples

Couples of certain ethnic background suggesting an increased risk for
    specific disorder

Couples considering prenatal diagnosis for any disorder

Couples who may be carriers for a genetic disorder based on family
    history of disorder

Abnormal fetal ultrasound finding

countries and ethnic groups. On the other hand, population screening for FAP is impractical in view of the cost of screening and the rarity of the disorder. Population screening may become more applicable and attractive as high-prevalence genes that affect common disease susceptibility are elucidated.

Genetic counseling

Genetic counseling is the process of communicating information and providing support regarding a genetic disorder. Core components of genetic counseling include:

- evaluation of a patient's risk of having a certain genetic disorder

- delivery of medical facts about the disorder, including its course and medical management

- explanation of the cause of the disorder and relevant inheritance information (i.e., risks to relatives)

- description of alternatives for dealing with risk, including genetic testing, and assistance in choosing an individualized plan.

The genetic counseling session is collaborative in nature because of the amount of education and personal decision making involved for the patient [20,21]. Family members are often seen with the patient because of the hereditary nature of the disorder. The most common issues covered in a genetic counseling session are found in Table 31.5.

Indications for counseling

Any patient with a GI condition for which a genetic etiology is suspected or known is a candidate for genetic counseling. Patients who undergo genetic counseling for most GI disorders with a known genetic etiology can generally be grouped by age or special populations; the common considerations

indicating a genetic consultation are summarized in Table 31.6, although the list is not exhaustive.

Counseling for conditions involving fetuses, newborns, or young children

Fetuses, newborns, or young children who present with congenital GI malformations may have chromosomal abnormalities or single-gene mutations. For example, 25% of fetuses with cystic fibrosis and 12% of fetuses with chromosomal disorders present with an echogenic bowel seen on ultrasonography during the second trimester. It is currently estimated that more than half of all birth defects have a genetic origin. Some types of GI dysfunction may be seen as part of a syndrome or display genetic heterogeneity (see Tables 31.1 and 31.2).

Table 31.7 Database resources for teratology information

Database name	URL
OTIS (Organization of Teratology Information Specialists)	www.otispregnancy.org/
REPROTOX (Reproductive Toxicology Center)	www.reprotox.org/
TERIS (Teratogen Information System)	http://depts.washington.edu/terisweb/teris/

Counseling for women of childbearing age

Gastroenterologists caring for women who are of childbearing age should be familiar with reproductive counseling, specifically regarding teratogens. A teratogen is defined as an environmental agent, such as a GI medication, that is capable of causing either structural or functional abnormalities in the developing fetus. In an assessment of potential risk to a pregnancy, an environmentally induced malformation depends on several measures. These may include the time of exposure during pregnancy, the dose of the drug, the duration of exposure to the drug, individual susceptibility, the potential interaction with other environmental agents, placental transport, species differences, and the pharmacokinetics and metabolism of the agent [22].

In counseling a woman whose pregnancy is at risk for teratogenicity, it is important to compare the risk of a major birth defect in the general population for any pregnancy (2%–5%, regardless of family history and exposures) with the potential for increased risk based on currently known teratogenic exposure(s). If discontinued before pregnancy, most drugs generally pose no increased risk to the developing fetus. Moreover, the developmental period when exposure occurs can be a predictor of the type of embryonic damage. Typically, medications taken during the preimplantation phase, or the first 2 weeks after conception, exhibit the all-or-none phenomenon. This should not be misinterpreted to mean that malformations cannot be induced at this stage. Rather, embryonic lethality resulting in an unrecognized pregnancy is more likely than a surviving fetus with anomalies [22]. The period of organogenesis (gestational day 18 through about day 60) is when most major and gross anatomical and functional development occurs, and therefore this is the time when fetal exposure to teratogens is most likely to result in severe malformations. During the second and third trimesters of pregnancy, damage to the genitourinary system and the brain is more likely.

The US FDA has developed a rating system that combines what is known regarding the teratogenicity of a given drug and the potential benefit of that drug to a pregnant woman [23]. Physicians' Desk Reference provides a similar rating scale. Several comprehensive resources provide detailed information on teratogenicity and pregnancy risk to clinicians (Table 31.7).

Counseling for adults and for cancer predisposition

Although some predominantly GI disorders of the young adolescent and adult population have been linked to genes or genetic loci, most GI disorders for which genetic testing is commercially available relate to cancer predisposition. A small but significant number of colon cancers (5%–10%) belong to a distinct class of inherited colorectal cancer predisposition syndromes (see Table 31.3) [24].

Collection of background information
Personal and family medical history

A personal medical history must be obtained from the patient. In addition, when investigating whether a patient has a genetic disorder, collection of family history information is critical. Table 31.8 lists important questions to ask when obtaining personal and family history. Information gathered is pertinent to determine the inheritance pattern of the disorder, to propose the differential diagnoses of genetically related GI disorders, to provide risk assessment, to determine which diagnostic test to order, to interpret genetic test results accurately, and to guide individualized medical intervention. When genetic tests are unavailable or declined by

Table 31.8 Suggested components of family and personal history

Family medical history

Full, three-generation pedigree and extended family as needed

Ethnicity of paternal and maternal sides

Congenital defects, bilaterality of disease, or occurrence of multiple disease-related symptoms in an affected relative

Diagnosis and age of affected relatives

Documentation of repeated miscarriages or infertility

Cause of early death(s) or deaths; if living, current ages of asymptomatic relatives

Personal medical history

Present symptoms relevant to genetic disorder under evaluation or chief complaint

Prenatal/neonatal history (e.g., prenatal exposures, maternal complications)

Childhood development and illnesses

Past surgeries, hospitalizations, or trauma

Current medications and nontraditional treatments

Other pertinent information (e.g., diet, social habits)

the patient, the family history remains valuable in providing targeted surveillance and aiding in management decisions [25].

A helpful tool in genetic counseling is a family tree or "pedigree." A pedigree is a schematic diagram of familial generations, including personal and family medical history, in which standardized symbols are used [26]. For examples see Figs 31.1–31.4. Pedigrees aid in determining the inheritance pattern of disorder.

Accuracy and perceptions

Generally, individuals report accurate medical diagnoses for first-degree relatives (parents, children, siblings) and second-degree relatives (grandparents, aunts, uncles, grandchildren), but reports for distant relatives may be less accurate [27,28]. Confirmation of the information provided by the patient through collection and review of medical records can be insightful. Subtle differences detected from pathology records or a repeated consultation of a previous histopathological report can change the diagnosis, affect appropriate medical recommendations, and necessitate different genetic testing or surveillance. For example, it is common for family members to know if a close relative has colonic polyps, but it is unusual for the patient to know whether the polyps are adenomatous, hyperplastic, or hamartomatous. Knowledge of the histology of polyps is pertinent when a family is evaluated for an inherited colon cancer disorder (see Table 31.3).

A review of the family history information during clinic visits can also provide an opportunity to learn about the patient's health beliefs. An example of beliefs would be "Aunt Mary got cancer because she has a stressful job," and an example of family dynamics would be "My brother and I haven't spoken since I was diagnosed with cancer."

Physical evaluation

Depending on the suspected disorder, a physical examination can be extremely important in determining the likelihood that the disorder is present. A good example is FAP. The presence of associated extracolonic manifestations, such as osteomas, fibromas, and congenital hypertrophic retinal pigment epithelium in a patient at risk makes the diagnosis much more likely. The family and personal history, environmental risk factors, and complete physical examination are collectively meaningful in an assessment of the probability that a genetic disorder is present.

Psychosocial issues

In view of the many psychological issues surrounding genetic diagnosis and testing, a thoughtful psychological assessment should be included. The primary aspect that differentiates genetics from other forms of medicine is that genetic information not only affects the patient, but also may have significant ramifications for the patient's family, especially children. The most important initial step for the provider is acceptance of the patient's responses and vulnerabilities [29,30]. An environment of trust and openness can then be provided so that short- and long-term psychological support can be given. The genetic diagnosis frequently delineates risks that differ widely from the patient's beliefs or perceived risks. Challenges for the provider thus also include the reconciliation of unexpected news with long-held beliefs and ideas. Referral to support groups may be helpful.

Determinations made and subsequent patient education

Risk assessment and medical management

Genetic risk assessment is the determination of a patient's risk for a genetic disorder based on an evaluation of personal and family history and environmental influences. A physician will then share with the patient the likelihood of a possible genetic component and its implications. An individual or family that fulfills one or more of the criteria listed in Table 31.6 is generally considered at increased risk of a contributing hereditary factor. Genetic testing may ultimately define the genetic risk with precision. The results of genetic testing can direct those with the inherited disorder in question to proper management.

When a specific diagnosis can be made, patient education consists of information about the nature and etiology of the disorder, its natural history and prognosis, the mode of inheritance, the occurrence or recurrence risks, the recommended prevention, screening, and treatment options, the availability of research studies, and the possibilities for prenatal diagnosis (Table 31.5). Helping patients understand the basic principles of genetics and disease can dispel myths. It is not uncommon for individuals with a strong family history of a disorder to develop their own beliefs about the inheritance, such as "the disease only affects males in my family" when the disease is actually autosomal dominant. An association with physical features is common, such as "everyone in my family with red hair gets cancer."

In a discussion of the quantitative risks of health problems associated with an inherited disorder, it is important to recognize that many patients do not understand statistical terminology. It may often be better, for example, to state that eight of ten individuals with HNPCC will acquire colon cancer in their lifetime, rather than that the lifetime risk of associated colon cancer is 80%. It may also be useful to compare risks with the risks in the general population. For example, although 6% of US citizens will acquire colon cancer in their lifetime, the risk of individuals with HNPCC for the development of colon cancer is increased approximately 13-fold. Risk communication geared toward the patient's educational background and personal experience will improve understanding and facilitate compliance with the recommended surveillance.

Risks to family members

Whether a specific disorder is diagnosed in an individual or the individual is at a high risk of having a hereditary contribution, the implications for family members should be discussed. If a genetic syndrome diagnosis can be made, family members' risks can be determined as the inheritance pattern will be known. Even without a clear genetic diagnosis, empirical risks to family members can often be shared.

The duty to warn at-risk relatives about the ramifications of inherited disorder has been heavily debated [31]. Two legal cases have concluded that, at minimum, there appears to be at least a duty to warn the patient about the familial implications of genetic disorder. In one of the cases, it was further declared that "reasonable steps be taken by the provider to assure that the information reaches those likely to be affected or is made available for their benefit" – *Pate v. Threlkel*, 661 So 2d 278 (Fla 1995) and *Safer v. Estate of Pack*, 677 A2d 1188 (NJ Super Ct App Div 1996). Positions from the American Medical Association and American Society of Clinical Oncology (ASCO) suggest that physicians should inform their patients of the risks to their family members, and allow the patients to communicate this risk information to their family members [32,33]. Documentation of the discussion regarding family members' risk should be placed in the patient's chart [31].

Role of genetic testing
The availability of genetic testing for many disorders adds a new dimension to clinical care and genetic counseling. The clinician must determine whether or not genetic testing is available and helpful. GeneTests (www.genetests.org), a federally funded and continually updated database, provides assistance in finding clinical and research laboratories that perform molecular analyses for single-gene inherited disorders. The clinician should involve the patient in the decision on whether or not genetic testing is helpful to them.

Position statements on genetic testing have emerged and serve as valuable references to guide clinicians in routine and special situations. For gastroenterological cancer conditions, ASCO has developed recommendations for when genetic testing should be offered. This organization states that genetic testing be offered when:
- the individual has personal or family history features suggestive of a genetic cancer susceptibility condition
- the test can be adequately interpreted
- the results will aid in the diagnosis or influence the medical or surgical management of the patient or family members at hereditary risk of cancer [33].

Informed consent
The informed consent process is uniformly accepted by professional genetic societies as an integral part of genetic testing and should be part of pretest counseling. Informed consent should include the benefits, risks, and limits of genetic testing (Table 31.9) and cover the issues listed in Table 31.10. For cancer-related conditions, ASCO has defined topics that

Table 31.9 Benefits, risks, and limitations of genetic testing

Benefits
Better definition of disease risk
Improved and individualized medical screening and management
Reduced uncertainty or anxiety; may provide explanation for disease in self or family
Information for oneself and extended family members
Family planning

Risks
Psychological distress
False sense of security and inappropriate medical management when results inaccurately interpreted
Increase emotional uncertainty because of disease penetrance
Change in family social dynamics
Potential for genetic discrimination by employers or insurance carriers

Limitations
Results indicate probability and not certainty of disease
Unproven efficacy of some interventions for mutation carriers
Uncertain clinical significance for some mutations
Negative result of no clinical value unless disorder mutation identified in the family
Not all mutations are detectable by standard laboratory methods

should be discussed for informed consent for genetic testing [33]. Guidelines are also available for genetic testing in special circumstances, such as presymptomatic testing in minors and potential adoptees [34–36].

Genetic testing for children
Genetic testing in children should be considered only if medical benefit is clearly possible [34,37]. If the outcome of genetic testing would not alter medical management in a child, it is considered best to allow the child to decide for him or herself about testing after the age of 18. FAP testing is an example where results impact medical management. Genetic testing is appropriate to perform in a child around the age 10–12 years as colon surveillance and preventive measures are indicated by that age in carriers, whereas screening is unnecessary in noncarriers [38]. In some situations, genetic testing for FAP may be appropriate in the first years of life because of the 0.7%–1.6% risk of hepatoblastoma in children [39]. When the testing of minors is being considered, both the parents and health-care professionals need to weigh the potential medical benefits against the psychosocial well-being of the child. The decision-making capacity of a child should also be considered, and whether advocacy for testing is truly in the child's interests. Age-appropriate education for the child undergoing testing is also a necessity. Continuing education and follow-up as the child matures can focus on information relevant for life decision making.

Table 31.10 Informed consent for genetic testing

The patient should have a working understanding of the following issues:

Medical issues

The syndrome in question, including inheritance, risks, screening guidelines, and disease management

Medical care better directed with genetic diagnosis

Compliance with surveillance guidelines necessary for benefit

Prevention improved with knowledge and compliance

Genetic issues

Interpretation and implications of a positive, a negative (dependent on whether familial mutation is known), and an indeterminate genetic test result

Risk to self and family members better defined if genetic testing successful

Methods of testing and the accuracy associated with each testing option

Alternatives to genetic testing

Psychological issues

Failure to detect a mutation in the first person tested in family: frustration, anxiety, disappointment, possible relief

Positive test: relief that a diagnosis can be made, coping with possible anger, anxiety, responsibility guilt, stress, self-image issues

Negative test in a member of a family with a known mutation: relief, decreased worry for self and offspring, survivor guilt

Social/economic issues

Failure to detect a mutation in the first person tested in family: no information for self, children, and other at-risk relatives

Positive test: possible insurance, employment, and social discrimination

Negative test in a member of a family with a known mutation: possible resolution of insurance problems, family relationships possibly positively or negatively affected

Special issues for testing in children

Protection of children's rights

Self-image problems

Possible problems with parent–child relationships, sibling–sibling relationships

Social stigmatization

Other issues

Cost of test, insurance coverage, and potential for genetic discrimination

Confidentiality of results

Testing of adopted persons

The American Society of Human Genetics (ASHG) recommends that the guidelines for the testing of adoptees (newborns and children) be consistent with those for genetic testing performed in all children of similar age (as discussed previously). Thus, the timing of genetic testing should be primarily justified for reasons such as the initiation of preventive or therapeutic medical management through early diagnosis [36]. Additionally, ASHG recommends that a relevant family history and medical history for the adoptee be accessible and updated so that this information can be shared by all parties involved, including the adoptee, the biological parents, and the adoptive parents when medically appropriate.

Genetic discrimination

Genetic discrimination is the act of being treated differently based on one's genetic makeup. Although the risks of genetic discrimination are low, it is a common question raised by patients and health-care providers. The National Human Genome Research Institute hosts a website with policies on genetic privacy (www.genome.gov/PolicyEthics/LegDatabase/pubsearch.cfm). The most important federal safeguard for genetic information is the Health Insurance Portability and Accountability Act of 1997, which states that a person with a genetic mutation who is asymptomatic is not considered to have a preexisting condition. This law also prohibits health insurers from using genetic information to exclude a person from group coverage or individually charging higher premiums within a group. In the context of employment, the Americans with Disabilities Act of 1990 includes "genetic or medically identified potential of or predisposition toward a physical or mental impairment that substantially limits a major life activity" as a definition of a disability. Most states have enacted some level of protection for genetic privacy and some states have legislative protection in place for employment, disability insurance, and life insurance.

Genetic test results

Results of genetic testing are usually presented in person to ensure a precise understanding of the test results, to provide support for the psychological consequences, and to outline appropriate medical care. If disclosure of results occurs by telephone, an in-person follow-up visit is often scheduled. Because testing has implications not only for the testing candidate but also for extended family members, a discussion during pretest or posttest counseling regarding how to share test results with other family members or children at risk is appropriate.

Logistical aspects

Who should be tested first?

In a family believed to have an inherited syndrome, initial genetic testing should be offered to the person most likely to carry the mutant gene. In a FAP family, for example, genetic testing would start with a person diagnosed with most clinical confidence as having the disorder. This individual is considered the ideal "testing candidate." Finding a mutation would allow testing in other family members with nearly 100% accuracy. A negative test result in this case would be interpreted as a failure to find a disease-causing mutation in that person, and would imply that genetic testing cannot be used in the family and that other family members must be managed on the basis of the clinical findings.

An important issue to keep in mind is that finding a mutation in the child of a living parent often indicates that a parent also has the mutation. This situation can be challenging when the parent has not consented to know his or her genetic status, has not learned about genetic testing, and possibly does not want such information at all. Assessing the family dynamics and encouraging family decision making regarding genetic testing should therefore be part of the pretest counseling, although ultimately genetic testing is the individual's choice.

Sample submission for genetic testing

The type of sample required for clinical genetic testing depends on the type of testing being performed. Contacting the laboratory that offers the test allows assurance that the correct sample type will be submitted. Most often a blood sample is required. In some instances, DNA may be obtained from cells in a buccal check swab. When the death of an individual key to the genetic diagnosis in a family is imminent, DNA banking is an option. A laboratory will store DNA, usually extracted from a blood sample, for a certain length of time for a specified cost so that it will be available for testing in the future.

Regulatory issues

Clinical genetic testing is controlled by specific regulations, and oversights are implemented to ensure that tests are performed properly. In the United States, the Clinical Laboratory Improvement Amendments of 1988 (CLIA) oversee all testing on human samples for health assessment or for the diagnosis, prevention, or treatment of disease [40]. Genetic test results to be returned to the patient should be performed in a CLIA-approved laboratory.

Genetic providers

Medical geneticists (PhD or MD), advanced practice nurses with genetic certification (MSN), and genetic counselors (MS) are specialty-trained clinical genetic practitioners who provide education, a diagnosis based on the clinical findings or results of genetic testing, therapeutic management and options, and psychosocial support throughout the duration of care for the patient at risk for or affected with a genetic disorder. Genetic providers also stay abreast of the socioethical, legal, ethnocultural, and financial issues that surround genetic testing.

Although the majority of genetic services are in obstetrical care, other subspecialties have quickly developed because of the expanding knowledge of the genetic etiology of human disease. Subspecialty areas include cancer, neurogenetics, hematology, psychiatric, and pediatric counseling. In genetics clinics, a consultation may require a multidisciplinary team comprising PhD/MD geneticists, surgeons, genetic counselors, nurses, nutritionists, and other practitioners of health-care disciplines to address the patient's complex needs and manage the pleiotropic effects of a genetic disorder. Some gastroenterologists may have specialty training or knowledge to provide genetic counseling, whereas others may find it valuable to consult with or refer to genetic practitioners. To find a genetics clinic, search the Clinic Directory at www.genetests.org.

Developing technology

From our experience, a frequently asked question during genetic counseling pertains to gene therapy. Gene therapy involves introducing genetic material into human cells with the goal of achieving a preventive or therapeutic effect [41]. To date, gene therapy has had limited success; it was initially considered useful, but has not been accomplished, for monogenic disorders such as cystic fibrosis and familial hypercholesterolemia. Gene therapy is under investigation for use in treatment of more complex genetic and infectious diseases. The main challenges are finding safe, reliable, and efficient vehicles through which genetic material can be transferred to the target cells in the body. An additional challenge involves ensuring that the therapeutic gene expresses itself in the target cells at the right time and in the right quantity to be beneficial to the patient.

Patients also express an interest in opportunities to participate in clinical trials. Lists of clinical trials currently underway can be found at the Clinical Trials website (www.clinicaltrials.gov) and Clinical Center website (www.cc.nih.gov) of the US National Institutes of Health.

Genetic tools and technologies

The cooperative effort of the Human Genome Project, together with extensive genetic work in numerous laboratories, has given rise to powerful new tools and technologies for genetic research and clinical application. Familiarity with these tools is useful for the practice of medicine as clinical genetic offerings continue to emerge.

Human Genome Project

The Human Genome Project was conceived in the 1980s, and an international multicenter program was organized in 1990. The program was designed to construct detailed genetic and physical maps of the human genome, to determine the complete nucleotide sequence of human DNA, to localize all genes within the human genome, and to sequence genomes of other model organisms. In 2004 the International Human Genome Sequencing Consortium completed sequencing and analysis of the human genome [42]. The genome contains 2.85 billion base pairs and appears to encode only 20 000–25 000 protein-coding genes. The number of protein-coding genes is significantly lower than the previously predicted 100 000 genes, but alternative splicing of RNA accounts for much of the protein complexity.

Data and research tools from the Human Genome Project are available to the public and can be accessed through the National Center for Biotechnology Information (NCBI) website (www.ncbi.nlm.nih.gov/genome/guide/human/) and the University of California Santa Cruz Genome browser website (http://genome.ucsc.edu/cgi-bin/hgGateway). At these websites, you can search for specific genetic markers or genes and also browse through a genomic region while using the information resources that you select. Most of the genetic loci that are displayed link to detailed descriptions of the marker or gene. The NCBI website also contains Online Mendelian Inheritance in Man (OMIM), a unique and comprehensive hyperlinked catalogue of human genes and associated diseases, originally developed by Victor McKusick in the 1950s.

Genetic markers

Short tandem repeats

One tool developed throughout the 1990s is a set of genetic markers placed in order along chromosomes and spanning the entire human genome. Many of these markers are unique regions of the genome that contain variable numbers of nucleotide repeats resulting in variable length of the DNA segments in the human population. These are referred to as *short tandem repeats* (STRs) or *variable number tandem repeats* (VNTRs). STRs can be repeats of any length, but the ones most utilized are the dinucleotide repeats (CACACA ...) and the tetranucleotide repeats (AGATAGATAGAT ...). Genotyping of individuals at these markers is used extensively in genetic linkage studies to search for new familial disease genes. This tool has thereby dramatically changed the pace of gene discovery because the entire genome is systematically scanned by using these markers. Linkage by means of these markers is used in the clinical setting to identify carriers of disorder genes when a specific mutation cannot be found.

Single-nucleotide polymorphisms and the International HapMap Project

A *single-nucleotide polymorphism* (SNP) is a site on the DNA where a single base pair varies from person to person. Linkage and association studies make use of SNPs as genetic markers. A cooperative effort resulted in identification of 1.4 million SNPs within the human genome [43], and by 2005 this had grown to 4.9 million validated SNPs. Researchers estimate that 4.3% of these SNPs are within exons. In addition, a small portion of SNP variants encode amino acid changes (0.12%–0.17%) and may have functional consequences. Thus, a small fraction of SNPs are not only markers but may contribute to certain disorders. Stemming from the SNP identification and mapping efforts is the International HapMap project, which was completed in 2005 [44]. The goal of this project "is to determine the common patterns of DNA sequence variation in the human genome, by characterizing sequence variants, their frequencies, and correlations between them, in DNA samples from populations with ancestry from parts of Africa, Asia, and Europe" [45]. SNPs that are close together on a chromosome are inherited in blocks, called haplotypes. A few SNPs within this block allow for identification of the haplotype. The HapMap is a map of these haplotype blocks, and the specific SNPs that identify the haplotypes are called tag SNPs. The vision is to be able to use a small set of SNPs, the tag SNPs, for functional studies of candidate genes and linkage studies, and to understand common variants responsible for disease risk.

The DNA microchip and microarrays

The DNA microchip is a research tool with anticipated use in clinical genetic diagnosis. A DNA microchip contains subnanoliter amounts of single-stranded DNA spotted on a solid surface, such as a silicon wafer or a glass microscope slide. Thousands of different DNA sequences can be spotted onto a single microchip and each fragment is analyzed as an independent data point. The DNA to be tested against the microchip is marked with a fluorescent label, and if the sequence is present in the test DNA it will bind to its complementary single-stranded DNA on the microchip. DNA microchips can be used to determine if genomic DNA from either normal or disease tissue has a genetic change. DNA microchips can also be used in a quantitative way to identify loss of or amplification of DNA in a sample (DNA microarray) and to investigate differences in gene expression levels (RNA microarray). RNA microarray has shown great potential clinically with some of the best recognized work in the field of breast cancer. It has been used to categorize breast cancers and to predict optimal treatment choices and prognosis [46]. This concept is being applied to many other cancers and disease conditions. It is also anticipated that RNA microarrays will be another tool for diagnosis of genetic disorders whereby an individual with a genetic disorder will have a distinct molecular profile in his or her tissues.

Summary and conclusions

The genetic revolution and its emerging implications to clinical medicine make it necessary for the gastroenterologist to have a basic understanding of genetics and to know when genetic testing is a part of disease management. Furthermore, the far-reaching effects of genetic diagnoses on patients require the physician to have not only a medical understanding of inherited disorder but also a familiarity with the process of genetic testing. Only then can proper education and advice be given to patients as inherited disorders and genetic testing are considered in the clinical setting.

References

1. Lichtenstein P, Holm NV, Verkasalo PK, et al. Environmental and heritable factors in the causation of cancer – analyses of cohorts of twins from Sweden, Denmark, and Finland. N Engl J Med 2000;343:78.

2. Burt R, Neklason DW. Genetic testing for inherited colon cancer. Gastroenterology 2005;128:1696.

3. Brooks AS, Oostra BA, Hofstra RM. Studying the genetics of Hirschsprung's disease: unraveling an oligogenic disorder. Clin Genet 2005;67:6.

4. Ho GT, Nimmo ER, Tenesa A, et al. Allelic variations of the multidrug resistance gene determine susceptibility and disease behavior in ulcerative colitis. Gastroenterology 2005;128:288.

5. Ahmad T, Tamboli CP, Jewell D, et al. Clinical relevance of advances in genetics and pharmacogenetics of IBD. Gastroenterology 2004; 126:1533.

6. Al-Tassan N, Chmiel NH, Maynard J, et al. Inherited variants of MYH associated with somatic G:C→T:A mutations in colorectal tumors. Nat Genet 2002;30:227.

7. Sieber OM, Lipton L, Crabtree M, et al. Multiple colorectal adenomas, classic adenomatous polyposis, and germ-line mutations in MYH. N Engl J Med 2003;348:791.

8. Qaseem A, Aronson M, Fitterman N, et al. Screening for hereditary hemochromatosis: a clinical practice guideline from the American College of Physicians. Ann Intern Med 2005;143:517.

9. Bisgaard ML, Fenger K, Bulow S, et al. Familial adenomatous polyposis (FAP): frequency, penetrance, and mutation rate. Hum Mutat 1994;3:121.

10. Spirio L, Olschwang S, Groden J, et al. Alleles of the APC gene: an attenuated form of familial polyposis. Cell 1993;75:951.

11. Burt RW, Leppert MF, Slattery ML, et al. Genetic testing and phenotype in a large kindred with attenuated familial adenomatous polyposis. Gastroenterology 2004;127:444.

12. Nagase H, Miyoshi Y, Horii A, et al. Correlation between the location of germ-line mutations in the APC gene and the number of colorectal polyps in familial adenomatous polyposis patients. Cancer Res 1992;52:4055.

13. Armour JA, Barton DE, Cockburn DJ, et al. The detection of large deletions or duplications in genomic DNA. Hum Mutat 2002;20: 325.

14. Schouten JP, McElgunn CJ, Waaijer R, et al. Relative quantification of 40 nucleic acid sequences by multiplex ligation-dependent probe amplification. Nucleic Acids Res 2002;30:e57.

15. Church J, Simmang C. Practice parameters for the treatment of patients with dominantly inherited colorectal cancer (familial adenomatous polyposis and hereditary nonpolyposis colorectal cancer). Dis Colon Rectum 2003;46:1001.

16. Huntsman DG. Early gastric cancer in young, asymptomatic carriers of germ-line E-cadherin mutations. N Engl J Med 2001;344:1904.

17. Baron JA. Epidemiology of non-steroidal anti-inflammatory drugs and cancer. Prog Exp Tumor Res 2003;37:1.

18. Potter JD. Colorectal cancer: molecules and populations. J Natl Cancer Inst 1999;91:916.

19. Hall J, Hamerton J, Hoar D, et al. Policy statement concerning DNA banking and molecular genetic diagnosis. Canadian College of Medical Geneticists. Clin Invest Med 1991;14:363.

20. Emery J. Is informed choice in genetic testing a different breed of informed decision-making? A discussion paper. Health Expect 2001; 4:81.

21. Bernhardt BA, Biesecker BB, Mastromarino CL. Goals, benefits, and outcomes of genetic counseling: client and genetic counselor assessment. Am J Med Genet 2000;94:189.

22. Finnell RH. Teratology: general considerations and principles. J Allergy Clin Immunol 1999;103:S337.

23. Shepard T, Lemire R. Catalog of Teratogenic Agents. Johns Hopkins University Press, 2004.

24. Burt RW. Colon cancer screening. Gastroenterology 2000;119:837.

25. Newell GR, Vogel VG. Personal risk factors. What do they mean? Cancer 1988;62:1695.

26. Bennett RL, Steinhaus KA, Uhrich SB, et al. Recommendations for standardized human pedigree nomenclature. J Genet Couns 1995;4: 267.

27. Love RR, Evans AM, Josten DM. The accuracy of patient reports of a family history of cancer. J Chronic Dis 1985;38:289.

28. Aitken J, Bain C, Ward M, et al. How accurate is self-reported family history of colorectal cancer? Am J Epidemiol 1995;141:863.

29. Lerman C. Psychological aspects of genetic testing: Introduction to the special issue. Health Psychology 1997;16:3.

30. Meiser B, Gleeson MA, Tucker KM. Psychological impact of genetic testing for adult-onset disorders. An update for clinicians. Med J Aust 2000;172:126.

31. Offit K, Groeger E, Turner S, et al. The "duty to warn" a patient's family members about hereditary disease risks. JAMA 2004;292:1469.

32. Report of the Council on Ethical and Judicial Affairs of the American Medical Association. CEJA Report 2-A-02, 2005 (http://www.ama-assn.org/ama1/pub/upload/mm/369/ceja_1203j.pdf).

33. American Society of Clinical Oncology policy statement update: genetic testing for cancer susceptibility. J Clin Oncol 2003;21:2397.

34. American Society of Human Genetics Board of Directors, American College of Medical Genetics Board of Directors. Points to consider: ethical, legal, and psychosocial implications of genetic testing in children and adolescents. Am J Hum Genet 1995;57:1233.

35. American Society of Human Genetics Social Issues Committee report on genetics and adoption: points to consider. Am J Hum Genet 1991;48:1009.

36. The American Society of Human Genetics Social Issues Committee and The American College of Medical Genetics Social, Ethical, and Legal Issues Committee. Genetic testing in adoption. Am J Hum Genet 2000;66:761.

37. Nelson RM, Botkjin JR, Kodish ED, et al. Ethical issues with genetic testing in pediatrics. Pediatrics 2001;107:1451.

38. MacDonald DJ, Lessick M. Hereditary cancers in children and ethical and psychosocial implications. J Pediatr Nurs 2000;15:217.

39. Hirschman BA, Pollock BH, Tomlinson GE. The spectrum of APC mutations in children with hepatoblastoma from familial adenomatous polyposis kindreds. J Pediatr 2005;147:263.

40. Schwartz MK. Genetic testing and the clinical laboratory improvement amendments of 1988: present and future. Clin Chem 1999;45: 739.

41. Blum HE, Wieland S, von Weizsacker F. Gene therapy: basic concepts and applications in gastrointestinal diseases. Digestion 1997;58:87.

42. International Human Genome Sequencing Consortium. Finishing the euchromatic sequence of the human genome. Nature 2004;431:931.

43. Sachidanandam R, Weissman D, Schmidt SC, et al. A map of human genome sequence variation containing 1.42 million single nucleotide polymorphisms. Nature 2001;409:928.

44. Altshuler D, Brooks LD, Chakravarti A, et al. A haplotype map of the human genome. Nature 2005;437:1299.

45. The International HapMap Consortium. The International HapMap Project. Nature 2003;426:789.

46. Cleator S, Ashworth A. Molecular profiling of breast cancer: clinical implications. Br J Cancer 2004;90:1120.

Index

Note: page numbers in *italics* refer to figures, those in **bold** refer to tables.

Abbreviations: CNS, central nervous system; CT, computed tomography; GERD, gastroesophageal reflux disease; HBV, hepatitis B virus; HCV, hepatitis C virus; MRI, magnetic resonance imaging; NSAID, nonsteroidal antiinflammatory drug; SIRS, systemic inflammatory response syndrome.

abdominal aortic aneurysm 285
abdominal mass, appendicitis 277, 278
abdominal pain 228–51, 402
  acute recurrent 241
  age 276
  aggravating factors 239–40
  auscultation 274–5
  character 239
  children 276
  chronic
    functional abdominal pain syndrome 244, 246–7
    intractable 247
    pharmacological management 248–50
    treatment 247–51
  classification 238
  clinical assessment 238–44, *245*, 246–7
  confounding factors 275–6
  diagnostic workup 242–4
  differential diagnosis 241–2
  digital rectal examination 275
  gastrointestinal symptoms 273–4
  gender 275
  history taking 238–40, 274
  immunosuppression 276
  intensity 239
  laparotomy 276–7
  location 271–2
  neuroanatomy 271–3
  neuronal pathways 272
  neuropathic 238
  nociceptive 238
  palpation 275
  physical examination 240–1, 274–5
  pregnancy 275–6
  rare causes 242, **243**
  red flags 243–4
  relieving factors 239–40
  site *235*, 238
  temporal characteristics 239
  treatment 247–51
abdominal palpation 240, 275
abdominal wall, irritable bowel syndrome 261
abdominal wall pain 42
  chronic 244
  etiology **245**

abetalipoproteinemia, steatorrhea 324
abscess, pericolonic 282
absolute risk reduction (ARR) 10–11
acetaminophen (paracetamol)
  content of analgesics 497, **497–8**
  dosage 116
  hepatic injury 400
  hepatotoxicity causing acute liver failure 492, 493, 495–9
    management 505
  labeling 499
  mortality from toxicity 495–6
  overdose
    diagnosis 496–7
    intentional 497
    management 496–7
    nonintentional 496, 498–9
  over-the-counter products 497, **498**, 499
  packaging 499
acetaminophen–cysteine adduct serum assay 496
acetyl coenzyme A 562–3, 566, 567
  pyruvate metabolism 568
achalasia 64
  dysphagia association 69
  GERD differential diagnosis 89
acid regurgitation, GERD 83
acid-fast bacilli (AFB) culture 447–8
action potentials 232–3
acupressure 251
  nausea and vomiting of pregnancy 546
acupuncture 251
  gas and bloating management 266
acute abdomen
  abdominal aortic aneurysm 285
  abdominal causes **272**
  acute cholecystitis 282–3
  appendicitis 277–8
  approach to patient 271–85
  causes 277–85
  colonic diverticulitis 281–2
  confounding factors 275–6
  extraabdominal causes **272**
  gastrointestinal symptoms 273–4
  history taking 274
  mesenteric ischemia 283–4, *285*
  perforated gastric/duodenal ulcer 278–9
  physical examination 274–5
  small intestine obstruction 279–81
acute fatty liver of pregnancy 432, 548–9
  acute liver failure 501
  treatment 549
acute liver failure (ALF)
  acetaminophen hepatotoxicity 492, 493, 495–9
  ammonia serum level lowering 506
  approach to patient 492–511

cerebral edema 502
  management **505**, 506
clinical features **494**
clinical presentation 501–3
coagulopathy 502, 508
complications 501–3
definitions 492
demographics 492, 493
drug idiosyncratic reactions 492, 493, 500–1
etiology *494*, 495–501
global assessment models 503–4
glutamine hypothesis 502
hemodynamic monitoring 507–8
hepatic encephalopathy 502, **505**
hepatocyte death 502
hepatotropic viruses 499–500
hyperventilation 506
incidence 492, 493
indeterminate 501
infections 502, 507
infiltrative disorders 501
inotropes 507–8
liver transplantation 509–10
management 505–11
mental status alteration 502
multiorgan failure 502–3
neurological features 505–7
nutritional therapy 507
outcome *494*
pregnancy 501
prognosis 503–4
renal failure 507
seizures 506–7
treatable causes 492, **493**
viral hepatitis 499–500
acute renal failure, cirrhosis 457–8
acute tubular necrosis (ATN), acute liver failure 507
adaptive thermogenesis 564
adefovir, HBV therapy 519
adenosine deaminase (ADA) ascitic fluid activity 447–8
adherence-to-protocol analysis 9
adhesions, abdominal 243
  small intestine obstruction 281
adipose tissue, mobilization 563
adopted persons, genetic testing 640
adrenal insufficiency, steatorrhea 324
aerophagia 39–40, 261
  management 264
affective–cognitive circuit 231
age
  dyspepsia 46
  gastrointestinal bleeding 124
AIDS *see* HIV infection
Alagille syndrome 432
alanine aminotransferase (ALT) 405–6, 413
  hepatocellular injury 414–15
  intrahepatic cholestasis of pregnancy 547

albumin
  extracorporeal dialysis *459*, 460
  intravenous in spontaneous bacterial peritonitis 456–7
  liver function 436
  plus vasconstrictors in hepatorenal syndrome therapy 460, 461
  serum concentration 404, **412**
  serum–ascites albumin gradient **443**, 444–5, 446, 447
alcohol consumption
  adequate intake 558
  cancer risk 562
  diarrhea 329
  folate excretion 611
  GERD 90
  gastropathy 129
  hemorrhagic gastritis 155
  hepatic injury 400
  osteoporosis 616
  serum enzyme levels 406–7
alcoholic hepatitis 435
  hepatorenal syndrome prevention 461
  peripheral parenteral nutrition 600
alcoholic pancreatitis, common bile duct stenosis 401
alcoholism
  thiamin deficiency 609
  weight loss 188
aldehydes 570
alkaline phosphatase 406, **412**, 414
  hepatocellular carcinoma 414
  jaundice diagnosis 435, 436
allelic heterogeneity 629–30
allodynia 235
allopregnanolone 472
alosetron, diarrhea therapy 347
alternative therapies *see* complementary and alternative medicine
alvimopan 300
Alzheimer type II astrocyte 469
Alzheimer disease, weight loss 188
Amanita phalloides fungal toxin, acute liver failure 501
ambulatory pH monitoring, noncardiac chest pain 76–7
amebic colitis 370
amebic dysentery treatment 370
amino acids 564
  changes in mutations 631
  codons 631
  infant requirements 565
  metabolism 565
  response to illness/injury 582
  starvation 581
γ-aminobutyric acid (GABA)
  hepatic encephalopathy 471–2
  pain inhibition 233
γ-aminobutyric acid (GABA) receptor antagonists 474
aminopyrine breath test 404–5

aminosalicylates, use in pregnancy 541–2
aminotransferases 405–6
    drug-induced liver injury 500
    hepatitis differential diagnosis 415
    jaundice diagnosis 435
ammonia, interorgan trafficking 470
ammonia serum levels 410–11
    hepatic encephalopathy 469–70, 474
    lowering
        acute liver failure 506
        hepatic encephalopathy 474
amoxicillin, H. pylori treatment 107
amygdala 231
amylin 193
anal fissures, gastrointestinal bleeding 140
analgesics
    acetaminophen content 497, 497–8
    over-the-counter 497
    visceral 50
anaphylaxis, iron dextran administration 608
anemia
    iron deficiency 606
    occult gastrointestinal bleeding 159–61
    pernicious 612
angina, intestinal 42
angiodysplasia, gastrointestinal bleeding 136, 139
angiography
    gastrointestinal bleeding 138
        acute upper 125–6
    mesenteric ischemia 283, 284
    pulmonary for hepatopulmonary syndrome 480
anorectal disease, pseudodiarrhea 305
anorectal manometry, constipation 384–5
anorexia, abdominal pain association 274
anorexia nervosa, complications 387
anorexia–cachexia syndrome 185
antacids
    dyspepsia 49
    GERD 49, 91, 93
        pregnancy 535, 536
    hypophosphatemia 606
    peptic ulcer disease 106
antegrade continent enema 391
anthracene laxatives, melanosis coli 340
anthraquinones 388, 539
antibiotics
    ascites prophylaxis 454
    combinations for H. pylori eradication 113
    diarrhea treatment 318, 319, 367–80
    inflammatory bowel disease treatment during pregnancy 544
    spontaneous bacterial peritonitis treatment 456, 457
anticholinergic drugs, peptic ulcer disease 106
anticoagulants
    gastrointestinal bleeding 155
    vitamin K deficiency 617
antidepressants
    chronic abdominal pain treatment 248–9
    dyspepsia 51
    functional gastrointestinal disorders 24–5

nausea and vomiting management 217, 218–19
    noncardiac chest pain 75
    tolerance 249
antidiarrheal agents 345–7
    infectious diarrhea 367
    mechanism of action 345–7
    pregnancy 537, 538
antiemetics 216–19, 220–2
    hyperemesis gravidarum 546, 547
antiepileptic drugs 50
    chronic abdominal pain 250
antihistamines 216, 217
    hyperemesis gravidarum 546, 547
    nausea and vomiting of pregnancy 221
anti-human hemoglobin antibody test 173
anti-liver/kidney microsomal antibodies (anti-LKM1) 408
antimicrobial drugs
    drug combinations 111
    H. pylori resistance 113–15
    peptic ulcer disease 106–8, 111
    with PPIs for H. pylori 112–13, 114
    resistance 113–15
antimitochondrial antibodies 408
antinauseant drugs 51
antinuclear antibodies 408
antioxidants 570
antireflux surgery
    dysphagia 72
        esophageal 73
    GERD 94–5
    pregnancy 536
antisecretory therapeutic trials, noncardiac chest pain 76
anti-smooth muscle antibodies (SMA) 408
antispasmodic drugs, dyspepsia 50–1
anti-TNF antibodies, inflammatory bowel disease treatment during pregnancy 543–4
α_1-antitrypsin
    clearance 342
    deficiency 410
    serum levels 410
anxiety
    dyspepsia 52
    functional gastrointestinal disorders 31
        gastrointestinal-specific 31
    irritable bowel syndrome 24
    noncardiac chest pain 75
anxiolytics, functional gastrointestinal disorders 24
aortoenteric fistula, gastrointestinal bleeding 136
APC gene mutations 629–30, 634
appendicitis
    abdominal mass 277, 278
    acute abdomen 277–8
    diagnosis 277
    imaging 277–8
    misdiagnosis in children 315
    nausea and vomiting induction 210
    pregnancy 275, 276
aprepitant 217–18, 221
arachidonic acid 567
area postrema, emetic stimulus receptor 206
arginine 580
argon plasma coagulator 126, 127
    intestinal obstruction ablative therapy 299
Arias disease 427
arsenic 401

arterial blood gases, hepatopulmonary syndrome 478–9
arterial embolization, gastrointestinal bleeding 138
arteriovenous shunts, hepatopulmonary syndrome 476–7
ascites
    antibiotic prophylaxis 454
    approach to patient 442–61
    bacterial infections 446–7
    chylous 448
    cirrhotic 435, 445, 448–55
        with acute renal failure 457–8
        hepatic hydrothorax 455
        natural history 448–9
        pathogenesis 448–9
        refractory 454–5
        uncomplicated 452–4
    constrictive pericarditis 445
    cytological examination 447
    definition 442
    diagnostic paracentesis 444
    evaluation 444
    fluid appearance 444
    fluid leakage 450
    hepatic venous pressure gradient measurement 446
    imaging 443
    infection evaluation 446–7
    jaundice 435
    malignancy evaluation 447
    new-onset 444–8
    pancreatic 448
    peritoneal tuberculosis 447–8
    tense 452, 453
    total protein level 444, 445–6
    treatment 449–52
    tumor markers 447
    see also spontaneous bacterial peritonitis
ascorbic acid 575, 577
    deficiency 409, 614
aspartate 580
aspartate aminotransferase (AST) 405–6, 412, 413
    hepatocellular injury 414–15
aspiration, dysphagia 70
aspirin
    dosage 116
    dyspepsia 46
    gastrointestinal bleeding 129, 155–6
assumptions, sensitivity to 18
asthma, GERD 84
athletes, elite
    diarrhea 321
    gastrointestinal bleeding 156
ATOX1 protein 574
ATP7A protein 574
ATP7B gene mutation 409
atrophic gastritis 612
attapulgite, diarrhea treatment 367
autogenic training 26, 27
autoimmune disorders, nodular regenerative hyperplasia of liver 530
autoimmune enteropathy
    celiac disease misdiagnosis 323
    steatorrhea 322
autoimmune hepatitis
    diagnosis 415
    pregnancy 433
autonomic nervous system, nausea and vomiting response 207
autosomes 624
azathioprine, use in pregnancy 542, 543
azithromycin 368

baclofen, GERD 95
bacteria
    dietary fiber fermentation 570
    duodenal aspirate growth 338
bacterial colitis 364
bacterial flora
    abnormal 258
    gas production 255
    irritable bowel syndrome 259
    methanogenic in constipation 378
bacterial infections
    acute liver failure 502, 507
    ascites 446–7
    diarrhea 312–13, 314–15
    nausea and vomiting induction 208, 209
    see also spontaneous bacterial peritonitis
bacterial overgrowth 258
    bile acid levels 403
    breath testing 262–3
    cobalamin deficiency 612
    gas and bloating 261
    intestinal pseudoobstruction 289
    irritable bowel syndrome 259–60
    spontaneous bacterial peritonitis 456
    steatorrhea 324
    tests 338
bacterial toxins
    endotoxins in jaundice 429
    enterotoxin intestinal secretion 306
    ileus 289
    secretory diarrhea 310
bacterial translocation, ileus/intestinal obstruction 291
balloon dilation, intestinal obstruction 299
balloon expulsion test 385
balloon tamponade, esophageal varices hemorrhage management 131–2
balloon therapy for obesity 201
barbiturates, functional gastrointestinal disorders 24
bariatric surgery 199–201
barium esophagram, GERD 88–9
barium studies
    constipation 382, 383
    gas and bloating 262
    ileus 294–6, 297
    intestinal obstruction 294–6, 297
    malabsorption 333, 335
barium swallow
    esophageal dysphagia 71–2
    oropharyngeal dysphagia 69, 70
Barrett esophagus, GERD 84
baseline risk 17
bed nucleus of the striata terminalis (BNST) 21
behavior therapy, obesity 197–8
behavioral abnormalities, weight loss 188
behavioral techniques, functional gastrointestinal disorders 27–8
Behçet disease, diarrhea 331
belching 39–40
Bendectin 546
benfotiamine 610
bentiromide test 337
benzodiazepine(s)
    chronic abdominal pain 250
    functional gastrointestinal disorders 24
benzodiazepine partial inverse agonists 474

benzodiazepine receptor antagonists 474
bethanechol, GERD 91
bicarbonate ions 308
    secretion 306
bile acids
    definition 422
    diarrhea 326
    dihydroxy 309
    function 422
    jaundice diagnosis 436
    malabsorption
        syndromes 326
        testing 340–1
    secretion 422
    serum 403
    stool weight 305
    synthesis 422
bile duct obstruction 414
    extrahepatic 413
    jaundice 425
    steatorrhea 321–2
bile duct stenosis in alcoholic
        pancreatitis 401
biliary atresia, cholestasis 431–2
biliary cirrhosis, primary 402
    pregnancy 433
biliary colic 274
    gallstone impaction 282
biliary cystadenocarcinoma, biliary
        cystadenoma differential
        diagnosis 531
biliary cystadenoma 531
biliary pain 241
biliary tract disease 41
biliopancreatic diversion 199
bilirubin 412, 423–5
    albumin-bound 403
    biliary obstruction 413
    clearance 424–5
    conjugated 425
    conjugation 424
    deconjugation 425
    excretion 424–5
    formation 423–4
    measurement 425
    metabolism 423
    stereoisomers 423
    structure 423
    tests 402–3, 425, 436
    unconjugated 424
    urine 403, 425
    urine tests 436
    see also hyperbilirubinemia
δ-bilirubin 403
    measurement 425
bilirubin encephalopathy 424
bilirubin uridine diphosphate
        glucuronosyltransferase
        deficiencies 426–7
BILN-2061, HCV treatment
        523
biofeedback methods 26–7
    constipation 388, 390–1
BioLogic-DT 511
biopsy
    inflammatory diarrhea 342
    liver 411
        hepatitis 415–16
        HCV 520–1
        jaundice 437–8
    malabsorption 335, 336
    watery diarrhea 339–40
biopsychosocial factor assessment,
        functional gastrointestinal
        disorders 30
biopsychosocial models 26
biotin 575, 577
    deficiency 614–15
birth defect risk 637
bisacodyl 388, 539

bismuth salts
    gas and bloating 265
    peptic ulcer disease 107
bismuth subsalicylate, diarrhea
        treatment 317, 347, 367
    pregnancy 537
bleeding 122–42
    acute lower gastrointestinal
        137–41
        causes 138–41
        colonoscopy 137
        diagnosis 137–8
        history 137
        physical examination 137
        therapy 138–41
    acute upper gastrointestinal
        124–37
        angiography 125–6
        causes 126–37
        diagnosis 125–6
        endoscopy 125
        esophageal varices 130–4
        history 125
        physical examination 125
        prognostic indicators 124–5
        therapy 126–37
    alcohol consumption 129
    anal fissures 140
    angiodysplasia 136, 139
    angiography 138
    aortoenteric fistula 136
    blood loss etiology 154–6
    chemical tests 156–7
    clinical presentation 122–4
    colitis 140–1
    Dieulafoy disease 136–7
    diverticular bleeding 138–9
    double-balloon enteroscopy 142
    erosive duodenitis 135
    esophageal ulcers 135
    esophagitis 135
    factitious 137
    fecal blood testing 157
    gastric antral vascular ectasia 136
    gastric erosions 128–34
    gastric varices 135
    hematocrit 123
    heme-porphyrin assay 157–8
    hemobilia 136
    hemorrhoids 140
    hemosuccus pancreaticus 136
    hepatic adenoma 529
    immunochemical tests 157
    inflammatory bowel disease 140
    intraoperative enteroscopy 142
    intussusception 141
    location 123–4
    Mallory–Weiss tears 135
    management in acute liver failure
        508
    Meckel diverticulum 140, 141
    neoplasms 135, 139–40
    nonintestinal sources 137
    NSAIDs 125, 141
    obscure 141–2
    occult 152–64
        anemia 159–61
        assessment 156–61
        blood loss etiology 154–6
        blood loss manifestations 156
        blood loss quantification 152,
            153
        diagnosis 156–61
        hemoglobin metabolism 152–3
        iron metabolism/deficiency
            153–4
        treatment 163–4
    patient assessment 122–3
    patient evaluation 158–61
    peptic ulcer disease 125, 126–8
    perianal disease 140

physical findings 156
portal hypertension 141
postpolypectomy bleeding 140
predictors of recurrent hemorrhage
        124
radiolabeled erythrocyte technique
        158
radionuclide scans 137–8
rectal ulcer 141
rectal varices 141
resuscitation 123
severity 124
specimen collection/sampling 158
symptoms 156, 161
testing 156–61
thrombocytopenia–hemangioma
        syndrome 527
vital signs 123
wireless capsule endoscopy 141–2
blinded comparisons 3
blinding 8
    double 8–9
    unmasking 8
bloating
    clinical syndromes 256–7
    dysmotility syndromes 258
    fiber supplements 258
    see also gas and bloating
blood, ingestion 156
blood loss
    etiology 154–6
    fecal 152, 153
    fecal tests 157
    infectious causes 155
    inflammatory causes 154–5
    manifestations 156
    nausea and vomiting 213
    quantification 152, 153
    vascular causes 155
blood transfusion, gastrointestinal
        bleeding 123
blood urea nitrogen (BUN),
        gastrointestinal bleeding
        123–4
body composition 557
    protein–energy malnutrition 588
body mass, protein–energy
        malnutrition 588
body mass index (BMI) 191, 192, 557,
        558
    associated disease risk 591
    determination in obesity 196
    protein–energy malnutrition 588
body weight 183
bolus movement, fine perception 64
bone marrow
    hemosiderin levels 157
    transplantation causing jaundice
        429–30
borborygmi, intestinal obstruction
        289, 291
bosentan, portopulmonary
        hypertension treatment 485
botulinum toxin
    dysphagia treatment 72
    noncardiac chest pain 75
bowel habit, constipation 379
bowel rest 599
bowel sounds see borborygmi
brain, glucose utilization in hepatic
        encephalopathy 470–1
Brainerd diarrhea 319, 329
brain–gut axis 21, 22
brainstem tachykinin NK$_1$ pathways,
        emesis 207
bran 388
    constipation 387
Bravo pH capsule 88
breath testing
    carbon-13 labeled 215
    carbon-14 D-xylose 338

carbon-14 triolein 337
cholyl-^{14}C-glycine 338, 340
gas and bloating 262–3
breathing retraining 26, 27
Bristol Stool Form scale 381
bromocriptine 474
Budd–Chiari syndrome
    acute liver failure 501
    pregnancy 433
budesonide, use in pregnancy 542,
        543
bulking agents 388
    constipation 387
bupropion, weight loss 198, 199
"burning feet" syndrome 615

CA19-9, cholangiocarcinoma
        detection 526
CA-125, ascites 447
cachexia 184, 185
calciferol 616
calcitonin gene-related peptide
        (CGRP) 233, 236
calcitriol 616
calcium
    ionized serum 572
    toxicity 604
    transport of lumenal 572
calcium, dietary 572
    adequate intake 557–8
    deficiency 603–4, 615
    recommended daily amount
        572
    sources 572
calcium antacids, GERD in
        pregnancy 535
calcium docusate 387–8
calcium ion channels 232
calcium supplements 603, 604
caloric balance 594
calorie intake 557
    parenteral nutrition 597
calprotectin
    fecal tests 342
    immunoassay 157
Cameron erosions 163
Campylobacter
    antibiotic treatment 369
    infectious diarrhea 360–1, 365
cancer
    chemoprevention 560–2
    genetic counseling 637
    genetic testing 639
    hereditary syndromes 625, 627
    predisposition 637
    see also chemotherapy; malignancy;
        named conditions and tumors
Candida albicans, odynophagia 67
cannabinoids, nausea and vomiting
        management 217, 218
capsule endoscopy
    gastrointestinal bleeding 161
    inflammatory diarrhea 342
carbohydrate 568–9
    bacterial degradation 308
    complex in
        maldigestion/malabsorption
        257–8
    fecal tests 340
    intolerance in irritable bowel
        syndrome 259
    malabsorption 321
        diarrhea 325
        fecal pH 340
        tests 340
    maldigestion 257–8
        breath testing 262
    metabolism 563
    osmotic diarrhea 308
    rapid intestinal transit 325
    response to illness/injury 582–3

carbon monoxide, hepatopulmonary syndrome 478
carbon-13 labeled breathing tests 215
carbon-14 D-xylose breath test 338
carbon-14 triolein breath test 337
α-carboxyglutamic acid (Gla) 580, 617
carboxyhemoglobin, hepatopulmonary syndrome 478
carcinoembryonic antigen (CEA), cholangiocarcinoma detection 526
carcinogens, colonic mucosa exposure 571
carcinoid syndrome, diarrhea 327, 347
cardiac disease
  nausea and vomiting 209, 212
  weight loss 186
cardiopulmonary dysfunction, differential diagnosis in liver disease 483
cardiovascular disease, abnormal liver chemistry 401
Carnett test 241, 244
carnitine 580
Caroli disease 428–9
carotene 615
carrier testing 635
cascara sagrada 539
catastrophizing 31
catheter-related sepsis
  home parenteral nutrition 599
  total parenteral nutrition complication 597–8
cecostomy 391
celiac artery, occlusion 284
celiac disease
  aminotransferase levels 415
  antibody tests 323
  associated conditions 323, 332
  diagnosis 323
  fertility 540
  gaseous symptoms 261
  misdiagnosis 323
  pregnancy 540
  serological testing 262, 332
  subclinical 332
celiac neurolysis 250
celiac sprue 321
  diagnosis 331
  steatorrhea 323–4
cellulose 569
central nervous system (CNS)
  alterations in dyspepsia 45–6
  emesis activation 206
    nausea and vomiting induction 209, 210
  homeostatic afferent inputs 22, 23
  niacin deficiency signs 610–11
  vomiting coordination 206–7
central pain amplification 23–4
central stress response 21–2
cerebral blood flow, hepatic encephalopathy 470–1
cerebral edema in acute liver failure 502
  management 505, 506
cerebral folate deficiency syndrome 611
cerebrovascular accident, oropharyngeal dysphagia 65
ceruloplasmin 409, 415, 574
  copper supplementation 609
charcoal, activated 264–5
chemotherapy
  diarrhea 320–1
  nausea and vomiting 205, 207, 209, 211–12
    management 218, 221

chenodeoxycholic acid 403, 422
chest pain, GERD 84
children
  abdominal pain 276
  acute infectious diarrhea 311
  appendicitis misdiagnosis 315
  congenital gastrointestinal malformations 636
  day-care diarrhea 315
  dietary reference intakes 560–1
  fatty acid oxidation disorders 549
  genetic testing 639
    results 640
  growth failure 600
  infectious diarrhea treatment 347, 368
  intestinal intussusception 291
  jaundice 431–2
  Munchausen syndrome by proxy 328
  rickets 615
  see also infants; neonates
Child–Turcotte–Pugh (CTP) score 451
chloride channel activators 389
chloride ions 307, 308
  intestinal transport 305, 306
  secretion 306
cholangiocarcinoma 429, 526
cholecalciferol 578
  deficiency 615–17
cholecystectomy
  acute cholecystitis 283
  liver chemistry abnormalities 401
  pregnancy 550
cholecystitis
  acalculous 433
    parenteral nutrition 598
  acute 282–3
  imaging 549–50
  nausea and vomiting induction 210
  pregnancy 549–50
cholecystoduodenal fistulae, intestinal obstruction 293
cholecystokinin
  age-related levels 188
  food intake 192
  functions 425
choledochal cystic disorders 428–9
choledocholithiasis, pregnancy 433
cholelithiasis see gallstones
cholescintigraphy 283
cholestasis
  anatomical causes 431–2
  benign recurrent intrahepatic 428
  biliary atresia 431–2
  chronic 430
    infants 431
  complications 438–9
  definition 422
  drug-induced 414
  enzyme markers 406–7
  extrahepatic 413–14, 428
  familial 427–8
  hepatocellular diseases 429
  infiltrative disorders 429
  intrahepatic 413, 414, 428
    of pregnancy 432, 547–8
  liver transplantation 433–4
  sepsis-associated 429
  tests 412
  total parenteral nutrition 430
  urine tests 436
cholesterol, liver disease 404
cholestyramine, intrahepatic cholestasis of pregnancy 547
cholic acid 403, 422
choline 580
cholinesterase inhibitors see neostigmine

cholyl-14C-glycine breath test 338, 340
chromium 574
chromosomal disorders 624–5
Churg–Strauss syndrome, diarrhea 331
chylous ascites 448
chymotrypsin 337
cimetidine
  GERD 91
  GERD in pregnancy 536
  peptic ulcer disease 104
cingulate cortex 231
ciprofloxacin, use in pregnancy 544
cirrhosis
  acute renal failure 457–8
  alcoholic 600
  ammonia serum levels 411
  ascites 445, 448–55
    with jaundice 435
    refractory 454–5
    uncomplicated 452–4
  hepatic hydrothorax 455
  hypoxemia 476
  obesity 194
  spontaneous bacterial peritonitis 456
  steatorrhea 321–2
cisapride
  dyspepsia 50
  dysphagia 73
  GERD 91
cisplatinum, nausea and vomiting induction 211
citric acid cycle 563, 569
clarithromycin, H. pylori treatment 107
Clichy criteria for acute liver failure 503, 504
clinical decision making 1–12
clinical effectiveness 16
clinical trials 19
  see also randomized controlled trial (RCT)
clonidine 50
  ascites therapy 452
  diabetic diarrhea 329
  diarrhea treatment 347
Clostridium difficile
  antibiotic treatment 370
  diarrhea 314–15, 331, 363
    enteral feeding 320
    treatment 318, 347, 370
  infectious diarrhea 365
  testing 366
  tissue culture cytotoxicity assay 366
  toxic megacolon 364
clotting factors
  acute liver failure 502
  liver chemistry abnormalities 403–4
CNS activators, peripheral neural activation 206
coagulation, impaired in liver disease 403–4
coagulopathy, acute liver failure 502, 508
cobalamin 575, 577
  absorption 577
  deficiency 612–14
    causing intestinal pseudoobstruction 289
    recommended daily allowance 577
  Schilling test 338
  supplementation 614
codons 630
coffee, dyspepsia 46
"coffee bean sign" 294

cognitive techniques/cognitive–behavioral therapy 28
  dyspepsia 52
  evidence base 29
  functional gastrointestinal disorders 28, 29
  integrated pharmacological approach 29–30
  noncardiac chest pain 75
cointerventions 9
colchicine 389
colectomy, subtotal 391–2
colitis
  amebic 370
  bacterial 364
  collagenous 330
  infectious 140
  ischemic 140
  lymphocytic 330
  NSAIDs 331
  radiation-induced 141
colon
  antegrade irrigation 391
  dysmotility 377
  flora in irritable bowel syndrome 259
  obstruction 291
  pseudoobstruction 299
  resection and diverticular bleeding 139
colon cancer
  dyspepsia 42
  see also colorectal cancer
colonic diverticulitis 281–2
colonic manometry, constipation 386
colonic neuropathy 377
colonic transit
  capsule study 384
  radiopaque marker studies 382, 383, 384
  scintigraphy 382, 383, 384
  time and dietary fiber intake 570–1
colonocytes, sodium ion transport 308
colonoscopy
  colorectal cancer screening 171, 177–8
  complications 178
  constipation 382, 383
  diverticular bleeding 138–9
  female patients 544
  gastrointestinal bleeding 137
  pregnancy 545
  sensitivity 177
  sigmoid volvulus 297–8
  virtual 296
  watery diarrhea 339–40
colorectal cancer
  dietary prevention 560–2, 570–1
  fecal DNA tests 178–9
  iron deficiency 155
  obesity 195
  oncogenesis 171
  predisposition 625
  pregnancy 544
  screening 158, 170
    colonoscopy 177–8
    complications 174
    doctor's office 175–6
    duty of care 180
    effectiveness 172–8
    endoscopic 176–8
    fecal blood 161–3
    fecal occult blood test 171, 172–3, 174–6, 178
    female patients 544
    goals 170
    guidelines 163
    home-based 175–6
    imaging 179
    incidence impact 175

mortality impact 174–5
one-step testing 171
participation 179–80
process *171*
recent developments 178–9
risk management 180
specificity 161–2
tests 171–2
two-step testing 171
test
compliance 162
validity 161–2
colorectal polyps
bleeding 161
obesity 195
common variable immunodeficiency
syndrome, bacterial
overgrowth 258
complementary and alternative
medicine
dyspepsia 51
ginger 221, 222, 546
medications
causing acute liver failure 500
causing hepatic injury 400
complementary DNA (cDNA) 633
compound heterozygosity 630
computed tomography (CT)
abdominal pain 275
abdominal wall in irritable bowel
syndrome 261
appendicitis 277–8
ascites 443
cholecystitis 549
cholelithiasis 549
colonography for colorectal cancer
screening 179
diverticulitis 282
enterography 214
gas and bloating 262
hepatic adenoma 530
hepatic hemangioma 528
high-resolution chest for
hepatopulmonary syndrome
480
ileus 294, *295*, 296, 297, 299
intestinal obstruction 294, *295*, 296,
297, 299
jaundice 436
liver cell dysplasia 531–2
malabsorption 333
mesenteric ischemia 283, 284
multidetector scanning 179
nausea and vomiting investigation
214
nodular regenerative hyperplasia
of liver 531
peptic ulcer disease 102
small intestine obstruction 281
concealed random allocation 8
confidence intervals 11
congenital malformations,
gastrointestinal 636
congestive heart failure 186
conscious sedation for endoscopy
545
constipation 373–93
abdominal pain association 274
anorectal manometry 384–5
approach to patient 373–93
balloon expulsion test 385
behavioral modification 538–9
biofeedback methods **388**, 390–1
chronic 379–82, **383**, 384–6
treatment 386–92
clinical evaluation 379–82, **383**,
384–6
colonic manometry 386
complications 392–3
defecography 385–6
definition 375

diagnostic tests 382, **383**, 384–6
diet 379–80, 387, **388**, 539
dietary fiber intake 571
digital rectal examination 381
drug-induced 387
economic impact 373–5
epidemiology 373–5
etiology 375–6
familial tendency 373
hormone disturbances 377–8
imaging 382, **383**, 386
lifestyle changes 386–7
medical history 379–81
neurotransmitter disturbances
377–8
objective measures 381
pharmacological treatments
387–90
physical examination 381
populations at higher risk 373
pregnancy 537–9
primary 376
psychological distress 375
quality of life 375
rectal barostat test 385
Rome III criteria **375**
sacral nerve stimulation 392
secondary 376
sexual abuse 375
slow-transit 376–8, 381
social impact 373–5
subtypes 375–6, 381
treatment 374, 386–92
Constipation Assessment Scale
381
continuous venovenous
hemofiltration (CVVH), acute
liver failure 507
contrast agents
hepatic adenoma 530
ileus 294–6, *297*
intestinal obstruction 294–6, *297*
nausea and vomiting
investigations 214
contrast enema, diverticulitis 281–2
convergence–facilitation theory of
referred pain 233, *235*
copper
absorption 574
deficiency 609
dietary 574
storage parameters in liver disease
409
supplementation 609
transport 574
urinary excretion 409
copper sulfate 609
Cori cycle 569
cortical inputs, central stress
response 21
corticosteroids
hyperemesis gravidarum 547
inflammatory bowel disease
treatment during pregnancy
542–3
nausea and vomiting of pregnancy
221
corticotropin-releasing factor (CRF)
21, 237
synthesis/secretion in pathological
stress 22
corticotropin-releasing factor (CRF)
subtype 1 receptor antagonists
21–2
cost(s) 15
baseline risk in treatment
population 17
direct 15, 16
economic analysis 19
health-care 19
incremental 17–18

indirect 15, 16
measurement 16
outcome data integration 16
of treatment 12
treatment benefits 18
cost–benefit analysis 15
cost–consequence analysis 15
cost-effectiveness analysis 14, 18
outcomes 18
cost-minimization analysis 14
cost-utility analysis 14–15, 17–18
dyspepsia 46
gastrointestinal bleeding 155–6
NSAID gastropathy 129
ulcer treatment 115–16
cricopharyngeal bars 70
cricopharyngeal myotomy,
dysphagia treatment 72
Crigler–Najjar syndrome 427
Crohn's disease
blood loss 155
cobalamin deficiency 612
diarrhea 329–30
differential diagnosis 315
fish oil supplementation 599
inflammatory bowel disease
599
intestinal obstruction 288, 292
pregnancy 540–4
^{51}Cr-albumin clearance 342
Cronkhite–Canada syndrome,
diarrhea 331
cryoprecipitate, acute liver failure
508
Cryptosporidium, infectious diarrhea
361, 366
Cushing reflex, acute liver failure
507
Cushing syndrome, obesity 194
cutaneous abdominal nerve 244,
245
cyanosis, hepatopulmonary
syndrome 478, 480
cyclic vomiting syndrome **209**, 212
management 222
cyclizine 51
cyclooxygenase 2 (COX-2) inhibitors
42
cyclooxygenase 2 (COX-2)-specific
NSAIDs 42
Cyclospora, infectious diarrhea 366
cyclosporine (ciclosporin) **542**, 543
CYP2C19 pathway 108, **109**, 110
CYP3A4 pathway **109**, 110
cystathionine synthase 611
cystic fibrosis
bile duct stenosis 401
chronic diarrhea 322
genetic counseling 636
cytochrome P450
drug interactions with antiulcer
drugs 108, **109**, 110
pathway induction by
acetaminophen 400, 495
cytokines
response to illness/injury 582
unintentional weight loss 184–5,
187, 188
cytomegalovirus (CMV)
acute liver failure 500
odynophagia 67

Dacron graft surgery, aortoenteric
fistula 136
daily reference value (DRV) 558–9
dairy products 615
decision analysis 14
defecography 385–6
deletions, large 632, 633
dementia, weight loss 188
dental erosion, GERD 84–5

deoxycholic acid 422
depression
dyspepsia 45
functional gastrointestinal
disorders 31
noncardiac chest pain 75
weight loss 188
dermatitis herpetiformis, steatorrhea
324
descending pain-inhibiting system
231
developed/developing countries,
acute infectious diarrhea 311
dexamethasone
chemotherapy-induced nausea
and vomiting 221
intestinal obstruction 300
intrahepatic cholestasis of
pregnancy 548
diabetes mellitus
dyspepsia 42
nerve root disease 242
obesity 195, *196*
weight loss 186
diabetic diarrhea 258, 329
diabetic neuropathy 238
diagnosis, prevalence 3
diagnostic tests
abnormal results 4
clinical research application to
patient 6–7
critical appraisal of article 2–7
necessity 2–3
negative study results 4
patient population 4
reproducible accuracy 7
sensitivity 4–5
specificity 4–5
study design 3–4
diaphragm disease 331
diaphragmatic breathing retraining
26, 27
diarrhea 304–47
abdominal pain association 274
acute infectious 311–19
definition 311
diagnosis 315, *316*, 317
epidemiology 311–15
high-risk groups 314–15
mortality 311
sporadic 312, **313**, **314**
transmission 312
treatment 317–18
alcoholic 329
antibiotic-associated 314–15
autoimmune inflammatory
310–11
bile acid 326
bloody 364–5
Brainerd 319, 329
cancer therapy 320–1
carbohydrate malabsorption
325
categories 306
chronic 321–45
classification 321
clinical evaluation 331–3, *334*,
335–45
definition 321
epidemic 319
epidemiology 321
idiopathic 319, 328–9
steatorrhea 321–5
congenital 329
day-care 315
definition 304, 360
diabetic 258, 329
electrolyte transport abnormalities
305–6
elixir 320
elusive 342–5

diarrhea (*cont'd*)
  endocrine tumors 327–8
  enteral feeding 320
    side effect 595
  epidemic chronic 319
  epidemiology 304, 360, 362
  evaluation 342–5
  factitious 328, 340
  fecal impaction 319–20
  fecal–oral transmission 312, 315
  fluid transport abnormalities 305–6
  foodborne 312–14
    transmission 361
  fructose 325
  hypokalemia 602
  ileostomy 326
  infectious 360–70
    acute 311–19
    approach to patient 360–70
    clinical features 361–4
    complications 363–4
    cost issues 366–7
    diagnostic evaluation 364–7
    epidemiology 360, 362
    etiology 360–1
    foodborne transmission 361
    history 364–5
    laboratory diagnosis 315, *316*, 317
    microbiology 360–1
    nosocomial 320
    ova tests 365–6
    parasite tests 365–6
    persistent 363
    person-to-person transmission 361
    physical examination 364–5
    prolonged 318–19
    stool culture 365
    transmission 361
    treatment 367–70
    waterborne transmission 361
  inflammatory 306, 309–11, 329–31
    autoimmune 310–11
    classification **311**
    history 341–2
    physical examination 341–2
    radiography 342
    screening tests 342, 365
    treatment 347
  irritable bowel syndrome 326–7
    induction 319
  magnesium-induced 325
  malabsorption 306, 308, **309**, 321–5
  malnutrition 317, 319
  medication-induced 320
  motility 305
  motor function abnormality 305
  neonatal 329
  niacin deficiency 610
  nosocomial 319–21, 363, 366–7
  oral rehydration therapy 594
  oral replacement solutions 317
  osmotic 308, **309**
  pathophysiology 305–11
  persistent 363
  postinfectious 319
  postvagotomy 326
  pregnancy 537, **538**
  recurrent 317
  runner's 321
  secretory 309, 327–9
    classification **310**
    treatment 347
  severe 342–5
  sexually transmitted 315
  sodium anion 325
  sodium loss 601
  sorbitol-induced 320, 325
  toddler's 325

transmission 312, 315, 361
traveler's 315, 361–3
  persistent 319
  treatment 368
treatment 345–7, 367–70
  acute infectious 317–18
  oral rehydration therapy 317, 594
tropical sprue 319
waterborne 312–14
waterborne transmission 361
watery 306, 325–7
  carbohydrate malabsorption 325
  functional 326–7
  history 338–9
  imaging 339–40
  nonabsorbable solute ingestion 325
  physical examination 338–9
  prior surgery 326
  radiography 339
  screening tests 339
  stool tests 340
  weight-reducing agents 320
diarrhea spiral 305
diazepam, contraindications in pregnancy 545
diazo method of bilirubin measurement 425
diet
  constipation 379–80, 387, **388**, 539
  diarrhea 330
  gas and bloating 261
    management 263–4
  GERD 90
  gastrointestinal cancer chemoprevention 560–2
  guidelines 557, 558–9
  healthy people 557–62
  low-carbohydrate 196–7
  meal replacements 197
  nausea and vomiting 216
  obesity 196–7
  stool consistency 305
  whole-food 592
dietary reference intakes (DRIs) 559, **560–1**
  life stage groups 565, **566**
Dieulafoy disease, gastrointestinal bleeding 136–7
diffusion impairment, hepatopulmonary syndrome 476–7
digestion rate, fiber influence 570
digital rectal examination
  abdominal pain 275
  constipation 381
  fecal impaction 392
1,25-dihydroxyvitamin D 578, 579, 603, 616
dimenhydrinate 51
diphenoxylate atropine, diarrhea treatment 367
  pregnancy 537
diphenylmethanes 539
direct costs 15
disaccharidase deficiency 325, 340
discounting 16
disseminated intravascular coagulation (DIC), hepatic hemangioma 527
diuretics
  ascites treatment 449, 453
  complications of therapy 449
  hepatic hydrothorax 455
  potassium-sparing 605
diverticular bleeding 138–9
diverticulitis 281–2
  CT-guided drainage 282
DNA microarray 642

DNA microchips 642
DNA polymerase 630
DNA replication 630
DNA sequencing 633
DNA structure 630
docosahexaenoic acid (DHA) 568
domperidone
  dyspepsia 50
  gastroparesis management 220
  nausea and vomiting management **218**, 219–20
L-dopa 474
dopamine
  acute liver failure 507
  hepatic encephalopathy 472
dopamine antagonists, nausea and vomiting management 216, **217**
dopamine receptor agonists
  GERD 91
  hepatic encephalopathy 474
dorsal column 230
dorsal motor nucleus of the vagus (DMNV) 206–7
dorsal root ganglion 228
double-balloon enteroscopy 142
doxylamine, hyperemesis gravidarum **546**, 547
drainage, CT-guided 282
droperidol, hyperemesis gravidarum **546**, 547
drug abuse, illicit, hepatic injury 400
drug-induced liver injury (DILI) 500–1
dry film method of bilirubin measurement 425
Dubin–Johnson syndrome 427
  pregnancy 433
  sulfobromophthalein test 403
duodenal aspirates, bacterial growth 338
duodenal bulb
  atypical ulcers 103
  deformity 102
duodenal eosinophilia 38
duodenal ulcer 99
  atypical 103
  complicated 102–3
  GERD 100–1
  H. pylori 100–1
  perforated 278–9
  recurrence 38
duodenitis
  dyspepsia 45
  erosive 135
duodenogastric reflux, dyspepsia 44
duodenum, sensory threshold 44
duplications, genetic 632, 633
dysentery 364–5
dysfibrinogen, hepatoma-associated 404
dyslipidemia, obesity 195, *196*
dyspepsia 38–54
  abdominal ultrasonography 47
  acid 99–100
  acid inhibitions 49
  age 46
  alarm features 46
  anxiety 52
  causes 41–2
  clinical practice 41
  clinical presentation 38–41
  CNS alterations 45–6
  cytoprotection 49–50
  depression 45
  diagnosis 46–7
  disturbed sensory function 44
  drug-induced 42
  duodenitis 45
  duodenogastric reflux 44
  endoscopy 47, 48

  food intolerance 46
  functional 38, 41, 54
    pathogenesis 42–6
    postprandial distress subtype 210
  gastric acid 44–5
  GERD differential diagnosis 89
  gastrointestinal bleeding 125
  gastroparesis 210
  genetics 46
  health-care seeking behavior 41
  H. pylori 47
  incidence 41
  intractable 52
  malignancy 41, 42, 47–8
  management 47–52, **53**
  nausea and vomiting induction 210
  new-onset 52
  nonulcer 38
  NSAIDs 46, 47
  patients failing to respond 51–2
  placebo response 48–9
  postinfectious 45
  postprandial distress subtype 210
  prevalence 41
  prognosis 54
  psychiatric disorders 42
  psychological distress 41
  psychological treatments 52
  psychosocial factors 45–6
  quality of life 38
  recurrent/relapsing 52
  reflux-like 39
  stress 45–6
  subgroups 39
  symptoms
    pattern 46
    severity *43*
  therapeutic approach 48–52, *53*
  uninvestigated 47–8, 52
  see also peptic ulcer disease
dysphagia 62–6, 67–73
  approach to patient 63–6
  aspiration 70
  esophageal 63, 65–6, 68–9
    approach to patient 71–2
  GERD 83–4
  medical history 67–9
  mucosal damage 64
  oropharyngeal 63, 64–5, 67, 68
    approach to patient 69–71
    evaluation 69–70
  physical examination 67–9
  symptoms 62–3
    mechanisms 64
  treatment 72–3
dyspnea, liver disease 483
dyssebacea 610
dyssynergic defecation 378, *379*, 381
  anorectal manometry 385
  biofeedback methods **388**, 390–1
  criteria **375**
  treatment 390–1

ear, nose and throat diseases, GERD 84–5, 94
early life events, adverse 22
eating disorders 42
economic analysis 14–19
  components **15**
  costs 19
    measurement 16
  forms 14–15
  outcomes measurement 16
  parameter estimates 17
  patient care 18–19
  results 17–18
  strategy comparison 15–16
  uncertainties 16–17

economic studies, evidence-based approach 15–19
effectiveness 16
efficacy 16
eicosanoids 567
eicosapentaenoic acid (EPA) 568
Elderly Bowel Symptom Questionnaire 381
elderly patients
  GERD treatment 93
  intestinal obstruction 292
  jaundice 431
  malignancy 431
  small intestine obstruction 281
  unintentional weight loss 183–4, 187–8
electrocardiogram (ECG), hypocalcemia 603, 604
electrocoagulation
  angiodysplasia 139
  multipolar 126, 127
electroencephalogram (EEG), hepatic encephalopathy 468
electrogastrography (EGG) 43, 215
electrolytes
  gastrointestinal tract 306, 307, 308
  stool measurement 343–5
  transport
    diarrhea-related abnormalities 305–6
    intestinal secretion 306
electromyography (EMG), feedback 27
emesis
  abdominal pain association 274
  anticipatory 221
  brainstem tachykinin NK_1 pathways 207
  chemotherapy-induced 205, 207, **209**, 211–12
emetic response activation 206
emotional memory 231
emotional motor system 21, 22
  outputs to gastrointestinal tract 23
encephalopathy
  bilirubin 424
  hyperammonemia 411
  post-TIPS portosystemic 451, 455
endocrine disorders, weight loss 186–7
endocrine system
  food intake 192–4
  nausea and vomiting response 207
endocrine tumors, diarrhea 327–8
endoscopic retrograde cholangiopancreatography (ERCP)
  biliary cystadenoma 531
  jaundice 437
  pregnancy 545
endoscopic therapy
  angiodysplasia 139
  esophageal varices hemorrhage management 131
  gastroparesis management 220
  ileus 299–300
  intestinal obstruction 299–300
  stress gastric erosions 129
endoscopic ultrasound, jaundice 437
endoscopy
  colorectal cancer screening 176–8
  conscious sedation 545
  constipation 382, **383**
  dyspepsia 47, 48, 54
  esophageal dysphagia 71
  gas and bloating 262
  GERD 85–6
    treatments 95
  gastrointestinal bleeding 122, 159–61
  ileus 297–8

infectious diarrhea 366
inflammatory diarrhea 342
intestinal obstruction 297–8
malabsorption 335
noncardiac chest pain 76
odynophagia 74
peptic ulcer disease 102
pregnancy 544–5
upper gastrointestinal 47
videocapsule 335
wireless capsule 141–2
endothelin receptor antagonists 485
energy
  homeostasis 191–2
  intake 192–4
  production 563
  requirement 557
    calculation **559**
  storage 191–2
  units 563
energy expenditure 192–4
  components 563–4
  physical activity 564
  starvation 581
energy metabolism 562–4
  response to illness/injury 582
enkephalinase inhibitors 346, 347
Entamoeba dispar 366
Entamoeba histolytica 366
entecavir, HBV therapy 519
enteral feeding/nutrition
  acute liver failure 507
  alcoholic cirrhosis 600
  diarrhea 320
  formulas 593–4
  gastroparesis 221
  growth failure in children 600
  inflammatory bowel disease 599
  intermittent 600
  pancreatitis 600
  tube 594–4
    complications 595–6
enteritis
  milk-induced 154
  radiation 163
enteroclysis
  gas and bloating 262
  nausea and vomiting investigations 214
enterocolitis
  neutropenic 331
  nongranulomatous chronic idiopathic 322
enterocytes
  brush border carbohydrate hydrolases congenital absence 325
  inflammatory diarrhea 309
enterohepatic circulation 422
enteroscopy 141, 142
enzyme preparations, gas and bloating management 264–5
enzyme-linked immunosorbent assay (ELISA), HCV diagnosis 520
eosinophil(s), esophagitis 86
eosinophilic enterocolitis, pericrypt 330
eosinophilic gastroenteritis
  diarrhea 330
  protein-losing enteropathy 330
  steatorrhea 322, 330
epidural access systems 250
epigastric hernia, pain 242
epigastric pain syndrome 39
epoprostenol, portopulmonary hypertension treatment 485
Epstein–Barr virus (EBV), acute liver failure 500
ergocalciferol 578

erythrocyte(s), radiolabeled 158
erythrocyte aspartate aminotransferase (E-AST) index 611
erythromycin
  gastroparesis management 220
  ileus 300
  nausea and vomiting management **218**, 219
erythropoiesis, ineffective 426
Escherichia coli
  antibiotic treatment 370
  enterohemorrhagic 364
  enteropathogenic 318, 319
  hemorrhagic 320
  infectious diarrhea 360–1, 365
  Shiga toxin-producing 370
esomeprazole, GERD 92
esophageal acid exposure time 42
esophageal adenocarcinoma 41, 66
esophageal body, motility alterations 64
esophageal cancer, GERD 84
esophageal dilation, esophageal dysphagia 73
esophageal manometry 72
  GERD 89
esophageal motility testing, noncardiac chest pain 75, 77
esophageal pH monitoring
  clinical indications 87–8
  GERD 86–8
esophageal rings, distal 65–6
esophageal sensation 64
esophageal sphincter, lower
  pressure/relaxation assessment 89
  pressure/relaxation management 95
esophageal strictures, GERD 65
esophageal ulcers, gastrointestinal bleeding 135
esophageal varices 130–4
  hemorrhage
    management 130–3
    prevention of recurrent 133–4
    prophylaxis 134–5
  rupture 130
  size 130
esophageal webs
  barium esophagram 89
  iron deficiency 156
esophagitis 38
  erosive 90
  GERD 85–6
  gastrointestinal bleeding 135
  grading systems 86, **87**
esophagus
  biopsy 86
  dysmotility 66, 67
  high-amplitude peristaltic contractions 66, 67
  hyper-/hypomotility 64, 66, 67
  nutcracker 66, 67
  secondary hypomotility 64
  spastic disorders 66, 67
  transit disruptions 66, 67
estimated average requirement (EAR) 559
evacuation disorders 376
  pathophysiology 378–9
  treatment 390–2
evidence-based medicine 1–2
  clinical research application to patient 6–7, 12
  critical appraisal of article about a diagnostic test 2–7
  economic studies 15–19
exercise, constipation 386–7
extracorporeal albumin dialysis (ECAD), hepatorenal syndrome therapy 459, 460

factitious diarrhea 328, 340
factor V, acute liver failure 508
factor VIIa, recombinant (rFVIIa)
  acute liver failure 508
  contraindications 508
  esophageal varices hemorrhage management 131
familial adenomatous polyposis (FAP) 629
  attenuated 629–30
  genetic diagnosis 635
  genetic testing 634
    children 639
familial microvillus atrophy 329
familial neonatal hyperbilirubinemia, transient 431
famotidine
  GERD 91
  peptic ulcer disease 104
fat
  dietary 196
  energy storage 191
  fecal excretion 337
  fecal testing 335–7
  malabsorption 321–5
  metabolism 563
  starvation effects 581
  storage 568
fatigue, iron deficiency 154, 156
fatty acid(s)
  biosynthesis 567
  essential 567
  oxidation in starvation 581
fatty acid oxidation disorders
  children 549
  pregnancy 548–9
fecal blood loss 152, *153*, 162–3
  screening 163
fecal blood testing 157, 158
  colorectal cancer 161–3
  compliance 162
  effectiveness 162–3
  occult 159
    colorectal cancer screening 171, 172–3, 174–6, 178
    doctor's office 175–6
    effectiveness 172–6
    home-based 175–6
    participation 179–80
  occult bleeding patterns 161
  validity 161–2
fecal DNA tests 178–9
fecal fat tests
  qualitative 335–6
  quantitative 336–7
fecal immunochemical tests for hemoglobin (FIT) 173
fecal impaction
  diagnosis 392
  diarrhea 319–20
  management 392
  manual disimpaction 392
fecal pH 340
fenfluramine 198
fentanyl, contraindications in pregnancy 545
ferritin 154
  serum levels 156–7, 158–9, 409–10, **412**
    iron deficiency 606–7
ferrous sulfate supplementation 163
fertility
  celiac disease 540
  inflammatory bowel disease 540–1
α-fetoprotein radioimmunoassay 410
fetus, congenital gastrointestinal malformations 636
fever
  infectious diarrhea 364–5
  thiamin deficiency 609

fiber, dietary 569–71
  cancer chemoprevention 562, 570–1
  constipation 387, 539
  fermentation 570
  maldigestion/malabsorption 258
  physiological effects 570
finger clubbing, hepatopulmonary syndrome 478, 480
fish oils 568
  supplementation 599
flatulence 256–7
flatus 255
  analysis 263
  fiber intake 258
flavin adenine dinucleotide, reduced (FADH₂) 569
flavin adenine dinucleotide (FAD) 575, 576
flavin mononucleotide (FMN) 575, 576
flavonoids 570
flow cytometry, ascites 447
fluid intake, constipation 386–7
fluid transport
  diarrhea-related abnormalities 305–6
  intestinal secretion 306
fluid volume, gastrointestinal tract 306–7
flumazenil, hepatic encephalopathy 474
fluoride 575
fluoroquinolones, H. pylori treatment 107
fluphenazine, chronic abdominal pain 250
focal fatty change in liver 531
focal nodular hyperplasia of liver 528–9
  hepatic adenoma differential diagnosis 529–30
folate 575, 576–7
  cancer chemoprevention 562
  deficiency 611–12
  metabolism 576–7
  recommended daily allowance 576
  sources 576
food allergy
  bloating in IBS 261
  diarrhea 330
  irritable bowel syndrome 263–4
food intake, endocrine system 192–4
food intolerance, dyspepsia 46
food poisoning 312–14, 361
foreign bodies, intestinal obstruction 293
founder mutations 635–6
free copper 409
free hepatic vein pressure (FHVP) 446
fresh frozen plasma (FFP), acute liver failure 508
fructooligosaccharides 569
fructose
  diarrhea 325
  exclusion 263
  intolerance 257
fruit intake, cancer chemoprevention 561–2
functional abdominal pain syndrome 244, 246–7
  biopsychosocial etiopathogenesis 246
  etiopathogenesis 246
  management 247
  physical examination 246
functional bowel disorders, gas and bloating 258–61

functional gastrointestinal disorders
  abnormal emotional motor system responses 24
  antidepressant therapy 24–5
  anxiety 31
  assessment batteries 32
  behavioral techniques 27–8
  beliefs about nature/cause 33
  biopsychosocial factor assessment 30
  centrally targeted therapies 24–6
  clinical interview 30–1
  cognitive techniques 28
  comorbidity 34
  depression 31
  integrated pharmacological and cognitive–behavior therapy approach 29–30
  management algorithm 32–4
  neurobiological model 21–4
  psychodynamic–interpersonal treatment 28–9
  psychological treatments 26–30
  psychological/psychiatric aspects of patients 30–2
  psychological/psychiatric comorbidity 33
  psychosocial assessment 34
  psychosocial factors in patient care 20–34
  quality of life 32
  respondent techniques 26–7
  screening 34
    questionnaires 31–2
  sexual abuse history 32, 46
  somatization 34
  symptom chronicity/severity 33
  trauma history 32
fundic relaxation
  dyspepsia 50
  impaired 43–4
fungal infections, acute liver failure 502
fungal toxins, acute liver failure 501
furazolidone, H. pylori treatment 107, 113
furosemide, ascites treatment 449

G proteins
  constipation 377–8
  polymorphism in dyspepsia 46
gabapentin 50
  chronic abdominal pain 250
α-galactosidase 264
β-galactosidase 264
gallbladder
  contraction regulation 425
  stasis with parenteral nutrition 598
gallbladder disease
  inflammation 282–3
  obesity 41, 194–5, 201
  pregnancy 276
  referred pain 273
gallstones 41
  cholecystitis 283
  cholesterol 549
  imaging 549–50
  impaction 282
  intestinal obstruction 293
  obesity 194, 195, 201
  parenteral nutrition 598
  pregnancy 433, 549–50
  weight loss complication 201
garlic powder, hepatopulmonary syndrome 480
Garren–Edwards gastric bubble 201
gas
  clinical syndromes 256–7
  production 255
  reflex inhibition of flow 260

  retention in irritable bowel syndrome 260
  transit 255–6
    irritable bowel syndrome 260–1
gas and bloating 255–66
  abdominal pain association 274
  abnormal gut flora 258
  dietary therapy 263–4
  dysmotility syndromes 258
  functional testing 262–3
  history taking 261–2
  laboratory testing 262
  management 263–6
  pathogenesis 257–61
  patient evaluation 261–3
  physical examination 261–2
  structural testing 262
gas–bloat syndrome 258
gastric acid
  dyspepsia 44–5
  nocturnal breakthrough 91
  sensitivity 44–5
gastric adenocarcinoma 41
gastric antral hypomobility, dyspepsia 43
gastric antral vascular ectasia 136
gastric arrhythmias 43
gastric emptying
  fiber influence 570
  quantification 214–15
  slow 43
  tests in gas and bloating 263
gastric erosions
  hemorrhage 128–34
  stress 129–30
gastric mechanosensory thresholds 44
gastric outlet obstruction, nausea and vomiting 291
gastric scintigraphy 214–15
  dynamic antral 215
gastric ulcer 99
  complicated 102–3
  perforated 278–9
  recurrence 38
gastric varices 135
gastrin, measurement 101
gastrinoma, diarrhea 327
gastritis
  atrophic 612
  histological 38
  histology 128
gastrocolic reflex 539
gastroduodenal pain 241
gastroesophageal reflux disease (GERD) 40
  acid suppression empirical trial 85
  alarm symptoms 86
  antacids 49
  antireflux surgery 94–5
  approaches to patient 83–95
  barium esophagram 88–9
  chest pain 84
  clinical course 89–90
  clinical manifestations 83–5
  diagnostic evaluation 85–9
  differential diagnosis 89
  duodenal ulcer 100–1
  ear, nose and throat diseases 84–5, 94
  elderly patients 93
  endoscopy 85–6
  endoscopy-negative 42
  erosive 90
  esophageal biopsy 86
  esophageal manometry 89
  esophageal pH monitoring 86–8
  esophageal strictures 65
  extraesophageal manifestations 84–5, 88
    treatment 93–4

  lifestyle modification 90, 93
  maintenance therapy 92–3
  misclassification as dyspepsia 39
  mucosal inflammation 64
  nocturnal gastric acid breakthrough 91
  noncardiac chest pain 63, 74, 76, 84
  nonerosive 89–90
  obesity 194
  peptic ulcer disease 100–1
  PPI empirical trial 85
  pregnancy 93, 534–6
    diagnosis 534
    management 535–6
    pathogenesis 534
  reflux symptoms 83–4
  surgical management 94–5
  treatment 90–5
gastrointestinal-specific anxiety 31
gastrointestinal disease, structural 41–2
gastrointestinal disorders
  nausea and vomiting induction 208, 209, 210
  pregnancy 540–4
  weight loss 185–6
  see also functional gastrointestinal disorders
gastrointestinal fistula, nutritional support 599–600
gastrointestinal function testing, nausea and vomiting 214–16
gastrointestinal manometry 215
  gas and bloating 263
gastrointestinal motor studies 214–16
gastrointestinal myoelectric activity studies 214–16
gastrointestinal symptom overlap 39, 40
gastrointestinal tumors/neoplasms, blood loss 155
gastroparesis
  dyspepsia 210
  enteral tube feeding 595–6
  investigations 214–15
  nasoduodenal/nasojejunal feeding 595
  nausea and vomiting
    induction 208, 209, 210
    investigations 214
    management 220–1
    surgical intervention 220–1
gastropathy
  alcohol consumption 129
  drug-induced 128–9
  portal 129
gastroplasty, vertical banded 199–200
gastrostomy
  percutaneous endoscopic 266
  surgical 595
gastrostomy tube 595
gate theory of pain 250
Gaviscon, GERD 91, 93
gender
  abdominal pain 275
  hepatic adenoma 529
gene therapy 641
generator potential 232
genetic counseling 636–41
  accuracy 638
  cancer predisposition 637
  congenital gastrointestinal malformations 636
  determinations 638–9
  family medical history 637–8
  indications 636–7
  medical management 638
  patient education 638–9
  perceptions 638

personal history 637–8
physical evaluation 638
psychosocial issues 638
risk assessment 638
women of childbearing age 637
genetic discrimination 640
genetic disorders 629
types 624–5
genetic heterogeneity 629
genetic markers 642
genetic predisposition 635
genetic providers 641
genetic screening
general population 635–6
neonates 635
genetic testing 634–6
carrier 635
children 639
classification 634–6
clinical management impact 634
definition 634
diagnostic 634
genetic providers 641
informed consent 639, **640**
initial 634
logistics 640–1
prenatal 635
presymptomatic 634–5
regulation 641
results 640
role 639
sample submission 641
genetic tools/technology 641–2
genetics
for gastrointestinal patients 624–42
molecular 630–1
ghrelin 194
Giardia (giardiasis)
malabsorption 322, 335
test 335, 366
treatment 370
Gilbert syndrome 426–7, 430
age 431
diagnosis 403
jaundice 431
ginger
nausea and vomiting of pregnancy 221, 546
postoperative nausea and vomiting management 222
Glasgow Coma Scale, hepatic encephalopathy 468, **469**, 502
globus sensation 62, **63**
glucagon, dysphagia treatment 73
glucagon-like peptide-1 193
glucagonoma, diarrhea 328
glucolipids 565
gluconeogenesis 569
glucose
ascites 447
oral replacement solutions 594
parenteral nutrition 596
production 569
starvation 581
storage 568
stress response 582
utilization by brain in hepatic encephalopathy 470–1
glucose–alanine cycle 569
glucose–galactose malabsorption 325
GLUT5 transporter defect 325
glutamate, hepatic encephalopathy 471
glutamate dehydrogenase 406
glutamine
dietary 580
synthesis stimulation 474

glutamine hypothesis, cerebral edema in acute liver failure 502
glutamine synthetase (GS), hepatic encephalopathy 469–70
γ-glutamyltransferase, liver disease 436
glutathione *S*-transferase (GST) 424
gluten-sensitive enteropathy *see* celiac disease
glycemic index 559–60
glycine, pain inhibition 233
glycogen 563, 568
glycogen storage disease
type I 529
type Ia 527
type II 529
glycogenolysis, hepatic 569
glycolysis 568–9
GNβ3 CC polymorphism 46
gold standard 3
graft-versus-host disease
diarrhea 331
nausea and vomiting **209**, 212
Graves disease, weight loss 186
guaiac tests 153, 156, 157
effectiveness 172–3, 178
specimen collection/sampling 158
test validity 161
Guillain–Barré syndrome, bacterial colitis 364
gut flora
abnormal 258
gas production 255
irritable bowel syndrome 259
methanogenic in constipation 378
modification in gaseous syndromes 265–6
gut motor function tests, gas and bloating 263

H₂ breath test 338
carbohydrate malabsorption 340
haloperidol, chronic abdominal pain 250
harms, treatment benefits 18
Harris–Benedict equation *557*, **559**
Hartnup disease 610
HBeAg 516, 517
maternal 550
HBsAg 407, 516, **517**
maternal carriers 550
HBV DNA 516, 518, 519
vertical transmission rate 550
HBV immunoglobulin for neonates 550
HCV RNA 520, 551
headache, cyclic vomiting syndrome 222
health-care costs 15, 19
health-care strategies, economic comparison 15–16
heart disease, ischemia 42
heartburn 38
diet 90
with dyspeptic symptoms 42
esophageal reflux 39
GERD 83
nonerosive 89
heater probe 126, 127
α-heavy-chain disease 322
Helicobacter pylori 41
antimicrobial drugs 106–8
antimicrobial resistance 113–15
biopsy 102
confirmation of cure 115
duodenal ulcer 100–1
dyspepsia 47, 48, 52
eradication 103, 111–12, 113–14
gastrointestinal bleeding 154
improved therapies 112–13

peptic ulcer disease 100, 279
pregnancy 537
therapy 110–15
postinfectious dyspepsia 45
probiotics 114
quadruple therapy 112–13
sequential therapies 113
test-and-treat strategy 48, 50, 52
testing 101–2
treatment
antimicrobial 106–8
failures 114, 115
patient compliance 115
peptic ulcer disease 110–15
quadruple therapy 112–13
side effects 114
test-and-treat strategy 48, 50, 52
triple therapy *111*, 112, **113**
hemolysis, elevated liver enzymes, and low platelet count (HELLP) syndrome 432–3
acute liver failure 501
pregnancy 545, 549
treatment 549
hematochezia 124
hematocrit, iron deficiency 606
heme 153, 423, 424
metabolism 425
heme-porphyrin assay 157–8
hemicellulose 569
hemobilia, gastrointestinal bleeding 136
hemochromatosis 401, 402
hemodynamic monitoring, acute liver failure 507–8
hemoglobin
heme metabolism 425
immunochemical tests 157
iron deficiency 606
metabolism 152–3
hemoglobinopathies 401
hemolysis, hyperbilirubinemia 426
hemolytic anemia 426
hemolytic–uremic syndrome, bacterial colitis 364
HemoQuant assay 158
hemorrhage *see* bleeding
hemorrhagic shock, motility dysfunction 290
hemorrhagic telangiectasia, gastrointestinal bleeding 155
hemorrhoidectomy, excisional in pregnancy 540
hemorrhoids
dietary fiber effects 571
gastrointestinal bleeding 140
pregnancy 539–40
hemosiderin 154
bone marrow levels 157
hemosuccus pancreaticus, gastrointestinal bleeding 136
HepatAssist device 511
hepatic abnormalities with parenteral nutrition 598
hepatic adenoma 529–30
diagnosis 529
focal nodular hyperplasia differential diagnosis 529–30
gender 529
imaging 530
malignant transformation 529, 530
hepatic encephalopathy 467–75
acute liver failure 502
management **505**
ammonia levels 469–70
lowering 474
classification 467
clinical grading 468, **469**
definition 467

diagnosis 468
EEG changes 468–9
inflammation 472–3
liver transplantation 475
manganese deposition 470
neuroimaging 469, 470
neuropathology 469
neuropharmacology 474–5
neurotransmitters 471–2
nutritional support 473–4, 600
pathophysiology 469–73
psychometric testing 468
SIRS response 472–3, 502
therapy 473–5, 600
total parenteral nutrition 600
hepatic failure, fulminant, ammonia serum levels 410–11
hepatic function tests 402–5
hepatic hemangioma 527–8
hepatic hydrothorax, cirrhosis 455
hepatic iminodiacetic acid (HIDA) scan 437
hepatic iron index 410
hepatic metabolism tests 404
hepatic osteodystrophy, cholestasis complication 438–9
hepatic sinusoids 445
hepatic vein occlusion, acute liver failure 501
hepatic venous pressure gradient (HVPG) measurement 446
hepatitis
alcoholic 435
hepatorenal syndrome prevention 461
peripheral parenteral nutrition 600
autoimmune 433
diagnosis 415
differential diagnosis 415
fibrosing cholestatic 434
granulomatous 429
pregnancy 550–1
see also viral hepatitis
hepatitis A virus 400
acute liver failure 499
diagnosis 407
pregnancy 550
serological tests 407
hepatitis B virus (HBV) 400
acute liver failure 499
antiviral therapy 518–20
approach to patient 516–24
course of infection *517*
diagnosis 516
fibrosing cholestatic 434
genotype 517
histology 517–18
interferon therapy 518
maternal 550
molecular tests 516–17
pregnancy 550–1
serological tests 407, 516, **517**
treatment 518–20
vertical transmission 550
viral load 517
hepatitis C virus (HCV) 400, 401
antiviral therapy 521–4
duration 522–3
approach to patient 520–4
diagnosis 407–8, 520
early virological response 521, 522, *523*
fibrosing cholestatic 434
fibrosis 520
genotype 520, 523
histology 520–1
liver biopsy 520
molecular tests 520
NS3-4A protease inhibition 523–4
pregnancy 551

hepatitis C virus (HCV) (*cont'd*)
serological tests 415, 520
side effects of therapy 521–2
sustained virological response
521, 522
treatment 521–4
vertical transmission rates 551
viral load 520
virological response to treatment
521, **522**
hepatitis D virus 400
diagnosis 408
hepatitis E virus 400
acute liver failure 499–500
diagnosis 408
pregnancy 433, 551
hepatobiliary disease, pregnancy
545–50
hepatobiliary dysfunction
serum markers 405–7
tests 411
hepatocarcinogenesis 532
hepatocellular carcinoma
alkaline phosphatase 414
diagnosis 526
evolution from preneoplastic
lesions 532
hepatic adenoma transformation
529, 530
liver cell dysplasia association
531–2
nodular regenerative hyperplasia
of liver association 530
hepatocellular diseases 429
hepatocellular injury
aminotransferases 414–15
markers in liver disease 405–6
tests 411
hepatocellular necrosis, tests **412**
hepatocytes
canalicular ATP-dependent export
pumps 424
extracorporeal circuit 511
unconjugated bilirubin uptake 424
hepatoma-associated dysfibrinogen
404
hepatopulmonary syndrome 475–81
arterial blood gases 478–9
arterial oxygenation changes
476–7
chest radiography 479
clinical manifestations 478
definition 475
diagnosis 476, 478–80, *481*
diffusion–perfusion defect 477
epidemiology 475–6
hypoxemia 476, 478
intrapulmonary vascular dilations
475, 479–80, *481*
liver transplantation 481
lung function tests 479
natural history 476
oxygen therapy 480
pathophysiology 476–8
prognosis 476
pulmonary vascular tree changes
476
pulmonary vasodilation 477–8
screening 480
treatment 480–1
hepatorenal syndrome 448–9
approach to patient 458–61
cirrhosis 457–8
liver transplant 459
prophylaxis 461
suspected 460–1
therapies 459–60
hepatotoxins, exposure to 400–1
hepcidin 573–4
hephaestin 573
HER-2 testing 634

herbal medicines
acute liver failure 500
see also complementary and
alternative medicine
hereditary cancer syndromes 625,
627
hereditary hemochromatosis
diagnosis 409–10
gene mutations 410
hepcidin levels 573
hereditary hypoceruloplasminemia
409
hereditary nonpolyposis colon cancer
(HNPCC) 629
genetic counseling 638
genetic test 635
herpes simplex virus (HSV)
acute liver failure 500
hepatitis 408
odynophagia 67
heteroduplex analysis 633
hexosaminidase B deficiency 305
HFE gene mutations 410
hippocampus 231
Hirschsprung disease 378, 384
management 392
histamine, hepatic encephalopathy
472
histamine H₁-receptor antagonists 51
hepatic encephalopathy 475
histamine H₂-receptor antagonists 47
drug combinations 111
dyspepsia 49
GERD 91–2, 93
pregnancy 535–6
noncardiac chest pain 93
peptic ulcer disease 104, 111
histoplasmosis, diarrhea 331
human immunovirus (HIV) infection
cobalamin deficiency 612
jaundice 429
odynophagia 73, 74
weight loss 186
Hodgkin disease
acute liver failure 501
jaundice 429
home parenteral nutrition 598–9
homocysteine 612
hookworm
blood loss 155
stool examination 160
hormones
disturbances in constipation
377–8
malabsorption disorder
blood/serum levels 341
response to illness/injury 582
Hospital Anxiety and Depression
Scale (HADS) 31
hospitalization, nausea and vomiting
216
hypercalcemia, dyspepsia 42
5-HT₃ receptor antagonists 25–6, 50,
51
chemotherapy-induced nausea
and vomiting 221
constipation 378
diarrhea therapy 347
hyperemesis gravidarum 547
nausea and vomiting 211
management 216–17, 221, 222
5-HT₄ agonists 73
constipation 378
laxative use 389
Human Genome Project 641–2
human leukocyte antigens (HLA),
liver disease 408–9
hydrogen breath testing, gas and
bloating 262–3
7α-hydroxy-4-cholesten-4-one
concentration 341

5-hydroxyindole acetic acid
(5-HIAA) 211
5-hydroxytryptamine (5-HT)
hepatic encephalopathy 471
pain inhibition 233
signaling alterations in
constipation 378
see also 5-HT₃ receptor antagonists;
5-HT₄ agonists
25-hydroxyvitamin D 616
hyperalgesia 235
visceral 237
hyperammonemia, hepatic
encephalopathy 469–70
hyperbilirubinemia 412–13, 424,
426–30
congenital 427–9
conjugated 427–30
differential diagnosis 435
hemolysis 426
hepatocellular diseases 429
ineffective erythropoiesis 426
infection 429
infiltrative disorders 429
intrahepatic cholestasis of
pregnancy 432
neonatal 431
renal disease 429
transient familial neonatal 431
unconjugated 402–3, 426–7
differential diagnosis 435
venoocclusive disease 429–30
hyperemesis gravidarum 211, 432,
545–7
management 221, 432, 546–7
hyperglycemia, stress response 582
hyperhomocysteinemia 612
hyperhomocystinuria 611
hyperinsulinemia, obesity 194
hyperkalemia **602**, 603
hypertension, obesity 195, *196*
hyperthyroidism
liver chemistry abnormalities 401
weight loss 186
hyperventilation, acute liver failure
506
hypervitaminosis A, hepatic injury
400
hyperzincemia 609
hypnosis 27, 29
dyspepsia 52
noncardiac chest pain 75
hypnotherapy, gas and bloating
management 266
hypobetalipoproteinemia,
steatorrhea 324
hypochromic microcytic anemia 156
hypokalemia 601, 602
hypomagnesemia 604–5
hypophosphatemia 605–6, 615
hypoproteinemia 608
hypotension, gastrointestinal
bleeding 123
hypothermia, raised intracranial
pressure therapy 506
hypothyroidism
dyspepsia 42
liver chemistry abnormalities 401
obesity 194
weight loss 186–7
hypoxemia
cirrhosis 476
hepatopulmonary syndrome 476,
478
ventilation/perfusion mismatch
476

ibuprofen, dosage 116
ileal disease, bile acid diarrhea 326
ileal resection, bile acid diarrhea
326

ileostomy
diarrhea 326
sodium loss 601
ileus
adynamic 293
approach to patient 287–300
auscultation 261
bacterial translocation 291
blood flow changes 290
causes 288
clinical manifestations 291
differential diagnosis 292–3
dysmotility 258
endoscopic therapy 299–300
epidemiology 287–8
epithelial changes 289–90
history taking 291–2
imaging 293–4, *295*, 296–8, 299
intestinal decompression 298–9
intestinal dysmotility 288–9, 290
laboratory tests 293
lumenal content changes 289
mechanisms 289
motility changes 288–9
motility studies 298
pathophysiology 288
pharmacotherapy 300
physical findings 292
postoperative 289, 300
sepsis-induced 289
surgery 299
treatment 298–300
illness, metabolic responses 581–3
illness behavior 231–2
iloprost, portopulmonary
hypertension treatment
485
immune system, function in
protein-energy malnutrition
590–1
immunoassays, gastrointestinal
bleeding 153
immunochemical tests, effectiveness
173, 178
immunoglobulin(s), liver chemistry
abnormalities 404
immunoglobulin A (IgA), liver
disease 404
immunoglobulin A (IgA)
antiendomysial antibody
assay 323, 332, 415
immunoglobulin M (IgM), liver
disease 404
immunological tests, liver disease
408–9
immunonutrition formulas 594
immunoproliferative small intestinal
disease 322
immunosuppression
abdominal pain 276
odynophagia 67
incontinence, fecal 305
incremental cost-effectiveness ratio
(ICER) 14, 16, 17–18
indirect costs 15
indocyanine green test 403
indomethacin, diarrhea treatment
347
infants
abdominal pain 276
amino acid requirements 565
chronic cholestasis 431
congenital gastrointestinal
malformations 636
dietary reference intakes **560–1**
HBV prophylaxis 550
Hirschsprung disease 378
intestinal intussusception 291
protein requirements 565
stool samples 336
see also neonates

infections
  acute liver failure 502, 507
  approach to patient 360–70
  ascites 446–7
  chronic causing diarrhea 331
  fungal in acute liver failure 502
  hyperbilirubinemia 429
  nausea and vomiting induction 208, **209**
  nosocomial causing diarrhea 319–20
  odynophagia 74
  pericolonic abscess 282
  steatorrhea induction 322
  weight loss 186
  see also bacterial infections; hepatitis A–E viruses; viral infections
infiltrative disorders 429
  acute liver failure 501
inflammation
  hepatic encephalopathy 472–3
  see also diarrhea, inflammatory
inflammatory bowel disease
  diarrhea 329–30
    differential diagnosis 315
  fertility 540–1
  fish oil supplementation 599
  gastrointestinal bleeding 140
  hepatobiliary manifestations 401
  nutritional support 599, 600
  pregnancy 540–4
  treatment 329–30
    during pregnancy 541–4
  see also Crohn's disease; ulcerative colitis
inflammatory mediators
  inflammatory diarrhea 309
  intestinal secretion 306
infliximab, inflammatory bowel disease treatment during pregnancy 543–4
informed consent, genetic testing 639, **640**
inheritance
  autosomal dominant 626, *627*, *628*
  autosomal recessive 628
  modes 625–6, *627*, *628*
injection sclerotherapy, hemorrhoids in pregnancy 540
injury, metabolic responses 581–3
inotropes, acute liver failure 507–8
insula 231
insulin
  resistance 582
  sensitivity 195
intention-to-treat analysis 9
interferon
  HBV therapy 518, 551
  pegylated for HCV 521, **522**, 523
International HapMap Project 642
international normalized ratio (INR) 617
  acute liver failure 502, 503, 508
interstitial cells of Cajal
  colonic neuropathy 377
  enteric neuromuscular transmission 289
intestinal colic, obstruction of small intestine 279–80
intestinal decompression 298–9
intestinal dysmotility 261, 262
  colonic 377
  hemorrhagic shock 290
  ileus 288–9, 290
  syndromes 258
intestinal failure, steatorrhea 324
intestinal fluid volume 306–7
intestinal lymphangiectasia 324
intestinal mucosa, ileus 289–90

intestinal obstruction
  ablative therapy 299
  approach to patient 287–300
  bacterial translocation 291
  blood flow changes 290
  causes 288
  clinical manifestations 291
  decompression 298–9
  differential diagnosis 292–3
  dysmotility 288–9
  endoscopic therapy 299–300
  epidemiology 287–8
  epithelial changes 289–90
  extrinsic lesions 292
  history taking 291–2
  imaging 293–4, *295*, 296–8, 299
  intrinsic lesions 292
  laboratory tests 293
  lumenal content changes 289, *290*
  mechanical 292
  metabolic consequences 291
  motility
    changes 288–9
    studies 298
  pain 291
  pathophysiology 288
  pharmacotherapy 300
  physical findings 292
  stents 299–300
  surgery 299
  systemic consequences 291
  treatment 298–300
  vomiting 291
intestinal physiology, normal 306–8
intestinal pseudoobstruction
  bacterial overgrowth 289
  epithelial changes 290
  gas and bloating 263, 266
  ileus 292
  intestinal obstruction 292
  motility studies 298
  pneumatosis intestinalis 294, *296*
  see also colon, pseudoobstruction
intestinal strangulation 280–1
intracranial pressure monitoring **505**, 506
intragastric balloon 201
intrapulmonary vascular dilations (IPVDs) 475, 479–80, *481*
intrathecal access systems 250
intrinsic factor 338
intussusception
  children 291
  gastrointestinal bleeding 141
  intestinal obstruction 293
  rectoanal 392
inversions, genetic 632
iodine 575
IPEX syndrome 322, 329
iron, dietary 573–4
  parenteral preparations 607–8
  recommended daily amount 573
iron deficiency 606–8
  blood tests 156, 159–60
  bone marrow tests 156
  colorectal cancer 155
  disorders 154
  esophageal webs 156
  fatigue 154, 156
  gastrointestinal bleeding 153–4, 155
  metabolic consequences 154
  physical findings 156
  pica 156
  symptoms 161
  vascular malformations 155
iron dextran 608
iron metabolism
  absorption 153, 573–4
  excretion 153–4
  gastrointestinal bleeding 153–4

iron storage 154
  parameters in liver disease 409–10
iron therapy
  iron dextran 608
  oral 163–4
  parenteral 164
  supplements 607–8
irritable bowel syndrome (IBS) 20
  abdominal wall factors 261
  antidepressants 24–5
  anxiety 24
  bacterial overgrowth 259–60
  carbohydrate intolerance 259
  carbohydrate rapid transit 325
  colonic flora 259
  constipation-predominant 376, 379
  depression 31
  diagnosis 40–1
  diarrhea 305, 326–7
  emotional motor system enhanced responsiveness 23–4
  gas and bloating 258–61
    management 263–4
  gas transit 260–1
  gut flora modification 265
  hypnosis 27
  infectious diarrhea-induced 319, 364
  methane production 260
  obesity 195
  pain 242
    sensitization 236, *237*
  pathophysiology 236, *237*
  postinfectious 329, 364
  psychodynamic therapy 28–9
  psychological treatments 26–30
  rapid small intestine transit 305
  serotonin 5-HT$_3$ receptor antagonists 25–6
  somatization disorder 31 2
  SSRI therapy 249
  therapies 22
    5-HT$_3$ receptor antagonists 25–6
    psychodynamic 28–9
    psychological 26–30
    SSRI 249
  vagal function 44
Irritable Bowel Syndrome Quality of Life measurement (IBS–QOL) 32
isoniazid 610
isosorbide mononitrate 133
itopride 50

JAG1 gene mutations 432
jaundice 402
  age of patient 430–1, 435
  approach to patient 430–9
  ascites 435
  bile duct obstruction 425
  children 431–2
  definition 422
  diagnosis 430–1, 434–8
  drug-induced liver injury 500–1
  elderly patients 431
  Gilbert syndrome 431
  history taking 434–5
  imaging 436–7
  invasive tests 437
  laboratory tests 435–6
  liver transplantation 433–4
  neonatal 423, 430–2
  noninvasive tests 436–7
  pharmaceutical drugs 431, 435
  physical examination 435
  postoperative 433
  pregnancy 432–3
  total parenteral nutrition 433
  viral hepatitis 431

  see also bilirubin; hyperbilirubinemia
jejunoileal bypass 199
jejunostomy feeding, pancreatitis 600
jejunostomy tube 595
jejunum, length 594
junctional permeability, secretory diarrhea 310

kaolin–pectin diarrhea treatment 367
  pregnancy 537
Kasabach–Merritt syndrome, hepatic hemangioma 527
Kayser–Fleischer rings 402, 501
kernicterus 424, 431
keto acids 565
ketogenesis, starvation 581
ketone bodies 566–7
  starvation 581
King's College criteria for acute liver failure 503, **504**
Krebs–Henseleit cycle 410

labyrinthine disorders, nausea and vomiting induction **209**, 210
lactase deficiency 257
  breath testing 262
  diarrhea 325
lactase supplements 264
lactate dehydrogenase 407
  ascites 447
lactation
  dietary reference intakes **560–1**
  GERD therapy 93
lactic acid cycle 569
lactic dehydrogenase, ascites 447
lactoferrin, fecal tests 342, 365
lactoferrin immunoassay 157
lactose, osmotic diarrhea 308
lactose intolerance 257
  breath testing 262
  diarrhea 325
  lactase therapy 264
  testing 340
lactose tolerance test 340
lactulose
  acute liver failure 506
  hepatic encephalopathy treatment 474
  laxative use 388, 389
  osmotic diarrhea 308
lamivudine, HBV therapy 519, 551
lansoprazole, GERD treatment 92
laparoscopic adjustable banding (LAGB) 199, 200
laparoscopy
  abdominal pain 275
  cholecystectomy 550
laparotomy, abdominal pain 276–7
large bowel pain 242
large deletions 632, 633
large-volume paracentesis (LVP)
  ascites treatment 449–50, 451
  refractory disease 454, 455
laryngitis, reflux 84
laxatives
  abuse 340
  constipation 374
  fecal impaction 392
  ileus 300
  osmotic 388–9, 539
  pregnancy 538, 539
  screen 340
  stimulant 388, 539
  use 380
leptin 193–4
  nausea and vomiting of pregnancy 211
leptospirosis 401
leucine aminopeptidase 407

leukocyte(s), stool samples 365
leukocyte elastase inhibition 410
leukocyte protein tests 157
leukocyte scintigraphy,
    inflammatory diarrhea 342
leuprolide acetate 50
    nausea and vomiting management
        218, 220
L-dopa 474, 611
lifestyle, constipation 386-7
life-years gained 16
lignins 569-70
likelihood ratios 5-6
limbic system 231
limited doses 9
linaclotide 390
linkage analysis 633
linoleic acid 567
linolenic acid 567
lipid emulsion infusion 597
lipids, dietary 565-8
    metabolism 566-7
        response to illness/injury 583
    pancreatitis 600
    parenteral nutrition 596-7
lipoprotein X 404
lipoproteinemia, steatorrhea 324
lipoproteins, liver disease 404
lithocholic acid 422
liver
    drug-induced injury 500-1
    focal fatty change 531
    focal nodular hyperplasia 528-30
    pain 241
    tumors 429
liver, abnormal chemistry 399-416
    differential diagnosis 412-13
    disease-specific markers 407-11
    drug-induced 399
    dye tests 403
    hepatic function tests 402-5
    jaundice 399
    physical findings 402
liver assist devices *see* liver support
    devices
liver biopsy 411
    hepatitis 415-16
    hepatitis C virus 520-1
    jaundice 437-8
liver disease 411-16
    ammonia serum levels 410-11
    α$_1$-antitrypsin serum levels 410
    cardiopulmonary dysfunction
        differential diagnosis **483**
    copper storage parameters 409
    disease-specific markers 407-11
    end-stage
        complications 467-86
        hepatic encephalopathy
            467-75
        hepatopulmonary syndrome
            475-81
        portopulmonary hypertension
            481-6
    α-fetoprotein radioimmunoassay
        410
    gastric varices 135
    hepatic function tests 402-5
    hepatic metabolism tests 404-5
    hepatocellular dysfunction
        markers 405-6
    immunological tests 408-9
    infiltrative process **412**, 414
    iron storage parameters 409-10
    metastases 429, 526
    nutritional support 600
    obesity 195
    pregnancy 432-3, 545-9
    tests 411-12
    see also acute liver failure (ALF);
        hepatic entries; hepatitis

liver mass
    approach to patient 526-32
    benign lesions 526-7
    biliary cystadenoma 531
    dysplastic nodules 531-2
    focal fatty change 531
    focal nodular hyperplasia 528-30
    hepatic adenoma 529-30
    hepatic hemangioma 527-8
    nodular regenerative hyperplasia
        530-1
    patient evaluation 526
    regenerative nodules 531-2
liver support devices
    artificial/bioartificial 510-11
    hepatic encephalopathy 475
liver transplantation
    acute liver failure 509-10
    ascites treatment 449
    auxiliary partial orthotopic 509-10
    cholestasis 433-4
    chronic rejection 434
    hepatic encephalopathy 475
    hepatopulmonary syndrome 481
    hepatorenal syndrome 459
    jaundice 433-4
    liver chemistry abnormalities 416
    living donor 510
    portopulmonary hypertension
        treatment 485-6
local anesthesia, "trigger"-point
    injections 244
locus heterogeneity 629
lomotil, diarrhea treatment 367
    pregnancy 537
long-chain 3-hydroxyacyl-CoA
    dehydrogenase (LCHAD)
    deficiency 548-9
long-chain fatty acids
    dietary 309
    metabolic defects in acute liver
        failure 501
loperamide, diarrhea treatment
    317-18, 367
    pregnancy 537
low-density lipoprotein (LDL) 579
lubiprostone **388**, 389
Lucy–Driscoll syndrome 431
Lundh meal test 338
lung function tests, portopulmonary
    hypertension 483
lymphadenopathy, dysphagia 68
lymphoma
    acute liver failure 501
    celiac disease association 323
    infiltrative disorders 429
    steatorrhea 322

Magenblase syndrome 256
magnesium, serum concentrations
    605
magnesium, dietary 572-3
    deficiency 604-5
    recommended daily amount 572
    supplements 605
magnesium compounds, laxative
    388, 389
magnesium ions
    absorption 321
    diarrhea 325
        osmotic 308
    stool measurement 344
magnesium sulfate, GERD in
    pregnancy 535
magnetic resonance
    cholangiopancreatography
        (MRCP), jaundice 436-7
magnetic resonance defecography
    386
magnetic resonance imaging (MRI)
    cholecystitis 549-50

cholelithiasis 549-50
colorectal cancer screening 179
constipation 386
dynamic 386
gastric emptying 215
hepatic encephalopathy 469, 470
hepatic hemangioma 528
ileus 296
intestinal obstruction 296
jaundice 436-7
liver cell dysplasia 531, 532
malabsorption 333
nausea and vomiting investigation
    214
nodular regenerative hyperplasia
    of liver 531
pregnancy 276
malabsorption
    carbohydrate 257-8
        diarrhea 325
        fecal pH 340
        tests 340
    carbon-14 triolein breath test 337
    clinical evaluation 331-3, *334,*
        335-8
    clinical manifestations **333**
    diarrhea 306, 308, **309**, 321-5
    evaluation *334*
    fat 321-5
    giardiasis 322
    history 331-2
    hypocalcemia 603-4
    imaging 333, 335
    laboratory findings **333**
    mucosal 322-4
    pancreatic function tests 337-8
    pathophysiology **333**
    physical examination 331-2
    radiography 332-3, 335
    riboflavin deficiency 610
    screening tests 332, **334**
    steatorrhea 321-5
    stool tests 335-7
    thiamin deficiency 609
    vitamin E deficiency 617
    D-xylose absorption tests 337
malignancy
    acute liver failure 501
    anorexia–cachexia syndrome *185*
    ascites 447
    cachexia 184, *185*
    celiac disease association 323
    dyspepsia 41, 42, 47-8
    elderly patients 431
    hepatocarcinogenesis 532
    intestinal obstruction 292
    nausea and vomiting induction
        208, **209**
    nonendocrine causing diarrhea 328
    obesity 194
    weight loss 184-5, 189
    see also cancer; *named conditions and*
        tumors
Mallory–Weiss tears 135
malnutrition
    diarrhea 317, 319
    see also protein–energy
        malnutrition
Malone continent enema 391
manganese 574-5
    hepatic encephalopathy 470
mannitol, raised intracranial pressure
    therapy 506
manometry
    anorectal for constipation 384-5
    colonic 386
    dyssynergic defecation 378, *379*
    esophageal 72, 89
    gastrointestinal 215
        gas and bloating 263
    small bowel 298

mastocytosis, systemic
    diarrhea 328
    steatorrhea 322
meal replacements 197
"Meals on Wheels" acronym **187**,
    188
mean pulmonary arterial pressure
    (MPAP) *481,* 484, 486
Meckel diverticulum
    blood loss 155
    gastrointestinal bleeding 140, 141
Mediterranean lymphoma 322
meiosis 630
melanosis coli 340, 388
melanosis coli 340, 388
Mendelian disorders 625, **626, 627**
Ménétrier disease 42
Ménière disease, nausea and
    vomiting induction **209**, 210
Menkes syndrome 409
    protein 574
menorrhagia, iron deficiency 154
menstrual cycle, constipation 377
meperidine
    conscious sedation in pregnancy
        545
    pancreatitis pain control 248
6-mercaptopurine, use in pregnancy
    542, 543
mesalamine, use in pregnancy 542
mesenteric embolism 283-4
mesenteric ischemia 283-4, *285*
mesenteric vascular bundles, torsion
    290
mesenteric vascular ischemia,
    chronic 331
metabolic diseases, steatorrhea
    324-5
metabolic syndrome, obesity 195,
    196
metastases, liver 429, 526
metformin, weight loss **198**, 199
methane production in irritable
    bowel syndrome 260
methionine synthase 613
methotrexate, use in pregnancy **542**,
    543
methylmalonyl-CoA mutase 613
methylnaltrexone 390
metoclopramide
    dyspepsia 50
    GERD 91
    hyperemesis gravidarum **546**, 547
    ileus 300
    nausea and vomiting management
        218, 219
metronidazole
    H. pylori treatment 107
    inflammatory bowel disease
        treatment during pregnancy
        544
    protozoal infection treatment 370
mianserin, dyspepsia 51
micronutrients 571-80
    deficiencies 600-18
microsatellite instability (MSI) testing
    634
midazolam, contraindications in
    pregnancy 545
midodrine
    ascites therapy 452
    hepatorenal syndrome therapy
        460
migraine, cyclic vomiting syndrome
    222
milk
    allergy causing diarrhea 330
    raw 319
milk-induced enteritis 154
mineral deficiency, laboratory
    detection **591**
mineral oil stool softener 388

minerals, dietary 571–5
mirtazepine, nausea and vomiting management **217**, 218–19
misoprostol
    laxative use 389–90
    NSAID ulcer prevention 116
    peptic ulcer disease 106
mitochondrial disorders 625, *627*, **627**
mitochondrial isoenzyme of aspartate aminotransferase (mAST) 406
mitochondrial neurogastrointestinal encephalopathy syndrome (MNGIE) 625, **626**
mitochondrial trifunctional protein (MTP) 548–9
mitosis 630
Model for End-stage Liver Disease (MELD) score 416, 459, 503
    hepatopulmonary syndrome screening 480
models, sensitivity to assumptions 18
modified 3-day rule 320
Molecular Absorbent Recirculating System (MARS) 511
molecular genetics 630–1
monoamine oxidase A (MAO-A) 471, 472
monomeric formulas 593
mosaicism 625
motility
    changes in ileus 288–9
    diarrhea 305
    esophageal testing in noncardiac chest pain 75, 77
    small bowel manometry 298
    studies in ileus 298
    see also intestinal dysmotility
motion sickness, nausea and vomiting induction **209**, 210
motor function, disturbed in dyspepsia 42–4
multidrug resistance 3 (MDR3) gene 547
multiorgan failure, acute liver failure 502–3
multiple endocrine neoplasia (MEN) types 1 and 2 327
multiple symptom illness 32
multiplex ligation-dependent probe amplification (MLPA) 633
Munchausen syndrome by proxy 328
Murphy sign 402
    sonographic 283
muscle
    amino acid uptake 565
    cramps with liver chemistry abnormalities 401–2
muscle protein
    response to illness/injury 582
    starvation 581
mutations
    detection techniques 632–4
    founder 635–6
    frameshift 631–2
    missense 631
    new 629
    nonsense 631
    regulatory 632
    screening methods 633
    silent 631
    splice-site 632
    types 631–2
MYH gene mutations 634
MUTYH (MYH)-associated polyposis (MAP) 628
myofascial trigger points 244

myopathic dysmotility, auscultation 261
MyPyramid food guidance 559

N-acetylcysteine (NAC) 497, 505
NAPQI 495
narcotics, abdominal pain treatment 247, 248
nasendoscopy 70
nasoduodenal feeding 595
nasoenteric feeding tube 595
nasogastric decompression 298–9
    small intestine obstruction 280
nasogastric feeding tube 595
nasojejunal feeding 595
nausea 40
    antinauseant drugs 51
    dyspepsia 43
nausea and vomiting 205–22
    autonomic response 207
    causes 208, **209**, 210–12
    chemotherapy 205, 207, **209**, 211–12
        management 218, 221
    complications 213
    diet 216
    endocrine system response 207
    gastric outlet obstruction 291
    gastrointestinal events 207
    gastrointestinal function testing 214–16
    gastrointestinal motor/myoelectrical activity studies 214–16
    history taking 212–13
    hospitalization indications 216
    imaging investigations 214
    laboratory testing 213–14
    management principles 216–22
    medications 208, **209**, 216–20
    pathophysiology 206–8
    physical examination 213
    postoperative 205, **209**, 211–12
    pregnancy 205, **209**, 210–11, 545–7
        management 221
    serological tests 213–14
    socioeconomic impact 205
    structural evaluation 214
    thiamin deficiency 609
Nd:YAG laser 126, 127
neck masses, dysphagia 68
negative predictive value (NPV) 5
neonates
    bilirubin encephalopathy 424
    congenital gastrointestinal malformations 636
    genetic screening 635
    HBV immunoglobulin 550
    HBV prophylaxis 551
    HCV diagnosis 551
    hyperbilirubinemia 431
    jaundice 430–2
    kernicterus 424
neostigmine 266
    ileus 300
nerve root disease 242
neural blockade
    chronic abdominal pain 250
    local 244
neural tube defects, folate association 576, 612
neurokinin NK$_1$ antagonists 207
    nausea and vomiting management 217–18
neurokinin NK$_1$ receptor 236
neuroleptics, chronic abdominal pain 250
neurological disorders, weight loss 188
neurolytic therapy, chronic abdominal pain 250

neuropeptide Y (NPY) 192, *193*
neurotransmitters
    disturbances in constipation 377–8
    hepatic encephalopathy 471–2
neurotropins 390
neutropenic enterocolitis 331
neutrophils, esophagitis 86
niacin **575**, 576
    deficiency 610–11
nicotinamide adenine dinucleotide, reduced (NADH) 569
nicotinic acid 611
Nissen fundoplication 94
nitric oxide (NO), hepatopulmonary syndrome 478
nitric oxide synthase (NOS)
    endothelial (eNOS) 478
    inducible (iNOS) 472, 478
    neuronal (nNOS) 472
nitrogen
    balance 565, 594
    blood urea in gastrointestinal bleeding 123–4
    free amino acids 564
    response to illness/injury 582
2-nitropropane 401
nitrosative stress, hepatic encephalopathy 472
nizatidine
    GERD 91
    peptic ulcer disease 104
NK1 *see* neurokinin NK$_1$ receptor
N-methyl-D-aspartate (NMDA) receptor 233
nociception 231–2
    peripheral 232–3
    visceral 233–7
nociceptors 228
    functions 232–3
    silent 234
nodular regenerative hyperplasia of liver 530–1
nomograms 6
nonalcoholic fatty liver disease (NAFLD) 195, 416
nonalcoholic steatohepatitis (NASH) 195, *196*, 416
noncardiac chest pain 62–3
    approach to patients 74–7
    cardiac disease differential diagnosis 75–6
    differential diagnosis 75–6
    GERD 84
    histamine H$_2$ blockers 93
    investigations 74–5, 76–7
    management 75
    mechanisms 74–5
    medical history 76
    nonesophageal causes 75
    physical examination 76
    proton pump inhibitors 93
    psychological/psychiatric factors 75, 77
    symptom patterns 76
non-health-care costs 15, 16
non-Hodgkin lymphoma
    acute liver failure 501
    jaundice 429
nonpenetrance, genetic 629
nonsteroidal antiinflammatory drugs (NSAIDs)
    chronic abdominal pain 248
    dyspepsia 42, 46, 47
    gastrointestinal bleeding 125, 141, 155–6
    gastropathy 128–9
    ulcers
        giant peptic 103
        prevention 115–16
        risk 116
        treatment 115–16

nonsteroidal antiinflammatory drug (NSAID) colitis 331
norepinephrine (noradrenaline)
    acute liver failure 507
    hepatorenal syndrome therapy 461
    pain inhibition 233
norfloxacin, prophylactic in ascites 454
noxious stimuli 230, 231
NS3-4A protease inhibition 523–4
5′-nucleotidase 407
nucleotide oligomerization domain (NOD) proteins 309
nucleotides 630
nucleus tractus solitarius (NTS) 206
number needed to treat (NNT) 10–11, 12
nutrition 557–83
    see also diet
nutritional assessment 588, **589**, 590–1
    techniques 588, 590–1
nutritional deficiencies 588, **589**
nutritional states, altered 580–3
nutritional status, subjective global assessment 591, *592*
nutritional supplementation, approach to patient 588–618
nutritional support
    guidelines 592
    hospitalized patient with gastrointestinal disease 599–600
    routes 591–9
        choice 591–2
    see also enteral feeding/nutrition; parenteral nutrition; total parenteral nutrition

obesity 191–201
    behavior therapy 197–8
    BMI 191, **192**
        determination 196
    cirrhosis 194
    class **558**
    colorectal cancer 195
    complications 194–5
    diabetes mellitus 195, *196*
    dietary intervention 196–7
    dyslipidemia 195, *196*
    endoscopic therapy 201
    gallbladder disease 41, 194–5, 201
    GERD 90, 194
    history taking 194
    hypertension 195, *196*
    irritable bowel syndrome 195
    lifestyle modification 196–8
    liver disease 195
    malignancy 194
    metabolic syndrome 195, *196*
    over-the-counter products 199
    pancreatic disease 195
    pharmaceutical drugs 198–9
    physical activity 197
    physical examination 194
    prevalence 191, 557
    surgical therapy 199–201
    treatment 196–201
occupational exposure to hepatotoxins 400–1
octadecaneuropeptide (ODN) 472
octreotide 50
    chronic abdominal pain 250
    diarrhea treatment 321, 347
    esophageal varices hemorrhage management 130–1
    intestinal lymphangiectasia 324
    intestinal obstruction 300
    nausea and vomiting management **218**, 220
    peptic ulcer rebleeding prevention 127–8

odynophagia 62–3, 66–7, 73–4
  approach to patient 73–4
  with dysphagia 64, 68
  GERD 84
  investigation 74
  medical history 73
  physical examination 73
  symptoms 62–3
Ogilvie syndrome *see* colon,
    pseudoobstruction
oligomeric formulas 593
olsalazine, use in pregnancy 542
omeprazole
  GERD treatment 91, 92, 93
  GERD in pregnancy **536**
  pharmacology *105*
  safety 93
  test in noncardiac chest pain 76
ondansetron, hyperemesis
    gravidarum **546**, 547
operant behavior therapy 28
opiates
  epidural/intrathecal access
    systems 250
  laxative use 390
opioids
  chronic abdominal pain 248
  hepatic encephalopathy 472
  postoperative ileus 300
oral contraceptives, hepatic
    hemangioma 527
oral rehydration therapy 594
  short bowel syndrome 599
oral replacement solutions (ORS)
    594, 599
  diarrhea 317, 367
organic anion-transporting
    polypeptide (OATP) 424
orlistat 198–9
ornipressin, hepatorenal syndrome
    therapy 460
L-ornithine L-aspartate 474
orthodeoxia, hepatopulmonary
    syndrome 479
Osler–Weber–Rendu syndrome
  gastrointestinal bleeding 155
  hepatic hemangioma 527
osteomalacia 615
osteophytes, prominent vertebral 70
osteoporosis, alcohol consumption
    616
ostomy output 594
outcomes
  baseline risk in treatment
    population 17
  cost data integration 16
  cost-effectiveness analysis 18
  discounting 16
  generalizability of research
    findings 18–19
  incremental 17–18
  measurement 16
  time preferences 16
overweight 191, **192**
oxidative phosphorylation 569
oxidative stress, hepatic
    encephalopathy 472
oxygen therapy, hepatopulmonary
    syndrome 480
oxyntomodulin 193

packed erythrocyte transfusion,
    gastrointestinal bleeding 123
pain
  abdominal wall 42
  acute 238
  anatomical pathways 228, 229,
    230–2
  antidepressant therapy 24–5
  ascending pathways 230
  biopsychosocial continuum 231–2

cellular substrates 232–3
central 23–4
chronic 238
circuits 230–1
colonic obstruction 291
descending pathways 231
duration 239
epigastric 274
gate theory 250
inhibitory systems 233
intestinal obstruction 291
molecular substrates 232–3
neurobiology 228, *229*, 230–8
neurochemical substrates 232–3
neuropathic 238, *245*
nociceptive 238
noxious stimuli 230, 231
onset 239
pattern 239
perception 231
peripheral pathways 228, *229*, 230
poststroke 238
referred 233–4, *235*, 273
sensitization 234–7
somatic 23, 230
spinal connections 230
suffering 231–2
supraspinal structures 230–1
swallowing 66–7
visceral 23, 230, 233–7, 240
  distribution 271–2
  neuronal pathways 272
  referred pain 273
  stress 237–8
visceral afferents 232
see also abdominal pain; noncardiac
    chest pain
pain disorder, functional abdominal
    pain syndrome 246
pain scales 239
pancrealauryl test 337
pancreatic ascites 448
pancreatic cancer 41–2
  bile duct obstruction 321
  celiac neurolysis for pain control
    250
  obesity 195
pancreatic disease, obesity 195
pancreatic exocrine insufficiency
    331–2
  chronic diarrhea 322
pancreatic function tests 337–8
pancreatic pain 241
pancreatic polypeptide (PP) 192, 193
pancreatic stimulation tests 338
pancreatitis
  acute 600
  alcoholic 401
  chronic 41–2
    chronic diarrhea 322
    pain control 248, 250
  liver enzymes 414
  meperidine treatment 248
  nausea and vomiting induction
    210
panenteroscopy, laparoscopically
    assisted 160–1
panic disorder, noncardiac chest pain
    75
pantoprazole, GERD treatment 92
pantothenic acid **575**, 577
  deficiency 615
paraaminobenzoic acid (PABA) 337
parabrachial nucleus 231
paracentesis
  diagnostic 444
  large-volume for ascites treatment
    449–50, 451
  refractory disease 454, 455
parathyroid hormone (PTH) 615,
    616

parenteral nutrition 596–9
  complications 597 8
  gastroparesis 221
  home 598–9
  inflammatory bowel disease 599
  metabolic complications 598
  pancreatitis 600
  peripheral 598
    alcoholic hepatitis 600
  solutions 596
  see also total parenteral (central)
    nutrition
Parkinson disease
  oropharyngeal dysphagia 65, 71
  weight loss 188
Paterson–Kelly syndrome,
    esophageal webs 156
pathogen-associated molecular
    patterns (PAMPs) 289
  inflammatory diarrhea 309
pathogens, community-acquired **363**
Patient Health Questionnaire 15
    (PHQ-15) 32
patients
  application of clinical research
    results 12
  inconvenience of therapy 12
  lost to follow-up 10
  non-health-care costs 15
  numbers 11, 12
pellagra 610, 611
pelvic floor dysfunction 381
pelvic organs, pain 242
pelvic pain 242
penetrance, genetic 629
pentobarbital, raised intracranial
    pressure therapy 506
pentoxifylline
  hepatopulmonary syndrome
    prevention 478
  hepatorenal syndrome prevention
    461
peptic strictures
  barium esophagram 89
  GERD 83–4
peptic ulcer disease 38, 41, 47,
    99–116
  acid secretion 101
  antisecretory agents 104–6
  atypical ulcers 103
  bleeding cessation 126–8
  comorbidity **103**
  complications presentation 101
  confirmation of cure 115
  conventional therapy 110
  CT 102
  disease associations **103**
  drug combinations 110–12
  drug interactions with antiulcer
    drugs 108, **109**, 110
  embolization of bleeding 128
  endoscopic control of bleeding
    126–7, 128
  endoscopy 102
  etiology **103**
  evaluation 102–3
  follow-up 102–3
  GERD association 100–1
  gastrointestinal bleeding 125,
    126–8
  giant ulcers 103
  healing 110
  history 101
  idiopathic **103**
  laboratory evaluation 101–2
  mechanical ligation with clips
    127
  natural history 103–4
  pain 241
  patient compliance 115
  physical examination 101

pregnancy 537
radiological imaging 102
recurrent hemorrhage prevention
    127–8
surgery for rebleeding 128
thermal control of bleeding 126–7
treatment 104–8, **109**, 110–16
  failures 114, 115
  side effects 114
peptide tyrosine tyrosine (PYY)
    192–3
percutaneous endoscopic
    gastrostomy (PEG)
  pregnancy 545
  tube placement 595
percutaneous transhepatic
    cholangiography (PTC),
    jaundice 437
perianal disease, gastrointestinal
    bleeding 140
periaqueductal gray 231
pericarditis, constrictive in ascites
    445
pericolonic abscess 282
pericrypt eosinophilic enterocolitis
    330
peripheral nervous system
  emesis activation 206
  vomiting initiation response 207
peripheral parenteral nutrition 598
  alcoholic hepatitis 600
peripheral sensitization 234
peripheral veins, nutritional support
    route 598
"peripheral-type" benzodiazepine
    receptor (PTBR) 472
peritoneal disorders, nausea and
    vomiting induction **209**, 210
peritoneal tuberculosis, ascites
    447–8
peritoneovenous shunt (PVS)
  ascites treatment 451–2
  complications 452
peritoneum innervation/
    physiological properties 273
peritonitis 282
  spontaneous bacterial 442, 446–7
    approach to patient 455–7
    hepatorenal syndrome
      prevention 461
    management 453–4, 456–7
pernicious anemia 612
PFIC genes 428
pharmaceutical drugs
  acetaminophen content of
    analgesics 497, **497–8**
  cholestasis post liver
    transplantation 434
  chronic abdominal pain 248–50
  constipation treatment 387–90
  constipation-inducing 387
  diarrhea induction 320
  gas production 261
  gastrointestinal bleeding 155–6
  hepatic injury 399–400
  hepatitis B virus 551
  hepatopulmonary syndrome 480
  hepatotoxicity 429
  hyperemesis gravidarum 546–7
  idiosyncratic reactions causing
    acute liver failure 492, 493,
    500–1
  ileus 300
  integrated cognitive–behavioral
    therapy 29–30
  jaundice 431, 435
  nausea and vomiting 216–20
    induction 208, **209**
  obesity 198–9
  steatorrhea induction 322
  weight loss 187

pharyngeal diverticulum
  lateral 70
  retaining 68
pharyngolaryngeal cancer surgery,
    oropharyngeal dysphagia 65
phenolic acids 570
phenothiazines
  hyperemesis gravidarum 546
  nausea and vomiting of pregnancy
      221
phentermine 198, 199
phenytoin, seizures in acute liver
    failure 507
phosphate, sodium-dependent
    cotransporters (NPT) 573
phosphodiesterase inhibitors,
    portopulmonary hypertension
    treatment 485
phospholipids 565
phosphorus, dietary 573
  deficiency 605–6, 615
phototherapy, neonatal jaundice 423
phylloquinone 617
pica, iron deficiency 156
pill-induced injury, odynophagia 67,
    74
pirenzepine 49
placebo response, dyspepsia 48–9
plasma renin activity (PRA) 450
platelets, acute liver failure 508
pleiotropy 629
pleural effusion see hepatic
    hydrothorax
Plummer–Vinson syndrome,
    esophageal webs 156
pneumatosis intestinalis 294, 296
pneumoperitoneum, perforated
    gastric/duodenal ulcer 278,
    279
Polle syndrome 328
  see also Munchausen syndrome by
      proxy
polyethylene glycol (PEG), laxative
    use 388, 389, 539
polyglandular syndrome type I,
    steatorrhea 325
polymerase chain reaction (PCR) 633
polymeric formulas 593
polymers, injectable for GERD 95
polymorphonuclear leucocytes
    (PMNs)
  ascites 446, 447
  spontaneous bacterial peritonitis
      diagnosis 456
polyphenols 569, 570
ω-3 polyunsaturated fatty acids
    (PUFAs) 568, 579
ω-6 polyunsaturated fatty acids
    (PUFAs) 597
population, baseline risk 17
porphyrin 153
portacaval shunt, esophageal varices
    recurrent hemorrhage
    prevention 133–4
portal decompression, esophageal
    varices recurrent hemorrhage
    prevention 134
portal gastropathy 129
portal hypertension
  gastrointestinal bleeding 141
  hepatopulmonary syndrome 476
  portopulmonary hypertension
      complication 482
  pregnancy 433
portopulmonary hypertension
    481–6
  clinical manifestations 483
  definition 482
  diagnosis 481, 483–4
  epidemiology 482
  hemodynamic assessment 484

liver transplantation 485–6
lung function tests 483
natural history 482
pathophysiology/pathogenesis
    482–3
right heart catheterization 484
right ventricular systolic pressure
    481, 484
treatment 484–6
portosystemic shunting 482–3
positive predictive value (PPV) 5
positron emission tomography (PET),
    hepatic encephalopathy 469
postenteritis syndrome 318–19
postoperative nausea and vomiting
    (PONV) 209, 211–12
  management 221–2
postparacentesis circulatory
    dysfunction (PCD) 450
postpolypectomy bleeding 139–40
postprandial distress syndrome 39
posttest probability 4–6
posttraumatic fever 582
postural hypotension,
    gastrointestinal bleeding 123
potassium, dietary 571–2
  assessment 601
  deficiency 601–3
  oral products 602
potassium ion channels 232
potassium ions
  intestinal transport 305, 306
  secretory diarrhea 344
pouchitis, treatment 347
pramlintide 193
preeclampsia 432
pregabalin 50
  chronic abdominal pain 250
pregnancy
  abdominal pain 275–6
  acute fatty liver 432, 501, 548–9
  acute liver failure 501
  albumin serum levels 404
  antireflux surgery 536
  appendicitis 275, 276
  celiac disease 540
  cholecystectomy 550
  cholecystitis/cholelithiasis 549–50
  cobalamin deficiency 613
  coincident diseases 433
  colorectal cancer 544
  conscious sedation 545
  constipation 537 9
  Crohn's disease 540–4
  diarrhea 537, 538
  dietary reference intakes 560–1
  endoscopy 544–5
  fatty acid oxidation disorders
      548–9
  FDA drug categories 535
  folate deficiency 612
  gallbladder disease 276
  gallstones 549–50
  GERD 534–6
    treatment 93
  gastrointestinal chronic diseases
      540–4
  gastrointestinal complaints
      534–40
  HELLP syndrome 545, 549
  hepatic hemangioma 527
  hepatitis 433, 550–1
  hepatobiliary disease 545–50
  imaging 276
  inflammatory bowel disease
      540–4
  intrahepatic cholestasis 432, 547–8
  jaundice 432–3
  laxatives 538, 539
  liver chemistry abnormalities 401
  liver disease 432–3, 545–9

nausea and vomiting 205, 209,
    210–11, 545–7
  management 221
  nutritional demands 565
  peptic ulcer disease 537
  prenatal genetic testing 635
  recommended daily allowance
      565
  teratogen risk 637
  ulcerative colitis 540–4
prenatal testing 635
pretest probability 2–3
  estimation 3
probability (P) 11
probability theory 14
probiotics 114
  gut flora modification 265
  hepatic encephalopathy
      management 474
  inflammatory diarrhea treatment
      347
productivity costs 15, 16
progressive familial intrahepatic
    cholestasis (PFIC) 427–8
progressive muscle relaxation
    training 26, 27
prokinetic drugs
  dyspepsia 50, 51
  gas and bloating management 266
  GERD 91, 93
  nausea and vomiting management
      218, 219–20
prolactin, nausea and vomiting of
    pregnancy 211
proof-of-concept studies 7
propranolol, esophageal varices
    recurrent hemorrhage
    prevention 133
prostacyclin analogues,
    portopulmonary hypertension
    treatment 485
prostaglandins
  NSAID ulcer prevention 116
  peptic ulcer disease 106
protease inhibitor system 410
protein
  ascites total level 444, 445–6
  bioavailability 564
  composition 564–5
  enteric loss 342
  metabolism 563, 565
    response to illness/injury 582
  quality 564
  serum concentrations in
      protein–energy malnutrition
      590
protein, dietary
  digestion 564
  hepatic encephalopathy 473–4
protein truncation test (PTT) 633
protein–energy malnutrition 588,
    590–1
  subjective global assessment 591,
      592
protein-losing enteropathy
  diarrhea 330–1
  eosinophilic gastroenteritis 330
  intestinal lymphangiectasia 324
prothrombin time 403, 404, 412, 416
  liver function 436
  one-stage 617
proton pump inhibitors (PPIs) 47
  with antimicrobials for H. pylori
      112–13, 114
  drug combinations 111
  dyspepsia 49, 52
  GERD 91, 92, 93
    empirical trial 85
  GERD in pregnancy 536
  noncardiac chest pain 93
  NSAID gastropathy 129

NSAID ulcer
  prevention 116
  treatment 115
peptic ulcer disease 104–6, 111,
    279
  rebleeding prevention 127
  pharmacology 104–6
  stress gastric erosions 129
    prophylaxis 130
protozoal infections, diarrhea 361,
    366
  treatment 370
PRSS1 gene 629
pruritis
  cholestasis complication 438
  intrahepatic cholestasis of
      pregnancy 547–8
  liver chemistry abnormalities
      401–2
pseudodiarrhea 305
pseudohypocalcemia 603
pseudomembranous colitis, diarrhea
    314
pseudopancreatic cholera syndrome
    328–9
PST1 gene 629
psychiatric disorders
  dyspepsia 42
  noncardiac chest pain 75, 77
  weight loss 188
psychodynamic therapy
  evidence for 29
  irritable bowel syndrome 28–9
psychodynamic–interpersonal
    treatment 28–9
psychological distress
  dyspepsia 41
  noncardiac chest pain 75, 77
psychological treatments
  dyspepsia 52
  functional gastrointestinal
      disorders 26–30
  outcomes 29
  randomized controlled trials 29
psychosocial factors
  dyspepsia 45–6
  functional gastrointestinal disorder
      patient care 20–34
  screening 30–1
  stressors in adults 22–3
psychotherapy, dyspepsia 52
psyllium 388
  constipation 387
pteroylglutamic acid (PGA) 576
pulmonary angiography,
    hepatopulmonary syndrome
    480
pulmonary arterial hypertension
    (PAH)
  idiopathic 483
  portal hypertension association
      482
pulmonary disease
  GERD 84
  weight loss 186
pulmonary vasodilation,
    hepatopulmonary syndrome
    477–8
push enteroscopy 141
pyridoxal phosphate 611
pyridoxine 575, 576
  deficiency 611
  and doxylamine 546
pyridoxine antagonists 611
pyruvate metabolism 568

quality of life
  constipation 375
  dyspepsia 38
  functional gastrointestinal
      disorders 32

quality-adjusted life-year (QALY) 15, 16, 17–18

rabeprazole, GERD treatment 92
racecadotril 346–7
radiation enteritis 163
radiation enterocolitis 331
radiation-induced vomiting 211
  management 221
radiofrequency techniques, GERD 95
radiography
  constipation 382, **383**
  diverticulitis 281–2
  gas and bloating 262
  hepatopulmonary syndrome 479
  ileus 293–4, *295, 296, 297*
  inflammatory diarrhea 342
  intestinal obstruction 293–4, *295, 296, 297*
  malabsorption 332–3, 335
  nausea and vomiting investigations 214
  watery diarrhea 339
radiolabeled technetium–sulfur colloid, jaundice 437
radiological imaging
  odynophagia 74
  peptic ulcer disease 102
radionuclide scans
  gastrointestinal bleeding 137–8
  hepatic hemangioma 528
  lung perfusion in hepatopulmonary syndrome 479–80
radiotelemetry capsule 215
radiotherapy, diarrhea 320–1, 331
random allocation, concealed 8
randomized controlled trial (RCT) 1, 8
  double-blinded 8
  psychological therapies 29
ranitidine 49
  GERD 91
  safety 93
rearrangements, genetic 633
receptor potential 232
recombinant immunoblot assay (RIBA), HCV diagnosis 520
recommended daily allowance (RDA) 557, 558–9
  pregnancy 565
rectal barostat test 385
rectal pain 242
rectal resection, stapled 392
rectal ulcer, gastrointestinal bleeding 141
rectal varices, gastrointestinal bleeding 141
rectoanal coordination training 390
rectoanal inhibitory reflex 378, 384
rectoanal intussusception 392
rectocele repair 392
reference daily intake (RDI) 558–9
reference standard 3
reflex responses, homeostatic 23
reflex-arc theory of referred pain *235*
regurgitation, esophageal 69
relative risk reduction (RRR) 10–11
relaxation training
  functional gastrointestinal disorders 26–7
  noncardiac chest pain 75
renal cell carcinoma 401
renal dialysis, thiamin deficiency 609
renal disease
  hyperbilirubinemia 429
  weight loss 186
renal failure
  acute liver failure 507
  intrinsic 458

prerenal 457
  see also acute renal failure
renal impairment, ischemic hepatitis 415
renal replacement therapy
  acute liver failure 507
  hepatorenal syndrome 461
renin, plasma activity 450
resistant starches 569
respondent techniques, functional gastrointestinal disorders 26–7
resting energy expenditure (REE) **559**, 563–4
  response to illness/injury 582
resuscitation, gastrointestinal bleeding 123
retinol 578, 615
retrograde giant contraction 207
rheumatological disorders, weight loss 187
ribavirin, hepatitis C virus 521, 522, 523
riboflavin 575–6
  deficiency 610
rickets 615
rifabutin 108
rifamixin 368
right ventricular systolic pressure (RVSP) *481, 484*
rimonabant 199
RNA microarray 642
RNA polymerase 630
RNA structure 630
Rotor syndrome 427
  sulfobromophthalein test 403
Roux-en-Y gastric bypass 199, *200*
rumination 40
runners, long-distance
  diarrhea 321
  gastrointestinal bleeding 156

sacral nerve stimulation, constipation 392
salicylates, inflammatory diarrhea treatment 347
Salmonella
  antibiotic treatment 369–70
  infectious diarrhea 360–1, 365
Salmonella enteritidis, postinfectious dyspepsia 45
salt
  adequate intake 558
  see also sodium chloride
salt substitutes 572
sample size 11, 12
satavaptan 452
satiety testing 215–16
Schatzki ring 66
  barium esophagram 89
  GERD 83–4
Schilling test 338
scleroderma
  gastroparesis 208, **209**
  weight loss 187
sclerosing cholangitis, primary 413–14
  cholangiocarcinoma 526
sclerotherapy for esophageal varices
  hemorrhage prophylaxis 134–5
  recurrent hemorrhage prevention 133
scopolamine 216
screening 17–18
  functional gastrointestinal disorders 34
  genetic 635–6
  questionnaires 31
scrotal edema 450
scurvy 614
secretin test 338

sedatives, functional gastrointestinal disorders 24
seizures, acute liver failure 506–7
selective serotonin reuptake inhibitors (SSRIs)
  chronic abdominal pain treatment 249
  dyspepsia 51
  irritable bowel syndrome 24–5
  noncardiac chest pain 75
selenohomotaurocholic acid 340–1
selenium 574
Sengstaken–Blakemore tube, modified 132
sensitivity
  analysis 18
  diagnostic tests 4–5
sensorimotor dysfunction, esophageal dysphagia 73
sensory training, dyssynergic defecation **388**, 390–1
sensory–discriminative circuit 231
sepsis, catheter-related
  home parenteral nutrition 599
  total parenteral nutrition 597–8
serotonin *see* 5-hydroxytryptamine (5-HT)
serotonin 5-HT$_3$ receptor antagonists *see* 5-HT$_3$ receptor antagonists
serotonin and norepinephrine reuptake inhibitors (SNRIs) 25, 249
  dyspepsia 51
serum–ascites albumin gradient (SAAG) **443**, 444–5, 446, 447
sex chromosomes 624
sex-linked disorders 628
sexual abuse
  constipation 375
  history in functional gastrointestinal disorders 32, 46
sexually transmitted diseases, hepatic injury 400
Shigella
  antibiotic treatment 368, **369**
  infectious diarrhea 360–1, 365
shock, gastrointestinal bleeding 123
short bowel syndrome
  congenital 329
  nutritional support 599
  oral replacement solutions 594, 599
  steatorrhea 324
short tandem repeats 612
sibutramine 198
sigmoid colon, ischemia 284
sigmoid volvulus, colonoscopy 297–8
sigmoidoscopy, flexible
  colorectal cancer screening 171, 176–7, 178
  constipation 382, **383**
  pregnancy 545
  sigmoid colon ischemia 284
  watery diarrhea 339–40
sildenafil, portopulmonary hypertension treatment 485
simethicone 264–5
  dyspepsia 49
single nucleotide polymorphisms (SNPs) 642
single photon emission computed tomography (SPECT), gastric emptying 215
site-specific mutation analysis 633–4
small bowel enteroscopy 141
small bowel manometry, motility studies 298
small deletions and insertions 631–2

small intestine
  absorptive capacity 305–6
  necrosis side effect of jejunal feeding 595–6
  pain 241–2
small intestine obstruction 279–81
  cancer treatment 281
  diagnosis 280
  management 280–1
small-molecule chloride channel inhibitors 346
SmartPill 284
smoking cessation, GERD 90
smooth-muscle relaxants, dysphagia treatment 73
social skills training 28
sodium
  deficiency 601
  dietary 571
    assessment 601
  loss 571
  restriction
    ascites treatment 449, 453
    hepatic hydrothorax 455
  toxicity 601
sodium anion diarrhea 325
sodium benzoate, hepatic encephalopathy treatment 474
sodium chloride, sodium deficiency treatment 601
sodium chloride ions, absorption 306
sodium docusate 387–8
sodium ion channels 232
sodium ions *307*, 308
  intestinal transport 305, **306**
  osmotic diarrhea 308
  secretory diarrhea 344
  transport 308
sodium-dependent multivitamin transporter (SMVT) 577
somatic neuropathic pain syndromes 238
somatic vs germ-line mutations 630
somatization
  functional gastrointestinal disorders 31–2, 34
  noncardiac chest pain 75
somatosensory cortex 230, 231
  abdominal pain 271
somatostatin
  esophageal varices hemorrhage management 130–1
  peptic ulcer rebleeding prevention 127–8
somatostatinoma, chronic diarrhea 322
sorbitol
  diarrhea 320, 325
  exclusion 263
  intolerance 257
soy protein allergy, diarrhea 330
space sickness 210
specificity, diagnostic tests 4–5
spectrum bias 4
sphincter of Oddi, relaxation regulation 425
spinal cord electrical stimulation 250
SPINK1 gene 629
spinoreticular tract 230
spironolactone
  ascites treatment 449, 453
  magnesium deficiency 605
splenic pain 241
splenopneumopexy, esophageal varices recurrent hemorrhage prevention 134
splenorenal shunt, esophageal varices recurrent hemorrhage prevention 133–4

spontaneous bacterial peritonitis 442, 446–7
    approach to patient 455–7
    ascites 456
    diagnosis 456
    hepatorenal syndrome prevention 461
    infecting organism 456
    management 453–4, 456–7
    pathogenesis 456
    renal dysfunction 456–7
sprue
    tropical 319
    see also celiac disease
stapling, evacuation disorders 392
starch, resistant 569
start codon 630
starvation 580–1
steatorrhea 321–5
    bile duct obstruction 321–2
    cirrhosis 321–2
    dermatitis herpetiformis 324
    mixed causes 324–5
    mucosal malabsorption 322–4
    postmucosal obstruction 324
    Whipple disease 324
stents
    esophageal varices hemorrhage management 132–3
    intestinal obstruction 299–300
sterols 565
stiff fundus 43
stomach
    infiltrative diseases 42
    proximal distension 44
    sensory threshold 44
stool(s)
    appearance 335
    collection 335
    consistency 304–5
    culture in infectious diarrhea 365
    electrolyte measurement 343–5
    fat concentration 337
    fecal fat tests
        qualitative 335–6
        quantitative 336–7
    frequency 304, 305
    impaction treatment **388**, 391–2
    leukocyte presence 365
    malabsorption diseases 331–2
    osmolality 308, 344
    osmotic gap 343, **344**
    ova tests 365–6
    pancreatic function tests 337–8
    parasite tests 365–6
    sodium ion content 308
    watery diarrhea tests 340
    weight 304–5, 343
stool softeners 387–8, 539
stop codon 630
stress
    adult responsiveness to adverse early life events 22
    current 32
    dyspepsia 45–6
    gastric erosions 129–30
    pathological 22–3
    response 582
    visceral pain 237–8
stress system 21–4
    adverse early life events 22
stressors, controllability 28
strictures, intestinal obstruction 292–3
stroke, oropharyngeal dysphagia 65
study design 3–4
    assessment 8
    number of patients 11
    outcomes 11
subgroup analyses 12
substance P 233, 236

sucralfate 49–50
    GERD in pregnancy 535
    hypophosphatemia 606
    peptic ulcer disease 106
    stress gastric erosion prophylaxis 130
sucrase–isomaltase deficiency 257
    breath testing 262
    dietary management 263
sucrose intolerance, breath testing 262
sugars, simple, maldigestion/ malabsorption 257
Sugiura procedure, esophageal varices recurrent hemorrhage prevention 134
sulfasalazine, use in pregnancy 541–2
sulfobromophthalein test 403
sumatriptan 50
sunflower cataract 402
sunlight exposure 615, 616
superior mesenteric artery, emboli 283–4, *285*
surgery
    abdominal pain 276–7
    appendicitis 278
    gas and bloating management 266
    Hirschsprung disease management 392
    ileus 299
    intestinal obstruction 299
    investigational in acute liver failure 509–10
    postoperative jaundice 433
    pregnancy 276
    prior in watery diarrhea 326
    small intestine obstruction 280–1
    stool impaction treatment **388**, 391–2
surgical shunt, esophageal varices hemorrhage prophylaxis 134–5
    recurrent hemorrhage prevention 133–4
surveillance 17–18
swallowing 62
    compensatory/corrective strategies 72
    evaluation 70
    pain 66–7
    therapy techniques **71**
    see also dysphagia; odynophagia
syndrome X 75
systemic inflammatory response syndrome (SIRS) 472–3, 502
systemic lupus erythematosus (SLE)
    hepatic hemangioma 527
    weight loss 187

tachygastria 43
Tangier disease 324
T-cell lymphoma
    celiac disease association 323
    steatorrhea 322
tea 570
technetium-99m albumin scintigraphy 342
tegaserod 50, 266
    laxative use **388**, 389, 539
telbivudine, HBV therapy 519–20
TENS (transcutaneous electrical nerve stimulation) 250
teratogenicity 637
teratology, database resources **637**
terlipressin 452
    esophageal varices hemorrhage management 131
    hepatorenal syndrome therapy 460, 461
tetany 615
tetracyclines, *H. pylori* treatment 107

therapy
    benefits 18
    costs 12
    critical appraisal of article **2**, 7–12
    follow-up study 10
    potential benefits 12
    side effects 12
thermic effect of feeding (TEF) 563, 564
thermic effect of physical activity (TEPA) 563, 564
thermogenesis, adaptive 564
thiamin 575
    deficiency 609–10
thiamin hydrochloride 610
thinking, dysfunctional 28, 31
thiopental, raised intracranial pressure therapy 506
thoracocentesis, hepatic hydrothorax 455
thought distortions 28, 31
thrombocytopenia–hemangioma syndrome, hepatic hemangioma 527
thyroid medullary carcinoma, diarrhea 327
thyromegaly, dysphagia 68
thyrotoxicosis
    carbohydrate rapid transit 325
    steatorrhea 324
tight junctions, secretory diarrhea 310
time preferences 16
tinidazole, *H. pylori* treatment 107
tissue transglutaminase (tTG) antibodies 415
TLR-4 pathway 289
tocopherol(s) 579
α-tocopherol 617
α-tocopherol transfer protein (TTP) 579
tocopherol-associated proteins (TAP) 579
toddler's diarrhea 325
tolerable upper intake level (UL) 559
Toll-like receptors (TLRs) 289
    inflammatory diarrhea 309
topiramate, weight loss **198**, 199
TORCHES 431
torsion 293
total parenteral (central) nutrition (TPN) 596–8
    acute liver failure 507
    cholestasis 430
    complications 597–8
    essential fatty acid abnormalities 567
    gastroparesis 221
    growth failure in children 600
    hepatic encephalopathy 600
    inflammatory bowel disease 599
    jaundice 433
Toupet partial fundoplication 94
toxic megacolon 293, 364
toxins
    food poisoning 313–14
    fungal in acute liver failure 501
    nausea and vomiting induction 208
    see also bacterial toxins
tracheobronchial aspiration, dysphagia 68
transcobalamin II (TCII) 612, 613, 614
transcription 630–1
transferrin
    function defects 153
    iron deficiency 607
    liver disease 409
transferrin receptors 607

transjugular intrahepatic portosystemic shunt (TIPS)
    ascites treatment 450–1
        refractory disease 454–5
    complications 451, 455
    contraindications 451
    esophageal varices
        hemorrhage management 132–3
        recurrent hemorrhage prevention 133
    hepatic hydrothorax 455
    hepatopulmonary syndrome 480–1
    hepatorenal syndrome therapy *459*, 460
translation 630–1
translocations 632
transthoracic contrast-enhanced echocardiography (TT-CEE) 479
transthoracic echocardiography, portopulmonary hypertension 484
transtubular K+ concentration gradient (TTKG) 601
trauma history, functional gastrointestinal disorders 32
traveler's diarrhea 315, 361–3
    persistent 319
    treatment 368
treatment failures 9
trepostinil, portopulmonary hypertension treatment 485
tricarboxylic acid cycle 566, *567*
trichlorethylene 400
tricyclic antidepressants
    chronic abdominal pain treatment 249
    dyspepsia 51
    functional gastrointestinal disorders 24–5
    nausea and vomiting management **217**, 218–19
    noncardiac chest pain 75
triglycerides 565
    chylous ascites 448
    clearance 600
    energy source 563
    lipolysis in starvation 581
    structured 568
trimethoprim sulfamethoxazole, infectious diarrhea treatment 368
Tropheryma whipplei (Whipple disease) 324
tropical sprue 319
TRPV1 vanilloid receptor 232, 236
truncal vagotomy, diarrhea 326
trypsinogen, cationic 629
tryptophan
    absorption defect 610
    hepatic coma 471
trypsin inhibitor 629
tuberculosis
    diarrhea 331
    peritoneal 447–8
tumor markers, ascites 447

UGT-1A1 microsomal enzyme 424
    abnormalities 426–7
ulcerative colitis
    carbohydrate rapid transit 325
    congenital abnormality risk 541
    diarrhea differential diagnosis 315
    fish oil supplementation 599
    pregnancy 540–4
ulcerative jejunitis 322
ulcerative proctitis, diarrhea differential diagnosis 315

ultrasonography
    abdominal 47
    appendicitis 277
    ascites 443
    cholecystitis 283
    gas and bloating 262
    gastric emptying 215
    hepatic adenoma 530
    hepatic hemangioma 528
    ileus 296
    intestinal obstruction 296
    jaundice 436
    liver cell dysplasia 531–2
    malabsorption 333, 335
    nodular regenerative hyperplasia
        of liver 531
    pregnancy 276
urea synthesis stimulation 474
urobilinogens 425
ursodeoxycholic acid, intrahepatic
        cholestasis of pregnancy 432,
        547–8
urticaria pigmentosa, diarrhea 328

V₂ receptor agonists, ascites
        treatment 452, 453
vagal function, dyspepsia/irritable
        bowel syndrome 44
vagotomy, postoperative symptoms
        44
vanillin 570
variable expressivity 629
variable nucleotide tandem repeats
        (VNTRs) 642
variceal band ligation for esophageal
        varices
    hemorrhage management 131, 132
    hemorrhage prophylaxis 134–5
    recurrent hemorrhage prevention
        133
vasoconstrictors plus albumin,
        hepatorenal syndrome
        therapy 460, 461
vascular ectasia 139
vascular malformations, blood loss
        155
vasoconstrictors, ascites therapy 452
vasodilators, portopulmonary
        hypertension treatment 485,
        486

vasopressin
    hepatorenal syndrome therapy
        461
    nausea and vomiting 207
vegetable intake, cancer
        chemoprevention 561–2
venoocclusive disease,
        hyperbilirubinemia 429–30
ventilation/perfusion mismatch,
        hepatorenal syndrome 476
verification bias 4
vertebral osteophytes, prominent 70
vertical banded gastroplasty
        199–200
Vibrio cholerae, antibiotic treatment
        370
Vibrio vulnificus 364
videocapsule endoscopy,
        malabsorption 335
videofluoroscopy
    esophageal dysphagia 72
    oropharyngeal dysphagia 69, 70,
        71
villous adenoma, diarrhea 328
vinyl chloride 401
VIPoma, diarrhea 327
viral gastroenteritis, nausea and
        vomiting induction 208, 209
viral hepatitis 429
    acute liver failure 499–500
    age 431
    cholestasis 429
    jaundice 431
    see also hepatitis A–E viruses;
        individual hepatitis diseases
viral infections
    diarrhea 313
    gastroenteritis 208, 209
    hepatotropic 499–500
visceral afferents 232
visceral hyperalgesia 44
visceral sensitivity 23
Visceral Sensitivity Index (VSI) 31
vitamin(s) 575–80
    absorption mechanisms 575
    deficiency
        clinical laboratory tests 590
        fat-soluble 439
    fat-soluble 439, 565
    water-soluble 575

vitamin A 578
    deficiency 615
    hydrolysis 578
    synthesis 578
vitamin B-1 see thiamin
vitamin B-2 see riboflavin
vitamin B-3 see niacin
vitamin B-6 see pyridoxine
vitamin B-12 (cobalamin)
    deficiency causing intestinal
        pseudoobstruction 289
    Schilling test 338
    serum levels 409–10
    see also cobalamin
vitamin C see ascorbic acid
vitamin D 578–9
    deficiency 603, 615–17
    insufficiency 578, 579
    supplementation 603–4
    toxicity 617
vitamin E 579
    deficiency 617
vitamin K 579–80
    coagulation function 403
    deficiency 617–18
volvulus formation 293
    see also sigmoid volvulus
vomiting
    CNS coordination 206–7
    colonic obstruction 291
    cyclic vomiting syndrome 209,
        212
    functional 40
    oral rehydration therapy 594
    radiation-induced 211
        management 221
    sodium loss 601
    somatic muscular events 207
    see also nausea and vomiting
von Hippel–Lindau syndrome,
        hepatic hemangioma 527
VX-950, hepatitis C virus treatment
        523–4

waist circumference 192, 194
    determination in obesity 196
water, drinking
    acute infectious diarrhea 312
    untreated 319
water brash, GERD 84

watery diarrhea–hypokalemia–
        achlorhydria (WDHA)
        syndrome 327
wedged hepatic venous pressure
        (WHVP) 446
weight loss
    cachexia 184, 185
    complications 201
    diets 196–7
    GERD 90
    gastrointestinal disorders 185–6
    malignancy 184–5, 189
    unintentional 183–9
        clinical studies 184
        diagnosis 188–9
        etiology 183–8
        malignancy screening 189
        physical examination 188–9
        prognosis 189
        treatment 189
weight-reducing agents, diarrhea 320
West Haven encephalopathy criteria
        502
Whipple disease
    diagnosis 331
    steatorrhea 324
Wilson disease 409, 415
    acute liver failure 501
    protein 574
wireless capsule endoscopy 141–2

xerostomia 62
X-linked disorders,
        recessive/dominant 628
D-xylose absorption tests,
        malabsorption 337

Yersinia enterocolitica, antibiotic
        treatment 370
yogurt, gas and bloating
        management 263

zinc
    deficiency 608–9
    dietary 574
    supplements 609
zinc sulfate 609
Zollinger–Ellison syndrome,
        diarrhea 327
zonisamide, weight loss 198, 199